EMERGENCY MEDICINE
Board Review

Elsevier
1600 John F. Kennedy Blvd.
Ste 1800
Philadelphia, PA 19103-2899

EMERGENCY MEDICINE BOARD REVIEW ISBN: 978-0-323-679701

Notice

Practitioners and researchers must always rely on their own experience and knowledge in evaluating and using any information, methods, compounds or experiments described herein. Because of rapid advances in the medical sciences, in particular, independent verification of diagnoses and drug dosages should be made. To the fullest extent of the law, no responsibility is assumed by Elsevier, authors, editors or contributors for any injury and/or damage to persons or property as a matter of products liability, negligence or otherwise, or from any use or operation of any methods, products, instructions, or ideas contained in the material herein.

Library of Congress Control Number 2021936080

Content Strategist: Kayla Wolfe
Content Development Specialist: Deborah Poulson/Meghan Andress
Publishing Services Manager: Shereen Jameel
Project Manager: Rukmani Krishnan
Design Direction: Bridget Hoette

Printed in The United States of America

Last digit is the print number: 9 8 7 6 5 4 3 2 1

EMERGENCY MEDICINE Board Review

Editors

Amy Kaji, MD, PhD
Professor
Clinical Emergency Medicine
David Geffen School of Medicine at UCLA
Interim Chair
Department of Emergency Medicine
Harbor-UCLA Medical Center
Torrance, CA

Ryan Pedigo, MD, MHPE
Assistant Professor
Clinical Emergency Medicine
David Geffen School of Medicine at UCLA
Associate Residency Program Director
Department of Emergency Medicine
Harbor-UCLA Medical Center
Torrance, CA

ELSEVIER

Section Editors

Elijah James Bell III, MD, MS
Assistant Clinical Professor
Department of Emergency Medicine
University of California, Los Angeles
Los Angeles, CA

Thomas E. Blair, MD
Assistant Clinical Professor
Department of Emergency Medicine
David Geffen School of Medicine at UCLA
Los Angeles, CA

Illene Claudius, MD
Associate Professor
Department Emergency Medicine
David Geffen School of Medicine at UCLA
Harbor-UCLA Medical Center
Los Angeles, CA

Richelle J. Cooper, MD, MSHS
Professor of Emergency Medicine
David Geffen School of Medicine
Research Director
UCLA Department of Emergency Medicine
Ronald Reagan UCLA Medical Center

Steven Lai, MD
Assistant Clinical Professor
Department of Emergency Medicine
Ronald Reagan UCLA Medical Center/
OliveView-UCLA Medical Center
Los Angeles, CA

Lynne McCullough, MD, FACEP
Professor of Emergency Medicine
Medical Director, Ronald Reagan UCLA
Emergency Medicine Department
Chief of Staff
Ronald Reagan UCLA Medical Center/
OliveView-UCLA Medical Center
Los Angeles, CA

Rick McPheeters, DO
Health Sciences Clinical Professor
and Chief
Department of Emergency Medicine/UCLA
Kern Medical Bakersfield, CA

James T. Niemann, MD
Senior Faculty
Department of Emergency Medicine
Professor of Medicine
David Geffen UCLA School of Medicine
Harbor-UCLA Medical Center
Los Angeles, CA

Manpreet Singh, MD, MBE
Assistant Professor of Emergency Medicine
Department of Emergency Medicine
Harbor-UCLA Medical Center
Torrance, CA

Scott R. Votey, MD
Professor of Emergency Medicine
Department of Emergency Medicine
David Geffen School of Medicine at UCLA
Los Angeles, CA

Natasha Wheaton, MD
Associate Clinical Professor
Department of Emergency Medicine
Ronald Reagan UCLA Medical Center/
OliveView-UCLA Medical Center
Los Angeles, CA

To all of the emergency medicine residents at Harbor-UCLA and all of my mentors and teachers throughout my career who have been there to support and guide me and drive me to be a better physician and teacher.

—Amy Kaji, MD, PhD

To my wife Tiffany and new daughter Lucy, who have given me so much joy and love in my life.

—Ryan Pedigo, MD, MHPE

CONTRIBUTORS

Fredrick M. Abrahamian, DO, FIDSA, FACEP
Health Sciences Clinical Professor of Emergency Medicine
David Geffen School of Medicine at UCLA
University of California, Los Angeles
Los Angeles, CA

Omid Adibnazari, MD, BS
Physician
Department of Emergency Medicine
Harbor-UCLA Medical Center
Torrance, CA

Haig Aintablian, MD, MS
Physician
Department of Emergency Medicine
University of California, Los Angeles
Los Angeles, CA

Thomas Akie, MD, PhD
Resident Physician
Department of Emergency Medicine
University of California, Los Angeles
Los Angeles, CA

Manish Amin, DO
Health Sciences Associate Clinical Professor
Department of Emergency Medicine/UCLA
Kern Medical
Bakersfield, CA

Julie Elizabeth Anderson, DO
Chief Resident
Department of Emergency Medicine
Harbor-UCLA Medical Center
Los Angeles, CA

Catherine Danielle Antonuk, MD
Resident Physician
Department of Emergency Medicine
University of California, Los Angeles
Los Angeles, CA

Cameron Araghi, MD
Physician
Department of Emergency Medicine
Harbor-UCLA Medical Center
Torrance, CA

Jessa Baker, MD
Physician
Department of Emergency Medicine
Ronald Reagan UCLA Medical Center/OliveView-UCLA Medical Center
Los Angeles, CA

Kieron K. Barkataki, DO
Health Sciences Assistant Clinical Professor
Department of Emergency Medicine/UCLA
Kern Medical
Bakersfield, CA

Zahir Basrai, MD
Physician
Department of Emergency Medicine
VA Greater Los Angeles Healthcare System
Los Angeles, CA
Health Sciences Assistant Clinical Professor
Department of Emergency Medicine
David Geffen School of Medicine at UCLA
Los Angeles, CA

Joshua J. Baugh, MD, MPP, MHCM
Assistant Professor
Department of Emergency Medicine
Massachusetts General Hospital
Harvard Medical School
Boston, MA

Rebecca A. Bavolek, MD
HS Associate Clinical Professor
Department of Emergency Medicine
David Geffen School of Medicine at UCLA
Los Angeles, CA

Elijah James Bell III, MD, MS
Assistant Clinical Professor
Department of Emergency Medicine
University of California, Los Angeles
Los Angeles, CA

Lilly Agnes Bellman, MD
Health Sciences Clinical Instructor
Department of Emergency Medicine
Harbor-UCLA Medical Center
Torrance, CA
Pediatric Emergency Physician
Department of Emergency Medicine
California Pacific Medical Center
San Francisco, CA

Annum A. Bhullar, MA, MD
Physician
Department of Emergency Medicine
University of California, Los Angeles
Los Angeles, CA

Thomas E. Blair, MD
Assistant Clinical Professor
Department of Emergency Medicine
David Geffen School of Medicine at UCLA
Los Angeles, CA

Claudie Bolduc, MD, MPH
Physician
Department of Emergency Medicine
UCLA Health System
Los Angeles, CA

Steven Bolger, MD
Resident Physician
Department of Emergency Medicine
UCLA Medical Center, Los Angeles
Los Angeles, CA

Kendra Campbell, MD
Physician
Department of Emergency Medicine
Harbor-UCLA Medical Center
Torrance, CA

Angelique Campen, MD, FACEP
Assistant Clinical
Professor Emergency Medicine
UCLA Medical Center
Providence Saint Joseph Emergency Department
CMO and Founder, Vital Medical Services

John Campo, MD
Resident Physician
Department of Emergency Medicine
Harbor-UCLA Medical Center
Torrance, CA

Caleb P. Canders, MD
Physician
Ronald Reagan UCLA Medical Center/OliveView-UCLA Medical Center
Department of Emergency Medicine
University of California, Los Angeles
Los Angeles, CA

Robert Carey, MD
Resident Physician
Department of Emergency Medicine
Harbor-UCLA Medical Center
Torrance, CA

Manuel Amando Celedon, MD
Health Sciences Assistant Clinical Professor of Emergency Medicine
David Geffen School of Medicine at UCLA
Department of Emergency Medicine
VA Greater Los Angeles Healthcare System
Los Angeles, CA

Cindy D. Chang, MD
Resident Physician
Department of Emergency Medicine
Harbor-UCLA Medical Center
Torrance, CA

Bradley Chappell, DO, MHA, FACOEP
Medical Director
Department of Emergency Medicine
Harbor-UCLA Medical Center
Torrance, CA
Associate Clinical Professor
Department of Emergency Medicine
David Geffen School of Medicine at UCLA
Los Angeles, CA

Theresa H. Cheng, MD, JD
Physician
Department of Emergency Medicine
University of California, Los Angeles
Los Angeles, CA

Alan Chiem, MD, MPH
Director of Ultrasound
Department of Emergency Medicine
Ronald Reagan UCLA Medical Center/OliveView-UCLA Medical Center
Sylmar, CA
Associate Clinical Professor
Department of Emergency Medicine
David Geffen School of Medicine at UCLA
Los Angeles, CA

Wendy C. Coates, MD
Emeritus Professor of Emergency Medicine
Department of Emergency Medicine
David Geffen School of Medicine at UCLA
Harbor-UCLA Department of Emergency Medicine Dance Medicine Specialist
Los Angeles, CA

Eugenie Como, MD
Resident Physician
Department of Emergency Medicine
Ronald Reagan UCLA Medical Center/OliveView-UCLA Medical Center
Los Angeles, CA

Richelle J. Cooper, MD, MSHS
Professor of Emergency Medicine
David Geffen School of Medicine
Research Director
UCLA Department of Emergency Medicine
Ronald Reagan UCLA Medical Center
Los Angeles, CA

Illene Claudius, MD
Associate Professor
Department of Emergency Medicine
David Geffen School of Medicine at UCLA
Los Angeles, CA

Sara Crager, MD
Assistant Professor
Department of Emergency Medicine
University of California, Los Angeles
Los Angeles, CA
Assistant Professor
Division of Critical Care, Department of Anesthesia
University of California, Los Angeles
Los Angeles, CA

Alexander Daguanno, MD, BS
Resident Physician
Department of Emergency Medicine
University of California, Los Angeles
Los Angeles, CA

Ryan DeVivo, DO, MS
Physician
Department of Emergency Medicine
Harbor-UCLA Medical Center
Torrance, CA

Ryan C. Dollbaum, MD
Physician
Department of Emergency Medicine
University of California, Los Angeles
Los Angeles, CA

Pamela L. Dyne, MD
Professor of Clinical Medicine
Department of Emergency Medicine
David Geffen School of Medicine at UCLA
Los Angeles, CA
Attending Physician
Department of Emergency Medicine
Ronald Reagan UCLA Medical Center/OliveView-UCLA Medical Center
Sylmar, CA

Susannah Empson, MD
Physician
Department of Emergency Medicine
Harbor-UCLA Medical Center
Torrance, CA

Brandon Endo, MD
Clinical Instructor
Department of Emergency Medicine
University of California, Los Angeles
Los Angeles, CA

Jasmin England, MD, FAAP
Physician
Department of Pediatric Emergency Medicine
Children's Hospital of Orange County
Orange, California

Adam R. Evans, MD
Clinical Instructor
David Geffen School of Medicine
Ronald Reagan UCLA Medical Center/OliveView-UCLA Medical Center
Los Angeles, CA

Jennifer Fang, MD
Resident Physician
Department of Emergency Medicine
Harbor-UCLA Medical Center
Torrance, CA

Joanne Feldman, MD, MS
Assistant Clinical Professor
Department of Emergency Medicine
University of California, Los Angeles
Los Angeles, CA

Patricia Fermin, MD
Assistant Clinical Professor
David Geffen School of Medicine at UCLA
VA Greater Los Angeles Healthcare System
Los Angeles, CA

Allison Ferreira, MD
Assistant Clinical Professor
Department of Emergency Medicine
University of California, Los Angeles
Los Angeles, CA

Elizabeth Tang Ferreira, MD
Resident Physician
Department of Emergency Medicine
Ronald Reagan UCLA Medical Center/OliveView-UCLA Medical Center
Los Angeles, CA

Vanessa Franco, MD, PhD
Assistant Professor
Department of Emergency Medicine
University of California, Los Angeles
Los Angeles, CA

Joseph Friedrich, MD
Resident Physician
Department of Emergency Medicine
Harbor-UCLA Medical Center
Torrance, CA

Lauren Fryling, MD
Resident Physician
Department of Emergency Medicine
Harbor-UCLA Medical Center
Torrance, CA

Victor Galson, MD
Physician
Department of Emergency Medicine
Adventist Health Castle
Kailua, HI

Alexander Garrett, MD
Resident Physician
Department of Emergency Medicine
Harbor-UCLA Medical Center
Torrance, CA

Michael Ghermezi, MD, MS
Resident Physician
Department of Emergency Medicine
Harbor-UCLA Medical Center
Torrance, CA

Sarah Gracie Gonzalez, MD
Health Sciences Assistant Clinical Professor
Department of Emergency Medicine
Kern Medical/UCLA
Bakersfield, CA

Isaac Grabiel, DO
Physician
Graduate of Kern Medical/UCLA
Sanford Aberdeen Medical Center
Aberdeen, SD

Thomas Graham, MD
Professor of Emergency Medicine
Department of Emergency Medicine
UCLA School of Medicine, Los Angeles
Los Angeles, CA

Andrew Grock, MD
Faculty Physician
Division of Emergency Medicine
VA Greater Los Angeles Healthcare System
Los Angeles, CA
Assistant Clinical Professor of Emergency Medicine
David Geffen School of Medicine at UCLA
Los Angeles, CA

Alexandra Grossman, MD
Chief Resident
Department of Emergency Medicine
University of California, Los Angeles
Los Angeles, CA

Brittany Guest, DO
Physician
Department of Emergency Medicine
Ronald Reagan UCLA Medical Center/OliveView-UCLA Medical Center
Los Angeles, CA

Malkeet Gupta, MD, MS
Associate Clinical Professor
Department of Emergency Medicine
University of California, Los Angeles
Los Angeles, CA
Managing Partner, AVEMA Inc.
Department of Emergency Medicine
Antelope Valley Hospital
Lancaster, CA

Puneet Gupta, MD
Attending Physician
Department of Emergency Medicine
Harbor-UCLA Medical Center
Torrance, CA

David Haase, MD
Physician
Department of Emergency Medicine
University of California, Los Angeles
Los Angeles, CA

Tyler Haertlein, MD
Physician
Department of Emergency Medicine
University of California, Los Angeles
Los Angeles, CA

Cameron W. Harrison, MD
Physician
Department of Emergency Medicine
University of California, Los Angeles
Los Angeles, CA

Sean Heavey, MD
Resident Physician
Department of Emergency Medicine/UCLA
Kern Medical
Bakersfield, CA

Jagdipak S. Heer, MD
Health Sciences Associate Clinical Professor
Department of Emergency Medicine/UCLA
Kern Medical
Bakersfield, CA

Greg Hendey, MD
Professor and Chair
Department of Emergency Medicine
University of California, Los Angeles
Los Angeles, CA

Jonie Hsiao, MD
Assistant Clinical Professor
Department of Emergency Medicine
David Geffen School of Medicine at UCLA
VA Greater Los Angeles Healthcare System
Los Angeles, CA

Dennis Hsieh, MD, JD
Director, Social Medicine and Community Health
Harbor-UCLA Medical Center
Los Angeles County Department of Health Services
Torrance, CA
Assistant Professor
Department of Emergency Medicine
Harbor-UCLA Medical Center
Torrance, CA

Diane D. Hsu, MD
Physician
Department of Emergency Medicine
Harbor-UCLA Medical Center
Torrance, CA

Alex Huang, MD
Resident Physician
Department of Emergency Medicine/UCLA
Kern Medical
Bakersfield, CA

Caroline Humphreys, MD
Physician
Department of Emergency Medicine
Ronald Reagan UCLA Medical Center/OliveView-UCLA Medical Center
Los Angeles, CA

Daniel Ichwan, MD
Resident Physician
Department of Emergency Medicine
University of California, Los Angeles
Los Angeles, CA

James Jiang, MD
Resident Physician
Department of Emergency Medicine
University of California, Los Angeles
Los Angeles, CA

Jaime Jordan, MD, MAEd
Associate Professor
Department of Emergency Medicine
David Geffen School of Medicine at UCLA
Los Angeles, CA

Michael T. Jordan, MD
Resident Physician
Department of Emergency Medicine
Harbor-UCLA Medical Center
Torrance, CA

Samantha Phillips Kadera, MD, MPH, FACEP
Assistant Clinical Professor
Department of Emergency Medicine
Ronald Reagan UCLA Medical Center/OliveView-UCLA Medical Center
Los Angeles, CA

Sheetal Khiyani, MD
Physician
Department of Emergency Medicine
Harbor-UCLA Medical Center
Los Angeles, CA

Kellie Kitamura, MD
Assistant Clinical Professor
Department of Emergency Medicine
University of California, Los Angeles
Los Angeles, CA

Cynthia Koh, MD
Assistant Professor
Department of Emergency Medicine
VA Greater Los Angeles Healthcare System
Los Angeles, CA
Assistant Professor
Department of Emergency Medicine
University of California, Los Angeles
Los Angeles, CA

Casey Krebs, MD
Physician
Department of Emergency Medicine
Harbor-UCLA Medical Center
Torrance, CA

Vanessa Camille Kreger, MD, MPH
Resident Physician
Department of Emergency Medicine
University of California, Los Angeles
Los Angeles, CA

Jacqueline Kurth, MD
Physician
Department of Emergency Medicine
University of California, Los Angeles
Los Angeles, CA

Steven Lai, MD
Assistant Clinical Professor
Department of Emergency Medicine
Ronald Reagan UCLA Medical Center/OliveView-UCLA Medical Center
Los Angeles, CA

Carol Lee, MD
Assistant Clinical Professor
Department of Emergency Medicine
VA Greater Los Angeles Healthcare System
Los Angeles, CA

Randall W. Lee, MD
Instructor
George Washington School of Medicine and Health Sciences
Washington, DC
Attending Physician
Department of Emergency Medicine
George Washington University Hospital
Washington, DC

Matthew Levin, MD, BA
Resident Physician
Department of Emergency Medicine
University of California, Los Angeles
Los Angeles, CA

Lev Libet, MD
Health Sciences Assistant Clinical Professor
Department of Emergency Medicine/UCLA
Kern Medical
Bakersfield, CA

George Lim, MD
Assistant Clinical Professor
Department of Emergency Medicine
Division of Critical Care, Department of Anesthesia
University of California, Los Angeles
Los Angeles, CA

Yiju Teresa Liu, MD
Associate Professor
Department of Emergency Medicine
Harbor-UCLA Medical Center
Torrance, CA

Sarah Lopez, MD, MBA
Patient Safety Officer
Harbor-UCLA Medical Center
Los Angeles County Department of Health Services
Torrance, CA
Assistant Professor
Department of Emergency Medicine
Harbor-UCLA Medical Center
Torrance, CA

Scott Lundberg, MD
Clinical Professor
Department of Emergency Medicine
David Geffen School of Medicine at UCLA
Los Angeles, CA

Lynne McCullough, MD, FACEP
Professor of Emergency Medicine
Medical Director, Ronald Reagan UCLA Emergency Medicine Department
Chief of Staff
Ronald Reagan UCLA Medical Center/OliveView-UCLA
Medical Center
Los Angeles, CA

Alexandra McLeroy-Wallace, MD
Resident Physician
Department of Emergency Medicine
Ronald Reagan UCLA Medical Center/OliveView-UCLA Medical Center
Los Angeles, CA

Rick McPheeters, DO
Health Sciences Clinical Professor and Chief
Department of Emergency Medicine/UCLA
Kern Medical
Bakersfield, CA

Gregory J. Moran, MD
Professor
Department of Medicine
David Geffen School of Medicine at UCLA
Los Angeles, CA

Naseem Moridzadeh, MD
Resident Physician
Department of Emergency Medicine
Ronald Reagan UCLA Medical Center/OliveView-UCLA Medical Center
Los Angeles, CA

Mark Morocco, MD
Health Sciences Clinical Professor
Emergency Medicine UCLA Emergency Medical Center
Director of Development Past President, UCLA Medical Alumni Association
Los Angeles, CA

Brittney Mull, MD, MPH
Resident Physician
Department of Emergency Medicine
Harbor-UCLA Medical Center
Torrance, CA

James J. Murphy Jr., MD, MPH
Resident Physician
Department of Emergency Medicine
Ronald Reagan UCLA Medical Center/OliveView-UCLA Medical Center
Los Angeles, CA

Anna Nguyen, DO
Resident Physician
Department of Emergency Medicine/UCLA
Los Angeles, CA

James T. Niemann, MD
Senior Faculty, Department of Emergency Medicine
Harbor-UCLA Medical Center
Professor of Medicine
David Geffen UCLA School of Medicine
Los Angeles, CA

Rachel O'Donnell, MD
Health Sciences Assistant Clinical Professor
Department of Emergency Medicine
Kern Medical/UCLA
Bakersfield, CA

Adedamola Ogunniyi, MD
Associate Director, Residency Training Program
Department of Emergency Medicine
Harbor-UCLA Medical Center
Torrance, CA
Assistant Clinical Professor
David Geffen School of Medicine at UCLA
Los Angeles, CA

Chinwe Onu, MD
Resident Physician
Department of Emergency Medicine
Harbor-UCLA Medical Center
Torrance, CA

Kelly Painter, MD, FACEP
Clinical Faculty
Department of Emergency Medicine
Integris Southwest Medical Center
Oklahoma City, OK

Ryan Pedigo, MD, MHPE
Assistant Professor
Clinical Emergency Medicine
David Geffen School of Medicine at UCLA
Associate Residency Program Director
Department of Emergency Medicine
Harbor-UCLA Medical Center
Torrance, CA

Gregory Sampson Powell, MD, BS
Physician
Department of Emergency Medicine
St. Joseph Hospital of Orange
Orange, CA

Kian Preston-Suni, MD, MPH
Assistant Clinical Professor
Department of Emergency Medicine
David Geffen School of Medicine at UCLA
Los Angeles, CA
Attending Physician
Department of Emergency Medicine
VA Greater Los Angeles Medical Center
Los Angeles, CA

Daniel Quesada, MD
Health Sciences Assistant Clinical Professor
Department of Emergency Medicine/UCLA
Kern Medical
Bakersfield, CA

Katie Rebillot, DO
Health Sciences Clinical Instructor
Department of Emergency Medicine
David Geffen School of Medicine at UCLA
Torrance, CA

Chelsea E. Robinson, MD
Resident Physician
Department of Emergency Medicine
University of California, Los Angeles
Los Angeles, CA

Armando Darnell Rodriguez, MD, MS, BS
Assistant Clinical Professor
Department of Emergency Medicine
Ronald Reagan UCLA Medical Center/OliveView-UCLA Medical Center
Sylmar, CA

James Rosbrugh, MD
Health Sciences Assistant Clinical Professor
Department of Emergency Medicine
Kern Medical/UCLA
Bakersfield, CA

Matthew Rosen, MD
Resident Physician
Department of Emergency Medicine
Ronald Reagan UCLA Medical Center/OliveView-UCLA Medical Center
Los Angeles, CA

Amir A. Rouhani, MD
Associate Clinical Professor/Director of Simulation Education
Departments of Emergency Medicine and Internal Medicine
Ronald Reagan UCLA Medical Center/OliveView-UCLA Medical Center
David Geffen School of Medicine at UCLA
Los Angeles, CA

Carolyn Joy Sachs, MD, MPH
UCLA Department of Emergency Medicine
David Geffen School of Medicine at UCLA
Los Angeles, CA
Medical Director FNS
Sexual Assault Evaluation Program
Long Beach, CA

Eric Savitsky, MD
Professor of Emergency Medicine
Department of Emergency Medicine
University of California, Los Angeles
Los Angeles, CA

Shira A. Schlesinger, MD, MScPH
Assistant Professor of Emergency Medicine
Director of EMS & Disaster Preparedness Programs
Department of Emergency Medicine
Harbor-UCLA Medical Center
Torrance, CA

Vikram Shankar, MD
Physician
Graduate of Kern Medical/UCLA
Pine Ridge Hospital / Indian Health Services
Pine Ridge, SD

Supriya Sharma, MD
Fellow Physician
Department of Pediatric Emergency Medicine
Harbor-UCLA Medical Center
Carson, CA

Jackie Shibata, MD, MS
Assistant Professor
Department of Emergency Medicine
Ronald Reagan UCLA Medical Center/OliveView-UCLA Medical Center
Sylmar, CA

Rachel Shing, MD
Adjunct Clinical Professor
Department of Emergency and Rural Medicine
Oklahoma State University Center for Health Sciences
Tulsa, OK

Carolyn Shover, MD
Fellow Physician
Department of Critical Care Medicine
UCLA Medical Center
Los Angeles, CA

Elizabeth Siacunco, MD
Resident Physician
Department of Emergency Medicine/UCLA
Kern Medical
Bakersfield, CA

Jaskaran Singh, MD
Emergency Physician
Department of Emergency Medicine
Harbor-UCLA Medical Center
Torrance, CA

Manpreet Singh, MD, MBE
Assistant Professor of Emergency Medicine
Department of Emergency Medicine
Harbor-UCLA Medical Center
Torrance, CA

Luiz Souza-Filho, MD
Resident Physician
Department of Emergency Medicine
University of California, Los Angeles
Los Angeles, CA

Hannah Spungen, MD, MPH
Resident Physician
Department of Emergency Medicine
UCLA Health
Los Angeles, CA

Andrea Takemoto, MD
Assistant Professor
Department of Emergency Medicine
David Geffen School of Medicine at UCLA
Los Angeles, CA
Attending Physician
Department of Emergency Medicine
Ronald Reagan UCLA Medical Center/OliveView-UCLA Medical Center
Sylmar, CA

David Tanen, MD
Professor
Department of Emergency Medicine
Harbor-UCLA Medical Center
Torrance, CA

Ryan Tenold, DO
Resident Physician
Department of Emergency Medicine
Harbor-UCLA Medical Center
Torrance, CA

Michael Tetwiler, MD, MPH
Physician
Department of Emergency Medicine
Harbor-UCLA Medical Center
Torrance, CA

Joshua Tobias, MD
Clinical Faculty
Department of Emergency Medicine/UCLA
Kern Medical
Bakersfield, CA

Juliana Tolles, MD, MHS
Assistant Professor of Emergency Medicine
Department of Emergency Medicine
Harbor-UCLA Medical Center
Torrance, CA

Sabrina M. Tom, MD
Assistant Clinical Professor
Department of Emergency Medicine
David Geffen School of Medicine at UCLA
Los Angeles, CA
Attending Physician
Department of Emergency Medicine
Ronald Reagan UCLA Medical Center/OliveView-UCLA Medical Center
Sylmar, CA

Atilla Uner, MD, MPH
Clinical Professor of Emergency Medicine and Nursing
Department of Emergency Medicine
David Geffen School of Medicine at UCLA
Los Angeles, CA

Scott R. Votey, MD
Professor of Emergency Medicine
Department of Emergency Medicine
David Geffen School of Medicine at UCLA
Los Angeles, CA

Ashley Vuong, MD, MA
Resident Physician
Department of Emergency Medicine
Ronald Reagan UCLA Medical Center/OliveView-UCLA Medical Center
Los Angeles, CA

Hannah Wallace, MD, MPH
Resident Physician
Department of Emergency Medicine
University of California, Los Angeles
Los Angeles, CA

Matthew Waxman, MD, DTM&H
Clinical Professor
Department of Emergency Medicine
David Geffen School of Medicine at UCLA
Attending Physician
Ronald Reagan UCLA Medical Center/OliveView-UCLA Medical Center
Los Angeles, CA
Medical Director
NYCMedics Global Disaster Relief
New York, NY

Catherine Weaver, MD
Assistant Professor
Department of Emergency Medicine
University of California, Los Angeles
Los Angeles, CA

Daniel Weingrow, DO
Associate Clinical Professor
Department of Emergency Medicine
Ronald Reagan UCLA Medical Center/OliveView-UCLA Medical Center
Los Angeles, CA

Natasha Wheaton, MD
Associate Clinical Professor
Department of Emergency Medicine
Ronald Reagan UCLA Medical Center/OliveView-UCLA Medical Center
Los Angeles, CA

Denise Whitfield, MD, MBA
Assistant Professor of Clinical Medicine
Harbor-UCLA Department of Emergency Medicine
David Geffen School of Medicine at UCLA
Los Angeles, CA

Kelsey Wilhelm, MD, BS
Physician
Department of Emergency Medicine
Harbor-UCLA Medical Center
Torrance, CA

James Williams, MD
Resident Physician
Department of Emergency Medicine
Harbor-UCLA Medical Center
Torrance, CA

Kevin Wroblewski, MD
Resident Physician
Department of Emergency Medicine
Ronald Reagan UCLA Medical Center/OliveView-UCLA Medical Center
Los Angeles, CA

Andrea W. Wu, MD, MMM
Associate Clinical Professor
Department of Emergency Medicine
David Geffen School of Medicine at UCLA
Vice Chair, Director of Clinical Operations
Harbor-UCLA Medical Center
Torrance, CA

Anna Yap, MD, BA
Resident Physician
Department of Emergency Medicine
University of California, Los Angeles
Los Angeles, CA

Kathleen Yip, MD
Physician
Department of Emergency Medicine
VA Greater Los Angeles Healthcare System
Los Angeles, CA

Lisa Zhao, MD
Assistant Professor
Department of Emergency Medicine
VA West Los Angeles
Los Angeles, CA
Assistant Professor
Department of Emergency Medicine
Ronald Reagan UCLA Medical Center/OliveView-UCLA Medical Center
Sylmar, CA

PREFACE

Welcome to the first edition of *Emergency Medicine Board Review*. This title is a review book geared toward practicing emergency physicians and residents in training who are preparing for their training in-service examinations and certifying written board examinations. It is a comprehensive collection of chapters that summarize the topics covered in the American Board of Emergency Medicine's Emergency Medicine Model. The content is streamlined and presented in a high-yield format for easily "digestible" pieces of information alongside an abundance of clinical photographs, charts, and graphs to aid in understanding and recall of core concepts. In addition to the book content itself, the companion eBook includes access to more than 500 board-style, multiple-choice questions with answers and rationales to help you test and confirm your knowledge.

The authors and section editors of this text are all affiliated with the David Geffen School of Medicine at UCLA. We are indebted to each and every one of the authors and editors who have dedicated tremendous time and energy to this endeavor. We are also grateful to Meghan Andress, our managing editor from Elsevier, for helping all of us navigate the electronic editing process. Finally, we would like to express our gratitude to our Harbor-UCLA family of faculty, residents, and patients, who motivate us to always strive to be better physicians and teachers.

CONTENTS

SECTION ONE

BOARD REVIEW

Gastrointestinal

CHAPTER 1

BOARD REVIEW

Esophagus

CATHERINE DANIELLE ANTONUK, MD, and ELIJAH JAMES BELL III, MD, MS

Esophageal Perforation

General Principles

- Most esophageal perforations are caused by iatrogenic etiologies, such as endoscopy, dilation, biopsy, or variceal banding.
- However, 10% to 15% of all esophageal perforations are full-thickness perforations caused by sudden forceful vomiting, which is a condition known as Boerhaave syndrome. Usually seen in those with a history of extensive alcohol use, these full-thickness esophageal tears typically occur at the left posterior distal esophagus.
- Boerhaave syndrome can also be due to coughing, straining, seizures, childbirth, trauma, foreign body or caustic ingestion, and food impaction (causing a mucosal injury).

Clinical Presentation

- History: forceful emesis, coughing, or straining.
- Symptoms: acute, severe pain in the chest, neck, back, or abdomen that worsens with swallowing.
- The pain tends to be associated with dysphagia, hoarseness, dyspnea, and hematemesis.
- Signs: examination findings depend on the severity, location, and time since the injury.
- Patients may manifest subcutaneous emphysema or the Hamman crunch.
- Patients who have progressed to mediastinitis demonstrate tachycardia, tachypnea, and sepsis with hypotension and fever.

Diagnosis and Evaluation

- Chest radiograph (CXR) and computed tomography (CT) scan of the chest and abdomen may show subcutaneous air, pneumomediastinum, a widened mediastinum, the tubular artery sign (air tracking up the neck, along vessels), pleural effusion, retroperitoneal air, or air in the lesser sac (Fig. 1.1).
- Because CT does not localize the exact site of the perforation, a gastrografin, water-soluble contrast esophagram should be performed when Boerhaave syndrome is suspected.
- If the water-soluble contrast esophagram is negative, it must be followed by a barium esophagram, which has a higher sensitivity for detecting small perforations but is not used as the initial diagnostic study because it can cause a significant inflammatory response in the mediastinum.

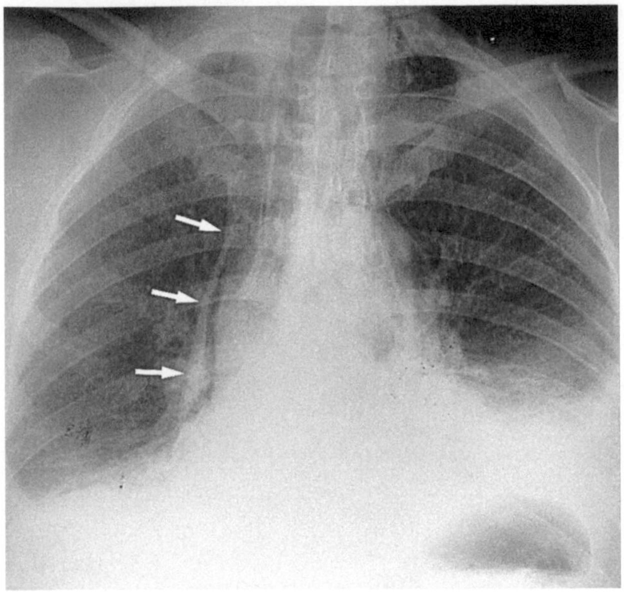

FIG. 1.1 Posteroanterior chest radiograph shows a right-sided pneumomediastinum *(arrows)* and a left pleural effusion. *(Courtesy Seth N. Glick, MD, Philadelphia. From Gore, R. M., & Levine, M. S. (2010). High-yield imaging: Gastrointestinal. Elsevier, Fig. 46.2.)*

Treatment

- These patients should immediately have nothing by mouth (NPO) and undergo resuscitation, broad-spectrum intravenous (IV) antibiotics, nutritional support, drainage of fluid collections, and specialist consultation with cardiothoracic surgery, because they may warrant primary repair of the esophageal defect, diversion, and, in some cases, esophagectomy.

Caustic Ingestions

General Principles

- Can be intentional (psychiatric patients) or accidental (more common in pediatric patients).
- It is helpful to determine if the agent was acidic or alkali because the tissue damage varies.
- More common in developed countries. Causing liquefactive necrosis, these ingestions (e.g., industrial-strength bleach, not household bleach) tend to damage the esophagus more than the stomach or duodenum.

- Acid ingestion is more commonly seen in developing countries. and it causes more gastric damage owing to coagulation necrosis, and has a higher mortality rate.

Clinical Presentation

- On initial presentation, patients may complain of nausea, vomiting, dysphagia, drooling, or choking. Young children may refuse to eat or drink. Lack of oral lesions does not exclude possibility of injury.
- History can be straightforward for pediatric patients found next to or in the vicinity of an open container of caustic chemicals. Adult patients may be less forthcoming, and it is crucial to obtain collateral history with any concern for intentional self-harm.
- Severity of injury will depend on the pH of the substance, the concentration and amount ingested, whether the substance was a solid or liquid, and the duration of mucosal contact.
- With esophageal perforation, mediastinitis and sepsis may ensue; with gastric perforation, peritonitis may develop.
- Complications include gastrointestinal (GI) bleeding, strictures, fistulization into adjacent organs and vessels, as well as later esophageal carcinoma.

Diagnosis and Evaluation

- Diagnosis is primarily based on the patient's history.
- Chest radiographs and CT scan may help identify complications of the ingestion, including esophageal or gastric perforation.
- Early endoscopy is recommended, provided there is no evidence of perforation.
- Zargar classification is used to grade injury severity.

Treatment

- Airway management is critical, especially in an actively vomiting patient, to protect the lungs from insult.
- There is no role for activated charcoal or ipecac syrup.
- Neutralization is generally contraindicated with one notable exception: the ingestion of hydrofluoric acid, which requires treatment with magnesium citrate.
- There is no evidence to support steroid or antibiotic use in the emergency department (unless there is evidence of esophageal or gastric perforation and mediastinitis and sepsis).
- Need for immediate medical and surgical management will depend on the severity of the injury and the presence of complications (e.g., perforation, bleeding).

Foreign Body Ingestion

General Principles

- Ingestion of foreign bodies is important to consider in pediatric, psychiatric, and prisoner populations. Elderly patients with dementia or dentures are also at increased risk.
- Objects that are more than 2.5 cm wide, more than 6 cm long, or have irregular or sharp edges may not pass the pylorus quickly or safely.

Clinical Presentation

- Adults may not necessarily describe specific symptoms, depending on the population; they may report retrosternal chest pain, dysphagia, vomiting, and choking.
- Pediatric patients may refuse to eat and may have a history of vomiting, gagging, and coughing. They may also have new wheezing, stridor, or drooling.

Diagnosis and Evaluation

- CXR (2-View) or kidney, ureter, bladder (KUB) is helpful to localize the foreign body, especially if radioopaque.
- CXR anteroposterior view—swallowed coins in the esophagus appear flat and round (Fig. 1.2), and coins in the trachea appear flat and round on the lateral CXR view. Disc or button batteries will appear round but with

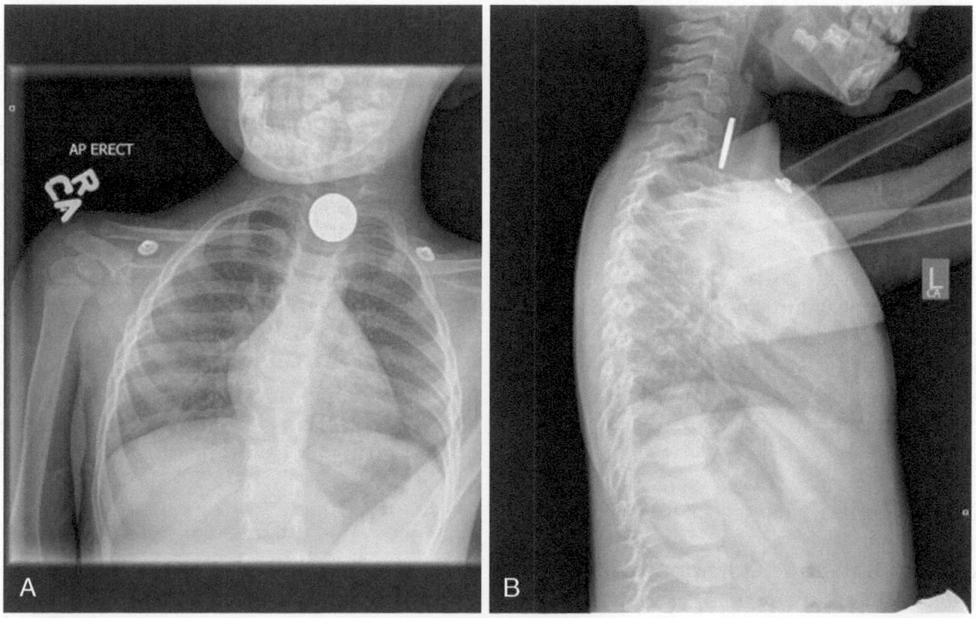

FIG. 1.2 Chest radiograph: Foreign body ingestion. (A) Anteroposterior radiograph of coin in the esophagus (note the typical en-face appearance of the coin in this view). (B) The edge of the coin seen on the lateral view. *(From Chung, S., Forte, V., & Campisi, P. (2010). A review of pediatric foreign body ingestion and management. Clinical Pediatric Emergency Medicine, 11(3), 225–230, Copyright © 2010 Elsevier Inc.)*

BOX 1.1 Foreign Body Ingestion: Indications for Emergent Interventions

Airway Compromise (Tracheal Compression)

Esophageal obstruction and patient inability to tolerate secretions

Objects which are:

1. Sharp, > 6 cm long or > 2.5 cm wide
2. High-powered magnet or multiple magnets
3. Superabsorbent polymer
4. Disc battery in the esophagus (immediate removal required)

a double line or "poker chip" appearance on PA and a step-off on lateral imaging.

- CT is more sensitive than plain films for fish/animal bones, glass, and plastic (e.g., radiolucent or organic material).
- With negative imaging but high clinical suspicion, endoscopy is the diagnostic test of choice.

Treatment

- Indications for emergent intervention are noted in Box 1.1.
- If the foreign body has passed the pylorus, the patient can typically be monitored by serial radiograph to confirm it has completely passed the GI tract in 48 to 72 hours.
  - Button batteries are an exception to this. Button batteries larger than 12 mm, composed of lithium, or multiple batteries warrant removal or inpatient monitoring. If the battery has not passed within 10 to 14 days, or if the patient develops GI symptoms, then intervention is also required. Multiple magnets similarly require removal, even if past the pylorus.
  - There is a national battery ingestion hotline (1-800-498-8666), which can further assist with management.

Food Impactions

General Principles

- Food impactions are typically caused by a meat bolus.
- Food impactions may be an early finding of an obstructive esophageal lesion (e.g., carcinoma, strictures, Schatzki ring) or underlying esophageal pathology, such as eosinophilic esophagitis.

Clinical Presentation

- History should be consistent with recent food ingestion.
- Patients will complain of symptoms similar to those of as foreign body ingestion, including nausea, dysphagia, choking, and chest pain.
- Drooling and inability to tolerate secretions are consistent with an esophageal obstruction.

Diagnosis and Evaluation

- Food impaction is a clinical diagnosis based on history and symptoms.
- Emergent endoscopy is indicated for symptoms of esophageal obstruction or airway compromise (tracheal compression).
- Patients who cannot pass the impacted food within 12 to 24 hours should receive an endoscopy.
- Older patients and those who have recurrent impactions should be referred for an outpatient endoscopy to rule out pathology, such as esophageal carcinoma.

Treatment

- Symptomatic management should start with carbonated drinks.
- Endoscopy should be pursued for the indications listed above.
- Meat tenderizers, such as papain, are contraindicated, because they are associated with esophageal perforation.
- Consider glucagon (1 to 2 mg in adults or 0.02 mg/kg to 0.03 mg/kg in children less than 20 kg) IV, which can aid in lower esophageal sphincter relaxation. Some studies suggest a benefit, whereas others do not, and rapid administration of this medication may also cause emesis, which can lead to aspiration. It should not, however, delay endoscopic therapy.

Esophagitis

General Principles

- Esophagitis can be infectious or medication-induced (from either direct mucosal injury or its systemic effects).
- With immunosuppression, there is an increased risk of infectious etiology (Candida, herpes).
- Patients may have oral lesions, but a lack of oral lesions does not exclude this condition.

Clinical Presentation

- Patients may complain of odynophagia or dysphagia.
- Pain may be retrosternal, burning, or stabbing.
- Patients with pill esophagitis may report new medications.
- Risk factors for this etiology include elderly age and taking medications with little to no water.

Diagnosis and Evaluation

- Diagnosis should be based on history; symptoms can determine severity (e.g., is the patient tolerating the secretions, is the patient hydrated).
- Examination of the oropharynx may show lesions.
- CXR or CT of the neck and chest is useful when there is a concern for perforation or abscess.
- Endoscopy with biopsy, culture, or both is indicated to rule out infection or if there are persistent symptoms after discontinuation of suspected culprit medications.

Treatment

- Administer the appropriate antimicrobial medications for infectious etiologies: antifungals for Candida (typically fluconazole 400 mg IV or PO) and acyclovir (400 mg PO TID or 5 mg/kg IV q8h) in immunocompromised patients with herpes or cytomegalovirus esophagitis (CMV).
- Pill esophagitis is treated by discontinuing the medication or changing its formulation to a liquid or a tablet form.

GERD

General Principles

- Symptomatic gastroesophageal reflux disease (GERD) is common; up to 40% of adults in the United States have monthly symptoms.

- Risk factors include advanced age, male, white, smoking, obesity, high-fat diet, alcohol use, chocolate, citrus drinks, soda, coffee, and certain medications.

Clinical Presentation

- Patients tend to complain of heartburn, retrosternal burning, bitter taste, and dysphagia.
- Symptoms tend to worsen at night, after eating, with exercise, when lying down, or when bending over.

Diagnosis and Evaluation

- GERD, in itself, is a clinical diagnosis based on history and response to treatment.
- In the emergency department, it is especially important to differentiate GERD from atypical manifestations of cardiopulmonary pathologies. Depending on clinical suspicion, electrocardiogram or other cardiac laboratory studies may be appropriate.

Treatment

- In stable patients without signs of dehydration or bleeding, lifestyle and dietary modification, as well as antacid medications, and outpatient GI referral are appropriate.
- Mild intermittent symptoms warrant a trial of H_2 antagonists. Moderate to severe symptoms that have failed an H_2 blocker may warrant a 6-week trial of proton pump inhibitors (PPIs).

Esophageal Dysmotility

General Principles

- Esophageal motility disorders include achalasia, diffuse esophageal spasm, nutcracker esophagus, as well as anatomic obstructions such as esophageal web, rings, strictures, and tumors.

Clinical Presentation

- Patients may complain of chest pain, dysphagia, regurgitation, and heartburn.
- Patients may also have weight loss owing to decreased oral intake.

Diagnosis and Evaluation

- Patient airway, breathing, and circulation—especially volume status—should be evaluated.
- The emergency physician will need to exclude conditions that result in chest pain and dysphagia.
- Obtaining an electrocardiogram should be considered, and CXR will help rule out esophageal perforation and may show evidence of obstructive pathology.

Treatment

- Patients capable of adequately hydrating themselves and who have no indications for admission can be referred to a gastroenterologist for further workup (e.g., barium swallow, esophagogastroduodenoscopy, esophageal manometry).

SUGGESTED READINGS

Harwood-Nuss'. (2009). *Clinical practice of emergency medicine*. Philadelphia: Lippincott Williams & Wilkins.

Tintinalli, J. E., Stapczynski, J. S., Ma, O. J., Yealy, D. M., Meckler, G. D., & Cline, D. M. (2015). *Tintinalli's emergency medicine: A comprehensive study guide* (8th ed.). McGraw-Hill.

Gallbladder

ANNUM A. BHULLAR, MA, MD, and ALAN CHIEM, MD, MPH

Cholelithiasis/Choledocholithiasis

General Principles

- Cholelithiasis refers to gallstones in the gallbladder, whereas choledocholithiasis refers to stones in the common bile duct.
- Present in 20% of women, 8% of men.
- Cholesterol stones are more common than calcium stones.
- Cholelithiasis risk factors include age, female gender, obesity, oral contraceptive use, family history ("*fat, female, forty, fertile, familial*").

Clinical Presentation

Most patients with cholelithiasis are asymptomatic, and only 25% of those with incidental gallstones become symptomatic after 10–15 years of follow-up. Thus physical examination may be normal. However, if symptomatic, patients may present with colicky right upper quadrant pain, often worse after meals, with radiation to the epigastrium or right scapula, associated with nausea and vomiting.

In contrast, most patients with choledocholithiasis are symptomatic with right upper quadrant or epigastric pain, nausea, and vomiting. Physical examination may demonstrate right upper quadrant and/or epigastric tenderness and jaundice.

Diagnosis and Evaluation

- Cholelithiasis: Results of laboratory tests (complete blood count, liver function tests, and lipase) are usually normal. Ultrasonography is the imaging modality of choice in the emergency department, and gallstones appear hyperechoic with shadowing. Ultrasonography has a sensitivity of 94% with gallbladder visualization, and specificity of 78%.
- Choledocholithiasis: Liver test results, including transaminases, are elevated and consistent with an obstructive, cholestatic pattern with an elevated direct bilirubin. Ultrasonography demonstrates common bile duct dilatation >5–7 mm. If unable to visualize with ultrasonography, and the suspicion remains high, magnetic resonance cholangiopancreatography (MRCP) or endoscopic retrograde cholangiopancreatography (ERCP) may be obtained.

Treatment

- For patients who present with uncomplicated biliary colic, pain control with outpatient referral to general surgery is appropriate. Definitive management is surgical cholecystectomy in those patients with persistent symptoms. Because most patients with choledocholithiasis are symptomatic and may develop cholangitis or pancreatitis, patients are usually admitted and undergo MRCP or ERCP with stone removal, followed by cholecystectomy. Alternatively, cholecystectomy can be performed with intraoperative cholangiography, common bile duct exploration, and/or ERCP.

Cholecystitis

General Principles

- Gallbladder outlet obstruction leads to gallbladder distension and elevated intraluminal pressures, leading to impaired perfusion to the gallbladder wall; as a result, wall ischemia and inflammation develop, facilitating bacterial translocation and infection.
- Most commonly due to the presence of gallstones, although a small percentage (<10%) may be acalculous.

Clinical Presentation

- Right upper quadrant, epigastric, and/or flank pain. Pain is initially colicky, then becomes constant. Pain may radiate to the right scapula (right-sided Kehr sign).
- Associated symptoms include nausea, vomiting, and anorexia.
- Examination may demonstrate a Murphy sign: increase in pain or inspiratory arrest during deep subcostal palpation of the right upper quadrant (65% sensitive, 87% specific).
- Complications of cholecystitis include progression to gangrenous cholecystitis (in up to 20%), perforation, emphysematous cholecystitis, cholecystenteric fistula, and gallstone ileus.
- Often an insidious presentation, acalculous cholecystitis is classically seen in the elderly, critically ill hospitalized patient, or postoperative patients with sepsis of unclear source.

Diagnosis and Evaluation

- Liver function test results may be mildly elevated but are sometimes within normal limits.
- Ultrasonography is the primary imaging modality, but it is operator-dependent and may offer limited visualization in obese patients. Findings include thickened gallbladder wall (>3–5 mm), pericholecystic fluid, immobile stone in the gallbladder neck, and a positive sonographic Murphy sign. See Fig. 2.1.
- Contrast-enhanced computed tomography (CT) scan may miss small radiolucent stones, such as noncalcified pigment stones. However, CT is highly sensitive for findings associated with cholecystitis (e.g., thickened

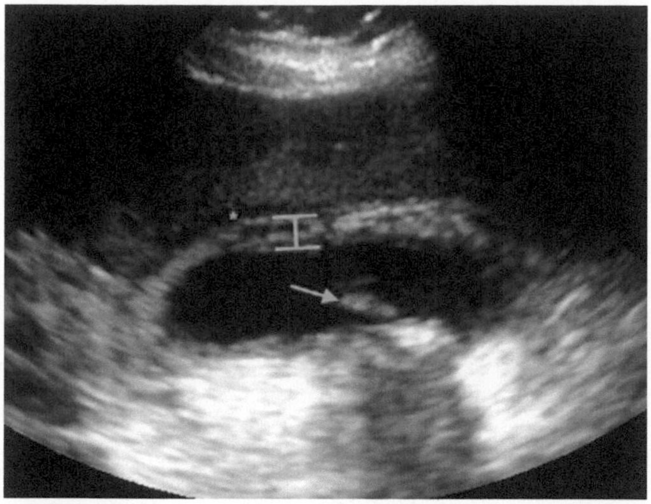

FIG. 2.1 Abdominal ultrasound image showing acute cholecystitis with pericholecystic fluid (*), gallbladder wall thickening (*bracket*), and a gallstone with shadowing (*arrow*). (Courtesy Alan Chiem, MD.)

gallbladder wall and pericholecystic fluid) and should be obtained if ultrasonography is nondiagnostic or equivocal for acute cholecystitis.
- Nuclear scintigraphy (hepatobiliary iminodiacetic acid scan) is also highly sensitive for cholecystitis. Failure to visualize the gallbladder 1 hour after administration of iminodiacetic acid is diagnostic.

Treatment

- Hospital admission; supportive care with intravenous fluid resuscitation (IVF), antiemetics, and pain control
- Antibiotic coverage with a single second- or third-generation cephalosporin is usually adequate, unless the patient appears septic.
- Diabetic and immunocompromised patients are at higher risk for complications, including sepsis, and emphysematous and gangrenous cholecystitis.
- Surgical consultation for definitive treatment (laparoscopic removal preferred to open removal). Indications for emergent cholecystectomy include gallbladder necrosis, emphysematous cholecystitis, and gallbladder perforation.
- For patients with acalculous cholecystitis who are poor surgical candidates and do not have indications for emergent surgery, insertion of a cholecystostomy tube may be an effective, less invasive alternative intervention.

Cholangitis

General Principles

- Ascending cholangitis is a life-threatening bacterial infection of the biliary tract secondary to bile duct obstruction.
- Gallstones are the most common cause of biliary obstruction, although blockages may be extrahepatic or secondary to malignant compression or strictures.
- Bacteria reach the obstructed gallbladder in either a retrograde fashion, through the lymphatics, or via the portal vein.

Clinical Presentation

- Charcot triad: fever + right upper quadrant pain + jaundice (all three occur only in ~50% of cases).
- Reynolds pentad: Charcot triad + hypotension + altered mental status (occurs in <5% of cases).
- Shock or multiple organ system dysfunction may be the presentation in immunocompromised or elderly patients.
- Examination classically demonstrates fever, tenderness in right upper quadrant, and scleral icterus. Tachycardia, hypotension, and altered mental status may also be present if cholangitis is severe.

Diagnosis and Evaluation

- Diagnosis requires (1) evidence of systemic inflammation (fever/chills or laboratory evidence of an inflammatory response with leukocytosis, elevated C-reactive protein) and (2) laboratory evidence of cholestasis (bilirubin > 2 mg/dL and/or liver enzymes > 1.5 times upper limit of normal), plus imaging with evidence of biliary dilation (ultrasonography, CT, MRCP, or ERCP).
- If the ultrasonography result is normal or equivocal but cholangitis is still suspected, then CT, MRCP, and/or ERCP are indicated. Endoscopic ultrasonography is an alternative in patients who cannot undergo ERCP.

Treatment

- Hemodynamic stabilization with fluids, vasopressors as needed, and broad antibiotic coverage for common pathogens such as *Escherichia coli*, *Klebsiella*, *Enterococcus*, *Bacteroides*, and *Clostridium*
  - Anaerobes: metronidazole
  - Gram-negative bacteria: β-lactams, fluoroquinolones, carbapenems (carbapenems also have anaerobic coverage)
- Gastrointestinal consultation for biliary drainage and decompression: ERCP and cholangiography are diagnostic and therapeutic, allowing for direct removal of stones. Although surgical decompression is reserved for patients in whom medical biliary drainage has failed, management of the underlying cause with elective cholecystectomy, if patient has gallstones, is indicated.

Gallbladder Tumors

General Principles

- Malignancies of the gallbladder are uncommon.
- Gallbladder carcinoma is more common in patients with gallstones, females, and obese patients.
- Cholangiocarcinoma or ductal carcinomas occur less frequently and are more common in males. The prognosis for both is poor: 5-year survival rates are only 5%–10%.

Clinical Presentation

Often asymptomatic or symptoms may mimic those with biliary colic. Incidental diagnosis on pathology after elective cholecystectomy is the most common presentation for early-stage cancer. If symptomatic, patients may present with painless jaundice, chronic abdominal pain, or a palpable mass of right upper quadrant (Courvoisier sign).

Diagnosis and Evaluation

Laboratory study results may be normal, but bilirubin and alkaline phosphatase levels may be elevated if there is any bile duct obstruction. Ultrasonography may demonstrate calcification, a mass, a gallbladder polyp >10 mm, or infiltration of the liver. CT, magnetic resonance imaging, and MRCP may better delineate the gallbladder mass. Cholangiocarcinomas may demonstrate dilatation of both intra- and extrahepatic bile ducts (Fig. 2.2). Biopsy and pathology are definitive for diagnosis.

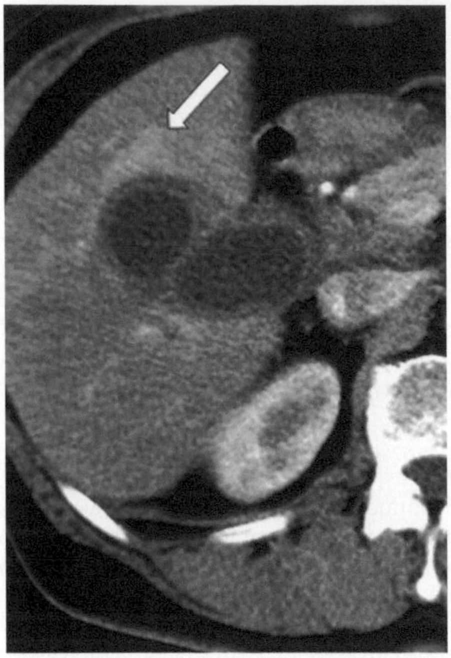

FIG. 2.2 Computed tomography image showing gallbladder carcinoma. (From Kim, S. W., Kim, H. C., Yang, D. M., Ryu, J. K., & Won, K. Y. (2016). Gallbladder carcinoma: Causes of misdiagnosis at CT. *Clinical Radiology, 71*(1), e96–e109.)

Treatment

Treatment depends upon the histologic type and the stage of the carcinoma.

SUGGESTED READINGS

Marx, J. A., Hockberger, R. & Walls, R. M. (2014). *Rosen's emergency medicine: Concepts and clinical practice* (8th ed.). Elsevier/Saunders.

Tintinalli, J. E., Ma O. J., Cline, D., Cydulka, R., Meckler, G., Handel, D., et al. (2012). *Tintinalli's emergency medicine manual* (7th ed.). McGraw Hill Education.

Small Bowel

CATHERINE DANIELLE ANTONUK, MD, and GEORGE LIM, MD

Epigastric, periumbilical, or diffuse abdominal pain can be due to small-intestinal pathology. Important conditions to consider are obstruction, ileus, intussusception, and hernia.

Small-Bowel Obstruction

General Principles

- Small-bowel obstructions (SBOs) are four times more common than large-bowel obstructions.
- Most common cause: adhesions, followed by hernias
  - Less common causes: strictures from inflammatory bowel disease, space-occupying neoplasms
  - Causes in children: volvulus, intussusception, hernias, and congenital abnormalities

Clinical Presentation

- Symptoms
  - Colicky abdominal pain
  - Nausea and vomiting
    - Bilious with proximal obstructions
    - Feculent with distal obstructions
  - No recent bowel movements or flatus
    - Partial obstructions may still permit bowel movements or flatus.
- Physical examination
  - Abdominal distension
  - Tympanitic
  - Focal or diffuse abdominal tenderness
  - Bowel sounds
    - Early presentations: high-pitched, active bowel sounds
    - Late presentations: diminished or absent bowel sounds
  - Peritoneal signs: guarding, rigidity, and rebound tenderness
    - Prolonged and increased intraluminal pressure may lead to intramural venous and capillary congestion, ultimately resulting in ischemia and necrosis.

Diagnosis and Evaluation

- Laboratory tests
  - Complete blood count may demonstrate leukocytosis.
  - Basic metabolic panel may demonstrate an anion gap acidosis.
  - Lactate level may be elevated with bowel ischemia but is nonspecific.
  - Laboratory values may also be deceptively normal.
- Imaging
  - Abdominal x-ray (flat, upright, and/or lateral decubitus) (Fig. 3.1)
    - Air-fluid levels, dilated loops of bowel, string of air pockets ("string of beads/stack of coins" sign) and no colonic gas except with early or partial obstruction
    - Five percent of patients have normal abdominal x-ray results.
  - Computed tomography (CT) of the abdomen/pelvis with intravenous (IV) or oral contrast (Fig. 3.2)
    - Most sensitive and specific
    - Dilated loops of bowel and air-fluid levels
    - Identifies a transition point
    - May determine underlying etiology and pathology
    - May provide insight into mucosal viability (particularly in setting of lactic acidosis)
- Mechanical SBO should be differentiated from ileus (see Ileus section) because of medical etiologies such as hypokalemia or opioid-induced constipation.

Treatment

- Nothing by mouth
- Surgical consultation
  - Nonoperative management is successful in 65% of patients with SBO due to adhesions.
  - Surgical intervention warranted in cases complicated by necrosis and perforation
- Administer IV fluids and correct electrolyte abnormalities from decreased oral intake, vomiting, and ineffective absorption.
- Gastric decompression with nasogastric or orogastric tube
  - Indicated for excessive vomiting and/or distention
  - May not be necessary for mild to moderate cases
- Antibiotics generally not indicated for uncomplicated SBO
  - In cases of perforation or necrosis, broad-spectrum antibiotics to cover intestinal flora
- Hospital admission

Ileus

General Principles

- Adynamic ileus is characterized by intestinal dysmotility without mechanical obstruction.
- Etiologies: opioid use, electrolyte abnormalities (calcium, potassium), and immobility

Clinical Presentation

- Symptoms
  - Diffuse, constant, and dull abdominal pain
  - Nausea and vomiting
  - Presence of flatus and scant bowel movements or even diarrhea

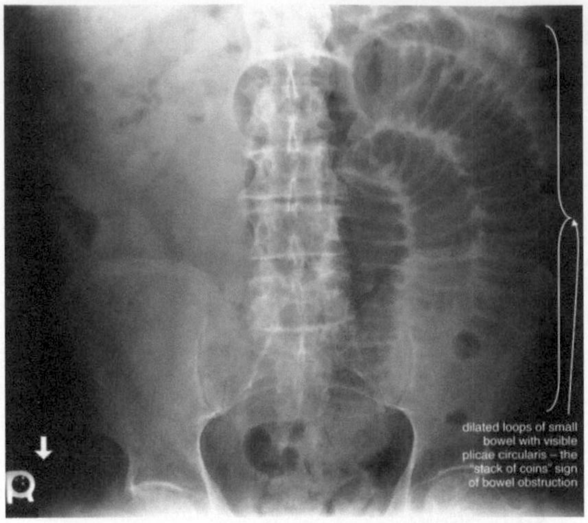

FIG. 3.1 X-ray; small-bowel obstruction. Dilated loops of small bowel characterized by the "string of beads/stack of coins" sign.

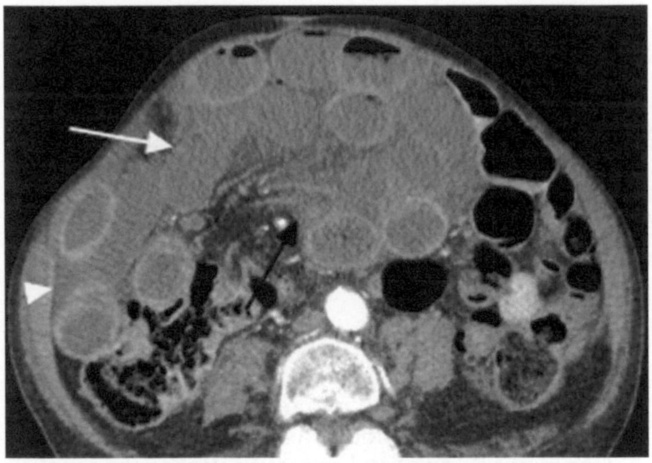

FIG. 3.2 Computed tomography; small-bowel obstruction. Closed-loop obstruction with hypoenhancing loops of bowel (*white arrow*) and mesenteric fluid (*arrowhead*).

- Physical examination
  - Abdominal distention
  - Decreased bowel sounds
  - Mild diffuse tenderness

Diagnosis and Evaluation

- CT of the abdomen/pelvis (has higher sensitivity and specificity than abdominal x-ray)
  - Dilated loops of bowel without transition point
  - Less prominent air/fluid levels (compared to SBO)

Treatment

- Because ileus is usually self-limited, treatment is supportive.
- Identification and treatment of the underlying etiology
  - Correct electrolytes.
  - Discontinue offending medication.
- Nothing by mouth; administer IV fluids
- Encourage early physical activity as tolerated (i.e. out of bed to chair, ambulation, physical therapy).

Intussusception

General Principles

- Intussusception is the telescoping of proximal bowel into distal bowel.
- Classified by location
  - Ileocolic (most cases)
  - Can occur anywhere in the small and large intestines (e.g., ileo-ileal, jejuno-jejuno, colo-colic)
- One of the most common causes of pediatric obstruction
  - 80-90% of affected patients are <2 years old.
  - 75% of pediatric intussusceptions are idiopathic without an identified lead point.
    - Among remaining 25%, Meckel diverticulum is the most common pediatric lead point.
- Patients of any age can develop intussusception.
  - Adults who develop this condition often have a pathologic lead point (e.g., malignant mass).

Clinical Presentation

- Symptoms
  - Severe, crampy, intermittent abdominal pain
  - Children often find comfort in the knees-to-chest position.
  - Nausea and vomiting, which eventually becomes bilious
  - Only 50% of cases have hematochezia with "currant jelly" stools as a rare late finding.
  - Pain-free but lethargic between episodes
    - Lethargy may be the most prominent manifestation (and so intussusception should be part of pediatric altered mental status differential diagnosis).
- Physical examination
  - Nontender or right upper/middle quadrant tenderness
  - Empty right lower quadrant (Dance sign) or right upper/middle quadrant "sausage-shaped mass" (classically taught, but rare in clinical practice)

Diagnosis and Evaluation

- Imaging
  - Ultrasonography (Fig. 3.3)
    - Specificity and sensitivity approach 100%.

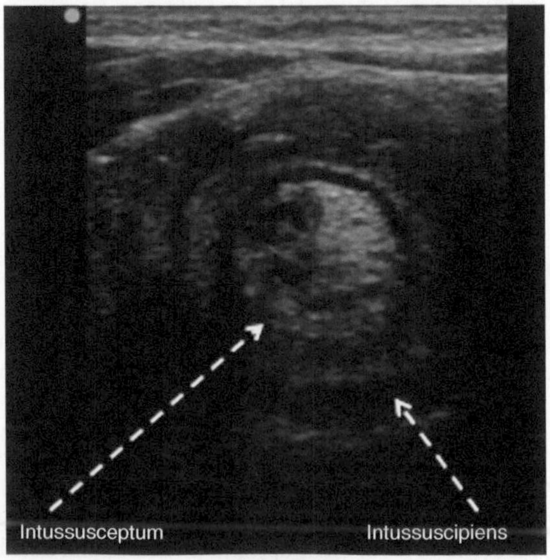

FIG. 3.3 Ultrasonography; ileocolic intussusception.

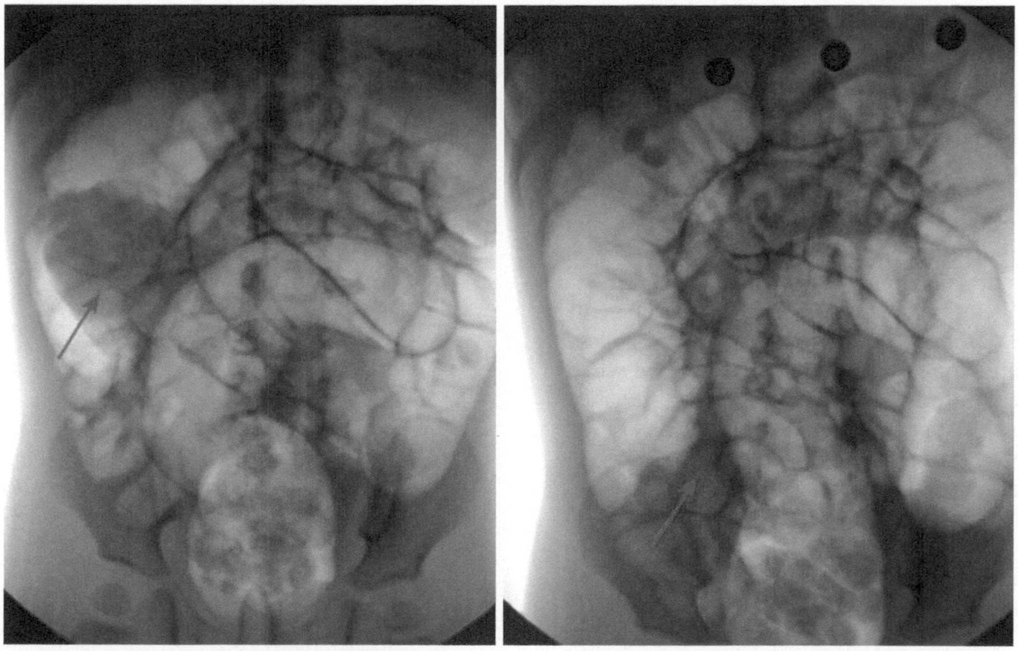

FIG. 3.4 Fluoroscopy; intussusception (*left*) and reduction (*right*). Air-contrast enema showing intussusception at hepatic flexure.

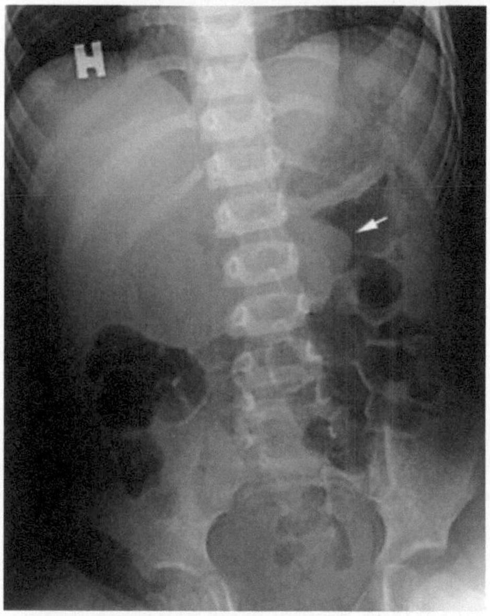

FIG. 3.5 X-ray; intussusception. Soft tissue mass against air-filled bowel loop called the "meniscus sign" (*arrow*).

    - Allows for diagnosis and subsequent ultrasound-guided hydrostatic reduction
    - Given 1% risk of perforation during the reduction, surgery should be consulted and be available for possible operative intervention.
  - Fluoroscopy (Fig. 3.4)
    - Similarly diagnostic and therapeutic as ultrasonography
  - X-ray and less commonly CT (Fig. 3.5)
    - Purely diagnostic

Treatment

- Nonoperative reduction with pneumatic or hydrostatic enema
  - Treatment of choice in stable patients without evidence of bowel perforation or shock
  - After successful, noninvasive reduction with enemas, 10% of cases recur, most within the first 3 days of intervention.
  - After 12–24 hours of observation and monitoring for recurrence, patients who are asymptomatic and tolerating a diet may be safely discharged home with return precautions.
- Surgical intervention
  - For patients with failed enemas, hemodynamic instability, or evidence of intestinal ischemia/perforation

Hernias

General Principles

- A hernia is a protrusion of a structure through overlying tissue.
- Classified by anatomic location, content (e.g., omentum, bowel), and status (e.g., reducible, incarcerated, strangulated)
- Most common are groin hernias.
- Other common hernias: ventral, lumbar, and pelvic
- Most important to determine whether hernia is reducible, incarcerated (nonreducible), or strangulated (compromised vascular supply)
  - Strangulated hernia is a true surgical emergency.

Clinical Presentation

- Symptoms and signs
  - Vary depending on the size and location of the hernia
  - Pain and discomfort with bulging of the hernia upon Valsalva maneuver
  - Incarcerated hernias can present as intestinal obstructions.
  - Patients with strangulated hernias can have discolored overlying skin with signs of systemic illness and shock.
  - Perform a thorough abdominal and genital examination (with particular attention to surgical scars) in the supine and upright positions.

- In thin patients, a hernia with its fascial defect may be readily palpated.

Diagnosis and Evaluation

- Physical examination is usually sufficient to make the diagnosis (e.g., bulge in the groin with increased abdominal pressure).
- Imaging
  - Obese patients and those with lumbar/pelvic hernias often warrant imaging to identify occult hernias.
  - Distinguish femoral from inguinal hernias or differentiate hernias from other pathology that can produce a mass such as lymphoma, hydrocele, or aneurysmal vessels.
  - CT most commonly used but ultrasonography and magnetic resonance imaging are also options
  - Laboratory tests are often unnecessary but may help to distinguish strangulation.

Treatment

- Reducible hernias
  - Outpatient surgical follow-up
- Incarcerated hernias
  - Reduce in the emergency department with adequate pain control, ice, and steady pressure back through the hernia ring while the patient is in the Trendelenburg position.
- Strangulated hernias
  - Should not be reduced due to risk of perforation and sepsis
  - Immediate surgery consultation
  - IV antibiotics

SUGGESTED READINGS

Tintinalli, J. E., Stapczynski, J. S., Ma, O. J., Yealy, D. M., Meckler, G. D., & Cline, D. M. (Eds.). (2016). *Tintinalli's emergency medicine: A comprehensive study guide* (8th ed.). McGraw-Hill Education.

Wolfson, A. B., Cloutier, R. L., Hendey, G. W., Ling, L. J., Rosen, C. L., & Schaider, J. J. (Eds.). (2015). *Harwood-Nuss' clinical practice of emergency medicine* (6th ed.). Wolters-Kluwer.

Large Bowel

CATHERINE DANIELLE ANTONUK, MD, and GEORGE LIM, MD

Any kind of abdominal pain can be of large-intestinal etiology. The large bowel can be a site of surgical emergencies (e.g., appendicitis, volvulus), acute infection (e.g., diverticulitis, diarrheal illness), or a chronic condition such as irritable bowel syndrome. It is important to manage these patients in the context of their intravascular volume status and ability to tolerate nourishment by mouth.

Appendicitis

General Principles

- Most common abdominal surgical emergency
- Most common nonobstetric surgical emergency in pregnancy
- Luminal obstruction of the appendix, usually by a fecalith, causes elevated intraluminal pressure leading to vascular insufficiency, thereby increasing risk of infection and perforation.

Clinical Presentation

- Initially poorly localized, visceral periumbilical pain from appendiceal inflammation
- Pain then localizes to McBurney point (right lower quadrant) from surrounding peritoneal inflammation
- Associated with fever, anorexia, and nausea/vomiting
- Sudden relief of previously severe abdominal pain can suggest appendiceal perforation.
- Pathognomonic signs
  - Rovsing sign (pain in right lower quadrant with palpation of left lower quadrant [LLQ])
  - Psoas sign (pain upon right hip extension)
  - Obturator sign (pain with internal rotation of flexed right hip)
- Signs and symptoms vary based on anatomic location of appendix.
  - Appendicitis in late pregnancy can present with right upper quadrant pain as the gravid uterus shifts the appendix upward.
  - Inflammation of the retrocecal appendix can cause flank or back pain.
  - In patients with congenital gut malrotation, appendicitis presents with left upper quadrant pain.

Diagnosis and Evaluation

- Appendicitis is a clinical diagnosis (for likelihood ratios of signs/symptoms, see Table 4.1).
- Laboratory test results and clinical scoring systems (i.e., Alvarado score, Table 4.2) are neither specific nor sensitive but in combination may assist diagnosis.
  - White blood cell (WBC) count, erythrocyte sedimentation rate (ESR), and C-reactive protein (CRP) may be elevated.
  - Urinalysis may show pyuria and/or hematuria (due to close proximity of the ureter to the appendix).
- Ultrasonography is the first-line imaging modality for pregnant women and children.
  - If nondiagnostic, magnetic resonance imaging or computed tomography (CT) is recommended.
  - Intravenous (IV) gadolinium is not administered in pregnancy or renal insufficiency because it crosses the placenta and can cause nephrogenic systemic fibrosis, respectively.
- CT is often the first-line imaging modality in males and nonpregnant females.
  - Intraabdominal fat can serve as natural contrast in CT studies, obviating the need for IV contrast.
- Imaging findings (Fig. 4.1)
  - Blind-ending, noncompressible appendix with diameter >6 mm
  - Thickened wall
  - Surrounding edema and fat stranding

Treatment

- Currently, definitive treatment remains surgery.
- Obtain early surgical consultation before imaging in classic, unequivocal cases.
- Antibiotics covering aerobic and anaerobic gram-negative bacteria
- Select patients (i.e. pediatrics) are treated only with antibiotics without surgery, however this decision should be made with a surgeon as these patients need careful return precautions and still may require surgery at a later date.

Diverticulitis

General Principles

- Diverticulosis is an increasingly common disease and incidence increases with age.
- Affects up to one-third of the population by age 50 years. Typically diagnosed by colonoscopy. Nearly a quarter of people with diverticulosis will develop diverticulitis.
- Diverticulitis is inflammation and infection of these diverticula.
- Potential complications: bacterial translocation, microperforation, and abscess
- In the United States, patients most commonly present with left-sided pathology (i.e., descending and sigmoid colon).
- 2-5% of cases are right-sided (usually in Asian patients).

TABLE 4.1 Likelihood Ratios Associated with Various Historical Factors

Symptom	Positive LR (95% CI)	Negative LR (95% CI)
Right lower quadrant pain*	7.31–8.46	0–0.28
No similar pain previously	1.50 (1.36–1.66)	0.323 (0.246–0.424)
Migration	3.18 (2.41–4.21)	0.50 (0.42–0.59)
Pain before vomiting†	2.76 (1.94–3.94)	NA
Anorexia	1.27 (1.16–1.38)	0.64 (0.54–0.75)
Nausea*	0.69–1.20	0.70–0.84
Vomiting	0.92 (0.82–1.04)	1.12 (0.95–1.33)

LR, Likelihood ratio
*In heterogeneous studies, the LRs are reported as ranges without CIs because a meta-analysis could not be performed.
†Only 1 study in meta-analysis.
The authors report no studies identified evaluating the precision of the clinical examination for appendicitis.
Reprinted from Yeh B. Does This Adult Patient Have Appendicitis? In Annals of Emergency Medicine, 2008;52(3):301–303.

TABLE 4.1 Likelihood Ratios Associated with Various Physical Examination Findings

Signs	Positive LR (95% CI)	Negative LR (95% CI)
Rigidity	3.76 (2.96–4.78)	0.82 (0.79–0.85)
Psoas sign	2.38 (1.21–4.67)	0.90 (0.83–0.98)
Fever	1.94 (1.63–2.32)	0.58 (0.51–0.67)
Rebound tenderness test*	1.10–6.30	0–0.86
Guarding*	1.65–1.78	0–0.54
Rectal tenderness*	0.83–5.34	0.36–1.15

*In heterogeneous studies, the LRs are reported as ranges without CIs because a meta-analysis could not be performed.
Reprinted from Yeh B. Does This Adult Patient Have Appendicitis? In Annals of Emergency Medicine, 2008;52(3):301–303.

TABLE 4.2 Alvarado Score for Acute Appendicitis[a]

Appendicitis Indicator	Alvarado Score Points
Signs	
Right lower quadrant tenderness	Yes: +2
Elevated temperature (37.3°C)	Yes: +1
Rebound tenderness	Yes: +1
Symptoms	
Migration of pain to right lower quadrant	Yes: +1
Anorexia	Yes: +1
Nausea or vomiting	Yes: +1
Laboratory Test Results	
Leukocytosis > 10,000 white blood cells	Yes: +2
Leukocyte left shift (>75% neutrophils)	Yes: +1

[a]A score of <5 is unlikely appendicitis. A score of 5 or 6 is possible appendicitis. Scores of 7 or 8 are likely appendicitis. A score of 9 is definite appendicitis.

CLINICAL PRESENTATION

- LLQ pain
- Fever
- Nausea/vomiting
- Diarrhea or constipation

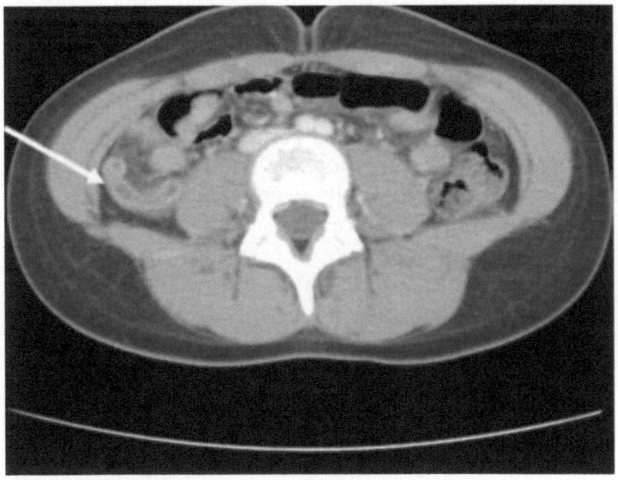

FIG. 4.1 Computed tomography scan; appendicitis. *Arrow* points to a dilated appendix with thickened walls.

- Anorexia
- Physical examination
  - LLQ/suprapubic tenderness
  - Possible peritoneal signs in cases of microperforation and abscess

Diagnosis and Evaluation

- CT with IV contrast is imaging of choice (Fig. 4.2).
  - Assesses severity, complications (i.e. abscess), and other differential diagnoses

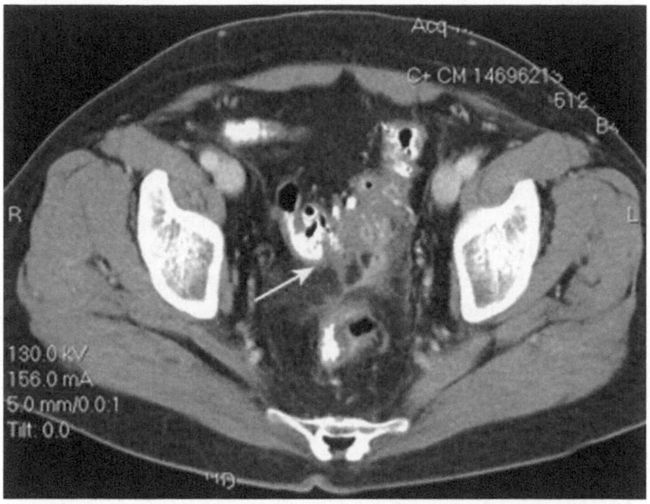

FIG. 4.2 Computed tomography scan; diverticulitis. Severe sigmoid diverticulitis. *Arrow* points to contrast extravasation and free air.

- Increasing incidence of diverticulitis among patients younger than 40 years with rising rates of obesity in the United States
  - Associated with increased complications and operative interventions

Treatment

- Uncomplicated diverticulitis in immunocompetent patients is managed as outpatient.
- Oral antibiotics covering anaerobes/gram-negative bacteria
- Bowel rest with a liquid diet
- Ensure ability to tolerate nutrition by mouth and adequate pain control.
- Uncomplicated diverticulitis in immunocompromised or otherwise high-risk patients requires admission.
- IV antibiotics
- Close observation for complications
- Complicated diverticulitis (by perforation, abscess, fistula, etc.) requires admission.
- IV antibiotics
- Possible percutaneous versus operative intervention
- All patients should be educated on dietary and lifestyle modifications.
- Some gastroenterology societies are now withholding antibiotics for a select group of patients; however, in the acute emergency department setting, it is more likely that patients are provided antibiotics.

Large-Bowel Obstruction

General Principles

- Most common etiology: neoplasms
- Second most common etiology: diverticulitis
  - Caused by mesenteric edema and eventual stricture
- Third most common etiology: sigmoid volvulus
- More common in elderly, bedridden, and/or psychiatric patients likely due to medications with anticholinergic side effects

Clinical Presentation

- Dependent on underlying cause and location of obstruction
- Focal or diffuse abdominal pain
- Nausea/vomiting (classically feculent)
- Absence of bowel movements and flatus
- In cases of neoplasm, history of unintentional weight loss, pencil-thin stools, and melena or hematochezia
- Physical examination
  - Abdominal distension
  - Focal or diffuse abdominal tenderness
  - Hyperactive bowel sounds (early presentation) or diminished/absent bowel sounds (late presentation)

Diagnosis and Evaluation

- Abdominal x-ray (flat, upright, and/or lateral decubitus)
- CT of the abdomen/pelvis is imaging modality of choice.
  - Higher sensitivity and specificity than x-ray
  - Identification of a transition point and underlying pathology

Treatment

- Nothing by mouth
- IV fluids
- Correction of electrolyte abnormalities
- Surgical consultation
  - Self-expanding intraluminal stents at times utilized to temporarily relieve obstruction until definitive surgical procedure (i.e., operative debulking or resection of neoplasms)
  - Closed-loop obstruction, bowel necrosis, or cecal volvulus requires emergent surgical intervention.
  - Strictures may only require endoscopic dilation and stenting.
- Broad-spectrum antibiotics if concern for bowel necrosis and perforation

Sigmoid Volvulus

General Principles

- Segment of sigmoid and attached mesentery twists on itself causing intestinal obstruction, compromised blood flow, and ultimately ischemia
- Common risk factors: advanced age (mean age 70 years), psychiatric disorder, and anticholinergic use. Also seen in children with significant intellectual disability and severe chronic constipation.

Clinical Presentation

- Progressively worsening LLQ pain
- Abdominal distention
- Obstipation/constipation
- Nausea/vomiting
- Physical examination
  - Empty left iliac fossa (good specificity but poor sensitivity)
  - Signs of peritonitis and shock if volvulus progresses to gangrene and perforation

Diagnosis and Evaluation

- Abdominal x-ray (Fig. 4.3)
  - Up to 60% of cases can be diagnosed.

4

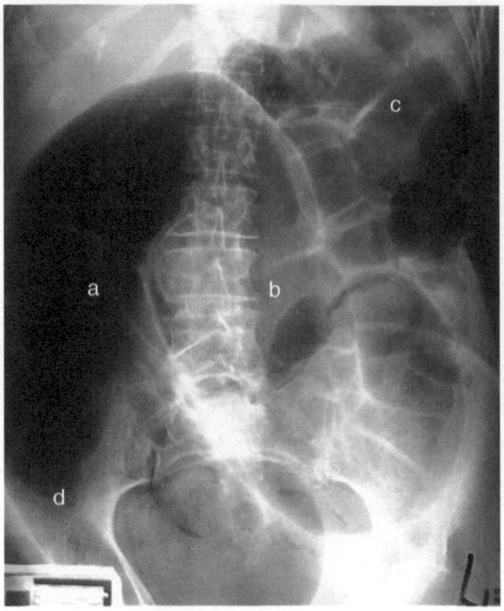

FIG. 4.3 X-ray; sigmoid volvulus. Dilated sigmoid loop seen at *a* and *b*. Dilated bowel at c and d.

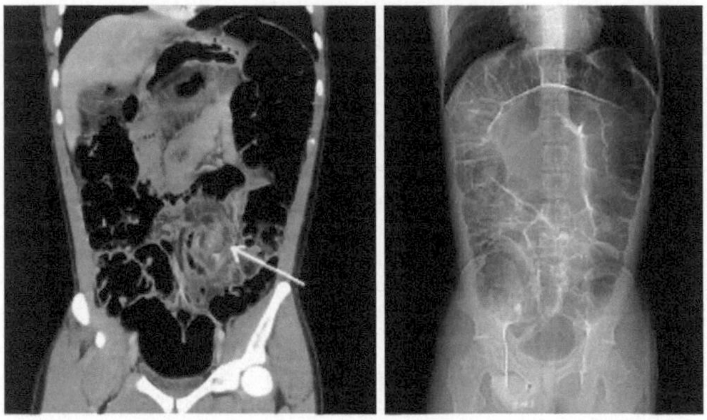

FIG. 4.4 Left image: Computed tomography scan; sigmoid volvulus. *Arrow* points to a dilated sigmoid with swirled mesentery. Right image: X-ray showing dilated bowel in the same patient.

  - Distended loops of bowel
  - Loss of haustral markings
  - "Bent inner tube" or "coffee bean" extending into the right upper quadrant
- CT has higher sensitivity and specificity (Fig. 4.4).
  - Evaluates for complications and other differential diagnoses
  - Classic signs: whirl pattern and bird-beak appearance of affected intestine

Treatment

- Uncomplicated sigmoid volvulus
  - Detorsion with flexible sigmoidoscopy with or without subsequent operative repair
- Complicated sigmoid volvulus
  - Cases with gangrene or perforation warrant immediate operative intervention.

Cecal Volvulus

General Principles

- Cecum twists around its mesentery.
- Risk factors
  - Developmental failure of posterior peritoneal fixation
  - Bowel restriction at a fixed point (i.e., pelvic mass, third trimester pregnancy, or adhesions)
- Unlike sigmoid volvulus, cecal volvulus tends to affect younger patients aged 30–60 years.

Clinical Presentation

- Variety of nonspecific symptoms
  - Abdominal pain
  - Nausea/vomiting
  - Constipation/obstipation
  - Lack of flatus or bowel movements
- Physical examination
  - Diffuse abdominal tenderness
  - Distension
  - Tympanitic bowel sounds
  - Signs of peritonitis and shock in cases of ischemia, gangrene, and perforation

Diagnosis and Evaluation

- Abdominal x-ray (Fig. 4.5)
  - Only a fraction of patients have the pathognomonic "coffee bean" finding in the left upper quadrant.
- CT has higher sensitivity and specificity (Fig. 4.6).
  - Evaluates for complications and other differential diagnoses
  - Classic findings: "bird-beak" sign and "whirl" sign

Treatment

- All typically require operative management
  - Type and extent of surgery depend on patient stability and pathologic mechanism.

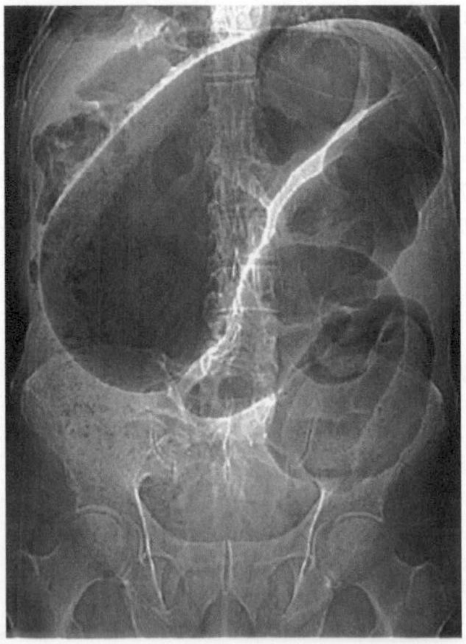

FIG. 4.5 X-ray; cecal volvulus. Classic "coffee bean" sign.

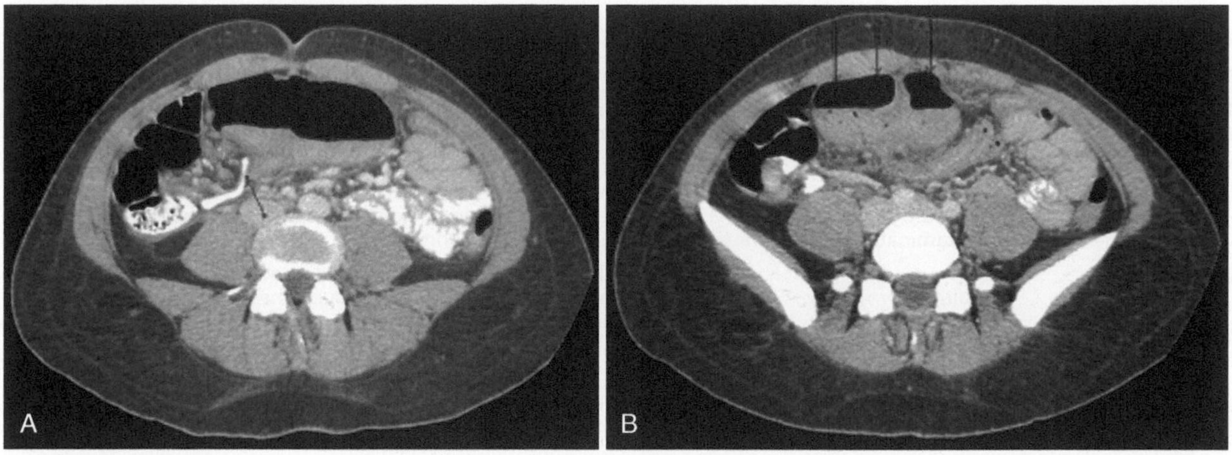

FIG. 4.6 Computed tomography scan; cecal volvulus. *Arrow* in (A) points to swirling of collapsed ileum and mesentery. *Arrows* in (B) point to dilated cecum.

Diarrheal Illness

General Principles

- Diarrhea is caused by four main mechanisms: increased secretion, decreased absorption, increased osmotic load, abnormal motility.
  - Increased secretion: excessive intestinal crypt secretion
  - Decreased absorption
    - Ninety percent of intraluminal fluid is normally reabsorbed by sodium- and glucose-dependent transport systems.
    - Various enterotoxins block sodium reabsorption, thereby increasing intestinal water loss; as glucose-dependent transports are often unaffected, treatment includes glucose-containing oral fluids.
  - Increased osmotic load: often iatrogenic (i.e., laxatives, colchicine)
  - Abnormal motility: seen in irritable bowel syndrome or various neuropathies

Viral

- Most common cause of diarrhea worldwide
- Diarrhea is mucoid and nonbloody.
- Treatment is only symptomatic management because the diarrhea is self-limiting.
- Common viruses that cause diarrheal illnesses and their key associations are listed in Table 4.3.

Bacterial

- Travel to developing countries within South Asia, Africa, and Latin America increases the risk of bacterial diarrhea by 80%.
- Certain travel activities can increase the risk: camping, living among local populations, eating food from street vendors, and practicing poor hand hygiene.
- Time of year also affects the risk of infection; rainy seasons are associated with more diarrheal illnesses.
- Bacterial diarrheal infections categorized as invasive or noninvasive
  - Invasive infections are caused by direct bacterial invasion of intestinal mucosa.
    - Classic symptoms: bloody diarrhea and fever
    - Common causes detailed in Table 4.4
  - Noninvasive bacterial diarrhea is due to toxins released from bacteria that disrupt the normal secretory and absorptive functions of the gut.
    - Patients typically have profuse watery, nonbloody diarrhea.
    - Common causes detailed in Table 4.5

Parasitic

- Travel to developing countries increases risk for parasitic diarrheal illness.
- Common causes detailed in Table 4.6

TABLE 4.3 *Viral Causes of Diarrhea*

Virus	Findings
Norovirus (Norwalk virus)	50%–80% of infectious diarrhea in the United States
Rotavirus	Most common cause of pediatric diarrhea More common in winter Vaccine available

Irritable Bowel Syndrome

General Principles

- Chronic and recurrent disorder of gut motility and sensation
- Believed to be both a neurologic and an intestinal condition

Clinical Presentation

- Nonspecific symptoms
  - Generalized abdominal pain
  - Bloating
  - Nausea/vomiting
  - Constipation or diarrhea
- Symptoms exacerbated by certain foods, hormone fluctuations, and psychological stress
- Abdominal examination is often unremarkable.

TABLE 4.4 *Invasive Bacterial Causes of Diarrhea*

Bacterium	Source/Risk Factor	Treatment/Findings
Enterohemorrhagic *Escherichia coli* (O157:H7)	Raw ground beef Unpasteurized milk	Supportive care Antibiotics/antispasmodics can increase risk of hemolytic uremic syndrome.
Campylobacter jejuni	Raw poultry Unpasteurized milk Contaminated food or water	Supportive care Severe symptoms: ciprofloxacin (Cetraxal), levofloxacin (Levaquin), or azithromycin (Zithromax)
Salmonella	Eggs Poultry Dairy Exposure to reptiles and turtles Contaminated food or water	Ciprofloxacin (Cetraxal), levofloxacin (Levaquin), or azithromycin (Zithromax) May have "rose spots" or "salmon patches" on skin Can cause bacteremia in children < 6 months of age and immunosuppressed.
Shigella	Contaminated food or water	Ciprofloxacin (Cetraxal), levofloxacin (Levaquin), or azithromycin (Zithromax)
Vibrio parahaemolyticus *V. vulnificus*	Undercooked/raw shellfish	Supportive care Severe symptoms: ciprofloxacin (Cetraxal), trimethoprim/sulfamethoxazole (Bactrim)
Yersinia enterocolitica	Undercooked pork Tofu Contaminated water	Supportive care Can mimic appendicitis

TABLE 4.5 *Noninvasive Bacterial Causes of Diarrhea*

Pathogen or Condition	Source/Risk Factors	Treatment/Findings
Staphylococcus aureus	Dairy Eggs	Supportive care Most common cause of food-borne illness Symptoms within 6 h
Bacillus cereus	Fried rice	Supportive care
Enterotoxigenic *Escherichia coli*	Contaminated water	Ciprofloxacin (Cetraxal), trimethoprim/sulfamethoxazole (Bactrim) Most common cause of travelers diarrhea
Vibrio cholera	Contaminated water Fish	Doxycycline (Doxy-100), azithromycin (Zithromax), or trimethoprim/sulfamethoxazole (Bactrim) "Rice water" diarrhea
Listeria	Deli meat Fresh, soft unpasteurized cheeses	Penicillin, ampicillin, or trimethoprim/sulfamethoxazole (Bactrim) Associated with preterm delivery
Scombroid	Unrefrigerated fish (especially tuna, mackerel, bonito)	H_1 and H_2 blockers Heat-stable toxin; histamine-like reaction within 30 min Symptoms: burning-peppery taste, flushing, headache, abdominal cramping, vomiting, diarrhea Elderly: severe cardiac, respiratory symptoms
Ciguatera	Reef fish contaminated by *Gambierdiscus toxicus* (ciguatoxin) (e.g., grouper, snapper, amberjack, barracuda)	Mannitol (Osmitrol, Resectisol) for severe cases Heat-resistant toxin affects sodium channels Symptoms: nausea, vomiting, diarrhea within 1–24 h Paresthesia, hot/cold reversal, muscle weakness may last years; worse with alcohol Severe: hypotension, bradycardia
Clostridioides difficile (previously *Clostridium difficile*)	Postoperative Recent antibiotics	Frequent, profuse, watery diarrhea Can cause toxic megacolon or perforation in 1%–3% of patients Diagnosis: stool *C. difficile* toxin, immunoassay Oral vancomycin is first-line for non-fulminant disease

TABLE 4.6 *Parasitic Causes of Diarrhea*

Parasite	Source/Incubation Time	Diagnosis/Treatment
Giardia	Contaminated water Sexually transmitted 1–4 week incubation	Frothy, foul, floating diarrhea Diagnosis: stool ova/parasite; will see cysts, trophozoites Treatment: metronidazole (Flagyl), paromomycin (Humatin) during pregnancy
Entamoeba histolytica	Contaminated water Sexually transmitted 3–4 week incubation	Diarrhea, possibly bloody Sometimes central nervous system, cardiac, pulmonary symptoms Treatment: metronidazole (Flagyl), paromomycin (Humatin) during pregnancy
Cryptosporidium	Contaminated water 1 week incubation	Watery diarrhea; common in AIDS Diagnosis: stool ova/parasite; will see oocytes Treatment: supportive for immunocompetent, Nitazoxanide (Alinia) for severe cases or immunocompromised

Diagnosis and Evaluation

- Clinical diagnosis with thorough history and physical

Treatment

- Symptomatic treatment
  - Patients may benefit from antispasmodics, antidepressants, or anxiolytics. Antispasmodic agents such as loperamide and diphenoxylate/ atropine should be avoided in young children.

SUGGESTED READINGS

Tintinalli, J. E., Stapczynski, J. S., Ma, O. J., Yealy, D. M., Meckler, G. D., & Cline, D. M. (Eds.). (2016). *Tintinalli's emergency medicine: A comprehensive study guide* (8th ed.). McGraw-Hill Education.

Wolfson, A. B., Cloutier, R. L., Hendey, G. W., Ling, L. J., Rosen, C. L., & Schaider, J. J. (Eds.). (2015). *Harwood-Nuss' clinical practice of emergency medicine* (6th ed.). Wolters Kluwer.

CHAPTER 5

BOARD REVIEW

Liver

ANNUM A. BHULLAR, MA, MD, and ALAN CHIEM, MD, MPH

Hepatitis

General Principles

- Inflammation of the liver, which can be secondary to viral infections, toxic exposures, medications, or autoimmune diseases

Clinical Presentation

- Symptoms may include:
  - Fever
  - Jaundice
  - Abdominal pain
  - Vomiting
  - Diarrhea
  - Clay-colored stools
  - Easy bruising
  - Bleeding
- Signs of hepatitis include scleral icterus, abdominal tenderness, hepatomegaly, and cirrhosis.

Viral Hepatitis

- Hepatitis A: Transmitted fecal-orally, usually from contaminated food or water. Vaccine is available. Presents initially with nausea, vomiting, abdominal pain, then bilirubinuria, clay-colored stools, and jaundice one week later (Fig. 5.1).
- Hepatitis B: Transmitted through sexual encounters, intravenous (IV) drug abuse, transfusions, and perinatally. Can lead to chronic infection, cirrhosis, and hepatocellular carcinoma (HCC).
- Hepatitis C: Transmitted through exposure to contaminated blood or IV drug use, and sexually. Can also lead to chronic infections, cirrhosis, and HCC. Acute infection is often asymptomatic.
- Hepatitis D: Dependent on hepatitis B coinfection. Can rapidly progress to liver failure and death.
- Hepatitis E: Transmitted fecal-orally, often seen in travelers, and may result in epidemics. High mortality among pregnant patients.
- Autoimmune hepatitis: Often seen in young females.

Drug-Induced

- Acetaminophen can lead to liver injury in doses more than 4 g/day for adults or more than 150 mg/kg/day in pediatric patients.
- N-acetylcysteine should be administered if acetaminophen level is more than 150 μg/mL four hours after ingestion.

Diagnosis (Typical Liver Function Abnormalities) and Evaluation

- Liver function tests (LFTs) in 100s: viral inflammation, nonalcoholic steatohepatitis (NASH)
- LFTs in 1000s: hepatocellular necrosis, extensive liver injury, fulminant disease
- Aspartate transaminase (AST):alanine transaminase (ALT)< 1: acute and chronic viral hepatitis

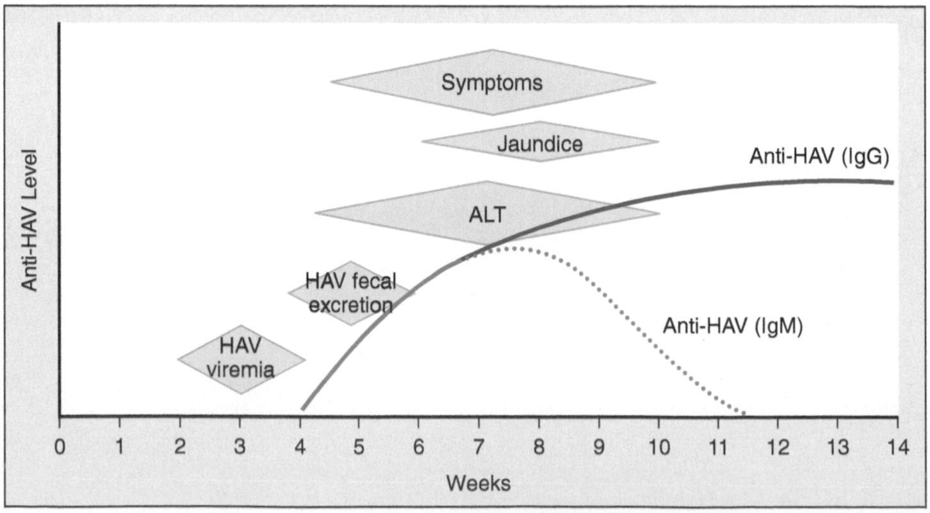

FIG. 5.1 Hepatitis A. (From Guss, D. A., & Oyama, L. C. (2010). Disorders of the liver and biliary tract. In J. A. Marx, R. S. Hockberger, & R. M. Walls (Eds.), *Rosen's emergency medicine: Concepts and clinical practice* (7th ed., p. 1154, Fig. 88.1). Mosby Elsevier.)

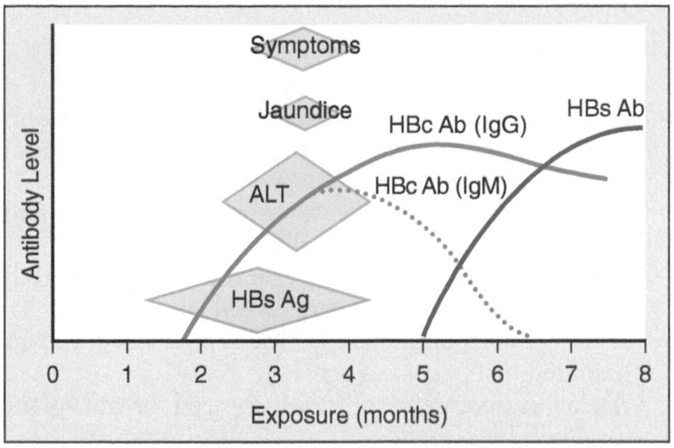

FIG. 5.2 Hepatitis B. (From Guss, D. A., & Oyama, L. C. (2010). Disorders of the liver and biliary tract. In J. A. Marx, R. S. Hockberger, & R. M. Walls (Eds.), *Rosen's emergency medicine: Concepts and clinical practice* (7th ed., p. 1154, Fig. 88.2). Mosby Elsevier.)

- AST:ALT > 2: alcoholic hepatitis
- Hepatitis B: (Fig. 5.2)
  - HBsAg: present in active infection
  - Anti-HBs: present if recovered from prior infection OR prior immunization
  - Anti-HBc: core antibody, if positive, immunity was from prior infection (not from vaccine)
    - Anti-HBc IgM: early marker of infection
    - Anti-HBc IgG: best marker of prior HBV infection
  - HBeAg: high infectivity period
  - Anti-HBeAg: low infectivity period

Treatment

- Supportive care
- Rest
- Oral fluids
- Avoidance of alcohol and hepatotoxic drugs
- Admit if encephalopathic, prolonged prothrombin time/international normalized ratio (INR), intractable vomiting, or fulminant hepatic failure.
- Hepatitis B: Suppress HBV DNA and eliminate HBsAg using antiviral agents, which may include pegylated interferon or nucleoside analogs such as entecavir and tenofovir. Patients should avoid alcohol use and be screened for hepatocellular carcinoma.
- Hepatitis C: Goal is to eradicate HCV RNA using direct antivirals, many of which are now interferon-free and ribavirin-free. Patients should avoid alcohol and marijuana use, mitigate risk factors for obesity and insulin resistance, and should have twice yearly ultrasound screening for hepatocellular carcinoma as well as upper endoscopy to check for esophageal varices.

Prophylaxis

- Hepatitis B exposure in *unvaccinated* patient: administer immune globulin within 14 days of exposure and initiate vaccination.
- Hepatitis B exposure in *vaccinated* patient: test for HBsAb. If low titers, administer immune globulin and booster.
- All pregnant women are screened for hepatitis B during their first prenatal visit: administer immune globulin and initiate vaccination if active infection.

Alcoholic Liver Disease

General Principles

- Most common cause of cirrhosis in the United States
- Usually occurs after 10 to 15 years of drinking
- Once the liver has become cirrhotic, the damage is not reversible. However, abstinence helps prevent further destruction.
- Genetic predispositions to liver damage exist.
- Mechanism of damage is due to toxic metabolites such as acetaldehyde, diminished NAD+/NADH ratio leading to fatty liver infiltration, and malnutrition.

Diagnosis and Evaluation

- History of heavy alcohol use
- AST greater than ALT
- Mild transaminitis with significant bilirubin elevation suggests alcoholic hepatitis.
- Often hypokalemic, hypomagnesemic
- Elevated PT/INR predictive of poor outcome

Treatment

- Supportive. IV fluids, electrolyte repletion, multivitamin
- Thiamine 50 to 100 mg IV/IM before glucose to prevent Wernicke's encephalopathy

Nonalcoholic Fatty Liver Disease (NAFLD)

General Principles

- Presence of hepatic steatosis without other etiology for hepatic fat accumulation
- Divided into nonalcoholic fatty liver (NAFL) and nonalcoholic steatohepatitis (NASH)
- NAFL refers to hepatic steatosis *without* hepatic inflammation.
- NASH refers to hepatic steatosis *with* hepatic inflammation, and can look similar to alcoholic steatohepatitis.
- Important cause of cryptogenic cirrhosis

Diagnosis and Evaluation

- Often asymptomatic. May have fatigue and right upper quadrant discomfort
- May have mild AST and ALT elevation or liver function tests may be normal
- May see hepatic steatosis on imaging
- Exclusion of significant alcohol consumption
- No other coexisting liver diseases
- Liver biopsy may be needed if diagnosis is unclear.

Treatment

- Weight loss
- Hepatitis vaccinations
- Abstaining from alcohol consumption
- Serial liver enzyme evaluations every 3 to 6 months
- Vitamin E
- Screen for hepatocellular carcinoma.

Cirrhosis

General Principles

- End-stage chronic liver disease that is characterized by destruction of hepatocytes, fibrosis, nodular regeneration, and, eventually, portal hypertension
- The most common cause is alcohol use or chronic viral hepatitis.
- Can also be caused by viral and autoimmune hepatitis, nonalcoholic fatty liver disease, biliary disease, vascular causes, Wilson disease, and hemochromatosis

Clinical Presentation

- Impaired coagulation leads to ecchymoses, GI bleeding, spider nevi (isolated telangiectasias).
- Portal hypertension leads to varices, ascites, caput medusa (dilated veins around umbilicus), splenomegaly, spontaneous bacterial peritonitis (SBP).
- Impaired bilirubin breakdown leads to jaundice, scleral icterus.
- Impaired estrogen and sex hormone breakdown leads to gynecomastia, palmar erythema, testicular atrophy, spider angiomata.
- Impaired ammonia breakdown leads to asterixis, encephalopathy, and fetor hepaticus (patient's characteristic breath also known as "breath of the dead").
- Hepatorenal syndrome: acute renal failure in patients with otherwise normal kidneys. Can occur with acute or chronic hepatic failure.
- Hepatopulmonary syndrome: shortness of breath and hypoxemia secondary to vasodilation in lungs of those with liver disease.

Diagnosis and Evaluation

- Thrombocytopenia (from splenic platelet sequestration)
- Elevated PT/INR
- Low albumin (decreased hepatic synthesis)
- Elevated alkaline phosphatase
- LFTs may initially be elevated at the beginning of cirrhosis, but may normalize as hepatic function is further impaired.
- May need abdominal ultrasound with Doppler studies and possibly biopsy for definitive diagnosis

Treatment

- Supportive care
- Diuretics: Aldosterone antagonists, such as spironolactone, inhibit excess water reabsorption, which reduces the incidence of hyponatremia and ascites development. They can be used alone or in conjunction with furosemide. However, note that patients who are cirrhotic are often volume-depleted in the intravascular space owing to low oncotic pressure.
- Consider albumin administration (6-8 g per L of ascites removed) IV after large-volume paracentesis (≥5L) to avoid fluid shifts and precipitating acute renal insufficiency.
- Administer vitamin K (10 mg), fresh frozen plasma, platelets prior to procedures in those with coagulopathy (INR > 1.5, platelet count < 50K).
- May be evaluated for liver transplant

Cirrhosis in Children

- Etiology in older children similar to adults
- Infants present with weight loss/ failure of weight gain
- Most common etiologies in infants are biliary atresia and genetic/metabolic disorders
- Biliary atresia is an obstruction of the biliary tract and can be congenital or perinatally acquired
  - Presents with conjugated hyperbilirubinemia shortly after birth or later in the neonatal period
  - Surgical portoenterostomy (Kasai procedure) recommended by 8 weeks of age
  - Delay in treatment can result in need for transplant or death by 2 years

Drug-Induced Cirrhosis

General Principles (Table 5.1)

- 50% of fulminant liver failure cases in the United States are from drug-induced liver disease.
- Damage may be secondary to direct cytotoxic effects or, more often, owing to toxic metabolites.

Clinical Presentation

- Often asymptomatic
- May have painless jaundice if cholestatic pathology
- May have moderate transaminitis
  - Medications causing hepatocellular necrosis: acetaminophen, phenytoin, statins, isoniazid
  - Medications causing cholestasis: oral contraceptives, anabolic steroids
  - Medications causing steatohepatitis: valproic acid, amiodarone
  - Medications causing chronic liver disease: nitrofurantoin, minocycline
  - Medications causing hepatic vein thrombosis: oral contraceptives
  - Medications causing ALT > AST: antiretroviral drug therapy

Treatment

- Stop the offending agent.
- Consider steroids if allergic mechanism.

Primary Biliary Cirrhosis

General Principles

- Autoimmune disease that causes slow destruction of biliary tract, which then leads to cholestasis and subsequent cirrhosis from buildup of bile and other toxins

Clinical Presentation

- Patients will often complain of pruritus or show jaundice before end-stage cirrhosis or complications develop.
- Often associated with other autoimmune syndromes; may have symptoms of scleroderma, Sjögren's or CREST (calcinosis, Raynaud's, esophageal dysmotility, sclerodactyly, telangiectasia)

TABLE 5.1 Drugs Causing Hepatic Injury

Agent	Injury Pattern
Acetaminophen	Cytotoxic
Amiodarone	Cytotoxic
Amphotericin	Cytotoxic
Anabolic steroids	Cholestatic, veno-occlusive
Azathioprine	Cytotoxic, cholestatic, veno-occlusive
Carbamazepine	Cytotoxic, cholestatic
Chlorpromazine	Cholestatic
Cis-platinum	Cytotoxic
Contraceptive steroids	Cholestatic, hepatic vein thrombotic
Cyclophosphamide	Cytotoxic
Erythromycin estolate	Cholestatic
Gold salts	Cytotoxic, cholestatic
Haloperidol	Cholestatic
Isoniazid	Cytotoxic
Ketoconazole	Cytotoxic
Lovastatin	Cytotoxic
Methotrexate	Cytotoxic
Methoxyflurane	Cytotoxic
Methyldopa	Cytotoxic
Phenobarbital	Cholestatic
Phenytoin	Cytotoxic
Quinidine	Cytotoxic
Salicylate	Cytotoxic
Tetracycline	Cytotoxic, fatty infiltrative
Valproic acid	Cytotoxic
Verapamil	Cholestatic

From Guss, D. A., & Oyama, L. C. (2010). Disorders of the liver and biliary tract. In J. A. Marx, R. S. Hockberger, & R. M. Walls (Eds.), *Rosen's emergency medicine: Concepts and clinical practice* (7th ed., p. 1163, Table 88.4). Mosby Elsevier.

Diagnosis and Evaluation

- Alkaline phosphatase and gamma-glutamyl transferase (GGT) elevation out of proportion to other liver enzymes is suggestive of biliary cirrhosis
- More than 90% have antimitochondrial antibodies
- Liver biopsy will show interlobular bile duct destruction

Treatment

- Ursodeoxycholic acid (Ursodiol) reduces cholestasis and improves LFTs.
- Cholestyramine (bile acid sequestrants) helps alleviate pruritus.
- Patient may ultimately need a liver transplant.

Spontaneous Bacterial Peritonitis (SBP)

General Principles

- Acute bacterial infection of the ascitic fluid in patients with liver disease
- Most commonly caused by *Streptococcus pneumoniae*. However, can also be secondary to gram-negative enteric organisms, such as *Escherichia coli*, *Klebsiella*, *Enterobacteriaceae*, *or* viridans streptococci. If enteric organisms are identified, consider secondary bacterial peritonitis owing to perforated diverticulitis or appendicitis.
- It is thought to be caused by portal hypertension leading to bowel edema causing bacterial translocation from the GI tract.

Clinical Presentation

- Often presents with:
  - Ascites
  - Fevers
  - Chills
  - Abdominal pain and tenderness
  - Shifting dullness

Diagnosis and Evaluation

- Paracentesis with ascitic fluid demonstrating:
  - Polymorphonuclear neutrophil (PMN) count greater than $250/mm^3$ and/or presence of bacteria on peritoneal fluid gram stain or culture
  - Suggestive of secondary peritonitis from perforated viscus (two of the following): ascitic fluid protein greater than 1 g/dL, lactate dehydrogenase higher than the upper limit of normal for serum, or glucose less than 50 mg/dL
  - With evidence of secondary peritonitis, imaging and surgical consult should be pursued to evaluate for perforated viscus, because the mortality rate is higher than for SBP.

Treatment

- Patients with SBP will require admission and any of the following antibiotic regimens:
  - Cefotaxime 2 g IV q8h
  - Ceftriaxone 2 g IV q24h (consider 2 g if >100 kg or severe infection)
  - Piperacillin/tazobactam 4.5 g IV q6h
  - Ertapenem 1 g IV qday

Hepatic Encephalopathy

General Principles

- Clinical state of disorientation caused by acute and chronic liver disease
- Normally, ammonia that is absorbed from the GI tract is metabolized into urea by the liver for excretion.
- When liver dysfunction occurs, ammonia levels increase and eventually cross the blood–brain barrier.
- Ammonia is metabolized to glutamine in the central nervous system (CNS), leading to cerebral dysfunction.
- Constipation causes increased ammonia production and can lead to encephalopathy, as can infection, GI bleeding, hypokalemia, or other acute insults.

Clinical Presentation

- Asterixis ("flapping" with wrist extension) caused by increased CNS glutamine
- Serum ammonia levels do **not** correlate well with degree of encephalopathy, but cerebral spinal fluid glutamine levels do.

- Four stages:
  - Grade 1: mild cognitive dysfunction, irritability, depression, poor sleep
  - Grade 2: lethargy, disorientation, asterixis, personality changes
  - Grade 3: somnolence, inability to follow commands, confused speech
  - Grade 4: coma

Diagnosis and Evaluation

- A clinical diagnosis that is supported by an elevated serum ammonia level

Treatment

- Initial treatment involves hemodynamic stabilization, electrolyte repletion, and addressing reversible insults.
  - Lactulose: osmotic cathartic, which traps ammonia in the stool
  - Neomycin: poorly absorbed aminoglycoside, which reduces colonic bacteria that is thought to be responsible for the production of ammonia
  - Rifaximin: decreases activity of urease-producing bacteria
  - Protein restriction

Hepatorenal Failure

General Principles

- Acute renal failure secondary to liver failure in a patient without evidence of other renal pathology (i.e., no prerenal, intrinsic, or obstructive etiology)
- It is a diagnosis of exclusion.
- Portal hypertension causes splanchnic arterial vasodilation leading to systemic vasoconstriction, especially to the kidneys, leading to decreased glomerular filtration and decreased sodium excretion.
- Often fatal

Clinical Presentation

- Rising serum creatinine with minimal proteinuria
- Often oliguric, resulting in volume overload
- May demonstrate uremic encephalopathy

Treatment

- Evaluate and treat any reversible etiologies such as dehydration, abdominal compartment syndrome from tense ascites, sepsis, drug-induced nephropathies, or obstructive uropathy.
- Albumin administration may help improve renal perfusion and has been shown to decrease mortality.
- Admit for further evaluation and treatment of reversible etiologies.
- Consider liver transplant.

Liver Abscess

General Principles

- Pyogenic abscesses are often associated with biliary tract obstruction or cholangitis but can be secondary to any bacteremia.
- Often no underlying cause is found. *E. coli*, *Klebsiella*, and *Pseudomonas* are the most common bacterial organisms.
- Amebic abscesses affect 10% of the world's population and are transmitted via the fecal-oral route, usually from contaminated water. *Entamoeba histolytica* can lead to invasive disease.

Clinical Presentation

- Patients are often ill appearing with fevers, right upper quadrant pain, nausea, and vomiting; however, in some cases, such as those with *Klebsiella* abscess in alcoholic patients, may present with only vague symptoms and have an indolent course.

Diagnosis and Evaluation

- Leukocytosis, elevated alkaline phosphatase (90%), and bilirubin greater than 2 mg/dL (50%)
- Either ultrasound and/or CT are the diagnostic imaging modalities of choice.

Treatment

- Fluid resuscitation, antipyretic, antiemetic, and pain control
- For amoebic abscess, metronidazole is the treatment of choice.
- Pyogenic abscess will need triple antibiotic coverage, with an aminoglycoside or third-generation cephalosporin (gram-negative), metronidazole or clindamycin (anaerobes), and ampicillin (streptococcus).
- Definitive treatment usually entails interventional radiology or surgical drainage of abscess.

Hepatic Cancer

General Principles

- Metastases to the liver from GI, lung, breast, or other primary tumors is more common than primary hepatic malignancy in the United States.
- HCC, the most common primary hepatic malignancy, is often secondary to chronic HBV/HCV infections.
- Chronic alcoholism, primary biliary cirrhosis, hemochromatosis, and drugs may also lead to HCC.

Clinical Presentation

- Nonspecific. May have nausea, vomiting, weight loss, cachexia, jaundice, right upper quadrant pain, or signs of cirrhosis

Diagnosis and Evaluation

- Alpha-fetoprotein can be elevated in HCC, although nonspecific.
- Ultrasound, CT, or MRI may help facilitate the diagnosis, but biopsy is necessary for definitive diagnosis of HCC.

Treatment

- Supportive management in the ED
- Surgical resection, chemo- and radioembolization, and liver transplant may be considered, based on the stage of disease.

SUGGESTED READING

Cline, D. M, Ma, J. O., Cydulka, R. K., Meckler, G. D., Handel, D. A., & Thomas, S. H. (Eds.). (2012). *Tintinalli's emergency medicine manual* (7th ed.). McGraw Hill Education.

Marx, J. A., Hockberger, R. S., Walls, R. M. (Eds.). (2014). *Rosen's emergency medicine: Concepts and clinical practice* (8th ed.). Elsevier/Saunders.

CHAPTER 6

BOARD REVIEW

Pancreas

DAVID HAASE, MD, and ALAN CHIEM, MD, MPH

Acute Pancreatitis

General Principles

- Acute pancreatitis involves inflammation of the pancreas. It is the leading cause of admission to the hospital for gastrointestinal (GI) disorders.
- The annual incidence ranges from 13 to 45 per 100,000 persons and has increased steadily in the United States along with the increase in obesity.
- Pancreatitis initially begins with acinar cell injury causing local inflammation, which can then progress to systemic inflammation and potentially multisystem organ failure.
- Gallstone pancreatic disease likely results from mechanical obstruction causing reflux into the intrapancreatic duct.
- Roughly two-thirds of cases are from gallstone disease and alcohol abuse; however, a variety of other etiologies as well as medications can be responsible (Box 6.1).
- Risk factors for pancreatitis include older age, comorbid illnesses, chronic alcohol abuse, and obesity. Treatment is generally supportive, depending on the etiology.

Clinical Presentation

- Severe, sharp, epigastric pain often radiating to the back
- Accompanied by nausea, emesis, anorexia, fever, and diaphoresis
- Pain usually peaks in 30 to 60 minutes and persists for days
- Physical examination: upper abdominal tenderness; unlikely findings in late-stage pancreatitis include Cullen's sign or Grey Turner's sign (skin discoloration around the umbilicus or flank, respectively)

Diagnosis and Evaluation

- Diagnosis of acute pancreatitis requires 2 of 3:
  - Umbilical or upper abdominal pain plus or minus radiation to the back
  - Serum levels of lipase or amylase three or more times the upper limit of normal
  - Findings from cross-sectional imaging
- Laboratory studies
  - Complete blood count, basic metabolic panel, lipase, amylase, liver function tests, triglyceride levels (if the etiology is unknown), and lactate dehydrogenase
    - Lipase is more specific than amylase (levels not reflective of disease severity)
    - False-positive results of elevated lipase occur in inflammatory bowel disease, diabetic ketoacidosis, bowel obstruction, and renal insufficiency
- Imaging Modalities
  - Ultrasound of the right upper quadrant to identify biliary pathology
    - Helps determine need for gallstone removal via ERCP in patients with gallstone pancreatitis (e.g., ductal dilatation suggestive of choledocholithiasis)
  - CT scan with contrast only if there is diagnostic uncertainty or other pathology suspected. CT will also demonstrate complications of pancreatitis, such as psuedocyst, phlegmon, and necrosis.

BOX 6.1 *Causes of Acute Pancreatitis*

Toxic – Metabolic
- Alcohol – #2 most common, often chronic alcoholics 12 to 24 hrs after last drink
- Drugs
- Hyperlipidemia – levels usually > 1000 mg/dL
- Hypercalcemia
- Uremia
- Scorpion venom

Mechanical – Obstructive
- Biliary stones–#1 most common
- Congenital–pancreas divisum, annular pancreas
- Tumors – ampullary, neuroendocrine, pancreatic carcinoma
- Post-ERCP
- Ampullary dysfunction or stenosis
- Duodenal diverticulum
- Trauma

Infectious
- Viral – mumps, coxsackie, HIV, CMV, EBV, varicella
- Bacterial – TB, *Salmonella*, *Campylobacter*, *Legionella*, Mycoplasma
- Parasitic – *Ascaris*

Vascular
- Vasculitis
- Embolism
- Hypoperfusion, ischemia
- Hypercoagulability

Other
- Idiopathic
- Hereditary
- Diabetes mellitus, DKA
- Autoimmune

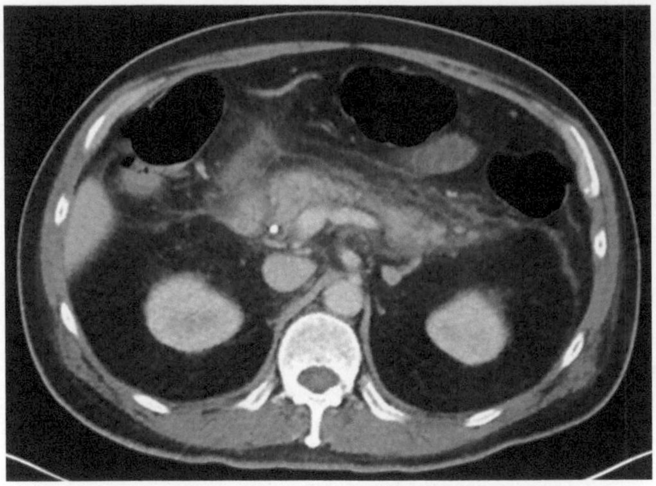

FIG. 6.1 CT image of acute pancreatitis with visible stranding. (From Arshad, A. & Marudanayagam, R. (2016). Upper gastrointestinal emergencies. *Surgery, 34*(11), 558–562.)

- Findings: pancreatic enlargement, peripancreatic stranding, and fluid collection (Fig. 6.1)
- Mortality risk stratification: Ranson criteria (requires 48 hours to complete)
  - Five points assessed on admission: age > 55, WBC > 16 K, blood glucose > 200 mg/dL, lactate dehydrogenase > 350 U/L, aspartate aminotransferase > 250 U/L
  - Six points assessed 48 hours later: drop in hematocrit by more than 10%, BUN increases by more than 5 mg/dL, serum calcium less than 8 mg/dL, pO2 less than 60 mm Hg, base deficit more than 4 MEq/L, fluid needs more than 6 L
  - Score of 3 or more on admission criteria may warrant ICU admission
- APACHE II and BISAP are two other scoring systems used to estimate mortality risk.
- Patients with respiratory failure or persistent hypotension should be admitted to the ICU.
- No formal guidelines for discharge from the ED, but patients who are older, have comorbid conditions, or have oral intolerance, persistent pain, or gallstones likely should be admitted.

Treatment

- Fluid resuscitation
  - Start an initial bolus of isotonic fluid followed by goal-directed therapy with a continuous infusion and frequent reexamination for improvement or progression to distributive shock (10%–20% of cases).
- Pain control
  - Nonopioid medications or judicious use of opioids
- Initially NPO
  - With clinical improvement, early feeding within 24 hours is encouraged over prolonged periods of NPO.
- Consult GI for gallstone pancreatitis, as an ERCP may be required. General surgery consultation for consideration of a subsequent laparoscopic cholecystectomy.
- Routine antibiotics are not recommended unless septic from another underlying infection or infected necrotizing pancreatitis.
- For severe hypertriglyceridemia, IV insulin may be used to bring the triglyceride level down to 500 mg/dL, unless there is hypocalcemia, lactic acidosis, or clinical deterioration, in which case plasma exchange should be considered.

Complications

- Acute peripancreatic fluid collection
  - Usually develops early with spontaneous resolution
- Pancreatic pseudocyst
  - Encapsulated fluid outside the pancreas with a defined wall without necrosis
  - In general, develops 4 weeks after the initial presentation of pancreatitis
  - Treated with supportive measures and at times endoscopic drainage or surgery
- Necrosis
  - Acute necrotic collection without a wall involving the parenchyma or surrounding structures
  - Initially sterile but may become infected in roughly one-third of patients
  - Often presents with sepsis and requires empiric antibiotics and operative washouts and debridements
  - Hemorrhagic pancreatitis is a rare complication and may require transfusions and surgical intervention.
- Walled-off pancreatic necrosis
  - Areas of walled-off necrosis can form with liquid or solid elements.

Chronic Pancreatitis

General Principles

- Progressive inflammatory damage leading to permanent impairment

Clinical Presentation

- Might be painless or present with epigastric abdominal pain radiating to the back
- Late findings with symptoms of pancreatic insufficiency (fat malabsorption or diabetes)

Diagnosis and Evaluation

- Usually normal lipase/amylase, with focal areas of infiltrate or calcification on imaging; unless there is an acute exacerbation

Treatment

- Cessation of alcohol and eating small low-fat meals is recommended.
- Persistent pain is treated with enzyme replacements, a PPI or H2 blocker, and analgesics.
- Complications include pseudocysts, obstruction of the bile duct or duodenum, and pancreatic ascites or pleural effusions.

Pancreatic Cancer

General Principles

- Often caught in the late stage of disease; 85% adenocarcinoma, 10% neuroendocrine
- High mortality associated with complications from metastasis

Clinical Presentation

- Abdominal pain, nausea, back pain, and weight loss

Diagnosis and Evaluation

- Diagnosed with CT of abdomen with IV contrast; showing up as an area of hypoattenuation

Treatment

- ED treatment focused on pain management and controlling complications

SUGGESTED READINGS

Lankisch, P. G., Apte, M., & Banks, P. A. (2015). Acute pancreatitis. *Lancet*, 386(9988), 85–96.

Waller, A., Long, B., Koyfman, A., & Gottlieb, M. (2018). Acute pancreatitis: Updates for emergency clinicians. *Journal of Emergency Medicine*, *55*(6), 769–779.

Wu, B. U., & Banks, P. A. (2013). Clinical management of patients with acute pancreatitis. *Gastroenterology*, *144*(6), 1272–1281.

Anorectal Emergencies

CAROLYN JOY SACHS, MD, MPH, and LUIZ SOUZA-FILHO, MD

Hemorrhoids

General Principles

- Hemorrhoids, the most common etiology of rectal bleeding seen in the emergency department (ED), are caused by the displacement of vascular cushions leading to excessive engorgement of the hemorrhoidal venous plexus.
- They are aggravated by constipation, excessive straining, and frequent diarrhea.
- Hemorrhoids may be described as either internal (above dentate line) or external (below dentate line).
- Although most hemorrhoids do not prompt an ED visit, those that become thrombosed, inflamed, prolapsed, ulcerated, or ischemic/necrotic often cause significant pain and may require urgent intervention.

Clinical Presentation

- Hemorrhoidal bleeding is usually self-limited. It is often described as bright red blood coating stool, slowly dripping blood, or blood noted on toilet tissue.
- Hemorrhoids do not typically cause pain unless they are thrombosed or strangulated. A palpable or painful anal mass is also a common presenting symptom of external hemorrhoids or prolapsed internal hemorrhoids.
- Foul-smelling discharge may be present in cases of mucosal necrosis from strangulation.

Diagnosis and Evaluation

- A simple anal examination will suffice to detect external hemorrhoids, whereas anoscopy must be used to view internal hemorrhoids, which appear as bluish-purple bulging distal rectal or anal canal veins. Prolapsed internal hemorrhoids may be seen externally and can be differentiated from external hemorrhoids via reduction attempts and anoscopy. Thrombosed hemorrhoids are typically tender, firm to touch, and range from dark red to purple in color.

Treatment

- Grades 1, 2, and 3 internal hemorrhoids (Table 7.1) and external hemorrhoids without acute thrombosis with a tolerable level of pain can be managed conservatively with warm water soaks, topical analgesics, steroidal creams, bulk laxatives, and stool softeners.
- Grade 4 internal hemorrhoids (see Table 7.1) causing severe pain, bleeding, or strangulation should be evaluated in the ED by a surgeon.
- Acute (<48 hr) severely symptomatic external thrombosed hemorrhoids may benefit from thrombus excision in the ED for symptomatic relief.

Anal Fissure

General Principles

- An anal fissure is a superficial linear tear of the anal canal below the dentate line. It is most commonly caused by the passage of a large, hard stool. Anal fissures are less commonly associated with frequent diarrhea, inflammatory bowel disease (IBD), obstetric trauma, localized malignancies, or infectious processes.

Clinical Presentations

- Symptoms: painful defecation, bright red blood per rectum, constipation

Diagnosis and Evaluation

- Physical examination:
  - Linear mucosal tear along the posterior midline in more than 80% of cases
  - Chronic fissure: more than 6 weeks, fibrotic raised edges, distal sentinel skin tag (often confused for external hemorrhoid), possible hypertrophic anal papillae and sentinel skin tag

TABLE 7.1 *Classification of Internal Hemorrhoids by Severity*

Type	Prolapse	Mode of Reduction	Treatment
First-degree	None	N/A	Medical management
Second-degree	During defecation	Spontaneous	Medical management
Third-degree	May be spontaneous or during defecation	Manual	Medical management Optional surgical repair
Fourth-degree	Permanently	Irreducible	Surgical repair

N/A, not applicable.
(From Marx J. A., Hockberger R. S., & Walls R. M. (2009). *Rosen's emergency medicine: Concepts and clinical practice* (7th ed., Table 94.2, p.1246). Elsevier.)

- Nonhealing fissure, multiple fissures, or nonposterior-midline should prompt investigation of other etiologies (e.g., IBD).

Treatment

- Acute uncomplicated fissure: warm baths, stool softeners, dietary fiber supplementation. Topical analgesics or hydrocortisone creams may reduce severe symptoms.
- Chronic or nonhealing: can add topical nitrate or calcium channel blocker, specialty referral for sphincterotomy vs. alternative therapies, such as botulinum injection.

Rectal Prolapse

General Principles

- Circumferential protrusion of part or all layers of rectum through the anal canal
- Three types:
  - Mucosal prolapse
  - Complete prolapse
  - Intussusception of the upper rectum through the lower rectum (partial prolapse)
- Associated with increased intraabdominal pressures and/or pelvic floor muscle weakness

Clinical Presentation

- Mucosal prolapse: Thin-walled mucosal protrusion red-purple in color, painless, possible mucus or blood, everted anal edges, more common in children. It is rare to have more than 5 cm protrusion.
- Complete prolapse: Large red ball-like mass protruding from anus with concentric folds.
- Normal anus (in contrast to mucosal prolapse): Rarely, a prolonged complete prolapse can strangulate, with ischemic whitish or mottled discoloration of prolapsed mucosa, ulceration, venous engorgement, or thrombosis.
- Partial prolapse: Stool seepage or constipation; mucous discharge or bleeding may be present, possible detection of mass after defecation or strenuous activity

Diagnosis and Evaluation

- History and physical examination as detailed above in Clinical Presentation. Circumferential prolapsed internal hemorrhoids can be distinguished from rectal prolapse by having only mucosal involvement and radial sulci between hemorrhoid bundles, in contrast to the full-thickness and concentric rings of the prolapsed rectum (Fig. 7.1).

Treatment

- Children: Manual reduction after analgesia and/or sedation. Digital rectal examination (DRE) after reduction. Postreduction constipation prevention and referral for further evaluation of possible underlying conditions (i.e., Hirschsprung's disease).
- Adults: Manual reduction with analgesia and sedation, if necessary. For complete prolapse, application of granulated sugar over entire prolapsed portion is effective in reducing edema to facilitate reduction. Postreduction DRE to ensure reduction and rule out rectal mass. All patients should be referred to specialist for further evaluation and possible surgery. Surgery should evaluate complete prolapse unable to be reduced, recurrence after reduction, or if any signs of ischemia or gangrene.

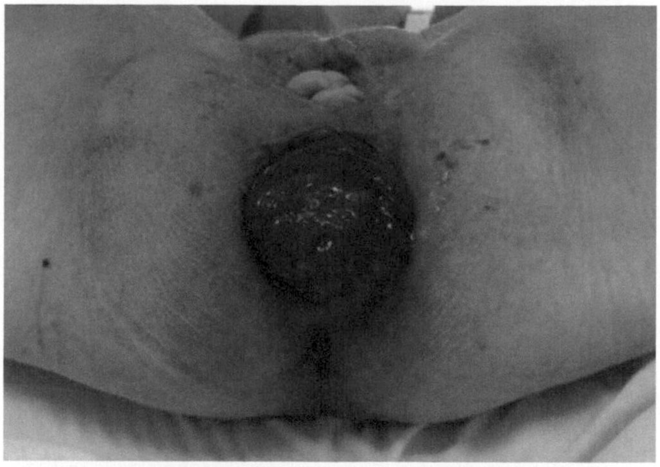

FIG. 7.1 Prolapse of the rectum. (From Davis, B.R. (2015). Transperineal repair of the rectal prolapse. In *Atlas of pelvic anatomy and gynecologic surgery* (4th ed., pp. 1143–1148, Fig. 102.2). Elsevier.)

Anorectal Infections

General Principles

- Infection of anal crypts secondary to mucosal breakdown from chronic constipation, diarrhea, or other mechanical insults provides the initial insult leading to anorectal abscess and fistula.
- Diffuse inflammation of the rectum (known as proctitis) can be caused by bacterial or viral invasion, radiation, autoimmune disorders, vasculitis, or ischemia.

Clinical Presentation

- Perianal abscess: Superficial painful and tender indurated or fluctuant mass. Located close to anal verge, often posterior-midline
- Perirectal abscess: Subcategorized anatomically into ischiorectal, intersphincteric, submucosal, post-anal, and supralevator (Fig. 7.2). Less often have cutaneous manifestations (if present, more laterally located along medial buttocks). More often have fever, leukocytosis, lymphadenopathy, sepsis. Rectal pain invariably present; worse with defecation or just prior to defecation. Sometimes associated with rectal purulent discharge.
- Anorectal fistula: Painless, blood-stained mucus, anal itching, malodorous discharge. Symptoms of abscess as outlined above if the fistula tract becomes blocked. The fistulous opening may be noted on an external examination or DRE. A frequent complication of anorectal abscess drainage. Can be the manifestation of IBD, malignancies, radiation, sexually transmitted infection, or other infectious processes.
- Proctitis: Anorectal pain, fever, itching, discharge, diarrhea, bleeding, lower abdominal and pain/cramping, tenesmus. May have anal cutaneous manifestations

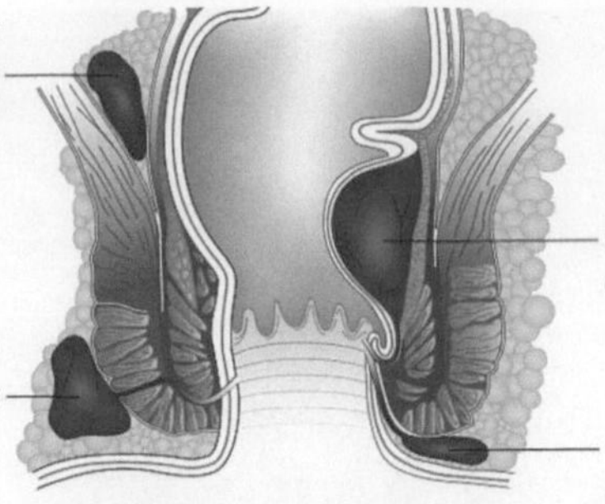

FIG. 7.2 Location of common anorectal abscesses. (Modified from Gordon P. H., & Vivatvonghs S. (1992). *Principles and practice of surgery for the colon, rectum, and anus*. Quality Medical Publishing.)

when caused by HSV, or syphilis. Unprotected anal receptive intercourse is the biggest risk factor for infectious causes.

Diagnosis and Evaluation

- Perianal abscess: Usually diagnosed by history and physical examination (see Clinical Presentation), but ultrasound (US) may be helpful.
- Perirectal abscess: May be palpable through rectal wall on DRE or externally. Pain out of proportion, constitutional symptoms, or symptoms of deeper infection. US may detect submucosal or intersphincteric abscesses, but is often unable to identify deeper abscesses.
- If there is concern for deeper abscess, contrast-enhanced CT or MRI should be ordered.
  - Anorectal fistula: May have a visible fistulous opening on examination or a palpable fibrous tract. The diagnosis can be confirmed with imaging; US and MRI are both more sensitive than CT.
  - Proctitis: Anoscopy may reveal mucosal inflammation, bleeding, erythema, ulcerations, or discharge.

Treatment

- Perianal abscess: ED incision and drainage under local anesthesia or procedural sedation. Antibiotics reduce recurrence.
- Perirectal abscess: Surgical consultation
- Anorectal fistula: Analgesics, IV fluids, antibiotics. Surgical consult necessary for decision on possible admission vs. later planned surgical drain placement, fibrin glue, fistulotomy, fistulectomy, or more complex procedures.
- Proctitis: For radiation proctitis, antiinflammatory agents and oral sucralfate can be prescribed from the ED. Specialist consultants may offer Botox injections, short-chain fatty acid enemas, hyperbaric oxygen, or sclerosing therapy. For proctitis related to systemic processes, such as IBD or infectious proctitis (Table 7.2), treat the underlying condition.

TABLE 7.2 *Sexually Transmitted Diseases of the Anorectum*

Disease/Condition (With Specific Pathogen When Known)	Findings	Treatment
Ulcerative		
LGV	Unilateral inguinal adenopathy Fever, malaise Mucoid or bloody discharge	Doxycycline 100 mg PO bid × 21 days *For pregnant patients or those allergic to tetracyclines:* Erythromycin 500 mg PO qid × 21 days
HSV infection	Rectal pain, tenesmus, constipation Bloody mucoid discharge Vesicles and ulcerations Fever, malaise, myalgias, parethesias	*First episode:* PERIANAL: acyclovir 400 mg PO tid or Famciclovir 250 mg PO bid × 7–10 days or Valacyclovir 1 g PO daily for 7–10 days PROCTITIS: acyclovir 800 mg PO tid × 7–10 days. *Recurrent:* acyclovir 400 mg PO tid for 5 days or Acyclovir 200 mg PO 5 times per day for 5 days or Acyclovir 800 mg PO bid for 5 days or Famciclovir 125 mg PO bid for 5 days or Valacyclovir 500 mg PO bid for 3–5 days or Valacyclovir 1 g PO daily for 5 days
Early (primary) syphilis (*Treponema pallidum*)	Chancre Tenesmus, pain, mucoid drainage Inguinal lymphadenopathy	Benzathine penicillin G 2.4 million units IM once. *Alternatives:* Doxycycline, Erythromycin
Chancroid (*Haemophilus ducreyi*)	Inflammatory lesion progresses to ulcer Inguinal adenitis - bubo	Azithromycin 1 g PO once or Ceftriaxone 250 mg IM once or Ciprofloxacin 500 mg PO bid × 3 days or Levofloxacin 500 mg PO for 7 days or Erythromycin 500 mg PO tid × 7 days
CMV infection	Tenesmus, diarrhea, weight loss	Ganciclovir with appropriate disposition
Idiopathic (usually HIV+)	Excentric, deep, poor healing, multiple lesions	Symptomatic relief or surgical referral
Nonulcerative		
Condylomata acuminata (HPV)	Keratinized vegetative growths in anus or skin Asymptomatic, or pruritus ani, or bleeding	Podophyllin, topical, or cryotherapy Consider home therapy with podofilox 0.5% solution or gel for limited involvement

TABLE 7.2 *Sexually Transmitted Diseases of the Anorectum—cont'd*

Disease/Condition (With Specific Pathogen When Known)	Findings	Treatment
Gonorrhea (*Neisseria gonorrhoeae*)	Pruritus ani Tenesmus Purulent yellow discharge	Cefixime 400 mg PO once or ceftriaxone 500 mg IM dose For persons weighing ≥150 kg (300 lbs), Ceftriaxone 1 g IM For patients with allergy to cephalosporins, a single 240 mg IM dose of gentamicin plus a single 2 g oral dose of azithromycin is an option or Ceftriaxone 125 mg IM once or Ofloxacin 400 mg PO once or Ciprofloxacin 500 mg PO once or Levofloxacin 250 mg PO once *For pregnant patients:* Spectinomycin 2 g IM once plus Erythromycin 500 mg PO qid × 7 days
Chlamydial infection (*Chlamydia trachomatis*)	Mucoid or bloody discharge Tenesmus	Azithromycin 1 g PO once or Doxycycline 100 mg PO twice per day × 7 days or Ofloxacin 300 mg PO bid × 7 days Ceftriaxone 500 mg IM as a single dose for persons weighing <150 kg (300 lb) 1 g ceftriaxone IM for persons weighing ≥150 kg (300 lb) Alternative regimens for uncomplicated gonococcal infections of the cervix, urethra, or rectum if ceftriaxone is not available or in case of allergies: Gentamicin 240 mg IM as a single dose plus azithromycin 2 g orally as a single dose OR Cefixime 800 mg orally as a single dose. If treating with cefixime, and chlamydial infection has not been excluded, providers should treat for chlamydia with doxycycline 100 mg orally twice daily for 7 days. During pregnancy, azithromycin 1 g as a single dose is recommended to treat chlamydia. *For pregnant patients:* Erythromycin 500 mg PO qid × 7 days
Syphilis (secondary)	Maculopapular rash Condyloma latum	Benzathine penicillin G 2.4 million units IM once. *Alternatives:* Doxycycline, Erythromycin

CMV, cytomegalovirus; *HIV,* human immunodeficiency virus; *HPV,* human papillomavirus; *HSV,* herpes simplex virus; *LGV,* lymphogranuloma venereum. (From Marx, J. A., Hockberger, R. S., & Walls, R. M. (2009). *Rosen's emergency medicine: Concepts and clinical practice* (7th ed., Table 94.5, p.1253). Elsevier.)

Rectal Foreign Bodies and Trauma

General Principles

- Patients frequently under-report history of foreign body placement owing to embarrassment and/or injury caused by an assault; thus having a foreign body and/or assault on the differential diagnosis is essential for prompt identification and extraction to prevent complications and to aid a victim who may have suffered from forced sodomy.

Clinical Presentation

- Abdominal pain, cramping, anorectal bleeding, discharge, discomfort
- Anoscopy may reveal signs of trauma, such as hematoma, abrasions, lacerations, perforation.
- Perforation may manifest with peritoneal signs if above peritoneal reflection or signs of retroperitoneal injury if below peritoneal reflection. Perforation can rapidly lead to sepsis.

Diagnosis and Evaluation

- DRE: most foreign bodies are in the rectal ampulla and palpable on examination.
- External anal injury may be visible after forced anal penetration (Fig. 7.3); injuries can be described in terms of a clock face for location.
- Anoscopy: Indicated if concern for sharp object or when patient presents with a complaint of anal pain after assault; may identify internal injury.
- X-ray: may show location, shape, and number of object(s); can show free air in peritoneum or along psoas muscles, if retroperitoneum.

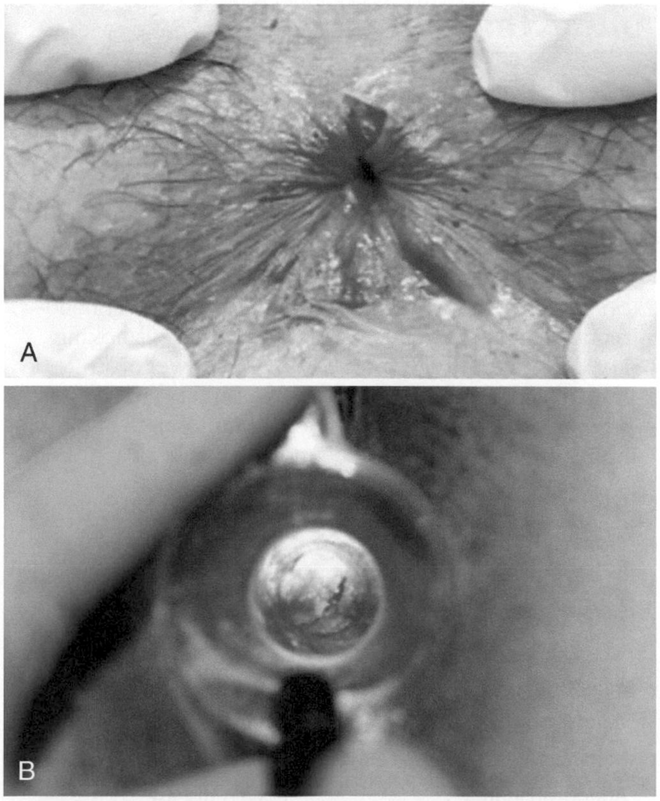

FIG. 7.3 Anorectal lacerations secondary to sexual trauma. **A,** Anal laceration visible on external examination. **B,** Internal rectal laceration detected via anoscopy. (Courtesy Malinda Wheeler, R. N., *FNP,* forensic nurse practioner and property of *FNS,* Forensic Nurse Specialists Incorporated, Long Beach, California Inc.)

- CT: use for radiolucent objects, concern for perforation, or ill-appearing patients.
- Any patient reporting nonconsensual anal penetration should be offered a forensic sexual assault examination, psychological support, and law enforcement reporting in accordance with local protocol (https://www.rainn.org/articles/reporting-law-enforcement).

Treatment

- Distal objects: Easily accessible foreign bodies without signs of perforation or other serious injuries, and with low risk of injury during extraction, can be removed in the ED. Use the lithotomy or knee-to-chest position, ask the patient to bear down, and use lubrication. Suprapubic pressure and obstetric forceps may be used to facilitate removal. Some objects may create a vacuum during traction, which can be overcome by injecting air beyond the object using a 3-way catheter. Foley catheters around or behind the object may also facilitate extraction.
- Proximal objects: Difficult to access, excessively large, have a high risk of injury (glass or sharp object), signs of perforation, failed removal in the ED, or injury during ED extraction are all indications for surgical or GI consultation. If the patient is ill-appearing, if there is a risk of sphincter injury during extraction, prolonged extraction, or other serious injuries, such as perforation, initiate IV fluids, order laboratory tests, and broad-spectrum antibiotics in addition to specialty consultation.

Anorectal Malignancies

General Principles

- Anorectal malignancies can be categorized by anatomic region (Table 7.3).
- Anal canal neoplasms (proximal to dentate line and including transitional zone of epithelium)
- Anal margin neoplasms (distal to dentate line arising from anoderm)
- Some factors associated with the development of anorectal neoplasms include: Anal intercourse, smoking, HPV infection, HIV infection. Large bowel obstruction is also a common presentation of anorectal neoplasms. The anal canal is the third most common site of melanoma; pigmentation may be more difficult to appreciate.

Clinical Presentation

- Anal margin neoplasms:
  - Low-grade malignant potential and slow to metastasize (to femoral and inguinal nodes)
  - Tend to be circumferential and frequently cause noticeable cutaneous manifestations visible on external examination, such as pruritus and bleeding.
- Anal canal neoplasms
  - Higher malignant potential, earlier metastasis (to perirectal, mesenteric, paravertebral nodes), poorer prognosis
  - May cause abscesses, fistulas, rectal prolapse, bloody mucous discharge, clear watery diarrhea, and profuse discharge (classic for villous adenoma).
  - Early signs are nonspecific, including pain, pruritis, bloody stools. Occasionally asymptomatic. Late signs include rectal fullness, change in stool caliber, palpable lump, bloating, anorexia, weight loss, tenesmus, large bowel obstructive signs.

TABLE 7.3 *Anorectal Malignancies*

Anal Canal	Anal Margin
Melanoma, SCC	Squamous cell carcinoma
Adenocarcinoma	Bowen disease
Transitional cell carcinoma	Melanoma
Villous adenoma	Basal cell carcinoma
Kaposi's sarcoma	Paget's disease

Perianal Hidradenitis Suppurativa

General Principles

- Hidradenitis suppuritiva is a condition characterized by obstruction of hair follicles and apocrine sweat glands.
- Areas typically affected include the groin, axilla, inframammary, and (notable for this chapter) perineum.

Clinical Presentation

- Inflamed glands, superficial abscesses, fistulous tracts, malodorous discharge, edema, fibrotic tissue in perianal region. Likely history of similar lesions in groin, axilla, inframammary region.

Diagnosis and Evaluation

- History and physical examination are usually sufficient.
- Imaging, such as CT, may be necessary with concern for deeper abscess or fistulous tract.

Treatment

- Small superficial abscesses can be drained in the ED. Larger or more extensive abscesses require surgical or dermatologic referral.
- Topical or oral antibiotics may be helpful.
- Other treatments are extensive and may be ordered by specialty consultants.

Pruritus Ani

General Principles

- Pruritus ani can occur from anorectal diseases (e.g., hemorrhoids, fistulas, abscesses, fissures).
- It can also arise from localized infection with parasites, fungi, bacteria, viruses, bed bugs, scabies, and other agents.
- Other secondary causes include certain foods, dermatologic conditions, and psychogenic disorders.

Clinical Presentation

- Often worse at night; multiple causes (as stated above)
- Early: normal-appearing skin
- Late or severe acute: thickened, erythematous, excoriated perianal skin

Diagnosis and Evaluation

- Assess for underlying cause
- Collect samples/cultures as necessary if concern for infectious cause
- Scotch tape test for pinworms

Treatment

- Treat underlying cause. Symptomatic relief with fiber supplementation, warm baths followed by thorough drying, zinc oxide ointment to facilitate healing, 1% hydrocortisone cream
- Infectious etiologies: Fungicidal creams, antibiotics, antivirals, antiparasitic medications, as necessary

SUGGESTED READINGS

Altomare, D. F., Binda, G. A., Canuti, S., Landolfi, V., Trompetto, M., & Villani, R. D. (2011). The management of patients with primary chronic anal fissure: A position paper. *Techniques in Coloproctology, 15*(2), 135–141.

Lohsiriwat, V. (2016). Anorectal emergencies. *World Journal of Gastroenterology, 22*(26), 5867–5878.

Marx, J. A., Hockberger, R. S., & Walls, R. M. (2009). *Rosen's emergency medicine: Concepts and clinical practice* (7th ed). Mosby Elsevier.

Talan, D. A., Mower, W. R., Krishnadasan, A., Abrahamian, F. M., Lovecchio, F., Karras, D. J., et al. (2016). Trimethoprim-sulfamethoxazole versus placebo for uncomplicated skin abscess. *New England Journal of Medicine, 374*(9), 823–832.

Tintinalli, J., Stapczynski, S., Ma, J., Yealy, D., Meckler, G., & Cline, D. (2016). *Tintinalli's emergency medicine: A comprehensive study guide* (8th ed., pp. 545–563). McGraw-Hill.

CHAPTER 8

BOARD REVIEW

Disorders of the Spleen

CALEB P. CANDERS, MD, and LUIZ SOUZA-FILHO, MD

A highly vascular organ in the left upper quadrant of the abdomen, the spleen filters red blood cells, stores platelets, and facilitates immune system maturity. Splenic disorders are often manifestations of other primary diseases.

Asplenia/Hyposplenia

General Principles

- Asplenia/hyposplenia is most commonly secondary to splenectomy related to trauma.
- Functional asplenia/hyposplenia, which refers to absent/reduced splenic function, can occur in various diseases, including sickle cell anemia, infiltrative disorders (sarcoidosis, amyloidosis, lymphoma, and leukemia), alcoholic liver disease, inflammatory bowel disease, and celiac disease.

Clinical Presentation

- Patients with impaired splenic function are at increased risk of severe and overwhelming infections from encapsulated microorganisms, including *Staphylococcus pneumoniae*, *Neisseria meningitidis*, and *Haemophilus influenzae* type B.
- Overwhelming postsplenectomy syndrome, characterized by bacteremia from encapsulated microorganisms without a clear primary source, is associated with high rates of disseminated intravascular coagulation (DIC) and mortality.
- Thrombocytosis, also common in asplenia/hyposplenia, may predispose patients to venous thromboembolic events.

Diagnosis and Evaluation

- Diagnosis should be anticipated in patients with certain diseases (e.g., sickle cell anemia, sarcoidosis, amyloidosis).
- Peripheral blood smears may show Howell-Jolly bodies or Heinz bodies.
- Ultrasonography, computed tomography (CT), and magnetic resonance imaging (MRI) can detect asplenia.

Treatment

- Patients with asplenia/hyposplenia should be vaccinated against encapsulated bacteria and influenza.
- Certain populations, such as children with sickle cell disease, may be maintained on prophylactic penicillin or other antibiotics.
- Patients with asplenia/hyposplenia who present with signs of bacterial infection should be promptly started on antibiotics with coverage against encapsulated organisms, such as ceftriaxone. There should be a low threshold to admit asplenic patients with fever and/or sepsis for close monitoring, supportive care, and parenteral antibiotic treatment.

Splenomegaly

General Principles

- Splenomegaly is defined as abnormal splenic enlargement, and its size correlates with height, weight, and sex.
- The diagnosis is often incidental and does not always require further emergent workup (Table 8.1).

Clinical Presentation

- The normal spleen is not usually palpable on physical examination. Thus patients with splenomegaly may have a spleen that is easily palpable below the left costophrenic border.
- Patients may have symptoms related to the increased size of the spleen, such as early satiety, abdominal or left shoulder pain (Kehr sign from diaphragmatic irritation), or chest pain. Other symptoms/findings (e.g., signs of liver disease or adenopathy and weight loss) depend on its underlying etiology.

Diagnosis and Evaluation

- Diagnosis can be made on physical examination, ultrasound, CT, or MRI. In isolation, it does not necessarily require further emergent workup. However, its presence may help to diagnose an underlying disease process.

Treatment

- Treatment depends on the underlying etiology. All patients should be educated to avoid contact sports and other activities that risk blunt abdominal injury.

Splenic Abscess

General Principles

- A splenic abscess is usually caused by septic emboli from infective endocarditis.
- Hematogenous seeding from other sites (e.g., pneumonia, pyelonephritis, arteriovenous malformation) can also occur. An abscess may also form at the site of a splenic infarct.

Clinical Presentation

- Most patients present with fever, left upper quadrant abdominal pain, or nausea. Other symptoms include chest and/or flank pain, shortness of breath, left shoulder pain or hiccups from a left pleural effusion, splenomegaly, and diaphragmatic irritation. Some patients have nonspecific symptoms and the diagnosis is often delayed or missed.

TABLE 8.1 Causes of Splenomegaly

Process	Examples
Congestive	Cirrhosis Congestive heart failure Portal/splenic/hepatic vein thrombosis
Infectious	Bacterial (tuberculosis, Salmonella) Viral (hepatitis, Epstein-Barr virus, cytomegalovirus) Fungal Parasitic (malaria, toxoplasmosis, schistosomiasis, leishmaniasis)
Inflammatory/ Autoimmune	Sarcoid Systemic lupus erythematosus Rheumatoid arthritis Serum sickness
Hematologic	Hemolytic anemia (any cause) Sickle cell disease Pegfilgrastim use
Infiltrative	Niemann-Pick disease Amyloid Hemophagocytic lymphohistiocytosis Gaucher disease Lysosomal storage disease Langerhans cell histiocytosis
Neoplastic	Leukemia Lymphoma Polycythemia vera Essential thrombocytopenia Monoclonal gammopathy of undetermined significance/multiple myeloma Primary splenic neoplasms Metastasis

Diagnosis and Evaluation

- CT and MRI are more accurate than ultrasonography.
- Patients diagnosed with a splenic abscess should also be evaluated for infective endocarditis.

Treatment

- Treatment includes antibiotic coverage against anaerobes and aerobes.
- Most patients undergo splenectomy, although percutaneous drainage can be successful in unstable patients. If left untreated, patients have high rates of mortality from sepsis.

Splenic Infarction

General Principles

- Splenic infarction is caused by occlusion of the splenic artery and its branches, which can be due to embolic disease (e.g., atrial fibrillation, endocarditis), hemoglobinopathies (sickle cell disease and sickle cell trait at high altitudes), thrombus formation from hypercoagulability, myeloproliferative disease, splenic artery torsion, or any disorder that causes marked splenomegaly.

Clinical Presentation

- Most patients present with acute left upper quadrant pain and tenderness. Other findings include fever, vomiting, and splenomegaly.

Diagnosis and Evaluation

- CT is the diagnostic modality of choice. Laboratory data, although nonspecific, may reveal a leukocytosis and elevated lactate.

Treatment

- Treatment aims to restore blood flow and relieve pain.
- Specific treatments depend on the underlying etiology. Anticoagulation may be warranted, for example, if the infarct is from valvular heart disease or a hypercoagulable state.

Splenic Artery Aneurysm

General Principles

- Splenic artery aneurysms are more common in women, patients over 50 years of age, patients with high-output cardiac states (e.g., arteriovenous fistulas, pregnancy), and those with connective tissue diseases. After the abdominal aorta and the iliac arteries, the splenic artery is the third most common site for an abdominal artery aneurysm.

Clinical Presentation

- Patients are usually asymptomatic or report nonspecific symptoms (e.g., nausea, vague pain). Alternatively, patients may have signs consistent with the etiology of their portal hypertension. Diaphragmatic irritation from the aneurysm or resulting splenomegaly can also cause left shoulder pain.
- A ruptured aneurysm presents as acute abdominal pain, peritonitis, and hemodynamic instability. If the splenic capsule tamponades the initial bleeding, there may be a period of stability, followed by rupture into the peritoneum, with more severe pain and hemodynamic collapse.

Diagnosis and Evaluation

- Duplex ultrasonography, CT, or MRI.

Treatment

- Management depends on the clinical condition and may include open repair, laparoscopic clipping, stenting, endovascular coil/ablation, or percutaneous embolization.
- Because rupture may be fatal, treatment is generally recommended to reduce the risk of aneurysmal rupture (increasing risk with size >2 cm, those that are expanding or growing rapidly, those that are symptomatic with pain, or if the patient is pregnant).

SUGGESTED READINGS

Kirkineska, L., Perifanis, V., & Vasiliadis, T. (2014). Functional hyposplenism. *Hippokratia, 18*(1), 7–11.

Rubin, L. G., & Schaffner, W. (2014). Care of the asplenic patient. *New England Journal of Medicine, 371*, 349–356.

Sjoberg, B. P., Menias, C. O., Lubner, M. G., Mellnick, V. M., & Pickhardt, P. J. (2018). Splenomegaly: A combined clinical and radiologic approach to the differential diagnosis. *Gastroenterology Clinics of North America, 47*(3), 643–666.

Disorders of the Stomach

CALEB P. CANDERS, MD, and LUIZ SOUZA-FILHO, MD

Gastroesophageal Reflux Disease

General Principles

- Gastroesophageal reflux disease (GERD) is characterized by dysfunction of the lower esophageal sphincter, with subsequent reflux of gastric contents into the esophagus.
- Agents or conditions that delay gastric emptying or decrease lower esophageal sphincter tone or esophageal motility can cause or exacerbate GERD (Box 9.1).

Clinical Presentation

- Heartburn and regurgitation are the two classic symptoms of GERD. Other symptoms include dysphagia, odynophagia, water brash, and globus pharyngeus.
- Atypical, extraesophageal symptoms, such as chest pain, chronic cough, wheezing, and hoarseness, may mimic cardiac or pulmonary diseases.

Diagnosis and Evaluation

- The diagnosis of GERD is usually based on the clinical presentation, if the symptoms are classic.
- For those patients without classic symptoms (e.g., isolated chest pain), it is important to exclude other diagnoses, such as acute coronary syndrome, before attributing the symptoms to GERD. An electrocardiogram and cardiac markers may be indicated in the emergency department (ED).
- Complications of GERD, such as Barrett esophagus or malignancy, should be considered, especially if the patient manifests alarm features suggestive of malignancy: dysphagia, odynophagia, anorexia, and unexplained weight loss.

Treatment

- Treatment is usually aimed at symptom relief and outpatient referral to primary care or gastroenterology. Treatment options include antacids, histamine-2 receptor blockers, and proton pump inhibitors (PPIs).
- Untreated, GERD can alter the gastrointestinal mucosa and cause malignant transformation or alteration of esophageal function.

BOX 9.1 *Conditions and Agents Associated With Gastroesophageal Reflux Disease*

Decreased Lower Esophageal Sphincter Pressure

Anticholinergics
Caffeine
Progesterone
Pregnancy
Nitrates
Nicotine
Ethanol
Benzodiazepines
Calcium channel blockers
Estrogen
Fatty foods

Decreased Esophageal Motility

Diabetes mellitus
Achalasia
Scleroderma

Delayed Gastric Emptying

Medications
Diabetic gastroparesis
Gastric outlet obstruction

Gastritis

General Principles

- Gastritis is defined as inflammation of the gastric mucosa and can be caused by *Helicobacter pylori* (most common cause), nonsteroidal antiinflammatory drugs (NSAIDs), alcohol, certain foods or medications, or it may be immune-mediated.

Clinical Presentation

- Common symptoms include dyspepsia, abdominal pain, nausea, and vomiting. Many are nonspecific and may be present for days to weeks.

Diagnosis and Evaluation

- Diagnosis of gastritis can only definitively be made by endoscopy.
- Diagnosis in the ED is often empiric and based on clinical symptoms and examination.
- Laboratory tests and imaging studies should only be used to assess for other diagnoses (e.g., pancreatitis, abdominal compartment syndrome).
- Response to treatment should not be relied on to rule out other more serious diagnoses. Angina may have responded to antacids, for example.

Treatment

- Treatment is similar to the treatment of GERD (see the previous section). Causative agents should be discontinued. Untreated gastritis can result in peptic ulcer disease.

BOX 9.2 Treatment of *Helicobacter pylori* Infection

Preferred Regimen
PPI
Amoxicillin
Clarithromycin

Penicillin-Allergic Patient
PPI
Metronidazole
Clarithromycin

Patients at Risk for Macrolide Resistance
PPI
Bismuth
Metronidazole
Tetracycline

PPI, proton pump inhibitor.

- If *H. pylori* gastritis is definitively diagnosed by biopsy or immunohistochemistry, the patient should be offered an antibiotic-based regimen to treat *H. pylori*, guided by the presence of risk factors for macrolide resistance and the presence of allergies. (Box 9.2)

Peptic Ulcer Disease

General Principles

- Peptic ulcer disease (PUD) is primarily caused by *H. pylori* infection or NSAID use. Rarely it is due to gastrin-secreting tumors, which induce increased acid production. These conditions impair the stomach's protective mucosa and cause ulceration.

Clinical Presentation

- Although peptic ulcers may be asymptomatic, the classical symptomatic clinical presentation of PUD includes vague epigastric pain, early satiety, and nausea and fullness. Pain relief with antacids is common.
- Complications of PUD include bleeding, gastric outlet obstruction, perforation, and penetration into another organ (e.g., pancreas) with fistulization. Hemorrhage, the most common complication, may present with hematemesis or melena and can be life-threatening, especially if there is ulceration into an artery. Perforation typically presents as acute epigastric pain that rapidly becomes generalized, with peritonitis.

Diagnosis and Evaluation

- Definitive diagnosis of PUD is made by direct visualization of the ulcer by upper endoscopy.
- Laboratory tests and imaging studies help to evaluate for complications in ill-appearing patients or to assess for other conditions.
- If perforation occurs, free air under the diaphragm may be seen on x-ray or computed tomography (CT).

Treatment

- Treatment is based on the presumed cause and if complications are present. If caused by NSAIDs, the NSAID should be discontinued and a PPI initiated. If caused by *H. pylori* infection, triple or quadruple therapy should be initiated.
- Hemorrhage can be managed via endoscopy, embolization, or (rarely) surgery.
- Perforation typically requires surgery.

Gastric Volvulus

General Principles

- Characterized by an abnormal rotation of the stomach along its long or short axis, resulting in varying degrees of gastric outlet obstruction, gastric volvulus is a rare condition with high mortality.
- It is most commonly seen in middle-aged patients with anatomic abnormalities, such as paraesophageal hernias. In infants and children, it is usually associated with abnormalities with the attachments of the gastric ligaments or with congenital diaphragmatic abnormalities.

Clinical Presentation

- If the gastric outlet is obstructed, patients can present with acute, severe abdominal pain, vomiting, and abdominal distension.
- Up to 70% of patients with acute gastric volvulus may present with the Borchardt triad, which includes abdominal or chest pain, vomiting, and the inability to pass a nasogastric tube.
- Chronic volvulus with partial obstruction may present with intermittent vomiting or vague symptoms, such as bloating and early satiety.

Diagnosis and Evaluation

- Gastric volvulus should be suspected if multiple attempts to pass a nasogastric tube fail.
- Radiographs may reveal a single, large, gas-filled stomach in the upper abdomen or chest and a paucity of air in the distal bowel. Barium swallow and CT studies can be diagnostic.
- Failure to detect gastric volvulus may lead to stomach ischemia, necrosis, perforation, sepsis, and death

Treatment

- Patients warrant admission with consults made to gastroenterology and general surgery.
- Treatment includes nasogastric tube placement, which can sometimes reduce the volvulus. If the nasogastric tube does not pass, endoscopic assistance and decompression may be necessary. Stable patients without gastric infarction may be candidates for endoscopic reduction; however, most patients require surgical reduction. Surgical repair of the anatomic defect (e.g., paraesophageal hernia) and gastric fixation are recommended to reduce the risk of recurrence.

Gastric Foreign Bodies

General Principles

- Ingestion of foreign bodies, both intentional and accidental, is a common ED complaint and can cause gastrointestinal obstruction or perforation.

BOX 9.3 Indications for Emergent Endoscopic Foreign Body Retrieval

Objects >2 cm wide or >6 cm long
Sharp-pointed objects in the esophagus (e.g., needles, toothpicks, chicken/fish bones, dentures)
Esophageal impaction with complete obstruction
Button batteries
Multiple magnets

- Most foreign body ingestions pass without endoscopic intervention. The approach to management depends on whether the ingested foreign body is associated with a high risk of complications (long object >5 cm, sharp objects, batteries, magnets, and multiple objects), location of the object, and the presence and severity of symptoms.
- "Body stuffing" refers to the unplanned, rapid ingestion of illicit drugs and poses the additional risk of rapid intoxication, which can be fatal. "Body packing" refers to the deliberate ingestion of drugs (often to traffic the drugs).

Clinical Presentation

- The constellation of signs and symptoms depends on the ingested material and can include postprandial vomiting, vague abdominal discomfort, distension from obstruction, or peritonitis secondary to perforation. "Body stuffers" may present with a specific toxidrome.

Diagnosis and Evaluation

- Plain radiographs are often diagnostic but they can be falsely negative, especially if the object is radiolucent. CT should be obtained if there is a high index of suspicion. Oral contrast should not be used in patients who are vomiting or at high risk for perforation. Patients who are not tolerating liquids or have ongoing symptoms of complete obstruction require endoscopic evaluation and treatment.

Treatment

- Treatment depends on the type of material ingested and clinical presentation. Most blunt objects pass through the gastrointestinal tract without complication. Early endoscopic retrieval is generally recommended in objects >2 cm wide or >6 cm long (Box 9.3).
- In patients who are observed, serial imaging may be performed until objects are passed into the stool. Immediate surgical or endoscopic retrieval is indicated in patients with signs of obstruction, perforation, or severe toxicity.

BOX 9.4 Medications Commonly Associated With Impaired Gastric Motility

α_2 agonists (e.g., clonidine)
Calcium channel blockers
Muscarinic cholinergic receptor antagonists
Phenothiazines
Cyclosporine
Tricyclic antidepressants
Dopamine agonists
Octreotide
Glucagon-like peptide-1 agonists

Gastroparesis

General Principles

- Gastroparesis is characterized by delayed gastric emptying, and may be idiopathic, iatrogenic, postoperative, or associated with diabetes (Box 9.4).

Clinical Presentation

- Common symptoms include nausea, vomiting, abdominal pain, early satiety, bloating, and weight loss. Patients may also present with symptoms of the underlying etiology (e.g., autonomic dysfunction).

Diagnosis and Evaluation

- Definitive diagnosis of gastroparesis depends on scintigraphy demonstrating objective delayed gastric emptying (in the absence of a mechanical obstruction). Thus the initial diagnosis is not often made in the ED, but rather, the patient may carry the diagnosis.
- ED evaluation should instead focus on ruling out other alternative diagnoses, such as bowel obstruction or diabetic ketoacidosis. Patients with suspected gastroparesis who do not have an established diagnosis should be referred for outpatient workup (e.g., scintigraphy).

Treatment

- Initial conservative management focuses first on dietary modification (small, frequent meals that are low in fat), hydration, and glycemic control for diabetic patients. Prokinetic and antiemetic medications are often initiated, including metoclopramide (first-line), domperidone, and erythromycin.

SUGGESTED READINGS

Chung, K. T., & Shelat, V. G. (2017). Perforated peptic ulcer: An update. *World Journal of Gastrointestinal Surgery*, 9(1), 1–12.
Light, D., Links, D., & Griffin, M. (2016). The threatened stomach: Management of the acute gastric volvulus. *Surgical Endoscopy*, 30(5), 1847.
Marx, J. A., Hockberger, R. S., & Walls, R. M. (2009). *Rosen's emergency medicine: Concepts and clinical practice* (7th ed., pp. 1137–1152). Mosby Elsevier.

CHAPTER 10

BOARD REVIEW

Assorted Gastrointestinal Topics

CAMERON W. HARRISON, MD, and ARMANDO DARNELL RODRIGUEZ, MD, MS, BS

Gastrointestinal Bleeding

General Principles

- Gastrointestinal bleeding is a very common presentation to the emergency department (ED), with over 1 million hospitalizations annually in the United States.
- Mortality rates remain significant and stable, with a rate of 13%–14% over the last 20 years.
- It is thought that as the population becomes older and acquires more comorbid conditions, such as liver failure, or conditions requiring the use of anticoagulants, there is a higher risk for gastrointestinal bleeding.
- Gastrointestinal bleeding has a wide range of clinical presentations, from the critically ill with massive hematemesis and shock to one with subacute bleeding and stable vital signs.
- Despite the variability in presentations, the foundations of ED management are to provide appropriate resuscitation while determining the cause of bleeding to facilitate definitive treatment (Table 10.1).
- Upper gastrointestinal bleeding (UGIB)
  - Defined as having a source proximal to the ligament of Treitz in the distal duodenum
    - Notably, UGIB is more common than lower gastrointestinal bleeding (LGIB).
    - UGIB has higher morbidity and hospitalization rates when compared with LGIB.
  - UGIB has a relatively high mortality rate of 13%–14%.
  - Classically, patients present with melena or coffee-ground emesis.
  - Peptic ulcer disease is the most common cause of UGIB.
- Lower gastrointestinal bleeding
  - Results from blood loss distal to the ligament of Treitz
  - In contrast to UGIB, LGIB has a mortality rate of 4%.
  - 80% of LGIB resolves spontaneously but should be considered a medical emergency until proven otherwise.
  - Patients with LGIB classically present with hematochezia or bright red blood per rectum.
- Diverticular bleeding is the most common cause of LGIB.

TABLE 10.1 *Differential Diagnoses for Upper and Lower Gastrointestinal Bleeding*

Upper Gastrointestinal Bleeding	Lower Gastrointestinal Bleeding
Peptic ulcer disease	Hemorrhoids
Gastroduodenal erosions	Arteriovenous fistula
Esophagitis	Colon cancer
Esophageal or gastric varices	Mesenteric ischemia
Mallory-Weiss tears	Anal fissures
Caustic ingestions	Foreign bodies
Boerhaave syndrome	Diverticular disease
Aortoenteric fistula	Infectious diarrhea
	Inflammatory bowel disease
	Intussusception
	Meckel diverticulum

Clinical Presentation

- Because both UGIB and LGIB may have more indolent courses, both types of patients may present primarily with symptomatic anemia with fatigue, lightheadedness, chest pain, and shortness of breath.
- UGIB
  - Passage of black tarry stools, or melena
  - Hematemesis, but emesis may be blood-streaked or appear similar to "coffee-grounds"
- LGIB
  - Painful or painless hematochezia, noted on the toilet paper or in the toilet bowl
  - Change in caliber of stools and abdominal mass with obstructive symptoms

Diagnosis and Evaluation

- Determining the general location of the bleed is critical in building an appropriate differential diagnosis and in determining the correct treatment. Although it is ideal for locating the source of bleeding as UGIB or LGIB, sometimes these presentations are not mutually exclusive, and finding the location of the bleeding is challenging. For this reason, it is imperative to first assess hemodynamic stability. Patients being evaluated in the ED for gastrointestinal bleeding warrant cardiac monitoring with pulse oximetry with frequent blood pressure measurements. They should also have two large-bore peripheral IVs placed for resuscitation efforts.
- History of present illness
  - Clinicians should also inquire about long-term alcohol use to gauge the risk of possible liver dysfunction and an increased possibility of a variceal bleed.

- It is critical to ask patients about long-term steroid, nonsteroidal antiinflammatory drug (NSAID), or anticoagulant use because such use pertains to risk for bleeding and the possible need for coagulopathy correction.
- Patients with rectal bleeding should also be screened for a history of aortic aneurysms and/or aortic grafting, which would increase the risk for aortic-enteric fistula as a cause of bleeding.

- Physical examination
  - Tachycardia and hypotension are always concerning for significant volume loss and hemorrhagic shock, which requires aggressive resuscitation.
  - Clinicians should look for evidence of a bleeding source from the oropharynx and nares (swallowed blood).
  - It is pertinent to look for ascites, jaundice, or other stigmata of liver disease because this would significantly change management.
  - A rectal examination may reveal a diagnosis, including a rectal fissure, bleeding hemorrhoid, or other sources of bleeding.
- Laboratory tests
  - Initial laboratory workup should include complete blood count, metabolic panel, coagulation studies, type, and cross.
  - Of note, the initial hemoglobin may not be decreased in the setting of an acute bleed.
  - A high BUN-to-creatinine ratio may be a sign of blood absorption from the intestines in the setting of UGIB.
- Diagnostic studies
  - Consider an ECG and a troponin in patients susceptible to demand/silent ischemia.
  - Placing a nasogastric tube for lavage was previously thought to help determine the presence of UGIB, but this practice has fallen out of favor owing to low sensitivity and specificity.
  - Bedside anoscopy may allow visualization of hemorrhoids or other lesions inside the anal canal.
- Imaging
  - CT of the abdomen/pelvis should be utilized if perforated viscus, small bowel obstruction, mesenteric ischemia, or a mass lesion/cancer is suspected.
  - Abdominal x-rays are usually not helpful for evaluation of gastrointestinal bleeding.
  - Radionuclide scintigraphy is usually not feasible in the ED.
  - Although rarely used, angiography may be used to identify more brisk bleeding and for therapeutic embolization.
  - Ultimately, the most common modality for diagnosing and treating gastrointestinal bleeding is endoscopy.

Treatment

- Correction of blood abnormalities
  - Transfusion is indicated in the setting of continuous bleeding despite treatment, brisk bleeding, signs of end-organ dysfunction, or hemoglobin less than 7 g/dL.
    - Hemoglobin threshold may be raised in patients with certain comorbid conditions (i.e. coronary artery disease [CAD]).
  - Platelet transfusion for a platelet count of less than 50,000/μL
  - Fresh frozen plasma or prothrombin complex concentration (PCC) for an INR greater than 1.5, either intrinsically or from warfarin use
  - Patients taking novel anticoagulants may require administration of PCC or specific antidotes (idarucizumab to reverse direct thrombin inhibitors, and andexanet alfa for factor Xa inhibitors).
- Medications
  - Proton-pump inhibitors, such as pantoprazole, are usually given for UGIB.
    - Most useful to prevent rebleeding in peptic ulcer disease
    - The dose for this is 80 mg IV bolus followed by 8 mg/hr on a continuous drip or 40 mg BID.
  - Medications used in the treatment of variceal bleeding
    - Octreotide or somatostatin to constrict the splanchnic circulation, which theoretically decreases variceal bleeding
    - Octreotide is most commonly used at a dose of 50 μg IV bolus, followed by an infusion of 50 μg/hr.
  - Ceftriaxone is an antibiotic that has a proven mortality benefit in these patients.
    - These patients are very susceptible to pneumonia, urinary tract infections, and spontaneous bacterial peritonitis secondary to bacterial translocation, which is possibly why this drug has proven beneficial.
    - Dose: 1 g IV
- Procedures
  - A Sengstaken-Blakemore tube is a device intended to function as a balloon tamponade for bleeding esophageal varices when endoscopy is not available.
    - This device has significant complications and is reserved as a heroic measure for critically ill patients who are actively exsanguinating and unstable for endoscopy.
- Consult gastroenterology
  - Endoscopy is frequently utilized in gastrointestinal bleeding.
  - Upper endoscopy is usually performed in patients with significant UGIB or patients thought to have variceal bleeding.
  - Stable patients with persistent LGIB benefit from colonoscopy.
- Surgical or interventional radiology consultation may be required for unstable LGIB.
  - Patients with suspected aortoenteric fistula need an emergent vascular surgery consultation.
- The disposition varies significantly, depending on the presentation, comorbid conditions, and etiologies of UGIB. Although not commonly used, the Glasgow-Blatchford Bleeding Score is a screening tool that originates from a well-validated study that used multiple physiologic and laboratory values (e.g., hemoglobin, BUN, systolic blood pressure) to calculate a score to predict the likelihood that a patient will need therapeutic intervention. A patient score of zero is most likely safe for discharge and considered low risk.

Spontaneous Bacterial Peritonitis

General Principles

- Spontaneous bacterial peritonitis (SBP) is defined as an infection of ascitic fluid without a surgically treatable intraabdominal source.

- This diagnosis is almost exclusive to patients with ascites secondary to cirrhosis.
- Risk factors for the disease are a high Child-Pugh score, lower albumin counts, and a history of SBP.
- The primary pathophysiologic mechanism of SBP is bacterial translocation into the peritoneal cavity from the intestines.
- Up to 30% of cirrhotic patients with ascites develop SBP every year.
- Any delay in diagnosis and treatment can have significant adverse effects on survival.
- One study noted an increase of 3.3% for in-hospital mortality for every hour that treatment was delayed.
- Untreated SBP has a mortality rate approaching 50%.
- Given the high mortality associated with delayed treatment along with its subtle presentation, many organizations recommend diagnostic paracentesis for every cirrhotic patient with ascites being admitted to the hospital.

Clinical Presentation

- Classically, patients present with a triad of fever, abdominal pain, and altered mental status.
- Patients may also present with nonspecific signs of sepsis, such as leukocytosis, hypotension, and metabolic acidosis.
- Bacterial overgrowth in the intestine may lead to diarrhea and precipitate SBP.
  - Up to 13% of patients may be asymptomatic.
- The physical examination classically presents as a diffusely tender abdomen.
  - Rebound tenderness may be elicited as well.
  - Many of the signs of an acute abdomen are absent secondary to the ascitic fluid acting as a physiologic barrier to the visceral organs.

Diagnosis and Evaluation

- The gold standard for diagnosing SBP is analysis of ascitic fluid via paracentesis. The sampling is ideally completed before the administration of antibiotics, although treatment should never be delayed.
- The sample is sent for albumin, cell count and differential, glucose, protein, LDH, amylase, Gram stain, as well as aerobic and anaerobic culture.
- Diagnosis is made if the polymorphonuclear (PMN) cell count is greater than 250/mm^3 which is considered a positive result.
  - Must also meet criteria for transudative ascites, which includes a serum-ascites albumin gradient (SAAG) greater than 1.1.
  - If the paracentesis is traumatic, then subtract one PMN for every 250 red cells/mm^3.
- Bowel or gallbladder perforation, both examples of secondary bacterial peritonitis, can present in a very similar fashion with similar PMN counts.
  - An elevated amylase may indicate pancreatitis or bowel perforation.
  - Consider gallbladder rupture if the fluid is dark orange or brown; send ascites fluid for a bilirubin level.

Treatment

- If SBP is suspected, but obtaining ascitic fluid will be delayed, start antibiotics. Antibiotic coverage should include intestinal flora, including *E. coli* and *Klebsiella*. Generally sensitive to broad-spectrum antibiotics, *Staphylococcus* or *Streptococcus* species can also cause SBP.
- First line: Cefotaxime 2 g IV q8h.
  - Alternatively, ceftriaxone can be used at a dose of 2 g IV.
  - Both cefotaxime and ceftriaxone achieve appropriate ascitic fluid levels.
- If patient is asymptomatic, oral antibiotics have been demonstrated to be effective against SBP.
  - However, literature is insufficient to suggest that outpatient management is safe to treat this potentially fatal condition.
  - Given this lack of data, it is common practice to admit patients with SBP.
- Albumin should be administered intravenously in patients with renal dysfunction and SBP.
  - Criteria (any one of the following):
    - Creatine > 1 mg/dL
    - BUN > 30 mg/dL
    - Total bilirubin > 4 mg/dL
  - Dosing
    - Day 1: 1.5 g/kg within 6 hours of diagnosis
    - Day 3: 1.0 g/kg

SUGGESTED READINGS

Koulaouzidis, A., Bhat, S., Karagiannidis, A., Tan, W. C., & Linaker, B. D. (2007). Spontaneous bacterial peritonitis. *Postgraduate Medical Journal*, 83(980), 379–383. Retrieved from http://dx.doi.org/10.1136/pgmj.2006.056168.

Orman, E. S., Hayashi, P. H., Bataller, R., & Barritt, A. S., IV. (2014). Paracentesis is associated with reduced mortality in patients hospitalized with cirrhosis and ascites. *Clinical Gastroenterology and Hepatology*, *12*(3), 496–503.e1. Retrieved from http://dx.doi.org/10.1016/j.cgh.2013.08.025.

Pauwels, A., Mostefa-Kara, N., Debenes, B., Degoutte. E., & Lévy, V. G. (1996). Systemic antibiotic prophylaxis after gastrointestinal hemorrhage in cirrhotic patients with a high risk of infection. *Hepatology*, *24*(4), 802–806. Retrieved from http://dx.doi.org/10.1002/hep.510240408.

Cardiovascular

CHAPTER 11

BOARD REVIEW

Cardiopulmonary Arrest

JOHN CAMPO, MD, and SHIRA A. SCHLESINGER, MD, MScPH

Cardiac arrest is the loss of effective function of the heart resulting in an unresponsive patient with no palpable pulse or effective breathing. When cardiac arrest occurs unexpectedly, it is termed sudden cardiac arrest (SCA). Rapid interventions, starting with CPR and defibrillation, attempt to prevent progression to irreversible cardiac death.

Cardiac Arrest

General Principles

- According to the American Heart Association, more than 325,000 individuals suffer out-of-hospital cardiac arrest each year.
- The majority of cardiac arrests are attributable to cardiac causes, although 50% of victims have no previously diagnosed heart disease.
- Many disease processes can lead to SCA (Box 11.1)
- In patients with known heart disease, the risk of SCA increases 6- to 10-fold.
- Despite substantial advances in the treatment of other cardiac diseases, outcomes for patients suffering out-of-hospital cardiac arrest (OHCA) remain poor, with less than 10% surviving neurologically intact.
- Significant regional variability in survival, ranging from 3% to 22% in counties across the country

Clinical Presentation

- Cardiac arrest is the sudden loss of cardiac function, regardless of presence or absence of electrical activity in the myocardial cells. Neurologic survival depends on maintaining or returning cerebral blood flow as quickly as possible. Unfortunately, most victims of OHCA do not receive high-quality CPR prior to the onset of anoxic brain damage.
- Roughly 70% of OHCA occurs at home, and more than 50% of OHCA are not witnessed.
- Only one-third of OHCA patients receive bystander cardiopulmonary resuscitation (CPR) prior to the arrival of emergency medical services (EMS).
- Cardiac arrests are commonly categorized as shockable or nonshockable, depending on the heart's electrical rhythm. Early rhythm identification is important to cardiac arrest treatment.
  - Ventricular fibrillation (VF) and pulseless ventricular tachycardia (pVT) are the two "shockable" dysrhythmias that occur in cardiac arrest.
  - Pulseless electrical activity (PEA) and asystole are not amenable to defibrillation.
  - PEA includes any rhythm detectable on cardiac monitoring other than VF/VT for which there is no palpable pulse.

BOX 11.1 *Potential Etiologies of Sudden Cardiac Arrest*

Ischemic Heart Disease

- Thrombotic or embolic coronary artery occlusion resulting in myocardial infarction
- Nonatherogenic coronary artery disease: arteritis, dissection, congenital coronary artery anomalies
- Coronary artery spasm

Nonischemic, Structural Heart Disease

- Hypertrophic or dilated cardiomyopathy
- Valvular heart disease
- Congenital heart disease
- Arrhythmogenic right ventricular dysplasia
- Myocarditis
- Acute pericardial tamponade
- Acute myocardial rupture
- Aortic dissection

Cardiac Conduction Abnormalities

- Primary electrical disease (idiopathic ventricular fibrillation)
- Brugada syndrome
- Long QT syndrome
- Preexcitation syndrome
- Complete heart block
- Familial sudden cardiac death syndrome
- Chest wall trauma (commotio cordis)
- Severe metabolic derangements (potassium, calcium, magnesium, phosphorus, acidosis)

Noncardiac Etiologies

- Pulmonary embolism
- Intracranial hemorrhage
- Drowning/suffocation
- Environmental hypothermia
- Hypoxia/hypercapnia (due to toxidromes, obstructive/bronchospastic pulmonary disease, or hypoventilation)
- Hypovolemic/distributive shock (anaphylaxis, sepsis, hemorrhage)
- Central airway obstruction by a foreign body or airway edema
- Sudden infant death syndrome (etiology unknown)
- Sudden unexplained death in epilepsy (SUDEP)

  - PEA can be further categorized based on the QRS morphology as shown in Table 11.1.
  - Asystole refers to absence of detectable electrical activity in cardiac monitoring.

Evaluation and Treatment

- The chain of survival (Fig. 11.1) was developed to illustrate the series of events that together maximize the

TABLE 11.1 Selected Differential Diagnosis and Emergent Treatments of PEA by QRS Duration

QRS Narrow	Emergent Treatment Modality
Cardiac tamponade	Pericardiocentesis
Tension pneumothorax	Needle thoracostomy
Mechanical hyperinflation	Manual chest decompression
Pulmonary embolism	Thrombolysis/embolectomy
Distributive/hypovolemic/hemorrhagic shock	Intravenous fluids and vasopressors/hemorrhage control and transfusion
Acute myocardial infarction with myocardial rupture	
QRS Wide	
Severe hyperkalemia	Calcium chloride
Sodium-channel blocker toxicity (e.g., tricyclic antidepressant toxicity)	Sodium bicarbonate
Acute myocardial infarction with pump failure	Extracorporeal cardiopulmonary resuscitation and cardiac intervention
Agonal rhythm	

chances of survival from SCA. It remains an effective way of demonstrating the critical interplay of bystander, prehospital, and hospital stages of care.

- However, the only interventions that have been definitively shown to increase survival from OHCA in the general population are immediate performance of chest compressions and early defibrillation for shockable rhythms.

General Treatment Measures

- CPR should be performed immediately when suspecting cardiac arrest.
- The American Heart Association (AHA) now advocates "hands-only CPR" for untrained laypersons, responding to a perceived reluctance of bystanders to provide conventional "mouth-to-mouth" resuscitation, and to studies demonstrating equivalent or improved outcomes in patients receiving compressions-only CPR after witnessed cardiac arrest.
- Dispatch-assisted CPR allows 911 operators to provide verbal instruction and coaching for hands-only CPR to callers when the victim is reported as unconscious and without normal breathing.
- Chest compressions should be performed at a rate of 100 to 120 compressions per minute, with a depth of at least 2 inches (5 cm) for adults, or one-third the anterior-posterior diameter for children, allowing for complete chest recoil between compressions.
- In the first minutes of a witnessed cardiac arrest, it is reasonable for rescuers to defer airway management to focus on maximizing compression quality and performing defibrillation, if indicated.
- Some prehospital protocols advise passive oxygenation with high-flow O_2 during the first minutes of cardiac arrest management, particularly for shockable rhythms.
- When a bag-valve mask device is used for ventilation/oxygenation in adults, compressions and breaths should be performed at a ratio of 30:2, with each breath delivering 500 to 600 mL over 1 second, or
- If an endotracheal tube or a supraglottic airway device is placed in an adult, breaths should be delivered every 6 seconds, while continuous compressions are performed.
- Efforts should be taken to avoid hyperventilation because this may cause gastric inflation, aspiration, and increased intrathoracic pressure, in turn decreasing venous return to the heart, impeding cerebral blood flow and decreasing the likelihood of return of spontaneous circulation (ROSC).
- Further rhythm-specific interventions are described in the advanced cardiac life support (ACLS) guidelines of the American Heart Association.

Shockable Rhythms

- Cardiac rhythm should be analyzed and treated as soon as a defibrillator is available.
- Successful termination of the rhythm by defibrillation, and ultimately patient survival, is highest early after the onset of the dysrhythmia.
- Even for OHCA occurring in public spaces, only 8% have an automated external defibrillator applied.
- CPR should be performed until the rescuer is ready to perform defibrillation and continued immediately after, without pausing for rhythm or pulse check.
- The purpose of defibrillation is to cause simultaneous global depolarization of unsynchronized or malfunctioning cardiac myocytes, producing a uniform refractory period after which natural pacemaker cells may reinitiate a rhythm.
- All currently manufactured defibrillators use biphasic energy waveforms, which send current in two directions. Research has indicated a higher likelihood of effective defibrillation at lower energy settings with biphasic waveforms compared with monophasic.

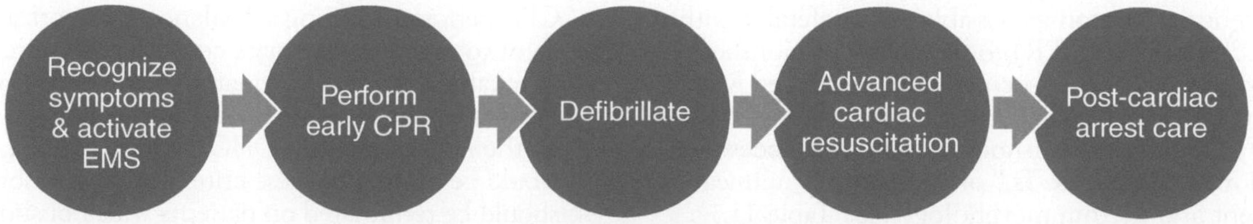

FIG. 11.1 Chain of survival recovery.

- Initial biphasic energy doses should be set per the manufacturer's guideline (usually 120 to 200 J).
- Epinephrine (1 mg intravenous or intraosseous, every 3 to 5 minutes) may be given if VF or pVT continues despite effective CPR and at least two defibrillation attempts.
- The AHA defines shock-refractory VF/pVT as persisting or recurring after one or more shocks, and the (2015) ACLS guidelines discuss use of medications to augment care, although no antiarrhythmic drugs have been shown to increase survival or improve neurologic outcomes in survivors of VF/pVT. The potential benefit of these drugs is in achieving termination of the dysrhythmia.
- Treatment includes administration of amiodarone 300 mg IV bolus for VF/pVT refractory to fewer than two shocks and to at least one dose of epinephrine, followed by a second bolus of 150 mg for continued refractory rhythm. Amiodarone is a class III antiarrhythmic that prolongs the refractory period of cardiac myocytes by prolonging phase 3 of the cardiac action potential.
- Lidocaine 1–1.5 mg/kg IV has been shown to have equivalent efficacy to amiodarone in survival to hospital discharge and can be repeated with a second dose of 0.5–0.75 mg/kg IV for ongoing refractory rhythm. In contrast to amiodarone, lidocaine is a class 1b antiarrhythmic that blocks sodium channels in nonnodal cardiac myocytes, which may assist in suppressing reentry tachycardias in the ventricles.
- Magnesium infusion may be appropriate in patients with torsades de pointes, a form of pVT, but is not indicated for general use in cardiac arrest. Magnesium functions in torsades by decreasing the influx of calcium into the cardiomyocyte, prolonging the refractory period in the ventricular myocytes.
- Esmolol (a beta-blocker) and procainamide (a class 1a, sodium channel blocker, antiarrhythmic) have been used by some authors with mixed or negative results of trials.
- A newer, as of yet unsanctioned, treatment for VF/pVT refractory to three or more shocks is dual sequential defibrillation, in which defibrillation is performed from two separate machines in quick succession, with the goal of terminating an otherwise refractory rhythm. More promising were a few studies of select patients with SCA of presumed cardiac etiology and initial shockable rhythm that demonstrated increased rates of neurologically intact survival when extracorporeal CPR (ECPR) was used for patients transported to the hospital. Several prehospital studies and programs incorporating ECPR into care protocols are ongoing. However, a recent review of currently available literature showed no improvement in patient outcomes when this modality was used.

Nonshockable Rhythms

- Treatment for asystole and PEA consists of high-quality CPR with early epinephrine administration.
- In contrast to treatment of VF/pVT, early administration of epinephrine (as soon as possible and preferably within the first 3 minutes of CPR) to patients with nonshockable rhythms has been associated with increased ROSC and survival rates, especially in pediatric cardiac arrest.
- Further treatment of nonshockable rhythms focuses on correction of the "Hs & Ts," often guided by clinical assessment and rhythm morphology (see Table 11.1). The "Hs & Ts" are as follows: Hypovolemia, Hypoxia, Hydrogen ion excess (acidosis), Hypokalemia, Hyperkalemia, Hypothermia, Tension pneumothorax, Tamponade (cardiac), Toxins, Thrombosis (pulmonary embolus), Thrombosis (myocardial infarction).

Return of Spontaneous Circulation (ROSC) and Post-ROSC Care

- Return of spontaneous circulation is the resumption of cardiac activity sufficient to demonstrate a palpable pulse. Post-ROSC care goals include prevention of rearrest, minimization of long-term neurologic injury, and identification and treatment of the cause of the cardiac arrest.
- Cardiogenic shock is common post-ROSC; immediate care should include infusion of 1 to 2 L intravenous crystalloid fluids (normal saline or lactated Ringer solution), as well as initiation of a vasopressor or inotrope to maintain adequate blood pressure.
- Hyperventilation should be avoided because increased intrathoracic pressure impedes venous return to the heart, and decreased partial pressure of carbon dioxide produces cerebral vasoconstriction, resulting in worse neurologic outcomes.
- Ventilation using waveform capnography should target an end-tidal CO_2 level of 40 mm Hg to decrease neurologic injury and rates of rearrest.
- Supplemental oxygen should be provided with a target PaO_2 between 80 and 120 mm Hg to avoid both hypoxia and hyperoxia, because these have been noted to worsen outcomes.
- An electrocardiogram (ECG) should be performed on all patients with ROSC and emergent coronary catheterization performed if the ECG demonstrates an ST-elevation myocardial infarction (STEMI).
- History, physical examination, and laboratory and diagnostic tests may identify other specific causes of the arrest, prompting interventions directed at the underlying etiology.
- Targeted temperature management (TTM) is believed to be neuroprotective after cardiac arrest, by decreasing inflammatory response to the anoxic cells, free radical formation, and cellular apoptosis. Although the exact ideal temperature goal for TTM has not been clarified, based on existing evidence, current recommendations state that TTM should be initiated on patients who are unable to follow commands post-ROSC with a goal temperature of 32°C to 36°C maintained for the first 24 hours to maximize neurologically intact survival.

Termination of Resuscitation

- Despite the best efforts of prehospital EMS personnel, physicians, and nurses, many patients with SCA will not survive. For patients with an initial rhythm of asystole on EMS arrival, survival to hospital discharge is less than 2%. For patients with an initial shockable rhythm during OHCA, evidence demonstrates that the highest likelihood of neurologically intact survival exists when ROSC is attained in the prehospital setting, because manual CPR performed during ambulance transport is insufficient to maintain adequate cerebral perfusion. For nonshockable rhythms, termination of resuscitation criteria have been validated in several studies and are advocated by the AHA for use in OHCA where ongoing treatment would be futile. Per these criteria, resuscitation efforts should be terminated on patients with nonshockable rhythms when all of the following criteria are met:

- The arrest was not witnessed by EMS personnel, AND
- There is no transient or sustained ROSC during a minimum of three full rounds of high-quality CPR, AND
- No automated external defibrillator shocks or defibrillations were administered by EMS personnel or bystanders.

SUGGESTED READINGS

American Heart Association. *CPR & ECC guidelines*. Retrieved from https://eccguidelines.heart.org/circulation/cpr-ecc-guidelines/.

Panchal, A. R., Bartos, J. A., Cabanas, J. G., Donnino, M. W., Drennan, I. R., Hirsch, K. G., et al. (2020). 2020 American Heart Association guidelines update for cardiopulmonary resuscitation and emergency cardiovascular care. Part 3: Adult basic and advanced life support. *Circulation, 142(16_Suppl_2)*, S366–S468. doi:https://doi.org/10.1161/CIR.0000000000000916. Retrieved from https://www.ahajournals.org/doi/10.1161/CIR.0000000000000261.

Panchal, A. R., Berg, K. M., Kudenchuk, P. J., Del Rios, M., Hirsch, K. G., Link, M. S., et al. (2018). 2018 American Heart Association focused update on advanced cardiovascular life support use of antiarrhythmic drugs during and immediately after cardiac arrest: An update to the American Heart Association guidelines for cardiopulmonary resuscitation and emergency cardiovascular care. *Circulation, 138*, 740–749. Accessed August 20, 2019. Retrieved from https://www.ahajournals.org/doi/10.1161/CIR.0000000000000613.

Cardiac Arrhythmias

CAMERON ARAGHI, MD, and ANDREA W. WU, MD, MMM

Supraventricular Tachycardia

Supraventricular tachycardia (SVT) is an umbrella term applied to tachyarrhythmias with a ventricular rate >100/min and a QRS duration of 0.12 seconds or less. Rhythms may be regular or irregular. There are a variety of etiologies for SVT and presentations may vary, ranging from asymptomatic to shock. Immediate attention should be addressed to the clinical stability of the patient followed by a determination of the type of arrhythmia.

SVT WITH REGULAR QRS

- Sinus tachycardia
- Reentrant tachycardia
  - Atrioventricular (AV) nodal reentrant tachycardia (AVNRT)
  - Atrioventricular reentrant tachycardia (AVRT), orthodromic
- Atrial flutter with "fixed" AV conduction ratio (e.g., 2:1, 3:1)
- Atrial tachycardia with "fixed" AV conduction ratio

SVT WITH IRREGULAR QRS

- Atrial fibrillation
- Atrial flutter with variable AV conduction ratio (e.g., 2:1 alternating with 3:1)
- Multifocal atrial tachycardia
- Atrial tachycardia with variable AV conduction ratio

Atrial Fibrillation

Atrial fibrillation (A fib) is the most common sustained tachyarrhythmia in the general population; prevalence is greatest in patients greater than 70 years of age. It is more common in males than females but females have a greater risk of stroke.

Mechanism

The electrophysiologic mechanism is likely multifactorial. The multiple wavelet hypothesis with multiple reentry foci within the atrial musculature and the focal initiation and maintenance with triggered activity and localized reentry in the pulmonary veins are two theories. The chaotic atrial rhythm may be paroxysmal or sustained.

Causes

- Systemic hypertension
- Coronary artery disease
- Cardiomyopathy
- Valvular heart disease
- Hyperthyroidism
- Hypoxia
- Drugs (alcohol, sympathomimetics)

Most cases are asymptomatic. The most common symptom is palpitations. Other presentations include chest pain, dyspnea, and syncope. In patients with underlying heart disease, pulmonary edema or hypotension/shock may occur in the setting of atrial fibrillation with a rapid ventricular response (RVR). The hemodynamic consequences of atrial fibrillation include loss of synchronous atrial contraction ("atrial kick" contribution to diastolic left ventricular filling) and a decrease in ventricular diastolic filling time, resulting in a fall in cardiac output. A decrease in diastolic filling time leads to impaired coronary blood flow.

ECG Recognition

- See Fig. 12.1.
  - Absence of P waves, undulating wavy baseline
  - Irregularly irregular R-R interval typically at a rate of 120–160/min
  - If R-R intervals are regular without P waves, consider atrial fibrillation with complete heart block and an escape rhythm. This condition may be seen in patients with chronic A fib who have been overmedicated with a β-blocker or calcium channel blocker.
- Patients with A fib are predisposed to the development of atrial thrombi and subsequent systemic embolization. This has implications for both long-term and short-term care. The decision to cardiovert A fib in the ED should take into account the duration of A fib: cardioversion should not be considered if A fib duration has exceeded 48 hours unless the patient is hemodynamically unstable. The decision to initiate long-term anticoagulation in a patient with A fib should incorporate risk guides such as the CHA_2DS_2VASc (Table 12.1) to help inform this decision. Long-term anticoagulation is recommended for score of 2 or greater.

Treatment

- Treatment depends on the patient's clinical condition, hemodynamic stability, underlying cause of illness, comorbidities, and ventricular rate (Fig. 12.2).
- Ventricular rate control is the typical approach in the ED setting. In general, ventricular rate of 110 beats/min or less is the initial goal. Drugs commonly used to manage A fib and other SVTs are shown in Fig. 12.3.

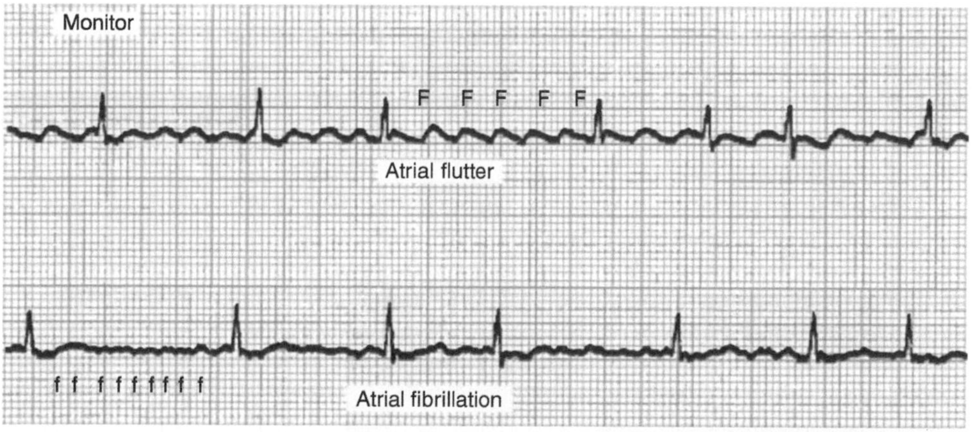

FIG. 12.1 Electrocardiogram demonstrating F waves in atrial flutter (*top*) and f waves in atrial fibrillation (*bottom*). (From Goldberger, A. L. (2006). Supraventricular arrhythmias. In A. L. Goldberger (Ed.), *Clinical electrocardiography: A simplified approach* (7th ed., pp. 163–174). Elsevier.)

TABLE 12.1 ***CHA_2DS_2VASc Score and Risk Criteria***

Score Points	Risk Criteria
1	Congestive heart failure
1	Hypertension
2	Age ≥75 y
1	Diabetes mellitus
2	Stroke, transient ischemic attack, thromboembolic event
1	Vascular disease (prior myocardial infarction, peripheral artery disease)
1	Age 65–74 y
1	Sex category (female sex)

Rate Control

- Class 2 antiarrhythmics: β-blockers, such as metoprolol or esmolol. Caution in concomitant pulmonary disease, hypotension. Preferred agent if cause is thyrotoxicosis.
- Class 3 antiarrhythmics: amiodarone can be considered for patients with decompensated heart failure with the caveat that drug-related hypotension and unintended pharmacologic cardioversion may occur.
- Class 4 antiarrhythmics: calcium channel blocker such as diltiazem. Caution in patients with heart failure, hypotension.
- Digoxin: possible option for hypotensive patients. However, has delayed onset of action, making its use in the ED limited.
- Although calcium channel blockers may hasten a decrease in ventricular response rate more rapidly than β-blockers, there is no evidence that one drug is more effective than the other with respect to a meaningful, patient-centered clinical outcome.
- Most patients presenting with atrial fibrillation and RVR have a history of chronic atrial fibrillation and recent inability to adhere to a prescribed drug regimen. After the target ventricular rate has been achieved, such patients can usually be discharged home without an extended observation period. Patients with newly diagnosed A fib ("new onset" A fib) can be admitted to an observation unit after rate control for the initiation of workup and management plan although outpatient is an option in selected patients with minimal symptoms. A fib with RVR in a patient with chronic A fib previously well rate-controlled and compliant with medications should suggest a compensatory response such as in blood loss, sepsis, or pulmonary embolism, and treatment should be directed to the underlying cause.

Rhythm Control (Cardioversion)

- Pharmacologic cardioversion is generally reserved for hemodynamically stable patients with A fib of ≤48 hours' duration and should be considered an elective rather than urgent intervention.
  - Class 1 antiarrhythmics: procainamide
  - Class 3 antiarrhythmics: amiodarone or ibutilide. Patients given ibutilide should be monitored for 24 hours due to the risk of torsades de pointes and polymorphic ventricular tachycardia.
- Procainamide, amiodarone, and ibutilide have similar cardioversion success rates (40%–50%). Amiodarone treatment generally requires a higher dose and longer infusion duration (up to 24 hours) for cardioversion rather than rate control.
- The Ottawa Aggressive Protocol for management of A fib and atrial flutter (A flutter) incorporates an infusion of procainamide followed by electrical cardioversion if drug therapy alone is unsuccessful. A successful conversion rate of about 90% has been reported in eligible patients.

Electrical Cardioversion

- Biphasic cardioversion at 100–200 J
- Indicated in unstable patients: consideration for risk of embolic events (time of onset, anticoagulation, if patient has known thrombus). Heparin should ideally be started before cardioversion and continued if successful.
- Stable patients: Cardioversion can be considered in patients with an onset of less than 48 hours or in those currently taking anticoagulant medications.
- Higher risk of ventricular arrhythmia postcardioversion in patients with hypokalemia or digitalis toxicity

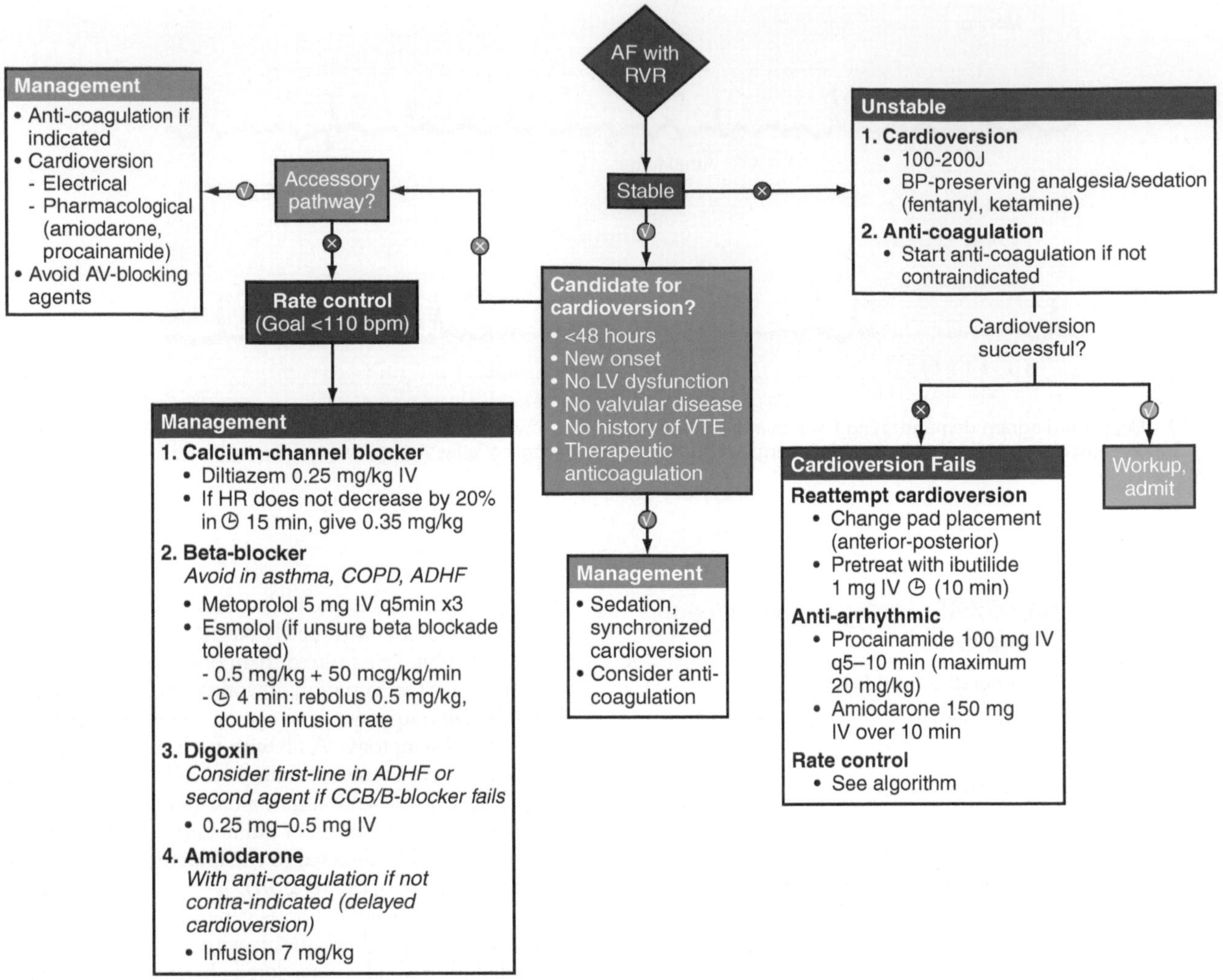

FIG. 12.2 Algorithmic approach to management of atrial fibrillation with rapid ventricular rate (*RVR*). *ADHF*, acute decompensated heart failure; *AF*, atrial fibrillation; *AV*, atrioventricular; *BP*, blood pressure; *bpm*, beats per minute; *CCB/B-blocker*, calcium channel blocker/beta-blocker; *COPD*, chronic obstructive pulmonary disease; *HR*, heart rate; *IV*, intravenous; *LV*, left ventricular; *VTE*, venous thromboembolism. (From Algorithm of atrial fibrillation with rapid ventricular rate (RVR). Fadial, T. (2019). *Atrial fibrillation with RVR management algorithm.* [image] Available at: https://ddxof.com/atrial-fibrillation/.)

Atrial Flutter

A flutter is common in patients with structural heart disease and is due to an intraatrial reentrant pathway.

ECG Recognition

- In patients with normal interventricular conduction, A flutter is characterized by a narrow complex tachycardia with an atrial rate that is typically around 300/min.
- The ventricular rate may be regular with a fixed AV conduction block (typically 2:1) or irregular if a variable conduction block exists (see Fig. 12.1).
- A ventricular rate of approximately 150 with inverted P waves in lead III suggests A flutter with a fixed 2:1 block.
- The typical sawtooth P wave pattern is most commonly seen at higher conduction ratios (e.g., 3:1 or higher) (see Fig. 12.1).
- Patients are usually asymptomatic or complain of palpitations. A flutter is typically better tolerated than A fib at comparable rates, likely because of continued atrial contraction during A flutter.

Treatment

Same principles and agents as A fib, including anticoagulation and decisions to cardiovert. Cardioversion of A flutter usually can occur at lower voltages (50–100 J synchronized cardioversion).

Multifocal Atrial Tachycardia

- Mechanism: multiple ectopic atrial foci due to increased automaticity
- Causes: most commonly due to respiratory failure, severe heart failure, or drug toxicity (sympathomimetics)

ANTIARRHYTHMIC DRUG ACTIONS

Vaughn-Williams Class		Drug	ECG changes	Channels			Receptors				Clinical effects			
				Ca⁺⁺	Na⁺	K⁺	α	β	ACh	Ado	Pro-Army	Extra cardiac	LV FX	Heart rate
I	A	Quinidine	A		M	M	L		M		H	M		
		Procainamide			M	M					M	H		
		Disopyramide (Norpace)			M	M			M		L	M	↓↓	
	B	Lidocaine (Xylocaine)	B		L						L	M		
		Mexiletine (Mexitil)			L						L	M		
	C	Propafenone (Rythmol)	C		H			M			M	L	↓↓	↓
		Flecainide (Tambocor)			H						H	L	↓↓	
II		β-Adrenergic antagonists						H			L	L	↓	↓↓
III		Dronedarone (Multaq)		L	L	H	M	M	M		L	H	↓	↓
		Amiodarone (Cordarone)		L	L	H	M	M	M		L	H		↓
		Sotalol (Betapace)				H		H			H	L	↓	↓
		Ibutilide (Corvert)			△	H					H	L		
		Dofetilide (Tikosyn)				H					H	L		
IV		Verapamil (Calan, Isoptin)		M							L	L	↓↓	↓
		Diltiazem (Cardizem)		M							L	L	↓	↓
Misc		Adenosine (Adenocard)								△	L	L		↓

Antagonist relative potency
L = Low
M = Moderate
H = High

△ = Agonist
● = ECG Changes related to Ca^{++} channel block
● = ECG Changes related to Na^{+} channel block
● = ECG Changes related to K^{+} channel block

FIG. 12.3 List of commonly used antiarrhythmic drugs and their effects. *ACh*, acetylcholine; *Ado*, adenosine; *ECG*, electrocardiogram; *LV FX*, left ventricular function. (From Romero, K., & Woosley, R. L. (2012). Clinical pharmacology of antiarrhythmic drugs. In E. M. Antman & M. S. Sabatini (Eds.), *Cardiovascular therapeutics: A companion to Braunwald's heart disease* (pp. 343–364). Elsevier.)

- Symptoms: usually related to the underlying disease or cause

ECG Recognition

- Irregular R-R rate at 100–160; may mimic A fib
- Varying P wave morphology; need to identify three consecutive P waves of different morphology in the same ECG lead
- Variable P-R interval
- QRS complexes are narrow unless there is a chronic or rate-related bundle branch block.

Treatment

The management of multifocal atrial tachycardia is similar to that of A fib. Attention should be directed to rate control if necessary. β-Blockers should be avoided because the underlying illness, such as chronic obstructive pulmonary disease or severe heart failure, is likely to be worsened with these agents. Calcium channel blockers are preferred.

Reentrant Supraventricular Tachycardia

Reentrant SVT is the term usually used to describe AVNRT and AVRT. Both involve a reentrant "circuit" with pathways characterized by slowed conduction and unidirectional block. These rhythms are typically initiated by a premature atrial depolarization.

AV Nodal Reentry Tachycardia

- See Fig. 12.4.
  - Reentry circuit within the AV node
  - Narrow complex (unless patient has a chronic bundle branch block or develops aberrant conduction, also called related bundle branch block)
  - Rate normally between 130 and 180 beats per minute but may be greater

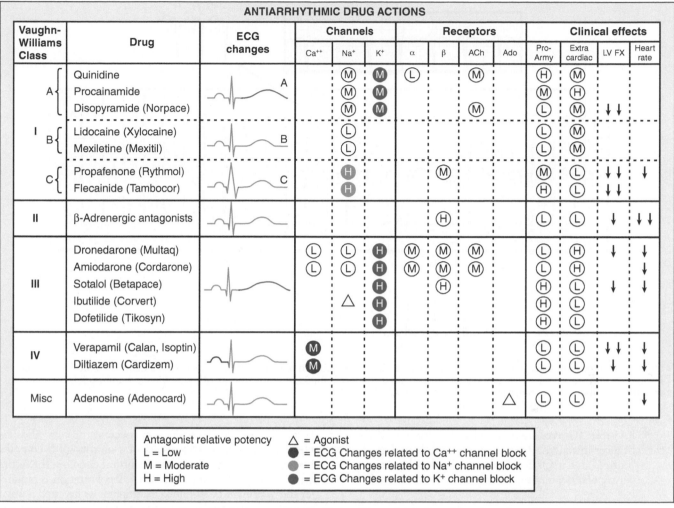

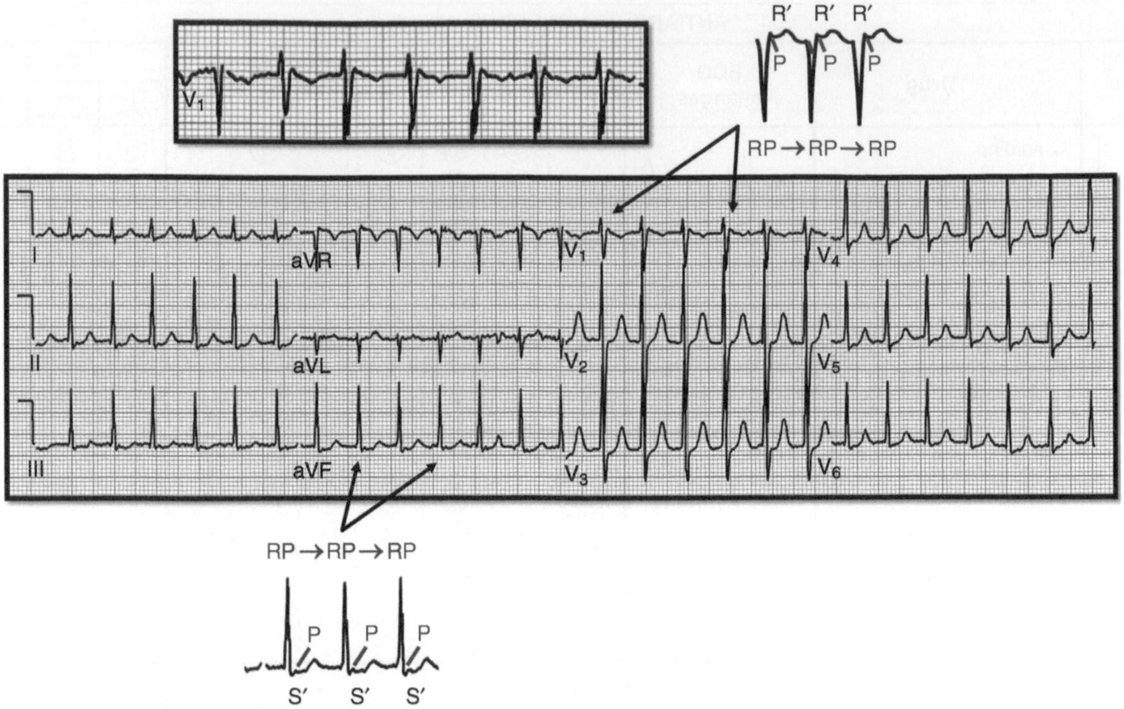

FIG. 12.4 Atrioventricular nodal reentrant tachycardia. Electrocardiograph of supraventricular tachycardia demonstrating location of P waves. (From DeSimone, C. V., Naksuk, N., & Asirvatham, S. J. (2018). Supraventricular arrhythmias: Clinical framework and common scenarios for the internist. *Mayo Clinic Proceedings, 93*(12), 1825–1841.)

- If visible, P waves are inverted in inferior limb leads. In most instances, P waves are not visible and are "buried" in the QRS complex (atrial depolarization and ventricular depolarization occur at the same time).

AV Reentrant Tachycardia

AVRT is SVT that results from a sustained reentrant "loop" that incorporates the AV node for one limb and an extranodal pathway for the other. The extranodal pathway may be "concealed," meaning AV conduction is normal, with a narrow QRS complex during normal sinus rhythm, or "manifest," as observed on the baseline ECG in patients with Wolff-Parkinson-White (WPW) syndrome during normal sinus rhythm; the delta wave represents preexcitation of the ventricle (Fig. 12.5). The depolarization of the ventricle via an accessory pathway is referred to as preexcitation. AVRT with narrow QRS complexes is the most common rhythm disturbance in patients with WPW. This is because the bypass tract conducts only "orthodromic," meaning the signal is conducted antegrade through the AV node fast His-Purkinje system and then retrograde through the bypass tract to the atria. Because the conduction occurs through the fast His-Purkinje system, this results in a narrow QRS complex. Because the atria are part of the reentrant circuit in the setting of an extranodal bypass tract, atrial depolarization is required for the rhythm to be sustained. Retrograde or inverted P waves are typically observed in the inferior leads during the tachycardia. AVNRT and AVRT are often indistinguishable on the surface ECG. "Antidromic" AVRT refers to when the antegrade conduction occurs through the bypass tract and the retrograde conduction occurs through the AV node. Because most of the depolarization occurs through slow myocyte-to-myocyte conduction, this is a wide complex tachycardia.

Clinical Presentation of AV Nodal Reentry Tachycardia and AV Reentrant Tachycardia

- Typically presents with sudden onset of palpitations. May have chest pain, dyspnea, or anxiety; rarely presents with hemodynamic instability

Treatment

- Vagal maneuvers (modified Valsalva, carotid massage, diver reflex)
- Adenosine

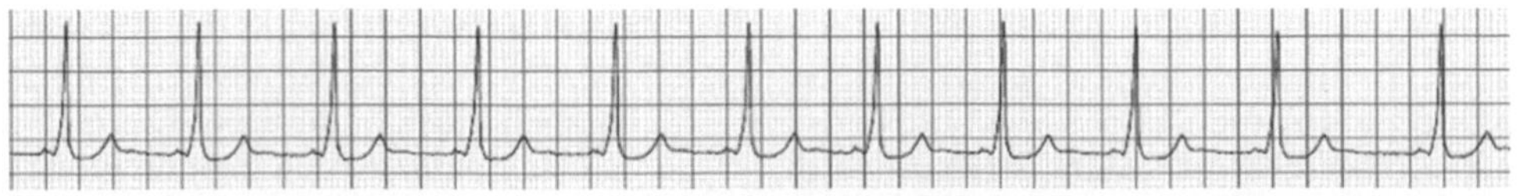

FIG. 12.5 Cardiograph with delta waves and shortened PR interval in patient with Wolff-Parkinson-White syndrome. (From Martin, R. J., Fanaroff, A. A., & Walsh, M. C. (2020). *Fanaroff and Martin's neonatal-perinatal medicine: Diseases of the fetus and infant* (11th ed.). Elsevier.)

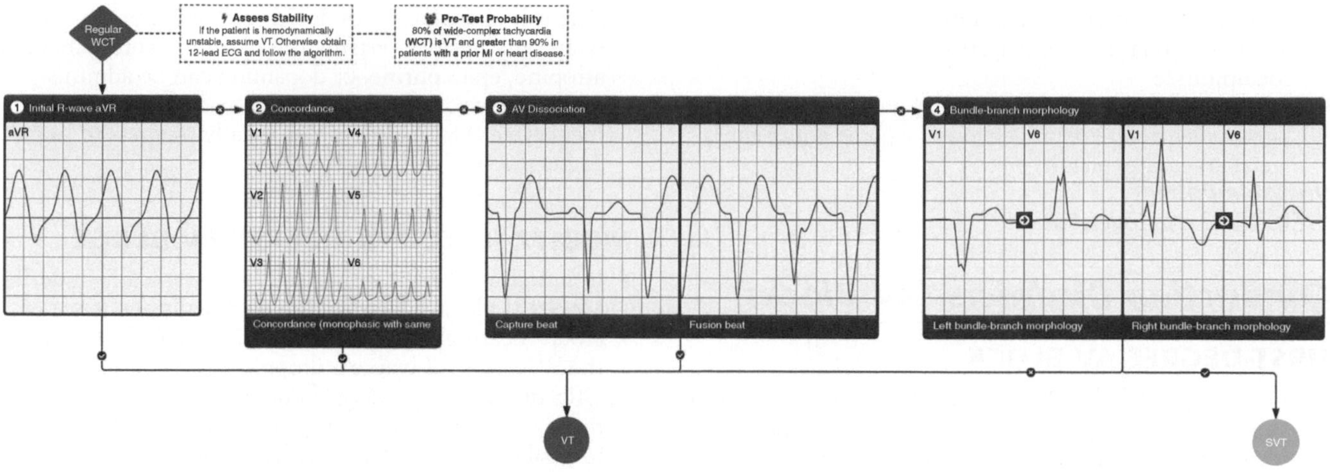

FIG. 12.6 Electrocardiographic findings in ventricular tachycardia. Algorithm for regular wide complex tachycardia. *AV,* atrioventricular; *ECG,* electrocardiogram; *MI,* myocardial infarction; *SVT,* supraventricular tachycardia; *VT,* ventricular tachycardia; *WCT,* wide complex tachycardia. (From Fadial, T. (2019). Wide complex tachycardia algorithm. Available at https://wikem.org/wiki/File:Wide_Complex_Tachycardia.png.)

- Class 1 agents: procainamide
- Class 2 agents: metoprolol
- Class 4 agents: diltiazem
- Electrical cardioversion if unstable, 100–200 J biphasic

Regular Wide Complex Tachycardia

- Regular wide complex tachycardias are characterized by regular R-R intervals with QRS duration of 0.12 sec or greater.
  - Mechanisms
    - Ventricular tachycardia (VT)
    - A regular SVT with aberrant conduction (also called rate-related bundle branch block)
    - A regular SVT in a patient with a chronic bundle branch block
    - Antidromic AVRT or antidromic atrial flutter in WPW syndrome

ECG Differential Diagnosis

VT due to structural heart disease, usually coronary artery disease with prior myocardial infarction, is the most common cause of a regular wide QRS tachycardia. Frequently reported ECG findings supporting a diagnosis of VT include a monophasic R wave in lead aVR, precordial QRS concordance (meaning the QRS all upward or all downward in the same direction in leads V_1–V_6), evidence of AV dissociation (capture and/or fusion beats, dissociated P waves), and specific QRS morphologies in V_1 and V_6 (Fig. 12.6).

Treatment

A conservative approach is recommended: a regular wide QRS complex tachycardia is VT until proven otherwise.

Hemodynamically Stable Patient

- The American Heart Association Emergency Cardiovascular Care Guidelines recommendation for regular and monomorphic WCT
  - Adenosine: will terminate AVNRT and some forms of VT (adenosine responsive, triggered)
  - Antiarrhythmics: procainamide, amiodarone, or lidocaine
  - Consider synchronized electrical cardioversion if drug treatment fails.
- These recommendations specifically exclude the use of β-blockers and calcium channel blockers because of possible adverse effects in patients with WPW syndrome and antidromic conduction.

Unstable Patient

- Synchronized electrical cardioversion

Irregular Wide Complex Tachycardia

An irregular WCT is usually due to atrial fibrillation in a patient with a chronic or rate-related bundle branch block. However, WPW syndrome with antidromic bypass conduction to the ventricles should be considered. In the latter, extremely high conduction rates (>250/min), are typical because the AV is not involved in AV conduction. Polymorphic VT is characterized by irregular wide polymorphic QRS complexes (Fig. 12.7). Torsades de pointes is a specific type of polymorphic VT that occurs in the setting of QT prolongation and is specifically treated with magnesium.

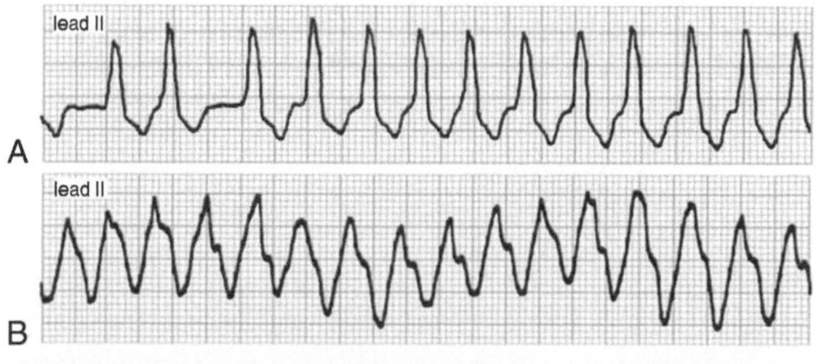

FIG. 12.7 (A) Atrial fibrillation with aberrancy. (B) Polymorphic ventricular tachycardia. (From Goldberger, A. L., Goldberger, Z. D., & Shvilkin, A. (2018). *Goldberger's clinical electrocardiography: A simplified approach* (9th ed.). Elsevier.)

Hemodynamically Stable Patient
- Avoid AV nodal blocking agents
- Procainamide
- Magnesium if polymorphic/torsades de pointes
- Correct electrolyte derangements (such as potassium)
- Electrical cardioversion

Unstable Patient
- Electrical cardioversion

Conduction Disorders (AV Blocks)

FIRST-DEGREE AV BLOCK

- In first-degree AV block, conduction time from the atria to the ventricles is prolonged. Electrocardiographically, it is defined as a PR greater than 0.20 s. The most common causes are AV nodal disease, increased parasympathetic (vagal) tone, and medications (agents that slow conduction through the AV node). Additional causes include electrolyte disorders (hyperkalemia), myocarditis, and myocardial ischemia. First-degree AV block alone does not cause symptoms. Treatment is directed to management of causes (correcting electrolytes, withholding medications). First-degree AV block alone does not progress to higher degrees of block. Patients with a first-degree AV block accompanied by a right bundle branch block and block of one of the left bundle fascicles (left anterior superior or left posterior inferior) are at greater risk of progressing to complete heart block.

MOBITZ I SECOND-DEGREE AV BLOCK (WENCKEBACH)

- Typically, the Mobitz I second-degree AV block is due to AV node disease resulting in decremental conduction delay through the AV node. Electrocardiographically, classic or typical Wenckebach block manifests in grouped QRS complexes with pauses between groups, PR prolongation from beat to beat (the largest PR interval increase is usually seen between the first and second beat in the group), gradual shortening of the R-R interval before a "dropped" QRS complex. Mobitz I block is often seen in the setting of inferior ST-elevation myocardial infarction due to occlusion of the proximal right coronary artery leading to ischemia of the AV node and increased vagal tone. It may also be seen in infections (Lyme carditis, infectious endocarditis with perivalvular abscess, myocarditis), infiltrative myocardial disease (amyloidosis, cardiac sarcoidosis), or idiopathic degenerative processes (Lev and Lenègre diseases), or result from overmedication (β-blockers, calcium channel blockers, digoxin). Type I block is usually asymptomatic unless it results in a bradycardia leading to hypotension, syncope, or symptoms of decreased cardiac output. In symptomatic cases (usually the result of acute ischemia), atropine, epinephrine, or dopamine can be administered, followed by transcutaneous pacing if drugs are ineffective. Mobitz I does not usually progress to higher degrees of block.

MOBITZ II SECOND-DEGREE AV BLOCK

- Infranodal conduction system disease typically underlies Mobitz II block. Electrocardiographically, evidence of group "beating" is seen and the PR interval is fixed, as is the R-R interval before a dropped QRS complex. The QRS duration is prolonged due to infranodal disease resulting from myocardial necrosis. Type II block is not reversible and frequently precedes complete heart block. Mobitz II block, with or without symptoms, is an indication for permanent pacemaker. In the ED, symptomatic patients should be managed with transcutaneous pacing. This rhythm disturbance rarely responds to atropine, epinephrine, or dopamine.

COMPLETE HEART BLOCK

- Depolarizations from a supranodal pacemaker are not conducted distally. Ventricular depolarization results from a lower pacemaker and QRS complexes are the result of depolarizations initiated by a lower "escape" pacemaker. Complete heart block results from diffuse conduction system disease due to myocardial necrosis, an infiltrative process, or drug toxicity. Electrocardiographically, "AV dissociation" is present. The atria are depolarized in the usual fashion and regular P waves are observed at the intrinsic rate of the SA node. The ventricles are depolarized independently at the intrinsic rate of the escape pacemaker, e.g., approximately 60/min with a nodal pacemaker, 30–40 with a ventricular pacemaker. Management is limited to temporary followed by permanent cardiac pacing.

SUGGESTED READINGS

Burns, E. (2019). Supraventricular tachycardia (SVT). Available at: http://litfl.com/supraventricular-tachycardia-svt-ecg-library/. Accessed June 03, 2019.

Desimone, C. V., Naksuk, N., & Asirvatham, S. J. (2018). Supraventricular arrhythmias: Clinical framework and common scenarios for the internist. *Mayo Clinic Proceedings*, 92, 1825–1841.

deSouza, I., Peterson, A., & Marill, K. (2015). Differentiating types of wide-complex tachycardia to determine appropriate treatment in the emergency department. *Emergency Medicine Practice*, *17*, 1–22.

January, C. T., Wann, L. S., Alpert, J. S., Calkins, H., Cigarroa, J. E., Cleveland, J. C., Jr., Conti, J. B., Ellinor, P. T., Ezekowitz, M. D., Field, M. E., Murray, K. T., Sacco, R. L., Stevenson, W. G., Tchou, P. J., Tracy, C. M., & Yancy, C. W. (2014). 2014 AHA/ACC/HRS guideline for the management of patients with atrial fibrillation. A report of the American College of Cardiology/American Heart Association Task Force on Practice Guidelines and the Heart Rhythm Society. *Journal of the American College of Cardiology*, *64*, e1–e76.

CHAPTER **13**

BOARD REVIEW

Congenital Heart Disease

LILLY AGNES BELLMAN, MD, and CINDY D. CHANG, MD

Ductal-Dependent Congenital Heart Disease

Congenital heart disease (CHD) occurs in about 1 in 100 live births. Of those, about 10% have a critical congenital lesion (often ductal-dependent) that requires acute (often surgical) intervention to avoid significant morbidity or mortality within the first months of life. Many of these babies are asymptomatic at time of nursery discharge and thus present initially in the emergency department.

General Principles

- The initial presentation of CHD depends on the lesion as well as the transition from fetal to newborn circulation.
  - The **ductus arteriosus** (connection from the pulmonary artery to the aorta) along with the foramen ovale supplies the fetal systemic circulation, bypassing the lungs. In normal circumstances, these connections close (via multiple mechanisms including decrease in prostaglandins, O_2 exposure, and changes in pulmonary vascular resistance) within the first hours to days of life.
  - **Ductal-dependent CHD** (DDCHD) lesions require a patent ductus arteriosus (PDA) to support extrauterine systemic circulation. Thus, the pathologic state presents itself as the PDA closes.
  - **Cyanosis:** bluish discoloration of the skin
    - **Central** cyanosis involves the oral mucosa (look under the tongue). It becomes apparent when at least 5 g/dL hemoglobin is deoxygenated (typically SpO_2 of <80–85%).
    - **Peripheral** cyanosis or **acrocyanosis** of the extremities secondary to peripheral vasoconstriction can be due to such extrinsic factors as cool ambient temperatures or secondary to compensatory mechanisms in response to circulatory shock state.
    - Both central and peripheral cyanosis may be seen in initial presentation of DDCHD.

Three Main DDCHD Pathophysiologies (*Table 13.1*)

- Pulmonary (right) blood flow obstruction
- Systemic (left) blood flow obstruction
- Complete mixing lesions

In normal circulation, the pulmonic and systemic circulations are connected in series. In these abnormal physiologies, however, the two circuits are connected in parallel via the ductus arteriosus and other shunts in order for both sides of circulation to receive blood flow (Table 13.1). Changes in **pulmonary vascular resistance** (PVR) and **systemic vascular resistance** (SVR) can thus significantly change the relative balance of the pulmonic and systemic circulations. It is important to consider how such emergency department interventions as O_2 administration (decreases PVR) may affect this circulatory balance. The effects of oxygen on DDCHD patients are discussed in the treatment section.

Clinical Presentation

- Infants may present with vague symptoms including irritability, poor feeding (especially long, slow feeds), sweating with feeds, and poor weight gain. At the time of decompensation, they often are in respiratory distress, may be cyanotic, or have circulatory collapse.
- Family medical history of CHD is notable because up to 20% of critical CHDs have a genetic component. Some genetic conditions have predispositions for CHD lesions such as atrioventricular canal defect in trisomy 21.
- Differential diagnosis includes sepsis, hematologic disorders (severe anemia or methemoglobinemia), and inborn errors of metabolism.

Diagnosis and Evaluation

Emergency physicians have a toolbox of bedside tests that can help evaluate a child with suspected DDCHD (Table 13.2). Integration of the information from age, general appearance, bedside tests, and radiology findings can help identify the pathophysiologic category and guide resuscitative interventions (Fig. 13.1). In this figure and later in the text, the concept of **"color"** refers to the general appearance. A "gray baby" is one who appears dusky with poor perfusion and has variable SpO_2. A "blue baby" is centrally cyanotic and hypoxic. A "pink baby" has a normal color, perfusion, and oxygen saturation.

Physical Examination

- Consider the vital signs; an afebrile, yet tachycardic, or tachypneic child should raise clinical suspicion for CHD.
- Perform the examination with particular attention to the patient's general appearance (color, respiratory effort), peripheral perfusion, quality of femoral pulses, brachiofemoral delay (when palpated simultaneously, the brachial or radial pulse is felt before the femoral pulse), and hepatomegaly.
- **Auscultation** of the heart, noting presence of murmur and lungs for crackles which may indicate pulmonary edema. Lack of cardiac murmur does NOT exclude CHD.

Four-Limb Blood Pressure Examination

- A positive test with blood pressure differential between upper and lower extremities is concerning for a left-sided obstructive lesion such as coarctation of the aorta. (see Table 13.2).

TABLE 13.1 *Example Congenital Heart Disease Lesions by Physiology*

Pulmonary (Right) Blood Flow Obstruction	Systemic (Left) Blood Flow Obstruction	Complete Mixing Lesions	Pulmonary Overcirculation[a]
Tricuspid atresia Pulmonary atresia Pulmonary stenosis Ebstein anomaly "Blue" tetralogy of Fallot	Hypoplastic left heart syndrome Coarctation of the aorta Aortic stenosis, atresia, or arch interruption	Total anomalous pulmonary venous return Truncus arteriosus Double-outlet right ventricle Dextro-transposition of the great arteries with ventricular septal defect (or patent ductus arteriosus)	Patent ductus arteriosus Ventricular septal defect Atrial septal defect Arteriovenous malformation Atrioventricular canal "Pink" tetralogy of Fallot

[a]Often called congestive heart failure.

TABLE 13.2 *Emergency Department Toolkit of Bedside Tests*

Hyperoxia Test

Traditional

1. Draw arterial blood gas while on room air.[a]
2. Place patient on 100% O_2 via non–rebreather mask for 5–10 min.
3. Repeat arterial blood gas and compare against prior.

Passed: Hyperoxia test result: $PaO_2 > 150$ after hyperoxia: suggestive of respiratory disease
Failed: Hyperoxia test result: $PaO_2 < 150$ after hyperoxia: <100 highly suggestive of critical congenital heart disease

Pulse Oximetry Method

Monitor response to 100% O_2 on the SpO_2. SpO_2 that remains <85% despite 5–10 min of 100% O_2 therapy highly suggestive of critical congenital heart disease.

Pulse Oximetry Screen

- Preductal (right upper extremity) or either lower extremity SpO_2 <90%
- Preductal and either lower extremity SpO_2 <94%
- Difference in SpO_2 >3% between preductal and either lower extremity

Four-Limb Blood Pressure Examination

- Systolic blood pressure differential >10 mm Hg between preductal right upper extremity and postductal (either lower extremity)
- Positive test suggests left-sided obstructive lesion such as coarctation of the aorta.

[a]May consider drawing only the posthyperoxia arterial blood gas.
PaO_2, partial pressure of arterial oxygen; *SpO_2,* oxygen saturation.

Pulse Oximetry

- Measure preductal (right upper extremity) and postductal (lower extremity) O_2 saturations
- A positive pulse oximetry screen (see Table 13.2) is strongly suggestive of DDCHD.
- This screen is performed after at least 24 hours of life and before nursery discharge in most states (recommended by the American Heart Association and the American Academy of Pediatrics) and triggers echocardiography, catching many cases of critical CHD early. Because newborn physiology continues to change for the first month of life, the timing of the pulse oximetry screening can still miss CHD in infants, particularly those with such left-sided obstructive lesions as coarctation of the aorta.

Chest Radiography

- Evaluate the cardiac silhouette as well as the lung fields on chest x-ray (CXR) as part of the evaluation of suspected DDCHD. CXR can also help identify noncardiac causes of respiratory distress.
  - Lung fields
    - **Dark lungs:** indicator of obstructed pulmonary blood flow
    - **White lungs:** indicator of pulmonary edema from pulmonary overcirculation or obstruction to pulmonary venous return
  - Heart appearance
  - Cardiomegaly
  - Some lesions are associated with classic appearances of the heart on CXR (Table 13.3).

Hyperoxia Test

- Helps determine whether hypoxia is due to a primary respiratory problem or secondary to a shunting process suggestive of a cardiac lesion
- Instructions for how to conduct a hyperoxia test are in Table 13.2.

Electrocardiography

- The pediatric electrocardiography findings change along with the circulatory physiology in the first month of life. Initially, right-sided forces dominate, shifting to left dominant after ~1 month of age.
  - Note the axis. An extreme superior axis (−90 to −180 degrees), also known as northwest axis, can suggest an atrioventricular canal defect.
  - Hypertrophy (must use age-based values)
    - Left ventricular hypertrophy in an infant is always abnormal.

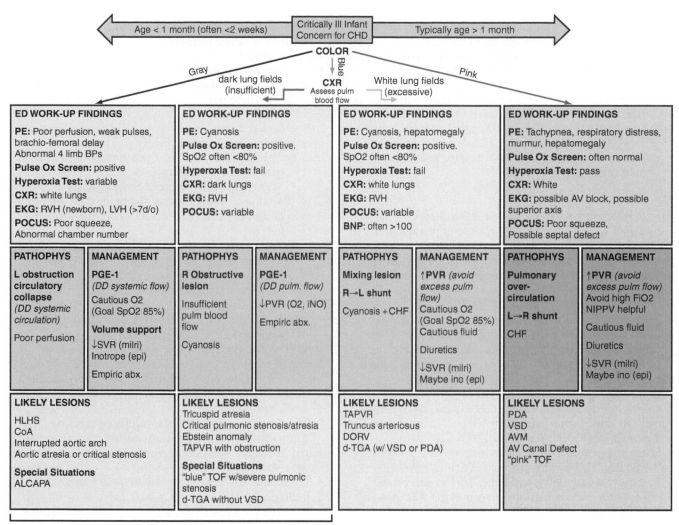

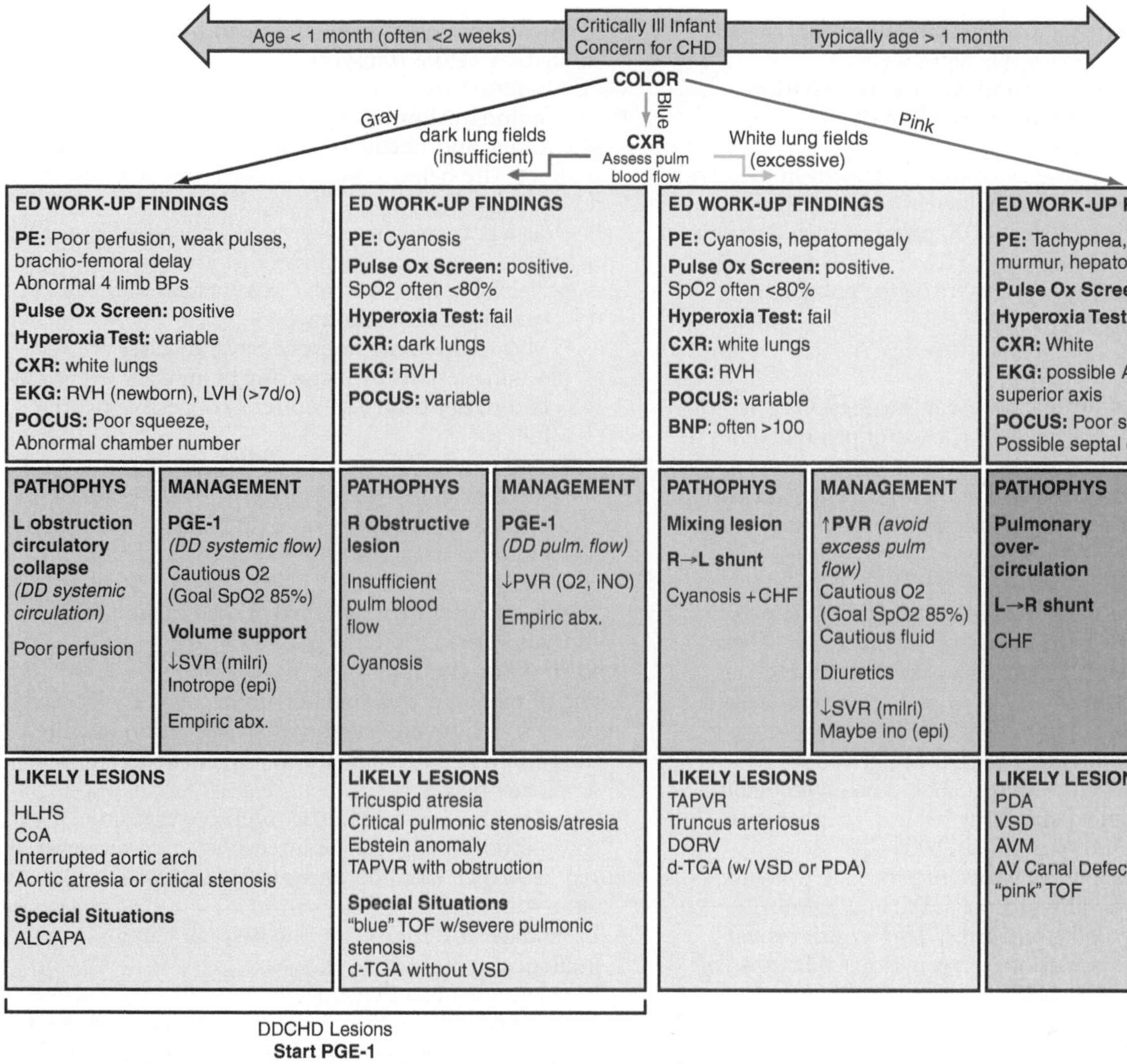

FIG. 13.1 Approach to an ill child with concern for congenital heart disease. This algorithmic approach of categorizing infants with concern for congenital heart disease starts by considering a patient's age, general appearance (color), and, in the case of a "blue" baby, the appearance of the lung fields on a chest x-ray. Pathophysiology and management are placed next to each other demonstrating how they inform each other. Special situations refer to pathologies that present clinically similarly to a pathophysiologic category but may not have that physiology. For example, anomalous left coronary artery from the pulmonary artery is an abnormality of the coronary vasculature not a left-sided obstruction but presents with circulatory collapse. *abx*, antibiotics; *ALCAPA*, anomalous left coronary artery from the pulmonary artery; *ASD*, atrial septal defect; *AV canal*, atrioventricular canal; *AVM*, arteriovenous malformation; *BPs*, blood pressures; *BNP*, B-type natriuretic peptide; *CHD*, congenital heart disease; *CHF*, congestive heart failure; *CoA*, coarctation of the aorta; *CXR*, chest x-ray; *DD*, ductal dependent; *DORV*, double-outlet right ventricle; *d-TGA*, dextro-transposition of the great arteries; *ED*, emergency department; *EKG*, electrocardiogram; *epi*, epinephrine; *HLHS*, hypoplastic left heart syndrome; *ino*, inotrope; *L*, left; *LVH*, left ventricular hypertrophy; *milri*, milrinone; *NIPPV*, noninvasive positive pressure ventilation; *PDA*, patent ductus arteriosus; *PE*, physical examination; *PGE-1*, prostaglandin E1; *POCUS*, point-of-care ultrasonography; *pulm*, pulmonary; *PVR*, pulmonary vascular resistance; *R*, right; *RVH*, right ventricular hypertrophy; *SVR*, systemic vascular resistance; *TAPVR*, total anomalous pulmonary venous return; *TOF*, tetralogy of Fallot; *VSD*, ventricular septal defect. (Adapted from Fig. 1 in Strobel, A. M., & Lu, L. N. (2015). The critically ill infant with congenital heart disease. *Emergency Medicine Clinics of North America*, *33*(3), 501–518. doi:10.1016/j.emc.2015.04.002.)

TABLE 13.3 ***Classic Chest X-ray Heart Shapes and Associated Congenital Heart Disease Lesions***

Classic Heart Shape	Lesion
Boot-shaped	Tetralogy of Fallot
Egg on a string	Transposition of the great arteries
Box-shaped	Ebstein anomaly
Snowman in snowstorm	Total anomalous pulmonary vascular return

- Right ventricular hypertrophy persistent after age 1 month is concerning.

Point-of-Care Ultrasonography

- Point-of-care ultrasonography (POCUS) can identify features suggestive of CHD as well as cardiogenic shock. POCUS does NOT serve as a comprehensive echocardiogram, which is still needed to definitively identify lesions.
- POCUS in this setting should focus on:
  - Global function or "squeeze"

- Gross heart appearance noting number of chambers or if there are any obvious septal defects
- Inferior vena cava size and respiratory variation
- Lungs for B-lines (pulmonary edema)

Laboratory Evaluation

- Perform a comprehensive laboratory workup given the broad differential diagnosis for an undifferentiated sick infant.
- **B-type natriuretic peptide > 100 pg/mL** is highly sensitive and specific for new diagnosis CHD in infants presenting with respiratory distress (lesions involving pulmonary overcirculation).

Treatment

Appropriate timely critical care can be lifesaving in children with DDCHD, particularly the use of prostaglandin E1 (PGE-1) (Alprostadil). Resuscitation interventions in the context of DDCHD must be used with care and attention to how they might affect physiology in a way distinct from a normal cardiovascular system.

Vascular Access

- Two lines of vascular access are important to support resuscitation with both fluids and medications. These can be a peripheral IV, umbilical venous catheter, or intraosseous access.

Prostaglandin E1

- Potentially lifesaving drug for DDCHD; maintains patency of ductus arteriosus. It should be given empirically to "blue babies" and "gray babies" younger than 1 month of age with presumed DDCHD.
- Must be given as a continuous infusion due to rapid metabolism in the lungs. Start at 0.05 μg/kg/min, Increase by 0.05 μg/kg/min every 10-15 minutes to effect (monitor circulation, oxygenation). Max 0.4 μg/kg/min. Monitor for **apnea**, hypotension, fever, seizure.

Fluid Management

- Cautious administration of 10 mL/kg boluses with frequent reevaluation
- Left-sided obstructive lesions (often the "gray babies") benefit from preload support.
- Too much fluid can worsen cardiac and respiratory status in the setting of pulmonary overcirculation.

Vasoactive Medications

- **Epinephrine** and **dopamine** are the inotropes of choice to improve contractility and support systemic circulation, although at the cost of increasing SVR, which can be problematic in the left-sided obstructive lesions
- **Milrinone** (often in combination with an inotrope) can help with lusitropy (cardiac relaxation and filling) and afterload reduction. This can be helpful in left-sided obstructive lesions to improve peripheral perfusion.
- Discussion of the optimal balance of vasoactive medications with a pediatric intensivist is crucial, especially if the infant could have a long transport.

Airway Management Considerations

- Mechanical ventilation may be needed in babies on PGE-1 infusions because apnea is a relatively common adverse effect. If these infants are to be transferred for definitive cardiology evaluation and treatment, consider intubation before transport.

O_2 Considerations

- O_2 administration has multiple effects on CHD physiology and needs to be used thoughtfully because it affects the balance of pulmonary and systemic blood flow.
  - O_2 is a potent pulmonary vasodilator (decreases PVR) and also constricts the PDA.
    - Helpful in the "blue baby" presentation with pulmonary circulation obstruction
    - May temporarily improve SpO_2 in cases of mixing lesions by increasing pulmonary overcirculation, but then also worsens congestive heart failure
    - Too much O_2 can worsen systemic circulation in "gray baby" presentation with systemic (left) circulation obstruction by increasing pulmonary circulation at the expense of the systemic circulation.
    - A safe goal in an undifferentiated infant with suspected DDCHD SpO_2: 85%

Inhaled Nitric Oxide

- Potent pulmonary vasodilator (to decrease PVR) used in cases with severe pulmonary hypertension in which the patient remains difficult to oxygenate despite high supplemental O_2
- Often reserved for use in the intensive care unit or with consultation of a pediatric intensivist or cardiologist

Rapid Sequence Intubation (RSI) Medication Considerations

- **Etomidate** or **fentanyl** are the best choices for induction.
  - Relatively hemodynamically neutral
  - Etomidate carries theoretical risk of adrenal suppression, making it a controversial choice when sepsis is on the differential diagnosis.
- Avoid **ketamine** as an induction agent.
  - Increases in SVR can compromise systemic circulation, especially in infants with left-sided obstruction physiology.
- **Rocuronium** is a good choice for paralytic.

Ventilation Considerations

- Positive pressure ventilation changes hemodynamics including lowering preload, SVR, and increasing PVR.
  - The decrease in preload can be offset with judicious intravenous (IV) fluids and low positive end-expiratory pressure settings on the ventilator.
  - Positive pressure ventilation can in turn help with heart squeeze.

Antibiotics

- Empiric antibiotics should be started because the differential diagnosis in the undifferentiated sick infant includes sepsis.

Disposition

- Infants with DDCHD often need urgent or emergent surgery and therefore require definitive care in a pediatric center with heart surgery capabilities, so it is crucial to initiate contact with an appropriate center as soon as DDCHD is suspected.

Pulmonary Overcirculation (or Congestive Heart Failure) as the Presentation of Congenital Heart Disease

After the first month of life, many CHD lesions present with pulmonary overcirculation, commonly (albeit technically incorrectly) referred to as congestive heart failure (CHF). Most pediatric cardiologists reserve the term CHF to describe complex pathophysiologic anatomic and neurohormonal changes that ultimately affect heart function, and in this line of thinking pulmonary overcirculation is a risk for but does not necessarily result in CHF. For the purpose of this chapter, because it is often used in emergency department vernacular, we use the terms pulmonary overcirculation and CHF interchangeably and mainly discuss the presentation of CHD as CHF.

It is important to consider CHF in the differential diagnosis of infants and children presenting with respiratory distress.

General Principles

Pathophysiology

- Signs and symptoms of CHF occur because anatomic anomalies (abnormal connections, valvular abnormalities) affect usual blood flow through the pulmonic and systemic circulation resulting in fluid backup or overcirculation.
  - **Pulmonary overcirculation** resulting in pulmonary edema occurs when there is excessive blood flow to the lungs. This can be secondary to either excessive volume (left-to-right shunting lesion such as ventricular or atrial septal defect), pressure build-up (such as in an obstructive lesion or regurgitant valve lesion), or a combination of both.
  - **Peripheral venous congestion** occurs on the systemic side of circulation secondary to volume or pressure backup in CHD. This can manifest with hepatomegaly and peripheral edema.
  - **Genetic cardiomyopathies, infectious myocarditis,** and **cardiotoxic drugs** cause direct cardiac injury resulting in cardiac dysfunction and resultant CHF. Pediatric cardiologists argue that these are the true cases of CHF. These are beyond the scope of this chapter.
  - **Noncardiac causes** of CHF in children include other fluid overload states such as renal failure as well as **high-output heart failure** conditions in which significant increase in cardiac output is needed to meet the body's anatomic or metabolic demands and can result in overload of the heart. These include vascular malformations, severe anemia, hyperthyroidism, and thiamine deficiency and are beyond the scope of this chapter.

Clinical Presentation

- Infants may present with vague symptoms including poor feeding, poor weight gain or failure to thrive, fussiness particularly around feeding, and fast breathing. Symptoms tend to occur between 1 and 6 months of age.
- Infants in CHF are often described as being "quietly tachypneic" with rapid respiratory rates (often >60 breaths/min) in the absence of significant distress.
- Feeding difficulties are common and include sweating with feeds, crying with feeds, and very long, slow feeds.
- Older children present more classically with dyspnea on exertion, orthopnea, and swelling in the extremities.
- Differential diagnosis for the infant presenting in respiratory distress includes respiratory illnesses like bronchiolitis and pneumonia.

Diagnosis and Evaluation

The same principles presented in the previous section on DDCHD also apply to CHF presentations. In this section we highlight the main components that are more suggestive of CHF.

Physical Examination

- "Quiet tachypnea" or tachypnea without significant respiratory distress
- Lung auscultation with crackles in the lung fields suggestive of pulmonary edema
- Cardiac auscultation demonstrating an S3 or S4 gallop; some cases may have a murmur.
- Hepatomegaly
- Edema (may be facial or gravity-dependent around the sacrum, the lowest part of the body in supine infants, or in the extremities of older children)

Chest Radiography

- White lung fields indicative of pulmonary edema
- Cardiomegaly

Electrocardiography Findings

- Atrioventricular nodal block (by age-based intervals)
- Ventricular hypertrophy (by age-based values)

Point-of-Care Ultrasonography

- Global decreased "squeeze"
- May identify large septal defects
- Plump-appearing inferior vena cava
- B-lines in lung fields
- Formal echocardiography is essential for definitive diagnosis and quantification of CHF.

Laboratory Evaluation

- Workup evaluating an infant in respiratory distress can include complete blood count with differential, BMP, blood gas analysis, and consideration of viral testing.
- **B-type natriuretic peptide >100 pg/mL** is highly sensitive and specific for new diagnosis CHD in infants presenting with respiratory distress (lesions involving pulmonary overcirculation).

Treatment

- The main principles of emergency department management include measures to increase PVR and decrease SVR (see DDCHD section for discussion on physiology and interplay of PVR and SVR in more detail). Diuretics are helpful in reducing acute volume overload. In the patient with CHF who is decompensating, inotropic support may be required. Long-term therapies (for patients

with true CHF) include afterload reduction with angiotensin-converting enzyme inhibitors, angiotensin II receptor blockers, diuretics, and β-blockers, and occasionally digoxin, and should be discussed with a pediatric cardiologist.
- Minimize **supplemental O_2** (O_2 decreases PVR and can worsen pulmonary overcirculation).
- In patients with more severe respiratory distress, **non-invasive positive pressure ventilation** methods such as high-flow nasal cannula or continuous positive airway pressure where FiO_2 can be controlled are ideal and help via alveolar recruitment and decreasing preload and afterload.
- Judicious use of **IV fluids;** 10 mL/kg normal saline boluses can be given with close reassessment for worsening of tachycardia, hepatomegaly, or respiratory distress.
- **Diuretic** therapy often with loop diuretics such as furosemide (Lasix) is the mainstay of initial management for pulmonary overcirculation.
- **Vasoactive** medications and **inotropes** are reserved for patients with hemodynamic decompensation (hypotension for age) or poor perfusion.

Disposition

- Consultation with a pediatric cardiologist and definitive care in a facility with pediatric critical care capabilities. These children may require cardiac surgery but not usually emergently.

Tetralogy of Fallot and Hypercyanotic Episodes

General Principles

- Tetralogy of Fallot (TOF) accounts for approximately 10% of CHD cases and is one of the most common congenital heart lesions that require surgical intervention in the first year of life.
  - TOF consists of four major anatomic features:
    - Ventricular septal defect (VSD)
    - Pulmonary stenosis with right ventricular outflow obstruction
    - Overriding aorta
    - Right ventricular hypertrophy

Clinical Presentation

- TOF represents a spectrum of CHD presentations. The degree of severity in how and when a child with TOF presents depends upon the degree of right ventricular outflow obstruction and the size and resistance of the VSD and ductus arteriosus. Infants with severe pulmonary stenosis have a right-to-left shunt across the VSD and may have ductal-dependent pulmonary blood flow. These babies present with cyanosis early in their newborn period and are sometimes referred as "blue tets." On the other end of the spectrum, "pink tets" are children with a mild pulmonary stenosis component, and/or have predominantly a left to right shunt (accross the VSD or large PDA) and present later in life with signs and symptoms of CHF.

Hypercyanotic "Tet Spells"

- Uncorrected TOF or other CHD lesion involving interventricular shunts or obstructions to pulmonary blood flow may present with **hypercyanotic spells**, also known as "**tet spells.**" These episodes are characterized by hypoxemia and hypercarbia triggered by agitation, pain, exertion, fever, or hypovolemia.

Tet Spell Pathophysiology

- During hypercyanotic spells, there is:
  - Increased pulmonary outflow obstruction (↑PVR)
  - ↓ SVR, which leads to increased right-to-left shunting across the VSD
    - Both of these mechanisms lead to a positive feedback loop of hypoxia which then further increases PVR, perpetuating the problem.
- Infants may present with severe cyanosis, sweating, hyperpnea (rapid and deep respirations), inconsolability, loss of consciousness, and occasionally seizures.
- Older children present with cyanosis, shortness of breath, agitation, and sometimes syncope. They also reflexively learn to squat during these episodes, which increases SVR and decreases the right-to-left shunt across the VSD to recover from the hypercyanotic episode.

Diagnosis and Evaluation

Physical Examination

Cardiac Auscultation

- Systolic ejection murmur at the left mid-upper sternal border due to right ventricular outflow tract obstruction; may be very soft during hypercyanotic episodes due to markedly increased obstruction.
- Loud, single S_2

Electrocardiography Findings

- Right axis deviation
- Right atrial enlargement
- Right ventricular hypertrophy (age-based values)

Chest Radiography Findings

- "Boot-shaped" heart with an upturned apex due to right ventricular hypertrophy
- Normal heart size
- Pulmonary vascularity may be normal or decreased depending on degree of obstruction.

Treatment

Hypercyanotic Tet Spells (Severe Right Ventricular Outflow Obstruction)

- **Maneuvers:** neonates, toddlers, or children may present with tet spells. Patients should be placed immediately in a "knees-to-chest" position to increase SVR and decrease the right ventricular outflow obstruction.
- **Oxygen:** provides pulmonary vasodilation
- **Additional therapies** (Table 13.4) include fluid bolus, pain control, anxiolysis, and in the most severe cases, vasoactive medications
- After resolution of the spell, perform targeted evaluation to identify the trigger of the episode.

Antibiotic Prophylaxis for Dental Work

- Patients with unrepaired cyanotic CHD should have prophylactic antibiotics to prevent bacterial endocarditis before dental procedures or before surgical correction.

TABLE 13.4 *Hypercyanotic Spell Management*

Therapy	Administration/Dose	Effect
Nonpharmacologic	Calming measures and knees-to-chest positioning	Intrinsic Knees-to-chest position ↑SVR Calming ↓PVR
Supplemental O_2	Face mask	Pulmonary vasodilation ↓PVR
IV fluid bolus	Normal saline 10-20 mL/kg	Increase preload
Opioid	Morphine 0.05-0.1 mg/kg IV/IM (max 4 mg) Fentanyl 1 μg/kg IV/IM or 1.5-2 μg/kg IN (max 50 μg).	Pain control Relaxation of pulmonary infundibulum, ↓obstruction
Benzodiazepine	Midazolam 0.1 mg/kg IV/IM or 0.2–0.3 mg/kg IN (max 6 IV, max 10 mg IM).	Anxiolysis
β-Blocker	Propranolol 0.1-0.25 mg/kg IV (max initial dose 1 mg) Esmolol 100 μg/kg IV and 50–75 μg/kg per minute IV drip if single dose is ineffective	Rate control
Vasopressor	Phenylephrine 5–20 μg/kg IV, followed by IV drip 0.1 to 0.5 μg/kg/minute, titrate to effect	↑SVR If other methods fail

IV, intravenous; IM, intramuscular; IN, intranasal; PVR, pulmonary vascular resistance; SVR, systemic vascular resistance.

A general emphasis on maintaining good oral health is paramount.

Disposition

- Consultation with a pediatric cardiologist and definitive care in a facility with pediatric critical care capabilities. If possible, consulting with the patient's primary cardiologist or surgeon is ideal.

SUGGESTED READINGS

Akkinapally, S., Hundalani, S.G., Kulkarni, M., Fernandes, C.J., Cabrera, A.G., & Shivanna, B., et al. (2018). Prostaglandin E1 for maintaining ductal patency in neonates with ductal-dependent cardiac lesions. *Cochrane Database of System Reviews*, 2, CD011417. doi:10.1002/14651858.CD011417.pub2. 29486048.

Doyle, T., Kavanaugh-McHugh, A., & Fish, F.A. (2019). Management and outcome of tetralogy of Fallot. *UpToDate*. https://www.uptodate.com/contents/management-and-outcome-of-tetralogy-of-fallot?sectionName=Tet%20spells&topicRef=5769&anchor=H11096360&source=see_link#H11096360.

Horeczko, T., & Inaba, A.S. (2018). Cardiac disorders. In Walls, R. M., Hockberger, R. S., & Gausche-Hill, M. (Eds.), *Rosen's emergency medicine: Concepts and clinical practice* (9th ed.) (pp. 2099–2125). Elsevier.

Strobel, A.M., & Lu, L.N. (2015). The critically ill infant with congenital heart disease. *Emergency Medicine Clinics of North America*, 33(3), 501–518. doi:10.1016/j.emc.2015.04.002.26226862

CHAPTER 14

BOARD REVIEW

Valvular Disorders

CAMERON ARAGHI, MD, and ANDREA W. WU, MD, MMM

Mitral Stenosis

General Principles

The normal cross-sectional area of the mitral valve is 4–6 cm^2. Mitral stenosis is characterized by a decrease in orifice size and obstruction of inflow to the left ventricle from the left atrium during diastole. Most commonly this is the result of a diseased mitral valve apparatus secondary to rheumatic heart disease resulting in fusion, thickening, fibrosis, and calcification of the valve leaflets. Obstruction to left atrial outflow results in increased left atrial pressure and a transmitral pressure gradient. Decrease in ventricular filling and consequently preload can lead to decreased stroke volume and cardiac output, particularly with an increase in heart rate (exercise, stress, onset of atrial fibrillation). High left atrial pressures stimulate atrial remodeling, which results in hypertrophy and predisposition to arrhythmia (atrial fibrillation) as well as thrombus formation. The chronic elevation in the left atrial pressure has an upstream effect on the pulmonary veins, which in turn can lead to a passive increase in pulmonary artery pressure, pulmonary hypertension, and ultimately right-sided heart failure.

Causes

- Post–rheumatic heart disease (RHD): most common cause worldwide but declining prevalence
- Mitral annular calcification due to chronic degenerative changes: most often seen in patients >75 years of age
- Radiation-associated valve disease
- Congenital abnormalities
- Secondary to systemic disease (systemic lupus erythematosus, rheumatoid arthritis)

Clinical Presentation

- History: RHD, exercise intolerance, dyspnea on exertion, orthopnea, hemoptysis, hoarse voice, and, in some cases, symptoms of right heart failure
- Physical examination: opening snap early in diastole, middiastolic apical murmur (rumble) with presystolic accentuation, and loud S1 early in disease. Signs of right ventricular failure, such as peripheral edema, jugular venous distention may also be found.
- Chest x-ray may demonstrate evidence of atrial enlargement with straightening of the left side of the heart border or a double density sign with severe left atrial enlargement. Electrocardiogram (ECG) may show left atrial enlargement and evidence of pulmonary hypertension and right ventricular enlargement, e.g., large R wave in V_1 with right axis deviation. Left ventricular enlargement is not seen with mitral stenosis alone.

Diagnosis

The auscultatory findings of mitral stenosis are subtle and are often missed, especially during tachycardia. The diagnosis should be suspected in a patient with a history of heart valve disease and ECG findings of left atrial and right ventricular enlargement. The diagnosis is most often made with echocardiography performed during evaluation of dyspnea or newly diagnosed heart failure.

Treatment

- Emergency department (ED) treatment is focused on sustaining hemodynamic stability and addressing precipitants such as volume status, anemia, atrial fibrillation, ischemia, infection, etc. Diuretics may be needed in the setting of pulmonary congestion or edema. Atrial fibrillation is common in mitral stenosis and a rapid ventricular response rate is not well tolerated, often leading to acute pulmonary edema. Immediate rate control is required. Rhythm control carries a high risk of systemic embolization.
- Various surgical interventions exist for the appropriate patient, including valvulotomy, repair and replacement.

Mitral Regurgitation

General Principles

Acute mitral insufficiency differs from chronic mitral insufficiency in both etiology and presentation (Table 14.1).

Acute Mitral Insufficiency

- Usually the result of sudden rupture of chordae tendineae or dysfunction or rupture of a papillary muscle. Acute mitral insufficiency is generally more severe and abrupt in presentation because the left atrium (LA) and left ventricle (LV) are unable to adapt to the sudden physiologic changes (Table 14.1). There is an abrupt elevation in the LA pressure with resultant elevation in pulmonary venous pressure, leading to acute pulmonary congestion.
- If a significant amount of LV volume is ejected back into the LA during systole, systemic outflow from the LV will decrease. Regurgitation is worsened in the setting of increased systemic vascular resistance (afterload). As cardiac output decreases, the heart rate increases but cardiac output often remains low, often resulting in cardiogenic shock.
- Common causes include endocarditis, chordal rupture in myxomatous valve disease, and papillary muscle rupture

TABLE 14.1 Findings in Acute and Chronic Mitral Regurgitation

	Acute	Chronic
Cardiac output	↓	N
Ejection fraction	N or ↓	N or ↑
Left ventricular end-diastolic pressure	↑↑	N
Left atrial compliance	N	↑
Left ventricle size	N	↑
Systolic murmur	Soft, early decrescendo	Holosystolic
S3	Rarely present	+/−

N, Normal.
(Adapted from Stout, K. K., & Verrier, E. D. (2009). Acute valvular regurgitation. *Circulation, 119*, 3232–3241.)

after myocardial infarction. Stress cardiomyopathy (takotsubo cardiomyopathy) and myocarditis are less common etiologies.

Chronic Mitral Regurgitation

- In contrast to acute insufficiency, chronic mitral regurgitation is insidious in nature and, over time, manifests by effects on the LV and LA, usually resulting in LA and LV dilatation and hypertrophy (Table 14.1). Eventually in severe mitral regurgitation (MR) the LV decompensates and heart failure ensues. Common causes include RHD and dilated cardiomyopathy.

Causes

- Primary MR (structural disruption of the valve)
  - Degenerative mitral valve disease
  - RHD
  - Infective endocarditis
  - Cleft mitral valve
  - Mitral annular calcification
  - Medications: ergotamine, bromocriptine, pergolide, cabergoline
  - Iatrogenic: complication of atrioventricular canal defect repair
- Secondary MR (functional): due to abnormalities of the LV
  - Post–myocardial infarction
  - Dilated cardiomyopathy
  - Trauma
  - Hypertrophic cardiomyopathy

Clinical Presentation

- Chronic MR usually presents with typical symptoms of congestive heart failure.
- Acute MR typically presents with pulmonary edema and often cardiogenic shock.
- Apical holosystolic murmur radiating to the axilla in chronic MR, may be decrescendo in acute MR
- ECG may demonstrate ischemia or evolving infarction in acute regurgitation. Chronic MR may show evidence of left atrial enlargement and left ventricular hypertrophy (LVH).
- The posteromedial papillary muscle with chordal attachments to the posterior mitral leaflet is more prone to rupture, causing acute MR. Blood supply is via only the right or circumflex coronary artery (depending on dominance). Rupture occurs in the setting of an inferior ST-elevation myocardial infarction, typically within a week of acute ischemia. The anterolateral papillary muscle (anterior leaflet) usually has a dual blood supply from the left anterior descending and left circumflex coronary arteries and is less prone to rupture.
- Papillary muscle rupture may present with unilateral pulmonary edema involving the right lung. It may be misdiagnosed as pneumonia. This location is believed to be related to the position of the posterior leaflet to the pulmonary veins.

Diagnosis

- Clinical diagnosis in the ED, which can be assisted by point-of-care ultrasonography (POCUS)
- Echocardiogram and cardiac catheterization for definitive diagnosis

Treatment

Acute MR treatment is focused on treatment of pulmonary edema and immediate consultation for potential surgical intervention. Temporizing measures such as intraaortic balloon counterpulsation or left ventricular assist device may be considered. Chronic MR is treated for symptoms of heart failure via medical therapy; surgical intervention is typically not indicated emergently.

Aortic Stenosis

General Principles

Aortic stenosis (AS) occurs when the cross-sectional area of the aortic valve (normally 3–4 cm^2) is reduced more than 50% of the inherent size. Severe AS typically occurs when the size is less than 1 cm^2 and evidenced by a transvalvular jet velocity of 4 m/s. Worldwide, RHD is the most common etiology, with concomitant mitral valve disease frequently seen. Degenerative calcific disease (aortic sclerosis) is more common in the developed world, most commonly affecting patients ≥70 years of age. The stenotic process is slow with a prolonged asymptomatic period until critical AS develops. Compensatory LVH aids in maintaining cardiac output and left atrial hypertrophy is commonly seen.

Causes

- Congenital abnormality (bicuspid aortic valve)
- Degenerative calcification
- RHD

Clinical Presentation

Presentation depends on the severity of stenosis and state of LV function. Early AS may be asymptomatic and incidentally recognized via echocardiography performed to evaluate a systolic murmur. Symptomatic patients may present with dyspnea, angina, syncope, or heart failure. It is not uncommon for patients who are compensated and asymptomatic at baseline to present critically ill after a secondary illness (sepsis, trauma, etc.) precipitates physiologic stress.

Diagnosis

- Auscultation reveals a late-peaking crescendo-decrescendo holosystolic murmur best heard at the second right

intercostal space that radiates to the carotids. The second heart sound will be reduced in intensity. Pulsus parvus et tardus (diminished volume and late upstroke of the carotid upstroke when timed to ventricular systole) may be appreciated. ECG and chest x-ray may reveal LVH and left atrial enlargement.
- Clinical diagnosis in the ED, which can be assisted by POCUS
- Echocardiogram for definitive diagnosis

Treatment

In the minimally symptomatic patient, management of systemic hypertension decreases afterload and preserves cardiac output. There is a limited role for medical management of the more symptomatic patient. Decreasing metabolic demand should be considered when treating concomitant disease (arrhythmia, heart failure, anemia, infection). Intravenous nitroglycerin has been used in the emergency setting for the treatment of decompensated heart failure. It was classically taught that this should be avoided, but the data do not support this. Intravenous nitroprusside, when administered in a setting with advanced monitoring capabilities, can increase cardiac output in the setting of severe stenosis and is well tolerated. Definitive treatment is valve replacement either via the transcatheter approach or open.

Aortic Insufficiency

The most common etiology for aortic insufficiency (AI) worldwide is RHD. AI occurs when valve coaptation during diastole is compromised, leading to retrograde flow from the aorta into the LV. In chronic AI, the LV gradually dilates to maintain a near-normal end-diastolic pressure. LV remodeling and compensatory hypertrophy facilitate maintenance of a normal stroke volume and cardiac output. Over time, LV dysfunction occurs and leads to failure. Acute aortic regurgitation presents with a more severe clinical presentation of ventricular failure and pulmonary congestion (Table 14.2).

TABLE 14.2 Findings in Acute and Chronic Aortic Insufficiency

	Acute	Chronic
Cardiac output	↓	N
Pulse pressure	N or ↓	↑
Systolic pressure	↓	↑
Left ventricular end-diastolic pressure	↑	N
Diastolic murmur	Soft, early	Decrescendo holodiastolic
S1	Soft	N
S2	Soft	N
S3	Present	Often absent

N, normal.
(Adapted from Stout, K. K., & Verrier, E. D. (2009). Acute valvular regurgitation. *Circulation, 119*, 3232–3241.)

Causes

- RHD
- Bicuspid valve
- Infective endocarditis (acute presentation)
- Aneurysm
- Aortic dissection (acute presentation)
- Trauma
- Aortic root abnormality (aortitis, aneurysm)

Clinical Presentation

Chronic AI

- The classic finding of chronic AI includes a wide pulse pressure, which is associated with numerous physical examination findings related to the arterial pulse (Corrigan pulse, Quincke pulse, de Musset sign, etc.).
- Auscultation reveals a soft, high-pitched, blowing, early diastolic decrescendo murmur best heard at the third left sternal intercostal space (Erb point). To facilitate recognition, the patient should be sitting and leaning forward. Listen at end-expiration.

Acute AI

- Because there is rapid equilibration of aortic diastolic pressure and LV pressure and a narrow pulse pressure, the classic findings of chronic AI are absent. A soft, faint early diastolic murmur may be present. Most patients with acute AI have a sinus tachycardia and the murmur of acute AI may be mistaken for a systolic murmur. Timing of the murmur may be facilitated by palpation of the carotid artery during cardiac auscultation. Early closure of the mitral valve causes a soft S1 and absence of aortic valve closure causes a soft or indistinct S2. Crackles may be heard and the neck veins distended in acute severe AI.

Diagnosis

- Clinical diagnosis in the ED, which can be assisted by POCUS
- Echocardiogram for definitive diagnosis

Treatment

Acute AI requires emergent surgical intervention. Depending on the etiology, this may include aortic root and/or aorta repair. Medical management is limited, but in severe acute aortic regurgitation, intubation, dobutamine may be necessary to increase contractility and stroke volume. β-Blockers are relatively contraindicated because the reflex tachycardia needed to maintain cardiac output could be decreased. Symptomatic patients with chronic AI are now being managed primarily with transcatheter aortic valve replacement performed electively.

SUGGESTED READINGS

Blaufuss Medical Multimedia Laboratories. (2019). Heart sounds tutorial. Available at: http://blaufuss.org/.

Kanwar, A., Thaden, J. J., & Nkomo, V. T. (2018). Management of the patient with aortic stenosis. *Mayo Clinic Proceedings*, 93, 488–508.

Stout, K. K., & Verrier, E. D. (2009). Acute valvular regurgitation. *Circulation*, *119*, 3232–3241.

Zack, J., & Long, B. (2017). Acute valvular emergencies: Pearls and pitfalls. Available at: http://www.emdocs.net/acute-valvular-emergencies-pearls-pitfalls/.

Diseases of the Myocardium

JAMES WILLIAMS, MD, and MANPREET SINGH, MD, MBE

A variety of disease processes affect the heart musculature. Myocyte damage can occur as a result of ischemia, toxins, infection, or genetic mutations. Ischemic heart disease is a leading cause of death in the United States.

Heart Failure

Cardiac failure refers to impaired cardiac function leading to insufficient delivery of oxygen and nutrients to the tissues. Clinically this leads to fluid retention and volume overload.

CONGESTIVE HEART FAILURE

Congestive heart failure (CHF) is a low-output state that results from impaired systolic function (heart failure with reduced ejection fraction) or impaired diastolic function (heart failure with preserved ejection fraction). The net effect is impaired forward flow, impaired tissue perfusion, elevated diastolic filling pressures, pulmonary vascular congestion, and fluid retention. There are a range of causes of low-output heart failure, including ischemic heart disease, valvular heart disease, myocarditis, cardiomyopathies, and hypertension (due to either impaired left ventricle filling or excessive afterload).

Clinical Presentation

- Dyspnea on exertion, orthopnea, paroxysmal nocturnal dyspnea, lower extremity edema.
- Physical examination may show rales, tachypnea, hypoxia, lower extremity edema, S3, or jugular venous distension.
- May have murmur depending on etiology of CHF such as aortic stenosis, mitral stenosis, or mitral regurgitation.

Diagnosis

- Echocardiography to assess systolic and diastolic dysfunction as well as chamber size.
- May need left-sided heart catheterization to evaluate for underlying ischemic heart disease.
- B-type natriuretic peptides, troponin, complete blood count, basic metabolic panel (BMP), urinalysis, and liver function tests can be helpful to evaluate for ischemia, cause of CHF, and to rule out other causes of volume overload states.
- Human immunodeficiency virus (HIV) and thyroid-stimulating hormone (TSH) testing can be considered.

Treatment

- Diuretics (furosemide) to promote diuresis and remove excess volume.
- Supplemental oxygen if hypoxemic or noninvasive ventilation if dyspneic.
- Nitrates can be used in acute heart failure to reduce preload and afterload unless contraindicated, such as in sexually enhancing drug use (phosphodiesterase 5 inhibitors such as sildenafil, which potentiate the effects of nitrates).
- Angiotensin-converting enzyme inhibitor and other antihypertensives reduce afterload and promote forward flow.
- β-Blockers are contraindicated in setting of decompensated CHF but promote diastolic filling and increase cardiac output after acute CHF symptoms resolve.

HIGH-OUTPUT HEART FAILURE

High-output heart failure is a rare entity that results from excessive cardiac output over a prolonged period of time. There are several causes including chronic anemia, wet beriberi (thiamine deficiency), hyperthyroidism, pregnancy, atrioventricular malformations, or arteriovenous fistulas.

RIGHT-SIDED HEART FAILURE

Right-sided heart failure may arise as a consequence of left-sided heart failure or of underlying pulmonary pathology. Causes of right-sided heart failure may include pulmonary hypertension, obstructive sleep apnea, pulmonary embolism, chronic obstructive pulmonary disease, or chronic lung disease. Cor pulmonale refers to remodeling and hypertrophy of the right ventricle due to pulmonary disease.

Clinical Presentation

- Symptoms may include dyspnea on exertion, fatigue, weight gain, peripheral edema.
- May not have signs of left-sided heart failure such as rales or orthopnea.
- May have pedal edema, hepatomegaly, jugular venous distension.

Diagnosis

- Echocardiography may show evidence of elevated right-sided pressures.
- Catheterization of the right side of the heart may be necessary to confirm diagnosis.
- Electrocardiogram (ECG) may show right axis deviation, right atrial enlargement, right ventricular hypertrophy.
- Multifocal atrial tachycardia can be seen in chronic obstructive pulmonary disease and is characterized by P waves of three or more different morphologies.

Treatment

- Treatment is focused on the underlying cause.
- Diuresis (furosemide) to decrease preload; however, patients are highly preload-dependent and may need fluid if hypotensive or critically ill.
- Pulmonary vasodilators for pulmonary hypertension.
- Oxygen as needed.
- Rapid sequence intubation (RSI) may precipitate cardiac arrest due to sudden reduction in preload in these highly sensitive patients.

Cardiomyopathies

Cardiomyopathies are a diverse group of diseases that affect heart muscle and impair cardiac function through their effects on cardiac conduction, diastolic function, and systolic function. Generally cardiomyopathies are divided into restrictive, hypertrophic, and dilated cardiomyopathies.

HYPERTROPHIC CARDIOMYOPATHY

Hypertrophic cardiomyopathy is the result of an autosomal dominant disorder that affects cardiac sarcomere proteins and leads to left ventricular hypertrophy. This may result in asymmetric septal hypertrophy and narrowing of the left ventricular outflow tract (LVOT).

Clinical Presentation

- May present with syncope, presyncope, chest pain particularly in setting of exertion.
- In most dramatic cases, presents with sudden cardiac death.
- May have family history of sudden cardiac death.
- May have systolic murmur on examination, changed with maneuvers that affect LVOT diameter; increases with Valsalva maneuver and standing.

Diagnosis

- Echocardiography with focal septal thickening >15 mm.
- ECG often shows left ventricular hypertrophy or "dagger-like Q waves" in lateral leads.

Treatment

- β-Blockers improve diastolic filling and mediate catecholamine effects on LVOT obstruction.
- Implantable cardioverter defibrillator for patients with exercise-induced syncope, survivors of sudden cardiac death, ventricular arrhythmias, or family history of sudden cardiac death.
- Septal myomectomy or ablation for those who do not respond to medical therapy.

DILATED CARDIOMYOPATHY

Dilated cardiomyopathy is characterized by ventricular dilation with a left ventricular ejection fraction <40%. Causes of dilated cardiomyopathy include ischemic heart disease, viral myocarditis, HIV, alcohol use, cocaine or methamphetamine use, toxins such as the chemotherapy agent doxorubicin, and peripartum cardiomyopathy. Chagas disease due to the protozoon *Trypanosoma cruzi* is a leading cause globally. About 25% of cases are genetically linked. Most cases are ultimately deemed idiopathic.

- Signs and symptoms are identical to CHF symptoms and treatment is the same. Implantable cardiac defibrillators may be needed for those with severely reduced ejection fraction. Dilated cardiomyopathy has a poor prognosis and is a leading indication for heart transplant.

RESTRICTIVE CARDIOMYOPATHY

Restrictive cardiomyopathy results from progressive myocardial infiltration leading to impaired ventricular filling. Causes include sarcoidosis, hemochromatosis, scleroderma, or glycogen storage disease. ECG demonstrates low voltage due to the infiltrative process.

TAKOTSUBO CARDIOMYOPATHY

Known also as stress cardiomyopathy or broken heart syndrome, takotsubo cardiomyopathy is believed to be due to catecholamine release during periods of significant emotional or physiologic stress. Takotsubo cardiomyopathy generally presents in menopausal women and symptoms may include chest pain or shortness of breath. ECG often shows ST-segment elevation on initial presentation. Diagnosis is made by ECG or left ventricular angiogram showing apical ballooning. Most patients have spontaneous recovery and return to their baseline function.

Acute Coronary Syndromes

Acute coronary syndromes refers to a range of presentations resulting in ischemic chest pain due to impaired coronary blood flow and includes unstable angina, non–ST-segment elevation myocardial infarction (NSTEMI), and ST-segment elevation myocardial infarction (STEMI).

UNSTABLE ANGINA

Pathophysiologically, unstable angina represents plaque rupture or vasospasm with reduced myocardial blood flow but no myocardial necrosis. Unstable angina is a harbinger of impending myocardial infarction (MI).

Clinical Presentation

- New onset of angina.
- Angina occurring at rest or with minimal exertion.
- Change in prior pattern of stable angina such as increase in duration, severity, or frequency or symptoms.
- Angina lasting 20 minutes or with cessation of precipitating activity.
- Historical factors that increase likelihood of cardiac chest pain include radiation to the arm, diaphoresis, nausea/vomiting with chest pain, and exertional chest pain.

Diagnosis

- ECG may show T-wave inversions or ST-segment changes.
- Cardiac biomarkers are within normal limits.

Treatment

- Same as for NSTEMI as outlined below.

NSTEMI

- NSTEMI represents myocardial ischemia with concurrent rise in serum biomarkers but no ST-segment elevation on ECG. There are five types of NSTEMI.
  - Type 1: myocardial infarction due to coronary plaque rupture and thrombus formation.

- Type 2: myocardial ischemia due to mismatch in oxygen supply and myocardial demand.
- Type 3: sudden cardiac death.
- Type 4: myocardial infarction associated with coronary instrumentation such as percutaneous coronary intervention (PCI).
- Type 5: myocardial infarction associated with coronary artery bypass grafting.
- Type 1 NSTEMI represents the true acute coronary syndrome. NSTEMI is generally differentiated from unstable angina by the presence of elevated cardiac biomarkers, and the two cannot be differentiated until serial troponins are obtained.

Diagnosis

- Troponin level is elevated, often with typical pattern of rise and fall.
- ECG shows T-wave changes, ST-segment depression but no STEMI.
  - ST depression >0.5 mm in two contiguous leads.
  - T-wave changes concerning for myocardial ischemia are those at least 2 mm deep and in two continuous leads.

Treatment

- Nitroglycerin as needed for chest pain; can also consider opioids if nitroglycerin is contraindicated (i.e., hypotension, inferior MI, or use of phosphodiesterase inhibitors within 24 hours) but opioids may have interactions with P2Y12 platelet inhibitors such as clopidogrel.
- Can start nitroglycerin drip if no response to sublingual nitroglycerin.
- Aspirin 162–325 mg chewed.
- Clopidogrel.
- Heparin or low-molecular-weight heparin.
- Oxygen only if hypoxemic.
- Thrombolytics are never used for NSTEMI.
- Indications for immediate revascularization include refractory ischemic chest pain, ventricular arrhythmias or cardiac arrest, and cardiogenic shock.

WELLENS SYNDROME

Wellens syndrome refers to a pattern of inverted or biphasic T waves in V_2 through V_4 in patients with ischemic chest pain and represents a critical stenosis of the proximal left anterior descending artery (LAD). Appropriate management is with cardiac catheterization because patients are at high risk of massive MI in the near future. Patients with Wellens syndrome should not receive a treadmill stress test because this may precipitate MI.

STEMI

STEMI is the result of complete coronary occlusion due to plaque rupture and thrombus formation with ensuring transmural MI. The diagnosis of STEMI is made based on ECG criteria.

Complications may include ventricular arrhythmias, heart block, ventricular free wall rupture, cardiogenic shock, ventricular septal rupture, acute mitral regurgitation, and right-sided heart failure. Later complications may include heart failure, left ventricular aneurysm formation, and pericarditis.

Diagnosis

- Two continuous leads with ST elevation ≥1 mm in all leads but V_2 and V_3 but ≥2 mm in V_2 or V_3 for men >40 years, ≥1.5 mm for women, and ≥2.5 mm for men <40 years
  - Septal: V_1, V_2
  - Anterior: V_3, V_4
  - Inferior: II, III, aVF
  - Lateral: V_5, V_6, I, aVL
- May show reciprocal changes, which can be remembered with PAILS mnemonic (where ST elevations in one region most commonly cause reciprocal changes in the next region in the mnemonic).
  - Posterior-anterior-inferior-lateral-septal
- Several other "STEMI equivalents"
  - Posterior MI
    - Prominent R wave in V_1/V_2, ST depression, upright T wave
    - Posterior ECG with ≥0.5 mm ST-segment elevation
  - Left main coronary artery occlusion
    - ST elevation in aVR ≥1 mm with lateral ST depression or diffuse ST depression
  - De Winter T waves
    - ST depression and prominent T waves in precordial leads
    - Proximal LAD occlusion
  - Modified Sgarbossa criteria: used to diagnose STEMI in setting of left bundle branch block (LBBB) or paced rhythm
    - Concordant ST elevation ≥1 mm in leads with positive QRS complex
    - Concordant ST depression ≥1 mm in V_1 through V_3
    - Excessively discordant ST elevation ≥5 mm or ≥25% of the depth of the preceding S wave
- Anteroseptal STEMI suggests LAD occlusion.
- Anterolateral suggests left circumflex occlusion or LAD diagonal branch occlusion.
- Inferior STEMI suggests right coronary artery (RCA) occlusion.
  - May also have hypotension due to impaired preload
  - May have bradycardia or heart block due to infarction of sinoatrial/atrioventricular node
- Posterior STEMI suggests left circumflex or right coronary artery occlusion.
- Progression of ischemia: hyperacute T waves→ST-segment elevation→ST-segment normalization and T-wave inversion→pathologic Q-wave formation.

Treatment

- Revascularization is the most important step in management.
  - PCI within 90 minutes if catheterization laboratory immediately available.
  - Fibrinolytics if PCI unavailable within 120 minutes and no contraindication.
- Aspirin 162–325 mg chewed.
- Nitroglycerin for chest pain unless contraindicated (i.e., hypotension, inferior MI with concern of RV infarction, or use of phosphodiesterase inhibitors within 24 hours).
- Clopidogrel; dose depends on whether PCI is anticipated.
- GPIIb/IIIa inhibitors: can be given in catheterization laboratory.
- Oxygen as needed, although hyperoxia can also be harmful.
- Atorvastatin.

- Acute mitral regurgitation requires immediate surgery to repair valve.
- Free wall rupture is treated with surgical repair.
- Intraaortic balloon pump and vasopressors can be used to assist in treatment of cardiogenic shock.

MYOCARDITIS

Myocarditis is infection and necrosis of the myocardium, most often due to viral infections such as coxsackievirus, adenovirus, and influenza. Less common causes of myocarditis include toxoplasma, cytomegalovirus, Lyme disease, and parvovirus B19. Chagas disease is the most common cause globally.

Clinical Presentation

- May present with fever, chest pain, dyspnea, flu-like syndrome, new-onset CHF, or arrhythmias.
- Suspect if tachycardia is out of proportion to fever.
- Consider if septic-appearing individual who gets worse after receiving intravenous fluids.

Diagnosis

- Suspect on basic of clinical syndrome.
- ECG, troponin, echocardiography are informative.
- Endocardial biopsy is gold standard but rarely used.

Treatment

- Supportive care, management of CHF and arrhythmias.
- Antivirals such as interferon alfa or ribavirin may be useful in acute phase.
- Intravenous immunoglobulin may be used in pediatric patients.
- May need left ventricular assist device or cardiac transplant ultimately.

VENTRICULAR ANEURYSM

Ventricular aneurysm formation is the result of focal weakening of the ventricular wall that leads to ballooning of the ventricular wall. Aneurysm may be seen after transmural MI or less commonly because of Chagas disease and is the result of focal fibrosis of the myocardium.

Clinical Presentation

- May present with CHF symptoms, mitral regurgitation.
- Often have history of MI.
- More commonly seen in women than men.

Diagnosis

- Made on echocardiography or left ventricular angiography.
- ECG may show persistent ST elevations after MI.

Treatment

- Management of CHF as above.
- Can be complicated by left ventricular thrombus formation, which can lead to systemic embolization and stroke and requires anticoagulation.
- Indications for surgical repair include ventricular arrhythmias and CHF symptoms refractory to medical management.

SUGGESTED READINGS

Amsterdam, E. A., Wenger, N. K., Brindis, R. G., Casey, D. E., Jr., Ganiats, T. G., Holmes, D. R., Jr., Jaffe, A. S., Jneid, H., Kelly, R. F., Kontos, M. C., Levine, G. N., Liebson, P. R., Mukherjee, D., Peterson, E. D., Sabatine, M. S., Smalling, R. W., & Zieman, S. J. (2014). 2014 AHA/ACC guideline for the management of patients with non-ST-elevation acute coronary syndromes: A report of the American College of Cardiology/American Heart Association Task Force on Practice Guidelines. *Journal of the American College of Cardiology*, 64(24), e139–e228.

Thygesen, K., Alpert, J. S., Jaffe, A. S., Chaitman, B. R., Bax, J. J., Morrow, D. A., White, H. D., and The Executive Group on behalf of the Joint European Society of Cardiology (ESC)/American College of Cardiology (ACC)/American Heart Association (AHA)/World Heart Federation (WHF) Task Force for the Universal Definition of Myocardial Infarction. (2018). Fourth universal definition of myocardial infarction. *Journal of the American College of Cardiology*, 72(18), 22231–22226.

Yancy, C. W., Jessup, M., Bozkurt, B., Butler, B., Case, D. E., Jr., Drazner, M. H., … Wilkoff, B. L. (2013). 2013 ACCF/AHA guideline for the management of heart failure. *Journal of the American College of Cardiology*, 62(16), e147–e239.

CHAPTER **16**

BOARD REVIEW

Pericardial Diseases

MANPREET SINGH, MD, MBE, and JAMES T. NIEMANN, MD

Acute Pericarditis

General Principles

- The pericardium consists of two layers: (1) the visceral pericardium, which is a serous membrane adherent to the epicardium, and (2) the parietal pericardium, which is a fibrous layer that surrounds the heart.
- The space between the two layers is filled with a small amount of serous fluid, usually less than 50 mL, which is usually not seen on bedside ultrasound. Inflammation of the pericardium results in fluid accumulation.
- Pericardial inflammation can result from myriad local or systemic processes. The most common causes of pericarditis are listed in Table 16.1.

Clinical Presentation

- Patients with pericarditis typically present with acute, sharp, pleuritic, retrosternal chest pain.
- Pain may radiate to the trapezius or shoulder due to accompanying diaphragmatic inflammation.
- Pain is worse when the patient is supine and during coughing or inspiration and may be lessened when the patient is sitting and leaning forward.

Diagnosis and Evaluation

- The major finding on physical examination is a pericardial friction rub, which is heard in >80% of cases.
  - A friction rub is best heard with the diaphragm of the stethoscope at the apex at end-expiration with the patient sitting and leaning forward. A pericardial friction rub has been likened to the sound of Velcro.
  - It may be heard only during early systole (single component rub), during early systole and early diastole (two-component rub) or early systole, and early and late diastole (three-component rub).
  - A single component rub may be mistaken for a systolic murmur.
  - The rub may vary in intensity over time and become less audible as fluid accumulates.
- The cardiac silhouette is usually normal on chest x-ray (CXR) unless a large effusion is present. An infiltrate or mass on CXR should suggest an infectious or oncologic etiology for pericarditis.
- The electrocardiogram (ECG) usually shows diffuse ST-segment elevation (most prominent in the lateral precordial leads) and PR segment depression. The ST-T wave amplitude ratio in lead V_6 is >0.25.
  - Arrhythmias other than sinus tachycardia are uncommon.
  - The ECG finding of ST elevation may mimic ST-elevation myocardial infarction (STEMI) or early repolarization.
  - *In STEMI*, ST elevation is limited to those leads reflecting the distribution of a single coronary artery (II, III, aVF; V_1 to V_3, etc.), reciprocal ST depression is usually but not always observed, loss of R wave voltage is present, and the PR segment is isoelectric.
  - *In early repolarization*, ST elevation is usually limited to the precordial leads, there is no PR segment depression, and the ST-T wave ratio is <0.25.
  - The ECG in pericarditis evolves over time with gradual return of the ST segment to baseline, T-wave inversion, and later return to normal.
- Cardiac ultrasound shows an anechoic space anterior to the RV wall and posterior to the LV free wall.
- Laboratory assessment should include complete blood count, blood urea nitrogen/creatinine, C-reactive protein, erythrocyte sedimentation rate, and troponin. Serum troponin may be elevated if there is associated epimyocarditis or myocarditis. Blood cultures should be obtained if a bacterial infection is suspected. Serologic studies (antinuclear antibody, rheumatoid factor, etc.) and acute and convalescent viral titers can be obtained for etiologic diagnoses.
- At least two of the following clinical criteria are required for the diagnosis of acute pericarditis:
  - Typical chest pain
  - Pericardial friction rub
  - Suggestive ECG findings
  - New or worsening pericardial effusion on ultrasonography

TABLE 16.1 *Common Causes of Acute Pericarditis*

Idiopathic
Infectious causes • Viral: coxsackievirus and echovirus; cytomegalovirus, Epstein-Barr virus, HIV • Bacterial: *Streptococcus pneumoniae, Mycobacterium tuberculosis* • Fungal: histoplasmosis
Autoimmune causes • Systemic lupus erythematosus • Rheumatoid arthritis • Familial Mediterranean fever
Neoplastic • Metastatic from lung, breast, lymphoma
Metabolic • Hypothyroidism • Uremia
Drugs • Hydralazine, isoniazid, phenytoin • Antineoplastic drugs (usually with myocarditis)

Treatment

- Nonsteroidal antiinflammatory drugs (NSAIDs) are the mainstay of treatment. Colchicine can be used as an adjunct to NSAIDs. The combination of drugs improves remission rates at 1 week and reduces recurrence rates in acute pericarditis. Duration of therapy is not standardized.
- Resolution of symptoms and resolution of an elevated erythrocyte sedimentation rate or C-reactive protein may serve as guideposts.
- Most patients with acute pericarditis can be managed in the outpatient setting. Patients with a large pericardial effusion on presentation, evidence of tamponade, or elevated troponin on presentation should be admitted for management.
- Troponin elevation suggests associated myocarditis, and admission or observation for worsening cardiac function and arrhythmias is recommended.

TABLE 16.2 *Causes of Pericardial Disease and Cardiac Tamponade*

Likely to progress to cardiac tamponade
• Neoplastic disease • Idiopathic or infectious pericarditis, especially tuberculosis • Iatrogenic hemopericardium • Postcardiotomy syndrome • Hemopericardium in aortic dissection • Renal failure
Less likely (rarely) progressing to cardiac tamponade
• Autoimmune disease • Hypothyroidism • Postinfarction (Dressler syndrome)

(Adapted from Ristic, A.D., Imazio, M., Adler, Y., Anastasakis, A., Badano, L. P., Brucato, A., Caforio, A. L. P., Dubourg, O., Elliott, P., Gimeno, J., Helio, T., Klingel, K., Linhart, A., Maisch, B., Mayosi, B., Mogensen, J., Pinto, Y., Seggewiss, H., Seferović, P. M., ... Charron, P. (2014). Triage strategy for urgent management of cardiac tamponade: A position statement for the European Society of Cardiology Working Group on Myocardial and Pericardial Diseases. *European Heart Journal, 35*(34), 2279–2284.)

Cardiac Tamponade

General Principles

- In most cases fluid accumulation occurring with pericardial inflammation does not have significant hemodynamic consequences. Intrapericardial pressure remains at or near intrapleural pressure and less than right-sided heart pressures. However, intrapericardial pressure may exceed right-sided heart pressures if there is a rapid accumulation of a large volume of fluid or if the parietal pericardium is noncompliant or nondistensible.
- The pericardial pressure-volume curve may be J-shaped with rapid fluid accumulation or flat with a late upward deflection with slower accumulation.
  - When intrapericardial pressure equals or exceeds right-sided heart pressures, venous return decreases, right-sided heart filling is impaired, and physiologic "tamponade" exists. The point at which this occurs depends on intrapericardial fluid volume, the elasticity of the parietal pericardium, and filling pressure of the right side of the heart, which depends on intravascular volume.
- Although there are many causes for pericarditis, only a limited number make up most of tamponade (Table 16.2). Incidence varies with the study population and practice setting. In developed countries, the most common cause for nontraumatic tamponade is metastatic malignancy.

Clinical Presentation

- The most common symptom is dyspnea with a sensitivity of approximately 85%. Hypotension is not common if pericardial fluid accumulation has occurred over days to weeks.
- The most common findings on physical examination include tachycardia and elevated jugular venous pressure, each with a sensitivity of approximately 75%. Diminished heart sounds on auscultation has the lowest sensitivity, about 25%. Pulsus paradoxus >10 mm Hg has a sensitivity of about 98% and specificity of 70%.
  - Pulsus paradoxus is an exaggeration of the normal physiologic decrease in systole pressure with inspiration. It is believed to be due to ventricular interdependence and respiratory variation in right- and left-sided heart filling. Pulsus paradoxus is measured with a manual sphygmomanometer with the patient supine. It is the difference between intermittent and persistence of the first Korotkoff sound during normal breathing. Detection may not be possible in the setting of a tachycardia. Although physical findings have respectable sensitivities, specificity is poor and dependent upon the study population. If found in a patient with large cardiac silhouette on CXR or large effusion on ultrasonography, diagnostic importance of these physical findings is increased.
- CXR may show an enlarged cardiac silhouette.
- The ECG typically demonstrates sinus tachycardia and may show low-voltage QRS complexes (≤5 mm amplitude in the limb leads and ≤10 mm in the precordial leads), and electrical alternans (beat-to-beat variation in QRS amplitude).

Diagnosis and Evaluation

- Focused ultrasonography plays an important role in diagnosis. Tamponade is usually suggested by the presence of pericardial fluid and ultrasonographic evidence of right atrial and/or right ventricular diastolic collapse. However, more than a third of patients with a pericardial effusion without clinical features of tamponade have collapse of at least one chamber on echocardiography. Clinical as well as ultrasonography data should be considered in making the diagnosis of tamponade (Table 16.3).

Treatment

- If the patient is hypotensive (systolic blood pressure <100 mm Hg), volume loading with 500 mL of normal saline may improve cardiac index and blood pressure. Emergency or urgent pericardiocentesis is usually required to restore normal cardiac filling and hemodynamic stability. Pericardiocentesis is optimally performed in the cardiac catheterization laboratory. If undertaken in the emergency department, it should be performed under ultrasound guidance (see Chapter 149, Cardiovascular Procedures).

TABLE 16.3 *Clinical Considerations in Evaluation for Possible Subacute Pericardial Tamponade*

- Is the patient symptomatic?
- Are there physical findings for pericardial tamponade?
- What is the most likely cause of the pericardial effusion?
- What is the size of the pericardial effusion?
- Is there chamber collapse on ultrasonography examination?
- Are there other supporting signs for tamponade on ultrasonography (respiratory variations in velocities and flows, superior vena cava flow pattern, inferior vena cava size)?

(Adapted from Argulian. E., & Messerli, F. (2013). Misconceptions and facts about pericardial effusion and tamponade. *American Journal of Medicine, 126,* 858–861.)

Constrictive Pericarditis

General Principles

- Constrictive pericarditis is characterized by fibrotic, thickened, scarred, and frequently calcified pericardium that is inelastic, restricting ventricular diastolic filling. The diseased pericardium prevents the normal inspiratory decrease in thoracic pressure from being transmitted to the cardiac chambers. As a result, venous pressure does not decrease and systemic venous return does not increase during inspiration. In most instances (>50%), a specific etiology is not defined during evaluation and the cause is considered "idiopathic."
- Pericardial scarring may be a long-term sequela of acute or chronic pericarditis (usually viral or bacterial). Tuberculosis is a common cause in underdeveloped countries. Constrictive pericarditis has been reported post pericardiotomy and after mediastinal radiation therapy.

Clinical Presentation

- Patients usually present with signs and symptoms mimicking subacute or chronic right-sided heart failure: dyspnea, pedal edema, right upper quadrant pain from hepatic congestion, and abdominal distention from ascites.
- Physical findings include jugular venous distention, hepatosplenomegaly, ascites, and lower extremity edema. These latter findings may suggest primary liver disease. Kussmaul sign (i.e., a paradoxical increase in jugular venous pressure during inspiration) may be observed. On auscultation, a "pericardial knock" may be heard at the apex during early diastole and reflects ventricular noncompliance with filling.

Diagnosis and Evaluation

- The ECG is nondiagnostic. CXR may show pericardial calcifications with a normal cardiac silhouette. B-type natriuretic peptide level is within normal range.
- Constrictive pericarditis should be suspected in the patient with a history of pericarditis who presents with signs or symptoms of right-sided heart failure, the patient with unexplained right-sided heart failure and a normal B-type natriuretic peptide level, or the patient who presents with findings suggesting hepatic disease without an apparent etiology.
- Cardiac ultrasonography demonstrates normal cardiac chamber size and normal wall motion (if no prior myocardial injury).
  - Abnormal septal motion may be observed and is due to ventricular interdependence during the respiratory cycle.
  - A thickened pericardium may be observed but the absence of thickening on ultrasound examination does not exclude the diagnosis.
- Cardiac computed tomography or magnetic resonance imaging are the imaging modalities of choice.
- Cardiac catheterization is usually performed to confirm the diagnosis.

Treatment

- Pericardiectomy is the treatment of choice for patients who have late (chronic) constrictive pericarditis with symptoms.
- Acutely, treatment as in pericarditis with NSAIDs and colchicine is reasonable to attempt to prevent the need for surgical intervention.

SUGGESTED READINGS

Imazio, M., Gaita, F., & LeWinter, M. (2015). Evaluation and treatment of pericarditis. A systematic review. *Journal of the American Medical Association, 314,* 1498–1506.

Miranda, W. R., & Oh, J. K. (2017). Constrictive pericarditis: A practical clinical approach. *Progress in Cardiovascular Diseases, 59,* 369–379.

Roy, C. L., Minor, M. A., Brookhart, M. A., & Choudhry, N. K. (2007). Does this patient with a pericardial effusion have cardiac tamponade? *Journal of the American Medical Association, 297,* 1810–1818.

16

CHAPTER 17

BOARD REVIEW

Disorders of Circulation

JOHN CAMPO, MD, and SHIRA A. SCHLESINGER, MD, MScPH

Circulatory disorders encompass a broad group of conditions that affect large, medium, and small sized blood vessels. This chapter discusses aortic aneurysm and dissection, and thromboembolic events of arterial and venous structures.

Abdominal Aortic Aneurysm (AAA)

General Principles

- An aneurysm is a localized dilation of an artery resulting in an increased diameter of the artery at least 50% greater than normal. Aneurysms can occur in any artery and are classified by location (i.e., cerebral, aorta, femoral, popliteal). AAA are the most common clinically significant variety requiring emergency care, and are the focus of this section.
- A *true aneurysm* involves all three layers of the vessel (Fig. 17.1).
- A *false* or *pseudoaneurysm* involves a defect of the intima and media of the arterial wall, with leakage contained by the adventitia.

Clinical Presentation

- Most AAA are asymptomatic and are detected incidentally on imaging.
- Symptomatic patients may complain of abdominal, back, or flank pain; sensation of abdominal fullness or abdominal pulsation.
- Physical examination may reveal a pulsatile abdominal mass.
- Emergency department presentation may include emergent symptoms from AAA complications or rupture. Potential complications include limb ischemia from associated thromboembolism, brisk gastrointestinal bleeding from erosion into the intestine (aortoenteric fistula), high-output heart failure from erosion/rupture into the vena cava (aortocaval fistula), chronic intestinal complaints from compression of adjacent intestinal (most frequently duodenal), or vascular structures resulting in early satiety, weight loss, or chronic progressive abdominal pain.
- The triad of severe abdominal pain, hypotension, and palpation of a pulsatile abdominal mass classically describes a ruptured AAA. However, many patients will have only one or two elements of this triad.

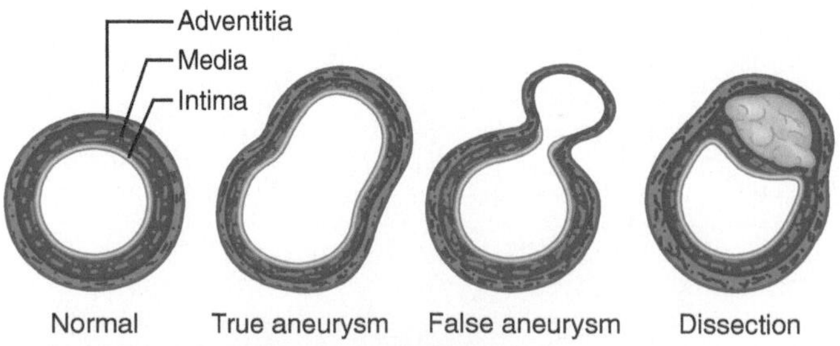

FIG. 17.1 Types of aortic aneurysms. (Adapted from LaRoy, L. L., Cormier, P. J., Matalon, T. A., Patel, S. K., Turner, D. A., & Silver, B. (1989). Imaging of abdominal aortic aneurysms. *American Journal of Roentgenology, 152*(4), 785–792.)

Diagnosis and Evaluation

- Bedside abdominal ultrasound is the initial test for determining presence of AAA.
  - The abdominal aorta is aneurysmal if measured more than 3 cm between the outer walls.
  - Bedside ultrasound is inexpensive and noninvasive, with high sensitivity (98%) and specificity (99%) for detecting AAA when performed properly (Fig. 17.2). It cannot, however, reliably identify ruptures as most occur retroperitoneally.
  - Point-of-care ultrasound (POCUS) is of significant benefit in hemodynamically unstable patients, where it can be performed without delaying other resuscitative interventions.
- Computed tomography (CT) with angiography is the test of choice for defining the location and extent of the aneurysm, determining the presence of rupture, aortoenteric or aortocaval fistula, and for operative planning.
  - Many asymptomatic AAAs are detected on CTs ordered for other indications—most commonly in the

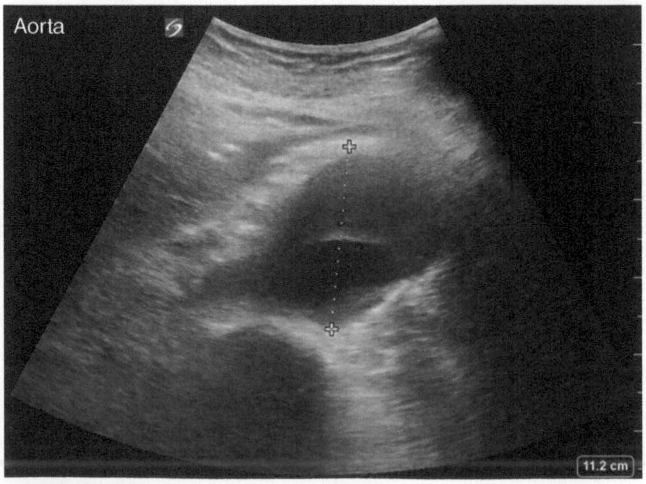

FIG. 17.2 Ultrasound showing abdominal aortic aneurysm (AAA). (Courtesy Lilly A. Bellman, MD.)

setting of nonspecific abdominal or flank pain with suspected diagnoses of renal colic or diverticulitis.
  - Although angiography is helpful for fine detail and operative planning, detection with nonangiographic studies do *not* necessitate repeat CT in all cases. It is advisable to discuss with the radiologist and/or vascular surgeon risks and benefits of repeating the CT in individual cases.
- Whereas cross-table lateral radiographs were previously advised for screening and diagnosis in asymptomatic and unstable patients, this is no longer recommended given that the sensitivity is less than 70% for detection of AAA.

Treatment

- Emergency management of symptomatic or ruptured AAA is directed at treating shock, expediting surgical management, and optimizing the patient for surgery.

Treating Shock

- A minimum of two large-bore IVs should be started, with strong consideration to placement of a large-bore central venous catheter (such as an introducer sheath catheter).
- Order cross-matching of 6 to 10 units of packed red blood cells, along with platelets and fresh frozen plasma per your hospital's massive transfusion protocol. Ensure that unmatched type O blood is readily available until cross-matched blood is prepared.
- A strategy of permissive hypotension targeting a systolic blood pressure of 70 to 90 mm Hg should be pursued, as tolerated, to minimize clot dislodgement and decrease degree of hemorrhage.
- Plasma or packed red blood cells may be used as the resuscitative fluid.

Expediting Surgical Management

- In hemodynamically unstable patients more than 50 years of age in the United States with AAA on bedside, vascular surgery consult should be initiated immediately. Do not delay for advanced imaging.
- Immediate or emergent repair is indicated for ruptured aneurysms and for abdominal/back pain likely attributable to an aneurysm.
- Elective repair should be considered in male patients with asymptomatic fusiform aneurysms 5.5 cm or greater and in women with aneurysms more than 5.0 cm, and for saccular aneurysms of any size. One study found a 3-year risk of rupture approaching 75% for aneurysm more than 5.5 cm, compared with 15% of aneurysms 3 to 5.5 cm.
- Conservative management with risk factor reduction (control of hypertension and other atherosclerotic risk factors, smoking cessation) and surveillance should be initiated in asymptomatic patients with aneurysms less than 5 cm. These patients should be referred for outpatient vascular surgery evaluation and initiation of surveillance. Recommended surveillance intervals differ based on size of the aneurysm at first detection.

Aortic Dissection

General Principles

- Aortic dissection occurs when the layers of the aortic walls are separated owing to a tear in the intima.
- Blood flowing under high pressures separates the intima from the media, creating a false lumen with proximal or distal propagation of the dissection.
- Dissections are characterized based on the portion of aorta involved. Two classification systems have been developed to describe the area affected (Fig. 17.3).
- In the emergency department, the Stanford classification is most useful.

Clinical Presentation

- Acute onset, severe, tearing, or sharp chest or back pain.
- Progression of dissection disrupts organ perfusion by arterial occlusion of vessels at their origin from the aorta or distal to it. End-organ ischemia may produce additional signs/symptoms (i.e., myocardial ischemia, stroke, paraplegia, acute kidney injury, limb and/or mesenteric ischemia).
- Bimodal age distribution:
  - Young *with* risk factors
    - Connective tissue disease (e.g., Marfan syndrome, Ehlers-Danlos, collagen vascular disease)
  - Pregnancy, especially third trimester
  - Recent cardiac catheterization
  - Bicuspid aortic valve
  - Aortic coarctation

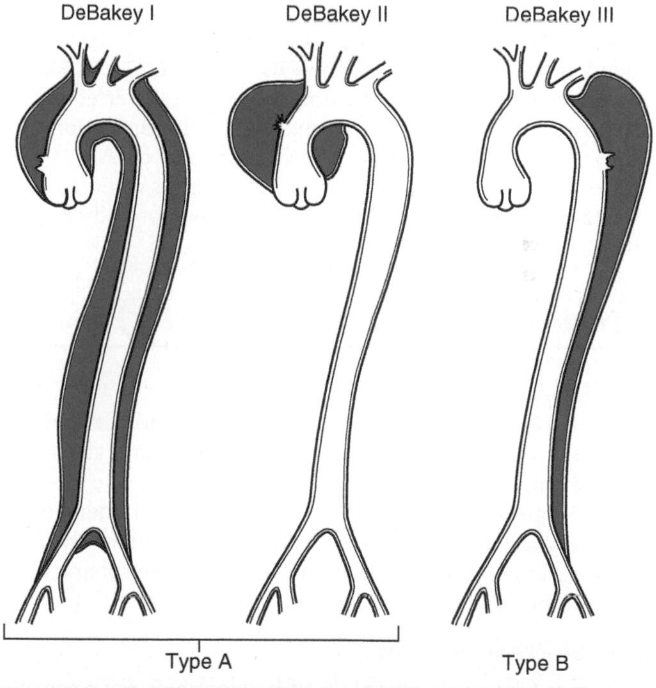

FIG. 17.3 Classification schemes of acute aortic dissection. DeBakey classification: Type I dissection originates in the ascending aorta and extends at least to the aortic arch and often to the descending aorta (and beyond). Type II dissection originates in the ascending aorta and is confined to this segment. Type III dissection originates in the descending aorta, usually just distal to the left subclavian artery, and extends distally. Stanford classification: Type A dissection involves the ascending aorta (with or without extension into the descending aorta). Type B dissection does not involve the ascending aorta. (From Mitchell, R. N., & Halushka, M. K. (2021). Blood vessels. In V. Kumar, A. K. Abbas, & J. C. Aster (Eds.), *Robbins & Cotran pathologic basis of disease* (10th ed., pp. 485–526, Fig. 11.23). Elsevier.)

17

- Elderly males with chronic hypertension
- Atherosclerotic risk factors (smoking, hypertension, hyperlipidemia, diabetes mellitus)

Diagnosis and Evaluation

- Although the D-dimer is in the Aortic Dissection Detection Risk Score, this novel clinical strategy still requires validation before being implemented into clinical practice.
- Chest radiographs can be normal, but may demonstrate widened mediastinum, irregular aortic contour, inward displacement more than 1 cm of calcification of the aortic knob ("calcium sign"), or apical capping.
- CT with angiography is the test of choice in patients with signs/symptoms concerning for acute aortic dissection, and is important for operative planning.
- In hemodynamically unstable patients, transthoracic echocardiography or transesophageal echocardiography may be useful.

Treatment

- Initial treatment is heart rate reduction to fewer than 60 beats/minute via intravenous beta-blockers, such as an esmolol drip, in order to decrease shear forces generated by myocardial contraction and minimize progression.
- If systolic blood pressure remains above 120 mm Hg after goal heart rate is achieved with beta-blockers, nitroprusside or nicardipine should be added to decrease systolic blood pressure to 120 mm Hg or lower within the first hour. These agents should not be initiated until heart rate is controlled, as their use may produce reflex tachycardia, thereby increasing shear forces exerted on the intimal layer and further extending the dissection.
- Emergent operative repair is indicated for type A dissections. For type B dissections, surgery is reserved for those that have persistent pain or signs of end-organ damage.

Arterial Dissection (Nonaortic)

General Principles

- Dissection may also occur in the cerebral and cervical (carotid and vertebral) arteries, with potentially devastating consequences.
- Neurologic sequalae occur secondary to thromboembolism formation and resultant ischemia. Alternatively, rupture in the cerebral vasculature may cause subarachnoid hemorrhage.

Clinical Presentation

- Patients frequently complain of headache or neck pain.
- Horner syndrome (ptosis, miosis, anhidrosis) may be seen with dissection of the internal carotid artery.
- Patients may present with signs and symptoms of acute anterior or posterior stroke, coinciding with the affected vessel.

Diagnosis and Evaluation

- The primary neuroimaging modalities for diagnosis of cerebral and cervical arterial dissections are CT or magnetic resonance imaging with angiography.

Treatment

- Signs of ischemic stroke should be treated with thrombolytics similar to other causes of ischemic infarct, that is, if presentation is within 3 hours of symptom onset. Beyond this timeframe, anticoagulation or antiplatelet therapy may be started, without thrombolysis.
- Patients with recurrent ischemia may benefit from endovascular repair.

Arterial Thromboembolism (Table 17.1)

General Principles

- Acute occlusion of an artery produces a sudden decrease in perfusion resulting in end-organ ischemia.
- The most common cause of acute occlusion is rupture of an atherosclerotic plaque with associated thrombosis.
- Embolic phenomena may result from other underlying conditions, including ventricular aneurysm, atrial fibrillation, or coagulopathy.

Clinical Presentation (Table 17.2)

- Clinical presentation depends on the organ system supplied by the affected artery.
- Certain systems are more susceptible.
- In this section, we focus on acute limb ischemia and mesenteric ischemia as the most frequently debilitating conditions.

TABLE 17.1 *Etiologies of Acute Arterial Occlusion*

Embolic Sources	Thrombotic Sources
Atrial fibrillation	Atherosclerotic plaque rupture
Endocarditis	Thrombosis of vascular aneurysm
Valvular disease	Arterial dissection
Prosthetic valves	Thrombophilia
Atrial myxoma	
Arterial aneurysm	
Vascular damage following trauma or intervention (e.g., angioplasty, bypass graft)	

TABLE 17.2 *Clinical Manifestations of Arterial Thromboembolism*

Organ System	Clinical Presentation
Brain	Focal neurologic deficits, with symptoms dependent on location of arterial occlusion (see stroke syndromes in Chapters 85)
Eyes	Sudden unilateral visual loss, either complete or partial (see Chapter 43)
Heart	Acute myocardial infarction
Intestine	Severe abdominal pain out of proportion to tenderness evident on examination (mesenteric ischemia)
Limb	Pain, decreased and/or absent pulse, acute motor or sensory deficits, abnormal temperature, and paralysis in the affected limb

- Coronary artery thrombosis is covered in Chapter 15, whereas thromboembolic phenomenon of the cerebral vasculature is covered in Chapter 84 Ischemic Strokes and Transient Ischemic Attacks (TIAs).

Diagnosis and Evaluation

- Laboratory derangements may include leukocytosis, elevated D-dimer, and metabolic acidosis secondary to lactate elevation.
- CT angiography and catheter-based arteriography are two suitable modalities for definitive diagnosis of acute limb ischemia. Of the two, CT angiography is more accessible and appropriate to emergency department use.
- CT angiography of the abdomen and pelvis is the test of choice for diagnosing acute mesenteric ischemia.

Treatment

- Initial management for both acute limb ischemia and acute mesenteric ischemia requires systemic anticoagulation with unfractionated heparin.
- Antibiotics should be started in cases of mesenteric ischemia owing to the risk of infection from bacterial translocation and microperforation.
- For patients with acute limb ischemia with minimal pain and no muscle weakness or sensory loss, either thrombolysis or urgent surgical revascularization may be acceptable for treatment. If the patient endorses pain at rest, muscle weakness or sensory loss in the setting of suspected acute thromboembolism, emergent surgical revascularization should be performed.
- Management options for acute mesenteric ischemia of embolic etiology include open surgical embolectomy, percutaneous clot aspiration, and catheter-directed thrombolysis.
- Treatment for mesenteric thrombosis involves mesenteric bypass or angioplasty with stenting. Overall outcomes for mesenteric ischemia are poor regardless of etiology, with mortality rates exceeding 60%.

Venous Thromboembolism

General Principles

- Pulmonary embolism and deep venous thrombosis (DVT) are subtypes of the phenomenon of venous thromboembolism.
- Venous stasis, hypercoagulability, and endothelial injury are the fundamental mechanisms driving venous thromboembolism formation. This chapter focuses on DVT.
- For information specific to pulmonary embolism, refer to Chapter 115 pulmonary embolism.

Clinical Presentation

- Unilateral limb pain and swelling is caused by obstructed venous return.
- Clinical signs include edema, warmth, erythema, and tenderness of the affected extremity.

Diagnosis and Evaluation

- The recommended diagnostic approach starts with determination of pretest probability based on clinician gestalt and clinical decision tools (i.e., Wells Score for DVT).
- Diagnostic algorithms guide further evaluation based on this pretest probability using ultrasound and D-dimer (Fig. 17.4).

Treatment

- Approximately 10% of untreated DVTs progress to pulmonary embolism.
- Anticoagulation should be initiated immediately in the absence of contraindications.
- Contraindications to anticoagulation include active bleeding, severe bleeding diathesis, recent high bleeding risk surgery, major trauma, or recent intracranial hemorrhage.
- In the setting of contraindications to anticoagulation, an inferior vena cava filter may prevent propagation of thrombosis and onset of pulmonary embolism in patients with lower extremity DVTs.

Special Population

- Patients with massive iliofemoral DVTs (phlegmasia cerulea or alba dolens) should be treated immediately, because it is a potentially life-threatening complication that can result in arterial ischemia. These patients typically present with localized cyanosis of the affected limb in addition to obvious unilateral, lower extremity swelling and pain. Early initiation of unfractionated heparin and consideration of thrombolysis and/or thrombectomy is necessary to prevent progression to gangrene.

17

SUGGESTED READINGS

Diercks, D. B., Promes, S. B., Schuur, J. D., Shah, K., Valente, J. H., Cantrill, S. V., American College of Emergency Physicians Clinical Policies Subcommittee on Thoracic Aortic Dissection. (2015). Clinical policy: Critical issues in the evaluation and management of adult patients with suspected acute nontraumatic thoracic aortic dissection. *Annals of Emergency Medicine*, *65*, 32–42.

Wolf, S. J., Hahn, S. A., Nentwich, L. M., Raja, A. S., Silvers, S. M., Brown, M. D., American College of Emergency Physicians Clinical Policies Subcommittee on Thromboembolic Disease. (2018). Clinical policy: Critical issues in the evaluation and management of adult patients presenting to the emergency department with suspected acute venous thromboembolic disease. *Annals of Emergency Medicine*, *71*, e59–e109.

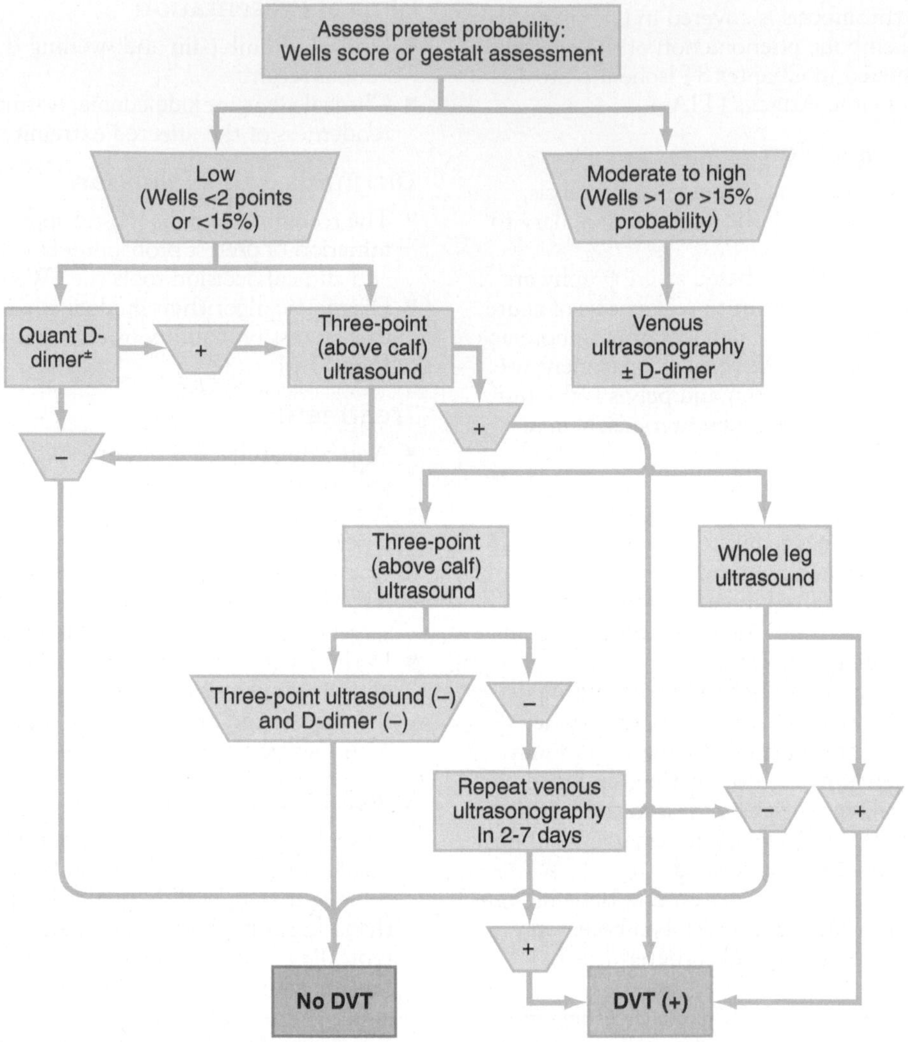

FIG. 17.4 Diagnostic algorithm to guide the diagnosis and exclusion of acute deep vein thrombosis. *DVT,* deep vein thrombosis; Quant, quantitative; −, test negative; +, test positive. (From Kline, J. A. (2018). Pulmonary embolism and deep vein thrombosis. In R. M. Walls, R. S. Hockberger, & M. Gausche-Hill (Eds.), *Rosen's emergency medicine: Concepts and clinical practice* (9th ed., pp. 1027–1035, Fig. 78.4). Elsevier.)

Endocarditis

CHINWE ONU, MD, and KIAN PRESTON-SUNI, MD, MPH

Infective endocarditis (IE) is a challenging condition due to its vague symptoms, varied presentations, and relative infrequency. As the population ages, IE is increasingly associated with indwelling devices and prosthetic valves. Despite advances in management over the last several decades, mortality remains high, at nearly 20%. A high index of suspicion should be maintained for patients with risk factors who present with infectious symptoms.

General Principles

- IE was classically categorized by duration of onset, being either subacute or acute. It is now better recognized as involving either a native or prosthetic valve, and this distinction guides therapy. Whereas skin flora, including coagulase-negative *Staphylococcus*, is associated mainly with early postoperative prosthetic valve infections, the predominant cause of both native and prosthetic valve IE is *S. aureus* (Table 18.1).
- Risk factors for IE are related to structural abnormalities and likelihood of experiencing bacteremia (Table 18.2).

Pediatric Considerations

- IE is rare in children; nearly all cases occur in children with risk factors. These are predominantly congenital heart disease, indwelling central venous catheter, and rheumatic heart disease. Risk for IE is highest in cyanotic heart disease, especially in lesions receiving surgical intervention.

TABLE 18.1 Epidemiology of Infective Endocarditis

Microorganism	%
Staphylococcus aureus	32
Viridans group streptococci	18
Enterococci	11
Coagulase-negative staphylococci	11
Streptococcus bovis	7
Other streptococci	5
Non-HACEK, gram-negative bacteria	2
Fungi	2
HACEK	2
Other organisms	3
Polymicrobial	1
Culture negative	8

HACEK, *Haemophilus*, *Aggregatibacter* (previously *Actinobacillus*), *Cardiobacterium*, *Eikenella*, *Kingella*.
(From Kosowsky, J. M., & Takhar, S. S. (2018). Infective endocarditis, rheumatic fever, and valvular heart disease. In R. M. Walls, R. S. Hockberger, & M. Gausche-Hill (Eds.), *Rosen's emergency medicine: Concepts and clinical practice* (9th ed., pp. 1000–1002). Elsevier.)

TABLE 18.2 Risk Factors for Endocarditis

Cardiac	Noncardiac
Prosthetic valve	Indwelling central venous catheter
Degenerative valve lesions (i.e., aortic stenosis)	Intravenous drug use
Implanted cardiac device	Recent dental or surgical procedure
Unrepaired congenital heart defect	Hemodialysis
Rheumatic heart disease	Immune suppression
Previous endocarditis	Poor dentition

Risk factors are related to abnormal physical structure and transient bacteremia.

Pathophysiology

- Normal, healthy heart valves resist bacterial adhesion and infection. Endocarditis starts with damage to the endothelium.
- Endothelial injury due to turbulent blood flow from congenital or acquired valve lesion, direct mechanical injury from medical instrumentation, or debris from impurities in illicit intravenous drugs.
- Platelet and fibrin disposition; injured endothelium initiates thrombus formation.
- Vegetation formation; bacteremia leads to secondary infection of thrombus.
- Vegetation progression leads to worsening valvular function and endocardial damage, impairing cardiac function.
- The mitral valve (41%) and aortic valve (38%) are most commonly affected; however, right-sided endocarditis typically associated with intravenous drug use and indwelling central venous lines usually involves the tricuspid valve.

Clinical Presentation

- Signs and symptoms are often vague and related to infection, ranging from malaise, fatigue, and fever to frank sepsis (Table 18.3).
- Impaired valve function may cause findings related to heart failure and valvular insufficiency.
- Embolic phenomenon can cause a range of complications, although the classically taught findings are all relatively uncommon.

TABLE 18.3 Signs and Symptoms of Infective Endocarditis

Symptoms	Signs
Fever	Fever (80%–90%)
Dyspnea	New or worsening of old murmur (70%)
Fatigue	Stroke, both ischemic and hemorrhagic (20%)
Weight loss	Metastatic infection: meningitis, pulmonary abscess, osteomyelitis, etc.
Back pain	Splenomegaly (11%)
	Hematuria (25%)
	Splinter hemorrhage (8%)
	Osler nodes (3%)
	Janeway lesions (5%)
	Roth spots (2%)
	Petechiae
	Acute limb ischemia

Diagnosis and Evaluation

- The presenting signs and symptoms of IE vary, and the diagnosis is often challenging.
- Routine laboratory and imaging findings are generally nonspecific. Echocardiography is helpful when positive.
- Blood cultures are the mainstay of diagnosis but are not helpful in the emergency department (ED).
- No study in the ED can exclude the diagnosis of endocarditis.

Laboratory Tests

- Blood cultures: essential for inpatient diagnosis and narrowing antimicrobial therapy after admission. Obtain at least three sets of blood cultures before administration of antibiotics, from different sites, ideally spaced 30–60 minutes apart if time allows.
- Complete blood count often shows anemia, may show thrombocytopenia.
- Chemistry often shows findings of renal insufficiency.
- Erythrocyte sedimentation rate and C-reactive protein tests are generally not useful.
- Urinalysis may show proteinuria, hematuria, red blood cell casts.

Ultrasonography

- Any patient with risk factors for endocarditis and consistent signs and symptoms should receive a transthoracic echocardiogram (TTE) to evaluate for findings of IE (Box 18.1) or alternative diagnosis.
- TTE has a modest sensitivity of 40%–90% and specificity greater than 90%, although sensitivity is lower for prosthetic valve infections.
- Transesophageal echocardiogram (TEE) can be difficult to obtain in the ED but has superior sensitivity (90%–100%) and specificity (90%–100%). TEE is also better able to visualize prosthetic valve infections and intracardiac complications, including paravalvular abscess and valvular leaflet perforation (Fig.18.1).

Electrocardiogram

- Electrocardiograms are often low-yield, but they can identify new conduction abnormalities, including heart block and new arrhythmia.
- Heart block is often noted after admission, can be progressive, and is associated with paravalvular abscess.

Radiography

- Chest x-rays are most useful in identifying alternative diagnoses. They can also show related conditions including pulmonary septic emboli and pulmonary edema, although findings are usually nonspecific.
- Noncontrast computed tomography or magnetic resonance imaging of the head may be useful, given that one-third of patients with IE suffer embolic events resulting in neurologic complications.

BOX 18.1 Duke Criteria (Clinical) for Diagnosis of Infective Endocarditis

Definite Endocarditis

Endocarditis is considered definitely present if any one of the following combinations of clinical findings is present:

- Two major clinical criteria
- One major and any three minor clinical criteria
- Five minor clinical criteria

Possible Endocarditis

Possible endocarditis is defined as the presence of any one of the following combinations of findings

- One major and one or two minor clinical criteria
- Three minor clinical criteria

Rejected Endocarditis

The diagnosis of endocarditis is considered rejected if any of the following occurs:

- A firm alternate diagnosis is made
- Resolution of clinical manifestations occurs after 4 days or less of antibiotic therapy
- Clinical criteria for possible or definite endocarditis not met

Major Criteria

Positive blood cultures (of typical pathogens) from at least two separate cultures

Evidence of endocardial involvement by echocardiography, such as the following:

- Endocardial vegetation
- Paravalvular abscess
- New partial dehiscence of prosthetic valve
- New valvular regurgitation

Minor Criteria

Predisposing heart condition or intravenous drug use

Fever: temperature ≥ 38°C (100.4°F)

Vascular phenomena: arterial emboli, septic pulmonary infarcts, mycotic aneurysm, conjunctival hemorrhages, Janeway lesions

Immunologic phenomena: Osler nodes, Roth spots, rheumatoid factor

Microbiologic evidence: single positive blood culture (except for coagulase-negative *Staphylococcus* or an organism that does not cause endocarditis)

Echocardiographic findings: consistent with endocarditis but do not meet above major clinical criteria

(From Kosowsky, J. M., & Takhar, S. S. (2018). Infective endocarditis, rheumatic fever, and valvular heart disease. In R. M. Walls, R. S. Hockberger, & M. Gausche-Hill (Eds.), *Rosen's emergency medicine: Concepts and clinical practice* (9th ed., pp. 1000–1002). Elsevier.)

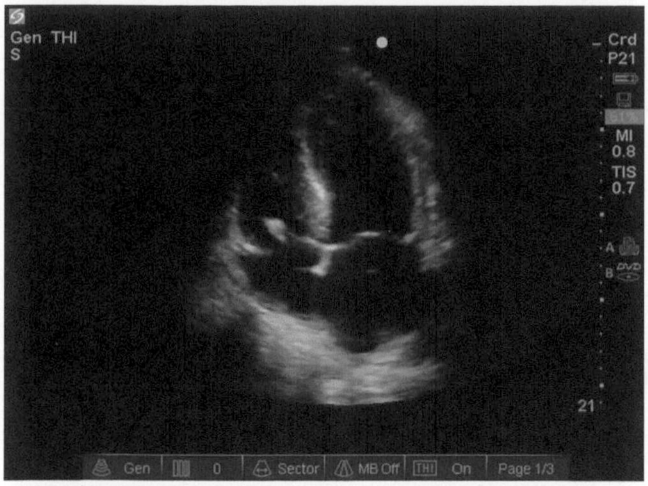

FIG. 18.1. Tricuspid vegetation seen on bedside transthoracic echocardiogram. (From Scott, C. (2016). Man with acute respiratory distress. *Annals of Emergency Medicine, 67,* 300.)

- Over three-quarters of patients with IE have cerebral abnormalities on magnetic resonance imaging, although many of these are of unclear clinical significance.

Diagnostic Criteria

- The Duke criteria are widely used for diagnosis of IE and incorporate the physical examination, microbiology, and imaging studies (see Box 18.1).
- Sensitivity of the criteria for IE is around 80% with 99% specificity, although sensitivity is lower for prosthetic valve and cardiac device infection.

Pediatric Considerations

- The Duke criteria have been validated in children with IE, with sensitivity similar to that seen in adult populations.

Treatment

Antibiotic Therapy

- Broad-spectrum empiric antibiotics should be started after obtaining cultures according to the local antibiogram and hospital recommendations.
- Empiric coverage of methicillin-resistant *S. aureus* should be included, for example, with vancomycin.
- Bactericidal antibiotics have shown benefit in penetrating vegetations; examples include the β-lactams (i.e., oxacillin) and gentamicin.
- Rifampin is beneficial in IE affecting prosthetic valves.

Consults

- Infectious disease consultation is useful for assistance with microbial therapy regimen selection. Cardiothoracic surgery should be consulted for patients presenting with acute valvular insufficiency causing heart failure. Surgery has been shown to reduce mortality for left-sided infections with severe valvular disease when performed <48 hours after presentation, although generalizability of these findings has been questioned.
- Recommendations for surgical intervention include large vegetations (>10 mm in diameter), new-onset heart failure, paravalvular abscess, septic emboli, and difficult-to-treat organisms.
- Additional echocardiographic findings associated with need for surgery include pseudoaneurysm, valve dehiscence, and valve perforation.

Anticoagulation

- There are no recommendations for routine anticoagulation in native valve endocarditis.
- Patients with prosthetic valves who are receiving anticoagulant therapy and who have cerebral emboli should have anticoagulation suspended, because anticoagulant therapy increases the risk of hemorrhagic conversion.
- Continuation of anticoagulant therapy in prosthetic valve infections without contraindications is controversial.

SUGGESTED READINGS

Hoen, B., & Duval, X. (2013). Clinical practice. Infective endocarditis. *The New England Journal of Medicine, 368,* 1425–1433.

Kosowsky, J. M., & Takhar, S. S. (2018). Infective endocarditis, rheumatic fever, and valvular heart disease. In R. M. Walls, R. S. Hockberger, & M. Gausche-Hill (Eds.), *Rosen's emergency medicine: Concepts and clinical practice* (9th ed., pp. 1000–1002). Elsevier.

Wang, A., Gaca, J. G., & Chu, V. H. (2018). Management considerations in infective endocarditis: A review. *Journal of the American Medical Association, 320,* 72.

CHAPTER 19

BOARD REVIEW

Hypertension

DAVID TANEN, MD, and JAMES WILLIAMS, MD

Hypertension is a commonly encountered condition in the emergency department and a leading risk factor for cardiovascular disease and stroke. Presentations range from asymptomatic to life-threatening end-organ dysfunction.

General Principles

- The 2017 American College of Cardiology-American Heart Association Hypertension Guideline defined hypertension as a systolic blood pressure (BP) of 130 mm Hg or more or a diastolic BP of 80 mm Hg or more.
- Hypertension can be divided into primary (essential) hypertension and secondary hypertension. Most hypertension is attributed to primary hypertension, which is the result of a complex meshwork of neurohormonal and lifestyle factors. The sympathetic nervous system and renin-angiotensin-aldosterone system both play important roles in mediating BP through their effects on arterial vasoconstriction, glomerular filtration, and salt reabsorption.
- Secondary causes of hypertension are listed in Box 19.1. Secondary causes of hypertension should be considered in individuals with onset of hypertension at a young age or hard-to-control hypertension.
- Long-term effects of poorly controlled hypertension are the result of chronic vasoconstriction that result in end-organ dysfunction. Examples of end-organ dysfunction due to chronic hypertension include hypertensive retinopathy, chronic kidney disease, and heart failure. Moreover, hypertension plays an important role in the pathogenesis of arterial atherosclerosis and is consequently a leading risk factor for myocardial infarction as well as stroke.
- In addition to the chronic effects of untreated hypertension, hypertension may also contribute to acute end-organ dysfunction, so-called *hypertensive emergency*. Examples of end-organ dysfunction are listed in Box 19.2.
- Appropriate hypertension management depends on the presence or absence of acute end-organ dysfunction. In the absence of acute end-organ dysfunction, chronic hypertension should be treated in the ambulatory setting with oral antihypertensive medications that can be initiated in the emergency department (ED) if appropriate. Multiple classes of oral antihypertensive medications exist and are outlined in Table 19.1.

BOX 19.1 *Secondary Causes of Hypertension*

Endocrine
Cushing disease
Hyperaldosteronism
Pheochromocytoma
Thyroid disease
Parathyroid disease
Glucocorticoid excess

Pulmonary
Obstructive sleep apnea

Renal
Chronic kidney disease
Nephritic syndrome
Nephrotic syndrome
Polycystic kidney disease
Renal artery stenosis
Fibromuscular dysplasia

Toxic
Sympathomimetic abuse

Vascular
Coarctation of the aorta
Atherosclerosis

(From Levy, P. D., & Brody, A. (2018). Hypertension. In R. M. Walls, R. S. Hockberger, & M. Gausche-Hill (Eds.), *Rosen's emergency medicine: Concepts and clinical practice* (9th ed., pp. 1007–1020). Elsevier.)

BOX 19.2 *Examples of End-Organ Damage in Acute Hypertensive Emergency*

Cardiovascular
Heart failure
Acute coronary syndrome
Aortic dissection

Central Nervous System
Acute ischemic stroke
Hemorrhagic stroke
Hypertensive encephalopathy
Hypertensive retinopathy

Renal
Acute kidney injury

Asymptomatic Hypertension

- Most patients presenting to the ED with hypertension are asymptomatic without evidence of acute end-organ dysfunction. In this case, no further evaluation is warranted beyond a history and physical and patients should be managed in the outpatient setting regardless of the numeric reading.
- First-line treatment for asymptomatic hypertension may include thiazide diuretics, calcium channel blockers

TABLE 19.1 Commonly Prescribed Oral Antihypertensive Medications

Medication Class	Examples
Thiazide diuretics	Hydrochlorothiazide
Angiotensin-converting enzyme inhibitor	Lisinopril Benazepril Captopril
Angiotensin receptor blockers	Losartan Valsartan
Dihydropyridine calcium channel blockers	Amlodipine Nifedipine
Adrenergic receptor blockers	Metoprolol Propranolol Atenolol Carvedilol Labetalol
α_2-Adrenergic receptor blockers	Clonidine
Direct-acting vasodilator	Hydralazine

such as amlodipine, or angiotensin-converting enzyme inhibitors.

Hypertensive Emergency

- Examples of end-organ dysfunction that may be seen with acutely elevated BP are listed in Box 19.2. Those who have evidence of end-organ dysfunction such as hypertensive encephalopathy should receive timely parenteral antihypertensive therapy.
- Examples of parenteral antihypertensives are listed in Table 19.2. The goal of treatment is to rapidly lower BP to a target goal while maintaining perfusion to the brain and the tissues.
- For adults without a compelling condition (i.e., aortic dissection, severe preeclampsia or eclampsia, or pheochromocytoma crisis), it is currently recommended that systolic BP be reduced by no more than 25% with the first hour; then, if stable, to 160/100 mm Hg within the next 2–6 hours; and then cautiously to normal over the next 24–48 hours. This recommendation is based on the principal of cerebral autoregulation, which preserves cerebral blood flow between mean arterial pressures ranging from 60 to 160 mm Hg. In chronic hypertension, there is a shift in the lower limit of the cerebral autoregulation curve, which tends to be about 25% below the baseline mean arterial pressure.
- There are multiple options for intravenous therapy for management of hypertensive emergency, and the ideal choice of agent and target BP depends on the exact diagnosis and goal of treatment.

TABLE 19.2 Intravenous Antihypertensive Therapies

Medication Class	Examples
ACE inhibitor	Enalaprilat
Calcium channel blocker	Nicardipine Clevidipine
Direct-acting vasodilator	Hydralazine
Adrenergic Inhibitors Alpha-1 antagonists Beta-blockers	 Phentolamine Esmolol, metoprolol, labetalol
Loop diuretic	Furosemide
Dopamine-1 receptor agonist	Fenoldopam
Nitric oxide donors	Sodium nitroprusside Nitroglycerin Isosorbide dinitrate

Hypertensive Encephalopathy

Clinical Presentation

- The result of impaired cerebral autoregulation and increased vascular permeability, the presentation of hypertensive encephalopathy may include headache, vomiting, altered mental status, seizures, or coma.
- Papilledema or retinal hemorrhages may be present on examination. Neurologic findings are often global and do not localize to a single vascular territory, which helps differentiate hypertensive encephalopathy from acute stroke.

Diagnosis

- Computed tomography (CT) may demonstrate cerebral edema but often shows normal results.
- Diagnosis is clinical and the combination of markedly elevated BP along with a normal or nonspecific head CT should prompt consideration of this diagnosis.
- Differential diagnosis also includes posterior reversible encephalopathy syndrome, which has a similar presentation with vision changes, seizures, altered mental status, and headache. Although changes of posterior reversible encephalopathy syndrome may be seen on a standard head CT, magnetic resonance imaging is more sensitive and is the preferred diagnostic modality.

Treatment

- Goal of treatment is to reduce cerebral edema and improve autoregulatory control.
- Intravenous therapy with nicardipine or labetalol should be initiated promptly, with the goal of reducing systolic BP, as noted above. Rapidly decreasing the BP beyond these goals risks decreasing cerebral perfusion and precipitating cerebral ischemia.

Acute Coronary Syndrome

- Hypertension may complicate acute coronary syndrome and may cause myocardial infarction as a result of impaired coronary perfusion and increased myocardial demand due to increased afterload. The goal of treatment is to reverse these processes.
- Appropriate BP management in the setting of acute coronary syndrome may include intravenous nitroglycerin to promote vasodilation and decrease afterload or nicardipine. β-blockers such as esmolol and metoprolol can also help decrease myocardial oxygen demand but,

due to the decrease in inotropy and chronotropy, should be avoided if cardiogenic shock is suspected.

Renal Hypertensive Emergency

- Chronic kidney disease is a common result of long-standing hypertension, but severely impaired renal function can be seen in the setting of acutely elevated BP as well. Many antihypertensive agents can lower the glomerular filtration rate. In this setting, fenoldopam, a dopamine agonist that preserves renal blood flow, or an intravenous calcium channel blocker are appropriate antihypertensive agents.

Sympathetic Crisis

- There are multiple causes of sympathetic crisis, such as pheochromocytoma, sympathomimetic overdose, clonidine withdrawal, and tyramine ingestion in those on a monoamine oxidase inhibitor. These processes lead to hypertension through excessive α_1-mediated vasoconstriction.
- Use of a β-blocker is contraindicated in these settings due to fear for unopposed alpha effects and worsening hypertension. Benzodiazepines can be used in the setting of sympathomimetic overdose. Use of an α_1 inhibitor, such as phentolamine, is preferred in the setting of sympathetic crisis.

Acute Ischemic Stroke

- Long-standing hypertension is a risk factor for acute ischemic stroke, and elevated BP can be seen in the setting of acute ischemic stroke.
- Initial BP >185/110 mm Hg is a contraindication to thrombolytic therapy. For reperfusion-eligible patients, BP should be lowered slowly to <185/110 mm Hg before thrombolytic therapy and maintained at <180/105 mm Hg for at least the first 24 hours after thrombolytics. For patients who do not undergo reperfusion therapy, if the BP is >220/120 mm Hg, the benefit of immediate lowering of BP is not clear. In the initial 24 hours after an acute stroke, so-called permissive hypertension <220/120 mm Hg may be protective of the ischemic penumbra. BP therapy should be initiated only if the BP is > 220/120 mm Hg and should aim to reduce the mean arterial pressure by no further than 15% in the first 24 hours.

Aortic Dissection

- Prompt control of hypertension and tachycardia reduces the intimal shear stress in aortic dissection and is essential to prevent further injury. BP should be controlled to a systolic BP < 100-120 mm Hg and heart rate < 60 beats/min.
- Esmolol should be administered as a bolus and a continuous infusion uptitrated to a heart rate < 60 beats/min. If hypertension persists, additional agents such as nitroprusside or nicardipine can be administered to reduce the BP to < 120 mm Hg during the first hour of management.

Intracerebral Hemorrhage

- Hypertension is associated with spontaneous intracerebral hemorrhage. Prompt administration of antihypertensive therapy in cerebral hemorrhage helps limit further bleeding and reduces surrounding edema but also risks cerebral hypoperfusion if not properly titrated. In general, systolic pressures of 140–160 mm Hg are targeted.
- Nicardipine or labetalol are generally the first-line agents. Nimodipine is given in the setting of subarachnoid hemorrhage to reduce cerebral vasospasm and secondary brain injury, which may develop days after the initial bleed.

Acute Heart Failure

- The goal of treatment of hypertension in acute heart failure is to decrease afterload and promote forward flow. Nitroglycerin is the preferred agent in acute heart failure due to its effects on both preload and afterload. Patients with evidence of volume overload should also receive loop diuretics to initiate diuresis. β-blockers should be avoided because they impair cardiac contractility and may precipitate shock in the setting of decompensated heart failure.

Eclampsia/Preeclampsia

- The agents of choice for lowering BP in these conditions are hydralazine or labetalol due to their safety profile, with a target systolic blood pressure of <140 mm Hg during the first hour.

SUGGESTED READINGS

Whelton, P. K., Carey, R. M., Aronow, R. M., Casey, D. E., Jr., Collins, K. J., Dennison Himmelfarb, C., et al. (2018). 2017 ACC/AHA/AAPA/ABC/ACPM/AGS/APhA/ASH/ASPC/NMA/PCNA Guideline for the prevention, detection, evaluation, and management of high blood pressure in adults. *Journal of the American College of Cardiology*, *71*, e127–e248. https://www.acc.org/guidelines.

Wolf, S. J., Lo, B., Shih, R. D., Smith, M. D., & Fesmire, F. M. (2013). Clinical policy: Critical issues in the evaluation and management of adult patients in the emergency department with asymptomatic elevated blood pressure. *Annals of Emergency Medicine*, *62*, 59–68. https://www.acep.org/patient-care/clinical-policies.

CHAPTER **20**

BOARD REVIEW

Implantable Cardiac Devices

ALEXANDRA GROSSMAN, MD, and MANPREET SINGH, MD, MBE

Pacemakers

General Principles

- Permanent cardiac pacemakers are usually implanted for one of two reasons: (1) bradyarrhythmia caused by advanced atrioventricular (AV) blocks and sinus node disease, and (2) cardiac resynchronization therapy for systolic heart failure in patients with an ejection fraction (EF) less than 35% and left bundle branch block (LBBB).
- Pacemaker systems are composed of three basic units: the pulse generator or power source, the electronic circuitry, and the lead system.
  - The pacemaker lead is connected to the pulse generator and the distal electrode is in contact with the endocardium.
  - In the typical multilead system of dual chamber pacing, one lead is placed in the right ventricle in contact with the endocardium and a second lead placed in contact with the endocardium of the right atrium.
  - For biventricular pacing used in cardiac resynchronization therapy, a lead is advanced through the coronary sinus until the electrode overlies the left ventricular epicardium.
- The pacemaker function and programming can be identified by a five-letter code (Table 20.1): (I) chamber paced, (II) chamber sensed, (III) sensing response, (IV) programmability, (V) antitachycardia function.
  - The first three letters are most important in the emergency setting because they represent the antibradycardia functions.

Terminology and Normal Pacemaker Function

- **Pacing** refers to the depolarization of a cardiac chamber triggered by a discharge from the pulse generator. It is detected by the presence of a "spike" or stimulus artifact on an electrocardiogram (ECG).
- **Sensing** indicates a pacemaker's ability to detect native cardiac depolarizations when they are occurring.
- **Response to sensing** indicates what a pacemaker does when it senses intrinsic cardiac depolarization. If a pacemaker is set as *inhibited*, detection or sensing of native cardiac depolarization inhibits the pacemaker from firing (most common). If set as *triggered*, then the opposite occurs (i.e., sensing depolarization triggers it to fire).
  - For example, in a VVI pacemaker, the ventricle is being both sensed and paced. If no native ventricular activity is sensed by the pacemaker, then it will pace the ventricle at a preprogrammed rate. If native ventricular depolarization is sensed, then the pacemaker is inhibited and does not fire.
- **Synchronous vs. asynchronous:** Pacemakers can exist in either synchronous or asynchronous modes. Nearly all modern pacemakers are *synchronous*, meaning the pacer senses intrinsic cardiac activity and paces in response to that. However, they can be turned *asynchronous* in certain situations in which no sensing occurs and the cardiac chamber is continuously paced regardless of the native activity (essentially becoming AOO, VOO, or DOO).
- Note that DDD is the most common and optimal pacemaker mode. In this mode, both the atria and ventricle are paced and sensed.
- Accordingly, if no intrinsic atrial impulse is sensed, the pacemaker will initiate atrial depolarization if the programmed pacing rate is exceeded (manifested by a spike preceding the p-wave on ECG).
- If an atrial impulse is sensed, but is not followed by a native ventricular depolarization, then it will pace the ventricle when the programmed AV interval is exceeded.
- If both atrial and ventricular impulses are sensed, then no pacing occurs.
- The ability to pace both the atria and ventricles makes this the preferred method of pacing owing to improved atrioventricular synchrony (to be discussed later).

Clinical Presentation

- Pacemaker complications can be due to either malfunction of the components of the pacing system or secondary to the implant itself.

TABLE 20.1 *Pacemaker Function and Programming Identification*

(I) Chamber Paced	(II) Chamber Sensed	(III) Sensing Response	(IV) Programmability	(V) Antitachycardia Function
A (atrium)	A (atrium)	T (triggered)	P (simple)	P (pacing)
V (ventricle)	V (ventricle)	I (inhibited)	M (multi)	S (shock)
D (dual = A+V)	D (dual = A+V)	D (dual = T+I)	R (rate adaptive)	D (dual I= shock+ pace)
0 (none)	0 (none)	0 (none)	C (communicating)	
			0 (none)	

Pacing malfunction typically arises from one of three potential problems: power source failure, pacemaker lead defect (displacement, lead fracture, or insulation failure), or disruption of the interface between the pacing electrode and the myocardium. The latter can commonly be caused by electrolyte disturbances, medications, myocardial fibrosis, and ischemia.

- Pacemaker failure clinically presents with syncope, dizziness, weakness, or extracardiac muscle twitches. Electrocardiographically, it can be divided into three main categories:
  - **Oversensing** occurs when the pacer incorrectly interprets other electric signals as native cardiac depolarization and is inappropriately inhibited (i.e., oversensing). These electric signals may be myopotentials from skeletal muscle contraction, retrograde P-waves, large T-waves, or output failure from a generator or lead defect.
  - **Undersensing** occurs when the pacemaker fails to recognize native cardiac conduction and subsequently paces the heart inappropriately. On ECG, this will appear as a pacer spike at an inappropriate location. Undersensing is usually caused by lead disruption, change in native beat morphology, or low-voltage cardiac waves.
  - **Failure to pace** occurs when there are no stimuli (no spikes) or subthreshold stimuli (spikes, no QRS). This can occur owing to either output failure or failure to capture. Output failure is generally caused by oversensing, wire fracture, lead displacement, or pulse generator failure.
- Failure to capture is generally caused by electrode displacement, wire facture, myocardial process (ischemia, edema, infiltrative process), or electrolyte disturbance (i.e., hyperkalemia).
- **Pacemaker-mediated tachycardia (PMT)** is an arrhythmia that can occur in patients with dual-chamber devices when the pacemaker stimulates the ventricles to beat inappropriately fast.
  - It is a form of AV-nodal reentrant tachycardia in which the AV node forms the retrograde circuit and the pacemaker forms the antegrade circuit, resulting in continued pacemaker-mediated ventricular depolarizations.
  - This is manifested on ECG by a regular, wide-complex tachycardia with a pacing spike prior to each QRS complex.
  - PMT is treated by placement of a magnet over the pacemaker, which converts it from a synchronous to an asynchronous mode, subsequently terminating the dysrhythmia.
- **Implant-related complications** can be caused by the procedure itself (i.e., postprocedural hematoma, pneumothorax) or related to the device.
  - Examples of the latter include infection, lead dislodgement or malposition, subclavian or brachiocephalic venous thrombosis, and tricuspid regurgitation.
  - Twiddler's syndrome is a specific cause of lead dislodgement that occurs when a patient either deliberately or subconsciously twists the pulse generator in its pockets, causing the leads to coil around the generator.

Diagnosis and Evaluation

- Key historical information that should be obtained include the original indications for pacemaker placement, timing of placement and revisions, and recent programming changes.
- The type of pacemaker should be identified by asking the patient for his/her pacemaker identification card.
- Patients should also be asked about pacemaker-related symptoms, including presyncope/syncope, palpitations, shortness of breath, and weakness.
- Examination should focus on cardiac auscultation and physical inspection of the implant site and ipsilateral arm.
- The implant site should be examined for signs of infection or bleeding, including erythema, warmth, tenderness, swelling, and bruising.
- Swelling to the ipsilateral arm or neck may be indicative of venous thrombosis and should prompt further testing with imaging of the venous system (see below).

Diagnostic Testing

- A chest x-ray should be obtained to visualize the pulse generator and its associated leads. By distinguishing the location of pacing leads, the type of pacemaker as well as complications such as lead migration, dislodgement, or fracture can be identified.
- For example, Twiddler's syndrome, as discussed above, can be diagnosed by visualizing coiled leads around the pulse generator on x-ray.
- Additionally, identification of the manufacturer code on the pulse generator can assist in identifying the device manufacturer.
- 12-lead ECG should be performed in all patients. The presence of a pacemaker spike immediately followed by a p-wave or QRS-complex indicates successful pacing and capture of the atrium and ventricle, respectively.
- Pacemaker spikes may be absent if native cardiac depolarization is adequate and the heart rate is above the pacemaker's programmed threshold for pacing or with pacemaker malfunction.
- The ECG should be examined for failure to capture, to pace, and to sense. Note that a normal paced rhythm will produce a wide QRS with a left bundle-branch block pattern, reflecting the spread of depolarization that originates from the pacemaker lead in the right ventricle.
- ECG should also be evaluated for evidence of myocardial ischemia using the modified Sgarbossa's criteria.
- Laboratory tests, including a basic metabolic panel and troponin, should be sent to evaluate for electrolyte derangements and myocardial ischemia, respectively.
- Hyperkalemia is an important cause of p-acing malfunction because it elevates the pacing threshold or the amount of energy needed to stimulate myocardial depolarization, thereby resulting in failure to capture.
- "Interrogation" of the pacemaker device should be performed in all patients with suspected pacemaker malfunction or symptoms suggestive of arrhythmia. Interrogation provides information regarding battery life, pacing parameters, and lead status.
- As the pacemaker also maintains continuous telemetry monitoring, it can also be used to diagnose tachyarrhythmias in the symptomatic patient.
- Devices used to assess pacemaker function are manufacturer-specific.

Management

- Reversible causes of pacemaker malfunction (i.e., acute coronary syndromes (ACS), electrolyte abnormalities) should be treated accordingly.
- Application of a magnet over the pacemaker can be performed to terminate pacemaker-mediated tachycardia or inappropriate sensing, because it converts the pacemaker from a synchronous to an asynchronous mode.
- In the asynchronous mode, the pacemaker will continuously fire at a specified programmed rate, regardless of the native cardiac activity.
- Magnets have additional functions if an automatic implantable cardioverter-defibrillators (AICD) is also present (to be discussed below).
- Advanced cardiac life support (ACLS) can be performed as normal with compressions and defibrillation. However, external transcutaneous pads should be placed as far away from the device as possible, ideally in an anteroposterior orientation.
- Note that pacemaker capture may not return immediately after defibrillation owing to global myocardial ischemia (which increases the pacing threshold). Subsequently, temporary pacing (transcutaneous or transvenous) may be required.

Implantable Cardioverter-Defibrillators (ICDs)

General Principles

- Automatic implantable cardioverter-defibrillators are placed for primary and secondary prevention of sudden cardiac arrest caused by ventricular tachycardia or fibrillation. Similar to the components of pacemakers, they are composed of a power source, electric circuitry, and a lead system, which senses and has the capability to pace the myocardium.
- An electric coil placed between the pulse generator and right ventricular lead delivers a shock to the myocardium in the setting of a ventricular arrhythmia.
- The lifespan of an AICD largely depends on the frequency of shocks.

Clinical Presentation

- Patients may present to the emergency department (ED) following discharge of a shock, ICD malfunction, or an implant-related complication (see above).
- Patients may present following a single shock episode or, commonly, for frequent shocks. Shock discharge can occur both appropriately (in response to VT/VF) or inappropriately in the setting of ICD malfunction. ICD malfunction with inappropriate shocks have several causes, including misinterpretation of supraventricular tachycardia as a ventricular arrhythmia and oversensing of t-waves or other signals as wide QRS complexes.
- Increased shock frequency should raise concern for recurrent VT/VF episodes ("electrical storm," characterized by the recurrence of hemodynamically unstable ventricular tachycardia and/or ventricular fibrillation. The most accepted definition refers to three or more separate episodes of the arrhythmia occurring over a single 24-hour time period, leading to ICD therapies), which can be precipitated by electrolyte abnormalities, myocardial ischemia, or drugs/medications.
- Patients may present with signs and symptoms of ventricular arrhythmia, including syncope/near-syncope, dizziness, weakness, or cardiac arrest. This can be caused by failure of the ICD to recognize ventricular arrhythmias (undersensing) or the delivery of a shock with a strength too low to terminate the arrhythmia.

Diagnosis and Evaluation

- In addition to elucidating the characteristics and frequency of shocks, ask patients about symptoms, such as chest pain, dyspnea, weakness, presyncope/syncope, and lightheadedness, which may point to an acute coronary syndrome, volume overload, electrolyte imbalance, or other arrhythmia.
- Physical examination should include auscultation of the heart and lungs along with assessment of volume status.
- Similar to the evaluation of the patient with a pacemaker, workup should include ECG, chest x-ray, and laboratory studies (electrolytes, troponin) to identify triggers of ventricular arrhythmia, including myocardial ischemia, heart failure, or a metabolic abnormality.
- A patient who presents with a single isolated shock without associated concerning symptoms can be discharged with close outpatient follow-up with an electrophysiologist. All patients who have received more than one shock, however, require telemetry monitoring and interrogation of their device in the ED.

Management

- As discussed above, all patients who have received more than one shock should have their device interrogated in the ED.
- Receipt of three or more appropriate shocks within a 24-hour period should be managed by addressing underlying causes (e.g., ischemia, electrolytes) and administrations of antiarrhythmics.
- With frequent *inappropriate* shocks, a magnet can be applied which disables the antitachycardia function and subsequently terminates shock output. Beta blockers, amiodarone, lidocaine, procainamide, and magnesium are commonly used to treat persistent ventricular arrhythmias after the AICD is disabled.
- In the setting of cardiac arrest, ACLS should be performed as per guidelines, including transthoracic defibrillation and manual chest compressions.

Cardiac Assist Devices

General Principles

- Ventricular assist devices (VADs) are used in the patient with end-stage heart failure as a bridge to cardiac transplant, as a bridge to recovery from reversible cardiac pathology, or as a "destination" in patients who do not qualify for cardiac transplant.
- VADs can be placed in either the left and/or right ventricle (left ventricle assist device or "LVAD," biventricular assist device or "BiVAD") and support cardiac function by mechanically pumping blood from the ventricle into its respective outflow vessel.

- The VAD system is composed of an inflow cannula, pumping chamber, outflow cannula, driveline, and system controller.
  - The inflow cannula, which is located within the ventricle, pulls blood from the ventricle into the pumping chamber.
  - In the pumping chamber, an impeller generates blood flow and pumps blood to the aorta via an outflow cannula.
  - The pump is attached to an external system controller, which houses the power source and system monitor through a subcutaneous driveline that exits the skin near the epigastric region.
- The vast majority of VADs are "continuous-flow" devices, meaning that blood flow occurs continuously through the pump, unlike the pulsatile nature of the normal, physiologic cardiac cycle. Patients with an LAVD require lifelong anticoagulation to prevent device clotting.

Clinical Presentation

Patients with a VAD can present with complications related to the device itself or to associated medical therapies as well as a myriad of unrelated issues.

- **Circuit or pump thrombosis** can result in complications, including pump malfunction, hemolysis, and systemic embolization. Patients can subsequently present with a wide range of symptoms, including bleeding, scleral icterus, dark urine, stroke, massive pulmonary embolism, and sudden cardiac arrest.
  - Keys to this diagnosis include low flow and high power on the system as well as a significantly elevated lactate dehydrogenase (LDH).
  - Laboratory studies may also show evidence of hemolysis, including low hemoglobin, low haptoglobin, and coagulopathy.
  - Management includes immediate consultation with an LVAD specialist and possible anticoagulation.
  - Severe thrombosis may result in pump stoppage, which is a true emergency. If hemodynamically unstable, patients may require systemic thrombolysis or emergent pump exchange.
- **Suction events** typically occur in the setting of low flow from dysrhythmia, hemorrhage, or other hypovolemic states that result in decreased left ventricle preload.
  - The underfilled left ventricle collapses and subsequently obstructs inflow to the LVAD. This is diagnosed by low flow, speed, and power on the controller.
  - Management includes volume repletion and correcting the underlying etiology.
- **Pump failure** is a life-threatening emergency and the second most common cause of death in patients with an LVAD. Common causes include loss of power, disconnected or kinked leads, or massive thrombus.
  - The controller may show low flow, low voltage, or power loss. A low-flow alarm should always be evaluated by first checking the power.
  - Be aware that even a short time of noncirculating flow within the LVAD drastically increases the risk of thrombus formation. Subsequently, if the device has been off for only a short period of time or the patient is unstable, it can be restarted.
  - However, if the device has been off for an unknown amount or an extended period of time (>1 hr) and the patient is stable, the device should not be restarted without LVAD specialist consultation owing to the high risk of thromboembolic events.
- **Bleeding diatheses.** Patients are at increased bleeding risk because they are on lifelong anticoagulation and develop an acquired von Willebrand disease from device-related shear stress.
  - They frequently present with intracranial or gastrointestinal hemorrhage.
  - Bleeding should be managed as per standard of care with blood products and resuscitation.
  - Reversal of anticoagulation should be done only when necessary owing to the risk of thrombosis and pump failure.
- **Infection** usually occurs within the first two months after implantation; the driveline and pump pocket are the two most common sites.
  - Broad-spectrum antibiotics should be administered.
- **Dysrhythmias** can be primary (cardiac in origin) or secondary (related to the LVAD). Common secondary causes include hypovolemia and decreased preload.
  - Dysrhythmias may result in poor perfusion leading to suction events, thrombus formation, and hemodynamic instability.
  - Note that patients may have minimal symptoms owing to continued forward flow from the LVAD, which, if untreated, can result in right ventricular failure.
  - Management should focus on reversal of the underlying cause (if applicable) and electrical/chemical therapy as needed.

Diagnosis and Evaluation

- Initial evaluation of patients with a VAD differs from those without in several ways, particularly in the assessment of vital signs. Continuous flow cannot typically produce a palpable pulse, therefore blood pressure is determined by measurement of the mean arterial pressure (MAP), rather than systolic and diastolic pressures as occurs with physiologic pulsatile flow.
- The MAP is the most important hemodynamic measurement in these patients and should be kept between 70 and 90 mm Hg. It can be determined by inflating a sphygmomanometer and placing a doppler probe over the radial artery; upon deflation of the cuff, the number that the signal returns is the MAP.
- Notably, some patients do have baseline pulses owing to residual ventricular function and blood pressure can be checked in the standard form. In patients who do not normally have a palpable pulse, the presence of one may indicate VAD thrombosis; therefore, all patients should be asked about their baseline pulse.
- Physical examination should also include auscultation of the chest and inspection of the device components as well as any other systems pertinent to their presentation.
- On auscultation of the chest, one should hear the mechanical hum of the device, which indicates that the device is powered and functioning.
- The driveline exit site should be inspected using sterile gloves and mask for signs of infection, such as erythema, warmth, or purulent drainage.

- Lastly, the external controller should be examined to identify any alarms and the system's functional parameters, including pump speed, pump flow, pulse index, and pump power. Most devices contain alarms for low battery or issues with flow or speed.
- Diagnostic testing should include a coagulation panel, haptoglobin, lactate dehydrogenase, and hemoglobin/hematocrit owing to the risk of bleeding diatheses (discussed below).
- An ECG, which is typically not specific, should be obtained in all patients to evaluate for an arrhythmia.
- Chest radiography can give information regarding the position and types of devices present.
- Echocardiogram can also be employed to assess cardiac function as well as for complications such as pulmonary embolism, valvular insufficiency, and thrombosis.

Management

- Early consultation with the patient's LVAD coordinator or specialist is critical and should be done for all patients presenting to the ED.
- Complications, such as bleeding, thrombosis, pump failure, and dysrhythmias, should be managed as above.
- In the unresponsive and hypotensive patient, external chest compressions can be performed if needed. However, prior to initiation of compressions, every attempt should be made to confirm the absence of circulation and correct pump malfunction.
  - Note that if the MAP is greater than or equal to 50 mm Hg or the end tidal CO_2 is greater than 20 with an audible hum, perfusion is likely adequate and chest compressions are not necessary.
  - Defibrillation can also be performed, as indicated, with pads positioned away from the device.

SUGGESTED READINGS

Madhavan, M., Mulpuru, S. K., McLeod, C. J., Cha, Y. M., & Friedman, P. A. (2017). Advances and future directions in cardiac pacemakers: Part 2 of a 2-part series. *Journal of the American College of Cardiology*, 69(2), 211–235.

Malone M., & Panchal A. (2020). Defibrillator malfunction: It's electric! Boogie, woogie, woogie!. In C. Kaide & C. San Miguel (Eds.), *Case studies in emergency medicine*. Springer.

Martindale, J., & deSouza, I. S. (2014). Managing pacemaker-related complications and malfunctions in the emergency department. *Emergency Medicine Practice*, 16(9), 1–21.

Mulpuru, S. K., Madhavan, M., McLeod, C. J., Cha, Y. M., & Friedman, P. A. (2017). Cardiac pacemakers: function, troubleshooting, and management: Part 1 of a 2-part series. *Journal of the American College of Cardiology*, 69(2), 189–210.

Robertson, J., Long, B., & Koyfman, A. (2016). The emergency management of ventricular assist devices. *American Journal of Emergency Medicine*, 34(7), 1294–1301.

Tracy, C. M., Epstein, A. E., Darbar, D., DiMarco, J. P., Dunbar, S. B., Estes, N. M., Ferguson, T. B., Hammill, S. C., Karasik, P. E., Link, M. S., Marine, J. E., Schoenfeld, M. H., Shanker, A. J., Silka, M. J., Warner Stevenson, L., Stevenson, W. G., & Varosy, P. D. (2013). 2012 ACCF/AHA/HRS focused update incorporated into the ACCF/AHA/HRS 2008 guidelines for device-based therapy of cardiac rhythm abnormalities: A report of the American College of Cardiology Foundation/American Heart Association Task Force on Practice Guidelines and the Heart Rhythm Society. *Journal of the American College of Cardiology*, 61(3), e6–e75.

SECTION THREE

BOARD REVIEW

Cutaneous

Cancers of the Skin

STEVEN BOLGER, MD, and GREG HENDEY, MD

Skin cancer comprises a small percentage of all presentations to the emergency department (ED), and early detection and referral can reduce associated morbidity and mortality. Skin cancer is the most common type of cancer in the United States with one in five Americans developing skin cancer in their lifetime. For all of the cancers of the skin discussed, the important part is recognition and then referral for biopsy and definitive diagnosis.

Melanoma

- Melanoma is the most important type of skin cancer to diagnose because of its potential for metastasis and associated mortality.
- There are four main types of melanoma: superficial spreading melanoma (Fig. 21.1), nodular melanoma (Fig. 21.2), lentigo maligna melanoma, and acral lentiginous melanoma.

Clinical Presentation

- Risk factors for the development of melanoma include personal or family history of melanoma, exposure to sunlight, history of sunburns, presence of fair skin, and more than 50 nevi or presence of atypical nevi on a patient's body.

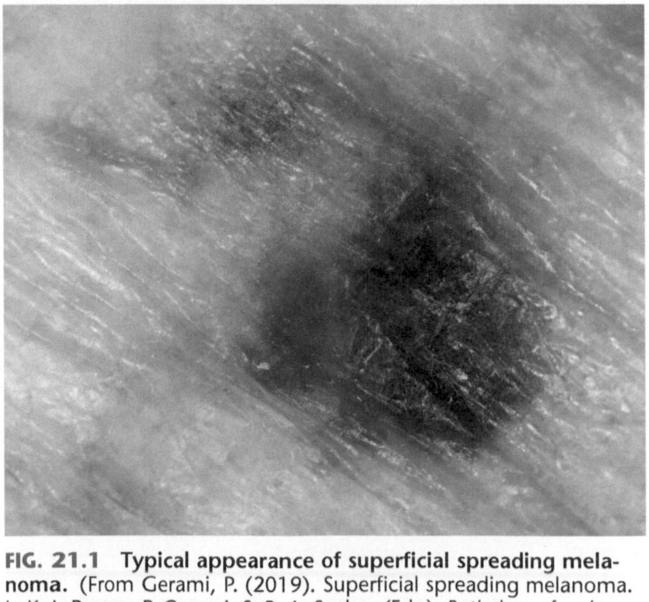

FIG. 21.1 Typical appearance of superficial spreading melanoma. (From Gerami, P. (2019). Superficial spreading melanoma. In K. J. Busam, P. Gerami, & R. A. Scolyer (Eds.), *Pathology of melanocytic tumors* (pp. 158–167, Fig. 13.1a). Elsevier.)

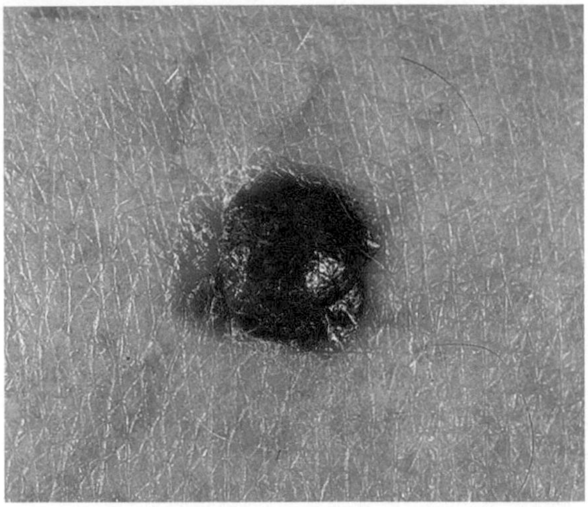

FIG. 21.2 Typical appearance of nodular melanoma. (From Habif T. P., Dinulos J. G. H., Chapman J.M. S., & Zug K. A. (2018). Benign melanocytic neoplasms and melanoma. In *Skin disease: Diagnosis and treatment* (4th ed., pp. 495–520, Fig. 1834c). Elsevier.)

- Early signs of melanoma include **A**symmetry, irregular **B**orders, variability of **C**olor, **D**iameter 6 mm or larger, and recent **E**volution or change in appearance. A helpful mnemonic for these characteristics is **ABCDE**.
- The observation that nevi in one patient tend to resemble each other and that melanoma often deviates from this pattern is the "Ugly Duckling" concept. This clinical feature is helpful in the identification of nevi that are suspicious for melanoma.
- The incidence of melanoma in the United States is increasing owing to an increased awareness and early detection and referral with an associated decrease in mortality. Emergency medicine physicians play an important role in referring patients to primary care or dermatology for further evaluation.

Basal Cell Carcinoma

- Basal cell carcinoma (BCC) is a common type of skin cancer arising from the basal layer of the epidermis and is the most common malignancy in Caucasians.
- Although BCC has a low risk of metastasis, the malignancy can be locally invasive and cause destruction of skin and surrounding structures.
- The two most common subtypes of BCC are nodular and superficial.

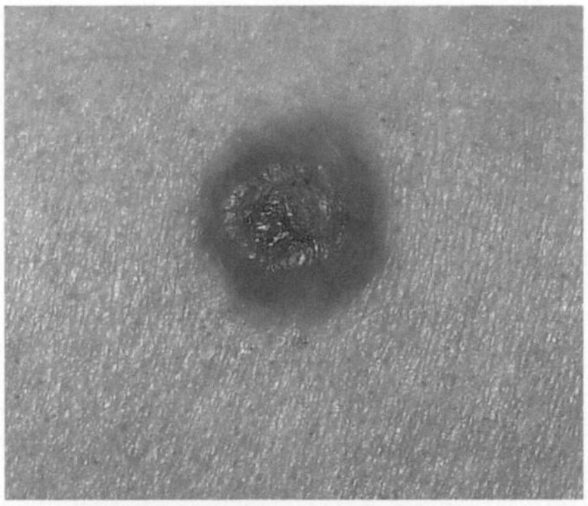

FIG. 21.3 Nodular basal cell carcinoma with central ulceration. (From Rigel D., Friedman R., Robinson J. et al. (2011). Basal cell carcinoma. In *Cancer of the skin* (2nd ed., pp. 99–123, Fig. 11.4). Elsevier.)

Clinical Presentation

- Nodular BCC accounts for 60% of all cases and presents with pink or flesh-colored papules on the face or neck (Fig. 21.3).
  - The lesions are typically pearly or translucent and ulcerated with a telangiectatic vessel within the papule.
- Superficial BCC accounts for 30% of all cases and consists of slightly scaly macules, patches, or plaques which are light red to pink in color.
  - Spots of brown or black pigment can be present, which may lead to confusion with melanoma.
- The most significant risk factor for BCC is exposure to ultraviolet radiation through sunlight.
- Other less-common risk factors include chronic arsenic exposure, radiation therapy, and long-term immunosuppressant therapy.

Squamous Cell Carcinoma

- Squamous cell carcinoma (SCC) is a relatively common form of skin cancer that can occur on any surface of the skin.
- Sun-exposed areas are the most common locations for SCC in patients with fair skin, and areas that are shaded from the sun are the most common locations in patients with dark skin.

Clinical Presentation

- SCC presents as well-demarcated and scaly patches or plaques, which are usually erythematous, but can also be pigmented or skin-colored (Fig. 21.4).
- Lesions tend to grow slowly over the course of years.
- Actinic keratoses are rough, scaly, and erythematous macules that develop on the surfaces of skin exposed to sun and can progress to SCC.
  - Although only 1% of all actinic keratoses progress to SCC, approximately 60% of all SCCs arise from actinic keratoses.
- Oral SCC presents as an ulcer, nodule, or indurated plaque, most commonly involving the floor of mouth and lateral or ventral tongue (Fig. 21.5).

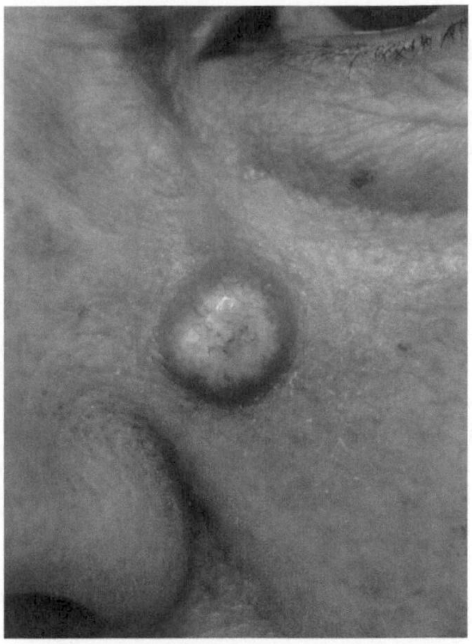

Fig. 21.4 Squamous cell carcinoma of the face. (From Gawkrodger, D. J., & Ardern-Jones, M. R. (2016). Skin cancer—Squamous cell carcinoma. In *Dermatology: An illustrated colour text* (6th ed., pp. 106–107, Fig. 53.6). Elsevier.)

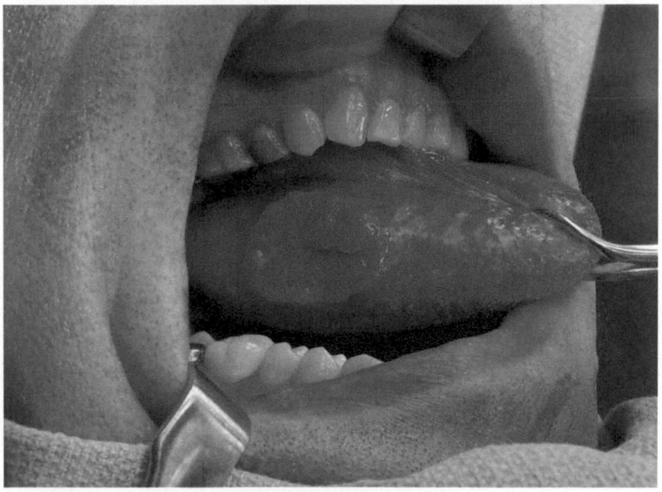

FIG. 21.5 Oral squamous cell carcinoma of the tongue. (From Ward, B. B., & Helman, J. I. (2017). Squamous cell carcinoma of the oral and maxillofacial region. In R. J. Fonseca (Ed.), *Oral and maxillofacial surgery* (3rd ed., pp. 670–689, Fig. 28.9). Elsevier.)

- Oral SCC is often associated with a history of tobacco or heavy alcohol use.

Kaposi Sarcoma

- Kaposi sarcoma (KS) is a malignancy characterized by endothelial cell proliferation that frequently affects multiple organ systems. Human herpesvirus 8 (HHV-8) is the underlying etiology. There are four types of KS: classic, endemic, organ transplant-associated, and epidemic or AIDS-related.

21

Clinical Presentation

- Classic KS has an indolent course, with cutaneous lesions primarily affecting the lower extremities of elderly men of Mediterranean or Jewish descent.
- Endemic KS is more aggressive than classic KS and may involve dissemination to lymph nodes, bone, or skin.
  - This form of KS occurs in equatorial Africa and affects both children and adults.
- Organ transplant-associated KS occurs after solid organ transplantation with manifestations similar to epidemic KS; it regresses with resolution of immunosuppression.
- Epidemic or AIDS-related KS is the most common malignancy in patients who are HIV-positive, and it is one of the AIDS-defining illnesses (Fig. 21.6).

Diagnosis

- The diagnosis of KS is based on clinical features, including lesions consisting of macules, plaques, or nodules, which can be erythematous, violaceous, brown, or black.
- The lesions are typically found on the skin, but may also be present in the oral mucosa, gastrointestinal tract, and respiratory tract.
- Patients should be referred to primary care or dermatology for biopsy to confirm diagnosis and further evaluation.

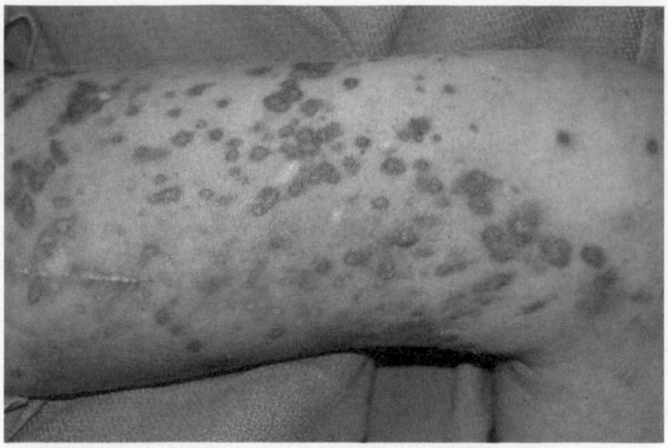

FIG. 21.6 Multiple plaques present on the lower extremity owing to AIDS-related Kaposi sarcoma. (From Brinster, N. K. Liu, V., Diwan, A. H., & McKee, P. H. (2011). Kaposi's sarcoma. In *Dermatopathology: High-yield pathology* (pp. 497–499, Fig. 1). Elsevier.)

SUGGESTED READINGS

Jeffes, E. W., III., & Tang, E. H. (2000). Actinic keratosis. Current treatment options. *American Journal of Clinical Dermatology*, *1*(3), 167–179.

Nadkarni, A., Domeisen, N., Hill, D., & Feldman, S. R. (2016). The most common dermatology diagnoses in the emergency department. *Journal of the American Academy of Dermatology*, *75*(6), 1261–1262.

Vangipuram, R., & Tyring, S. K. (2019). Epidemiology of Kaposi sarcoma: Review and description of the nonepidemic variant. *International Journal of Dermatology*, *58*(5), 538–542.

CHAPTER 22

BOARD REVIEW

Ulcerative Lesions

RYAN C. DOLLBAUM, MD, and ATILLA UNER, MD, MPH

Chronic skin wounds, defined as wounds that fail to heal within 30 days, are increasing in prevalence with a larger aging population. They can be a major source of pain and disability, fluctuate between various stages of healing, and may never fully heal.

Diabetic Foot Ulcers

Foot ulcers develop in 15%–20% of those with chronic diabetes. Moreover, ulcer precedes lower extremity amputation in 85% of cases. Therefore, early identification and treatment are important in preventing morbidity and mortality.

Pathophysiology

- Patients with diabetes are predisposed to development of skin and soft tissue infections due to:
  - Sensory, autonomic, and motor neuropathy: recurring trauma
  - Atherosclerotic vascular disease: diminished perfusion
  - Hyperglycemia: impaired healing/immunity and nerve damage
  - Impaired foot architecture: imbalance of intrinsic/extrinsic muscles

Clinical Presentation

- Location: most commonly over pressure points of the foot, such as the plantar surface beneath the first and fifth metatarsal heads, great toe, and heel.
- Appearance: cutaneous, punched-out ulcer with thick rim of callus.
- Symptoms: often asymptomatic but patient may complain of paresthesias such as burning, numbness, itching.
- Complications: Infection (most often polymicrobial, although severe infections are often associated with methicillin-resistant *Staphylococcus aureus* [MRSA]), cellulitis (see Chapter 24), lymphangitis, sepsis, and deep space infection (such as necrotizing fasciitis).

Diagnosis and Evaluation

Physical Examination

- Determine circumference and depth of cutaneous ulcer (probing with sterile instrument).
- Evaluate for purulence, surrounding cellulitis (redness, warmth, pain), lymphangitic streaking, and crepitus.

Imaging

- X-rays may aid in determining the presence of focal demineralization, periosteal elevation, and cortical disruption if osteomyelitis is suspected.
- Magnetic resonance imaging is more than 95% sensitive for soft tissue and bone inflammation.
- Radionuclide bone scan may be useful if suspicion for infection remains high and magnetic resonance imaging is either unavailable or contraindicated.

Laboratory Tests

- Complete blood count to assess for leukocytosis with increased band count.
- Blood cultures if sepsis is suspected.
- Wound cultures are often unreliable.
- Erythrocyte sedimentation rate values >70 mm/hr in conjunction with increased clinical suspicion correlate with increased likelihood of osteomyelitis; normal values do not exclude the diagnosis.

Treatment

- First-line therapy is either a penicillinase-resistant synthetic penicillin or a first-generation cephalosporin.
- Due to the prevalence of MRSA in the diabetic population, severe skin and soft tissue infections as well as all purulent infections should be treated with an antibiotic effective against MRSA.
- Criteria for admission and parental antibiotics:
  - High suspicion for osteomyelitis
    - Exposed tendon or bone *or* ability to probe to bone
  - Moderate to severe metabolic disturbances
  - Concern for deep space or necrotizing infection

Venous Stasis Ulcers

Approximately 85% of chronic lower extremity skin ulcers are a result of chronic venous insufficiency (CVI); 20% of those with CVI eventually develop ulcers.

Pathophysiology

CVI results from venous valve dysfunction, which causes venous pump failure, venous hypertension, and reflux. Prior deep venous thrombosis accounts for significant burden of valvular dysfunction resulting in CVI.

Clinical Presentation

- Location: medial aspect of the distal leg and bony prominences.
- Appearance: large, shallow ulcer with punched-out appearance.
  - Acute/early: dependent edema, erythema, and orange-brown hyperpigmentation.
  - Chronic/severe: weeping erythema and ulceration.

TABLE 22.1 *Treatment of Venous Stasis Ulcers*

Reduce Venous Hypertension	Alleviate Symptoms	Manage Secondary Bacterial Infection
Leg elevation, compression stockings	• Low- to mid-potency steroid (i.e. hydrocortisone 1% or triamcinolone 0.1%) twice daily for erythema and pruritis • Oral antihistamine for pruritis and nighttime sedation	First-generation cephalosporin, B-lactam inhibitor, OR fluoroquinolone for 7–10 days

- Symptoms: aching pain with dependency and relieved by walking/elevation, mild to severe pruritis.

Diagnosis and Evaluation

- Clinical diagnosis based on presence of venous stasis (i.e., edema, varicose veins, scarring, hyperpigmentation).
- Assess for signs of secondary infection including cellulitis and lymphangitis.

Treatment

- Treatment options for venous stasis ulcers are presented in Table 22.1.

Decubitus (Pressure) Ulcers

Pressure ulcers are often the result of chronic medical conditions, poor health, and nutritional deficiencies. Early identification of risk factors and rapid implementation of therapy are essential in reducing morbidity and mortality.

Definition

- Localized damage to the skin and underlying soft tissue, usually over a bony prominence as a result of intense and/or prolonged pressure.

Pathophysiology

- Sustained pressure over bony prominence leads to ischemia and tissue necrosis.
- Shear and friction forces impair capillary blood flow and contribute to local tissue hypoxia.
- Excess moisture leads to maceration and further skin breakdown.

Clinical Presentation

- Location:
  - Sacrum, ischial tuberosity, greater trochanter (~70%)
  - Heel and lateral malleolus (~15%–25%)
  - Occiput
- See Fig. 22.1 for a classification of pressure ulcers.

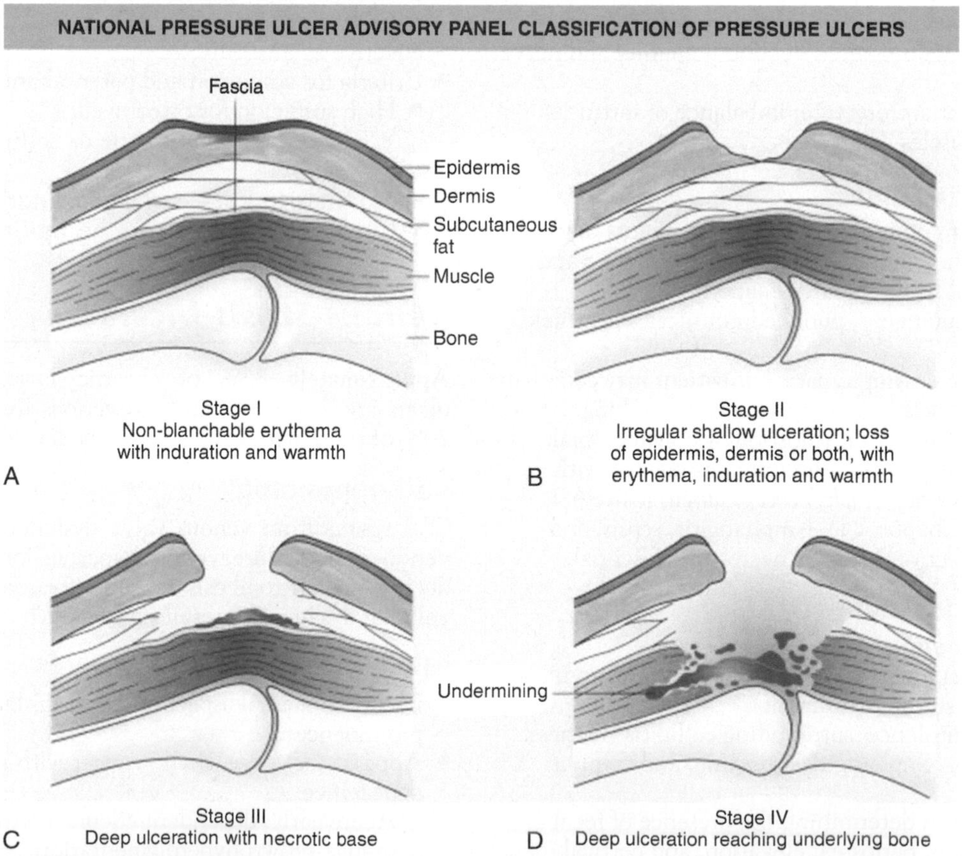

FIG. 22.1 Stages of pressure ulcers.(From Jean L. Bolognia, Julie V. Schaffer, Karynne O. Duncan, Christine J. Ko, Ulcers in "https://www.clinicalkey.com/#!/browse/book/3-s2.0-C20090416568" Dermatology Essentials, 86, 834–848, Fig 86.14).

Diagnosis and Evaluation

- Wound cultures are not indicated unless infection is suspected.
- Stage III and IV ulcers should be assessed thoroughly for sinus tracts and subcutaneous extension.
- Stage IV pressure ulcers are highly susceptible to osteomyelitis.

Treatment

- Continuous off-loading of pressure from site of ulceration.
- Saline/tap water are appropriate for wound cleaning.
- Dressing that promotes a moist wound-healing environment.
- Repositioning at least once every 2 hours for prevention.
- Surgical consult for stage III/IV ulcers (debridement, direct wound closure, skin grafts, and flap reconstruction).
- Consider admission for placement and reporting of care facility if there is high suspicion for neglect or malpractice given extent, severity, or recurrence of wounds.

SUGGESTED READINGS

Alavi, A., Sibbald, R. G., Mayer, D., Goodman, L., Botros, M., Armstrong, D. G., Woo, K., Boeni, T., Ayello, E. A., & Kirsner, R. S. (2014). Diabetic foot ulcers. Part I. Pathophysiology and prevention. *Journal of the American Academy of Dermatology, 70*(1), 1.e1–e18.

Alavi, A., Sibbald, R. G., Mayer, D., Goodman, L., Botros, M., Armstrong, D. G., Woo, K., Boeni, T., Ayello, E. A., & Kirsner, R. S. (2014). Diabetic foot ulcers. Part II. Management. *Journal of the American Academy of Dermatology, 70*(1), 21.e1–e24.

Hartoch, R. S., McManus, J. G., Knapp, S., & Buettner, M. F. (2007). Emergency management of chronic wounds. *Emergency Medicine Clinics of North America, 25*(1), 203–221.

Lipsky, B. A., Berendt, A. R., Cornia, P. B., Pile, J. C., Peters, E. J., Armstrong, D. G., Deery, H. G., Embil, J. M., Joseph, W. S., Karchmer, A. W., Pinzur, M. S., & Senneville, E. (2012). Executive summary: 2012 Infectious Diseases Society of America clinical practice guideline for the diagnosis and treatment of diabetic foot infections. *Clinical Infectious Diseases, 54*(12), 1679–1684.

Dermatitis

KEVIN WROBLEWSKI, MD, and VANESSA FRANCO, MD, PhD

Dermatitis is a group of skin disorders characterized by inflammation of the skin, which classically presents with a rash. Multiple underlying etiologies can result in different types of dermatitis, and the appearance of some types vary with age as well. History and physical examination can help differentiate among them. Most types of dermatitis are largely managed by allergen avoidance, moisturizing, and steroids.

Atopic Dermatitis/Eczema (*Fig. 23.1*)

Basic Information

- A chronic inflammatory skin condition characterized by a recurrent pruritic rash.
- Associated with environmental exposures (e.g., food, detergents).
- Associated with a personal or family history of atopic diseases (allergies, asthma).

Clinical Presentation

- Less than 2 years of age: widely distributed, erythematous, pruritic, weeping, scaly, or crusted lesions on face, scalp, trunk, and extremities.
- Older children and adults: erythematous or dry, lichenified plaques in a flexor distribution (especially the antecubital fossa and volar wrists).

Diagnosis and Evaluation

- Pruritic rash, flexor distribution, history of atopy, often begins before 2 years of age. Diagnosis is typically clinical.

Treatment

- Avoid offending agents.
- Topical emollients.
- Short course of topical corticosteroids (low potency for face).
- Treat secondary infection.

Contact Dermatitis (*Figs. 23.2 and 23.3*)

Basic Information

Allergic

- Delayed (type IV) hypersensitivity reaction caused by an exposure to an allergen.
- Common exposures: poison ivy, oak, and sumac (urushiol oil), mango skin, nickel in jewelry.

Irritant

- Caused by physical or chemical irritation of the skin.
- Often involves the hands of mechanics, housecleaners, health-care workers, and food handlers.
- Common exposures: soaps, bleach, solvents, gloves in health-care workers; nickel is a common cause in jewelry wearers.

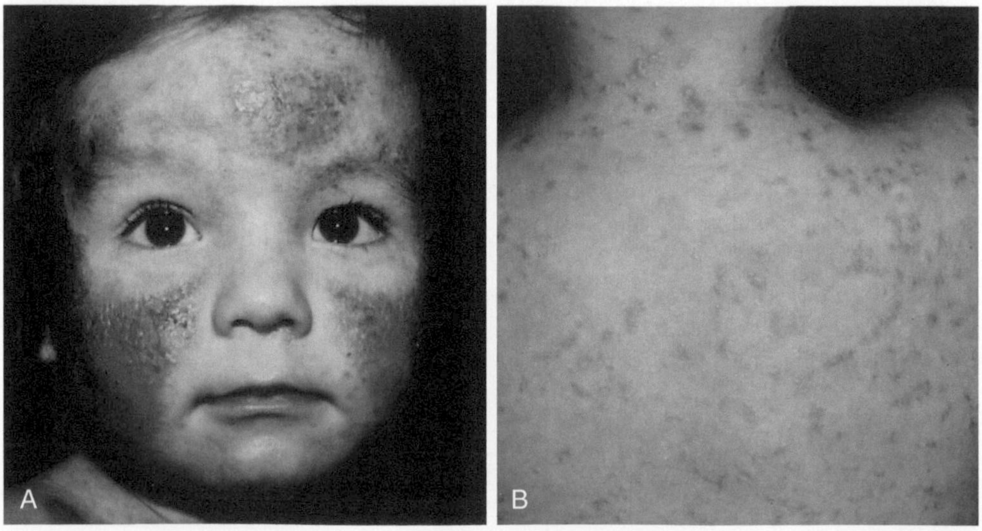

FIG. 23.1 **A** and **B**, Images of atopic dermatitis. In a young child, this condition often appears as a weeping, crusting, erythematous pruritic rash on the face, and trunk. (From Zitelli, B., McIntire, S., & Nowalk, A. (2017). *Zitelli and Davis' atlas of pediatric physical diagnosis* (7th ed., pp. 275–340, Fig. 8.11ab). Elsevier.)

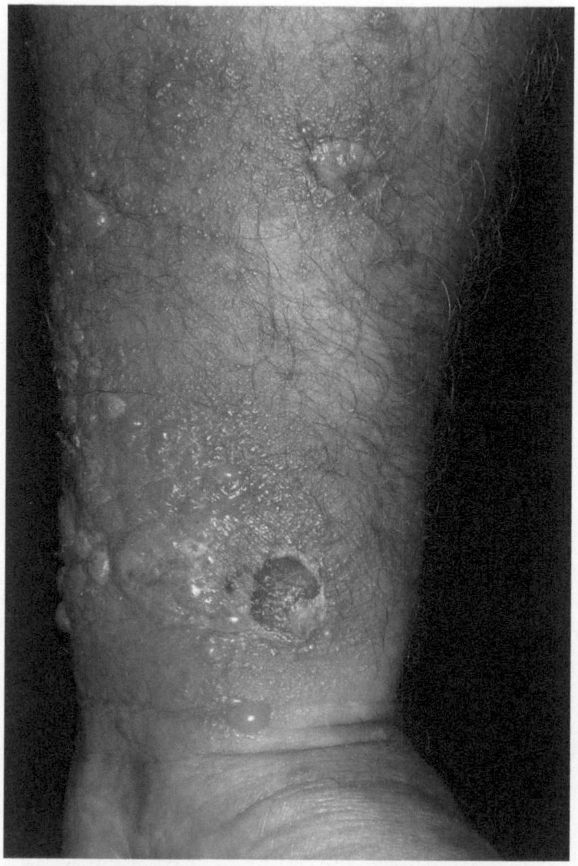

FIG. 23.2 Erythematous and vesicular appearance of a severe allergic contact dermatitis. (From Habif, T. P. (2016). *Clinical dermatology: A color guide to diagnosis and therapy* (6th ed., pp. 126–149, Fig. 4.13). Elsevier Saunders.)

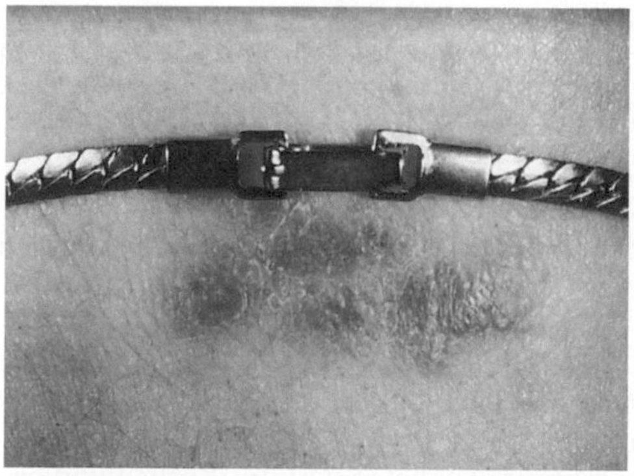

FIG. 23.3 Allergic dermatitis that is localized to a specific exposure site. (From Cohen, B. A. (2013). *Pediatric dermatology* (4th ed., p. 77). Elsevier.)

- Frequent handwashing or use of socks through multiple wet-dry cycles (eg, sweating) can cause a specific type of dermatitis called dyshidrotic eczema, which appears similar to contact dermatitis but doesn't involve contact with a specific agent. These patients should minimize wetting of extremities and use emollients.

Clinical Presentation

- Both allergic and irritant types can be characterized by pruritis, erythema, vesicles, or bullae.

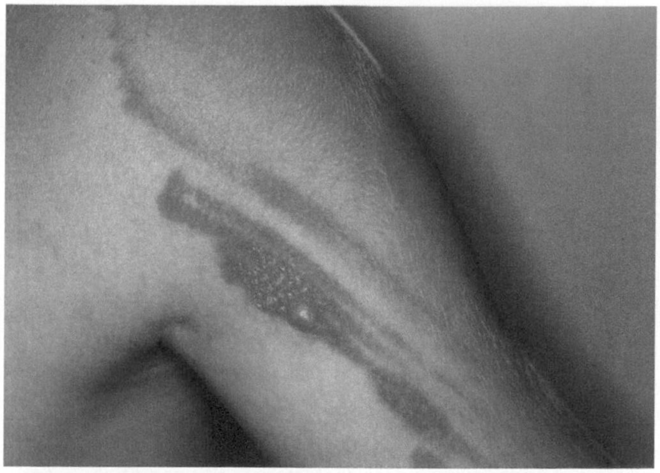

FIG. 23.4 Phytophotodermatitis. A phototoxic inflammatory skin reaction characterized by a pruritic erythematous rash that can later develop blistering and scarring. (Courtesy Jean L. Bolognia, MD. From Lim, H. W., Hawk, J. L. M., & Rosen, C. F. (2018). Photodermatologic disorders. In J. L. Bolognia, J. V. Schaffer, & L. Cerroni (Eds.), *Dermatology* (4th ed., p. 1548, Fig. 17.5), Elsevier.)

Allergic

- Linear distribution of erythema (can be serous blisters).
- Commonly seen on extremities, location of jewelry, and belt line.
- Classically localized, but can be diffuse.

Irritant

- Red, dry, chapped skin with fissuring.
- Commonly involves the hands and web spaces of fingers.
- A history of recent exposure to a botanical agent (such as citrus fruits) followed by exposure to ultraviolet light (from the sun) should raise suspicion for phytophotodermatitis, a specific form of contact dermatitis. (Fig. 23.4).

Diagnosis and Evaluation

Allergic

- Patch testing may be done to determine allergen.

Irritant

- Diagnosis of exclusion.

Treatment

- The management of both types involves topical emollients, topical corticosteroids (low potency for face), and avoidance of the offending agent.
- Refractory case or more than 20% body surface area require systemic corticosteroids (should be done in conjunction with discussion with dermatology).

Psoriasis (*Fig. 23.5*)

Basic Information

- A chronic immune-mediated inflammatory condition involving skin, joints, or both.
- Typically involves extensor surfaces.
- Multiple subtypes; chronic plaque psoriasis is most common.
- Associated with multiple comorbid conditions; 30% have psoriatic arthritis.

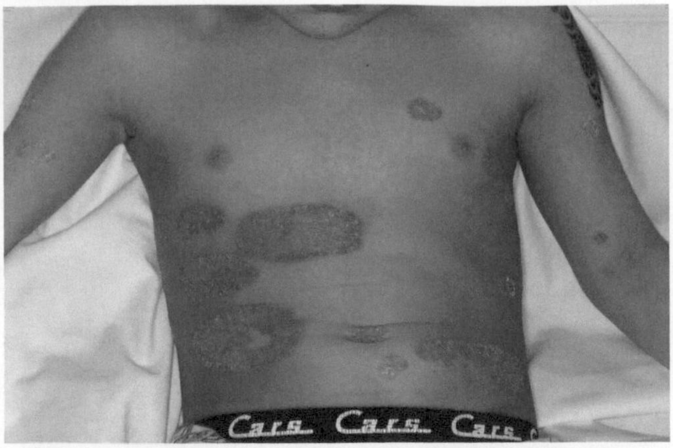

FIG. 23.5 Chronic plaque psoriasis. Silver scaling over a sharply demarcated erythematous base characterizes this condition. (From Tollefson, M. M. (2014). Diagnosis and management of psoriasis in children. *Pediatric Clinics of North America, 61*(2), 261–277.

Clinical Presentation

- Sharply demarcated erythematous plaques with overlying silvery scales.
- Typically involves extensor surfaces, elbows, knees, scalp, and gluteal cleft.
- Guttate psoriasis is a rapid onset diffuse form of small psoriatic lesions on the trunk and proximal extremities that is often associated with acute infections, such as streptococcal pharyngitis.

Diagnosis and Evaluation

- A clinical diagnosis based on history, morphology, and distribution of skin lesions.

Treatment

- Ultraviolet phototherapy, topical vitamin D3.
- Topical corticosteroids and emollients.
- May require referral for additional intensive treatment.

Seborrheic Dermatitis *(Fig. 23.6)*

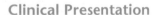

Basic Information

- A chronic inflammatory condition usually involving areas rich in sebaceous glands, such as the scalp and face.
- Dandruff is the mildest form; "cradle cap" in infants.
- Associated with *Malassezia furfur* (yeast).

Clinical Presentation

- Yellow, waxy scales on an erythematous base.
- Areas rich in sebaceous glands: scalp, face, upper trunk, and intertriginous areas.

Diagnosis and Evaluation

- Infants: thick white or yellow greasy scales on scalp or behind ears.
- Adolescents/adults: flaky, greasy, erythematous patches on the scalp, ears, eyebrows, chest, back.

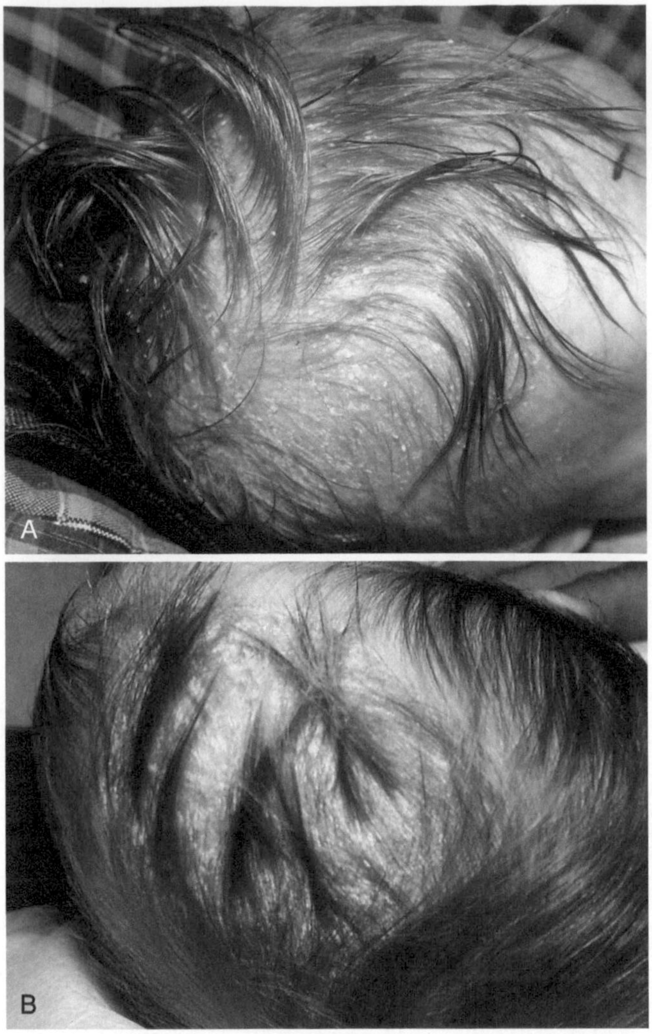

FIG. 23.6 Yellow waxy, oily rash concentrated around the sebaceous glands is characteristic of seborrheic dermatitis. (From Zitelli, B., McIntire, S., & Nowalk, A. (2017). *Zitelli and Davis' atlas of pediatric physical diagnosis* (7th ed., pp. 275–340, Fig. 8.24). Elsevier.)

- Consider evaluation for an acquired immunodeficiency syndrome, such as HIV, in patients with substantial seborrheic dermatitis beyond infancy.

Treatment

- Infants: self-resolves, can remove thick plaques with baby oil.
- Adolescents/adults: ketoconazole 2% shampoo or selenium sulfide shampoo (for scalp), ketoconazole 2% cream (for face or body).
- May consider low-potency topical corticosteroid in addition to antifungal.

SUGGESTED READINGS

Boehncke, W. H., & Schon, M. P. (2015). Psoriasis. *Lancet, 386*(9997), 983–994.

Weidinger, S., Beck, L. A., Bieber, T., Kabashima, K., & Irvine, A. D. (2018). Atopic dermatitis. *Nature Reviews. Disease Primers, 4*(1), 1.

Weston, W. L., & Howe, W. (2018). *Overview of dermatitis*. UpToDate. Available at: https://www.uptodate.com/contents/overview-of-dermatitis-eczema.

CHAPTER 24

BOARD REVIEW

Skin Infections

KEVIN WROBLEWSKI, MD, and ALAN CHIEM, MD, MPH

Skin and soft tissue infection comprise a common disorder with multiple causative organisms, including bacterial, viral, fungal, and parasitic etiologies. Many of these infections have classic clinical presentations, whereas others have significant overlap and can be more difficult to distinguish clinically. Although skin infection affects otherwise healthy individuals, a number of predisposing factors place certain individuals at greater risk. These risk factors include skin barrier disruption (e.g., abrasions, ulcers, insect bites), dermatitis (e.g., eczema, psoriasis), venous or lymphatic insufficiency, obesity, and immunosuppression (e.g., diabetes, HIV/AIDS).

Bacterial

CELLULITIS

General Principles

- Develops as a result of bacterial entry via disruption in the skin barrier.
- Involves the deeper dermis and subcutaneous tissue.
- Common organisms: group A *Streptococcus* (["Strep"], majority) and *Staphylococcus aureus* (["Staph"], both methicillin-sensitive [MSSA] and methicillin-resistant [MRSA]).
- Can present with or without systemic manifestations.

Clinical Presentation

- Erythema, edema, warmth, and tenderness of the affected site (Fig. 24.1).
- Poorly demarcated borders.
- Plus or minus purulent drainage.
- Almost always unilateral.

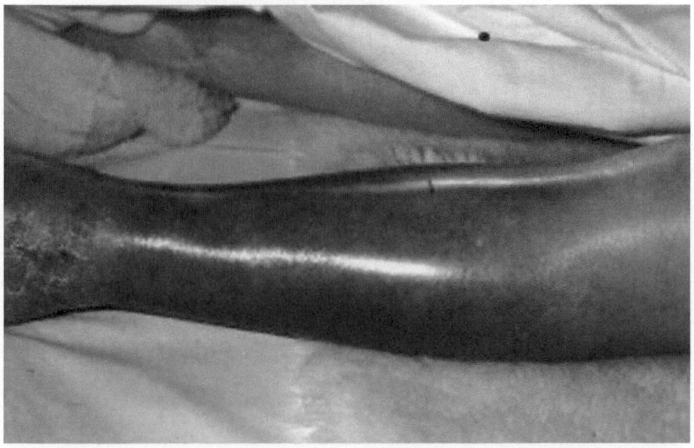

FIG. 24.1 Confluent erythematous limb with poorly demarcated borders as commonly seen with cellulitis. Cellulitis commonly affects the legs of individuals with venous stasis as is seen here. (From Lowe, G., & Tait, C. (2009). Limb pain and swelling. *Medicine, 37*(2):96–99, Fig. 1b.)

Diagnosis and Evaluation

- Clinical diagnosis based on history and examination.
- Ultrasonography if concern for abscess.
- Magnetic resonance imaging if high concern for osteomyelitis.

Treatment

- Nonpurulent (cover for *Streptococcus* and MSSA): cephalexin.
- Purulent (cover for MRSA): trimethoprim-sulfamethoxazole (TMP-SMX), clindamycin, or doxycycline.
- If central line infection or septic (cover for MRSA), admit: vancomycin. Daptomycin may also be considered for severe infections from MRSA.
- Animal bites and scratches (polymicrobial *including Staphylococcus*, *Streptococcus*, *Pasteurella multocida* and *Capnocytophaga canimorsus*): amoxicillin-clavulanate or clindamycin plus fluoroquinolone or TMP-SMX.
- Diabetic foot infections: in addition to *Staphylococcus* and *Streptococcus*, also cover for *Pseudomonas aeruginosa*.

ERYSIPELAS

General Principles

- Involves the upper dermis and superficial lymphatics.
- Most common organisms: β-hemolytic *Streptococcus*.
- Can present with or without systemic manifestations.
- Severe systemic symptoms should prompt further evaluation.

Clinical Presentation

- Hallmark is a raised erythematous lesion with well-demarcated borders (Fig. 24.2).
- Nonpurulent.
- Almost always unilateral or localized.
- Often involves the face of children or the elderly.

Diagnosis and Evaluation

- Clinical diagnosis based on history and examination.

Treatment

- Typically can be treated in outpatient setting.
- Penicillin or ampicillin for first-line therapy.
- If penicillin allergy: clindamycin or (if the patient can tolerate cephalosporins) cephalexin.
- If systemic symptoms or in high-risk groups (infants, the elderly): cefazolin or ceftriaxone; consider admission for facial infection.

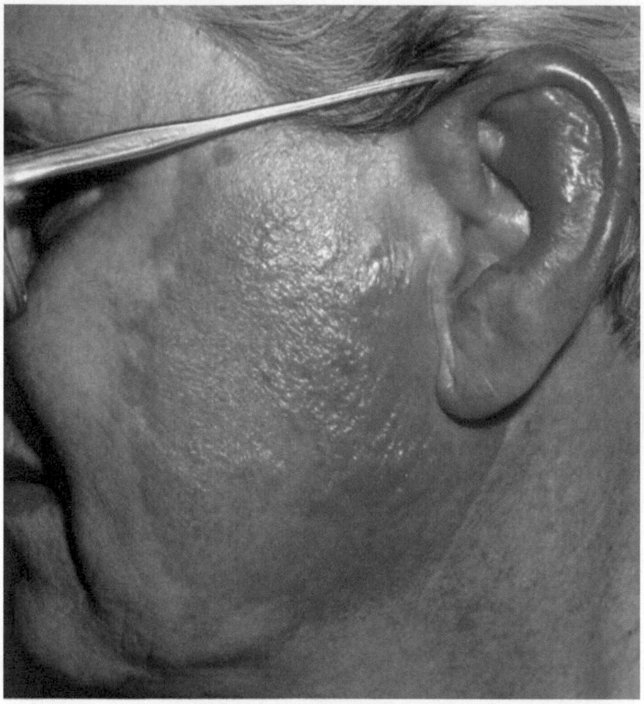

FIG. 24.2 Confluent erythematous patch with well-demarcated borders commonly seen in erysipelas. Erysipelas often involves the face of children and the elderly, and commonly involves the ear as seen here. (From James, W., Elston, D., Treat, J., Rosenbach, M., & Neuhaus, I. (2019). *Andrews' diseases of the skin: clinical dermatology* (13th ed., Fig. 14–16a). Elsevier.)

ABSCESS

General Principles

- A collection of purulent material within the deep dermis or subcutaneous tissue.
- Most common organism is *S. aureus* (MSSA or MRSA).
- MRSA risk factors: recent hospitalization or long-term care facility, recent surgery, hemodialysis, intravenous (IV) drug use, and immunocompromised. However, MRSA is also common in immunocompetent patients without risk factors, and is community-acquired.
- Systemic symptoms are uncommon.
- Patients may have history of the same or have an abscess on more than one site.

Clinical Presentation

- Painful, tender, fluctuant, erythematous nodule (Fig. 24.3).
- Plus or minus surrounding cellulitis.

Diagnosis and Evaluation

- Clinical diagnosis based on history and examination.
- Ultrasonography can help evaluate.

Treatment

- Incision and drainage.
- Antibiotics: (TMP-SMX), clindamycin, or doxycycline.
- If septic or indwelling medical device: vancomycin and admission.

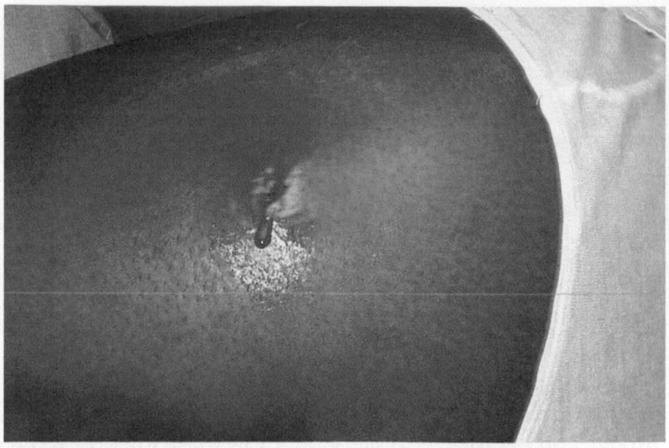

FIG. 24.3 A raised, erythematous fluctuant mass characteristic of an abscess. This example has spontaneous drainage. (From Roberts, J. (2018). *Roberts and Hedges' clinical procedures in emergency medicine and acute care* (7th ed., Fig. 37.1). Elsevier.)

NECROTIZING FASCIITIS AND CLOSTRIDIAL MYONECROSIS

See Chapter 59. Systemic Bacterial Infections.

IMPETIGO

General Principles

- Superficial bacterial infection.
- Contagious and easily spread.
- Most common organisms: *S. aureus* (majority) and group A *Streptococcus*. (still quite common).

Clinical Presentation

- Vesicles, pustules, and bullae with adherent golden (often described as honey-colored) crust (Fig. 24.4).

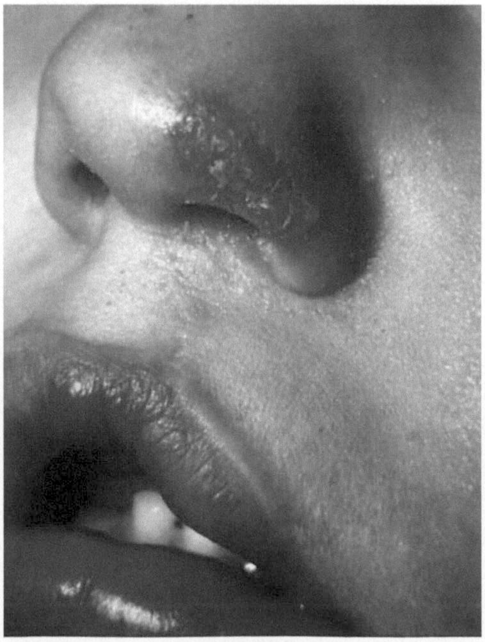

FIG. 24.4 The characteristic honey-colored crusted lesion of impetigo. Commonly seen around the mouth and nose of children as demonstrated here. (From Zitelli, B., McIntire, S., & Nowalk, A. (2017). *Zitelli and Davis' atlas of pediatric physical diagnosis* (7th ed., Fig. 13.22). Elsevier.)

- Commonly seen on the face or extremities of children (2 to 5 years of age).

Diagnosis and Evaluation

- Clinical diagnosis based on history and examination.

Treatment

- Mild (limited to a few lesions or a small area): topical mupirocin.
- Moderate (numerous lesions): oral cephalexin or dicloxacillin.

Fungal

CANDIDA

General Principles

- *Candida* is a common organism of the human microbiome, but can overgrow and lead to infection.
- Common *Candida* infections include diaper dermatitis, intertrigo, and vulvovaginitis.
- Vulvovaginitis is often preceded by recent antibiotic use.

Clinical Presentation

- *Candida* diaper dermatitis: erythematous papules and plaques with satellite lesions over the buttocks and areas in contact with the diaper (Fig. 24.5).
- Intertrigo: erythematous papules and plaques with satellite lesions of the intertriginous areas (such as mammary folds, pannus, genitals, gluteal cleft).
- Diaper dermatitis and intertrigo could be an irritant contact dermatitis, but erythematous papules and plaques with satellite lesions suggest primary or concomitant fungal infection.
- Vulvovaginitis: thick, white, cottage cheese-like vaginal discharge; often with pruritus, pain, and/or dysuria.

Diagnosis and Evaluation

- Clinical diagnosis based on history and examination.
- Wood's lamp examination and potassium hydroxide preparation can help identify a fungal etiology.

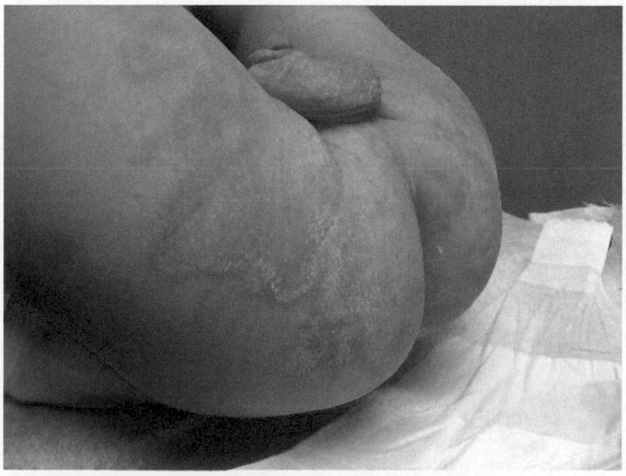

FIG. 24.5 *Candida* diaper dermatitis. This condition is apparent by the plaque with well-defined borders and satellite lesions. (From Zitelli, B., McIntire, S., & Nowalk, A. (2017). *Zitelli and Davis' atlas of pediatric physical diagnosis* (7th ed., Fig. 8.46). Elsevier.)

Treatment

- *Candida* diaper dermatitis: for mild infections, can use topical antifungal cream or nystatin powder. For more severe infection, treat with a topical combination cream containing nystatin, zinc oxide, moisturizer, and steroid.
- Intertrigo: topical azole antifungal cream (e.g., ketoconazole) and proper hygiene; keep the area dry.
- Vulvovaginitis: oral fluconazole (single dose). Pregnant patients: topical clotrimazole or miconazole (oral azoles are contraindicated in first trimester).

TINEA INFECTIONS

General Principles

- A cutaneous dermatophyte infection of the body, specifically epidermis.
- Other forms of tinea affect the scalp (capitis), groin (cruris), feet (pedis), nail (unguium), or other skin on the body (corporis).
- Trichophyton rubrum is the most common cause of tinea corporis.

Clinical Presentation

- Tinea corporis presents as annular (ring-shaped) lesions; oval, erythematous, scaly plaque with central clearing and raised border (Fig. 24.6).
- Tinea capitis presents with erythematous papule or plaque with broken hair follicles or alopecia plus or minus kerion (an abscess caused by a fungal infection).

Diagnosis and Evaluation

- Clinical diagnosis based on history and examination.
- Segmented hyphae seen on potassium hydroxide preparation.

Treatment

- Topical azoles (e.g., ketoconazole) or allylamines (e.g., naftifine).
- Topical nystatin is not effective.

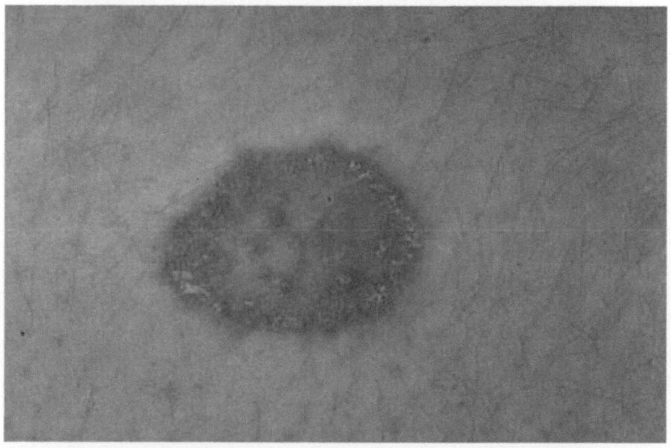

FIG. 24.6 An erythematous lesion with a scaly border, consistent with tinea corporis. With time, the lesion characteristically develops central clearing and appears as an erythematous ring, hence the term "ringworm." (From Hay, R. J. (2015). Dermatophytosis (ringworm) and other superficial mycoses. In J. E. Bennett R. Dolin, & M. J. Blaser (Eds.), *Mandell, Douglas, and Bennett's principles and practice of infectious diseases* (updated 8th ed., (pp. 2985–2994.e2, Fig. 268.1). Elsevier.)

- Oral anti-fungals (e.g., griseofulvin) are needed for scalp and nail infections.
- Do not incise and drain a kerion.

Viral

MOLLUSCUM CONTAGIOSUM

General Principles

- Localized skin infection caused by poxvirus.
- Transmitted by direct skin contact.
- Commonly seen in children, often involving the hands and face.
- In adults, especially if in the genital region, this condition is sexually transmitted.

Clinical Presentation

- Flesh-colored papules with central umbilication (Fig. 24.7).

Diagnosis and Evaluation

- Clinical diagnosis based on history and examination.
- Biopsy can confirm diagnosis when necessary.

Treatment

- Usually self-limited, no treatment necessary.
- Genital lesions treated with cryotherapy, podophyllin, or podophyllotoxin.

HUMAN PAPILLOMAVIRUS: WARTS

General Principles

- Human papillomaviruses (HPV) infect epithelial skin and mucous membranes and have many subtypes.
- HPV 6 and 11 cause anogenital warts (condyloma acuminatum).
- HPV 1 causes plantar warts.
- HPV types 16 and 18 also cause up to 70% of cervical cancers.

Clinical Presentation

- White or skin-colored hyperkeratotic papules (Fig. 24.8).
- Can be dome-shaped, cauliflower-shaped, or flat.
- Often with thrombosed capillaries that appear as black dots.
- Typical locations: genitals, hands, soles of the feet.

Diagnosis and Evaluation

- Clinical diagnosis based on history and examination.
- Biopsy can confirm diagnosis when necessary.

Treatment

- Approximately 30% self-resolve without therapy.
- Cryotherapy or topical agents (e.g., podophyllin).
- Surgical excision for severe cases.

HERPES SIMPLEX VIRUS (HSV)-1: ORAL HERPES AND HERPETIC WHITLOW

General Principles

- Highly prevalent (50%–90% have antibodies or past infection) in adults.
- Typically HSV-1 causes facial and oral infection, whereas HSV-2 causes genital infections, but there is significant overlap.
- HSV lies dormant in the sensory ganglia of the face (V1-V3) with recurrent, painful vesicular lesions during reactivation.

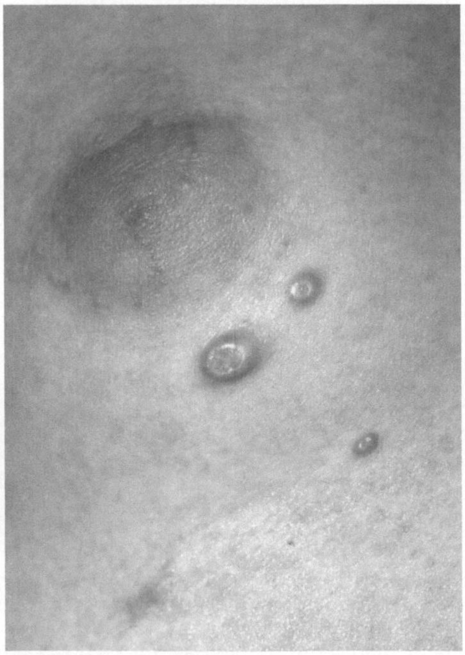

FIG. 24.7 Firm, skin-colored papule with classic dimpling is classic for molluscum contagiosum. (From James, W., Elston, D., Treat, J., Rosenbach, M., & Neuhaus, I. (2019). *Andrews' diseases of the skin: Clinical dermatology* (13th ed., Fig. 19.32). Elsevier.)

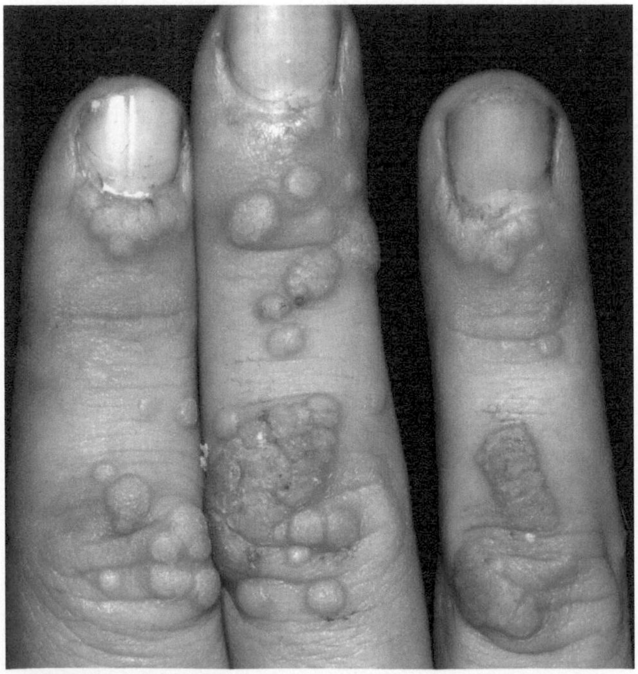

FIG. 24.8 Common warts of the back of the hands. Characteristic of multiple subtypes of human papillomavirus (HPV). (From Habif, T. P. (2015). *Clinical dermatology A color guide to diagnosis and therapy* (6th ed., Fig. 12.6). Elsevier.)

- Reactivation is associated with recent stress, illness, or temperature change, sunlight, or medications (e.g., steroids).

Clinical Presentation

- In primary infection, a flu-like illness may be present for 1 to 2 weeks.
- In infections owing to reactivation, patients appear well and without systemic signs of infection.
- Most commonly seen as grouped vesicular lesions typically in the perioral region (V3), especially involving the oral mucosa and/or vermillion border.
- Classically differs from varicella zoster virus (VZV) infection in age distribution (younger in HSV vs. elderly in VZV), nondermatomal distribution (HSV) vs. dermatomal distribution (VZV), and HSV is less likely to have systemic symptoms and/or cranial nerve or central nervous system involvement than VZV.
- HSV keratitis is the most common corneal viral infection in the United States, and a major cause of blindness due to corneal scarring worldwide.
  - Typically spread from oral (V3) to ophthalmic (VI) branch of trigeminal ganglion.
  - Presents with eye pain, blurry vision, tearing, and/or conjunctival infection.
- Herpetic whitlow is an HSV infection of the pulp or lateral aspect of the distal phalanx.
  - Typically occurs through direct inoculation.

Diagnosis and Evaluation

- Clinical diagnosis and history of recurrent infection is typically sufficient.
- Patients with potential eye involvement should receive a full ophthalmic examination, including slit lamp and fluorescein to look for dendritic lesions.
- Aspiration of vesicular fluid for culture or Tzanck smear may be helpful, but sensitivities are less than 60%.
- Polymerase chain reaction of the fluid is highly sensitive and specific, if clinical diagnosis is in question.

Treatment

- There is no curative agent for HSV infection.
- Uncomplicated oral herpes infection and herpetic whitlow typically self-resolve in 2 to 4 weeks.
- Oral acyclovir, topical acyclovir or penciclovir, and/or topical steroids have limited efficacy, with reduced healing times of 1 to 2 days.
- Herpetic whitlow should not be incised and drained.
- In severe infections or infections involving immunocompromised patients, oral or IV antivirals should be administered.
- Oral and ophthalmic antiviral agents are indicated for HSV keratitis, as well as urgent ophthalmology follow-up.

Parasitic

SCABIES

General Principles

- Caused by infestation of the skin by the mite *Sarcoptes scabiei*.
- Symptoms can be delayed up to 6 weeks from time of infection.
- Easily spread, therefore environmental measures and treatment of cohabitants are recommended.

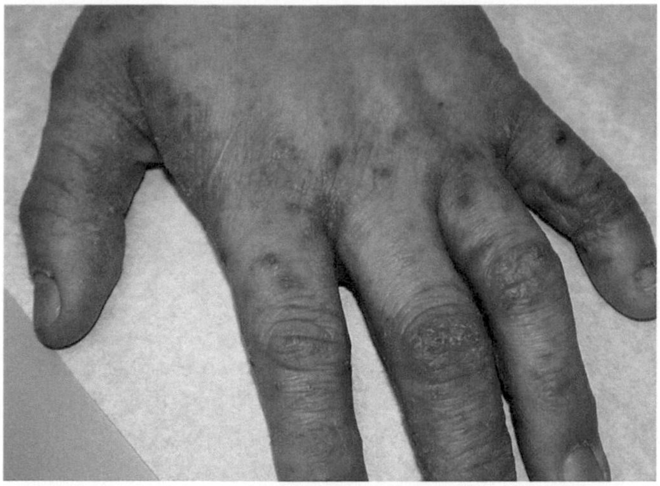

FIG. 24.9 Classic scabies involving the web spaces of the hands. (From Hills, J. L., et al. (2007). Head lice and scabies. In L. B. Zaoutis & V. W. Chiang (Eds.), *Comprehensive pediatric hospital medicine* (pp. 976–980, Fig. 154.4). Mosby.)

Clinical Presentation

- Erythematous papules or raised linear lesions involving the interdigital webs and extensor surfaces (Fig. 24.9).
- More generalized distribution of lesions in infants and children, often involving flexural surfaces, lower back, buttocks, and groin.
- Extremely pruritic.

Diagnosis and Evaluation

- Clinical diagnosis based on history and examination.
- Skin scrapings can be obtained and samples visualized under a microscope to confirm the diagnosis, but clinical diagnosis is often sufficient.

Treatment

- Topical permethrin 5% or oral ivermectin are first-line therapy.
  - Avoid ivermectin in children under age 5 years as well as in pregnant or lactating patients.
- Cohabitants should be treated as well.
- Clothes and bed sheets should be washed in hot water and dried at high temperature.
- Habitats should be cleaned and vacuumed.

LICE

General Principles

- Three species of lice affect humans:
  - Pediculosis humanus capitis: head louse, "lice".
  - Pediculosis humanus corporis: body louse, "bed bugs".
  - Pediculosis humanus pubis: crab louse, "crabs" (not discussed in this chapter).
- Transmission is by direct contact (lice do not jump or use pets as vectors).

Clinical Presentation

- Pediculosis capitis: nits (louse eggs) or adult lice look like white, blue, or black dots at the base of hair shafts

24

and cause intense pruritus, commonly affecting children.

- Pediculosis corporis: cause erythematous macules and wheals, and pruritus.

Diagnosis and Evaluation

- Diagnosed by clinical presentation and visual inspection.

Treatment

- First-line therapy is thorough bathing and hot-water washing of infested clothing and linen.
- A single 8- to 10-hour application of permethrin can be added, in addition to the above therapy for body louse.
- A 10-minute application of permethrin to dry hair (for hair louse) and to the genitals and perianal areas (for pubic louse) on day 1 and day 9 is effective.
- Children do not need to be excluded from school.
- Household members should be examined.
- Prophylactic treatment of individuals who share bedding with affected individual.

SUGGESTED READINGS

Life-threatening dermatoses. In A. B. Wolfson, R. L. Cloutier, G. W. Hendey, L. J. Ling, C. L. Rosen, & J. J. Schaider (Eds.). *Harwood – Nuss' clinical practice of emergency medicine* (6th ed.). Wolters Kluwer.

Skin and soft tissue infections. In A. B. Wolfson, R. L. Cloutier, G. W. Hendey, L. J. Ling, C. L. Rosen, & J. J. Schaider (Eds.). *Harwood – Nuss' clinical practice of emergency medicine* (6th ed.). Wolters Kluwer.

Childhood Exanthems

ALEXANDRA McLEROY-WALLACE, MD, and ALAN CHIEM, MD, MPH

Many classic illnesses seen in childhood are associated with fever and rash. Most of these are viral in origin and can be diagnosed based on history and physical examination alone. Although the majority are self-limited, it is important to distinguish them from one another to properly monitor for associated complications.

Measles (Rubeola)

Basic Information

- Highly communicable viral illness (90% of susceptible individuals exposed will develop measles) transmitted as a respiratory infection (droplets).
- Patients actively shed virus beginning 2 to 3 days from initial infection (often before symptoms present) until 3 to 4 days following the appearance of the rash.

Presentation

- Average incubation period of 10 to 14 days (range 7 to 21) followed by:
  - High fever (103°F–105°F)
  - Toxic appearance (milder in those partially vaccinated, receiving postexposure immunoglobin, and with residual maternal antibodies).
- Classic triad of "3C's": cough, coryza, conjunctivitis (bilateral and nonexudative), followed in 2 to 4 days by maculopapular rash on the head/neck with spread to the trunk.
- Koplik spots (Fig. 25.1): 1 to 3 mm white or gray-blue spots on an erythematous base found on buccal mucosa, hard and soft palate, which precedes the rash by about 48 hours.
  - Pathognomonic for measles, but absence does not rule out measles.
- Complications occur in 30%-40% of cases, especially in very young, very old, pregnant, immunocompromised (particularly T-cell deficiency), or individuals with poor nutritional status. Mortality is low in the United States (0.2% of infected), but is up to 25% in developing countries, disproportionately affecting malnourished children under 12 months of age. Those with vitamin A deficiency are at highest risk.
- Gastrointestinal tract: diarrhea, the most common complication (~8%), and stomatitis.
- Otitis media (5%–10%): almost exclusively in children.
- Pneumonia and pneumonitis (6% including viral and superimposed bacterial): this is the most common cause of measles-associated death (60%, highest among young children).
- Neurologic
  - Acute encephalitis (0.1% of cases) occurs within a few days of rash; approximately 15% mortality and residual neurologic damage in up to 25% of those who develop this complication. Seizures are reported in 0.6%–0.7%.
  - Acute disseminated encephalomyelitis is a postinfectious autoimmune demyelinating disease occurring in about 1 per 1,000 cases.
  - Subacute sclerosing panencephalitis (SSPE) is a rare (5 to 10 per million measles cases), late (5 to 10 years after infection) complication presenting with progressive neurologic deterioration, ataxia, myoclonus, and death.

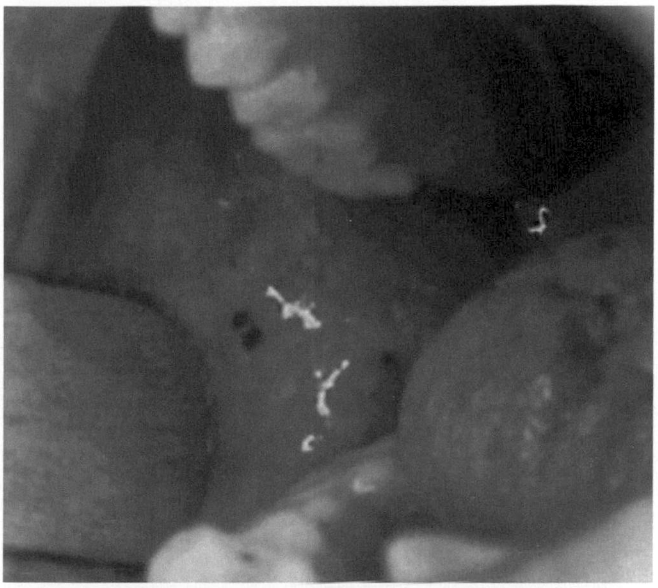

FIG. 25.1 Koplik spots. (From Patel, L. M., et al. (2011). Cutaneous signs of systemic disease. *Clinical Dermatology,* 29(5), 511–522.)

- "Atypical measles" occurs in those who received inactivated measles vaccine (an inactivated ["killed"] measles virus [KMV] was given in parts of the United States 1963–1967) and are subsequently exposed.
  - Presentation is similar, except rash typically starts on the ankles/wrists and can have vesicular component and edema of the extremities.
  - Revaccination with live vaccine is recommended for prevention.

Diagnosis

- Primarily clinical presentation.
- RT-PCR from nasopharyngeal, throat and urine specimens and serum serology (positive IgM + IgG is definitive) should be obtained from every patient with clinically suspected measles.

- Viral cultures should be submitted to the state public health laboratory or Centers for Disease Control and Prevention (CDC).
- Subacute sclerosing panencephalitis is confirmed by measles antibodies in cerebrospinal fluid and markedly elevated serum antibodies.

Treatment

- Live measles, mumps, and rubella vaccine is highly effective for prevention (95%–99% when given in one or two doses beginning at 12 months of age or older), but has no role in acute treatment.
- Immunocompromised individuals, pregnant women, and infants less than 1 year of age should receive immunoglobulin (0.25 to 0.5 mL/kg intramuscular) within 6 days of exposure; the live vaccine is not recommended in these groups.
- Notify the health department and/or CDC (most important to limit spread of an outbreak).
- Treatment is supportive care and management of complications. Place patients on respiratory droplet precautions.
- Children should be kept out of school for at least 4 days following appearance of rash.
- Vitamin A has been found to reduce mortality by up to 19% when administered as at least two doses of 200,000 IU for children older than 1 year or 100,000 IU for infants.

Rubella (German Measles)

Basic Information

- Mild febrile illness with incubation period 12 to 23 days.
- Highly communicable via respiratory droplets one week prior and up to four days after rash onset.
- Infection during pregnancy can lead to congenital rubella syndrome (a devastating congenital syndrome); infants with this syndrome may shed virus for more than 1 year.

Presentation

- Fever, malaise, and headache accompanied by:
  - Lymphadenopathy that is postauricular, cervical, and occipital;
  - Pink to red maculopapular rash spreading cranial to caudal, which may coalesce on the trunk.
- Congenital rubella syndrome: hearing loss, cataracts, retinopathy, mental retardation, cardiac abnormalities, premature delivery, fetal death.

Diagnosis

- Primarily clinical presentation.
- As with measles, suspected cases should be reported to the CDC or health department, and samples (throat, the best source; nasal, or urine polymerase chain reaction or serum IgM/IgG) submitted for confirmation.

Treatment

- Supportive care.
- Prevented by measles, mumps, and rubella vaccine, given at 12 to 15 months of age, with a second dose at age 4 to 6 years.
- Avoid contact with susceptible pregnant women.

Roseola (Exanthem Subitum aka Sixth Disease)

Basic Information

- Viral illness caused by human herpesvirus-6 with an incubation period of 5 to 15 days.
- Most common childhood exanthem in children 6 months to 2 years of age.

Presentation

- High fever for 3 to 5 days, then maculopapular rash after defervescence.
- Rose-colored maculopapular rash that rarely coalesces, beginning on the trunk and spreading to the neck and extremities.
- Children are generally well appearing despite fever, unlike with measles.
- May be associated with febrile seizures because fever typically has an abrupt onset rising to 39°C –41°C.

Diagnosis

- Clinical presentation

Treatment

- Antipyretics, supportive care

Erythema Infectiosum (Fifth Disease aka "Slapped Cheek")

Basic Information

- Caused by parvovirus B19 respiratory droplet infection with an incubation period of 4 to 14 days.
- Generally occurs in children ages 4 to 10 years of age.
- Tends to occur in epidemics, often in school outbreaks in late winter/early spring.
- Patients with sickle cell disease are at risk for aplastic crisis.
- Immunocompromised patients can develop chronic red cell aplasia.
- Pregnant patients exposed to parvovirus B19 should be monitored closely for the development of nonimmune fetal hydrops.

Presentation

- 20%–30% of patients are asymptomatic.
- Mild upper respiratory viral syndrome with low-grade fever, myalgia, arthralgia.
- "Slapped-cheek" rash (Fig. 25.2): striking erythema of the cheeks appears abruptly.
- Patients are no longer contagious at the time that the rash appears and may attend school.
- May be followed by a lacy erythematous rash on the extremities spreading to the trunk that may recur up to several weeks with heat and sunlight exposure.
- Adults are more likely to develop diffuse arthralgia and arthritis with a less-classic rash.

Diagnosis

- Clinical presentation with suspected exposure (e.g., school-aged children and close contacts).
- Serology not necessary, but IgM/IgG can be used to identify exposed pregnant women.

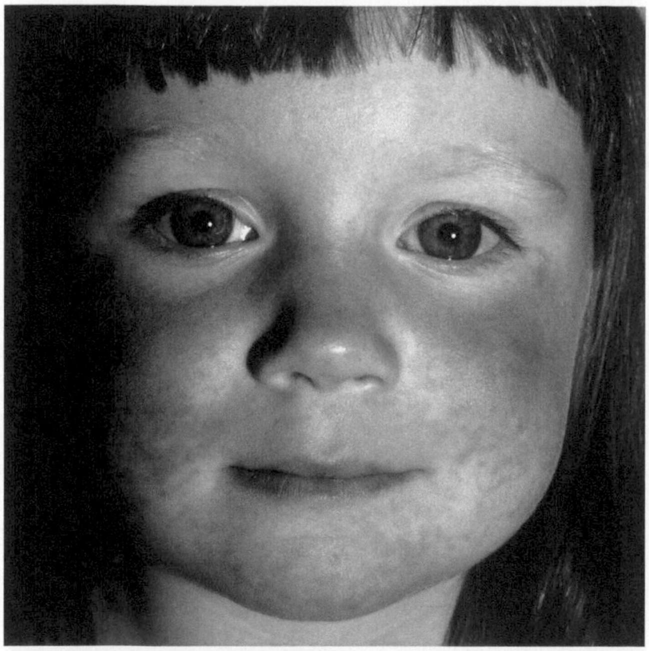

FIG. 25.2 Slapped cheek facial rash. (From Dinulos, J. G.H. (2018). Exanthems and drug reactions. In T. P. Habif, J. G. H. Dinulos, M. S. Chapman, & K. A. Zug (Eds.), *Skin disease: Diagnosis and treatment* (4th ed., pp. 282–305, Fig. 10.8). Elsevier.)

Treatment

- Immunocompetent individuals require only supportive treatment.
- Those who develop aplastic crisis may require transfusions and/or immune globulin (IVIG).
- Isolate pregnant women.

Scarlet Fever

Basic Information

- Caused by group A β-hemolytic Streptococci.

Presentation

- Abrupt onset fever, malaise, pharyngitis with characteristic "strawberry tongue" (Fig. 25.3).
- Followed in 12 to 24 hours by a rough "sandpaper" rash starting on the chest with linear petechia in the skin folds (Pastia lines) and circumoral pallor.
- Resolution of symptoms typically culminates with desquamation of the affected areas.
- Late complications:
  - Rheumatic heart disease (2 to 4 weeks postinfection).
  - Post-streptococcal glomerulonephritis (PSGN); typically 1 to 3 weeks after streptococcal pharyngitis, and 3 to 6 weeks following group A β-hemolytic Streptococci skin infection.

Diagnosis

- Clinical, with throat culture for diagnostic confirmation of group A streptococcus.

Treatment

- Penicillin VK, intramuscular benzathine penicillin one-time dose 1.2 million units (for patients more than 30 kg, 0.6 million units if less than 30 kg), or erythromycin if penicillin-allergic. Oral penicillin is also an option.

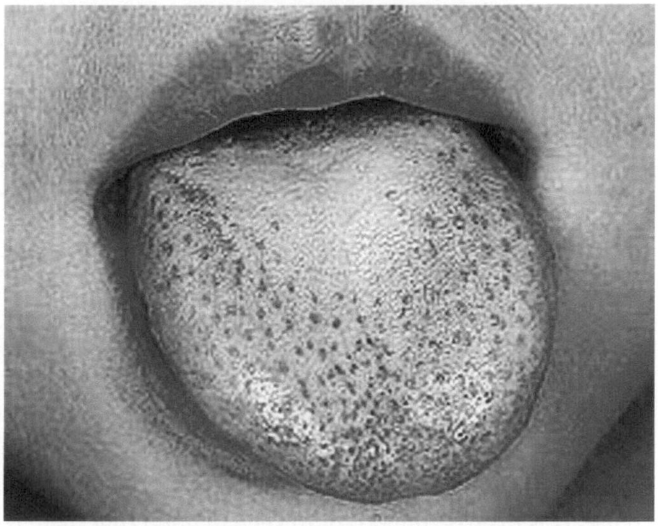

FIG. 25.3 Characteristic strawberry tongue of scarlet fever

  - Protects against development of rheumatic heart disease, but does not prevent PSGN.
  - Children can return to school 24 hours after initial antibiotic dose.

Coxsackieviruses

Basic Information

- Coxsackie A/B and echovirus are enteroviruses spread by contact with nasopharyngeal secretions, fecal material, or vesicular fluid.
- Highly contagious, particularly in the first week of illness; outbreaks often in the summer and early fall among groups with close contact (schools, daycare, military barracks).

Presentation

- Hand-foot-mouth (typically caused by coxsackie virus A16): febrile disease with vesicular lesions of the palms, soles, and/or oropharynx, typically in children younger than 10 years of age.
- Herpangina (coxsackie A): febrile illness with vesicular rash on the buccal mucosa and soft palate causing severe dysphagia.
- Other associated conditions include upper respiratory illness, interstitial pneumonia, diarrhea and gastroenteritis, hemolytic-uremic syndrome, aortitis, pancreatitis, and orchitis.

Treatment

- Supportive care and management of complications primarily related to dehydration.

SUGGESTED READINGS

Bonfante, G., & Dunn, A. (2016). Rashes in infants and children. In Tintinalli, J. E., Stapczynski, J. S., Ma, O. J., Yealy, D. M., Meckler, G. D., & Cline, D. M. (Eds.), (2015). *Tintinalli's emergency medicine: A comprehensive study guide* (8th ed., pp. 934–1041). McGraw-Hill Education.

Chapter 130, Viral Illnesses. (2013). In Marx, J., Hockberger, R., & Walls, R. (Eds.), *Rosen's emergency medicine: Concepts and clinical practice* (8th ed., pp. 1718–1741). Elsevier Saunders.

www.CDC.gov

Maculopapular Lesions

ALEXANDRA McLEROY-WALLACE, MD, and ALAN CHIEM, MD, MPH

A vast number of skin lesions can be classified as "maculopapular," ranging in etiology from infectious to allergic to autoimmune, and even malignancy. Identifying rashes can often greatly aid in the diagnosis of systemic illness and it is worth spending some time to differentiate these lesions based on appearance, pattern of distribution, and time course. It is likewise important to keep in mind that there is a virtually endless list of medications, infections, and exposures that can trigger dermatologic reactions and the ones listed below merely represent the most common etiologies.

Definitions

- Macule: flat lesion with color different from the surrounding skin, <1 cm.
- Papule: elevated skin lesion less than 1 cm in diameter.
- Patch: a macule with surface changes (e.g., scale) >/= 1 cm.
- Plaque: elevated skin lesion more than 1 cm in diameter and depth.
- Morbilliform: a macular rash with areas of confluence.

Erythema Multiforme

Basic Information

- A rare, acute immunogenic response occurring predominantly in young adults in response to:
  - Infection (90%): vast majority attributed to herpes simplex virus (HSV), followed by *Mycoplasma pneumoniae* (in children) and other infections triggering cell-mediated response.
  - Medications (less than 10%): nonsteroidal anti inflammatory drugs (NSAIDs), sulfonamides, antiepileptics, among many others.
  - Other (less than 1%): malignancy, inflammatory bowel disease, menstruation.

Clinical Presentation

- Painless erythematous macules, papules, vesicles, or bullae found primarily on the extensor surfaces, which may spread centripetally, characterized by:
  - **Targetoid lesions** with dark central papule or vesicle surrounded by a pale zone and a halo of erythema (Fig. 26.1) that may vary from patient to patient and often evolve over the course of illness.
  - **Multiforme** refers to the many varied appearances of the rash; typically the rash will be similar within a patient, but may evolve over time.
  - Commonly involves distal extremities; may involve palms or soles.
  - Mucosal involvement: oral lesions appear in up to 70% of patients.

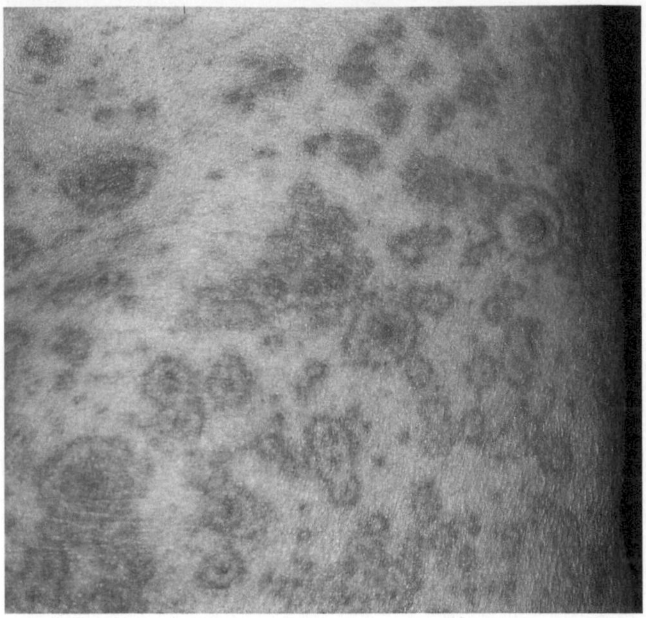

FIG. 26.1 Targetoid lesions of erythema multiforme. (From Avarbock, A., & Jorizzo, J. L. (2017). Erythema multiforme, Stevens–Johnson syndrome, and toxic epidermal necrolysis. In J. P. Callen, J. L. Jorizzo, J. J. Zone, W. W. Piette, M. A. Rosenbach, & R. A. Vleugels (Eds.), *Dermatological signs of systemic disease*, (5th ed., pp. 87–92, Fig. 11.1). Elsevier.)

  - Rarely accompanied by prodrome of malaise, low-grade fever, arthralgia, myalgia.
  - Recurrence: in rare cases, individuals experience multiple episodes yearly.

Diagnosis

- Clinical: there are no laboratory tests to confirm erythema multiforme. However, histopathologic studies and positive HSV or M. *pneumoniae* polymerase chain reaction can help to differentiate from Stevens-Johnson syndrome, fixed drug eruption, bullous pemphigoid, urticaria, and so forth.

Treatment

- Majority are self-limited, typically resolving in 2 to 3 weeks. Additionally:
  - Discontinue any inciting agents.
  - Symptomatic treatment with antihistamines or topical corticosteroids for pruritus.
  - It is appropriate to treat with antivirals or antibiotics when HSV or M. *pneumoniae* are suspected, although this will not alter the clinical course.
  - Corticosteroids in severe refractory cases are controversial.

- Those with extensive disease and mucosal involvement limiting oral hydration may require hospital admission for hydration, close monitoring, and specialty consult, as needed.
- Substantial blistering of lesions, extensive mucous membrane involvement, ill-appearance, and prodromal phase of fever and malaise should prompt consideration of Stevens Johnson Syndrome.

Erythema Nodosum

Basic Information

- A delayed hypersensitivity reaction, pathogenesis of which is not fully understood, but which has been associated with a large number of etiologies, including:
  - Medication: penicillins (especially amoxicillin), sulfonamides, oral contraceptives.
  - Infection: tuberculosis, coccidioidomycosis, histoplasmosis, β-hemolytic streptococci, *Yersinia enterocolitica, Chlamydia* spp. Viral hepatitis.
  - Malignancy: leukemia, Hodgkin lymphoma, metastatic carcinoid tumor.
  - Miscellaneous: sarcoidosis, inflammatory bowel disease, Behçet disease, pregnancy, idiopathic (40%).

Clinical Presentation

- An inflammatory reaction of the dermis and adipose tissue causing tender purple-red subcutaneous nodules, generally on the anterior shins (Fig. 26.2).
  - May be preceded by fever/arthralgia, fatigue, upper respiratory infection symptoms.
  - 3 to 6 times more common in women.

Diagnosis

- Skin lesions with mildly elevated serum white blood cell count, erythrocyte sedimentation rate, C-reactive protein (CRP), and appropriate diagnostics to evaluate for suspected precipitant (e.g., consider antistreptolysin O) titer, chest X-ray to assess for sarcoidosis or tuberculosis, depending on patient characteristics).

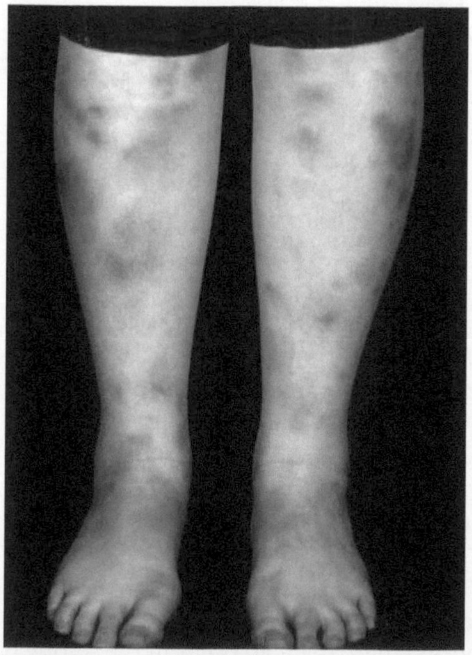

FIG. 26.2 Typical presentation of erythema nodosum. (From James, W. D., Elston, D. M., Treat, J. R., Rosenbach, M. A., & Neuhaus, I. M. (2019). *Andrews' diseases of the skin*: (13th ed., pp. 485–495, Fig. 23.1). Elsevier.)

Treatment

- Treat the underlying etiology. Lesions usually resolve spontaneously in 3 to 8 weeks.
- For symptomatic relief: bed rest, leg elevation, compression garments, NSAIDs.
- Potassium iodide (KI), typically 300 mg divided three times daily for 3 to 4 weeks. Some small non-randomized control studies have found KI to be effective in some cases, attributed to immunomodulatory effects on neutrophils.

Henoch-Schönlein Purpura

Basic Information

- Acute IgA-mediated vasculitis of small vessels of the skin, gastrointestinal (GI) system, and renal tracts.
- Approximately 50% of cases are preceded by an upper respiratory infection, most commonly streptococcus, although many other respiratory pathogens have been implicated.
- Typically occurs in children ages 3 to 15 years of age, but can occur in adults.
- Symptoms may be relapsing and remitting for several weeks.

Clinical Presentation

- Classic tetrad
  - Skin: symmetrically distributed erythematous eruptions on the buttocks and lower extremities that develop into *palpable purpura* (Fig. 26.3) over the course of 2 to 3 weeks.
    - This is the presenting symptom in 50% of patients.
    - Notably, there is *no* associated thrombocytopenia or coagulopathy.
  - Joints: arthritis, arthralgia favoring the lower extremities (60% of patients).
  - Gastrointestinal: colicky abdominal pain, caused by submucosal hemorrhage and edema of the intestinal wall (up to 70% of patients).
    - May be associated with bloody stools or ileoileal intussusception (3%–4% of patients).
  - Renal: microscopic hematuria in an otherwise well-appearing patient (40%–50% of patients).
    - 35% of males have severe scrotal edema.

Diagnosis

- Purpura or petechiae with lower limb predominance without thrombocytopenia or coagulopathy, PLUS one of the following:
  - Acute onset colicky abdominal pain.
  - Histology showing proliferative glomerulonephritis with IgA deposition.
  - Acute onset arthralgia or arthritis.
  - Proteinuria or hematuria.
- Ultrasound showing intraluminal hematomas, duodenal thickening, and/or intussusception in those patients with severe abdominal pain and/or GI bleeding

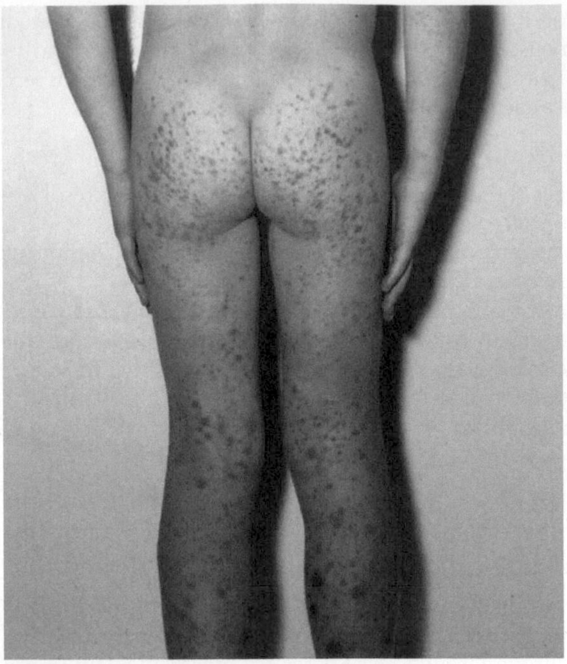

FIG. 26.3 Palpable Henoch-Schönlein purpura. (From Florentino, D. F. (2002). Cutaneous vasculitis. *Journal of the American Academy of Dermatology*, 48(3):311–344, Fig. 4.)

- Check urinalysis. and consider nephrology consult and/or admission if nephrotic syndrome or gross hematuria, as well as hypertension or abnormal renal function.

Treatment

- NSAIDs (ibuprofen or naproxen) for abdominal and joint pain EXCEPT in the case of significant intestinal bleeding or severe renal involvement.
- The vast majority of patients can be treated conservatively with supportive care (hydration, rest, analgesia, leg or scrotal elevation for edema) as outpatients.
- Admission and early oral or intravenous corticosteroids, 1 to 2 mg/kg/day (60 mg maximum) should be considered in cases of severe disease, particularly:
  - Persistent nephrotic disease (although steroids have not been proven to prevent glomerulonephritis).
  - Abdominal or pulmonary hemorrhage, or abdominal complications.
  - Severe soft tissue and scrotal edema.
- Other considerations: immunomodulators (primarily cyclophosphamide), plasmapheresis, and intravenous immunoglobulin (IVIG) have been studied with mixed outcomes with regard to severe and persistent renal disease and may be discussed with consultants.
- 50% of patients will have spontaneous remission within the first month, with complete recovery in up to 94% of patients by two years, although approximately 25% experience recurrence within the first year.
- Discharged patients will need weekly follow-up with primary care.

Pityriasis Rosea

Basic Information

- This is a benign rash of unclear etiology occurring primarily in children and young adults.

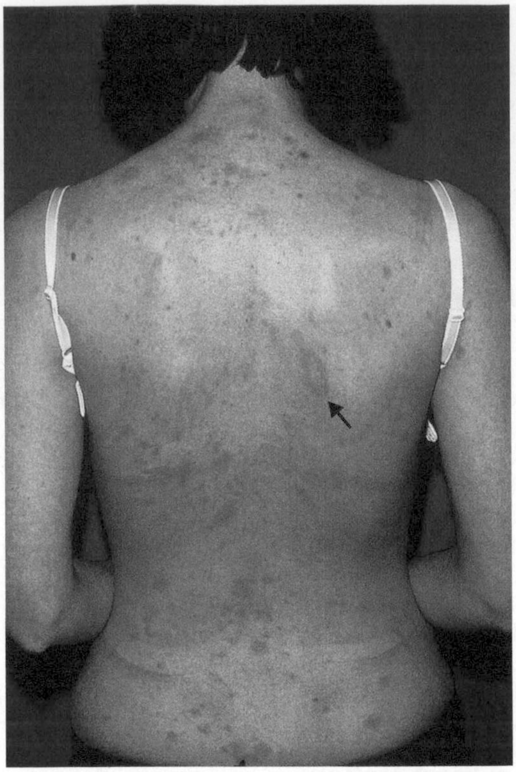

FIG. 26.4 Christmas tree pattern rash of pityriasis rosea demonstrating Herald patch (*arrow*). (From Calonje, E. (2020). Spongiotic, psoriaform, and pustular dermatoses. In E. Calonje, T. Brenn, A. J. Lazar, & S. D. Billings (Eds.), *McKee's pathology of the skin*: With clinical correlations (5th ed., pp. 201–240, Fig. 6.55). Elsevier.)

Clinical Presentation

- Multiple pink or pigmented oval papules or plaques measuring 1 to 2 cm each in a distribution described as a "Christmas tree" pattern on the trunk and proximal extremities.
- Like many rashes, can appear atypically in darker-skinned patients.
- 50%–90% of cases are preceded by a "Herald patch" (a larger lesion 2 to 6 cm, otherwise resembling the smaller lesions [Fig. 26.4]).

Diagnosis

- Identification of the rash in an otherwise well-appearing child or young adult.

Treatment

- Self-limited; lasts 8 to 12 weeks.
  - Direct sunlight/UV-B exposure has been recommended.
  - Low to moderate potency topical steroids (such as hydrocortisone or triamcinolone) for symptomatic treatment of severe pruritus has been proposed, but is controversial.

Purpura Fulminans

Basic Information

- This is a life-threatening emergency with shock and multiorgan failure that can occur in the setting of disseminated intravascular coagulation (DIC).
- Predilection for patients with clotting disorders, particularly protein C and S deficiency.

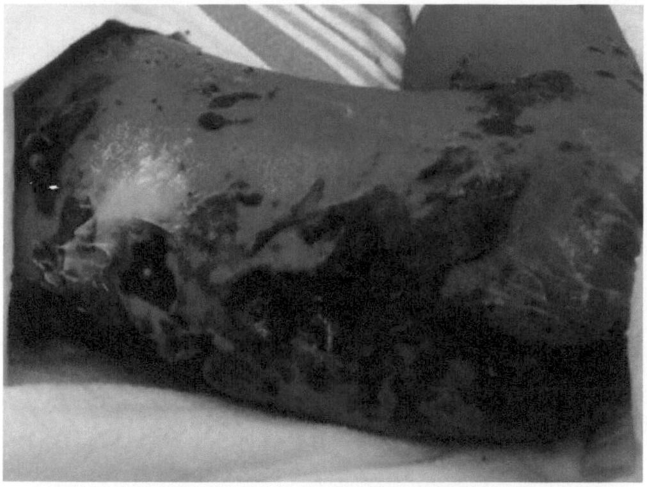

FIG. 26.5 Hemorrhagic bullae of purpura fulminans. (From Konda S, Zell D, Milikowski C, Alonso-Llamazares J. Purpura Fulminans Associated with Streptococo pneumoniae Septicemia in an Asplenic Pediatric Pacient. *Actas Dermosifiliogr.* 2013;104: 623–7. Copyright© 2011 Elsevier España, SL and AEDV. All rights reserved.)

- Three types:
  - Infectious: most commonly associated with group A streptococcus and meningococcus (10%–20%) and varicella, among many others.
  - Neonatal: manifestation of protein C deficiency occurring in 1 of 1,000,000 live births.
  - Idiopathic: "postinfectious" (7 to 10 days following illness) or traumatic (rarest form).

Clinical Presentation

- Rapidly developing retiform purpura, hemorrhagic bullae, and skin necrosis (Fig. 26.5) in the setting of fever, circulatory collapse, and DIC.

Diagnosis

- Petechiae or bruising in a neonate or patient who is septic should raise suspicion for this diagnosis, particularly when associated with necrotizing fasciitis.
- Confirmation of low levels of protein C, S, and/or antithrombin III.
- Laboratory findings consistent with DIC.

Treatment

- Treatment is primarily aimed at identifying and treating the underlying disorder, resuscitation, and hemodynamic support.
- In some cases, transfusion of platelets and plasma, factors C and S may be indicated. Heparin is also used in some case.
- Broad-spectrum antibiotic therapy should cover for *Neisseria meningitides*, *Streptococcus*, *Staphylococcus*, and *Clostridia*, plus clindamycin to inhibit endotoxins.
- Often requires surgical debridement, skin grafting, and even amputation.

Urticaria

Basic Information

- Also called hives or wheals.
- Caused by mast cell-mediated release of histamine, bradykinin, kallikrein, or acetylcholine.
  - Allergic: reaction to medication, cold, heat, plants, food, pollens, and so forth.
  - Infection: occult candida, dermatophytes, bacteria, viruses, parasites.
    - Especially hepatitis, mononucleosis, coxsackievirus.
  - Autoimmune: systemic lupus erythematosus, rheumatoid arthritis, or other vasculitis or rheumatologic disorder.
  - Malignancy (lymphoma, carcinoma).

Clinical Presentation

- Well-circumscribed edematous plaques wtih pale centers and red borders.
- Rash may be transient, developing and resolving in minutes to hours and may coalesce.
- Typically intensely pruritic.
- May be associated with angioedema.
- Well-circumscribed edematous plaques with pale centers and red borders, which may be transient, developing and resolving in minutes to hours, may coalesce, are typically intensely pruritic, and may be associated with angioedema.

Diagnosis

- A careful history and timeline in an attempt to determine the causative factor.
- Early identification of any associated hemodynamic instability or angioedema.

Treatment

- Remove the inciting factor. Two-thirds of new-onset urticaria is self-limited and treatment can focus on symptom relief.
- Antihistamines (diphenhydramine, hydroxyzine, loratadine, fexofenadine, or cetirizine).
- Corticosteroids: dexamethasone, methylprednisolone, or prednisone for severe or refractory cases.

Drug Rashes

Basic Information

- Immunogenic or nonimmunogenic reaction to pharmaceuticals.
- Especially common in patients with a history of atopic dermatitis, asthma, or eczema.
- Penicillin is the most common cause.

Clinical Presentation

- Highly variable dermatologic reaction appearing within a week of the offending drug that can appear exanthematous, eczematous, or vasculitic.
- Can produce different appearances in different patients or a different appearance in the same patient on different occasions.
- Can worsen even after the drug is discontinued if metabolites are still in the individual's system.
- Two types:
  - Photosensitive reaction which may be either:
    - Phototoxic: more common, benign, and not dose-related;
    - Photoallergic: must discontinue the drug.
  - Fixed drug eruption: pigmented, erythematous, or violaceous often pruritic rash that appears and recurs

in the same anatomic site after repeat exposures to the same drug

Treatment

- Stop the drug.
- Topical calamine, cool compresses, or tepid water baths with oatmeal (e.g., Aveeno) or cornstarch.
- Diphenhydramine.

SUGGESTED READINGS

Habif, T. (2015). *Clinical dermatology: A color guide to diagnosis and therapy* (6th ed.). Elsevier.

Marx, J., Hockberger, R., & Walls, R. (2013). *Rosen's emergency medicine: Concepts and clinical practice* (8th ed., pp. 1558–1576, 2180–2181). Elsevier.

Papular and Nodular Lesions

ANNA YAP, MD, BA, and KELLY PAINTER, MD, FACEP

Definitions

- Papular lesions: circumscribed, less than 1 cm, elevated, solid
- Nodular lesions: solid or cystic, palpable, more than 1 cm, usually dermal or subcutaneous

Select Types of Papular and Nodular Lesions

INFANTILE HEMANGIOMA

Basic Information

- Benign neoplasms of vascular endothelium
- Most common tumors of childhood
- Characterized by a growth phase and an involution phase

Clinical Presentation

- Most appear within the first few months of life.
- Can appear anywhere on the body, but there is a predilection for the head and neck.
- Superficial (cutaneous) type is most common; it is characterized by a raised, bright red papule or nodule (Fig. 27.1). A deep (subcutaneous) type of hemangioma grows under the skin; it is often blue or purplish in color.
- By 9 years of age, 90% involute but may cause permanent scarring.

Diagnosis and Evaluation

- Diagnosis is clinical, although biopsy is definitive if necessary.
- Considered high risk if they cause functional impairment, such as lesions in the periorbital region affecting vision, or if they are very large (> 5 cm) and rapidly growing.
- Most common complication is ulceration, which can be painful and may lead to bleeding, infection, or scarring.

Treatment

- Vast majority require no emergent intervention and can be referred to primary care for surveillance.
- High-risk hemangiomas may require treatment with topical or oral beta-blockers or intralesional steroids. Patients with high-risk lesions should be referred to a specialist.

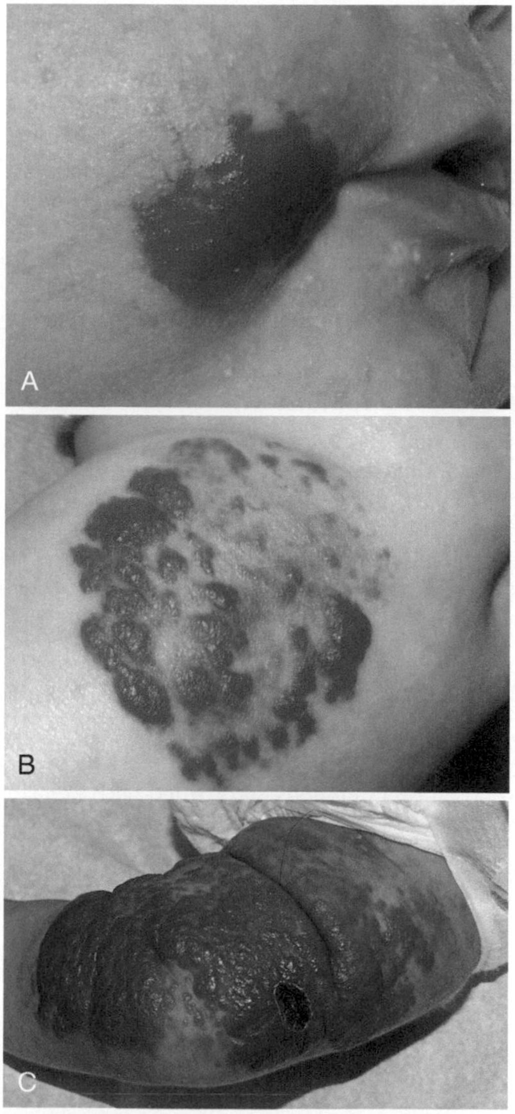

FIG. 27.1 Superficial infantile hemangiomas can be more discrete (**A** and **B**) or have a more diffuse distribution (**C**). (From Bolognia J., Schaffer J., & Cerroni L. (2017). *Dermatology,* (4th ed., Fig. 13-3ac). Elsevier.)

LYMPHANGIOMA

Basic information

- Benign mass of lymph channels
- Typically seen in the newborn or pediatrics

Clinical Presentation

- They are usually pink to reddish-blue in color, soft, and compressible.
- Most often seen on the tongue, lips, and buccal mucosa.
- Large lymphangiomas of the head or neck are called cystic hygromas, usually found at birth, and may sometimes obstruct the airway.

Treatment

- Referral to a surgeon for elective resection or percutaneous chemoablation.
- If the mass is obstructing the airway, the safest approach is a controlled airway in the operating room. Otherwise, prepare for a difficult intubation and consult anesthesia, if available.

Lipoma/Angiolipoma

Basic Information

- Most common benign soft-tissue neoplasm, consisting of encapsulated fat

Clinical Presentation

- Soft, superficial, subcutaneous mobile tumor.
- Typically painless.
- Most commonly on the trunk and upper extremities, ranging in size from 1 to more than 10 cm.
- Angiolipomas closely resemble lipomas, except they are usually painful, tender, and typically are multiple lesions 0.5 to 2 cm in diameter, usually on the forearm or chest wall.

Diagnosis and Evaluation

- Clinical diagnosis
  - Ultrasound can distinguish lipoma from cyst.

Treatment

- Uncomplicated lesions require no treatment.
- Referral to a surgeon for excision is indicated if firm, rapidly enlarging, or causing significant pain.

Epidermoid (Sebaceous) Cyst

Basic Information

- Most common cutaneous cysts, filled with keratinaceous material

Clinical Presentation

- Skin-colored dermal nodules.
- Occurring anywhere on the body.
- May range from a few millimeters to several centimeters in diameter; may grow in size.

Diagnosis and Evaluation

- Freely mobile on palpation.
- Typically, softer than a lipoma.
- If infected, will be erythematous and likely fluctuant and painful.

Treatment

- Noninfected lesions do not require any emergent therapy.
- Fluctuant cysts require incision and drainage; antibiotics may be necessary if there is surrounding cellulitis. If the patient desires permanent removal, excision of the sac by a specialist is required after resolution of infection.

Keloid (Fig. 27.2)

Basic Information

- Hypertrophic scar that crosses borders, caused by fibroblast growth and overproduction of collagen. More frequently seen in people of African and Asian descent.

Clinical Presentation

- Occur at site of previous open injury, extending to involve the adjacent normal skin.
- Pain, pruritus, hyperhidrosis, and functional impairment may be present.

Treatment

- No emergent treatment is indicated. May refer to primary care or dermatology for intralesional steroids, silicone gel, or cryotherapy.
- Patients with a history of keloids who present with a laceration should be advised to keep the wound moist and covered, avoid any tension on the wound, and use sunblock.

Neurofibroma

Basic Information

- Neurofibromas are common, benign, peripheral nerve sheath tumors. They can be cutaneous or found along peripheral nerves under the skin and nerve roots adjacent to the spine.

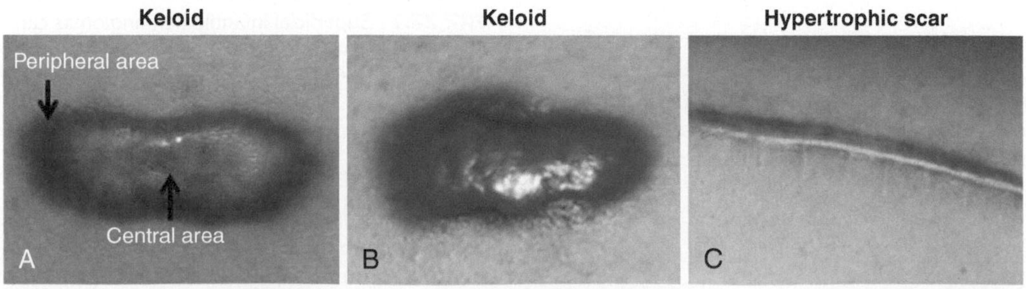

FIG. 27.2 Keloids can have an active peripheral area with a central area of regression (**A**) or a whole lesion can be active (**B**). Hypertrophic scar within the initial wound (**C**). (From Zhen G., Xiaoli, W., Nan, S., Lu, Z., Wei, L. (2010). Differential expression of growth differentiation factor-9 in keloids. *Burns*, 36(8), 1289–1295, Fig. 1.)

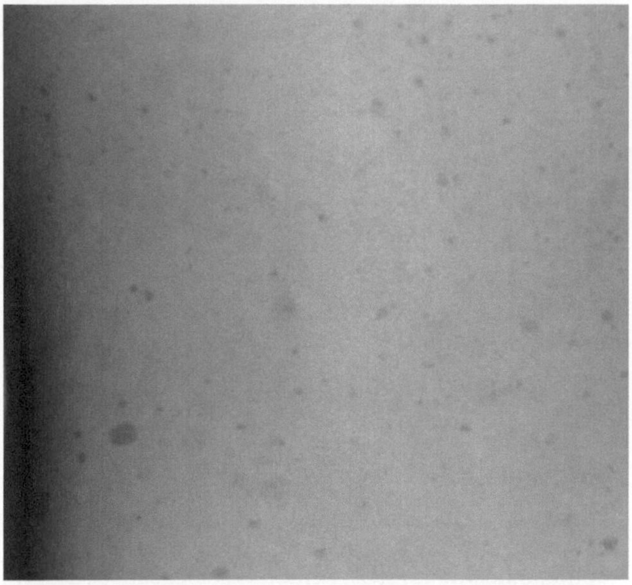

FIG. 27.3 Cutaneous neurofibromas in a young boy. From Hernández-Martín, A., Duat-Rodríguez, A. (2016). An update on neurofibromatosis type 1: Not just café-au-lait spots, freckling, and neurofibromas. An update. Part I. Dermatological clinical criteria diagnostic of the disease. Actas Dermo-Sifiliográficas, 107, 454–464.

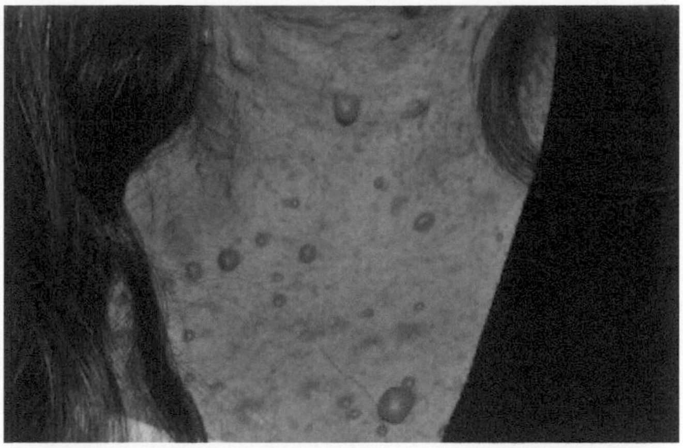

FIG. 27.4 Multiple pedunculated cutaneous neurofibromas in an adult woman. From Hernández-Martín, A., Duat-Rodríguez, A. (2016). An update on neurofibromatosis type 1: Not just café-au-lait spots, freckling, and neurofibromas. An update. Part I. Dermatological clinical criteria diagnostic of the disease. Actas Dermo-Sifiliográficas, 107, 454–464.

Clinical Presentation

- Cutaneous neurofibromas are soft, skin-colored or hyperpigmented papules or nodules, most commonly occurring just before or during adolescence (Fig. 27.3).
- May occur with no cause, or may be associated with the genetic disorder neurofibromatosis.
- These are painless, benign lesions representing mainly a cosmetic problem for adults because of their neurofibromatosis and multiple lesions (Fig. 27.4).
- Pruritus during growth of new lesions (owing to mast cells in the neurofibroma releasing histamine) may be a distressing symptom.

Treatment

- Pruritus may not respond to antihistamines and can be treated with gabapentin.
- Outpatient referral for surgical removal if painful, bleeding, or disfiguring.
- Cutaneous (dermal) neurofibromas do not typically become cancerous. Deeper lesions (diffuse neurofibromas) may undergo malignant deterioration. Malignancy is more common in patients with multiple lesions, such as those with neurofibromatosis, and typically presents with pain. If patients with neurofibromas present with back pain, headache, or neurologic symptoms, a thorough investigation is warranted because deeper neurofibromas can become malignant.
- Sudden growth of a tumor can be caused by bleeding in the tumor or may indicate malignant deterioration.

SUGGESTED READING

American Academy of Family Physicians, Luba, M. C., Bangs, S. A., Mohler, A. M., & Stulberg, D. L. (2003). Common benign skin tumors. *American Family Physician*, 67, 729–738. Available at: https://www.aafp.org/afp/2003/0215/p729.html.

Bullous and Vesicular Diseases

ALEXANDER DAGUANNO, MD, BS, and SAMANTHA PHILLIPS KADERA, MD, MPH, FACEP

This chapter reviews bullous and vesicular dermatologic diseases with emphasis on the emergency diagnosis and management of several rare but life-threatening conditions.

Stevens-Johnson Syndrome (SJS) and Toxic Epidermal Necrolysis (TEN)

General Principles

- Severe, life-threatening mucocutaneous reactions characterized by extensive necrosis and separation of the epidermis from the dermis.
- Occurs at any age; twice as common in women.
- Increased risk with HIV, malignancy, genetic factors, immunologic disease (especially systemic lupus erythematosus), UV light exposure, and radiation therapy.
- Disease continuum distinguished by percentage of body surface area affected (Box 28.1).

BOX 28.1 *Body Surface Area Affected in SJS and TEN*

SJS: ≤10% body surface area
SJS/TEN: 10%–30% body surface area
TEN: ≥30% body surface area

SJS, Stevens-Johnson, syndrome; *TEN*, toxic epidermal necrolysis.

Common Precipitants

- Drugs: allopurinol, lamotrigine, phenobarbital, carbamazepine, antibiotic sulfonamides, sulfasalazine, nevirapine, oxicam NSAIDs, penicillins, anticancer drugs, fluroquinolones, doxycycline.
- Infections: mycoplasma pneumonia.
- One-third of cases do not have an identifiable trigger.

Clinical Presentation

- Prodrome: fever (often >39°C), flu-like symptoms, photophobia, oral ulcers.
- Cutaneous manifestations: erythematous macules (often with purpuric centers) → bullae and vesicles → skin sloughing a few days later (Fig. 28.1).
  - Severe pain that does not consistently correlate with severity of wound appearance.
  - Spreads from face → thorax → extremities.
  - Spares scalp; rarely involves palms and soles.
- **Positive Nikolsky sign**: skin sloughing with gentle pressure to skin.
- **90% of cases involve mucous membranes:** vermillion border, oral mucosa, pharynx, conjunctival, cornea, urethra (leading to urinary retention), and so forth.
- **Severe complications can occur,** including massive fluid loss, electrolyte imbalance, hypovolemic shock, bacteremia, multiorgan dysfunction.

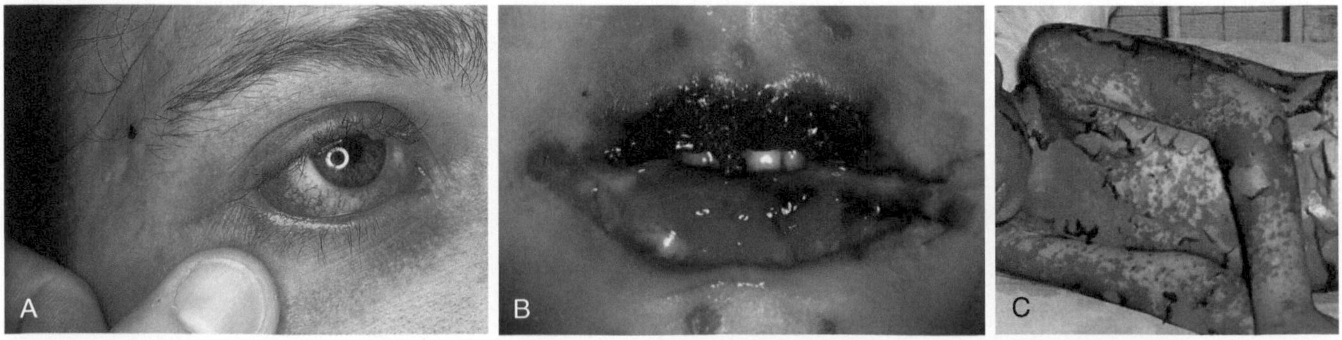

FIG. 28.1 Mucous membrane and skin involvement as seen with Stevens-Johnson syndrome and toxic epidermal necrolysis. (**A**, Avarbock, A., & Jorizzo, J. L. (2017). Erythema multiforme, Stevens–Johnson syndrome, and toxic epidermal necrolysis. In J. P. Callen, J. L. Jorizzo, J. J. Zone, W. W. Piette, M. A. Rosenbach, & R. A. Vieugels (Eds.), *Dermatological signs of systemic disease* (5th ed., Fig. 11.4.) Elsevier. **B,** From Sargenti Neto, S., Fernando Barbosa de Paulo, L., Rezende Rosa, R., & Durighetto, A. F. (2013). Stevens-Johnson syndrome: An oral viewpoint. *International Journal of Pediatric Otorhinolaryngology, 77*(2):284–286, Fig. 2. **C,** From Muñiz, A. E. (2008). Erythema multiforme major and minor. In: J. M. Baren, S. G. Rothrock, J. A. Brennan, & L. Brown (Eds.), *Pediatric emergency medicine* (pp. 836–840, Fig. 121.4.). Elsevier Saunders.)

Diagnosis

- Clinical (no universally accepted criteria); see "Clinical Presentation" above.
- Associated laboratory findings include anemia, lymphopenia, electrolyte abnormalities, hypoalbuminemia, elevated serum urea nitrogen, hyperglycemia, mild transaminitis.
- *Always obtain blood cultures and chest x-ray given high risk of infection.*
- Consult to dermatology in the emergency department (ED) is indicated, given disease severity and similarity to other bullous dermatologic conditions (i.e., staphylococcal scalded skin syndrome).

Management

- Requires admission to hospital; consider ICU or burn unit if ≥ 40 years of age, a history of cancer, body surface area (BSA) 30% or greater, tachycardia more than 120 bpm, uremia, hyperglycemia, or metabolic acidosis.
- Immediately stop culprit drug (if known or suspected).
- Supportive care: wound care, fluid resuscitation (2 mL per kg × %BSA over first 24 hr), pain control, antibiotics for infections (not prophylactic).
- No indication for corticosteroids. Adjunctive therapies may be indicated (e.g., cyclosporine, intravenous immunoglobulin, immunosuppressives), but use should be directed by dermatology consultants.

Bullous Pemphigoid and Pemphigus Vulgaris

- Bullous pemphigoid and pemphigus vulgaris are rare autoimmune diseases affecting adults, both characterized by formation of blisters and/or bullae. They are often confused for each other given their similar presentation. Table 28.1 provides a side-by-side comparison of these two disease entities.

TABLE 28.1 Clinical Features of Bullous Pemphigoid and Pemphigus Vulgaris

	Bullous Pemphigoid	Pemphigus Vulgaris
Pathophysiology	Autoimmune blistering disease; targets basement membrane causing *subepithelial blisters*	Autoimmune blistering diseases; target desmogleins causing *intraepithelial blisters*
Population	Almost always age > 60 years Female > Male	Typically age 40–60 years Male = Female
Early Symptoms	Pruritic/eczematous papules or urticarial lesions (lasts weeks)	Mucosal blisters [often oral] with severe pain and odynophagia
Late Symptoms	Numerous tense bullae (1–3 cm each) on erythematous base; bullae rupture to form moist erosions or crusts without scarring	Cutaneous findings with flaccid, painful blisters on erythematous base
Affected Areas	Localized or widespread; often affects trunk, flexor surfaces, axillae, inguinal folds	Localized or widespread; often affects conjunctiva, nose, vaginal and rectal mucosa
Mucosa	Sometimes affected (10%–30%)	*Almost always* affected
Nikolsky Sign	Negative [skin remains intact with gentle pressure]	Positive [skin erodes with gentle pressure]
Severity	Usually not life threatening	May be life-threatening; high risk of secondary infections (esp. HSV)
ED Diagnosis	Clinical + dermatology consult	Clinical + dermatology consult
Definitive Diagnosis	Biopsy and histopathology (i.e., dermatology referral)	Biopsy and histopathology (i.e., dermatology referral)
Primary Treatment	Potent topical corticosteroid or systemic corticosteroid *After diagnosis confirmed by biopsy	Systemic corticosteroids +/- antibiotics/antivirals for superimposed infection
Additional Management	Outpatient dermatology referral for biopsy; consider additional referrals as indicated (e.g. gastrointestinal, ophthalmology).	Usually requires admission and close follow up with dermatology for steroid taper; consider additional referrals as indicated
Examination	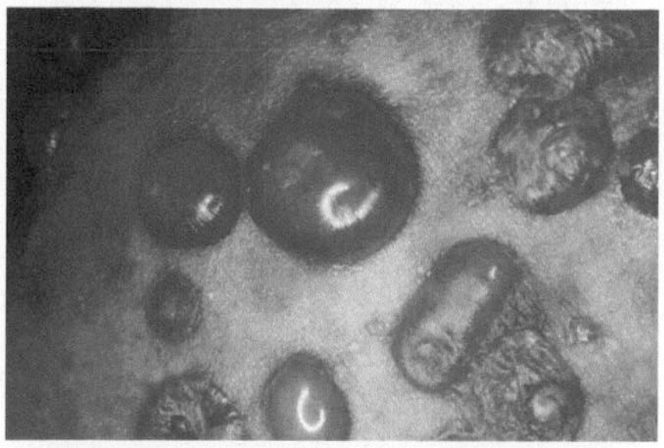 (From Paller, A. S., & Mancini, A. J. (2016). *Hurwitz clinical pediatric dermatology: A textbook of skin disorders of childhood and adolescence* (5th ed., Fig. 13.25.). Elsevier.)	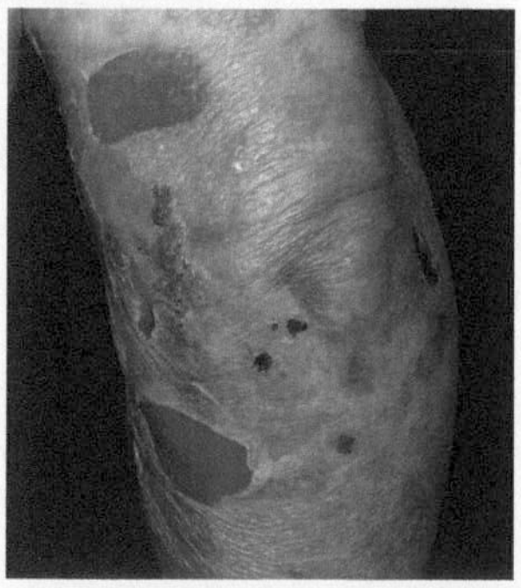 (From Dinulos, J. G. H. (2021). Vesicular and bullous diseases. In J. G. H. Dinulos (Ed.), *Habif's clinical dermatology: A color guide to diagnosis and therapy* (7th ed., pp. 631–668.e1, Fig. 16.19.). Elsevier.)

28

- Note that pemphigus vulgaris is often a paraneoplastic syndrome associated with certain malignancies. Patient may warrant additional oncologic workup.

Staphylococcal Scalded Skin Syndrome (SSSS)

General Principles

- Caused by specific strains of *Staphylococcus aureus* that produce exfoliative toxins which target desmoglein 1 in the epidermis, causing formation of flaccid, fragile bullae.
- Predominantly affects young children (most cases occur in children younger than 6 years); typically occurs in newborns between 3 and 7 days of age.
- Adults at risk for SSSS include those with renal impairment, diabetes mellitus, and those on immunosuppressive medications.

Clinical Presentation

- Irritable, febrile infant with diffuse blanching erythema that typically begins around the mouth; often with concurrent conjunctivitis.
- Flaccid blisters develop 1 to 2 days later, usually affecting sites under mechanical stress (flexural areas, buttocks, **hands, feet**), with superficial desquamation (Fig. 28.2).

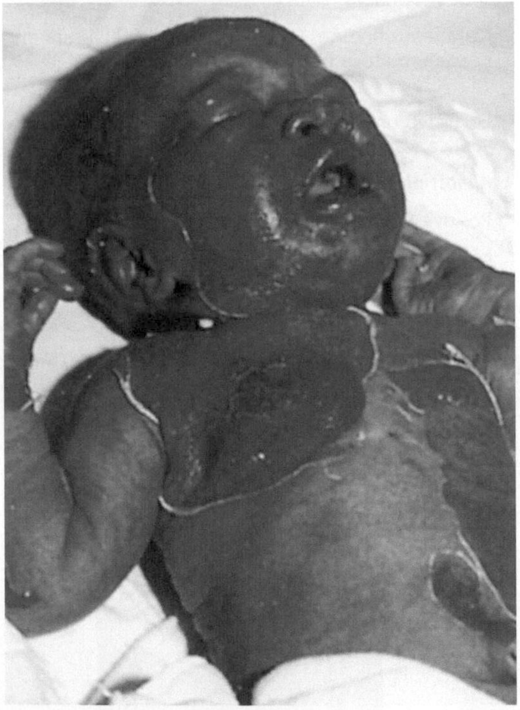

FIG. 28.2 Skin erythema and sloughing as seen with Staphylococcal scalded skin syndrome. (From Kliegman, R. M., St Geme, J. W., Blum, N. J., et al. (2020). Cutaneous bacterial infections. In R. M. Kliegman, J. W. St. Geme III, N. J. Blum, S. S. Shah, R. C. Tasker, K. M. Wilson, & R. E. Behrman (Eds.), *Nelson textbook of pediatrics* (21st ed., pp. 3549–3559.e1, Fig. 685.4). Elsevier.)

BOX 28.2 *Pearls for the Boards*

Positive Nikolsky Sign: BAD!

- Pemphigus (vulgaris, foliaceous, etc.): elderly
- Staphylococcal scalded skin syndrome: newborn
- SJS/TEN: any age after exposure to new drug

Tense Bullae in Elderly > 60: Bullous pemphigoid

Flaccid Bullae in Adults > 40: Pemphigus, most often pemphigus vulgaris

Systemic Symptoms + rash and desquamation after new medication: SJS/TEN

SJS, Stevens-Johnson syndrome; *TEN*, toxic epidermal necrolysis.

- **Positive Nikolsky sign.**
- **Does not affect mucous membranes** (though may appear hyperemic).

Diagnosis

- Clinical diagnosis based on presentation (above); can confirm with biopsy.

Management

- Cultures: blood, urine, nasopharynx, flaccid lesions (not intact bullae).
- Prompt administration of nafcillin or oxacillin; consider vancomycin in areas with high prevalence of methicillin-resistant *Staphylococcus aureus* or for patients who fail to respond to initial therapy.
- Supportive care with use of emollients to improve barrier function.
- Fluid and electrolyte repletion.
- Consider transfer to burn center if large surface area affected.

SUGGESTED READINGS

Harr, T., & French, L. E. (2010). Toxic epidermal necrolysis and Stevens-Johnson syndrome. *Orphanet Journal of Rare Diseases*, *5*, 39.

Mutasim, D. F. (2004). Management of autoimmune bullous diseases: Pharmacology and therapeutics. *Journal of the American Academy of Dermatology*, *51*, 859–877.

Patel, G. K., & Finlay, A. Y. (2003). Staphylococcal scalded skin syndrome: Diagnosis and management. *American Journal of Clinical Dermatology*, *4*, 165.

Metabolic/ Endocrine

CHAPTER **29** BOARD REVIEW

Acid–Base Disturbances

MATTHEW ROSEN, MD, and SARA CRAGER, MD

General Principles

- The body maintains an acid–base balance primarily through the bicarbonate-carbon dioxide buffer system (Fig 29.1).
- The pulmonary system regulates carbon dioxide (CO_2), and the kidneys regulate the excretion of nonvolatile acids by combining hydrogen ions (H^+) with urinary buffers (e.g., phosphate, ammonia). An arterial blood gas or venous blood gas measures the pH and partial pressure of CO_2 (pCO_2) (normal values in Box 29.1).
- The difference in pH between arterial and venous samples is minimal, so consider avoiding a painful arterial blood gas procedure for your patient and order a venous blood gas, unless an accurate assessment of the pO_2 or pCO_2 is important. The bicarbonate (HCO_3^-) reported for a blood gas is a calculated (not measured) value using the Henderson-Hasselbalch equation (Fig. 29.2).
- The nomenclature of acid–base disorders is provided in Box 29.2.

Clinical Presentation

- The clinical presentation will vary, depending on the severity and duration of the primary metabolic derangement and the patient's ability to compensate for the derangement.

$$pCO_2 + H_2O \leftrightarrow H_2CO_3 \leftrightarrow HCO_3^- + H^+$$

FIG. 29.1 The bicarbonate-carbon dioxide buffering system. *pCO2* = partial pressure of CO_2 in the blood. *H_2O* = water. *H_2CO_3* = carbonic acid. *HCO_3^-* = bicarbonate. *H^+* = hydrogen ion.

BOX 29.1 *Normal Arterial Blood Gas Values**

pH: 7.35 to 7.45
HCO_3^-: 21 to 27 mEq/L
pCO_2: 35 to 45 mm Hg

*For venous blood gas sampling, the pH is approximately 0.03 to 0.04 pH units lower, the HCO_3^- is 1 to 2 mEq/L higher, and the pCO_2 is 3 to 8 mm Hg higher.

$$pH = 6.10 + \log \frac{[HCO_3^-]}{[0.03 \times pCO_2]}$$

FIG. 29.2 The Henderson-Hasselbalch equation.

BOX 29.2 *Definitions of Acid–Base*

Acidemia: pH < 7.35
Alkalemia: pH > 7.45
Acidosis: a process that decreases the pH (increased [H^+]), by decreasing the [HCO_3^-] or increasing the pCO_2
Alkalosis: a process that increases the pH (decreased [H^+]), by increasing the [HCO_3^-] or decreasing the pCO_2
Metabolic acidosis: a disorder that decreases the [HCO_3^-] and decreases the pH
Metabolic alkalosis: a disorder that increases the [HCO_3^-] and increases the pH
Respiratory acidosis: a disorder that increases the pCO_2 and decreases the pH
Respiratory alkalosis: a disorder that decreases the pCO_2 and increases the pH
Compensation: the lungs or kidneys attempt to compensate, depending on the disorder. Compensatory mechanisms *usually do not return the pH to normal and never overcorrect;* an "overcorrected" pH suggests a mixed acid–base disorder.
Simple acid–base disorder: only one primary disorder is present: that disorder is appropriately compensated for. If appropriate compensation is not present, then there is more than one disorder.
Mixed acid–base disorder: presence of more than one acid-base disorder

Diagnosis and Evaluation

- A stepwise approach to the assessment of acid–base derangements is presented in Box 29.3.
- When confronted with an acid–base derangement, the body will attempt to compensate in order to minimize the impact of the disturbance on serum pH. It is important to assess the presence of an appropriate

BOX 29.3 *Approach to Acid–Base Disturbance*

1. Use the pH to determine if patient is acidemic or alkalemic.
2. Determine if the primary disorder is respiratory or metabolic.
3. Determine if there is appropriate compensation.
   a. If values are inadequate or excessive compared with the expected degree of compensation, a mixed disorder is likely present.
4. If there is a metabolic acidosis, determine if there is an increased anion gap.
   a. If there is an elevated anion gap, calculate the "delta–delta" (the ΔAnion Gap/ΔHCO_3^-).
5. Interpret the acid–base disturbance in the overall clinical context to identify underlying causes and appropriate management strategies.

BOX 29.4 *Evaluation of Compensation in Acid–Base Disturbances*

Metabolic Acidosis

For each 1 mEq/L a decrease in the [HCO_3^-], the pCO_2 decreases by 1.2 mm Hg.

There are several equally accurate ways to determine if compensation is appropriate for metabolic acidosis.

1. Winter's formula: $pCO_2 = (1.5 \times [HCO_3^-]) + 8 \pm 2$
2. $pCO_2 = [HCO_3^-] + 15$
3. pCO_2 should be similar to the decimal digits of the blood gas analysis (e.g., if the pH is 7.20, the pCO_2 should be approximately 20 mm Hg)

Limitations: the pCO_2 can fall no lower than 8 to 12 mm Hg.

Metabolic Alkalosis

pCO_2 increases by 0.7 mm Hg for every 1 mEq/L ↑ in HCO_3^-, usually does not increase above 55 mm Hg

Respiratory Acidosis

Acute: decrease in pH by 0.08 units and increase of [HCO_3^-] by 1 mEq/L for each 10 mm Hg ↑ in pCO_2

Chronic: decrease in pH by 0.03 units and increase of [HCO_3^-] by 4 mEq/L for each 10 mm Hg increase in pCO_2

Respiratory Alkalosis

Acute: increase in pH by 0.08 units and decrease of [HCO_3^-] by 2 mEq/L for each 10 mm Hg decrease in the pCO_2

Chronic: increase in pH by 0.03 units and decrease of [HCO_3^-] by 4 mEq/L for each 10 mm Hg decrease in the pCO_2

compensatory response to each category of primary acid–base disturbance (Box 29.4).

- For metabolic acidosis and alkalosis, the respiratory system will attempt to compensate by lowering or increasing the pCO_2, respectively. Respiratory compensation occurs quickly (within approximately 30 minutes) in comparison to the slower (3 to 5 days) metabolic renal response to a respiratory acidosis or alkalosis.

$$\text{Anion gap} = Na^+ - (Cl^- + HCO_3^-]$$

FIG. 29.3 Anion gap. The normal value for the serum anion gap is approximately 3 to 10 mEq/L (averaging 6 mEq/L). *Note:* the anion gap needs to be adjusted in patients with *hypoalbuminemia.* Adjusted anion gap = observed anion gap + 2.5 (4.2 – [serum albumin]).

- More than one metabolic process may be occurring at the same time in a patient (e.g., diabetic ketoacidosis [DKA] and contraction alkalosis); however, the lungs can only have one respiratory process in compensation leading to the most complex acid–base status, a triple disturbance.
- There are two types of triple disturbances.
  - Metabolic acidosis and metabolic alkalosis with a respiratory acidosis
  - Metabolic acidosis and metabolic alkalosis with a respiratory alkalosis
- Other important considerations when assessing an acid–base disturbance include the absence or presence of an elevated anion gap (Fig. 29.3) and osmolar gap.
- In patients with an anion gap metabolic acidosis, determine if there is an additional metabolic acid–base derangement by calculating the (ΔAnionGap/ΔHCO_3^-), or "delta–delta," which assesses whether the change in [HCO_3^-] is fully accounted for by the anion gap.
- A "delta–delta" less than 1 usually indicates a coexisting normal anion gap metabolic acidosis.
- A "delta–delta" more than 2 usually indicates a coexistent metabolic alkalosis. Values between 1 and 2 may indicate an uncomplicated elevated anion gap acidosis with impaired renal function or a chronic respiratory acidosis with a baseline compensatory metabolic alkalosis (an elevated). See Figs. 29.4–29.6 for a visual representation of "delta–delta".
- See Chapter 130, Toxic Alcohols for discussion of osmolar gaps.

29

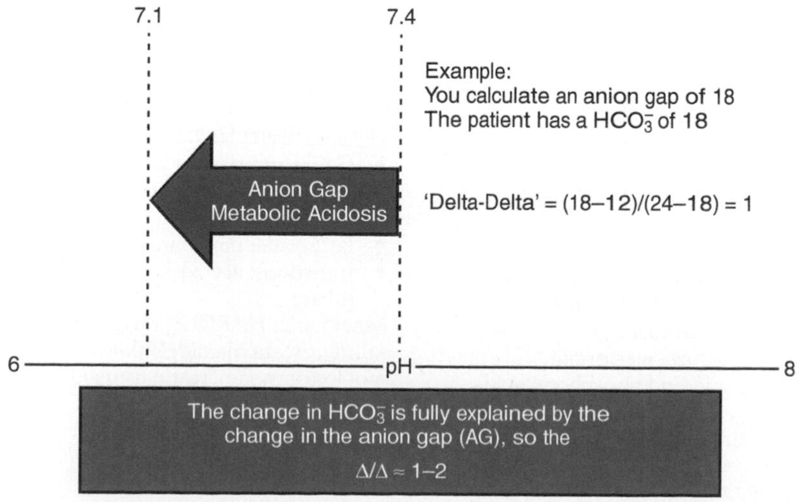
7.1
7.4
Example:
You calculate an anion gap of 18
The patient has a HCO3 of 18
Anion Gap
Metabolic Acidosis
'Delta-Delta' = (18–12)/(24–18) = 1
6
pH
8
The change in HCO3 is fully explained by the change in the anion gap (AG), so the
Δ/Δ ≈ 1–2

FIG. 29.4 "Delta–delta" = 1 – 2. The ratio is not precisely 1:1 owing to several factors, including the role of intracellular buffering of H^+.

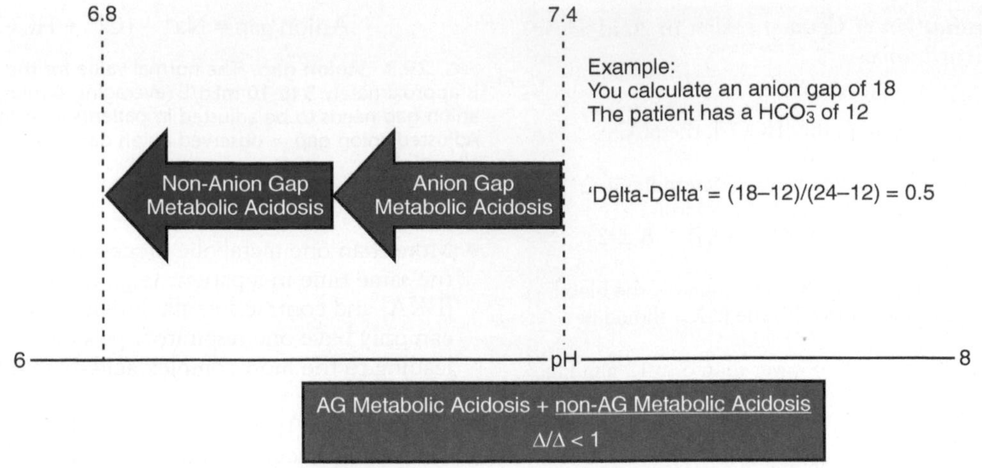

FIG. 29.5 **"Delta–delta" < 1.** If the [HCO_3^-] has decreased more than expected from the anion gap, there is a concurrent nonanion gap metabolic acidosis that is contributing to the lower [HCO_3^-].

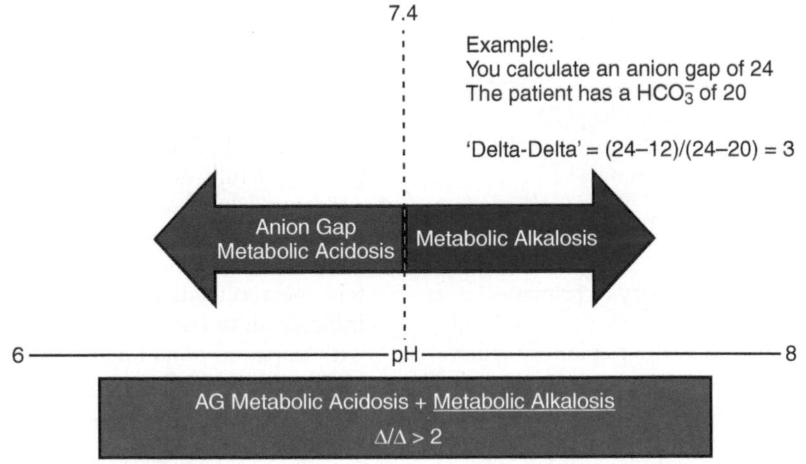

FIG. 29.6 **"Delta–delta" > 2.** If the HCO_3^- has decreased less than expected, then there is a concurrent metabolic alkalosis.

Treatment

- The goal of treatment is to reverse the underlying cause of the derangement and provide supportive care until the patient's derangement is corrected. Common etiologies of the four-primary acid–base disorders are listed in Box 29.5.

BOX 29.5 *Common Causes of Acid–Base Disturbances*

Metabolic Acidosis

Elevated Anion Gap

- Ketoacidosis: diabetic ketoacidosis (DKA), alcoholic ketoacidosis (AKA), starvation
- Lactic acidosis:
  - Tissue hypoperfusion/cellular poisons: shock, seizures, mesenteric/limb ischemia, hypoxia, carbon monoxide poisoning, cyanide, aspirin, iron toxicity
  - Decreased clearance: liver failure, metformin
- Renal failure (increased ammonia and phosphoric acid)
- Toxic acidic metabolites (e.g., methanol [formic acid], ethylene glycol [glycolic acid], aspirin [salicylic acid])

Mnemonic: *MUDPILES* (Methanol, Uremia, DKA/AKA, Paraldehyde, Isoniazid/Iron, Lactic Acidosis, Ethylene Glycol, Salicylates)

Normal Anion Gap

- Gastrointestinal or renal HCO_3^- loss: diarrhea, ostomies, fistulas, renal tubular acidosis (RTA), intrinsic renal disease, hyperparathyroidism
- Iatrogenic: rapid/large volume normal saline infusion
- Ingestions: acetazolamide, calcium chloride, magnesium sulfate

Mnemonic: *HARDUP* (Hyperchloremia [excess normal saline], Acetazolamide/Addison's, RTA, Diarrhea, Ureterosigmoidostomy, Pancreatic fistula/drainage)

Metabolic Alkalosis

- Volume contraction: vomiting, diuretics
- Volume expansion: hyperaldosteronism, hypercortisolemia, potassium depletion

BOX 29.5 *Common causes of Acid–Base Disturbances—cont'd*

- Hypoalbuminemia
- Hypercalcemia of malignancy
- Massive transfusion (due to citrate)

Respiratory Acidosis: "failure of ventilation"

Acute: airway obstruction, VQ mismatch, central nervous system (CNS) depressants, CNS catastrophe, neuromuscular disorders, thoracic trauma
Chronic: lung disease (e.g., chronic obstructive pulmonary disease), neurologic disease (e.g., amyotrophic lateral sclerosis, muscular dystrophy), obesity

Respiratory Alkalosis

- Hyperventilation: high altitude, anemia, VQ mismatch
- Central hyperventilation: CNS lesion (e.g., mass, stroke), increased intracranial pressure
- Toxic/pharmacologic: salicylates, caffeine, nicotine, catecholamines, thyroxine
- Pulmonary: pulmonary embolism, pneumonia, pulmonary edema, asthma
- Iatrogenic
- Endocrine: hyperthyroidism, pregnancy
- Bacteremia
- Hepatic encephalopathy
- Hyponatremia

SUGGESTED READING

Strayer, R. J. (2018). Acid–base disorders. In Walls, R. M. Hockberger, R. S. & Gausche-Hill, M. (Eds.), *Rosen's emergency medicine: Concepts and clinical practice* (9th ed., pp. 1509–1515). Elsevier.

CHAPTER 30

BOARD REVIEW

Adrenal and Pituitary Disorders

JOSHUA J. BAUGH, MD, MPP, MHCM, and SCOTT R. VOTEY, MD

Adrenal and pituitary disorders occur when insufficient or excess hormone is secreted from one of the organs in the hypothalamic-pituitary-adrenal (HPA) axis Figs. 30.1-30.2.

Adrenal Insufficiency

General Principles

- Adrenal insufficiency (AI) is classified as primary or secondary.
  - Primary AI refers to intrinsic disease of the adrenal glands resulting in decreased production of cortisol, aldosterone, and androgens.
    - The most common cause in the United States is autoimmune (Addison disease).
- Autoimmune AI is often part of an autoimmune polyendocrine syndrome (APS).
  - Type I APS: adrenal insufficiency + hypoparathyroidism + mucocutaneous candidiasis
  - Type II APS: adrenal insufficiency + DM1 or thyroid disorder + other autoimmune conditions
- Generally requires lifetime replacement of cortisol and often aldosterone
- Congenital adrenal hyperplasia is a life-threatening neonatal form of primary AI resulting from 21-hydroxylase deficiency that usually presents in the first week of life.
- Tuberculosis remains an important cause of adrenal insufficiency in the developing world.

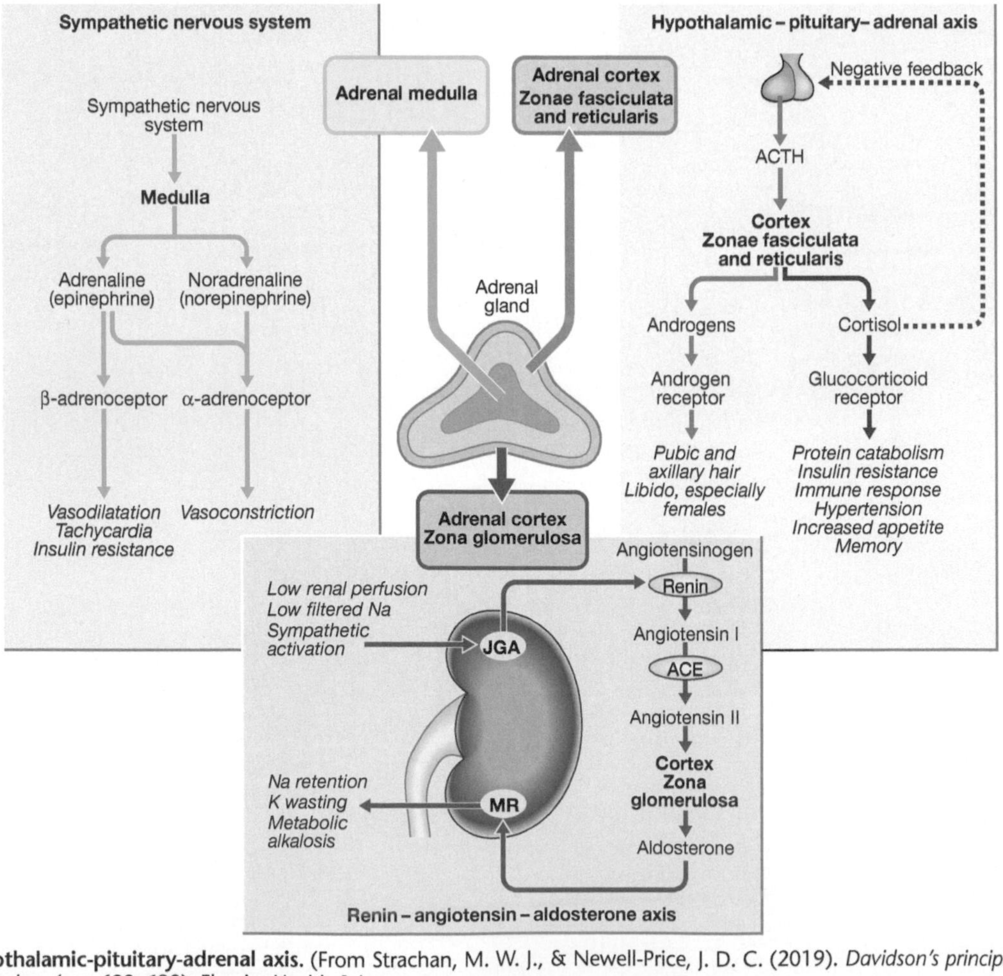

FIG. 30.1 Hypothalamic-pituitary-adrenal axis. (From Strachan, M. W. J., & Newell-Price, J. D. C. (2019). *Davidson's principles and practice of medicine: Endocrinology* (pp. 629–689). Elsevier Health Sciences.

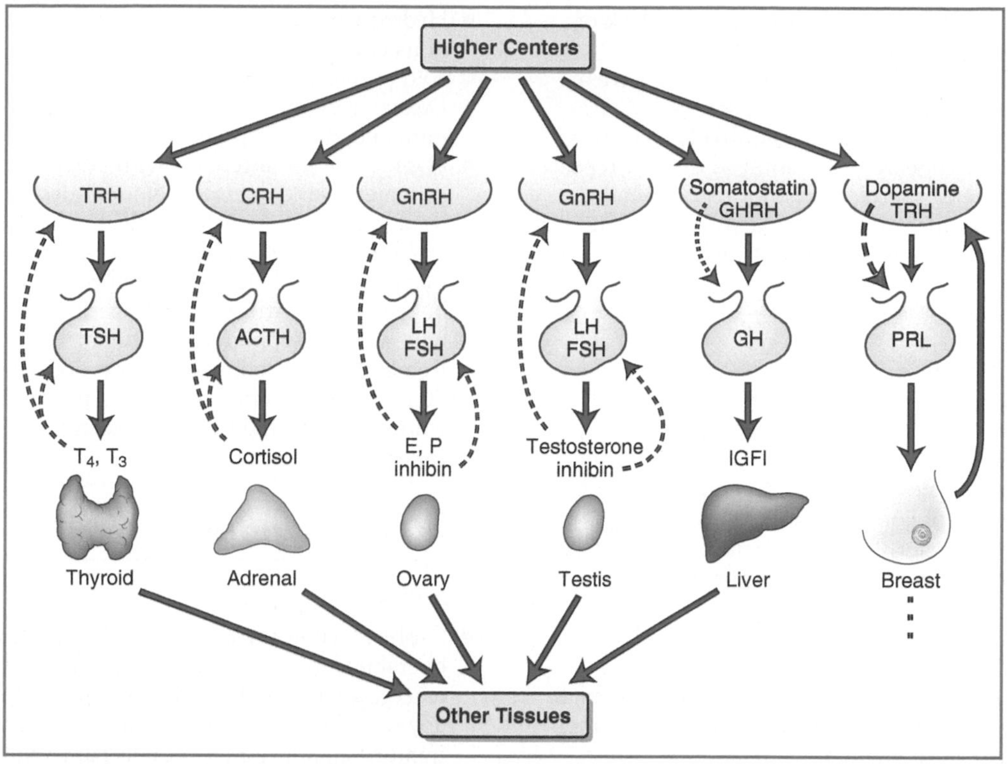

FIG. 30.2 Endocrine pathways. (From Nader, S. (2009). Other endocrine disorders of pregnancy. In Greene, M. F., Copel, J. A., & Resnik, R., et al. eds. *Creasy & Resnik's maternal-fetal medicine: Principles and practice* (8th ed., Fig. 62.2). Elsevier.)

- Secondary AI refers to adrenal insufficiency resulting from inadequate corticotropin (formerly adrenocorticotropic hormone, ACTH) or corticotropin-releasing hormone (CRH) production. The adrenal glands themselves generally remain functional.
- By far the most common cause of secondary AI is HPA-axis suppression resulting from chronic steroid therapy Table 30.1.
  - Prednisone more than 5 mg daily for more than 2 weeks creates a risk for secondary AI.
  - The duration of secondary AI after stopping steroid therapy generally ranges from weeks to months, but occasionally persists for a year or more.
  - Usually requires only cortisol replacement, because the adrenals continue to produce aldosterone in response to the renin-angiotensin-aldosterone system (RAAS) pathway, and the gonads continue to produce androgens unless there is concomitant hypothalamic dysfunction.
- Primary and secondary AI are both more common in patients with HIV.

Clinical Presentation

- Adrenal insufficiency may present acutely as an adrenal crisis or chronically. The signs and symptoms will depend on several factors, including whether the patient has preserved mineralocorticoid function, the rate and severity of loss of adrenal function, and whether the patient has a concomitant acute major stressor.
- Acute adrenal crisis is the most severe form of AI.
  - Adrenal crisis typically occurs in a patient with undiagnosed *primary* AI who experiences another physiologic stressor, such as sepsis or trauma. Patients with known primary AI may also develop adrenal crisis if they do not take additional glucocorticoids during an acute infection or other illness. Rarely, it can also occur after bilateral adrenal infarction or hemorrhage. It can also occur with the abrupt onset of *secondary* AI following pituitary infarct or hemorrhage.
  - Adrenal crisis is characterized by
    - Altered mental status
    - Hypotension (shock)
    - Anorexia, nausea, and vomiting
    - Abdominal pain that can mimic acute abdomen
  - Commonly occurring concomitantly with a physiologic stressor, acute adrenal crisis should be suspected if a patient's clinical presentation (hypotension) is

30

TABLE 30.1 *Causes of Primary and Secondary Adrenal Insufficiency (AI)*

Causes of AI	Primary	Secondary
Most common	Autoimmune (Addison)	Chronic corticosteroid use
Other causes	Tuberculosis, HIV, Waterhouse-Friedrichsen (sepsis), adrenal infarct, infiltrative (amyloid/sarcoid) traumatic adrenal hemorrhage, azole antifungals, etomidate	Hypothalamic/pituitary tumor, head trauma, pituitary apoplexy (infarction, usually of a tumor), infiltrative (amyloid/sarcoid), cranial radiation

more severe than expected, or if there is a lack of expected response to treatment.
  - 30%–70% of patients with septic shock have a component of adrenal insufficiency.
  - A single dose of etomidate is unlikely to cause clinically significant AI even in sepsis, but repeated doses can, and therefore are not recommended.
- Chronic AI has a more indolent course, and the findings may be subtle. Presentation typically includes:
  - Fatigue
  - Generalized weakness
  - Weight loss
  - Nausea and vomiting
  - Abdominal pain
  - Arthralgias
  - Postural hypotension
  - In primary chronic AI, hyperpigmentation may be seen as a result of corticotropin excess leading to melanin overproduction. Hyperpigmentation is not seen in secondary chronic AI because corticotropin levels are low.

Diagnosis and Evaluation

- In the ED, a presumptive diagnosis of AI can be made based on history, examination, and a chemistry panel that includes glucose Table 30.2.
- Volume depletion and electrolyte abnormalities in primary AI predominantly result from aldosterone deficiency.
- In secondary AI, aldosterone levels are high, but antidiuretic hormone may also be high, so the sodium and potassium concentrations are variable.
- Hypoglycemia from cortisol deficiency occurs in both primary and secondary AI.
- A corticotropin-stimulation test can be used to diagnose primary adrenal insufficiency.
- A baseline cortisol level is drawn followed by an intramuscular dose of corticotropin and a repeat cortisol level is measured at 30 and/or 60 minutes. In primary AI, there will not be a significant increase in the repeated cortisol level after stimulation.
- Use of cortisol levels and corticotropin-stimulation testing in critically ill patients is controversial. It is not clear that testing effectively delineates which critically ill patients will benefit from steroid therapy.
- Currently, little role is seen for cortisol levels and corticotropin-stimulation testing in the ED setting.

Treatment

- Goal of treatment is to treat the hypotension and to correct electrolyte abnormalities and cortisol deficiency.

TABLE 30.2 *Clinical and Laboratory Features that Support the Diagnosis of Adrenal Insufficiency (AI)*

Diagnostic Features	Primary AI	Secondary AI
Volume status	Very low	Mildly low
Sodium	Low	Variable
Potassium	High	Low-normal
Glucose	Low	Low

- Hydrocortisone 100 mg is the preferred therapy because of its combination of glucocorticoid and mineralocorticoid properties, <u>or</u>
- Dexamethasone 4 mg is an alternative, but it lacks mineralocorticoid properties.
- Hydrocortisone interferes with cortisol testing, whereas dexamethasone does not. Nonetheless, hydrocortisone is the preferred therapy for critically ill patients.
- Provide supportive care with fluids and pressors, as warranted.
- Electrolytes and glucose should be repleted, as needed. Take caution with treating hyperkalemia, because levels will fall with supportive treatment.
- Remember to administer a stress dose of hydrocortisone 50 to 100 mg every 6 to 8 hours to chronic steroid users who present to the ED with a significant acute illness or injury.

Cushing Syndrome

General Principles

- Cushing syndrome is a chronic state caused by an overabundance of cortisol. Cushing syndrome is not an emergency by itself, but it can affect responses to therapy for other conditions because it results in functional immunosuppression, as well as paradoxical adrenal insufficiency in the setting of physiologic stressors.
- Cushing syndrome is most commonly caused by iatrogenic chronic corticosteroid use. Rarer causes include:
  - Cushing disease owing to pituitary adenoma causing excess corticotropin, mostly in women aged 20 to 40 years.
  - Adrenal neoplasm producing excess cortisol.
  - Ectopic corticotropin from an extra-adrenal neoplasm, such as a small cell lung cancer.

Clinical Presentation

- Signs and symptoms depend on the severity and duration of the hypercortisolism, whether there is androgen excess, and the cause (weight loss rather than weight gain may be more common if the patient has small cell lung cancer).
- Truncal obesity, hypertension, striae, proximal muscle weakness, hirsutism, moon-facies.
- Can cause diabetes, osteoporosis, menstrual and sexual dysfunction, and depression.

Diagnosis and Evaluation

- The ED diagnosis of Cushing syndrome is made on the basis of the history and physical examination.
- Laboratory studies are generally unremarkable, but hypokalemia, hyperglycemia, and alkalosis can occur.
- Definitive diagnosis may be made by the patient's primary care physician with laboratory tests, such as late-night salivary cortisol, 24-hour urinary-free cortisol, and the overnight dexamethasone suppression test.

Treatment

- *Beware:* These patients are functionally immunosuppressed and do not mount a full response to infection. Treat infections broadly and aggressively.
- Goal of treatment is to normalize the hypothalamic-pituitary-adrenal function and reverse the signs/symptoms and complications of the excess cortisol (e.g., localize and treat the

corticotropin-secreting pituitary, the cortisol-secreting adrenal tumor, or the ectopic small cell lung tumor).

- May paradoxically require additional exogenous steroids if physiologically stressed.
- If the diagnosis suspected, but the patient not acutely ill, refer for outpatient testing.

Pheochromocytoma

General Principles

- Pheochromocytoma is a rare neuroendocrine tumor of the adrenal medulla that secretes catecholamines, causing excess sympathetic stimulation.
- It is found in less than 1% of those with hypertension, but not treating it can lead to significant morbidity.
- Rule of 10s: 10% extra-adrenal, 10% bilateral, 10% malignant, 10% familial, 10% pediatric.
- Associated with multiple endocrine neoplasia 2A and 2B; neurofibromatosis; Von Hippel-Lindau.

Clinical Presentation

- The classic triad of headache, hypertension, and tachycardia is seen in less than 50% of patients.
- The most common sign is intermittent or persistent hypertension.
- Can also have sweating, anxiety, dyspnea, heat intolerance, nausea, weakness. Symptoms are typically paroxysmal.
- May be triggered by physiologic stressors or medications

Diagnosis and Evaluation

- The differential diagnosis includes other hyperadrenergic states, such as drug toxicity, thyroid storm, and hypertensive emergency from other causes.
- The laboratory diagnosis is based on elevated fractionated plasma or urine metanephrines. ED testing is not practical.
- To diagnose in the ED, both magnetic resonance imaging (MRI) and computed tomography (CT) are highly sensitive for adrenal lesions.
- Intravenous (IV) contrast can precipitate hypertensive crisis. Be wary of giving contrast with CT imaging if concerned for pheochromocytoma

Treatment

- The principal acute treatment goal is hypertensive emergency management.
- Sodium nitroprusside IV infusion with or without phentolamine IV 2.5 to 5 mg boluses as needed (dosed every 5 minutes because of short half-life).
- Can give β-blockers, but pretreat with α-blockers (e.g., phenoxybenzamine) to prevent compensatory peripheral vasoconstriction.
- Peripheral calcium channel blockers, such as nicardipine, are also safe.
- Definitive treatment involves surgical excision of the tumor(s).

Pituitary Disease

General Principles

- Most pituitary diseases cause the loss of pituitary function, leading to hormone deficiencies, a condition known as hypopituitarism. Pituitary tumors, predominately nonsecreting macroadenomas, are the cause of approximately half of cases of hypopituitarism.
- Sudden hemorrhage into the pituitary, usually emanating from a pituitary adenoma, can result in panhypopituitarism. This condition, called *pituitary apoplexy*, is usually accompanied by headache and visual symptoms consisting of diplopia and/or visual field deficits.
- *Sheehan syndrome* is historically important, but now a rare cause of hypopituitarism. It occurs when postpartum hemorrhagic shock leads to pituitary infarction. Presentation is variable, but classically women do not lactate, and then develop hypothyroidism, adrenal insufficiency, and amenorrhea.
- Secreting adenomas can cause hormone excess resulting in Cushing syndrome, hyperthyroidism, acromegaly, or prolactinemia.
- There are numerous other causes of hypopituitarism, including infiltrative diseases, vasculitis, or sickle cell disease causing infarction, extrapituitary tumors, infections (fungal, meningitis, syphilis), empty-sella syndrome, autoimmune pituitary insufficiency, hypoperfusion from shock, internal carotid aneurysm, and traumatic brain injury.

Clinical Presentation

- Patients generally exhibit evidence of hormone deficiencies or excess, usually along multiple hormone pathways. The presentation will thereby depend on whether there is impaired or excess secretion of one, a few, or all of the pituitary hormones, as well as the severity of the hormone deficiency or excess, and the rapidity with which the pituitary is affected (apoplexy will likely present with a sudden onset, whereas an infiltrative disease will be gradual in onset).
- If there is a space-occupying lesion, patients may present with headache and visual symptoms, classically with bilateral loss of peripheral vision (bitemporal hemianopsia).
- If the posterior pituitary is involved, there may also be signs and symptoms of syndrome of inappropriate secretion of antidiuretic hormone (SIADH) or central diabetes insipidus (DI).

Diagnosis and Evaluation

- If high suspicion for pituitary disease, obtain an MRI (CT lacks adequate sensitivity).
- Also consider thyroid testing, prolactin level, cortisol level, and an electrolyte panel.

Treatment

- In the ED, providers should focus on addressing acute hormone imbalances (primarily thyroid hormone and cortisol), correcting electrolyte abnormalities, and providing supportive care, as indicated.
- Pituitary tumors may eventually require resection.
- Hormone deficiencies are treated chronically with hormone supplementation.

SUGGESTED READINGS

Field, A. G. (2015). Adrenal and pituitary disorders. In A. B. Wolfson, R. L. Cloutier, G. W. Hendey, L. J. Ling, C. L. Rosen, & J. J. Schaider (Eds.), *Harwood-Nuss' clinical practice of emergency medicine* (6th ed.). Wolters Kluwer.

Torrey, S. P. (2005). Recognition and management of adrenal emergencies. *Emergency Medicine Clinics of North America, 23*(3), 687–702.

Tucci, V., & Sokari, T. (2014). The clinical manifestations, diagnosis, and treatment of adrenal emergencies. *Emergency Medicine Clinics of North America, 32*(2), 465–484.

CHAPTER **31**

BOARD REVIEW

Fluid and Electrolyte Disorders

DANIEL ICHWAN, MD, and SCOTT R. VOTEY, MD

Background

Water balance is based on serum sodium and osmolality, which mediate thirst and antidiuretic hormone (ADH).

Sources of volume loss include:

- Gastrointestinal (GI): emesis, diarrhea, hemorrhage
- Renal
- Skin: sweat, burns, hemorrhage
- Third spacing: burns, peritonitis, pancreatitis
- Determining fluid status can be challenging, but it can be accomplished using a combination of symptoms, physical findings, and diagnostics.
- Pediatric dehydration can be suggested by sunken fontanelles, decreased capillary refill, lack of tears, or decreased wet diapers.
- An abnormally high or low serum concentration of key electrolytes can have significant clinical impact.
- Symptoms of electrolyte abnormalities can vary based on the specific electrolyte, acuity, cause, and severity of the abnormality.
- Sodium is the major determinant of serum osmolality.
- Abnormal sodium levels cause clinical manifestations when the resulting serum osmolality homeostasis causes fluids to shift into (hyponatremia) or out of (hypernatremia) brain cells.

Hyponatremia

General Principles

- Hyponatremia ($Na^+ < 135$ mEq/L) causes low serum osmolality. This low serum osmolality creates an osmotic gradient between the serum (lower osmolality) and brain cells (higher osmolality), causing fluids to shift *into* the brain to achieve an osmotic equilibrium resulting in cerebral edema and the clinical manifestations of hyponatremia.

Clinical Presentation

- Headache
- Nausea and vomiting
- Muscle cramps
- Weakness
- Altered mental status
- Seizures (usually [Na] < 120 mEq/L)

Diagnosis

- Sodium (Na) < 135 mEq/L. Serious neurologic manifestations generally occur at an Na < 120 mEq/L, but depends on the rapidity of the change.

Evaluation

- By determining the patient's volume status, the cause of hyponatremia can be diagnosed in a way that will direct treatment. Table 31.1 divides the major causes of hyponatremia and corresponding management.
- Determining a patient's volume status can be challenging, but the patient's comorbid conditions can be most helpful in determining the most likely etiology.
- Pseudohyponatremia (a falsely low measured sodium without the same clinical implications as true hyponatremia) can be caused by hypertriglyceridemia, and hyperproteinemia (e.g., multiple myeloma).

Treatment

- See Table 31.1.
- Hypertonic saline (3%) is indicated for severe hyponatremia ([Na] < 120 mEq/L) resulting in serious

TABLE 31.1 *Major Causes of Hyponatremia and Their Management*

	Hypovolemic Hyponatremia	Euvolemic Hyponatremia	Hypervolemic Hyponatremia
Major Causes	• Vomiting/diarrhea • Diuretics • Sweating • 3rd spacing	• SIADH: CNS/lung pathology, malignancies, pain, drugs (antidepressants, antieplipetic drugs, chemotherapy, 3,4-methylenedioxymethamphetamine (MDMA)) • Adrenal insufficiency • Hypothyroidism • Psychogenic polydipsia • Beer potomania	• Congestive heart failure • Cirrhosis • Acute kidney, injury (AKI)/ chronic kidney disease (CKD) • Nephrotic syndrome
Treatment	Address Underlying Cause		
	• Isotonic saline for volume resuscitation • Hypertonic saline (3%)	• Fluid restriction • Hypertonic saline (3%)	• Fluid restriction • Diuresis for hypervolemia • Hypertonic saline (3%)

neurologic impairment, such as seizure, altered mental status, or coma.

- Note that the threshold to correct the hyponatremia is lower in those with known intracranial pathology (traumatic brain injury, recent neurosurgery, neoplasm, and so forth).
- Therapy should ultimately be directed at the underlying cause.
- A dreaded complication of managing hyponatremia is osmotic demyelination syndrome, a delayed neurologic complication of rapid hyponatremia correction.
  - Increased risk if serum sodium is less than 105 mEq/L and those with hypokalemia, alcoholism, malnutrition, liver disease, and in chronic hyponatremia (developed over more than 48 hours).
  - Because the acuity is usually difficult to determine, a general approach to hyponatremia is to correct the sodium by no more than 4 to 6 mEq/L/day.
  - The exception to this rule is when there are significant central nervous system (CNS) manifestations (altered mental status and seizures). In this case, a bolus 100 mL of 3% saline over 10 minutes (up to 300 mL) should be given to manage increased intracranial pressure and prevent fatal brain herniation.

Hypernatremia

General Principles

- Hypernatremia causes high serum osmolality and the opposite pathophysiology of hyponatremia. The resultant high serum osmolality creates an osmotic gradient between the serum (higher osmolality) and brain cells (lower osmolality), causing fluids to shift *out of* the brain to achieve an osmotic equilibrium.
- Generally, hypernatremia can be caused by excessive sodium ingestion/retention or hypovolemia causing a higher sodium concentration (the same amount of salt in a lower volume). Such patients usually have an underlying condition that impairs their ability to respond to thirst (e.g., infant or bedbound elderly patient).
- Diabetes insipidus is the hypernatremic equivalent of the hyponatremic-causing syndrome of inappropriate secretions of antidiuretic hormone (SIADH).
- In diabetes insipidus, there is a decreased level or responsiveness of ADH and a subsequent urinary loss of volume, causing hypernatremia.
- In central diabetes insipidus, there is inadequate ADH production, usually owing to CNS pathology.
- In nephrogenic diabetes insipidus, the receptors on renal collecting duct cells do not respond appropriately to ADH.

Clinical Presentation

- Nausea and vomiting
- Weakness
- Thirst
- Altered mental status (usually Na > 155 mEq/L)
- Seizures, especially in infants

Diagnosis

- Na > 145 mEq/L

Evaluation

- By determining the patient's fluid status (e.g., calculate the free water deficit), the cause of hypernatremia can be diagnosed in a way that will direct treatment.

Treatment

- See Table 31.2.
- There is generally not as great a concern for too rapidly correcting hypernatremia as there is with hyponatremia.
- However, the general recommendation is to limit correction to less than 10 mEq/L/day in chronic (or unknown acuity) hypernatremia owing to the potential complication of cerebral edema and hemorrhage. The fluid prescription will be based on the calculated free water deficit, estimated ongoing losses, and the desired rate of correction.

Potassium Abnormalities

General Principles

- Potassium is the major intracellular cation.
- Because most potassium is intracellular, serum potassium levels may not be truly reflective of total body potassium.
- Serum potassium abnormalities can have a significant clinical impact, particularly on cardiac and muscle electrical conduction.
- Whereas potassium intake and excretion can cause significant imbalances, understanding the cellular

TABLE 31.2 *Major Causes of Hypernatremia and Their Management*

	Hypovolemic Hypernatremia	Excessive Na Ingestion/Retention
Major Causes	• Limited access to water • Urine loss: osmotic, loop diuretics • Inadequately diluted infant formula • Diarrhea, vomiting • Sweating, burns • Diabetes insipidus	• Iatrogenic • Cushing's, primary hyperaldosteronism • Salt water intake
Treatment	• Address underlying cause • D5W or 0.45% saline to correct water deficit in 1 day (acute) or < 10 mEq/L/d (chronic) • Consider desmopressin (also known as DDAVP, a synthetic antidiuretic hormone [ADH]) for central diabetes insipidus	

regulation of potassium homeostasis is important. Particularly, serum pH, insulin level, and beta-2-adrenergic activity can impact the serum potassium concentration.
- The potassium-hydrogen exchanger causes intracellular potassium shift in alkalosis and extracellular potassium shift in acidosis.
- Insulin and beta-2-adrenergic activity increases cellular Na-K-ATPase activity, which also causes intracellular potassium shift.

Hypokalemia

General Principles

- Potassium is important in determining membrane potential.
- Low serum potassium causes cell membrane hyperpolarization and the resultant muscle-related symptoms.
- Paradoxically, some cardiac cells are selective for potassium and transport sodium into cells in hypokalemia, which causes depolarization and increased cell excitability.

Clinical Presentation

- The mechanisms described above result in the manifestations of hypokalemia:
  - Weakness, paresthesia, paralysis
  - Hyporeflexia
  - Ileus, nausea, vomiting
  - Bradycardia, atrioventricular block
  - Atrial fibrillation, torsades des pointes, ventricular tachycardia, and fibrillation
  - Flattened T, prolonged QT
  - ST depression
  - U waves (Fig. 31.1)

Diagnosis

- Potassium [K] < 3.5 mEq/L

Evaluation

- Decreased potassium intake and increased potassium excretion are two major categories of total body hypokalemia. Intracellular shift reduces the measured serum potassium, but not the total body potassium.

Treatment

- Address underlying cause (Table 31.3)
- Correct hypomagnesemia to prevent ongoing renal potassium losses
- Initiate potassium-sparing diuretics if there are renal-related potassium losses
- Replete potassium
  - Stable: Administer oral potassium
  - Unstable (e.g., arrhythmias): Give intravenous (IV) potassium. Since IV potassium can be sclerosing to the vasculature, a max of 10mEq/h in peripheral veins and 20 mEq/h in central veins is recommended. Since rapid administration can cause significant arrhythmic effects, a total max of 40 mEq/h potassium repletion is recommended unless the patient is in cardiac arrest from hypokalemia.
  - Renal dysfunction can cause reduced potassium excretion so the amount of exogenous potassium repletion should be reduced in renal insufficiency to avoid hyperkalemia.
- If the hypokalemia is caused by redistribution for increased sympathetic tone (thyrotoxicosis), consider administering a beta blocker, such as propranolol.

Hyperkalemia

General Principles

- Hyperkalemia has similar manifestations as hypokalemia, with the exception of its electrocardiographic (ECG) manifestations. Although hyperkalemia causes depolarization of cells early in the disease course,

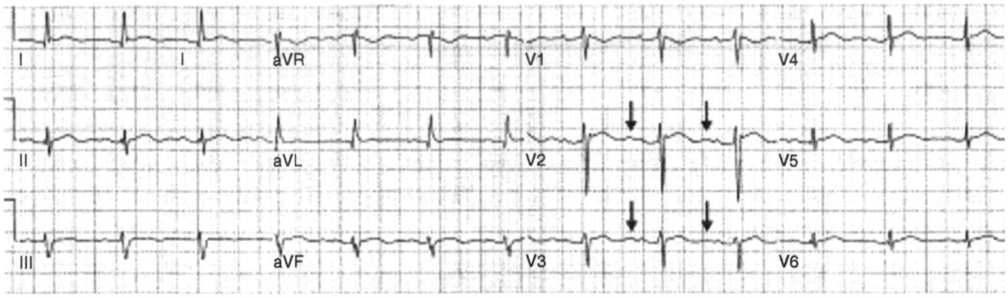

FIG. 31.1 U waves. (From Wald, D. O. (2006). ECG manifestations of selected metabolic and endocrine disorders. *Emergency Medicine Clinics of North America, 24*(1), 145–157, Fig. 1A.)

TABLE 31.3 *Major Causes of Hypokalemia*

Decreased K Intake	Intracellular K Shift	Increased K Excretion
• Fasting, eating disorders • Alcoholism	• Alkalosis • Insulin • Beta agonists • Hypokalemic thyrotoxic periodic paralysis	• **Gastrointestinal:** vomiting, diarrhea, malabsorption • Renal: **diuretics**, hyperaldosteronism, toxins, renal tubular acidosis, Bartter's, Gitelman's • Diaphoresis

persistent depolarization actually inactivates sodium channels in the cell membrane and causes decreased excitability and impaired conduction.

Clinical Presentation

- The following mechanisms result in the manifestations of hyperkalemia.
  - Weakness progressing to paralysis
  - Areflexia
  - Diarrhea, nausea, and vomiting
  - Sinoatrial and atrioventricular heart block, atrial paralysis
  - Ventricular fibrillation and asystole
  - ECG findings: [K] = 6.5-7.5: peaked T-waves, short QT, prolonged PR; [K] = 7-8: widened QRS, p-wave flattens, heart block; [K] > 8: sinusoidal, ventricular fibrillation and asystole (Fig. 31.2)

Diagnosis

- [K] > 5.5 mEq/L

Evaluation

- The causes of hyperkalemia are the opposite of those causing hypokalemia (Table 31.4).
- A notable common cause of measured (but not true) hyperkalemia is pseudohyperkalemia caused by hemolysis during phlebotomy.

Treatment

- Cardiac membrane stabilization to prevent life-threatening cardiac arrhythmias
  - Calcium gluconate 2-3 g IV
  - Calcium chloride 0.5 g to 1.0 g IV is more effective, but is irritating to peripheral veins.
  - Calcium may potentiate digoxin toxicity.
- Shift potassium intracellularly
  - Nebulized albuterol (beta-2-agonism)
  - Insulin + dextrose (to prevent hypoglycemia)
  - Sodium bicarbonate
  - Shifting potassium intracellularly in a patient with the intent of subsequent dialysis may cause rebound hyperkalemia if insufficient potassium is removed during dialysis. Following dialysis, intracellular potassium moves into the relatively hypokalemic serum and the serum potassium level rises.
- Definitively address the problem by removing potassium.
  - Furosemide IV to increase renal excretion
  - Bowel movement/GI cation exchanger (e.g., patiromer or zirconium cyclosilicate)
  - Dialysis
- If possible, discontinue medications that raise the serum potassium level, such as angiotensin-converting enzyme inhibitors, angiotensin II receptor blockers, aldosterone antagonists, and nonselective beta blockers.

Calcium Abnormalities

- Calcium homeostasis is regulated by parathyroid hormone (PTH), vitamin D, calcium, and phosphate. Calcium in the blood is bound to plasma proteins (particularly albumin), bound to anions (particularly phosphate), and unbound (ionized). Serum calcium should be corrected for albumin or an ionized calcium level should be obtained.

HYPOCALCEMIA

General Principles

- Hypocalcemia can be caused by any pathology affecting the homeostatic pathway, including the following:
  - Inadequate PTH (postsurgical hypoparathyroidisim, autoimmune hypoparathyroidism, and so forth)

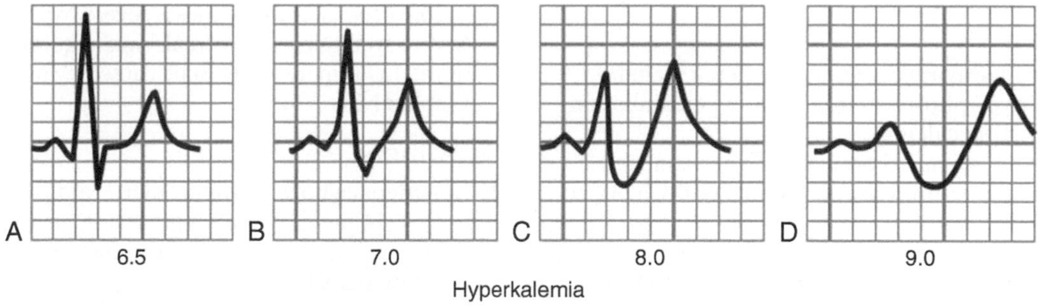

FIG. 31.2 Electrocardiograph changes of hyperkalemia. (From Campese, V. M., Adenuga, G. (2016). Electrophysiological and clinical consequences of hyperkalemia. *Kidney International Supplements*, *6*(1), 16–19, Fig. 1.)

TABLE 31.4 *Major Causes of Hyperkalemia*

Increased K Load	Extracellular Shift	Decreased K Excretion
• Potassium-containing foods or medications • Gastrointestinal bleeding	• Acidosis • Insulin deficiency • Beta blockade • Hyperkalemic periodic paralysis • Digitalis toxicity • Cell destruction (chemotherapy, rhabdomyolysis, crush injury, tissue necrosis)	• Drugs • Renal dysfunction • Aldosterone deficiency • Type 4 renal tubular acidosis (hyporeninemic hypoaldosteronism)

- Hypomagnesemia (causing PTH resistance)
- Vitamin D deficiency (causing decreased GI absorption of calcium)
- Increased calcium excretion
- Reduced bone resorption
- Decreased serum ionized calcium is detected by calcium-sensing receptors, leading to the release of parathyroid hormone, which decreases urinary calcium excretion, increases intestinal calcium absorption via vitamin D (made by the kidney), and increases bone resorption.

Clinical Presentation

- Hypocalcemia causes neuromuscular irritability, resulting in both specific and nonspecific manifestations.
  - Chvostek sign: tapping over facial nerve causes twitches of the mouth.
  - Trousseau sign: carpal spasm upon leaving a blood pressure cuff at suprasystolic pressure for 3 minutes
  - Nausea and vomiting
  - Fatigue
  - Tremors, tetany, paresthesia
  - Hyperreflexia
  - Delirium, hallucinations
  - Seizures
  - Hypotension
  - Prolonged QT, inverted T-waves
  - Rickets and osteomalacia if severe prolonged vitamin D deficiency or resistance

Diagnosis

- Total [Ca] < 8.5 mg/dL or ionized [Ca] < 2 mg/dL
- For total calcium, ensure that the level is corrected for hypoalbuminemia.

Evaluation

- The history and physical examination will reveal many causes of hypocalcemia. Other causes require specific laboratory testing (Table 31.5).

Treatment

- Address the underlying causes and replete calcium.
  - Treat any hyperphosphatemia from hypercatabolism before repleting calcium.
  - Replete magnesium (to prevent PTH resistance).
  - Asymptomatic or mild hypocalcemia: oral Ca 500 to 3000 mg ± vitamin D
  - Symptomatic (e.g., tetany carpopedal spasm, seizures, prolonged QT) or ionized Ca < 1.9: IV Ca gluconate 1 to 2 g over 10 to 20 minutes
  - Replete vitamin D if hypocalcemia is caused by vitamin D deficiency.
  - Consider calcitriol (vitamin D analog) for hypoparathyroidism.

HYPERCALCEMIA

General Principles

- The causes of hypercalcemia are the opposite of those causing hypocalcemia: increased GI calcium absorption, increased bone resorption, and decreased urinary calcium excretion.

Clinical Presentation

- The major manifestations of hypercalcemia (total [Ca] > 10.5 or ionized [Ca] > 2.7 mg/dL) can be remembered by the mnemonic "stones, bones, moans, and psychiatric overtones."
- Nephrolithiasis ("stones")
- Fractures ("bones")
- Abdominal pain ("moans")
- Nausea and vomiting
- Fatigue
- Polyuria, polydipsia, renal insufficiency
- Hyporeflexia
- Confusion, lethargy, coma ("psychiatric overtones")
- Shortened QT, coving ST-T, widened T wave, J waves
- Bradyarrhythmias, heart block

Diagnosis

- Normal [Ca] = 8 to 10 mg/dL with some variation in the reference range. Hypercalcemia is defined as a total [Ca] > 10.5 mg/dL. Hypercalcemia is considered mild if the total [Ca] is between 10.5 and 12 mg/dL and severe if the total [Ca] > 14 mg/dL.

Evaluation

- The patient's history and physical examination, with particular attention to any comorbid conditions, will often reveal the cause of hypercalcemia. Whereas primary hyperparathyroidism is the cause of more than 90% of hypercalcemia, it rarely causes severe hypercalcemia. Severe symptomatic hypercalcemia requiring treatment in the ED is more likely to be caused by malignancy (Table 31.6).

Treatment

- In patients who are asymptomatic and the total [Ca] < 14 mg/dL: avoid aggravating factors (medications, such as thiazides and lithium), prolonged bed rest, and dehydration.
- In symptomatic or total [Ca] > 14 mg/dL: administer IV NS to restore for euvolemia, plus calcitonin and bisphosphonates.
- In severe cases and if concomitant severe kidney disease, consider hemodialysis.

TABLE 31.5 *Major Causes of Hypocalcemia*

Decreased Vitamin D	Increased Ca Excretion or Reduced Bone Resorption	Hypomagnesemia
• Malnutrition • Malabsorption • Liver failure • Renal failure • Hyperphosphatemia	• Hypoparathyroidism, especially thyroid/ parathyroid surgery • Acute pancreatitis • Drugs: calcium chelators (massive transfusions), bisphosphonates	Causes parathyroid hormone resistance

TABLE 31.6 *Major Causes of Hypercalcemia*

Increased GI Ca Absorption	Increased Bone Resorption	Decreased Urinary Ca Excretion
• Granulomatous disease • Milk-alkali syndrome • Vitamin D toxicity	• Primary hyperparathyroidism • Malignancy: parathyroid hormone-related peptide (PTHrP), multiple myeloma • Renal failure • Adrenal insufficiency • Hyperthyroidism • Immobilization	• Familial hypocalcinuric hypercalcemia • Thiazides • Lithium • Excessive vitamin A

- In granulomatous disease and certain malignancies, consider steroids.
- Avoid phosphorus repletion in hypercalcemia to prevent calcium crystal deposition in tissues.

Magnesium Abnormalities

- Magnesium has similar effects on neuromuscular excitability and manifestations as calcium. Magnesium also has effects on the Na-K-ATPase, resulting in cardiac arrhythmias if there are extremes in magnesium abnormalities.

HYPOMAGNESEMIA

General Principles

- Most of the clinical manifestations of hypomagnesemia are similar to those of hypocalcemia (i.e., signs of neuromuscular irritability and cardiac dysrhythmias).
- Usually encountered in conjunction with other electrolyte abnormalities, such as hypokalemia.

Clinical Presentation

- The more severe signs of neuromuscular irritability are ataxia, tetany, and seizures.
- Vertical nystagmus is a finding occasionally seen in hypomagnesemia but not hypocalcemia.
- Prolonged PR, QRS, and QT/QT_c, ST depression, T-wave peaking then flattening
- Ectopy, atrial fibrillation, ventricular arrhythmias, including torsades des pointes

Diagnosis

- [Mg] $<$ 1.6 mg/dL. Severe symptomatic hypomagnesemia is uncommon until [Mg] $<$ 1.0 mg/dL.

Evaluation

- Hypomagnesemia is commonly caused by renal or gastrointestinal (chronic diarrhea) loss. The patient's history and physical examination, with particular attention to any comorbid conditions, will often reveal the cause of their hypomagnesemia (Table 31.7).

Treatment

- Treatment of hypomagnesemia consists of addressing the underlying cause and repleting magnesium (adjusting for renal dysfunction for similar reasons as in potassium repletion).
  - Asymptomatic: oral magnesium
  - Severe/symptomatic: intravenous magnesium
  - If life-threatening: magnesium sulfate 1.0 to 4.0 g IV over 10 to 60 minutes
  - Avoid magnesium-containing medications in patients with chronic kidney disease.

TABLE 31.7 *Major Causes of Hypomagnesemia*

Extrarenal Cause	Renal Loss
• Malnutrition, malabsorption • Burns • Pancreatitis • Proton pump inhbitors (PPIs) • Refeeding/ hyperalimentation	• Diuretics, nephrotoxic drugs • Renal disease • Alcoholism • Aldosteronism • Uncontrolled diabetes mellitus • Hypercalcemia • Familial syndromes

HYPERMAGNESEMIA

General Principles

- The major concern in hypermagnesemia is the decreased neuromuscular transmission causing CNS and neuromuscular activity depression.

Clinical Presentation

- There is a general relationship between levels and manifestations.
  - 5 to 7 mg/dL: nausea, flushing, drowsiness, diminished reflexes
  - 7 to 12 mg/dL: somnolence, areflexia, hypotension, bradycardia
  - $>$ 12 mg/dL: respiratory depression, heart block, cardiac arrest

Diagnosis

- [Mg] $>$ 2.6 mg/dL. Symptoms are uncommon until [Mg] $>$ 4 mg/dL.

Evaluation

- The causes of hypermagnesemia can be categorized into increased magnesium load or increased renal magnesium absorption (Table 31.8).

Treatment

- Involves temporizing life-threatening cardiac arrhythmias, followed by increasing magnesium excretion
  - If severe symptomatic: IV calcium gluconate or chloride 1-2 g over 5 minutes (antagonizes cardiac effects of Mg)

TABLE 31.8 *Major Causes of Hypermagnesemia*

Increased Mg Load	Increased Renal Mg Absorption
• Iatrogenic/Mg-containing drugs • Cell lysis	• Renal insufficiency • Hyperparathyroidism • Hypothyroidism • Lithium ingestion

- Normal renal function to moderate renal impairment: IV fluids and loop diuretics
- If renal failure or refractory hypermagnesemia: dialysis

SUGGESTED READINGS

Love, J. W., & Buckley, R. G. (2015). Disorders of calcium, phosphate and magnesium metabolism. In A. B. Wolfson, R. L. Cloutier, G. W. Hendey, L. J. Ling, C. L. Rosen, & J. J. Schaider (Eds.), *Harwood-Nuss' clinical practice of emergency medicine* (6th ed.). Wolters Kluwer.

Petrino, R., & Marino, R. (2016). Fluids and electrolytes. In J. E. Tintinalli, J. S. Stapczynski, O. J. Ma, D. M. Yealy, G. D. Meckler, & D. M. Cline (Eds.), *Tintinalli's emergency medicine: A comprehensive study guide* (8th ed.). McGraw-Hill.

CHAPTER 32

BOARD REVIEW

Glucose Metabolism Disorders

STEVEN BOLGER, MD, and SCOTT R. VOTEY, MD

Hyperglycemic Crises

General Principles

- Diabetic ketoacidosis (DKA) and hyperosmolar hyperglycemic state (HHS) result from insulin deficiency and associated increases in counterregulatory hormones, and are collectively referred to as hyperglycemic crises.
- Despite differences in diagnostic criteria, DKA and HHS are two different points along a common biochemical and clinical spectrum.

Clinical Presentation

DKA

- Patients typically present with abdominal pain, nausea, and vomiting due to ketonemia, and can develop altered mental status due to acidemia and hyperosmolarity.
- This may be the patient's first presentation of diabetes, but other precipitants include medication nonadherence, infection, pancreatitis, myocardial ischemia, stroke, and use of new medications such as corticosteroids and second-generation antipsychotics.
- Vital signs are notable for tachycardia, tachypnea, and sometimes hypotension.
- Physical examination may reveal signs of dehydration such as dry mucous membranes and poor skin turgor, odor of acetone on the patient's breath, abdominal distension, and abdominal tenderness. Patients with critical DKA may also develop altered mental status.

HHS

- Patients present similarly with evidence of dehydration on examination.
- Because of serum hyperosmolarity resulting from profound hyperglycemia, patients develop altered mental status ranging from lethargy to coma. Altered mental status is more common in HHS than in DKA. Patients can also develop other neurologic signs and symptoms including seizures, focal weakness, aphasia, dysphagia, and chorea.
- Triggers for HHS are similar to those for DKA and include the new onset of diabetes, medication nonadherence, infection, pancreatitis, and the use of medications including corticosteroids, diuretics, and second-generation antipsychotics.
- Impaired thirst, inability to consume fluids, and lack of access to fluids accelerate the development of HHS, so elderly, bedbound, and cognitively impaired patients are at higher risk for developing HHS.

Diagnosis

- Laboratory characteristics of DKA and HHS appear in Table 32.1.

DKA

- Typically characterized by the triad of:
  - Hyperglycemia >250 mg/dL. The glucose is commonly between 350 mg/dL and 500 mg/dL. Euglycemic DKA can occur with only minimal hyperglycemia and is uncommon, although the incidence has risen in conjunction with the use of sodium-glucose cotransporter-2 inhibitors for the treatment of type 1 and type 2 diabetes.
  - Anion gap metabolic acidosis (pH <7.3, HCO_3 ≤18)
  - Ketonemia

HHS

- Characterized by:
  - More severe hyperglycemia with glucose concentrations frequently >600 mg/dL resulting in elevated

TABLE 32.1 *Diagnostic Criteria and Classification: Diabetic Ketoacidosis*

	Mild	Moderate	Severe	HHS
Plasma glucose (mg/dL)	>250	>250	>250	>600
Arterial pH	7.25-7.30	7.00-<7.24	<7.00	>7.30
Serum bicarbonate (mEq/L)	15-18	10-<15	<10	>15
Urine ketone	Positive	Positive	Positive	Small
Serum ketone	Positive	Positive	Positive	Small
Effective serum osmolality	Variable	Variable	Variable mOsm/kg	>320
Anion gap	>10	>12	>12	<12
Alteration in sensorium or mental obtundation	Alert	Alert/Drowsy	Stupor/Coma	Stupor/Coma

(From Pasquel, F. J. & Umpierrez, G. E. (2016). Hyperglycemic crises: Diabetic ketoacidosis and hyperglycemic hyperosmolar state. In J. L. Jameson, L. J. De Groot, D. M. de Kretser, L. C. Guidice, A. B. Grossman, S. Melmed, J. T. Potts, Jr., & G. C. Weir (Eds.), *Endocrinology: Adult and pediatric* (7th ed.). Elsevier Saunders.)

plasma osmolality and associated neurologic abnormalities.
- The presence of an anion gap in HHS is variable, but the pH will typically be >7.3 and HCO_3 >18.

Evaluation

- The diagnostic evaluation and management of hyperglycemic crises should begin simultaneously with an *assessment* of airway, breathing, and circulation, initiation of cardiac monitoring and supplemental oxygen if needed, establishing intravenous (IV) access, and measuring a point-of-care glucose level. If available, measuring point-of-care potassium and venous pH may also help guide earlier initiation of treatment.

Laboratory Evaluation

- Complete blood count, basic metabolic panel, serum osmolality, serum ketones, venous blood gas, and urinalysis should be obtained.
- The anion gap should be calculated (anion gap = $Na^+ - [Cl^- + HCO_3^-]$); it is elevated in DKA and variable in HHS.
- Serum sodium should be corrected for hyperglycemia by adding factor of 1.6 to 2.4 mEq to the measured serum sodium for every 100 mg/dL glucose greater than 100 mg/dL.
- Chest x-ray and urine and blood cultures can be obtained in cases of suspected underlying infectious process. A lumbar puncture is indicated if a CNS infection is suspected.
- An electrocardiogram is generally indicated to evaluate for acute coronary syndrome or significant hyperkalemia or hypokalemia.
- Computed tomography of the brain should be considered in patients with focal neurologic deficits or altered mental status. Although a hyperglycemic crisis itself may cause these findings, it is important to identify patients who have an intracranial hemorrhage or an ischemic stroke in addition to hyperglycemic crisis.

Treatment

- The treatments of DKA and HHS overlap but have notable differences.

Management of DKA

Volume Resuscitation

- Patients with DKA require aggressive IV fluid replacement to correct both hypovolemia and hyperosmolality.
- The optimal rate of isotonic fluid infusion depends on the clinical state of the patient. Patients with hypovolemic shock should have isotonic fluid replacement begun as quickly as possible.
- Patients without evidence of shock should receive isotonic fluid infused at a rate of 15 to 20 mL/kg/hr for the first several hours with maximum of 50 mL/kg in the first 4 hours.
- After the second or third hour, the rate of isotonic fluid infusion depends on hydration status and urine output.
- Volume repletion alone initially reduces the serum glucose by 35 to 70 mg/dL/hr due to expansion of extracellular volume and increased urinary losses.
- Although normal saline induces a hyperchloremic metabolic acidosis that can transiently worsen acidemia, there is no clear evidence-based recommendation regarding choice of isotonic fluid for resuscitation in DKA.

Electrolyte Repletion

- Most patients with DKA have a significant potassium total-body deficit and require potassium replacement.
- The potassium deficit is due to activation of the renin-angiotensin system and urinary losses from osmotic diuresis.
- Despite a total-body potassium deficit, the initial measured serum potassium is often normal or high due to extracellular potassium shifts.
- Potassium should be repleted before insulin administration to avoid precipitating hypokalemia.
- If the initial serum potassium is <3.3 mEq/L, insulin should be held (insulin worsens hypokalemia by driving potassium into cells) and potassium chloride given at 20 to 30 mEq/hr until the potassium concentration is ≥3.3 mEq/L.
- If the initial serum potassium is between 3.3 mEq/L and 5.0 mEq/L, potassium chloride should be given at 10 to 20 mEq/hr.
- If the initial serum potassium is greater than 5.0 mEq/L, no potassium repletion is necessary. Test every 2 hours and start potassium replacement when the serum potassium falls below 5.0 mEq/L.

Insulin Administration

- Patients with DKA require insulin to lower serum glucose concentration, decrease ketone production, and augment ketone utilization. The choice of insulin is based on the severity of illness, institutional protocols and preferences, clinical experience, and cost.
- *Mild DKA* can be managed with subcutaneous, rapid-acting insulin rather than continuous insulin infusion. The initial dose of rapid-acting insulin is 0.3 unit/kg followed by hourly injections of 0.1 unit/kg until resolution of hyperglycemia and acidemia. Subcutaneous rapid-acting insulin has been shown to have similar efficacy compared with IV regular insulin, with the additional benefit of significant reduction of cost, primarily because of the high cost of treatment in intensive care units.
- *Moderate to severe DKA* is treated with regular insulin given as an IV bolus of 0.1 unit/kg followed by continuous infusion of regular insulin at 0.1 unit/kg/hr. An alternative regimen is a continuous infusion of regular insulin at a higher rate of 0.14 unit/kg/hr without a bolus.
- The serum glucose concentration should decrease by 50 to 70 mg/dL per hour. If the serum glucose does not fall by 50 to 70 mg/dL per hour, the insulin infusion rate should be doubled every hour until this goal is met.
- Dextrose should be added to the isotonic fluid, and the insulin infusion rate should be decreased to 0.02 to 0.05 units/kg/hr once the serum glucose decreases to 250 mg/dL.
- *Correction of acidemia* with sodium bicarbonate is controversial and only indicated in select patients with DKA.
  - Patients with arterial pH ≤6.9 with suspected decreased contractility and vasodilatation associated with the acidemia.
  - Patients with potentially life-threatening hyperkalemia including serum potassium level greater than 6.4 mEq/L.
- *Laboratory monitoring* is an essential component of the successful management of DKA.
  - The serum glucose should be measured every hour until stable.
  - The serum electrolytes, serum urea nitrogen, creatinine, and venous pH should be measured every 2 to 4 hours depending on disease severity.

- The serum bicarbonate levels and/or venous pH are adequate to assess response to therapy. Monitoring arterial blood gases is unnecessary except in cases of simultaneous ventilatory failure. Use of a venous blood gas avoids complications associated with additional arterial punctures.

Resolution

- Criteria for resolution of DKA are glucose <200 mg/dL with two of the following: serum bicarbonate ≥15 mEq/L, venous pH >7.3, or anion gap <12 mEq/L.
- Patients with known diabetes who were previously taking insulin should be restarted on their home insulin regimen including long-acting and short-acting insulin.
- Patients with new diagnosis of diabetes or no prior insulin regimen should be restarted on a regimen including long-acting and short-acting insulin.

DKA in Pediatric Patients

- According to the International Society for Pediatric and Adolescent Diabetes, the definition of DKA includes: (1) Hyperglycemia with blood glucose >200 mg/dL, (2) metabolic acidosis with venous pH <7.3 or plasma bicarbonate <15 mEq/L, and (3) the presence of ketones in blood or urine.

Treatment of DKA in Pediatric Patients

- ***Fluid therapy:*** Water losses in children with DKA range from 30 to 100 mL/kg with an average of 70 mL/kg. Initial volume expansion with 10 to 20 mL/kg isotonic fluid should be administered as an intravenous bolus. There are several differing fluid protocols used to rehydrate children with DKA, but there is no significant difference in acute or postrecovery neurologic outcomes in children with DKA treated with rapid versus slower hydration.
- ***Insulin*** should be administered as an infusion at a rate of 0.1 unit/kg/hr. An insulin bolus is unnecessary because the continuous insulin infusion rapidly achieves steady state. When serum glucose decreases to 250 to 300 mg/dL, dextrose should be added to the fluid infusion.
- ***The "two-bag method,"*** in which two intravenous fluid bags (one containing 0.45% or 0.9% normal saline and the other dextrose 5 or 10 in 0.45% normal saline) are administered simultaneously. This approach allows the rate of fluid and electrolyte administration to be held constant while the rate of dextrose infusion is titrated to maintain the patient's blood glucose in a specific range. Institutional protocols vary.
- ***Monitoring:*** The blood glucose should be monitored hourly, and a venous blood gas and basic metabolic panel should be obtained every 2 to 4 hours while the patient is receiving an insulin infusion. Fluid intake and urine output should be monitored closely.
- ***Resolution:*** Insulin infusion can be discontinued when all of the following conditions are met: (1) serum anion gap <12 mEq/L, (2) venous pH >7.3 or serum bicarbonate >15 mEq/L, (3) blood glucose <200 mg/dL, and (4) the patient is tolerating oral intake.

Cerebral Edema in Pediatric Patients with DKA

- Cerebral edema occurs in 0.3% to 0.9% of cases of DKA in children and the associated mortality rate is 20% to 25%.
- Children with elevated serum urea nitrogen or profound acidosis are at higher risk for cerebral edema.
- Neurologic examinations should be performed hourly to evaluate for cerebral edema.
- Patients who show signs of cerebral edema should be treated promptly with osmotic therapy with either mannitol (0.5 to 1 g/kg) or hypertonic saline (2.5 to 5 mL/kg over 10 to 15 minutes).

Management of HHS

Volume Resuscitation

- Patients with HHS have a significant volume deficit and require adequate fluid resuscitation before starting insulin therapy. The average fluid deficit in patients with HHS is 9 L which is significantly higher than in patients with DKA.
- The goal of volume resuscitation is to replace half of the fluid deficit over 12 to 24 hours and the remainder over the next 24 hours.
- Volume resuscitation lowers glucose by at least 25 to 50 mg/dL/hr and up to 200 mg/dL/hr, which is often sufficient to resolve associated hyperglycemia and hyperosmolality.

Electrolyte Repletion

- Patients with HHS commonly have hypokalemia similar to patients with DKA, and potassium should be repleted using the same algorithm used for DKA.

Insulin Administration

- Insulin therapy should not be initiated before adequate fluid resuscitation. The American Diabetes Association protocol recommends the same insulin regimen for HHS and DKA.

Insulin Pump Malfunction

- Commonly used in patients with type 1 diabetes mellitus, continuous subcutaneous insulin infusion via insulin pump has several advantages over daily self-administered insulin injections, including better glycemic control and ease of administration.
- Insulin infusion failure, most commonly due to kinks in the tubing or a dislodged needle, can result in hyperglycemia or DKA.

Hypoglycemia

General Principles

- Severe hypoglycemia can result in seizure, coma, and, rarely, death. A high level of clinical suspicion, a low threshold for point-of-care glucose testing, and prompt therapy are important to minimize morbidity.

Clinical Presentation

- The clinical presentation of hypoglycemia includes either or both of the following:
  - Sympathetic autonomic symptoms: nervousness, anxiety, tremulousness, sweating, palpitations, shaking, dizziness, and/or hunger.
  - Neuroglycopenic manifestations: confusion, weakness, drowsiness, speech difficulty, incoordination, and odd behavior progressing to seizure, coma, and/or, rarely, death.

Diagnosis

- In patients with history of diabetes, hypoglycemia has been defined as serum blood glucose ≤70 mg/dL. Glucose levels of 54 to 69 mg/dL are essentially a warning that clinically significant hypoglycemia of <54 mg/dL may occur.

- Severe hypoglycemia is characterized by altered mental or physical status requiring assistance for recovery.
- In patients without history of diabetes, patients must meet the Whipple triad for diagnosis of hypoglycemia: (1) signs or symptoms consistent with hypoglycemia, (2) a low plasma glucose level (typically <54 mg/dL), and (3) resolution of symptoms after the glucose level is increased.

Evaluation

- Only patients who meet the Whipple triad require evaluation of hypoglycemia.
- If the Whipple triad is positive, then review underlying comorbidities and medications taken by the patient, as well as other family members, and the nature and timing of symptoms, particularly in relation to food intake. If the cause of hypoglycemia is unclear, then further laboratory evaluation with plasma glucose, insulin, C peptide, proinsulin, and β-hydroxybutyrate, and the presence of an oral hypoglycemic agent is warranted.

Treatment

- Common diabetes medications that cause hypoglycemia are listed in Table 32.2.
- Patients with mild or moderate hypoglycemia should ingest 15 to 20 g of oral glucose in the form of glucose tablets, juice, or milk.
- Patients with severe hypoglycemia and/or impaired consciousness and IV access should receive one-half to one ampoule (50 mL) of dextrose 50% or 100 to 200 mL of dextrose 10%.
- Patients with impaired consciousness and no IV access should receive 1 mg of intramuscular glucagon.

TABLE 32.2 ***Common Oral Medications for Type 2 Diabetes Mellitus That Cause Hypoglycemia***

Class of Medication	Medications
Sulfonylureas	Glipizide
	Glyburide
	Glimepiride
Meglitinides	Repaglinide
	Nateglinide

- The glycemic response is transient, so glucose should be rechecked in 15 minutes.

Special Considerations

- Patients experiencing serious hypoglycemia due to the use of a sulfonylurea agent should be given octreotide 50–100 μg IV or subcutaneous every 6 hours to limit further insulin release.
- Patients whose hypoglycemia is due to a sulfonylurea agent or a long-acting insulin often require 24-hour observation with close monitoring of serum glucose because of the high risk for recurrent episodes of hypoglycemia.

Hypoglycemia in Pediatric Patients

- Hypoglycemia in pediatric patients occurs because of a variety of underlying etiologies, including inborn errors of metabolism, sepsis, ingestions (eg, sulfonylureas, ethanol, beta-blockers), cardiac disease, and hepatic failure.
- The threshold for confirming a diagnosis of hypoglycemia is <50 mg/dL, but to provide a margin of safety, the treatment goal is to maintain a plasma glucose >70 mg/dL.
- Patients who are conscious and able to swallow safely should be given rapidly absorbed carbohydrate such as glucose tablets, glucose gel, or fruit juice.
- Patient who are unconscious or unable to swallow safely should be given IV dextrose 0.20 to 0.25 g/kg (maximum dose 25 g).
- The volume of dextrose for pediatric hypoglycemia can be easily calculated using the rule of 50, which states that the product of the concentration of dextrose and volume per kilogram should equal 50. Pediatric patients can be given 5 mL/kg of dextrose 10% ($5 \times 10 = 50$) or 2 mL/kg of dextrose 25% ($2 \times 25 = 50$).
- Dextrose 50% should be avoided in pediatric patients because of the risk of phlebitis and thrombosis.

SUGGESTED READINGS

Kitabchi, A. E., Umpierrez, G. E., Miles, J. M., & Fisher, J. N. (2009). Hyperglycemic crises in adult patients with diabetes. *Diabetes Care*, *32*(7), 1335–1343.

Nugent, B. W. (2005). Hyperosmolar hyperglycemic state. *Emergency Medicine Clinics of North America*, *23*(3), 629–648, vii.

Wolfsdorf, J. I., Glaser, N., Agus, M., Fritsch, M., Hanas, R., Rewers, A., Sperling, M. A., & Codner, E. (2018). ISPAD clinical practice consensus guidelines 2018: Diabetic ketoacidosis and the hyperglycemic hyperosmolar state. *Pediatric Diabetes*, *19*(Suppl. 27), 155–177.

CHAPTER 33

BOARD REVIEW

Thyroid Emergencies

JOSHUA J. BAUGH, MD, MPP, MHCM, and SCOTT LUNDBERG, MD

Thyroid illness is common, but most cases of hyperthyroidism and hypothyroidism are mild and may not be readily apparent or clinically consequential in the emergency department (ED). However, severe excess or deficiency of circulating thyroid hormone can be deadly, and prompt recognition and treatment of these rarer cases is crucial for emergency physicians.

- Severe thyroid hormone imbalance frequently mimics other more commonly seen conditions such as sepsis and toxic ingestion, and thus requires a high index of suspicion (Fig. 33.1, Table 33.1).

Hyperthyroidism

General Principles

- Hyperthyroid states are caused by excess thyroid hormone, which generally involves elevated levels of triiodothyronine (T_3) and levothyroxine (T_4). Some diseases cause persistent hyperthyroidism, others produce a transient hyperthyroid state followed by a hypothyroid state.
- Graves disease is the most common cause of *persistent hyperthyroidism*, representing 85% of cases in the United States. It is an autoimmune condition caused by antibodies to the thyrotropin (TSH) receptor that stimulate excess thyroid hormone production.
- Iodine deficiency leading to multinodular toxic goiter is the most common etiology of persistent hyperthyroidism in the developing world.
- Rarer causes include toxic adenoma, TSH-producing pituitary tumor, surreptitious thyroid hormone ingestion, metabolically active thyroid cancer, ectopic production of thyroid hormone from *struma ovarii* (an ovarian teratoma containing thyroid tissue), and molar pregnancy (human chorionic gonadotropin in excess can stimulate the thyroid gland).
- *Transient hyperthyroidism*: Inflammation of the thyroid gland initially stimulates excess hormone release, and later results in decreased hormone production due to scarring. Etiologies include postviral thyroiditis, Hashimoto thyroiditis, drug-induced states, and infections of the thyroid.
  - Postviral thyroiditis is an autoimmune process that lasts 6–12 months for the full cycle.
  - Hashimoto thyroiditis: 10% start with thyrotoxicosis and can have "Hashimoto encephalopathy" involving altered mental status, seizure, myoclonus.
  - Drug-induced thyroiditis: amiodarone, lithium, interleukin, interferon alfa.
  - Infectious thyroiditis is usually bacterial.

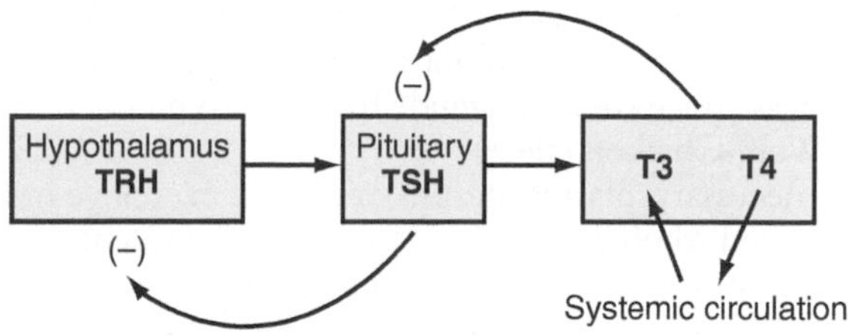

FIG. 33.1 Thyroid hormone axis. Note that T_3 is four times more potent than T_4, and T_4 is converted to T_3 in the bloodstream. *T3*, triiodothyronine; *T4*, levothyroxine; *TRH*, thyrotropin-releasing hormone; *TSH*, thyroid-stimulating hormone.

TABLE 33.1 Interpretation of Basic Thyroid Function Tests

Thyroid-stimulating Hormone	Free T_4	Condition
Normal	Normal	Euthyroid
Low	High	Primary hyperthyroidism
High	High	Secondary hyperthyroidism
High	Low	Primary hypothyroidism
Low	Low	Secondary hypothyroidism

Clinical Presentation

- Presentation varies with the severity and cause.
  - *Mild to moderate thyrotoxicosis* presents with tachycardia, hypertension, diaphoresis, anxiety, weight loss, heat intolerance, tremor, hyperreflexia, myalgias, hair loss, diarrhea, and proptosis with lid lag. Other physical findings may include a diffusely enlarged thyroid and a thyroid bruit.
  - *Graves disease* is 10 times more common in women. It causes the same manifestations as mild to moderate thyrotoxicosis plus unique problems, unrelated to the high thyroid hormone concentrations, such as ophthalmopathy with exophthalmos and periorbital edema (caused by local *inflammation* from antibody deposition), as well as infiltrative dermopathy (localized pretibial myxedema). Physical findings may include a diffusely enlarged thyroid and a thyroid bruit.
  - *Thyroid storm*, also known as hyperthyroid crisis, presents with hyperthermia, tachycardia, and central nervous system dysfunction (agitation, altered mental status, stupor, *coma*), often accompanied by gastrointestinal symptoms (nausea, vomiting, diarrhea, and abdominal pain) and

BOX 33.1 Complications of Hyperthyroidism

High-output cardiomyopathy
Atrial fibrillation (10%–20% of patients)
Prothrombotic state with increased risk for thromboembolism (e.g., pulmonary embolism)
Rhabdomyolysis
Amenorrhea, erectile dysfunction
Psychosis, tremor
Osteoporosis
Hypovolemia and hypokalemia

dyspnea. Thyroid storm is triggered by stressors (trauma, surgery, infection) and medications (iodine supplements, pseudoephedrine, salicylates) in patients with underlying hyperthyroidism.

- *Apathetic hyperthyroidism* is seen in elderly patients who present with subtle symptoms such as *lethargy*, weight loss, atrial fibrillation, and possibly congestive heart failure, but without overt manifestations of sympathetic overdrive.
- *Gestational thyrotoxicosis*: High levels of human chorionic gonadotropin can stimulate the thyroid gland and cause pregnancy complications. It is of particular concern in molar *pregnancies*.
- The *differential* diagnosis includes sepsis, sympathomimetic toxidromes, alcohol withdrawal, pheochromocytoma, and acute psychosis.

- Complications of hyperthyroidism appear in Box 33.1.

Diagnosis and Evaluation

- If hyperthyroidism is suspected, the best initial test is a serum TSH. The diagnosis of hyperthyroidism is diagnosed by an elevated free T_4/T_3, usually with a low TSH (unless pituitary-driven). Note that there are patients who have subclinical hyperthyroidism in whom the serum free T_4, T_3, and free T_3 are normal, but the TSH is low.
- A free T_3/T_4 is preferred over total T_3/T_4, because free hormone represents metabolically active hormone and thyroxine-binding globulin-bound hormone levels can be affected by other conditions.
- TSH-receptor antibodies can be sent to assess for Graves disease.
- Anti-thyroid peroxidase antibody levels may be diagnostic for autoimmune thyroiditis.
- Radionucleotide thyroid scan may be indicated (because the cause of the hyperthyroidism directs management) as an inpatient or outpatient, but is not necessary in the ED.

Treatment

- Treatment aims to reduce the activity of thyroid hormone at multiple points in the hormone production/action pathway.
- Initial therapy for *mild thyrotoxicosis* is an oral β-blocker, usually propranolol. Nonsteroidal antiinflammatory drugs may be used if there is painful thyroid inflammation. Avoid thionamide therapy unless there is a strong suspicion for Graves disease (e.g., patient with new-onset ophthalmopathy, a large nodular thyroid, and clinical symptoms of hyperthyroidism) or toxic multinodular goiter, because acute thyroiditis may soon progress to hypothyroidism.
- Suspected *Graves disease* or *multinodular goiter* without thyroid storm: start thionamide (e.g., methimazole 20 mg orally twice a day) and a β-blocker (e.g., propranolol 40 mg orally three times a day) therapy. Arrange for prompt endocrinology follow-up for further diagnostic testing and possible ablation.
- Effective management of *thyroid storm* requires multiple simultaneous interventions.
  - Supportive care with active cooling, intravenous (IV) fluids, and airway protection as needed.
  - Treat any precipitant concomitant conditions, such as infections. Have a low threshold for initiating antibiotics.
  - Administer a β-blocker, either propranolol 1–2 mg IV every 15 minutes, or 60 mg orally every 4 hours or esmolol 500 μg/kg IV bolus followed by 50 μg/kg/min IV drip. β-Blockade reduces hyperadrenergic symptoms and decreases conversion of T_4 to T_3 in peripheral circulation.
  - Start a thionamide to decrease T_3/T_4 production. Propylthiouracil (PTU) is more effective acutely, but methimazole has a better safety profile and is preferred for long-term use.
    - PTU: 600 mg orally followed by 200 mg every 4 hours. PTU can cause hepatotoxicity and agranulocytosis in long-term use. However, PTU is first-line treatment in the first trimester of pregnancy, or if the patient is acutely ill.
    - Methimazole: 40 mg orally followed by 20 mg every 4 hours.
  - Administer hydrocortisone 100–300 mg IV, then 100 mg every 8 hours. Glucocorticoids decrease thyroid hormone production and T_4 to T_3 conversion, and treat possible adrenal insufficiency. Data suggests their use improves survival.
  - Give an iodine load at least 1 hour *after* thionamide administration: Lugol solution (10 drops orally every 6 hours) or saturated solution of potassium iodide (5 drops orally every 6 hours). Iodine inhibits hormone release once the thionamide has stopped production (Wolff-Chaikoff effect).
  - If necessary, plasmapheresis or plasma exchange may be used when patient is refractory to treatment.
  - Consider administering cholestyramine, which promotes thyroid hormone excretion by reducing enterohepatic recirculation.
  - Some patients may need radioactive iodine ablation or surgical thyroid resection as definitive therapy.

Hypothyroidism

General Principles

- Hypothyroidism has an incidence of 0.5% in the United States; 95% are primary etiologies, and 5% are secondary causes.
- Hashimoto thyroiditis (autoimmune) is the most common etiology in the United States.
- Iodine deficiency is the most common cause, globally.
- Iatrogenic hypothyroidism from thyroidectomy is also a common cause.
- Other etiologies include congenital hypothyroidism, radiation, infiltrative thyroid disease, pituitary disease,

medications such as lithium or amiodarone, and the conditions that cause transient thyroiditis followed by hypothyroidism.

Clinical Presentation

- As with hyperthyroidism, hypothyroidism generally *presents* with mild symptoms, but can be acutely life-threatening in the setting of myxedema coma.
- *Mild to moderate hypothyroidism* presents with lethargy, hoarse speech, bradycardia, constipation, tingling, depression, decreased reflexes, nonpitting edema (pretibial, periorbital, nondependent), hair loss, dry skin, and amenorrhea.
- *Myxedema coma* presents with altered mental status, hypothermia, bradycardia, and edema.
  - Mortality is 30%–40%.
  - Episodes are typically precipitated by a physiologic stress or cessation of thyroid medications.
  - Can have hypoventilation, hypotension, coma, seizures from hypoglycemia or hyponatremia.
  - Edema is firm and nonpitting (as opposed to pitting edema from volume overload).
  - Frequently confused with sepsis, primary hypothermia, primary central nervous system dysfunction, toxic ingestion, or congestive heart failure (because of edema).
  - Normothermia suggests concomitant sepsis, because profound hypothermia is expected.

Diagnosis and Evaluation

- Diagnosed by low free T_4/T_3, and usually high TSH (unless secondary or central hypothyroidism, in which case there may be associated hypopituitarism and secondary adrenal insufficiency).
- May also have hyponatremia, hypoglycemia, elevated creatinine, elevated creatine kinase (CK), coagulopathy.
- If high suspicion for myxedema, treat empirically before thyroid testing because mortality is high.

Treatment

- *Mild to moderate symptoms:* First-line treatment is oral levothyroxine (T_4) starting at 50 μg daily, or 25 μg in the elderly. There is no need to adjust the dose or recheck levels for 3–4 weeks, which can be deferred to an outpatient provider.
- *Pregnancy*: Thyroid requirements increase in pregnancy. Levothyroxine doses should be increased in pregnant patients with known hypothyroidism, and hypothyroidism may also manifest for the first time during pregnancy. It is important to diagnose and treat hypothyroidism in pregnancy, because there is a high risk for birth defects if not treated. Interpretation of thyroid function tests in pregnancy can be complicated; thus, endocrinology consultation is recommended.
- *Myxedema coma*, an endocrine emergency, requires multiple simultaneous interventions, and the treatment should be instituted without waiting for laboratory confirmation.
  - Supportive care with IV fluids, adding chronotropic pressors as needed.
  - Patients may require endotracheal intubation. Beware of a difficult airway because of macroglossia.
  - Use passive rewarming. Generally avoid active rewarming because this can cause vasodilation and hypotension.
  - Treat hypoglycemia with 50 mL of 50% dextrose (D50) followed by a glucose infusion as needed.
  - Administer hypertonic saline 3% for hyponatremic seizures.
  - Administer hydrocortisone 100 mg IV 1 *hour before* thyroxine to treat high prevalence of concomitant adrenal insufficiency.
  - Prompt thyroid replacement is a crucial component of therapy. The choice of medications and doses should be individualized to the specific patient and their severity of illness. Endocrine consultation is appropriate to guide the specifics of therapy.
  - Begin thyroid replacement with levothyroxine (T_4) 4 μg/kg or 200–400 μg IV bolus. In the elderly, start with half the normal dose of IV thyroid medication.
  - Consider the addition of T_3 5–20 μg IV bolus if the patient is critically ill. T_3 increases the risk of cardiac complications, but the biologic activity of T_3 is greater and its onset of action is more rapid than T_4. Additionally, the conversion of T_4 to T_3 is impaired in hypothyroidism and with a concomitant illness.
  - Identify and treat precipitants.
  - Patients diagnosed with myxedema coma should be admitted to the intensive care unit.

Thyroid Masses

General Principles

- An *enlarged* thyroid can be caused by inflammation, goiter, benign lesions, and malignancy.

Clinical Presentation

- Patients may be asymptomatic or complain about cosmetic appearance. Alternatively, a thyroid *mass* can enlarge to an extent that it can mechanically obstruct the airway and other important structures in the neck.

Diagnosis, Evaluation, and Treatment

- *Imaging* is generally indicated in the ED only if there is a concern for airway compromise.
- If an enlarged thyroid is identified in the ED, the provider can order thyroid function tests.
  - If the thyroid function is normal or low, the patient should undergo thyroid ultrasonography as an outpatient.
  - If hyperthyroidism is present, the patient generally receives a radioactive iodine scan, as either an inpatient or an outpatient depending on the degree of thyroid hormone imbalance and clinical presentation.
- Most forms of thyroid cancer are treated on an outpatient basis with a combination of surgery, chemotherapy, and/or radioactive iodine.
  - Thyroglobulin levels are the usual tumor marker.
  - Many thyroid cancer patients are given supraphysiologic doses of thyroxine to suppress TSH production; a low TSH in these patients should not prompt medication adjustment unless recommended by an endocrinologist.

33

CHAPTER 34

BOARD REVIEW

Nutritional Deficiencies

RYAN C. DOLLBAUM, MD, and ADAM R. EVANS, MD

Nutritional disorders range from vitamin deficiencies to malabsorption and protein calorie malnutrition. Although patients with protein calorie malnutrition and other nutritional disorders are encountered in the emergency department (ED), it is uncommon for the nutritional disorder to be the cause of the presenting complaint or the focus of the ED evaluation and treatment. Symptomatic vitamin deficiencies were once common and their manifestations well known to physicians (Table 34.1), but in the developed world in the 21st century, only thiamine deficiency, the cause of Wernicke encephalopathy (WE) and Korsakoff syndrome (KS), remains sufficiently common to have broad clinical importance. Prompt identification and treatment of WE is pertinent to emergency medicine and may improve patient outcomes.

Wernicke Encephalopathy

General Principles

- WE is the acute neurologic syndrome caused by the severe depletion of thiamine (vitamin B_1) stores. Thiamine is a cofactor required for many enzymes in energy metabolism and plays an especially important role in cerebral energy use. Its deficiency in certain areas of the brain with high metabolic requirements, such as the cerebrum and cerebellum, leads to the classic neurologic signs and symptoms associated with the disease.
- Alcoholism is the most common cause of WE in the United States. Alcoholics are predisposed to vitamin B_1 deficiency because of malnutrition, diminished gastrointestinal absorption, and decreased hepatic storage.
- WE also occurs in association with other forms of chronic malnutrition, including in patients suffering from malabsorption, cancer, AIDS, starvation, end-stage renal disease on dialysis, and after bariatric surgery.

TABLE 34.1 Selected Vitamin Deficiencies

Vitamin	Deficiency, Clinical Presentation, or Syndrome
A	Vision loss, dry skin, growth retardation
Thiamine (B_1)	Wernicke-Korsakoff syndrome, beriberi; associated with alcoholism and severe nutritional deficiency
Riboflavin (B_2)	Cheilosis, corneal vascularization (the two C's of B_2)
Niacin (B_3)	Dermatitis, dementia, diarrhea (the three D's of B_3); associated with a corn-based diet
Pyridoxine (B_6)	Sideroblastic anemia, convulsions, peripheral neuropathy, Isoniazid use
Cobalamin (B_{12})	Megaloblastic anemia, neurologic disease, glossitis
C	Scurvy (bleeding, anemia, loose teeth)
D	Pathologic fractures; children: rickets; adults: osteomalacia, tetany
E	Hemolytic anemia, peripheral neuropathy, poor sensation, ataxia
K	Newborns: hemorrhagic disease of the newborn; adults: bleeding

Clinical Presentation

- The classic triad of WE consists of ophthalmoplegia, ataxia, and confusion, but only a minority (~10%) of patients experiencing WE present with all three manifestations. The range of neurologic and psychiatric manifestations is broad. The following list includes the more common abnormalities.
- Altered mental status is the most prevalent finding and may include memory impairment, profound disorientation, indifference, confabulation, and altered levels of consciousness ranging from mild confusion to coma. Depression and psychosis can occur.
- Oculomotor dysfunction is also common. Nystagmus, bilateral lateral rectus palsy, and conjugate gaze palsy are the most common ocular findings. Less common findings include ptosis, scotoma, retinal hemorrhage, and papilledema.
- Ataxia ranges from mild gait disturbance to complete inability to stand.
- Peripheral neuropathy and vestibular dysfunction are also common.
- Nonneurologic signs and symptoms include hypothermia, hypotension, abdominal pain, nausea, and vomiting.
- KS is the chronic neuropsychiatric sequela of WE characterized by anterograde and retrograde amnesia with relatively intact long-term memory. Confabulation is a common feature. Attention is often intact and patients are typically conversant and socially appropriate. KS occurs in approximately 80% of patients with WE. Recovery is rare.

Diagnosis and Evaluation

- The diagnosis of WE relies primarily on history and physical examination. Utilization of the Caine criteria improves the diagnostic sensitivity. WE is diagnosed based on the presence of two or more of the following factors, as outlined by Caine:

- Dietary deficiencies
- Oculomotor abnormalities
- Cerebellar dysfunction
- Either an altered mental state or mild memory impairment

- Laboratory testing and emergent neuroimaging are useful in patients with suspected WE only to the extent that they exclude other potential causes of the patient's symptoms.
  - Routine laboratory testing is not useful in the diagnosis of WE.
  - Blood thiamine levels are not routinely available in the ED and in any case do not reflect the brain thiamine level.
  - A low baseline erythrocyte thiamine transketolase level that increases by 25% after the addition of thiamine pyrophosphatase establishes the diagnosis, but this test is not readily available in the ED.
  - Magnetic resonance imaging, with a reported sensitivity of 53% and a specificity of 93%, is superior to computed tomography. The classic neuroimaging findings consist of atrophy of the mammillary bodies, but lesions may be seen in numerous other areas of the brain.

Treatment

- Prompt identification and treatment of WE is believed to improve patient outcomes. Treatment should not be withheld while awaiting laboratory or neuroimaging results.
- Thiamine replacement is the cornerstone of management. Despite this, there is little evidence on which to base the dose. A traditional recommended dose is thiamine 100 mg intravenously (IV) initially, followed by 100 mg IV daily. More recently, much higher doses of 250–500 mg IV or intramuscularly up to three times a day have been recommended. However, no regimen has established superiority in a randomized controlled trial, and the existing guidelines differ substantially in their recommendations. Oral administration of thiamine may be appropriate if the patient can be reasonably expected to absorb it.
- Intravenous glucose has long been believed to precipitate WE in susceptible patients, and standard practice has been to administer thiamine 100 mg IV before administering glucose. A countervailing view is that hypoglycemia should always be promptly corrected and not be delayed for the administration of thiamine. All that can be said with certainty in the face of this unresolved dilemma is that both prolonged hypoglycemia and thiamine deficiency are damaging to the brain and both should be treated without delay.
- Patients with thiamine deficiency often have concomitant deficiencies of other vitamins. Coadministration of vitamins B_6 and B_{12} may be helpful.

SUGGESTED READINGS

Day, E., Bentham, P. W., Callaghan, R., Kuruvilla, T., & George, S. (2013). Thiamine for prevention and treatment of Wernicke-Korsakoff syndrome in people who abuse alcohol. *Cochrane Database of Systematic Reviews*, (7), CD004033.

Donnino, M. W., Vega, J., Miller, J., & Walsh, M. (2007). Myths and misconceptions of Wernicke's encephalopathy: What every emergency physician should know. *Annals of Emergency Medicine*, *50*(6), 715–721.

Schabelman, E., & Kuo, D. (2012). Glucose before thiamine for Wernicke encephalopathy: A literature review. *Journal of Emergency Medicine*, *42*(4), 488–494.

Sharp, C. S., Wilson, M. P., & Nordstrom, K. (2016). Psychiatric emergencies for clinicians: Emergency department management of Wernicke-Korsakoff syndrome. *Journal of Emergency Medicine*, *51*(4), 401–404.

Shipton, M. J., & Thachil, J. (2015). Vitamin B12 deficiency. A 21st century perspective. *Clinical Medicine (London, England)*, *15*(2), 145–150.

Environmental

CHAPTER **35** BOARD REVIEW

Bites and Envenomations

THOMAS GRAHAM, MD, and BRANDON ENDO, MD

Envenomations by venomous reptiles, arthropods, and marine creatures are responsible for hundreds of thousands of deaths each year worldwide. The term *venomous* implies a specialized delivery system (fangs, stinger, spines, etc.) to deliver a toxin to incapacitate prey or to protect against predators. The term *poisonous*, in contrast, describes plants or animals that are harmful when consumed or touched, but do not have a specialized way of delivering their toxin.

Reptile Envenomations

General Principles

- Although venomous snake bites are responsible for roughly 10 deaths each year in the United States, thousands of such deaths per year are reported in Central and South America. Worldwide, mortality is believed to be in the hundreds of thousands. Venomous snakes are primarily represented by the pit viper family and the elapid (cobra) family.
- Pit vipers in the United States include rattlesnakes, cottonmouths (also known as water moccasins), and copperheads. There are many other representatives throughout the world. Pit viper envenomations are more common during warmer months, because reptiles are not active in cold environments.
- The elapid snakes (cobras, kraits, mambas, and many others, including the eastern and western coral snakes in North America) cause many thousands of deaths worldwide because of severe neurotoxicity. Coral snake envenomations are rare in the United States, but envenomations by exotic elapid snakes kept by zoos and hobbyists do occur and have caused deaths.
- The only two known venomous lizards, the Gila monster and the beaded lizard (*Heloderma* sp.), are native to North and Central America. Both have potent venom, and envenomate by latching tightly onto their victims and chewing their venom into the wound.

Clinical Presentation

- The clinical presentation of *pit viper envenomations* usually involves one or two puncture wounds corresponding to the fangs used to deliver the venom.
- Venom causes damage to vascular walls, muscle, and subcutaneous tissue. **In contrast to elapid envenomations, local effects predominate and can be severe, whereas systemic symptoms are less common.** Swelling may range from no edema (no venom delivered, the so-called dry strike) to marked edema. Ecchymosis is common, and patients often complain of severe pain at the site of the bite.
- When present, systemic symptoms include myokymia ("worms crawling under the skin" similar to fasciculations), bleeding from the bite and intravenous (IV) line sites, thrombocytopenia, a disseminated intravascular coagulation (DIC) like consumption coagulopathy, hypotension, and, rarely, death. Anaphylaxis is rare but can result in death.
- Some pit vipers, such as the Mojave green rattlesnake in the western United States, can cause neurotoxic effects similar to those caused by elapid snakes.
- **Elapid (cobra family) snake envenomations, in contrast to those of pit vipers, generally produce little or no pain or swelling at the bite site.** However, neurologic effects can cause weakness, vomiting, paresthesias, diplopia, respiratory muscle paralysis, and death. Systemic effects of elapid bites can be delayed by several hours from the time of the bite.
- Gila monster and beaded lizard bites cause maceration and crush injuries. Deaths are rare.

Diagnosis and Evaluation

- Distinguishing between venomous and nonvenomous reptiles can be challenging unless the snake or lizard responsible is brought into the emergency department (ED).
- Distinguishing characteristics of pit vipers are triangular heads, "cat's eye" (slit-like) pupils, fangs, a facial "pit" near the nostril to sense infrared radiation, a single row of subcaudal scales at the tail, and (in the case of rattlesnakes) rattles.
- Coral snakes have several brightly colored rings and mimic nonvenomous snakes. With very few exceptions, coral snakes have red bands touching yellow bands ("Red touch yellow, kill a fellow").

Treatment

- Prehospital care of snakebites in the United States is mainly directed at pit viper bites. Initial treatment involves removing the victim from danger, limiting their activity, removing any constrictive clothing or jewelry, and loosely immobilizing the affected limb in either a neutral or dependent position (not elevated at the level of the heart).
- **The most important intervention is to transport the victim to a medical facility that has access to antivenom.**
- Prehospital care that has not shown to be beneficial (and may be harmful) includes oral suction, incision and suction, electric shock, packing in ice, or tourniquets of any type.

- Wide area pressure dressings (the "Sutherland wrap") may be useful for elapid snake bites, where local effects are uncommon, but is not recommended for pit viper bites.
- ED treatment for pit viper envenomations involves the airway, breathing, circulation (ABCs), and rapid treatment of shock with IV fluids. The rare cases of anaphylaxis should be treated with epinephrine, antihistamines, and steroids. **The only effective treatment for pit viper envenomations is antivenom.**
- Crotalidae polyvalent immune Fab (ovine), or CroFab, is a Fab fragment antivenom synthesized from antibodies to pooled venom of several pit viper species. CroFab effectively treats envenomations by all North American pit vipers. Any pit viper bite with significant local swelling, or any systemic symptoms, should be treated with CroFab. It is uncommon for CroFab to cause anaphylaxis or serum sickness.
- Initial treatment involves 4-6 vials as an IV infusion. Repeat dosing after initial control is 2 vials every 6 hours for up to 18 hours (3 doses).
- Pediatric dosing is the same as adult dosing.
- There is a common "rebound" response after CroFab is administered. The antivenom is often cleared before the venom, leading to delayed presentations of local effects (swelling, pain, ecchymosis), and systemic effects (easy bleeding, thrombocytopenia, etc.) hours or days later.
- Treatment for lizard envenomations involves removing the lizard from the wound, wound care, and considering prophylactic antibiotics in high-risk wounds. Antivenom is not available.

Arthropod Envenomations

HYMENOPTERA

General Principles

- Of the insects, the order Hymenoptera is the most clinically important. Bees, wasps, hornets, and ants are responsible for more deaths in the United States than any other animals except for farm animals.
- These insects envenomate through a stinger. The composition of the venom is complex, and stings lead to significant local pain.
- The most common cause of death from these envenomations is anaphylaxis.
- Africanized honeybees, the so-called killer bees, are indistinguishable from native honeybees without laboratory analysis. Their venom is no more potent, but their threshold to swarm is much lower, leading to higher morbidity and mortality.
- The most clinically important North American ant is the imported fire ant (*Solenopsis invicta*), which causes significant injuries including mortality in humans and livestock due to mass stinging.
- Many species of centipedes, millipedes, and caterpillars can envenomate humans by biting or stinging, but generally do not cause severe systemic symptoms.

Clinical Presentation

- Hymenoptera envenomations cause one or more puncture wounds, often with a localized wheal or erythema, and significant local pain. The stinger may be retained in the wound, requiring removal.
- Localized hypersensitivity reactions can lead to swelling, pruritus, and erythema at the site of the sting. Usually this lasts only for a few hours. However, there may be exaggerated swelling that lasts a few days.
- Systemic allergic reactions can cause urticaria or edema remote from the sting location.
- Multiple stings on the order of 500 or more can cause systemic effects such as renal failure or multiorgan dysfunction, hypotension, and death in rare circumstances.
- Sensitized individuals can present with angioedema or anaphylaxis.
- Fire ant envenomations can result in multiple vesicles and sterile pustules.

Treatment

- Treatment of Hymenoptera envenomations is directed toward the specific exposure.
- For anaphylactic reactions, use epinephrine (0.01 mg/kg intramuscularly, maximum 0.5 mg), diphenhydramine 1 mg/kg IV push or intramuscularly (maximum 50 mg), methylprednisolone 125 mg IV or dexamethasone 10 mg IV, and consider H_2 blockers. IV steroids (e.g., methylprednisolone or dexamethasone) should be given unless contraindicated. Consider nebulized albuterol for any wheezing. Patients with anaphylaxis should be admitted for observation. Patients who manifest systemic symptoms should be prescribed an epinephrine auto-injector.
- Localized hypersensitivity reactions can be treated with cold packs, antihistamines, and topical steroids. Hypersensitivity reactions can sometime be difficult to discern from cellulitis. It is not common for the hypersensitivity reaction to become superinfected and become cellulitic, but if this is a concern, antibiotic administration (e.g., cephalexin) is reasonable.

ARACHNID (SPIDER AND SCORPION) ENVENOMATIONS

General Principles

- Mortality in the United States from any arachnid envenomation is very rare. Almost all spiders are venomous, but few cause clinical disease in humans. Many wounds seen in the ED are falsely blamed on spider bites.
- In the United States, the black widow spider (*Latrodectus mactans*) is a significant cause of morbidity. Venom composition includes latrotoxin, a potent neurotoxin. Females are large black spiders with shiny bodies and red or yellow hourglass-shaped markings on their ventral abdomen. They are nocturnal and build messy, disorganized webs.
- The brown recluse ("fiddle back") spider (*Loxosceles reclusa*) and other *Loxosceles* species native to the southeastern United States are believed to cause necrotic arachnidism, resulting in poorly healing wounds. These spiders are brown and relatively large, with a dark, fiddle-shaped marking on the dorsal cephalothorax, and three pairs of eyes instead of four.
- The hobo spider (*Eratagena agrestis* [formerly *Tegenaria agrestis*]) is native to the Pacific northwestern United States and may also cause necrotic arachnidism.

- Tarantula bites are painful but generally benign unless there is an allergic reaction. When threatened, tarantulas can flick hairs at aggressors, causing a local reaction.
- Scorpions cause significant mortality worldwide, but the only clinically relevant scorpion in the United States is the bark scorpion (*Centruroides sculpturatus*), native to the southwestern United States.

Clinical Presentation

- The clinical presentation of black widow spider bites involves one or two tiny fang marks, but very little else in the way of local effects. Back pain and abdominal pain predominate, and envenomations have been mistaken for acute abdominal emergencies.
- Brown recluse and other *Loxosceles* spiders can cause poorly healing wounds. Symptoms progress over several days from a stinging sensation to an erythematous ring around a violaceous center to a hemorrhagic bleb and underlying ischemia that may cause an overlying eschar and a poorly healing ulcerated wound persisting for weeks or months. Systemic effects are rare, but may include hemolytic anemia, DIC, and renal failure.
- Scorpion envenomations cause one or more tiny puncture wounds with severe local pain, but without significant edema or other local effects. *Centruroides* (bark scorpion) envenomations can cause neurotoxic effects such as restlessness, diaphoresis, hypersalivation, fasciculations, oculomotor dysfunction, and very rarely death. Anaphylaxis also rarely occurs.

Diagnosis and Evaluation

- Spider bites generally do not produce any initial local effects. Many cutaneous lesions are attributed to "spider bites," but are in fact due to other causes. Unless the patient saw the bite occur, it is important to consider alternative causes for the patient's presentation.
- Scorpion stings often result in severe local pain when the sting site is tapped or touched, the so-called positive tap test.

Treatment

- Pain control is the primary treatment for black widow envenomation. Opiates and benzodiazepines are effective first-line drugs. *Latrodectus* antivenom is available and indicated for intractable pain, cardiac ischemia, seizures, uncontrolled hypertension, and preterm labor in pregnancy. Anaphylaxis and serum sickness are rare potential complications of antivenom use.
- For brown recluse bites, local wound care is most important. Systemic symptoms are rare. Use of dapsone, nitroglycerine, and local steroid injection are not supported by evidence. Surgical debridement or excision of the wound is generally not recommended. *Loxosceles* antivenom has been developed, but is not commercially available.
- Treatment for United States scorpion stings involves pain control. The U. S. Food and Drug Administration approved a *Centruroides* Fab fragment antivenom in 2011 for the treatment of severe symptoms.

Marine Envenomations

General Principles

- Many marine creatures cause significant envenomations.
- The vertebrate fishes usually envenomate through a stinger (stingray) or spines (lionfish, scorpionfish, many others). The venoms of fish are almost all heat labile.
- The invertebrate *cnidarians* are a diverse phylum of aquatic animals that include corals, jellyfish, Portuguese man-of-wars, anemones, and many others. They cause injury through direct contact with human skin, envenomating with the numerous tiny stinging nematocysts arrayed on their tentacles. Box jellyfish envenomations (native to Australia) can be fatal.
- The sharp spines of sea urchins (phylum Echinodermata) injure by puncturing the skin.

Clinical Presentation

- Vertebrate fish envenomations usually present with puncture wounds and severe local pain. Stingray envenomations tend to occur when humans are walking in shallow surf, and generally result in a single puncture wound on the foot or ankle. Stingray spines can break off in the wound. Other venomous fish can cause multiple papular lesions where the spines contacted skin, causing severe local pain.
- Invertebrate envenomations such as those from jellyfish and Portuguese man-of-wars cause linear lesions on exposed skin of ocean swimmers. Intense local pain is common. With the exception of box jellyfish envenomations, systemic effects are rare.
- Sea urchin spines also cause puncture wounds, and the brittle spines commonly break off in the wounds.

Diagnosis and Evaluation

- The diagnosis is made on the basis of the history. Although the wounds occur underwater and patients rarely see the injury occur, the circumstances generally allow for a diagnosis to be made to a reasonable degree of certainty. X-rays for foreign body should be obtained when dealing with stingray or sea urchin envenomations to identify spines that have broken off in the wound, or if there is any concern for other foreign bodies.

Treatment

- The venom of almost all fish (stingray, lionfish, etc.) are heat labile, so treatment involves immersion in nonscalding hot water. Patients usually report immediate relief with a hot water bath.
- There is little clinical data to guide the treatment of invertebrate (jellyfish and other) envenomations. Leading authorities differ substantially in their recommendations. This may be in part because the invertebrates causing the envenomations differ, and optimal treatment may be organism specific. In particular, it is controversial whether to use seawater or fresh water, and whether the water should be hot or cold. While acknowledging the limitations in evidence, we recommend immediate copious irrigation with seawater to remove the stinging nematocysts as soon as the victim is removed from the site of exposure. This initial

treatment can be followed by copious irrigation with hot freshwater, because some aquatic invertebrate venom is known to be heat labile. Gently removing any adherent tentacles is recommended, but rubbing the wound should be avoided. Acetic acid (vinegar) has been recommended as a local treatment, as are commercially available antidotes (Stingose and others). Urinating on the wound and other various prehospital remedies have not been shown to have beneficial effects. Antivenom is available for significant Australian box jellyfish envenomations, which can be fatal.
- Prophylactic antibiotics are generally not necessary except for infection-prone wounds. When marine envenomations cause infection, consider covering normal skin flora (with cephalexin, for example) and adding doxycycline to cover *Vibrio* spp.

Nonvenomous Bites

General Principles

- Nonvenomous bites cause mechanical trauma without delivery of a toxin. Bites by nonvenomous creatures are underreported. However, it is estimated that 4.7 million Americans are bitten by dogs each year and roughly 750,000 seek medical attention.
- Dogs are the third most common cause of animal-related deaths in the United States (behind farm animals and Hymenoptera [bees, wasps, hornets, and ants]).
- Cats are believed to bite 400,000 people each year in the United States, and a significant percentage of bites result in serious infections.
- Human bites can result in serious infections.
- Patients present to the ED with the bites of numerous other mammals (rodents, rabbits, ferrets, horses, monkeys, and many others). The severity of injury varies, but primate and large-mammal bites often cause serious injuries.
- Bites to the hand can lead to morbidity due to joint infections, tendon sheath injuries, and other infections. Lacerations over the dorsal metacarpophalangeal joints should raise suspicion that they resulted from punching another person in the mouth, resulting in human tooth puncture wound: essentially a human bite. These clenched fist injuries or "fight bites" can lead to serious intraarticular infection that requires operative intervention. Patients are often evasive about the cause of these wounds.
- Rabies is a rhabdovirus transmitted by exposure to saliva of infected animals and if contracted is almost universally fatal.

Clinical Presentation

- Dog bites result in crush injuries and lacerations, sometimes with devitalized tissue.
- Cat bites result in puncture wounds that are difficult to cleanse.
- Bites by nonvenomous snakes (boas, pythons, many others) are grossly underreported and result in multiple puncture wounds in a linear pattern, corresponding to rows of tiny teeth.

Diagnosis and Evaluation

- The rabies status of the biting animal should be determined, if possible.
- Consider x-ray if there is any suspicion for fracture or foreign bodies.
- Animals with fragile teeth (e.g., nonvenomous snakes) often break one or more teeth in the wound, leaving behind a foreign body that is likely to cause infection unless identified and removed.
- If there is concern about a possible human bite over a joint, consider injecting the joint with methylene blue or a saline load and watching for extravasation through the wound. Consultation with a hand surgeon is recommended.
- Many local health departments mandate reporting of animal bites. Providers should be familiar with the laws where they practice.

Treatment

- Prehospital care of bite wounds involves direct pressure to control bleeding, avoidance of tourniquets unless necessary to prevent exsanguination. Irrigation of the wound with sterile water or saline may be appropriate if definitive care is expected to be delayed.
- ED care involves copious irrigation, wound closure if appropriate, and tetanus immunization if indicated.
- Suturing wounds, particularly distal extremity wounds, can result in a higher risk of infection. Wounds of the face and scalp are at lower risk of infection due to the excellent vascular supply. Shared decision-making can be important in deciding which wounds should be closed primarily. Improved cosmesis should be weighed against the increased risk of infection when wounds are sutured. Closing wounds by secondary intention after a short course of antibiotics is a reasonable strategy.
- Prophylactic antibiotics are frequently but not invariably indicated for animal bites. Consider antibiotics for bites on the hand or wrist, puncture wounds that are difficult to irrigate, wounds over a joint, sutured bite wounds, bites in older or immunocompromised patients, bites that cause crush injuries, or for any other infection-prone wounds. Treat for normal skin flora for all bites, plus *Pasteurella multocida* for dog and cat bites, and *Eikenella corrodens* for human bites. Amoxicillin-clavulanate (Augmentin) is a first-line choice for dog, cat, and human bites. If antibiotics are indicated for a wound due to a marine animal, consider adding *Vibrio* spp. coverage with doxycycline, in addition to covering normal skin flora.
- Human "fight bite" wounds are prone to serious infection. Careful irrigation of the wound is necessary, and the wounds should not be sutured. Consultation with hand surgery and consideration for admission for intravenous antibiotics is warranted, particularly if there is an accompanying metacarpal or phalangeal fracture in proximity to the wound.
- Rabies prophylaxis should be considered for bites by bats, foxes, skunks, coyotes, raccoons, and feral North American dogs or cats. Close contact with a bat should prompt rabies prophylaxis, even without a definite wound. Rabies is uncommon in North American domestic dogs and cats, rabbits, rodents, and ferrets. There are important geographic differences in the

prevalence of rabies and which animals are known to transmit rabies to humans around the world, and patients may have been bitten in another country. When deciding whether rabies prophylaxis is indicated, it is important to consider the nature of the attack, the animal involved, and the geographic location where the bite occurred.

SUGGESTED READINGS

Auerbach, P. S., & DiTullio, A. E. (2017). Envenomation by aquatic invertebrates. In P. S. Auerbach, T. Cushing, & N. S. Harris (Eds.), *Auerbach's wilderness medicine* (7th ed.). Elsevier.

Norris, R. L., Bush, S. P., & Cardwell, M. D. (2017). Bites by venomous reptiles in Canada, the United States and Mexico. In P. S. Auerbach, T. Cushing, & N. S. Harris (Eds.), *Auerbach's wilderness medicine* (7th ed.). Elsevier.

Diving Injuries

BRANDON ENDO, MD, and JOANNE FELDMAN, MD, MS

- Diving injuries can occur on descent, at depth, and on ascent. Pressure is the most important environmental factor contributing to dive-related injuries. Many of the common forms of diving-related injury are the result of barotrauma, which occurs when an air-filled body space fails to equilibrate with the ambient pressure.
- Given the relatively high density of water, small changes in depth cause a large change in pressure. One atmosphere of pressure is experienced at sea level. An additional atmosphere of pressure is experienced for every 10 meters (33 feet) of depth in seawater.
- Boyle's law: $P_1V_1 = P_2V_2$; given a constant temperature, the pressure and volume of an ideal gas are inversely related. As a diver descends, pressure increases, and the volume of air-containing structures proportionally decreases.
- Dalton's law: The total pressure exerted by a mixture of gas is the sum of partial pressures of each gas. Therefore, at depth, the partial pressure of each gas in an inhaled mixture will be greater than that at sea level due to the higher overall pressure.
- Henry's law: At equilibrium, the quantity of gas dissolved in solution is proportional to the partial pressure of the gas.

Descent Injuries

General Principles

- Upon descent, the increased pressure results in the volume of gas decreasing in air-containing body cavities. This combination of increased pressure and decreased volume can cause injury resulting in several distinct clinical syndromes that may occur individually or simultaneously.
- *Middle ear barotrauma* is the most common dive-related injury. As the diver descends, pressure is exerted on the tympanic membrane (TM), and the diver must force air through the eustachian tubes to equalize the internal pressure. At a depth of 4 feet of seawater (fsw), a pressure differential is created across the TM of ~90 mm Hg and the medial third of the eustachian tube collapses, preventing the diver's ability to further equalize pressure. If unaddressed, this can lead to pressure trauma of the TM and possible rupture.
- *Mask squeeze* occurs when negative pressure within the diver's mask causes damage to small blood vessels of the face and eyes. This can be avoided by adding air to the mask through the nose upon descent.
- In *sinus barotrauma*, occlusion of the sinus ostia and the resultant inability to maintain sinus pressure equilibrium leads to mucosal injury and edema. The frontal sinus is the most commonly affected, followed by the maxillary sinus. Sinus barotrauma often occurs in divers with an upper respiratory infection, allergic rhinosinusitis, or anatomic sinus abnormalities.
- *Inner ear barotrauma* is a rare but serious injury that results from the rapid development of a pressure differential between the middle ear and inner ear. This pressure gradient is typically caused by a rapid descent, often in association with a forceful Valsalva against an occluded eustachian tube. On descent, pressure is transmitted through the cochlear structures to the inner ear. A forceful Valsalva further increases pressure on the inner ear and can cause rupture of the oval window or round window.

Clinical Presentation

- *Middle ear barotrauma* presents with ear pain, vertigo, conductive hearing loss, hemorrhage, and sometimes TM rupture. If rupture occurs, caloric stimulation from cold water in the middle ear may cause vertigo and disorientation, which can be life-threatening in an underwater environment.
- *Mask squeeze* presents with facial pain, photophobia, petechial hemorrhages, ecchymosis, edema, subconjunctival hemorrhage, and occasionally hyphema. In severe cases visual changes, proptosis, or extraocular movement (EOM) deficits can occur due to the development of an orbital subperiosteal hematoma.
- *Sinus barotrauma* presents with facial pain. Maxillary barotrauma can present as maxillary teeth pain (from pressure on the posterior superior fifth cranial nerve), or cheek and upper lip numbness (from pressure on the infraorbital branch of the fifth cranial nerve).
- Symptoms of *inner ear barotrauma* include sudden-onset tinnitus, sensorineural hearing loss, and vertigo. Damage to the cochlea or vestibular structures may lead to permanent hearing loss.

Diagnosis and Evaluation

- Diagnosis of the various manifestations of barotrauma of descent (middle ear barotrauma, mask squeeze, sinus barotrauma, and inner ear barotrauma) is based on the history and physical examination. In patients with mask squeeze presenting with visual disturbances, proptosis, or EOM deficits, computed tomography (CT) or magnetic resonance imaging is recommended.

Treatment

- Treatment of *middle ear barotrauma* consists of analgesics and decongestants. Consider antibiotics with TM rupture.

- In most instances, treatment of *mask squeeze* is supportive. In the rare instances of an orbital subperiosteal hematoma with neurologic involvement, surgical drainage may be necessary.
- Treatment of *sinus barotrauma* consists of analgesics, decongestants, and antihistamines.
- Treatment of *inner ear barotrauma* consists of keeping the head of bed upright and avoiding activities that increase sinus or intracranial pressure (e.g., blowing nose). Some experts advocate urgent otolaryngology evaluation for consideration of surgical exploration and perilymph fistula closure.

At Depth

General Principles

- The increased partial pressures of nitrogen at depth cause intoxicating effects referred to as *nitrogen narcosis*. Nitrogen narcosis typically occurs below 100 fsw, and becomes profound below 150 fsw. Compressed air diving is not recommended below 120 fsw because of the risk of nitrogen narcosis.
- The higher partial pressures of oxygen that occur at depth can result in *oxygen toxicity* impacting the lungs and the central nervous system (CNS).
  - The limit for indefinite oxygen exposure without demonstrable lung injury is 0.5 atmospheres absolute. Higher pressures can be tolerated for shorter periods.
  - CNS oxygen toxicity is common when the partial pressures of oxygen exceed 1.4 atmospheres absolute, which is reached at a depth of 187 fsw, if breathing air. Deep divers breathe a helium-oxygen mixture formulated to reduce the proportions of oxygen (and nitrogen) below that of air to maintain partial pressures below dangerous levels.

Clinical Presentation

- *Nitrogen narcosis* presents with symptoms of euphoria, a false feeling of well-being, confusion, loss of judgment, impaired cognition, diminished motor control, and numbness or tingling.
- *Oxygen toxicity*
  - The acute pulmonary symptoms consist of chest pain and cough. In severe cases pneumonitis develops, resulting in shortness of breath and decreased arterial oxygen saturation.
  - The acute CNS symptoms consist of nausea, tinnitus and hearing loss, tunnel vision, muscle spasms resulting in twitching, and seizures.

Diagnosis and Evaluation

- The diagnosis of *nitrogen narcosis* is based on the history and physical examination. Nitrogen narcosis resolves upon ascent; therefore at sea level physical examination should be normal. If the patient has altered mental status, a broader differential must be considered and a diagnostic evaluation, often including a CT scan of the brain, is indicated.
- The diagnosis of *oxygen toxicity* is principally clinical. A chest x-ray can identify the presence of oxygen toxicity pneumonitis and exclude alternative diagnoses, such as pneumothorax. As with nitrogen narcosis, the patient with suspected CNS oxygen toxicity should undergo an altered mental status diagnostic evaluation.

Treatment

- The symptoms of *nitrogen narcosis* and CNS *oxygen toxicity* generally resolve with ascent. The treatment of pulmonary oxygen toxicity is supportive while avoiding high F_iO_2 therapy.

Ascent

General Principles

- *Reverse sinus barotrauma* and *reverse ear barotrauma* can occur when the volume of gas expands during ascent, causing local tissue ischemia. Sinus polyps can produce one-way valves and prevent equalization of air through sinuses during ascent.
- *Pulmonary barotrauma of ascent* is a lung expansion injury that can occur from an excessively rapid ascent with a closed glottis, or in divers with underlying lung disease (e.g., congenital cysts, cavitary lesions, obstructive pulmonary disease). A small depth change of 3–4 fsw can force air across the alveolar membrane. The greatest risk of pulmonary barotrauma occurs at depths of <10 fsw because of greater volume changes. Subcutaneous emphysema, pneumothorax, pneumomediastinum, and alveolar hemorrhage can also occur.
- *Decompression sickness* (DCS) is the spectrum of clinical symptoms that occurs when, with the reduction of pressure that occurs on ascent, dissolved nitrogen returns to a gas state, forming intravascular and extravascular bubbles. Small venous bubbles are typically filtered by the lungs asymptomatically. However, bubbles that are formed in the tissue (e.g., in joints) or move from the venous to arterial vasculature through cardiac or pulmonary shunts can have mechanical and biochemical effects resulting in direct damage to tissues, vascular obstruction with downstream ischemia, or an inflammatory cascade. DCS symptoms typically manifest within hours after diving (40% within 1 hour, 80% within 8 hours). DCS is categorized into type I (minor) or type II (serious).
- *Arterial gas embolism* (AGE) is one of the most common causes of death and disability among dive injuries. AGE occurs on ascent when bubbles enter the systemic arterial vasculature and embolize to smaller vessels, where they cause vascular obstruction. Two related mechanisms have been described. Most commonly AGE results from pulmonary barotrauma when expanding intraalveolar gas in the lungs injures alveoli and enters the pulmonary veins, returns to the left side of the heart, and moves on to the systemic circulation. This mechanism tends to occur in inexperienced divers who ascend rapidly or breath-hold on ascent, failing to exhale expanding gas. In the worst cases, the gas emboli are massive and result in cardiac arrest. AGE can also occur when bubbles form in the systemic venous circulation on ascent and pass from the right side of the heart to the left side of the heart via an atrial septal defect, ventricular septal defect, or patent foramen ovale. This second mechanism does not require barotrauma, and can occur in experienced divers, usually when ascending from a deep dive. These typically smaller emboli are only clinically

apparent when bubbles embolize to a critical structure such as the coronary, cerebral, spinal, or retinal arteries.

Clinical Presentation

- The symptoms of *reverse sinus* and *ear barotrauma* are similar to those of the corresponding barotrauma of descent syndromes.
- The symptoms of *pulmonary barotrauma of ascent* include shortness of breath, chest pain, and hemoptysis. Physical examination may reveal subcutaneous emphysema or signs of pneumothorax.
- *DCS type I* affects the musculoskeletal system, the skin, and the lymphatic system.
  - Musculoskeletal DCS symptoms, commonly known as "the bends," present as periarticular pain without erythema or swelling. Musculoskeletal DCS accounts for ~70% of DCS presentations, and elbows and shoulders are the most commonly affected joints.
  - Lymphatic obstruction can present as peripheral edema.
  - Cutaneous decompression illness presents as a purple marbling of the skin, most commonly in areas with large amounts of subcutaneous fat (trunk and thighs), accompanied by varying degrees of itching or pain.
  - *Cutis marmorata* presents as a reddish-blue reticular pattern on the skin. When accompanied by other DCS symptoms, it is usually neurologic in etiology and suggests a more severe (DCS type II) episode.
- *DCS type II* affects the CNS, the lungs, and the inner ear.
  - CNS DCS presents with weakness, numbness, headache, vision changes, dysarthria, behavior changes, and back or abdominal pain. Symptoms typically start as distal paresthesias and spread proximally to affect sensory and/or motor function. Distribution of these symptoms tends to be patchy and asymmetrical. Bowel or bladder symptoms may also be present.
  - Pulmonary DCS symptoms are called "the chokes" and present as substernal chest pain, cyanosis, dyspnea, and cough. The symptoms are believed to be the result of large pulmonary vascular air embolisms causing mechanical obstruction.
  - Inner ear DCS presents with nausea, dizziness, vertigo, and nystagmus. Known as "the staggers," it is distinguishable from inner ear barotrauma based on the symptoms starting on ascent rather than descent.
- Symptoms of AGE depend on the vessel to which the bubble embolizes.
  - Coronary artery emboli produce ischemic electrocardiographic changes, cardiac enzyme elevations, and arrhythmias.
  - Cerebral emboli frequently obstruct junctions between gray and white matter, producing a wide variety of neurologic symptoms. Although the mechanism is similar to a clot causing an embolic stroke, pure hemiplegia or unilateral brain syndromes are rare. Typical neurologic symptoms include loss of consciousness, mono- or multiplegia, paresthesias, seizure, aphasia, confusion, visual field deficits, vertigo, and headache.
  - Suspect AGE in any diver who loses consciousness on ascent or within 10 minutes of surfacing. Morbidity and mortality are significant: 4% die on the scene, 5% die in the hospital, and 50% do not have complete functional recovery.
- Creatinine kinase is elevated in nearly all cases, and the degree of elevation is inversely proportional to the likelihood of neurologic recovery.

Diagnosis and Evaluation

- The diagnoses of *reverse sinus* and *ear barotrauma* are based on the history and physical examination.
- The diagnosis of *pulmonary barotrauma of ascent* is based on the history, physical examination, and the chest x-ray. In more severe cases, a chest CT scan may be used to more fully elucidate the injuries.
- The diagnosis of DCS and AGE is clinical. Diagnostic testing and clinical imaging are indicated only to rule out other etiologies.

36

Treatment

- The treatment of *reverse sinus* and *ear barotrauma* consists of analgesics and decongestants.
- Treatment of *pulmonary barotrauma of ascent* usually requires only symptomatic treatment, but a pneumothorax may require aspiration or tube thoracostomy.
- The treatment for DCS and AGE is the same.
  - Oxygen 100% by nonrebreather mask replaces inert gases in the lungs. This creates a gradient that favors the removal of the inert gas that has precipitated as bubbles in the body tissue.
  - Intravenous fluid administration is believed to help eliminate gas bubbles in tissues and decrease intravascular inflammation. Target fluid administration to a urine output of 1–2 mL/kg/h.
  - Recompression with hyperbaric oxygen should be performed as soon as possible. Delay is associated with worse outcomes. Nonetheless, recompression therapy may be beneficial as late as 10–14 days after exposure.
  - Patients should be kept supine. Trendelenburg positioning is no longer recommended because it has not been shown to decrease risk of cerebral symptoms and may lead to worse cerebral edema.

Flying After Diving

- Commercial airline cabins are pressurized to ~8000 ft, which can put divers at risk for developing DCS during a flight if they fly too soon after diving. The most widely used guidelines set for recreational divers are:
  - Flying should be delayed by at least 12 hours for a single no-decompression dive.
  - Flying should be delayed by 18 hours for multiple days of diving or multiple dives in a day.
  - There is insufficient data for recommendations for dives requiring decompression stops.

SUGGESTED READINGS

Byyny, R. L., & Shockley, L. W. (2018). Scuba diving and dysbarism. In R. M. Walls, R. S. Hockberger, & M. Gausche-Hill (Eds.), *Rosen's emergency medicine: Concepts and clinical practice* (9th ed.). Elsevier.

Snyder, B., & Neuman, T. (2016). Diving disorders. In J. E. Tintinalli, J. S. Stapczynski, O. J. Ma, D. M. Yealy, G. D. Meckler, & D. M. Cline (Eds.), *Tintinalli's emergency medicine: A comprehensive study guide* (8th ed.). McGraw-Hill Education.

Van Hoesen, K. B., & Lang, M. A. (2017). Diving medicine. In P. S. Auerbach, T. Cushing, & N. S. Harris (Eds.), *Auerbach's wilderness medicine* (7th ed.). Elsevier.

Radiation and Electrical Injuries

CAROLINE HUMPHREYS, MD, and ERIC SAVITSKY, MD

Radiation Injuries

- Radiation is the process of energy transfer through space as electromagnetic waves or subatomic particles. Emergency physicians must know how to respond to many forms of radiation exposure, ranging from complications of radiation therapy in cancer patients, to nuclear power facility accidents and thermonuclear attacks.
- Radiation terrorism may take the form of a dirty bomb or radiation exposure device.
  - A dirty bomb (radiation dispersion device) is a conventional explosive attached to radioactive material that disperses the material when detonated.
  - A radiation exposure device is radioactive material positioned in a public space emitting ionizing radiation.
- The detonation of a nuclear weapon would cause widespread blast injury (including burns) in a wide area surrounding the detonation. Blast injuries are categorized into four types; each type has its own mechanism of injury (Table 37.1). Electromagnetic wave radiation will be immediately released and radioactive particulate matter will be dispersed into the environment.

TABLE 37.1 *The Four Types of Blast Injury*

Type of Blast Injury	Mechanism of Injury
Primary	Injury caused by the effect of the blast wave on the body. Injury occurs principally in the gas-filled organs, and results from extreme pressure differentials developed at body surfaces. Organs most susceptible are the middle ear, lungs, and bowel.
Secondary	Injury caused by flying debris and fragments, propelled mostly by the blast winds generated by an explosion. Most commonly produces penetrating injury to the body. At very close distance from the explosion, may cause limb amputation or total body disruption.
Tertiary	Injury results from victim being displaced through space by the blast wind and impacting a stationary object.
Quaternary	Injury suffered as a result of all other effects of bomb, including crush injury from a collapsed structure, inhalation of toxic gases and debris, exposure to radiation, exacerbation of prior medical illnesses, and thermal burns.

General Principles

- Radioactivity refers to the spontaneous loss of particles (α and β particles, neutrons) or energy (γ-rays and x-rays) from an unstable, decaying atom. Matter containing unstable atoms that emit ionizing radiation is said to be radioactive.
- A person or object exposed to ionizing radiation is exposed, but does not become radioactive (thereby endangering others) unless contaminated with radioactive particulate matter.
- Radioactive particles can be spread by direct contact, air, or water. A person or object contaminated by radioactive particles will continue to receive radiation exposure, and may spread these radioactive particles to the surrounding environment (secondary contamination).
- Radiation is classified as ionizing (high energy) and nonionizing (low energy).
  - Nonionizing radiation includes visible light, infrared light, radio waves, and microwaves, and can release heat, but is considered less dangerous to humans.
  - Ionizing radiation (α particles, β particles, neutrons, x-rays and γ-rays) may cause significant effects by damaging cells and DNA. Gamma (γ) rays are the principal cause of acute radiation syndrome.
- Radiation injury is determined by type, duration, and amount of radiation exposure.
- Radiation energy deposited into the body is termed a dose of radiation.
  - Gray (Gy) and rad units describe the absorbed dose of radiation per gram of tissue (1 Gy = 100 rad). Gray is the SI unit and rad is the unit used in the United States.
  - Sievert and rem units standardize the absorbed dose of radiation by potential to damage tissue (1 Sv = 100 rem). Sievert is the SI unit and rem is the unit used in the United States.
  - Rem and rad are often used interchangeably, which is acceptable, unless measuring effects of α particles and neutron radiation.

Clinical Presentation

- Clinical presentation is determined by the form of radiation exposure, as well as the patient's distance from the source, the time of exposure, and whether there was any shielding from the source.
- A radiation exposure device that covertly releases ionizing radiation may lead to victims presenting subacutely with nonspecific signs, including malaise, epilation (hair loss), gastrointestinal symptoms, and bone marrow suppression.

- Alternatively, a dirty bomb explosion will result in well-publicized blast injury and widespread radioactive contamination.
  - The type of radioactive material used in the bomb will determine ionizing radiation effects.
  - Radiation injury will be limited to the immediate blast location; the concentration of radioactive particles will diminish upon dispersal.
  - Significant injuries may result from blast injury, including burns.
- A nuclear power facility accident will likely also be well publicized and may result in workers being exposed to high levels of ionizing radiation, and widespread environmental radioactive contamination.
  - The general public is usually evacuated from the affected area, and exposed people may seek care hundreds of miles from the incident.
  - Most people seeking care will be asymptomatic but concerned about radioactive fallout and the need for specific treatment.
- A nuclear weapon attack will cause devastating widespread blast injuries (including burns) in the vicinity of detonation.
  - A large nuclear weapon (>50 kilotons) detonation will cause severe injuries from flying debris and burns. Survivors will present with sequelae of blast injury and burns in addition to radioactive particulate contamination, and will rapidly overwhelm health systems.
  - Most deaths will result from blast injury and burns, rather than from radiation. For reference, the 15-kiloton detonation over Hiroshima, Japan, in 1945 resulted in 75,000 deaths and 150,000 casualties. Most of the deaths were from blast injury.
  - Large amounts of electromagnetic wave (γ-ray) radiation will be immediately released, and radioactive particulate matter (α and β particles and neutrons) will be dispersed into the environment. Patients exposed to significant levels of ionizing radiation will develop dose-dependent signs and symptoms.
  - *Acute radiation syndrome* (ARS) refers to the sequence of body organ injuries that develop after high-level, whole-body exposure to ionizing radiation. Estimates from limited data on human exposure suggest the median lethal dose $LD_{50}/60$ (i.e., the dose that will kill 50% of an exposed population within 60 days) for whole-body exposure to ionizing radiation is 3.25–4 Gy, assuming no supportive medical care is provided. Doses >12 Gy are not survivable, even with aggressive medical care. Doses lower than a threshold of 1 Gy (100 rad) are not expected to cause clinically apparent ARS. ARS is defined by four phases:
    - *Prodromal (0–2 days)*: Presents with nausea, vomiting, diarrhea, anorexia, headache, lethargy, and weakness. The minimum whole-body absorbed dose that causes prodromal symptoms is 1–1.5 Gy.
    - *Latency (2–20 days)*: A transient period of seeming recovery—asymptomatic or minimally symptomatic
    - *Manifest illness (21–60 days)*: Characterized by bone marrow failure and multiple organ dysfunction; signs and symptoms may include bleeding, infection, diarrhea, and fatigue. Medical management greatly impacts patient outcomes during this phase.
    - *Recovery*: Variable; may span months to years, or death may occur.
  - The timing and duration of each phase is determined by radiation dose.
  - Survivable radiation injury is not life-threatening in the first few hours after exposure.
  - Body organs are sequentially damaged based on sensitivity to radiation. Most-to-least radiosensitive body systems are hematologic, gastrointestinal, cardiovascular, central nervous system.
  - There are also cutaneous manifestations of ARS, resulting in dose-dependent effects ranging from hair loss and erythema to desquamation to skin necrosis.
  - Survivors will be at increased risk for radiation-induced cancers, including leukemia and solid organ tumors.

37

Diagnosis and Evaluation

- Diagnosis of radiation injury is suggested by clinical history and supported by clinical and laboratory assessment.
- Consider radiation exposure in patients with a suggestive or known history of exposure and signs and symptoms that include malaise, epilation, nausea, vomiting, or diarrhea.
- Time to onset of symptoms is an important indicator of the severity of exposure and prognosis.
  - Time to emesis of <1 hour after exposure has 98% specificity for predicting an absorbed radiation dose of >2 Gy.
  - Absorbed radiation doses of 6–30 Gy (600–3000 rad) result in gastrointestinal symptoms within minutes of exposure.
  - Absorbed radiation doses >30 Gy (3000 rad) cause immediate additional skin, cardiovascular, and central nervous system signs and symptoms.
- Lymphocytes are the most radiosensitive cells in the body. The timing of initial symptoms coupled with the patient's absolute lymphocyte count provides early indication of radiation injury severity (Table 37.2).
- Once a radiation exposure incident injury is suspected, mobilize appropriate resources (e.g., health physicist or radiation safety officer) to confirm the diagnosis.
  - Definitive confirmation of radiation injury or radioactive contamination will involve radiation monitoring instruments and/or biologic dosimetry, among other techniques.
  - Radiation monitoring instruments (e.g., Geiger-Mueller counter) screen for radioactive contamination.

TABLE 37.2 *Lymphocyte Counts Within 24–48 Hours of Radiation Exposure*

Absolute Lymphocyte Count	Estimated Radiation Exposure
3000 cells/mm^3	<2.5 Gy
400–1200 cells/mm^3	2–3.5 Gy
<100 cells/mm^3	> 5.5 Gy

Treatment

- Radiation injury management depends on the context of the exposure. Most injuries and early deaths that follow a dirty bomb or nuclear weapon detonation are due to blast injury (including burns), and the primary treatment objective for exposed patients is to stabilize conventional injuries as the first priority.
- Do not delay lifesaving care for fear of secondary contamination. Unless the hospital is in the blast zone, radiation exposure risk will be limited to radioactive particulate contaminants on victims, clothing, or personal items.
- Request expert radiation assistance (e.g., health physicist or radiation safety officer) as soon as a radiation incident is suspected.
- Assume all patients with radiation exposure are contaminated until proven otherwise.
- Adhere to universal precautions (double gloves, face shields, gowns, double shoe covers) when caring for patients with radioactive contamination to prevent secondary contamination.
- Universal precautions are generally sufficient during treatment of hospitalized victims of nuclear or radiologic incidents, with the rare exception of highly radioactive embedded shrapnel.
- Stabilize immediate life threats and follow standard hazardous material decontamination principles. Ideally, patient decontamination is performed outside of the health-care facility so as to not contaminate the hospital.
- Decontamination involves removing contaminated clothing and cleaning patients with soap and water. Irrigate wounds copiously and remove foreign bodies.
- Avoid abrading intact skin because this may deposit radioactive material deeper into the dermis.
- Geiger-Mueller instruments can assess adequacy of decontamination (serial measurements may be required).
- Package contaminated clothing for future radioactive isotope identification. Collect decontamination effluent as radioactive waste.
- A nuclear power plant accident may result in environmental dispersion of radioactive isotopes, which can result in internal contamination, necessitating widespread distribution of a chelating agent to the affected population to prevent serious health effects.
- Routes for internal contamination include skin absorption, wound contamination, inhalation, and ingestion.
- Incorporation occurs when radioactive materials are absorbed into the bloodstream and distributed throughout the body. Rates of incorporation vary and treatment of internal contamination is directed at reducing the absorbed radiation dose. Additional treatments focus upon blocking absorption and/or enhancing elimination.
- Chelating agents need to be administered before, or shortly after, radioactive isotope exposure to be effective.
- Chelating agent selection depends upon the radioisotope(s) to which the patient has been exposed.
  - Potassium iodide (KI) is used to prevent thyroid cancer after exposure to radioactive iodine.
  - Specific medications mitigate negative effects of radionuclides (e.g., Prussian blue for radioactive cesium-137 and thallium).
  - These treatments are complex and require involving radiation experts, and many of these medications are not locally available and require federal agency support for access. Consultation with the Radiation Emergency Assistance Center and Training Site (REAC/TS) in Oak Ridge, Tennessee, is a good option.
- Management of a patient with ARS is primarily supportive, with a focus on symptom control (e.g., nausea, vomiting, pain), hematologic cell line monitoring and replacement, and infection control.
- Following initial triage and emergency care guidelines: transfer patients in need of intensive care to a facility with advanced care capabilities (i.e., burn and oncologic centers).
- High-level radiation can cause skin and soft tissue injury (radiation dermatitis).
- Monitor closely for fluid and electrolyte shifts.
- Serial monitoring and repletion of depleted hematologic cell lines with blood component transfusion and cytokine therapy may be required.
- Irradiated tissue exhibits delayed healing. Perform surgical interventions within the first 48 hours, or delay procedures for at least 6 weeks.
- Psychological effects of radiation exposure are significant. Concise, accurate, and timely communication with patients, family, and the public is very important and difficult to accomplish.

Electrical Injuries

General Principles

- The principal mechanisms of electrical injury include direct effects of electrical current, transformation of electrical energy into thermal energy, and secondary trauma.
- Electrical injury severity is determined by strength of electric current and duration of contact.
- Ohm's law ($I = V/R$) describes the relationship of current, voltage, and resistance: current is directly proportional to voltage and inversely proportional to resistance. I = current through conductor (amperes); V = potential electric difference (volts); R = resistance of conductor (ohms).
- Electrical injuries are classified as low-voltage (<1000 V), high-voltage (>1000 V), and lightning strikes. Household voltage is approximately 110 V in the United States and 220 V in much of the rest of the world; voltage in industrial power lines can exceed 100,000 V.
- Current is direct or alternating.
  - Alternating current is characterized by directional reversals of electron flow and is found in most electrical applications intended for public use, including outlets in homes and offices.
  - Direct current is characterized by unidirectional electron flow and is found in batteries, industrial applications (e.g., power lines), and lightning.

Clinical Presentation

- Signs and symptoms associated with both low- and high-voltage electrical injuries are highly variable and depend on the amount and duration of electric current flowing through the body.

- Alternating current can repetitively stimulate muscle contraction, resulting in tetany and protracted contact with electrical source.
- Direct current tends to jolt the victim away from the electrical source due to violent muscle contraction.
- Cardiac arrest may occur from low- or high-voltage electric circuit injury.
  - Ventricular fibrillation is more common after alternating current electrical injury, whereas asystole is more common after direct current electrical injury.
  - Atrial dysrhythmias and conduction system disorders may occur.
- A variety of central and peripheral nervous system disorders can accompany significant electrical injuries.
  - Intracranial hemorrhage can occur.
  - Signs and symptoms include loss of consciousness, weakness, paralysis, mental status disturbances, autonomic instability, and peripheral nerve dysfunction.
- Both low- and high-voltage exposures can injure deep tissue.
  - Arterial and venous thrombosis have been described after low- and high-voltage electrical injuries, but high-voltage electrical injuries tend to impart greater deep tissue injury and microvascular thrombosis.
  - Burn thickness and pattern varies in fatal low- and high-voltage electrical injuries.
  - The high resistance of bone to electrical current generates heat when a current passes through it, and the surrounding deep tissue is often injured. This may lead to tissue necrosis, rhabdomyolysis, and compartment syndromes. Acute renal failure is a known complication.
- As opposed to thermal burn injuries, external stigmata of electrical injury tend to be minimal, resulting in care providers underestimating injury severity.
  - Physical findings may include an entrance and exit wound.
  - Flash (arc) burns may be seen when electrical current fails to penetrate the skin.
  - Cutaneous thermal burns may occur if clothing catches fire during exposure.
- Children chewing on power cords may suffer a characteristic orolabial burn, classically complicated by delayed labial artery hemorrhage after eschar separation.

Diagnosis and Evaluation

- The clinical history is used to make diagnosis of low- or high-voltage electrical injury.
- Patients who are asymptomatic after low-voltage electrical exposure with normal physical findings do not require further medical evaluation.
- Patients with high-voltage electrical exposure (>1000 V) may benefit from inpatient observation, given the higher rate of complications. Consider telemetry observation for those who have arrhythmias in the field or in the emergency department, loss of consciousness, or if there are abnormal electrocardiogram changes.
- Physical findings (e.g., entrance and exit wound) may support the diagnosis, but physical findings often fail to reflect severity of deep tissue injury.
- Screen for secondary trauma. Patients who fall or are thrown after an electrical exposure may have sustained significant traumatic injuries.
- Complete hematologic and metabolic testing is indicated in symptomatic patients, including creatine phosphokinase and urinalysis.

Treatment

- First responders must confirm that patients are no longer in contact with the source of electrical current.
- Initiate immediate cardiopulmonary resuscitation and defibrillation (if indicated) in pulseless patients after electrical injury.
- Manage secondary traumatic injuries if any.
- If present, manage rhabdomyolysis and compartment syndrome as needed.
- Provide supportive burn care, including transfer to burn center as appropriate.

Lightning Injuries

General Principles

- Lightning strikes are the electrostatic discharge of an electrical potential that exceeds 10 million volts between the atmosphere and Earth. Lightning strikes have an approximately 30% fatality rate, with many survivors suffering permanent disabilities.

Clinical Presentation

- Mechanisms of lightning injury include electrothermal and blunt force effects. The specific mechanisms are complex and the resulting injuries are tremendously variable, but severe injury and death are common in lightning strike victims.
- Immediate deaths are typically due to respiratory arrest and cardiac dysrhythmias.
  - Sinus rhythm may spontaneously return after cardiac standstill caused by a lightning strike, provided respiratory support is immediately administered or breathing resumes.
  - In the setting of persistent apnea and hypoxemia, malignant degeneration of cardiac rhythm occurs.
  - Myocardial infarction may occur.
- Burns are often superficial because of the short duration of electrical energy exposure and flashover phenomena. A characteristic branching, fern-like, or dendritic pattern has been described, termed Lichtenberg figures. This rapidly resolving lesion is pathognomonic for lightning strikes (Fig. 37.1).
- Central nervous system dysfunction is common and may include loss of consciousness, paraplegia, seizures, amnesia, and hallucinations.
  - Autonomic instability is common.
  - The pupillary examination results may be unreliable owing to autonomic dysfunction. Dilated and unreactive pupils should not be equated with lack of neurologic function.
  - Basilar skull fractures and intracranial hemorrhages have been reported.
- *Keraunoparalysis* is a transient pulseless, paralyzed, cyanotic, or mottled extremity resulting from vasospasm after a lightning strike. The findings are typically transient, but may persist.

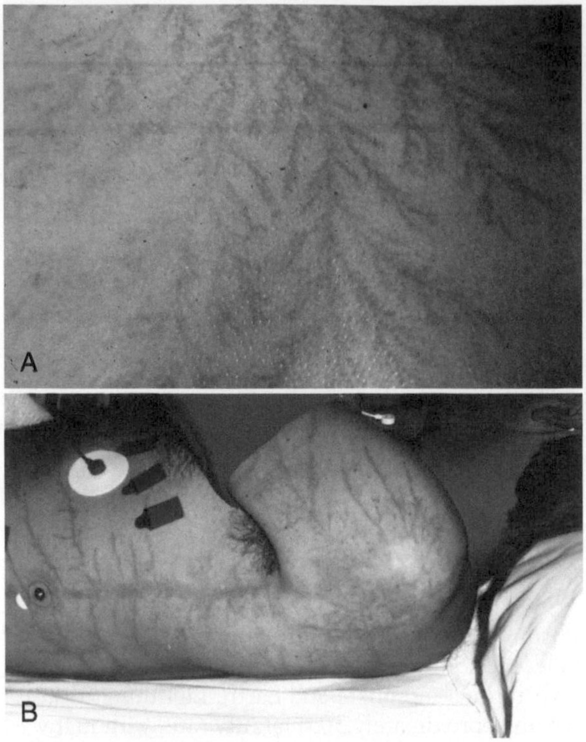

FIG. 37.1 (A) feathering marks; (B) ferning developed after the victim received a side flash lighting strike. (From Auerbach, P. S., Cushing, T., & Harris, N. S. (Eds.), *Auerbach's wilderness medicine* (7th ed.). Elsevier.)

- Many ocular abnormalities have been described, including hyphemas, cataracts, vitreous hemorrhages, and retinal and optic nerve injuries.
- Tympanic membrane rupture is seen in most lightning strike victims. Sensorineural hearing loss has also been described.
- A variety of musculoskeletal injuries can occur, including shoulder dislocations and fractures.
- Rhabdomyolysis with resultant secondary acute renal failure can occur.

Diagnosis and Evaluation

- Clinical history is often used to make the diagnosis of lightning injury.
- Physical findings (e.g., Lichtenberg figures) can establish the diagnosis, but they often fail to reflect the full extent of injuries.
- Patient should be screened for secondary trauma, with a low threshold for neuroimaging given frequent central nervous system and spinal injuries.
- Hematologic and metabolic testing, including creatine kinase and urinalysis, is indicated.

Treatment

- Initiate immediate cardiopulmonary resuscitation and defibrillation (if indicated) in pulseless patients after lightning injury.
- Manage secondary traumatic injuries as indicated.
- If present, manage rhabdomyolysis and compartment syndrome with standard measures.
- Provide supportive care.
- Unlike most multiple casualty incident triage priorities, patients with lightning injuries with cardiopulmonary arrest should be treated first ("reverse triage"), as they can have good outcomes if immediately managed.

Conducted Electrical Weapons

General Principles

- Conducted electrical weapons such as a stun gun or a Taser deliver incapacitating bursts of high-voltage, low-amperage direct current.
- Stun guns require direct contact, whereas Tasers fire projectiles and deliver electrical current through wires.

Clinical Presentation

- No significant physiologic sequelae have been documented when electric discharge is <15 seconds; however, exposure may precipitate secondary injuries. Case reports have described cardiac dysrhythmias and even cardiac arrest after being hit with conducted electrical weapons, although concurrent sympathomimetic drug use and/or underlying medical disorders were believed to be contributory.

Diagnosis and Evaluation

- Consider secondary trauma because these patients often fall after being "stunned" or have had a physical altercation before the electrical injury. However, prolonged observation or cardiac evaluation is not indicated in asymptomatic patients.
- Monitoring and symptom-based evaluation is warranted in patients with abnormal vital signs and/or systemic complaints, especially if they display evidence of a toxidrome or have significant medical comorbidities.

Treatment

- Supportive care for toxidromes, and treat the traumatic injuries.

SUGGESTED READINGS

Health Physics Society. (2017). *Radiation and risk: Expert perspectives*. Health Physics Society. https://hps.org/documents/radiation_and_risk.pdf

Gale, R. P., & Armitage, J. O. (2018). Are we prepared for nuclear terrorism? *New England Journal of Medicine*, *378*, 1246–1254. doi:10.1056/NEJMsr1714289

Koumbourlis, A. C. (2002). Electrical injuries. *Critical Care Medicine*, *30*(Suppl. 11), S424–S430. doi:10.1097/00003246-200211001-00007

Waselenko, J. K., MacVittie, T. J., Blakely, W. F., Pesik, N., Wiley, A. L., Dickerson, W. E., Tsu, H., Confer, D. L., Coleman, C. N., Seed, T., Lowry, P., Armitage, J. O., Dainiak, N., & the Strategic National Stockpile Radiation Working Group. (2004). Medical management of the acute radiation syndrome: Recommendations of the Strategic National Stockpile Radiation Working Group. *Annals of Internal Medicine*, *140*(12), 1037–1051.

CHAPTER 38

BOARD REVIEW

High-Altitude Illness

MATTHEW ROSEN, MD, and SCOTT R. VOTEY, MD

High-altitude illness (HAI) includes the clinical entities acute mountain sickness (AMS), high-altitude cerebral edema (HACE), high-altitude pulmonary edema (HAPE), and high-altitude retinal hemorrhage (HARH). Generally, HAI occurs only at elevations greater than 8000 feet.

- Elevations between 8000 feet and 10,000 feet are considered *moderate elevation*.
- *High elevation* is between 10,000 and 18,000 feet.
- *Extreme elevation* is >18,000 feet.

There are several risk factors for the development of HAI (Box 38.1).

Acclimatization is the body's ability to accommodate to the decreased partial pressure of oxygen at high elevations.

- The partial pressure of oxygen declines as the elevation increases, progressively causing hypoxemia and triggering a *hypoxic ventilatory response (HVR)*. The HVR increases minute ventilation, resulting in a respiratory alkalosis.
- In response, the kidneys excrete bicarbonate (acetazolamide facilitates this), resulting in normalization of the pH. Additionally, peripheral vasoconstriction occurs, leading to increased central blood volume, which in turn causes decreased antidiuretic hormone and increased diuresis.
- An increase in cardiac output is required to avoid tissue hypoxemia. This is achieved by increasing the heart rate (stroke volume is decreased secondary to the diuresis), although the heart rate eventually returns to normal with acclimatization.

BOX 38.1 *Factors That Increase the Likelihood of Developing High-Altitude Illness*

Rapid rate of ascent
Minimal previous high-altitude exposure
Higher sleep altitudes
Vigorous exertion at altitude before acclimatization
Sedative hypnotic use or alcohol intake (interferes with acclimatization)
Inadequate hypoxic ventilatory response[a]
Underlying medical problems (especially those that interfere with respiratory effort such as neuromuscular disease or chronic obstructive pulmonary disease[b])
Prior history of high-altitude illness

[a]The hypoxic ventilatory response is reduced by sedatives (e.g., alcohol, sleeping pills) as well as many other factors (including genetic and environmental factors).

[b]Whereas chronic obstructive pulmonary disease increases the risk for high-altitude illness, asthma does not.

BOX 38.2 *Pregnant Patients and Those With Chronic Conditions*

Travel to moderate elevation (8000–10,000 feet) is generally safe in pregnancy, but adherence to rate of ascent guidelines is recommended. Data is limited for travel to higher elevations and a pretravel evaluation is recommended.

Elevations that cause HAI are generally contraindicated in:
Sickle cell disease
Severe chronic obstructive pulmonary disease
Symptomatic pulmonary hypertension
Decompensated heart failure
Patients who experience angina with minimal effort

- With hypoxia, there is pulmonary vascular constriction and increased cerebral blood flow.

Patients with chronic medical conditions and those who are pregnant deserve special consideration (Box 38.2).

Acute Mountain Sickness and High-Altitude Cerebral Edema

- AMS and HACE are disease processes on the same spectrum.
- It is believed that AMS and HACE are due to increased cerebral blood flow and volume, with increased capillary pressures leading to vasogenic edema and brain swelling.
- Whether someone develops AMS or progresses to HACE depends on volume-buffering ability and the presence of increased intracranial pressure.

Clinical Presentation

- AMS presents much like a "hangover" with headache, nausea, anorexia, and fatigue.
- The physical examination is normal.
- The onset of AMS usually occurs within the first 6 hours of arrival at elevation. Symptoms of AMS may resolve or progress over the subsequent 24 hours.
- HACE typically develops from increasingly severe AMS, with the addition of altered mental status, ataxia, focal neurologic deficits (e.g., cranial nerve III and VI palsies), and rarely seizures.

Diagnosis and Evaluation

- Diagnosis is based on clinical signs and symptoms.
- Ultrasonography can be used to assess optic nerve sheath diameter as an indication of increased intracranial pressure.

TABLE 38.1 *Treatment of High-Altitude Illness*

Treatment	Indications	Notes
Acetazolamide	AMS/HACE prophylaxis AMS treatment	Side effects are common and include paresthesias, polyuria, nausea, tinnitus, transient myopia, dysgeusia.
Dexamethasone	AMS/HACE/HAPE prophylaxis AMS/HACE treatment	May have a role in prophylaxis against HAPE, but is not recommended in treatment of HAPE.
Nifedipine	HAPE treatment and prophylaxis	Adjunct to descent and supplemental O_2.
Phosphodiesterase inhibitors	HAPE treatment and prophylaxis	Sildenafil and tadalafil are effective in prophylaxis; there is less evidence for treatment.
β-Agonist (Salmeterol)	HAPE prophylaxis	Not enough studies to support its use for treatment, but may decrease risk of developing HAPE.

AMS, acute mountain sickness; *HACE*, high-altitude cerebral edema; *HAPE*, high-altitude pulmonary edema.

- Computed tomography of the brain may show cerebral edema, and magnetic resonance imaging may show intense T2 signal in the white matter.
- Consider usual alternative diagnoses for altered mental status and focal neurologic deficits, such as strokes (ischemic or hemorrhagic), hypoglycemia, sepsis, etc.
- Due to use of fire and combustion stoves to cook and keep warm at high elevation, consider carbon monoxide poisoning, which may present with symptoms similar to AMS.

Treatment

- AMS is treated with descent or acclimatization, acetazolamide, analgesics (avoid narcotics due to suppression of HVR), antiemetics (prochlorperazine may be preferred due to its ability to increase HVR), and dexamethasone (Table 38.1).
- Ibuprofen had efficacy comparable with acetazolamide in one study and may therefore be the analgesic of choice.
- HACE is treated with descent and/or hyperbaric bag (e.g., the Gamow bag, which simulates a descent of 4000 to 5000 feet), supplemental O_2, and dexamethasone.
- Prevention of AMS/HACE may be achieved by slow ascent, avoiding sedative hypnotics, lowering sleep altitude, acetazolamide, and dexamethasone.

High-Altitude Pulmonary Edema

- Hypoxemia leads to increased pulmonary blood volume and pulmonary vasoconstriction causing pulmonary hypertension. Pulmonary hypertension predisposes patients to HAPE.
- Some parts of the lungs are overperfused, causing endothelial injury and increased permeability leading to a *noncardiogenic pulmonary edema.*
- HAPE is the most common fatal manifestation of HAI.

Clinical Presentation

- Patients present with cough, dyspnea on exertion, and decreased functional capacity.
- If not recognized and treated, HAPE progresses to dyspnea at rest, cyanosis, rales, and frothy sputum.

Diagnosis and Evaluation

- Diagnosis and evaluation are based on clinical signs and symptoms.
- Chest radiograph may show alveolar infiltrates in a patchy distribution.
- Electrocardiogram may show right-sided heart strain (right axis deviation, tall R waves in precordium, and S waves in lateral leads).
- Ultrasonography may show evidence of elevated pulmonary pressures, and comet tails on lung ultrasonography.
- The differential diagnosis includes other causes of dyspnea such as bronchitis, pneumonia, pulmonary embolism, heart failure, asthma, and chronic obstructive pulmonary disease.

Treatment

- Descent (~3000 feet) is the most effective therapy. Use of a hyperbaric bag is an alternative when descent is not possible.
- Additional therapies include rest, supplemental oxygen, use of continuous positive airway pressure mask with or without supplemental oxygen, nifedipine, and phosphodiesterase-5 inhibitors (e.g., sildenafil).
- Acetazolamide and dexamethasone, although effective for the treatment of AMS and HACE, are of questionable benefit for the treatment of HAPE.
- Risk of developing HAPE may be reduced by using acetazolamide, nifedipine, dexamethasone, salmeterol, or a phosphodiesterase-5 inhibitor in high-risk individuals.

High-Altitude Retinal Hemorrhage

- Common among those reaching elevations >16,000 feet.
- HARH may be a sign of developing HACE or HAPE.
- HARH is managed conservatively.

Ultraviolet Keratitis

- Ultraviolet (UV) keratitis, also known as "welder's flash" or "snow blindness," is due to prolonged and excessive UV exposure leading to desquamation of the corneal epithelium.

- Usually presents with bilateral eye pain, foreign body sensation, lacrimation, photophobia, and chemosis, 6–12 hours after exposure.
- Diagnosis is based on a history of exposure, the expected symptoms, slit lamp examination showing superficial punctate keratitis, and symptomatic relief with a topical anesthetic.
- Treatment consists of oral analgesics, artificial tears/lubricant, consideration for topical antibiotics and, when severe, cycloplegics. Symptoms usually resolve in 1–3 days.

SUGGESTED READING

Harris, N. S. (2018). High altitude medicine. In Walls, R. M., Hockberger, R. S., & Gausche-Hill, M. (Eds.), *Rosen's emergency medicine: Concepts and clinical practice* (9th ed., pp. 1787–1800). Elsevier.

Drowning

CHELSEA E. ROBINSON, MD, and JOANNE FELDMAN, MD, MS

General Principles

- Peak incidence in three age groups:
  - Highest in children <5 years; evaluate for abuse and neglect
  - Second peak: children 15–24 years (alcohol, drug abuse, suicide attempts)
  - Third peak: the elderly
- Disorders associated with drowning: alcohol and other drugs, syncope, seizure, cardiac dysrhythmias, dementia, intentional (suicide, homicide, abuse, neglect)

Diagnosis

- Drowning is the process of experiencing respiratory impairment due to submersion or immersion in liquid.
- Terms such as near, wet, dry, active, passive, saltwater, or freshwater drowning are no longer used.

Clinical Presentation

- There are three outcomes for drowning: no morbidity, morbidity, and mortality.
- Primary organs impacted are the lungs and the brain.
  - Lungs: Patients aspirate water into lungs, which washes out surfactant and results in atelectasis, V/Q mismatch, and hypoxia. Patients may therefore present with shortness of breath, and physical examination may demonstrate crackles and wheezing.
  - Brain: The degree of hypoxic insult to the brain generally determines outcome. Patients who arrive to the emergency department (ED) awake and alert with stable vital signs have better prognosis than those with unstable vital signs or with altered mental status.
  - Some cerebral protection occurs in cold-water drowning, likely from rapid central nervous system cooling before hypoxic damage occurs.
  - Diving reflex may offer some neuroprotection.
    - Bradycardia, apnea, vasoconstriction, central shunting of blood flow on submersion
    - Strongest in infants <6 months; less protective as age increases
- Shallow water syncope occurs with prolonged breath-holding during submersion.
  - Loss of consciousness caused by cerebral hypoxia
  - Results from hyperventilation before breath-holding causing hypocapnia and decreased hypercapnic ventilatory drive, followed by excessively prolonged submersion with development of hypoxia and loss of consciousness during end of breath-hold.
  - These patients are typically young and healthy, but have a high mortality rate if not rescued.

Evaluation and Resuscitation

- Evaluation and resuscitation are begun simultaneously for patients with ventilatory distress or altered mental status.
- Monitor temperature; even warm-water drowning can result in hypothermia.
- Imaging
  - The initial chest radiograph does not correlate with arterial blood gas levels, outcome, or disposition.
  - Patients who go on to develop acute respiratory distress syndrome (ARDS) typically have an abnormal chest x-ray result within the first few hours, but not necessarily on arrival to the ED.
  - An initially normal head computed tomography scan has no prognostic value and is not recommended for the awake and alert, neurologically intact drowning victim.

Laboratory Testing

- Depending on the duration of submersion, metabolic and/or respiratory acidosis may be seen. However, electrolyte abnormalities are seldom significant and are usually transient.
- No studies have identified clinically significant electrolyte disturbances or hematologic abnormalities that guide therapy or provide prognostic information.
- Obtaining laboratory tests from a patient with altered mental status may help uncover a cause that led to the drowning incident, such as hypoglycemia or alcohol intoxication.

Treatment

Prehospital Considerations

- Rescuers without formal technical rescue training should avoid water entry and direct patient contact.
- After safely removing the victim from the water, ventilation is the most important treatment, in contrast to the typical cardiac arrest patient, for whom chest compressions are emphasized. Establishing an airway and providing supplemental oxygen are priorities in resuscitating drowning victims. However, if the patient does not respond to two rescue breaths that make the chest rise, then high-quality chest compressions should be initiated.
  - Otherwise, patients should be placed on high-flow oxygen by facemask if spontaneously breathing. If there are no spontaneous respirations or if the patient is in significant respiratory distress, then intubation and positive pressure ventilation are indicated.
  - Oxygen should be delivered at the highest concentration available.

- Pulses may be difficult to palpate if patient is hypothermic and has underlying atrial fibrillation or bradycardia. Thus, it is recommended that a search for pulses should occur for 1 minute before cardiopulmonary resuscitation (CPR) is begun. Ventricular fibrillation is rare, occurring in <10% of patients; therefore, the placement of an automatic external defibrillator on the patient should not delay oxygenation and ventilation.
  - Automatic external defibrillator use is not contraindicated in a wet environment.
- The Heimlich maneuver is not recommended in the resuscitation of a drowning patient.
- Trauma is an uncommon cause of drowning.
  - Evaluation for injury is not a top priority unless there is a history or signs on physical examination.
  - Incidence of cervical spine injury in drowning victims is low. Consider cervical spine immobilization only if there was a clear mechanism for cervical spine injury, focal neurologic deficit, or a significant distracting injury.
- Criteria for transport to ED:
  - Amnesia to event, confusion
  - Ongoing ventilatory distress
  - Witnessed apnea or required period of assisted ventilation

Initial Emergency Department Assessment and Stabilization

- Continue prehospital resuscitation
- Assess airway, breathing, circulation, and secure the airway if warranted (signs of neurologic deterioration or inability to protect airway).
- Remove wet clothing, determine temperature, and begin rewarming measures. If patient is hypothermic, begin passive and active external rewarming, and active internal core rewarming, as indicated. Frequent or continuous temperature monitoring is important to guide rewarming.
- Note that resuscitative efforts (CPR) should be continued until the core temperature reaches 32°C.
- Establish intravenous access.
- Assess for any other injuries. However, as stated above, there is no need for cervical spine precautions or routine computed tomography of the brain or cervical spine unless history of diving or trauma is provided or circumstances are unknown.
- Provide supplemental oxygenation to maintain oxygen saturation >94%.
- If initial Glasgow Coma Scale score is >13 and oxygen saturation >95%, the patient is at low risk for complications. Can monitor for 4–6 hours. Laboratory tests and imaging are unnecessary and not predictive of discharge.
- If initial Glasgow Coma Scale score is <13 and patient requires respiratory support, closely monitor need for intubation with frequent patient assessments and continuous pulse oximetry and cardiac monitoring. Temperature monitoring and management is also important in this patient group.

Ventilation

- Noninvasive positive pressure ventilation with continuous positive airway pressure/bilevel positive airway pressure can be used in the alert patient with respiratory distress. Continuous positive airway pressure and bilevel positive airway pressure can improve oxygenation and decrease ventilation-perfusion mismatch, but is not appropriate for drowning patients with altered mental status or vomiting.
- If unable to obtain an arterial partial pressure of oxygen (PaO_2) of >60 mm Hg in adults or >80 mm Hg in children, intubation is warranted. High positive end-expiratory pressure levels may be needed.
- Use a lung-protective ventilation strategy and follow an ARDS protocol.

Other Therapies

- There is no evidence to support empiric use of antibiotics in treatment of drowning patients.
- There is no evidence for routine corticosteroid use.
- There is insufficient evidence to support or discourage use of therapeutic hypothermia after cardiopulmonary arrest in drowning patients.

Prognosis and Disposition

- Patients who had symptoms at the scene but are asymptomatic on arrival to the ED can be observed for 4–6 hours, then discharged home if there is no increasing oxygen requirement.
- Symptomatic patients should be admitted for cardiopulmonary monitoring.
  - If patient does not require CPR on scene or in the ED, full recovery within 48 hours is likely.
  - Of victims requiring on-scene CPR, 20% of pediatric patients die in the hospital, 5% have significant hypoxic ischemic brain injury.
  - Victims undergoing CPR in the ED typically have a poor prognosis.
  - If patient is normothermic in the ED, but remains in cardiopulmonary arrest or asystole, termination of resuscitation efforts should be considered because recovery without profound neurologic complications is rare.
  - All drowning victims requiring ED resuscitation should be admitted to the intensive care unit.
- Freshwater drowning victims may have more severe hypoxemia, but no significant difference in serum lactate and no significant difference in outcome or length of stay in the intensive care unit compared with saltwater victims.

Other Considerations

- ARDS can develop if there is a significant aspiration event or cardiovascular collapse.
- Pneumonia, when it occurs, is typically a late complication. If it develops, consider covering *Aeromonas* species.

SUGGESTED READINGS

Cico, S. J., & Quan, L. (2020). Drowning. In J. E. Tintinalli, O. J. Ma, D. M. Yealy, G. D. Meckler, J. S. Stapczynski, D. M. Cline, & S. H. Thomas (Eds.), *Tintinalli's emergency medicine: A comprehensive study guide* (9th ed.). McGraw-Hill Education.

Michelet, P., Dusart, M., Boiron, L., Marmin, J., Mokni, T., Loundou, A., Coulange, M., & Markarian, T. (2019). Drowning in fresh or salt water: Respective influence on respiratory function in a matched cohort study. *European Journal of Emergency Medicine, 26*(5), 340–344.

Schmidt, A. C., Sempsrott, J. R., Hawkins, S. C., Arastu, A. S., Cushing, T. A., & Auerbach, P. S. (2016). Wilderness Medical Society practice guidelines for the prevention and treatment of drowning. *Wilderness & Environmental Medicine, 27*(2), 236–251.

Sempsrott, J., Schmidt, A. C., Hawkins, S. C., & Cushing, T. A. (2017). Drowning and submersion injury. In P. Auerbach, T. A. Cushing, & N. S. Harris (Eds.), *Auerbach's wilderness medicine* (7th ed.). Elsevier.

CHAPTER **40**

BOARD REVIEW

Temperature-Related Illness

RYAN C. DOLLBAUM, MD, and ANDREA TAKEMOTO, MD

Heat Illness

General Principles

- Heat-related illness varies greatly in its severity of presentation, from minor muscle cramps to heat stroke and death.
  - It affects both young and old, albeit often by different mechanisms. Prevention and awareness are key.
  - If illness has occurred, treatment is generally straightforward, and most victims recover rapidly.
- Heat is generated through cellular metabolism and skeletal muscle activity.
  - The primary mechanisms of heat dissipation are via radiation and evaporation, which can be augmented by conduction and convection if the ambient air or water is moving across the surface of the skin.
  - At ambient temperatures above 35°C (95°F) and with increasing humidity, heat dissipation mechanisms begin to fail and pathophysiologic mechanisms ensue.
    - Thermoregulatory response: a rise in blood temperature triggers the hypothalamus to increase blood flow to skin via sympathetic cutaneous vasodilation resulting in splanchnic hypoperfusion.
    - Acute phase response: inflammatory reaction of interleukins, cytokines, and proteins similar to those seen in sepsis.
    - Heat shock protein dysfunction: altered protein synthesis that induces end-organ dysfunction beginning at the cellular level.

Clinical Presentation

- Several heat illness syndromes are distinguishable by their symptoms.
  - Heat cramps: muscle pain in the setting of prolonged sweating and aldosterone-induced potassium wasting.
  - Heat edema: accumulation of interstitial fluid owing to increased hydrostatic pressure, vascular leak, and cutaneous vasodilation.
  - Heat syncope: syncope resulting from increased peripheral vasodilation, orthostatic pooling, dehydration, and impaired cardiac output.
  - Heat exhaustion: fatigue and generalized weakness in the setting of prolonged exposure to a hot environment and/or strenuous exertion; may progress to heat stroke if treatment is not initiated.
  - Heat stroke: life-threatening illness characterized by an altered level of consciousness with an elevated core body temperature above 40°C. There are two forms:
    - Classic: passive exposure to high environmental temperatures.
    - Exertional: pathologic hyperthermia induced by strenuous exercise.

Diagnosis

- The diagnosis of heat-related illnesses is clinical and is based on the symptoms and history of the patient.
- A core temperature should be obtained in all patients presenting with signs and symptoms of what may be a heat-related illness.
- Consideration must be given to the broad differential diagnosis of illnesses resulting in an elevated body temperature, including sepsis, hyperthyroidism, toxicities (including sympathomimetic and anticholinergic, serotonin syndrome, malignant hyperthermia, neuroleptic malignant syndrome), prolonged seizure, and alcohol withdrawal.

Evaluation

- Laboratory testing is generally only indicated for patients experiencing heat stroke, or to exclude other illnesses.

Treatment

- The mainstays of treatment are cooling and supportive measures.
  - Heat cramps: oral or intravenous (IV) fluid and electrolyte replacement.
  - Heat edema: extremity elevation and compression stockings.
  - Heat syncope: self-limited by definition; treatment involves rehydration and electrolyte replacement. However, it is imperative to consider alternative medical causes.
  - Heat exhaustion: cease physical activity, transport to a cool environment, and provide volume and electrolyte replacement.
  - Heat stroke: immediate and aggressive cooling until temperature normalizes to between 38°C and 39°C. Avoid shivering and hypothermic overshoot. The severity of heat illness and the resources available should guide the selection of cooling modalities.
    - Evaporative and convective cooling: application of cool, sprayed water and forced air current over the undressed body. This is moderately effective, and allows monitoring and resuscitation.
    - Conductive cooling: cold water immersion (usually in 0°C to 10°C water) results in rapid direct transfer of heat and is very effective, but use is limited by the inability to monitor and resuscitate immersed patients.

- Infusion of cold IV fluid is an adjunct to increase rate of cooling used in conjunction with either method.
- Invasive methods can be considered in refractory cases, which include cold water lavage of urinary bladder, peritoneum, or thorax, as well as extracorporeal membrane oxygenation (ECMO).

Hypothermia

General Principles

- Accidental hypothermia may occur anywhere, even in temperate or urban environments.
  - Cold and wet environments pose the greatest risk.
  - Patients undergoing evaluation and treatment for trauma and sepsis may lose their ability to thermoregulate and sustain iatrogenic hypothermia.
- Hypothermia results from heat loss by either conduction or convection.
  - Progressive tissue cooling results in decreased resting metabolism and inhibition of central and peripheral neurologic function.
  - Shivering increases metabolism via increased ventilation, cardiac output, and mean arterial pressure. Shivering increases as the core body temperature decreases down to 32°C, then begins to taper off and ceases altogether at approximately 30°C.
  - Below 30°C, cardiac output drops owing to abnormalities in electrical conduction.
    - Resultant dysrhythmias include bradycardia, PVCs, PACs, atrial fibrillation, and ventricular fibrillation.
    - At temperatures less than 28°C, the heart is especially susceptible to ventricular fibrillation, which may be triggered by acidosis, hypercarbia, hypoxia, or movement of the patient.

Clinical Presentation

- The clinical presentation of hypothermia correlates with the core body temperature.
  - Mild: 32°C to 35°C: tachypnea, tachycardia, impaired judgment, increased shivering, ataxia, and dysarthria (stumbles, mumbles, fumbles).
  - Moderate: 28°C to 32°C: hypoventilation, reduced cardiac output, lethargy, hyporeflexia, bradycardia, and arrhythmias (atrial fibrillation, junctional bradycardia).
  - Severe: less than 28°C: pulmonary edema, oliguria, areflexia, coma, hypotension, bradycardia, ventricular arrhythmias, including ventricular fibrillation and asystole.

Diagnosis

- The diagnosis of hypothermia is based on the core temperature. A core temperature should be obtained in all patients presenting with signs and symptoms suggestive of hypothermia.

Evaluation

- Obtaining an accurate core temperature is key to the diagnosis of hypothermia.
  - An esophageal temperature probe is the most accurate modality in clinical use. Commonly used in intubated patients.
  - Urinary catheter temperature probes are also accurate.
  - Rectal temperature measurement may be less accurate than esophageal or urinary probes. Should be deferred until the patient is in a warm environment.
  - Oral thermometers are often inaccurate at temperatures below 35.6°C.
- Other diagnostic tests include:
  - Electrocardiogram in cases of moderate to severe hypothermia
    - Elevation of the J point (junction of the QRS complex and ST segment), known as Osborn or J, waves tend to occur at temperatures at or below 32°C (Fig. 40.1).
    - Although neither sensitive, nor specific, these ECG changes are usually first identified in leads II and V_6 and tend to increase in amplitude with the severity of hypothermia.
  - Comprehensive laboratory testing is indicated for severe hypothermia because these patients are critically ill and may have severe organ dysfunction.

Treatment

- Resuscitation of hypothermic patients differs from the standard protocols for normothermic patients (Fig. 40.2). Aspects of resuscitation specific to hypothermia are reviewed here.
  - Initial assessment
    - Usual indicators of death (e.g., fixed, dilated pupils and apparent rigor mortis) are unreliable in hypothermic patients.
    - Assessment for signs of life may be difficult owing to absence of palpable pulses and slow, shallow breathing. Rescuers should feel for a carotid pulse for 1 minute prior to initiation of cardiopulmonary resuscitation (CPR).
    - Delayed, intermittent, and prolonged CPRs have all been shown to be effective in hypothermic patients owing to the reduced rate of oxygen consumption.
    - There is NO temperature below which resuscitation should be withheld. However, if there is a nonsurvivable injury, chest compressions cannot be performed owing to a frozen chest wall, or the airway is completely blocked by snow, resuscitative measures should be withheld.
  - Cardiac monitoring
    - If cardiac monitoring reveals electrical activity without a perfusing rhythm as demonstrated by either absence of pulses, end-tidal CO_2, or ultrasound, then CPR should be initiated.
    - If an automated external defibrillator is available and shock is advised (indicating either ventricular fibrillation or ventricular tachycardia), rescuers should proceed with defibrillation.
    - If initial defibrillation is attempted at a temperature below 30°C and is unsuccessful, a second attempt should not be performed until temperature has increased by at least 1°C to 2°C, or to 30°C.
  - Vascular access
    - Vascular access may be difficult owing to peripheral vasoconstriction; therefore the preferred methods for vascular access include femoral vein catheterization

40

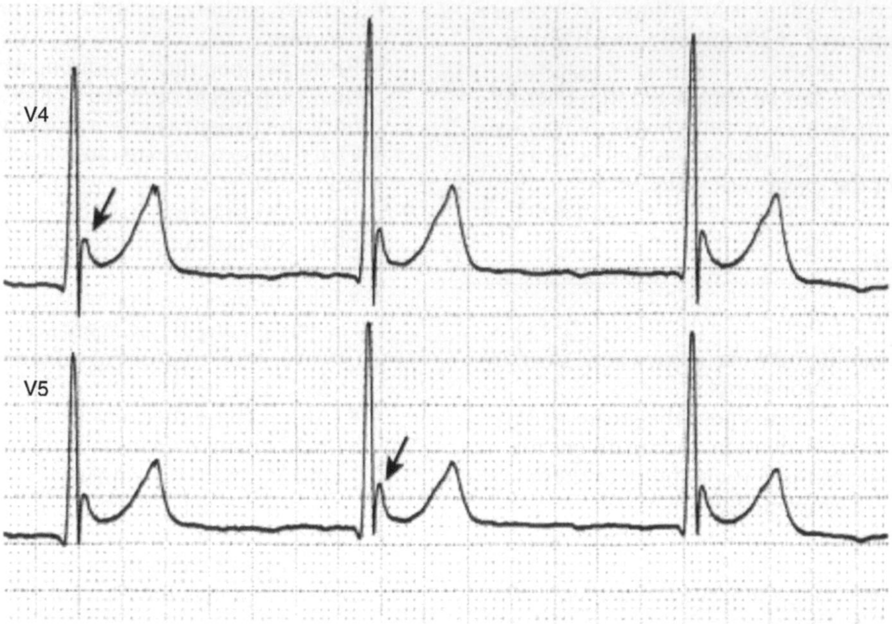

FIG. 40.1 Osborn or J wave. J waves in lateral leads during moderate hypothermia.

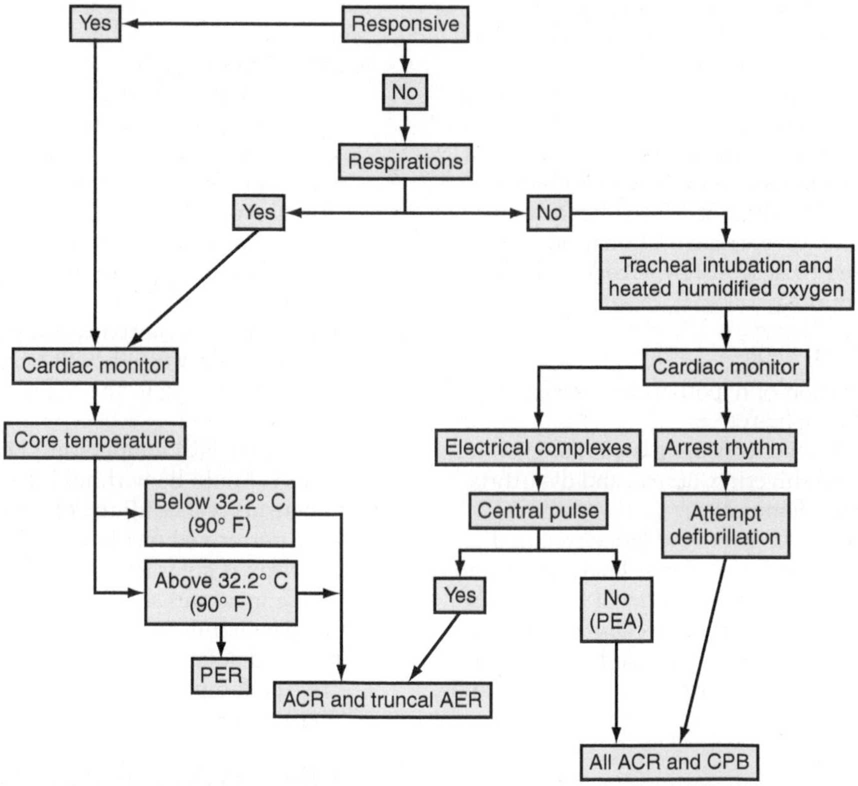

FIG. 40.2 Hypothermia resuscitation. (*PER*, passive external rewarming; *AER*, active external rewarming; *ACR*, active core rewarming; *PEA*, pulseless electrical activity; *CPB*, cardiopulmonary bypass.)

(in order to avoid possible dysrhythmia with internal jugular or subclavian access) and intraosseous (IO) access.

- Intravenous fluids warmed to between 40°C and 42°C should be infused in order to avoid volume depletion, a low central venous pressure, and resultant shock.
    - Limited evidence supports the use of vasoactive or antidysrhythmic drugs.
- Airway management
    - Any patients who are not spontaneously breathing or are unable to protect their airway should have an endotracheal tube or supraglottic device placed.

- After a definitive airway is established, decrease the rate of ventilation to half that of a normothermic patient to avoid hyperventilation relative to metabolic demand.
- Transport and triage
  - Moderately to severely hypothermic patients who are hemodynamically stable should be transferred to the closest receiving hospital.
  - Severely hypothermic patients with an altered level of consciousness or hemodynamic instability may benefit from transport to a hospital capable of ECMO.
- Duration of resuscitation
  - In the absence of a nonsurvivable injury, inability to perform chest compressions owing to a frozen chest wall, or airway blocked by snow, resuscitative measures should be continued until the patient's core temperature reaches 32°C to 35°C. Extended resuscitation efforts are justified by cases of neurologically intact survival from prolonged hypothermic cardiac arrest. These unusual outcomes have been attributed to the neuroprotective effects of hypothermia.
  - Serum potassium levels reflect the severity of cell lysis, and levels above 12 mEq/L predict futile resuscitation.
- Rewarming techniques for the emergency department (ED) management of hypothermia should be tailored to the severity of hypothermia and the available resources.
  - Passive external rewarming (PER)
    - PER should be applied to all hypothermic patients.
    - Limit further heat loss by removing any wet clothing, applying blankets or insulation, and maintaining the room temperature at approximately 28°C.
    - Warming occurs via cessation of heat loss combined with intrinsic heat production.
  - Active external rewarming (AER)
    - Used in cases of moderate hypothermia or refractory mild hypothermia (i.e., the patient is not rewarming at the goal rate of 0.5°C to 2°C/hr).
    - Apply warm blankets, heating pads, radiant heat, warm baths, or forced air.
    - AER should be applied to the trunk (axilla, chest, and back) to avoid a drop in core temperature, and associated acidemia and hypotension that can occur when AER is applied to cool extremities causing cold acidemic blood to be washed out of the extremities and into the central circulation.
  - Active internal rewarming (AIR)
    - Simple AIR measures consisting of intravenous administration of warmed crystalloid fluids (40°C to 42°C) and warmed humidified air (with supplemental oxygen, as needed) via face mask are appropriate for moderate hypothermia.
    - Administration of warm humidified air via endotracheal tube results in substantial transfer of heat to the central circulation as blood passes through the lungs, and it is appropriate for any hypothermic patient requiring intubation.
    - The more invasive AIR techniques, such as irrigation of the peritoneum or thorax (via pleural space) with warmed saline, should be reserved for severe hypothermia, particularly cases involving cardiac instability.
    - If the patient is in cardiac arrest or continues to be unstable despite use of PER, AER, and AIR, the treatment team should prepare for ECMO or transfer to a site with ECMO capability.
- In cases of refractory hypothermia, consider contributory causes, such as insufficient glycogen stores, sepsis, hypothyroidism, adrenal insufficiency, hypoglycemia, and intoxication.

Frostbite

General Principles

- Despite advances in clothing, protective equipment, and rescue times, dermal injuries owing to prolonged cold exposure remain prevalent. There are four phases of frostbite:
  - Prefreeze: tissue cooling with accompanying vasoconstriction and ischemia.
  - Freeze-thaw: ice crystals form, either intracellularly, during rapid freezing injury, or extracellularly, during a slower freeze. Freezing results in cell death. Thawing may result in reperfusion injury in adjacent tissues.
  - Vascular stasis: vessels alternate between constriction and dilation.
  - Late ischemia: progressive tissue ischemia and infarction from continued reperfusion injury, with inflammatory mediators, intermittent vasoconstriction, showers of emboli within microvessels, and thrombus formation in larger vessels.
- Refreezing dramatically increases inflammatory mediators associated with the freeze-thaw cycle, worsening vasoconstriction, platelet aggregation, thrombosis, and cellular injury.

Clinical Presentation (Fig. 40.3)

- Frostnip: superficial, nonfreezing cold injury, distinct from the diagnosis of frostbite but may precede it. Consisting of intense vasoconstriction of exposed skin, frostnip results in numbness and pallor, which dissipate rapidly upon rewarming or application of protective clothing.
- Frostbite is divided into four grades of severity in a classification schema similar to that of thermal burns:
  - First degree: numbness and erythema with areas of white or yellow discoloration. Firm, slightly raised plaques may develop in the area of injury.
  - Second degree: superficial skin vesiculation; clear or milky fluid present in blisters, surrounded by erythema/edema
  - Third degree: deeper hemorrhagic blisters; extension of injury into the reticular dermis beneath the dermal vascular plexus
  - Fourth degree: injury extends through dermis to the relatively avascular subcutaneous tissues, including muscle and bone.
- Chilblains (pernio) is a cold-related but nonfreezing injury presenting as burning, tenderness, and pruritic sensation associated with papules, plaques, nodules, and macules in an acral distribution after prolonged exposure to a cold, damp environment.

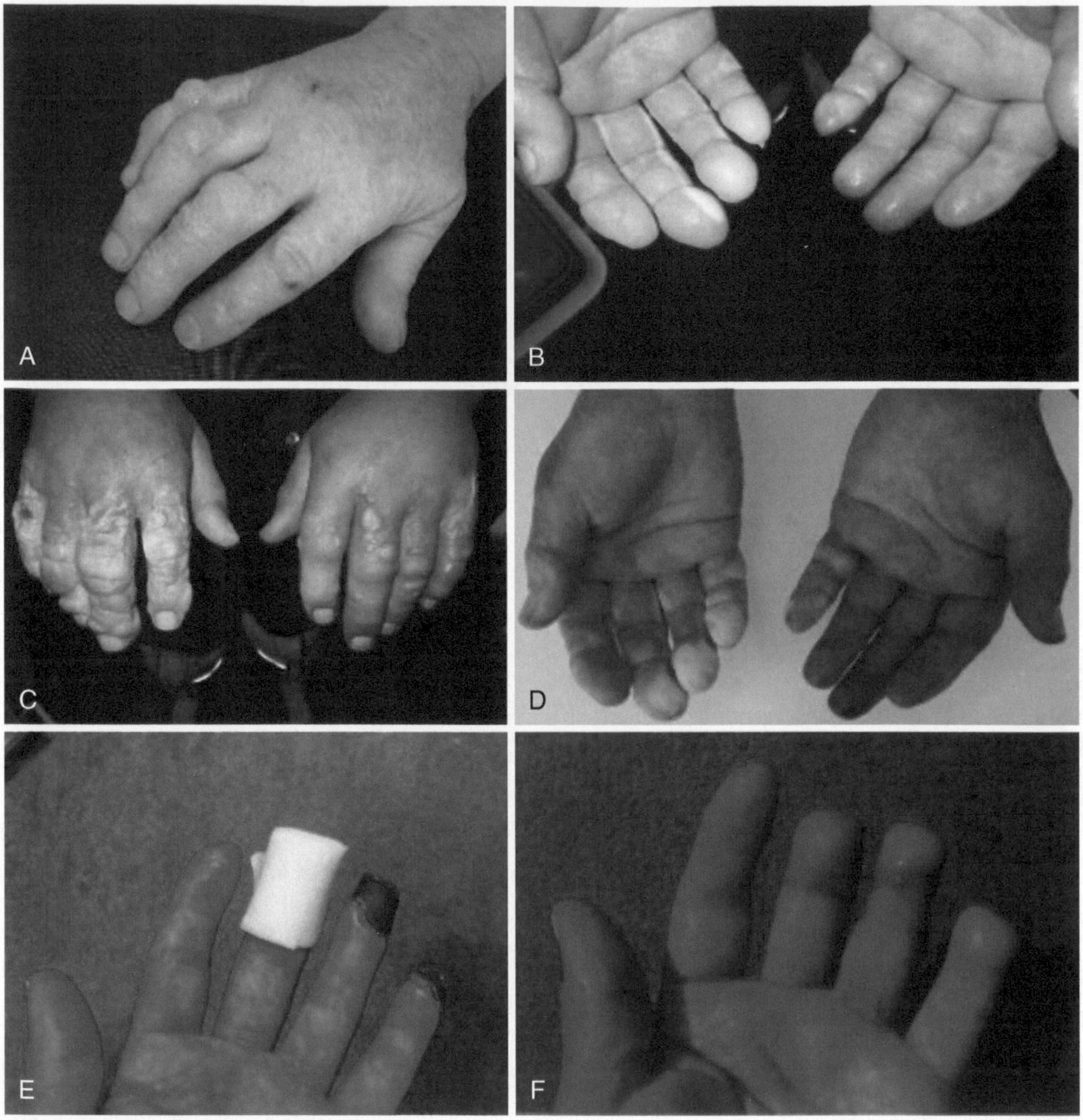

FIG. 40.3 Frostbite by severity and time since injury. **A**, Twenty-four hours following grade 2 frostbite injury with blister formation. **B**, Grade 2 right hand and grade 3 left hand at 36 hours. **C**, Grade 2 right hand and grade 3 left hand at 36 hours following soaks in povidone iodine. **D**, Grade 2 right hand and grade 3 left hand at 5 days. **E**, Grade 3 at 3 months; note the mummification. **F**, Grade 3 at 4 months.

Diagnosis

- Similar to thermal burns, the diagnosis of frostbite is based on the physical examination.

Treatment

- Treatment includes pain control, supportive measures, and rewarming.
  - Frozen extremities should be thawed only when there is no threat of refreezing.
  - Rewarm rapidly using warm water immersion. Water should be heated to 37°C to 39°C and maintained within this range until the affected area becomes soft and pliable to touch.
  - Slow rewarming via adjacent body heat from a rescuer or in a heated tent is also acceptable in field settings.
  - Nonsteroidal antiinflammatory drugs, which decrease the production of prostaglandins and thromboxanes released during the freeze-thaw cycle, may be used (e.g., ibuprofen up to 2400 mg/day divided into four doses).
  - Selectively drain tense, clear, or cloudy fluid-filled blisters and apply clean gauze.
  - Administer tetanus prophylaxis according to standard guidelines.
  - Tissue plasminogen activator may be considered in cases for potential proximal or multiple digit amputations.
    - Mitigates microvascular thrombosis in tissue injury.
    - Should be given within 24 hours of thawing.
  - Magnetic resonance imaging (MRI) may assist in determining the extent of tissue viability.
  - Ultimately, definitive management is surgical.

SUGGESTED READINGS

Cauchy, E., Davis, C. B., Pasquier, M., Meyer, E. F., & Hackett, P. H. (2016). A new proposal for management of severe frostbite in the austere environment. *Wilderness & Environmental Medicine, 27*(1), 92–99.

Gaudio, F. G., & Grissom, C. K. (2016). Cooling methods in heat stroke. *Journal of Emergency Medicine, 50*(4), 607–616.

Lipman, G. S., Eifling, K. P., Ellis, M. A., Gaudio, F. G., Otten, E. M., & Grissom, C. K. (2014). Wilderness Medical Society practice guidelines for the prevention and treatment of heat-related illness: 2014 update. *Wilderness & Environmental Medicine, 25*(Suppl. 4), S55–S65.

Mcintosh, S. E., Opacic, M., Freer, L., Grissom, C. K., Auerbach, P. S., Rodway, G. W., Cochran, A., Giesbrecht, G. G., McDevitt, M., Imray, C. H., Johnson, E. L., Dow, J., & Hackett, P. H. (2014). Wilderness Medical Society practice guidelines for the prevention and treatment of frostbite: 2014 update. *Wilderness & Environmental Medicine, 25*(Suppl. 4), S43–S54.

Zafren, K., Giesbrecht, G. G., Danzl, D. F., Brugger, H., Sagalyn, E. B., Walpoth, B., Weiss, E. A., Auerbach, P. S., McIntosh, S. E., Némethy, M., McDevitt, M., Dow, J., Schoene, R. B., Rodway, G. W., Hackett, P. H., Bennett, B. L., & Grissom, C. K. (2014). Wilderness Medical Society practice guidelines for the out-of-hospital evaluation and treatment of accidental hypothermia: 2014 update. *Wilderness & Environmental Medicine, 25*(Suppl. 4), S66–S85.

HEENT

Ear Emergencies

KENDRA CAMPBELL, MD, and RYAN PEDIGO, MD, MHPE

General Principles

- Ear emergencies can be traumatic or atraumatic and can involve the external, middle, and inner ear. They may span from simple to complex, bearing significant sequelae, both in terms of lasting cosmesis to life-threatening, including infections requiring surgical debridement.

The External Ear

BASIC INFORMATION

Anatomy of the External Ear

- The visible portion of the external ear is termed the pinna or auricle (Fig. 41.1).
- The layers of the pinna from deepest to most superficial include the cartilage, perichondrium, subcutaneous tissues, and skin. The lobule lacks cartilage.
- The cartilage of the ear has no direct blood supply and derives its nutrients solely via diffusion from the perichondrium. Therefore, any disruption to the close adherence of perichondrium to cartilage can result in chondronecrosis, fibrosis, and long-lasting deformity; a condition colloquially known as "cauliflower ear" (Fig. 41.2).
- Anesthesia to the external ear is best achieved by performing a regional block, as seen in Fig 41.3. Using a long, small-bore needle, 2 to 3 mL of anesthetic is

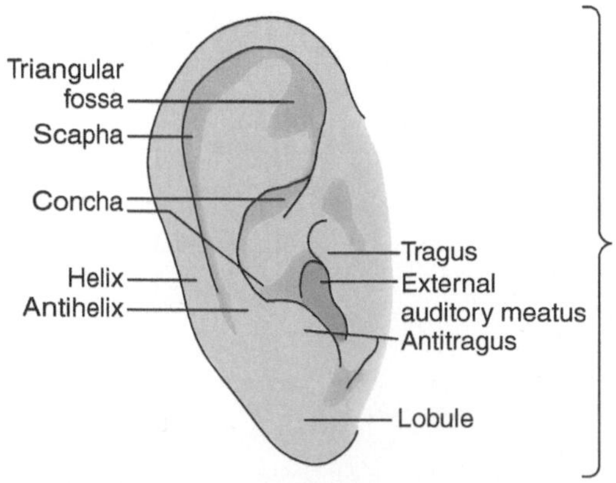

FIG. 41.1 Anatomy of the external ear. (From Harris, G. D. (2020). Auricular hematoma evacuation. In G. C. Fowler (Ed.), *Pfenninger and Fowler's procedures for primary care* (4th ed., Fig. 202.2). Elsevier.)

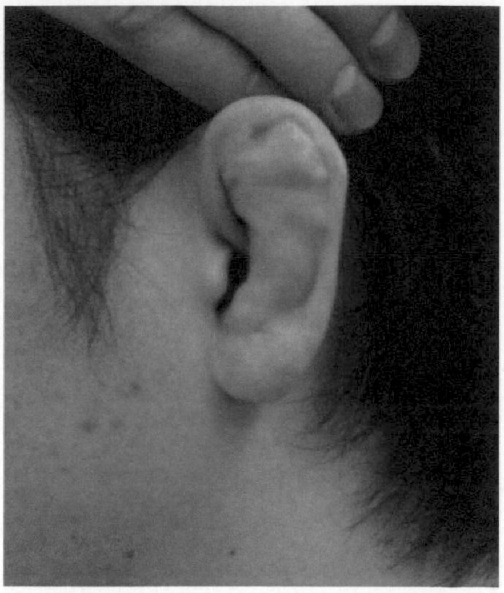

FIG. 41.2 "Cauliflower ear" as a result of an untreated auricular hematoma. (From Magee, D. J. (2014). Head and face. In D. J. Magee (Ed.), *Orthopedic physical assessment* (6th ed., pp. 84–147). Elsevier.)

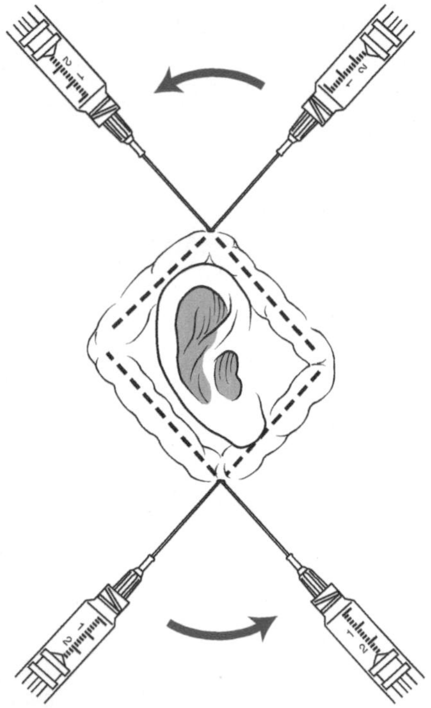

FIG. 41.3 Auricular block technique. (From Trott, A. T. (2012). Infiltration and nerve block anesthesia. In A. T. Trott (Ed.), *Wounds and lacerations: Emergency care and closure* (4th ed., Fig. 6.7). Elsevier.)

infiltrated along the illustrated tracts, using the mastoid process and tragus as landmarks.
  - The concha and external auditory meatus will not receive anesthesia using a regional block, but can be anesthetized with local injections.

External Ear Trauma

AURICULAR HEMATOMAS

Basic Information

- Auricular hematomas occur on the anterior surface of the pinna, arising from blunt or shearing forces (e.g., contact sports, motor vehicle accidents, and "high" ear piercings).
- In the pediatric or geriatric populations, auricular hematomas can be a sign of nonaccidental trauma.

Diagnosis

- Auricular hematomas are diagnosed clinically (Fig. 41.4).
- Hearing loss is not associated with isolated auricular hematomas; in these instances further investigation is warranted.

Treatment

- In the Emergency Department (ED), the task of the physician is to recognize the presence of a hematoma, drain the fluid collection, and prevent reaccumulation of fluid by applying compressive dressing. Hematomas over 7 days old require specialist intervention.
  - Incision and drainage provides greater exposure than needle aspiration, rendering complete clot evacuation certain and facile.

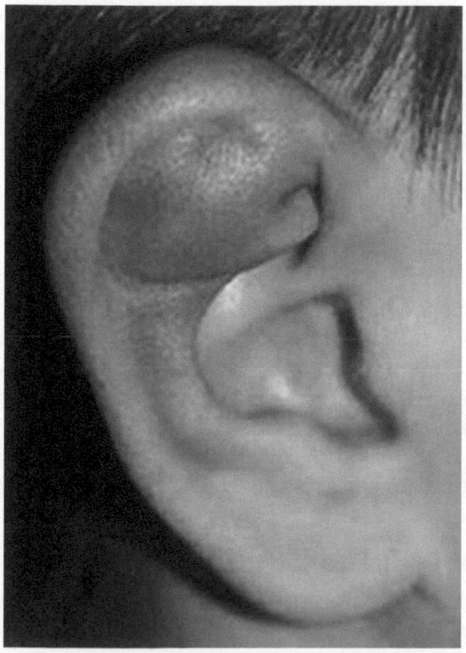

FIG. 41.4 Auricular hematoma. (From Handler E. B., Song, T., & Shih, C. (2013). Complications of otoplasty. *Facial Plastic Surgery Clinics of North America, 21*(4), 653–662.)

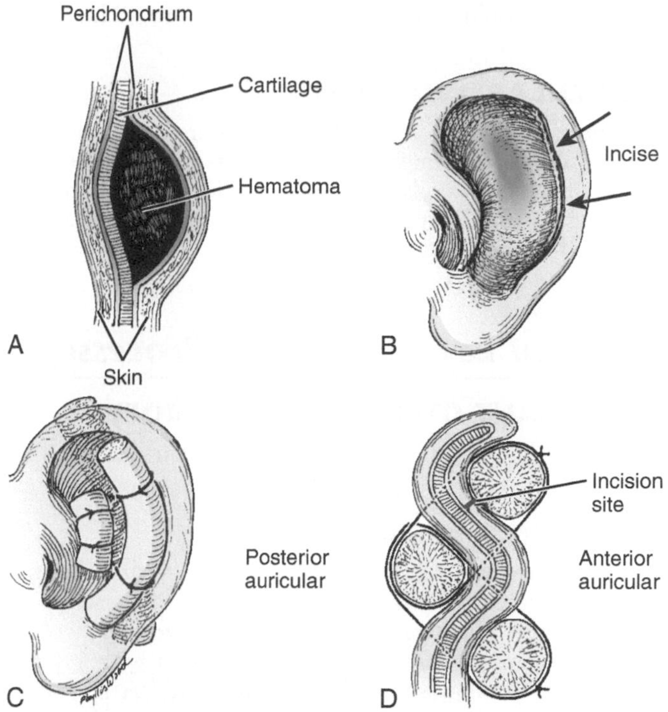

FIG. 41.5 Drainage of an auricular hematoma. A, Auricular hematoma. **B**, Incision along the anatomic fold of the ear. **C** and **D**, Suturing of dental rolls into folds. (From Shaye, D., Mazzorana, V., & Lindsay, R. W. (2017). Management of facial injuries. In P. S. Auerbach, T. A. Cushing, & N. S. Harris (Eds.), *Auerbach's wilderness medicine* (7th ed., pp. 420–440.e1). Elsevier.)

  - Care should be taken to incise over anatomic folds without cutting down to the cartilage, followed by complete clot evacuation and irrigation.
  - To prevent fluid reaccumulation, suture the opposing skin edges of the incision using mattress sutures, taking the suture material through the skin and cartilage (essentially suturing through and through the ear) and passing the suture material around dental rolls applied to the opposite side of the incision to create a pressure dressing (Fig. 41.5). In most instances, an elastic bandage should be wrapped around the head to ensure adequate compression.
  - Anti-*Staphylococcal* antibiotics should be prescribed for 7 to 10 days.
  - Specialist follow-up should be coordinated within 24 to 48 hours. Dental rolls should be removed in 1 week.

AURICULAR LACERATION

- Delayed primary closure should be considered for patients presenting greater than 24 hours after injury, if there is evidence of wound infection, or in patients with comorbid conditions, such as diabetes, placing them at higher risk for infection.
- Specialist consultation is necessary for lacerations that are: large and complex; extend to the external ear canal; complicated by middle and/or inner ear injury; or associated with skull base fractures.
- No data support the use of prophylactic antibiotics for auricular lacerations, even in the setting of exposed cartilage prior to repair.

- Patients should be reevaluated within 24 to 48 hours by a specialist.

AURICULAR AVULSION

- Subtotal and total auricular avulsions are emergencies requiring reattachment within 3 hours by specialists.
- Care for a fully avulsed auricle includes cleaning the detached auricle in cold saline and placing it in heparinized Ringer lactated solution.

External Ear Atraumatic Processes

MALIGNANT OTITIS EXTERNA (MOE)

- Osteitis/osteomyelitis of the skull base owing to otitis externa.

Clinical Presentation

- Classic presentation is an elderly patient with diabetes and severe unremitting otalgia that is often worse at night, otorrhea, hearing loss, and ear fullness.
- Younger patients are more likely to present with a history of immunosuppression, such as HIV/AIDS.
- *Pseudomonas aeruginosa* and *Aspergillus* spp. are the most commonly encountered bacterial and fungal causative agents.
- Physical examination may note an edematous, tender external ear canal, purulent otorrhea, periauricular lymphadenopathy, and exposed bone or granulation tissue in the canal. Cranial palsies reflect spread of infection through the skull base.
- MOE may lead to serious secondary complications, including cerebral abscess, meningitis, and venous sinus thrombosis.

Diagnosis

- History and physical examination in conjunction with laboratory and imaging testing.
- Pain out of proportion to the examination.
- Often leukocytosis and fever are absent, but erythrocyte sedimentation rate is usually elevated.
- Computed tomography (CT) is a reasonable test of first choice to delineate bony erosion and abscess formation.

Treatment

- Collaborative management with multiple services is often required.
- Ciprofloxacin is the preferred initial regimen until results of culture sensitivities; antibiotics are continued for 6 to 8 weeks.
- Amphotericin B is the initial therapy of choice for fungal MOE.
- Surgical intervention is no longer mandated, although drainage of any associated abscesses and/or debridement of granulation tissue may be necessary.

ACUTE OTITIS EXTERNA (AOE)

- Inflammation of the external ear canal, with or without inflammation of the pinna or tympanic membrane (TM). This is known colloquially as "swimmer's ear."

Basic Information

- In North America, 95% of cases are bacterial. Fungal infections are uncommon.
- Most common pathogen(s): polymicrobial, but most cases involve *P. aeruginosa* and/or *S. aureus*.
- Pathogenesis is multifactorial, including exposure when swimming and ear cleaning.

Diagnosis

- Rapid onset (under 48 hours) with signs and symptoms of ear canal inflammation.
  - Signs include tenderness with palpation or traction of the pinna and/or tragus, ear canal erythema/edema, otorrhea, TM erythema, cellulitis of the pinna and/or surrounding skin, regional lymphadenitis.
  - Symptoms include otalgia, fullness, and pruritus, jaw pain, hearing loss.
- AOE must be differentiated from "surfer's ear," an abnormal growth of bone that forms an exostosis in the external auditory canal, which occurs as a result of frequent exposure to cold and wet conditions.
- Complications of AOE include facial cellulitis, perichondritis, and MOE.

Treatment

- A multipronged approach is beneficial, composed of topical antibiotics to treat infection, analgesia for patient comfort, and measures to prevent recurrence.
  - Aminoglycoside or fluoroquinolone topical antibiotics for 7 to 10 days. Avoid aminoglycosides in tympanic membrane perforation or a history of neomycin skin contact sensitivity (occurs in 15% of the population).
  - Drops should be instilled for 3 to 5 minutes while the patient is lying on the unaffected side in the lateral decubitus position.
  - Symptoms persisting beyond day 14 are considered treatment failure.
  - Nonsteroidal antiinflammatory drugs or acetaminophen are effective for pain control.
- Swimming, use of earplugs, or hearing aids should be avoided until infection has resolved.

PERICHONDRITIS

- Infection involving the subcutaneous tissue and cartilage of the pinna.

Basic Information

- The most common cause of perichondritis is an infected hematoma, sometimes developing 3 to 4 weeks after the initial traumatic insult. Other inciting events include cosmetic piercings (namely "high" chondral piercings), insect bites, and burns.
- Early recognition of this entity is important because infection can progress rapidly, and failure to diagnose and treat can result in irreversible cartilage damage.

Clinical Presentation

- Patients may initially complain of pain at the infection site, which may progress to severe otalgia and frank purulence.
- The affected area will have erythema, warmth, and edema.

Diagnosis

- Clinical history and physical examination.

Treatment

- Remove any associated foreign body, such as an ear piercing.
- Antibiotics should target *P. aeruginosa* (the most common offending microorganism), skin flora, and *S. aureus*; ciprofloxacin is a reasonable choice. Some patients may require admission for intravenous (IV) antibiotics given comorbid conditions, local antibiograms, or poor social situation making follow-up difficult or impossible.
- Incision and drainage with culture is indicated for any associated abscess or hematoma.
- For outpatient management, early specialist follow-up is recommended.

The Middle Ear

- The middle ear is an air-filled cavity within the temporal bone. Important structures traversing the middle ear include the facial nerve, the ossicular chain, and the internal jugular vein. The internal carotid artery is also found in close proximity anteriorly.

MIDDLE EAR TRAUMA

Basic Information

- Red flags for middle ear traumatic pathology include:
  - Signs/symptoms of basilar skull fracture (such as hemotympanum, periorbital or retroauricular hematomas)
  - Cerebrospinal fluid leakage from the ears or nares
  - Acute traumatic facial nerve dysfunction
  - Acute hearing loss or vestibular symptoms (such as ataxia, nystagmus, and so forth)
  - In such cases, computed tomography (CT) imaging of the temporal bone without contrast should be obtained. Of note, head CT imaging is not sufficient to evaluate for temporal bone or middle ear pathology.

EAR FOREIGN BODY

Diagnosis

- History and physical examination with an otoscope, adequate light source, and patient cooperation.
- Laboratory studies and imaging are often not required, but CT imaging may be considered if the foreign body has been present for a prolonged period of time and/or if infection or erosion is suspected.

Treatment

- Many tools are available to facilitate removal. Although commercial irrigation devices exist, an 18- to 20-gauge angiocatheter in conjunction with a large syringe can suffice. Alligator forceps can be used to grasp objects.
- Avoid irrigation if organic material is suspected, because these objects may swell, making removal more difficult.
- If a live insect is encountered, one may instill alcohol, lidocaine, or mineral oil to euthanize the insect.
- Avoid instilling any fluid into the ear canal if TM perforation is suspected.
- Consider consultation or referral for objects that have been in the canal for 24 hours or longer, objects in contact with the tympanic membrane, or other types of objects, which may be more problematic to remove, such as ones with sharp edges.
- Consider antibiotics if trauma has occurred to the ear canal.

TRAUMATIC PERFORATION OF THE TM (TPTM)

Basic Information

- The most common mechanism is direct blunt trauma, but other causes include penetrating trauma, barotrauma, and primary blast injuries.
- TPTM is observed in approximately one-third of all severe traumatic head injuries and it occurs in up to 50% of temporal bone fractures.
- Complications of TPTM include otitis media, mastoiditis, and permanent hearing loss.

Clinical Presentation

- Hearing loss in the setting of trauma is the most common complaint, but other symptoms include otalgia, nausea, dizziness, tinnitus, and ataxia.

Diagnosis

- Otoscopic examination to assess the percentage of TM perforation
  - Protruding foreign objects or blood clots within the ear canal should not be removed until a specialist evaluates the patient.
- Patients with blast-related TM rupture should undergo a chest radiograph to evaluate for lung injury.

Treatment

- Most traumatic TM perforations heal spontaneously, but large perforations may require surgical repair.
- Antibiotic drops can be administered for contaminated perforations.
- Supportive management involves pain management with medications such as acetaminophen and warm, dry compresses over the ear.
- Water should be prevented from entering the ear owing to an increased risk of infection. Patients should therefore avoid swimming and wear ear protection while showering until the lesion has healed.
- Outpatient specialist evaluation is generally warranted, except for small, uncomplicated TPTM.

ACUTE OTITIS MEDIA (AOM)

- Rapid onset of inflammation or infection in the middle ear.

Basic Information

- AOM, which is more common in children, can be owing to either viruses or bacteria.
- Occurs in the setting of current or recent viral upper respiratory infection caused by Eustachian tube obstruction and secondary infection of the middle ear.
- The most common bacterial causes include *Streptococcus pneumoniae*, *Haemophilus influenzae*, and *Moraxella catarrhalis*.

- Tympanic membrane perforation can occur because of increased middle ear pressure.

Diagnosis

- Clinical diagnosis based on history and physical examination.
- Bulging of the TM, erythema of the TM, otalgia, and/or new otorrhea not attributable to AOE.
- Differentiating AOM from otitis media with effusion (OME) is important, given differences in management. OME is defined as a noninfectious middle ear effusion. In the case of OME, signs of infection should be absent, such as lack of TM erythema and otalgia.

Treatment (Table 41.1)

- First-line treatment for AOM is high-dose amoxicillin, 80 to 90 mg/kg/day divided BID. If a child has concurrent conjunctivitis or has taken amoxicillin in the last 30 days, amoxicillin/clavulanate should be prescribed instead.
- Observation for select populations can be considered (see Table 41.1). If symptoms worsen or fail to improve within 48 to 72 hours, rescue antibiotic therapy should be provided.
- Children with TM perforations in the setting of AOM should be treated with oral antibiotics, whereas those with existing tympanostomy tubes should be provided topical ciprofloxacin/dexamethasone.
- Children with preexisting conditions, such as cochlear implants, immunocompromised states, congenital facial deformities, or Down syndrome are not candidates for observational treatment.

ACUTE MASTOIDITIS (AM)

- Destructive bacterial infection of the mastoid bone, causing coalescence of air cells

Basic Information

- AM can occur as a complication of AOM, whereby fluid and inflammation extend to the mastoid air cells. In most cases this fluid accumulation resolves with or without antibiotic therapy, but rarely, can progress to AM.
- Extracranial and intracranial complications from AM include abscess formation, venous thrombosis, and meningitis. Subperiosteal abscesses are the most common complication of AM.
- AM should be distinguished from radiologic mastoiditis. On CT imaging, an incidental finding of fluid within the mastoid air space without evidence of bony septae destruction should be interpreted within the appropriate clinical context.
- The most common offending pathogen is *S. pneumoniae*.

Clinical Presentation

- Patients may present with otalgia, fever, retroauricular tenderness, edema, erythema, and proptosis of the auricle. Examination of the tympanic membrane may reveal signs consistent with AOM.
- In addition to extra- and intracranial abscess development, localized inflammation can cause cranial nerve deficits.

Diagnosis

- Clinical history and physical examination alone may be sufficient to diagnose uncomplicated cases.
- CT or magnetic resonance imaging may be required if intracranial involvement or venous sinus thrombosis is suspected or if neurologic deficits are observed.

Treatment

- Empiric therapy using parenteral antibiotics that cover the most likely causative pathogens should be promptly administered.
- Ear nose and throat (ENT) should be consulted, although many patients can be managed nonoperatively.

BULLOUS MYRINGITIS

- Inflammation of the TM and external ear canal causing blistering and bullae

Clinical Presentation

- Patients may present with severe otalgia, hearing loss, and fever. As the bullae rupture, otorrhea may occur.

Diagnosis

- Physical examination of the TM and ear canal with direct otoscopic visualization of the lesions

Treatment

- Management is focused on treating the underlying AOM infection. ENT referral may be required in severe cases, where debriding the bullous lesions is required.

The Inner Ear

Basic Information

- The inner ear is composed of the cochlea and vestibular system, which are responsible for hearing and balance, respectively.
- Pathology within the inner ear has many precipitants, including blunt and penetrating trauma, noise exposure, viral infections, ototoxic drugs, autoimmune disorders, tumors, and vascular abnormalities/disruption (e.g., cerebrovascular accidents).

TABLE 41.1 *Treatment for Acute Otitis Media*

Age	(+) Otorrhea	(+) Severe symptoms*	Bilateral AOM	Unilateral AOM
6 mo–2 yrs	Antibiotic therapy	Antibiotic therapy	Antibiotic therapy	Consider observation
≥ 2 yrs	Antibiotic therapy	Antibiotic therapy	Consider observation	Consider observation

*Severe symptoms include temperature 39°C or higher in the past 48 hours, persistent otalgia more than 48 hours, uncertain follow-up, or toxic appearance.

- Patients present with hearing loss and/or vestibular symptoms, such as ataxia.

VESTIBULAR NEURITIS

- Acute inflammation of the vestibular portion of the 8th cranial nerve caused by a viral or postviral syndrome

Basic Information

- Care should be taken to rule out more serious causes of vertigo, because there is considerable overlap with the symptomology of vestibular neuritis and cerebellar or brain stem insults (see Chapter 85 for more information).
- Vestibular neuronitis is characterized by acute-onset constant rotational vertigo, associated with nausea and vomiting, gait disturbance, nystagmus, and head motion intolerance, without hearing loss, lasting 24 to 72 hours.
- Labyrinthitis can exhibit all the above symptoms, but also includes hearing loss or tinnitus and is often associated with AOM.

Diagnosis

- History and physical examination consistent with a peripheral cause of vertigo.

Treatment

- Symptomatic management with antiemetics, benzodiazepines, and antihistamines can provide relief.
- A corticosteroid taper may improve recovery of vestibular function.

MENIERE DISEASE

- Chronic disease of the inner ear caused by endolymphatic hydrops.

Basic Information

- Characterized by intermittent "attacks" of rotational vertigo, fluctuating hearing loss, and tinnitus. Such episodes are often preceded by a sensation of ear fullness. Attacks last a few minutes to 2 hours.
  - Patients may also complain of postural instability, drop attacks, and nausea.
    - During initial disease stages, hearing is fully regained after attacks. However, as the disease progresses over time, hearing loss can become permanent.
    - Mean age of onset is in the fourth decade of life and its occurrence is rare after the age of 60 years.

Diagnosis

- Patients should be referred to a specialist for definitive diagnosis.

Treatment

- Initial therapy often involves salt restriction and avoidance of vasoconstrictors of the labyrinthine system, such as caffeine, nicotine, and alcohol.
- Benzodiazepines and antihistamines, such as meclizine, may be helpful during acute attacks.

Nasal Emergencies

VICTOR GALSON, MD, and RYAN PEDIGO, MD, MHPE

Epistaxis, rhinosinusitis, and retained foreign body are the primary nasal pathologies that result in emergency department presentation. Knowledge of the underlying anatomy and treatment strategies can lead to efficient disposition for these patients.

Epistaxis

General Principles

- Of the population, 60% will experience at least one episode of epistaxis, but only a minority require acute medical attention; an even smaller percentage require admission.
- Of epistaxis, 90% is anterior, usually from the Kiesselbach plexus on the anteroinferior nasal septum. Posterior epistaxis (10%) usually originates from a posterior branch of the sphenopalatine artery (Fig. 42.1).
- Causes of epistaxis include local, systemic, and idiopathic etiologies (Box 42.1).
- Hypertension does not cause epistaxis.

Clinical Presentation

- Anterior epistaxis typically:
  - Is unilateral
  - Ranges from minor to severe hemorrhage
  - Presents with a bimodal distribution of age ranges, most often in children younger than 10 and adults older than 50 years of age

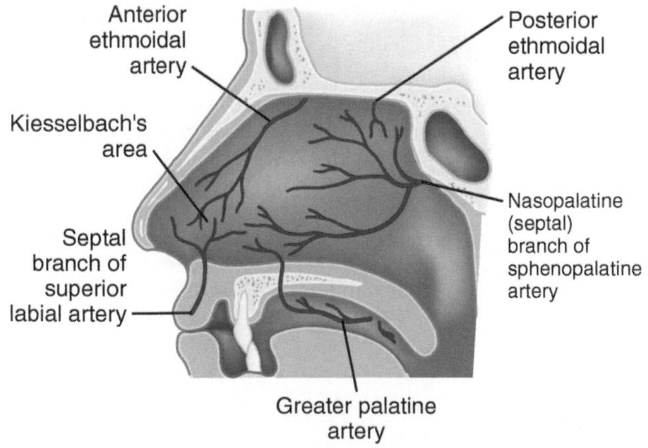

FIG. 42.1 Arterial supply to the medial wall of the nose. (From Pfaff, J. A., & Moore, G. P. (2018). Otolaryngology. In R. M. Walls, R. S. Hockberger, & M. Gausche-Hill (Eds.), *Rosen's emergency medicine: Concepts and clinical practice* (9th ed., pp. 820–832, Fig. 62.2). Elsevier.).

BOX 42.1 ***Causes of Epistaxis***

Local Causes
Nasal or facial trauma
Upper respiratory tract infections
Nose picking
Allergies
Low home humidity
Nasal polyps
Foreign body in the nose
Environmental irritants
Nasopharyngeal mucormycosis
Traumatic internal carotid artery aneurysm
Chlamydial rhinitis neonatorum
Neoplasms
Septal deviation
Surgery (postoperative epistaxis)

Idiopathic Epistaxis
Habitual
Familial

Systemic Causes
Atherosclerosis of nasal blood vessels
Anticoagulant therapy
Pregnancy
Barotrauma
Hereditary hemorrhagic telangiectasia (Rendu-Osler-Weber disease)
Blood dyscrasias (e.g., hemophilia, leukemia, platelet disorders)
Hepatic disease
Rupture of internal carotid artery aneurysm
Diabetes mellitus
Alcoholism
Vitamin K deficiency
Folic acid deficiency
Chronic nephritis
Chemotherapy
Blood transfusion reactions
Migraine headache
Chronic use of nasal vasoconstrictors
Cocaine use
Drug-induced thrombocytopenia

Adapted from Pfaff, J. A., & Moore, G. P. (2018). Otolaryngology. In R. M. Walls, R. S. Hockberger, & M. Gausche-Hill (Eds.), *Rosen's emergency medicine: Concepts and clinical practice* (9th ed., pp. 820–832, Box 62.1). Elsevier.

- Posterior epistaxis typically:
  - Demonstrates bleeding from bilateral nares
  - Is more severe
  - Is seen in older adults with comorbid conditions
  - Should be considered in cases where anterior packing does not achieve hemostasis

Diagnosis, Evaluation, and Treatment

- The primary diagnostic consideration is to determine the location of bleeding by physical examination. In stable patients, neither routine imaging nor laboratory testing is indicated, unless the patient has a known bleeding disorder or is anticoagulated. Identification and treatment of the bleed should proceed with a stepwise algorithm, such as the one suggested below.
  - If patient is hemodynamically stable, start with *direct nasal pressure*. If this fails, attempt again with a topical vasoconstrictor.
    - Patients should blow their nose to clear any clots.
    - Administer oxymetazoline or phenylephrine spray to bilateral nares.
    - Patient should apply constant pressure to cartilaginous part of nasal septum for 10 to 15 minutes.
  - If direct pressure fails, consider *chemical cauterization* if a small bleeding vessel is identified.
    - Examine bilateral nares with the floor of the nose parallel to the floor of the room, and with a nasal speculum opened vertically, so as not to obscure or put pressure on the nasal septum.
    - Perform chemical cauterization with silver nitrate, applied for no more than 5 seconds, and never to both sides of the nasal septum (avoid septal necrosis and perforation).
  - If cautery is not possible or successful, attempt to tamponade bleed with *anterior packing*. Options for anterior packing include:
    - Absorbable, thrombogenic agents, such as Gelfoam or Surgicel
    - Nonabsorbable nasal tampon, such as Merocel. Both thrombogenic agents and nasal tampons can be soaked in tranexamic acid (TXA) 500 mg for additional hemostasis.
    - Anterior balloon catheter, such as Rapid Rhino
  - If bleeding continues despite adequate anterior packing **or** a posterior bleed is initially suspected, proceed to *posterior packing*.
    - Commercially available double balloon catheter, after pretreatment with topical anesthetic (Fig. 42.2). This will tamponade both an anterior and posterior source.
    - Can also use Foley catheter, if needed, but will only be effective for a posterior bleed
- Patients with unilateral anterior packing can generally be discharged with close ear, nose, and throat (ENT) follow-up and packing in place for 48 hours. Prophylactic antibiotics are often requested by ENT, but this is not an evidence-based practice.
- Patients with posterior packing or unstable vital signs should be admitted. Posterior packing requires telemetry monitoring, owing to concern for vagal stimulation leading to bradycardia.

Rhinosinusitis

General Principles

- Sinusitis and rhinosinusitis are mostly interchangeable terms that describe the same condition: obstruction of the sinus ostia resulting in decreased mucus drainage. Sinusitis can be classified as acute (less than 4 weeks duration), subacute (4 to 12 weeks), chronic (more than 12 weeks), or recurrent acute.
- The causative agent can be viral, bacterial, fungal, or allergic, with viral etiologies comprising the vast majority of acute rhinosinusitis. Common bacterial pathogens include *Streptococcus pneumoniae*, nontypeable *Haemophilus influenzae*, and *Moraxella catarrhalis*; however, a bacterial infection is present in less than 2% of all cases of adult rhinosinusitis.
- Immunocompromised patients are at risk for an acute, invasive, and aggressive fungal sinusitis termed "mucormycosis" (previously termed zygomycosis).

Clinical Presentation

- Symptoms of rhinosinusitis include nasal congestion, nasal discharge, facial pressure or pain that is worse with leaning forward, ear pressure or pain, and hyposmia (decreased ability to smell).
- Physical examination findings include erythema, edema, or tenderness to palpation or percussion over the paranasal sinuses; however, no physical examination finding is specific for distinguishing viral from bacterial sinusitis.

Diagnosis and Evaluation

- Generally, identifying sinusitis and its etiology is a clinical diagnosis, and computed tomography should be obtained only with concern for complications or spread of infection (e.g., Pott puffy tumor, orbital cellulitis).
- Consider allergic rhinitis in patients with the following symptoms:
  - Clear, thin rhinorrhea
  - Nasal and/or ocular pruritus
  - Sneezing
- Consider bacterial sinusitis in patients with *any one* of the following:
  - *Persistent* symptoms for greater than or equal to 10 days, with no signs of improvement
  - *Severe* symptoms or high fever (39°C or higher) *and* purulent nasal discharge or facial pain, lasting for 3 to 4 days at onset of illness
  - *Worsening* sinusitis symptoms following a upper respiratory infection that lasted 5 to 6 days and was initially improving ("double sickening"). Consider invasive fungal infection (mucormycosis) with the following:
    - Early: gray, friable turbinates, which may be nonbleeding and numb owing to angioinvasion
    - Late:
      - Significant ulceration or necrosis
      - Involvement of orbits, vasculature, or brain resulting in severe headache, vision changes, or other neurologic deficits

Treatment

- Allergic rhinitis:
  - Decrease exposure to allergen.
  - Second-generation oral antihistamines
  - Nasal saline irrigation
  - Topical nasal steroids and/or topical nasal antihistamine sprays

EPISTAXIS MANAGEMENT: POSTERIOR PACKING WITH INFLATABLE DEVICES

A

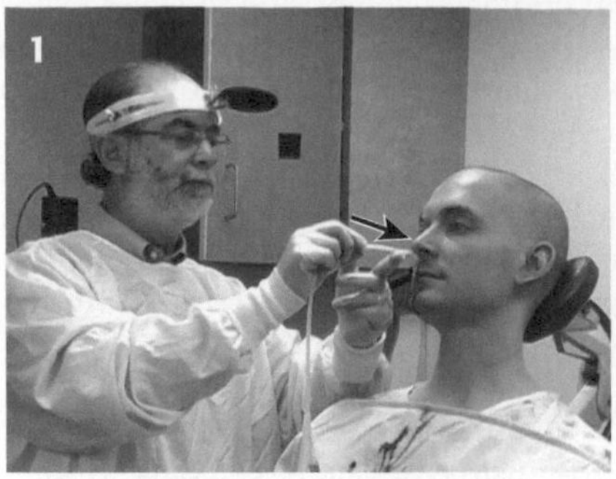

Insert a 12-Fr Foley catheter through the naris and into the posterior pharynx.

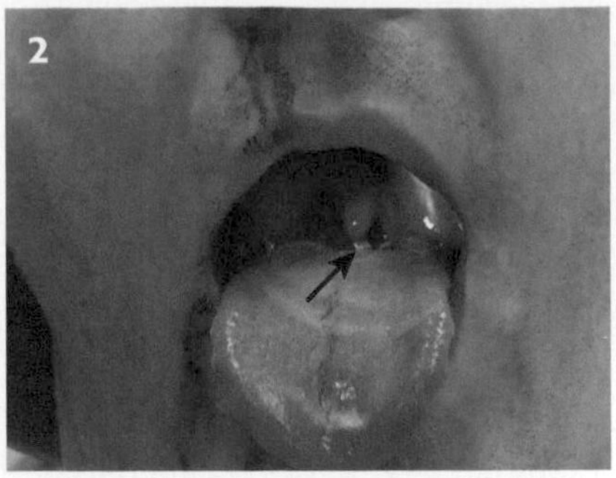

Look into the mouth to confirm that the catheter is properly positioned.

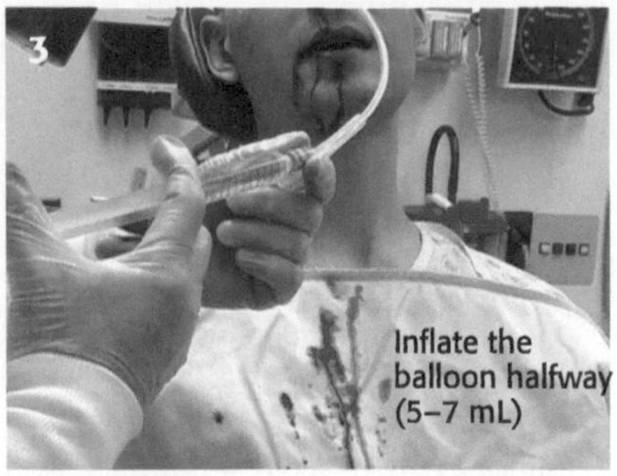

Inflate the balloon halfway with about 5–7 mL of water.

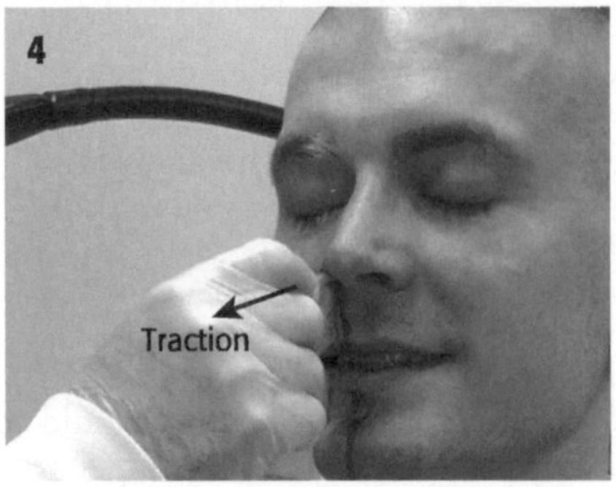

Slowly pull the catheter into the posterior nasopharynx up against the posterior aspect of the middle turbinate.

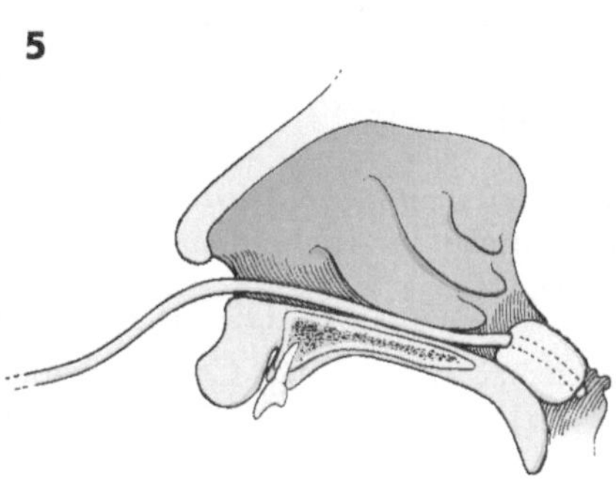

Foley catheter in proper position in the posterior nasopharynx. Inflate the balloon with another 5–7 mL of water.

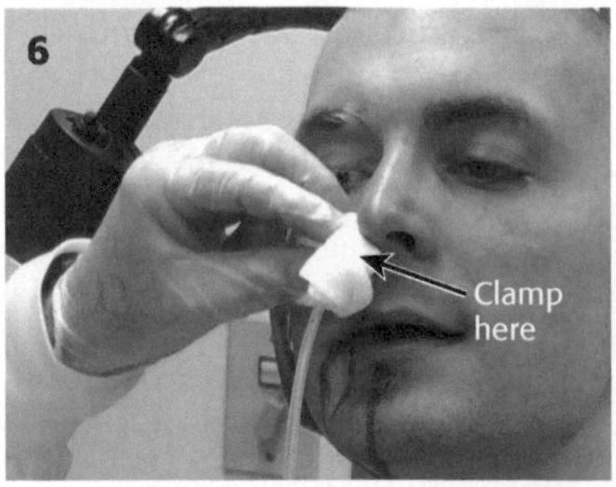

While maintaining traction, place anterior packing with layered gauze. Packing of the opposite side may be required to prevent septal deviation. Place a piece of gauze on the exposed catheter and secure with an umbilical clamp.

B

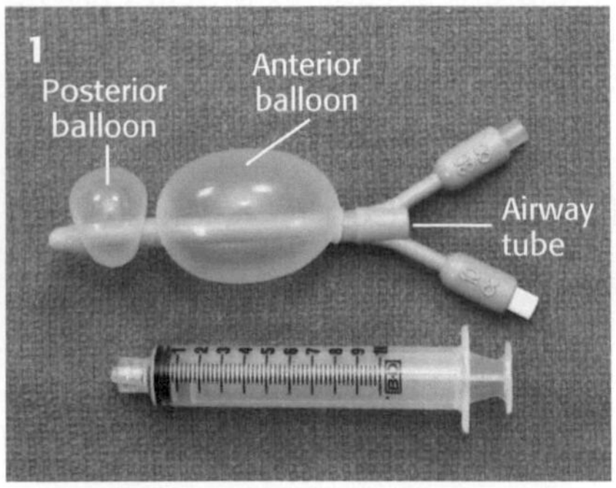

Double-balloon epistaxis catheters have both an anterior and posterior balloon, and some have an integral airway tube. These devices serve as an anterior and posterior pack. They are easily inserted and are often successful in the temporary control of posterior epistaxis in the ED.

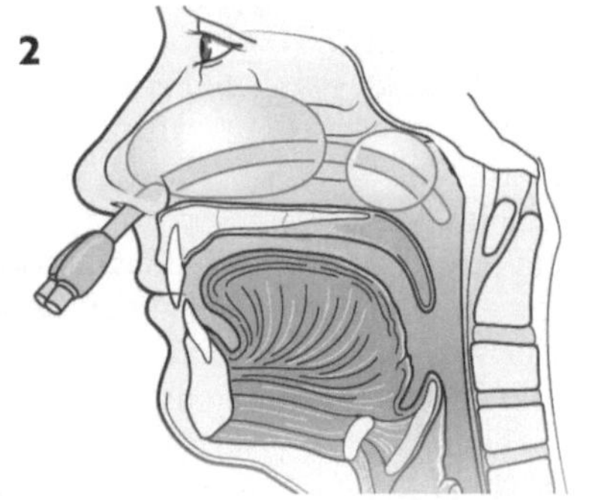

Insert the lubricated device along the nasal floor as far back as possible. Inflate the posterior balloon halfway with air, apply traction to pull the balloon up against the middle turbinate, and then complete the inflation. Maintain the position of the balloon and then inflate the anterior balloon with 30 mL of air.

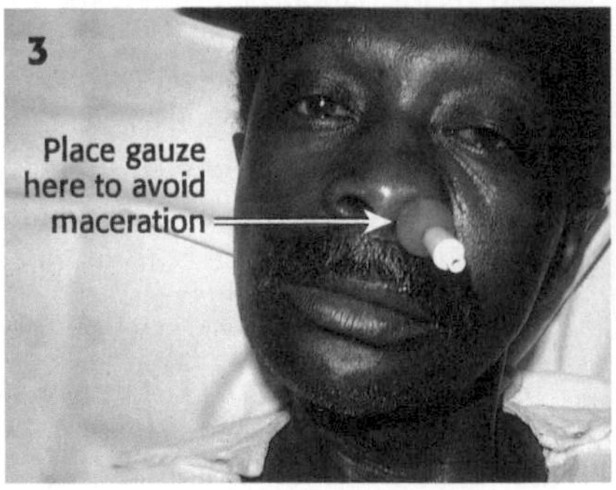

This patient with posterior epistaxis was successfully treated in the ED and discharged. Historically, most patients with posterior packs were admitted to the hospital; however, the ease and safety of balloon devices allow selected patients to be treated as outpatients. Consider admission for older adults and those with pulmonary or cardiovascular disease.

FIG. 42.2 Management of epistaxis—posterior packing with inflatable devices. (Adapted and reprinted from Pfaff, J. A., & Moore, G. P. (2018). Otolaryngology. In R. M. Walls, R. S. Hockberger, & M. Gausche-Hill (Eds.), *Rosen's emergency medicine: Concepts and clinical practice* (9th ed., pp. 826–828, Fig. 62.3). Elsevier.)

- Acute viral sinusitis:
  - Analgesics and antipyretics (e.g., acetaminophen, ibuprofen)
  - Nasal saline irrigation
  - Consider intranasal steroids
- Acute bacterial sinusitis:
  - First-line: amoxicillin-clavulanate for 5 to 7 days
  - Second-line: doxycycline or a fluoroquinolone
- Mucormycosis infection:
  - Consult ENT emergently for debridement in operating room (OR)
  - Amphotericin B intravenous (IV)

Nasal Foreign Bodies

General Principles

- Nasal foreign bodies are most commonly encountered in children less than 5 years of age, and often include marbles, beans, nuts, beads, or jewelry. Special consideration should be given to button batteries, or multiple magnets across the septum, which can lead to necrosis of the nasal septum and significant morbidity.

Clinical Presentation, Diagnosis, and Evaluation

- Most patients will present with either:
  - Direct history of placing a nasal foreign body; patients may have pain and discharge.
  - Persistent sinusitis, despite appropriate antibiotic treatment, especially with unilateral purulent or bloody nasal discharge. Consider radiography in this group, primarily to screen for a button battery or magnets.

Treatment

- Prior to an attempt at removal, consider pretreatment with a vasoconstrictive agent and/or topical anesthesia. Additional restraints or sedation may be necessary. Multiple effective techniques exist for removal of nasal foreign bodies without specialty consultation.
  - Positive pressure, with occlusion of unaffected nare, in order to expel foreign body. Pressure can be provided by the parent forming a seal over the patient's mouth and blowing, by a bag-valve mask, or by the patients themselves.
  - Balloon catheter, with the balloon tip passed proximally behind the foreign body, then inflated, followed by gentle retraction
  - Alligator forceps for directly visualized foreign bodies
  - Tissue adhesive glue on the end of a cotton swab
  - Suction catheter

Disposition

- Patients with simple foreign body removal: routine follow-up appointment with primary care doctor
- Prolonged foreign body placement or traumatic removals: obtain 24- to 48-hour ENT referral.
- Suspicion or presence of a button battery or multiple magnets unable to be removed in ED: ENT consultation from the ED

SUGGESTED READINGS

Melio, F. R. (2018). Upper respiratory tract infections. In Walls, R. M., Hockberger, R. S., & Gausche-Hill M. (Eds.), *Rosen's emergency medicine: Concepts and clinical practice* (9th ed., pp. 867–870). Elsevier.

Pfaff, J. A., & Moore, G. P. (2018). Otolaryngology. In Walls, R. M., Hockberger, R. S., & Gausche-Hill, M. (Eds.), *Rosen's emergency medicine: Concepts and clinical practice* (9th ed., pp. 826–828). Elsevier.

Thomas, S. H., & Goodloe, J. M. (2018). Foreign bodies. In Walls, R. M., Hockberger, R. S., & M. Gausche-Hill (Eds.), *Rosen's emergency medicine: Concepts and clinical practice* (9th ed., pp. 674–689). Elsevier.

CHAPTER 43

BOARD REVIEW

Ophthalmology

RYAN TENOLD, DO, and JULIANA TOLLES, MD, MHS

The eye is a complex sensory organ subject to a variety of pathology. Most diagnoses are based on a focused history and clinical examination.

Orbit

PRESEPTAL (PERIORBITAL) CELLULITIS

General Principles

- Bacterial infection of the preseptal soft tissue
- Critical to distinguish from orbital cellulitis, which involves tissues deep to the orbital septum

Clinical Presentation

- Eyelid erythema, tenderness, warmth, and swelling (Fig. 43.1)
- May have a low-grade fever

Diagnosis and Evaluation

- Clinical examination
- May obtain computed tomography (CT) of the orbit and complete blood count to help differentiate from orbital cellulitis

Treatment

- If no comorbid conditions, discharge home on oral antibiotics covering *Streptococcus* and *Staphylococcus*, including methicillin-resistant *Staphylococcus aureus* (MRSA).
- Hospitalize for intravenous (IV) antibiotics if less than 1 year of age or concern for orbital cellulitis.

ORBITAL CELLULITIS

General Principles

- Infection deep to the orbital septum
- Complications include orbital abscess, meningitis, osteomyelitis, and cavernous sinus thrombosis.

Clinical Presentation

- Distinguished from preseptal cellulitis by presence of **proptosis**, **ophthalmoplegia**, **pain with eye movements**, and **chemosis** (Fig. 43.2)
- An absolute neutrophil count (ANC) greater than 10,000 cell/μL, periorbital edema extending beyond eyelid margins, sudden onset, and recent antibiotic use also increase risk.

Diagnosis and Evaluation

- Contrast CT of the orbits or magnetic resonance imaging (MRI) of the orbits to evaluate for associated abscess or to help differentiate between preseptal vs. orbital cellulitis

Treatment

- IV antibiotics to cover MRSA, *Streptococcus*, and gram-negative bacilli
- If intracranial extension is suspected, add anaerobic coverage.

Eyelids

BLEPHARITIS

General Principles

- Inflammation of the eyelid margin that is often chronic
- May be associated with atopic dermatitis, psoriasis, or seborrheic dermatitis

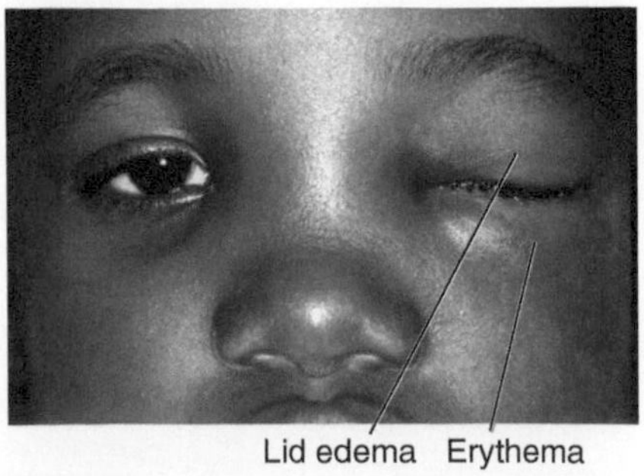

FIG. 43.1 Preseptal cellulitis. (From P. Kaiser, N. Friedman, & R. Pineda II. (2014). *The Massachusetts Eye and Ear Infirmary illustrated manual of ophthalmology* (4th ed., p. 12, Fig. 1.11). Elsevier.)

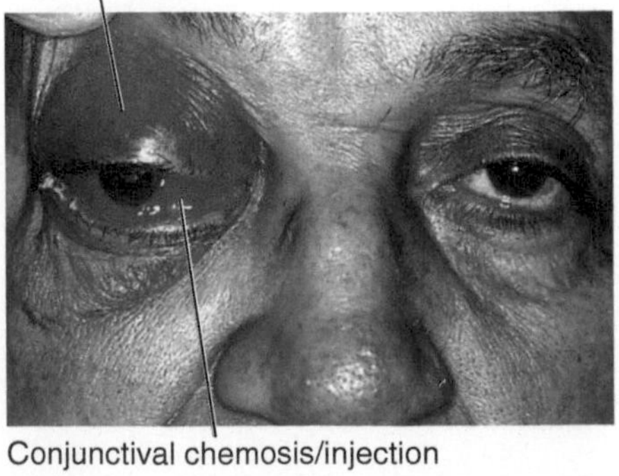

FIG. 43.2 Orbital cellulitis. (From P. Kaiser, N. Friedman, & R. Pineda II. (2014). *The Massachusetts Eye and Ear Infirmary illustrated manual of ophthalmology* (4th ed., p. 12, Fig. 1.12). Elsevier.)

Clinical Presentation

- Itching and burning of the eyelids often associated with a foreign-body sensation, photophobia, and pain
- Thickened, inflamed, crusted, red lid margins with tearing on examination

Diagnosis and Evaluation

- Slit-lamp examination
- Can be distinguished from preseptal cellulitis by involvement isolated to the lid margin

Treatment

- Warm compresses for 10 to 15 minutes, three to five times per day
- Clean lid margins with cotton swab soaked in mild baby shampoo twice per day.
- Treat bacterial superinfection with topical antibiotics covering *Staphylococcus* and *Streptococcus*.

HORDEOLUM (STYE)

General Principles

- Abscess of the internal or external eyelids caused by inflamed oil glands often caused by *Staphylococcus aureus*
  - Internal hordeola: meibomian glands
  - External hordeola: glands in eyelash follicle or lid margin (gland of Zeis or Moll)

Clinical Presentation

- Painful, swollen, erythematous nodule on the eyelid

Diagnosis and Evaluation

- Clinical examination

Treatment

- Warm compresses for 10 to 15 minutes, three to five times a day
- Cases that do not respond to conservative management may be started on topical antibiotics to cover *Staphylococcus* and referred to ophthalmology for incision and drainage.

CHALAZION

General Principles

- Chronic, sterile granulomatous inflammation of Zeis or meibomian gland

Clinical Presentation

- **Nontender**, rubbery nodule on eyelid
- May develop from a hordeolum
- More common on upper lid

Diagnosis and Evaluation

- Clinical examination

Treatment

- Warm compresses for 10 to 15 minutes, three to five times a day
- Nonurgent referral to ophthalmology for surgical excision

Lacrimal Sac

DACRYOCYSTITIS

General Principles

- Bacterial infection of the lacrimal sac, commonly caused by nasolacrimal duct obstruction

Clinical Presentation

- Unilateral pain, swelling, and erythema over the lacrimal sac medial to the eye with epiphora (overflow of tears) (Fig. 43.3A)
- Purulent material can be expressed through the puncta when manual pressure is applied to the sac.
- Complications include preseptal or orbital cellulitis, as well as meningitis.
- More common in infants and adults over the age of 50

Diagnosis and Evaluation

- Obtain cultures by applying gentle pressure to the nasolacrimal duct to express fluid.
- May use the "fluorescein dye disappearance test": place fluorescein dye in the affected eye. If it is still present after 5 minutes, this indicates an occluded duct and is consistent with dacryocystitis.

Treatment

- Warm compresses, massage, and systemic antibiotics with coverage for MRSA
- Admission for severe cases, and some may require drainage
- Pediatric patients require ophthalmologic consultation, empiric antibiotics, and consideration for admission as they are at increased risk for preseptal and orbital cellulitis.

Conjunctiva and Cornea

CONJUNCTIVITIS

General Principles

- Conjunctivitis can be classified by etiology as bacterial, viral, or allergic. Common bacterial pathogens include *Haemophilus influenzae*, *Streptococcus pneumoniae*, *S. aureus*, and *Moraxella catarrhalis*. The most common form of viral pathogen is adenovirus.

Clinical Presentation

- **Bacterial** conjunctivitis is characterized by mucopurulent discharge at lid margins and corners of the eye that appears within minutes of wiping the lids (Fig. 43.3B). Conjunctiva have diffuse injection that spares the limbus.
- **Viral** conjunctivitis is characterized by watery or mucoserous discharge and may be associated with symptoms of a viral syndrome, including fever, pharyngitis, upper respiratory tract infection, or adenopathy.
- **Allergic** conjunctivitis presents with bilateral conjunctival injection, profuse watery discharge, and **itching**. It may be associated with a history of allergy or hay fever.

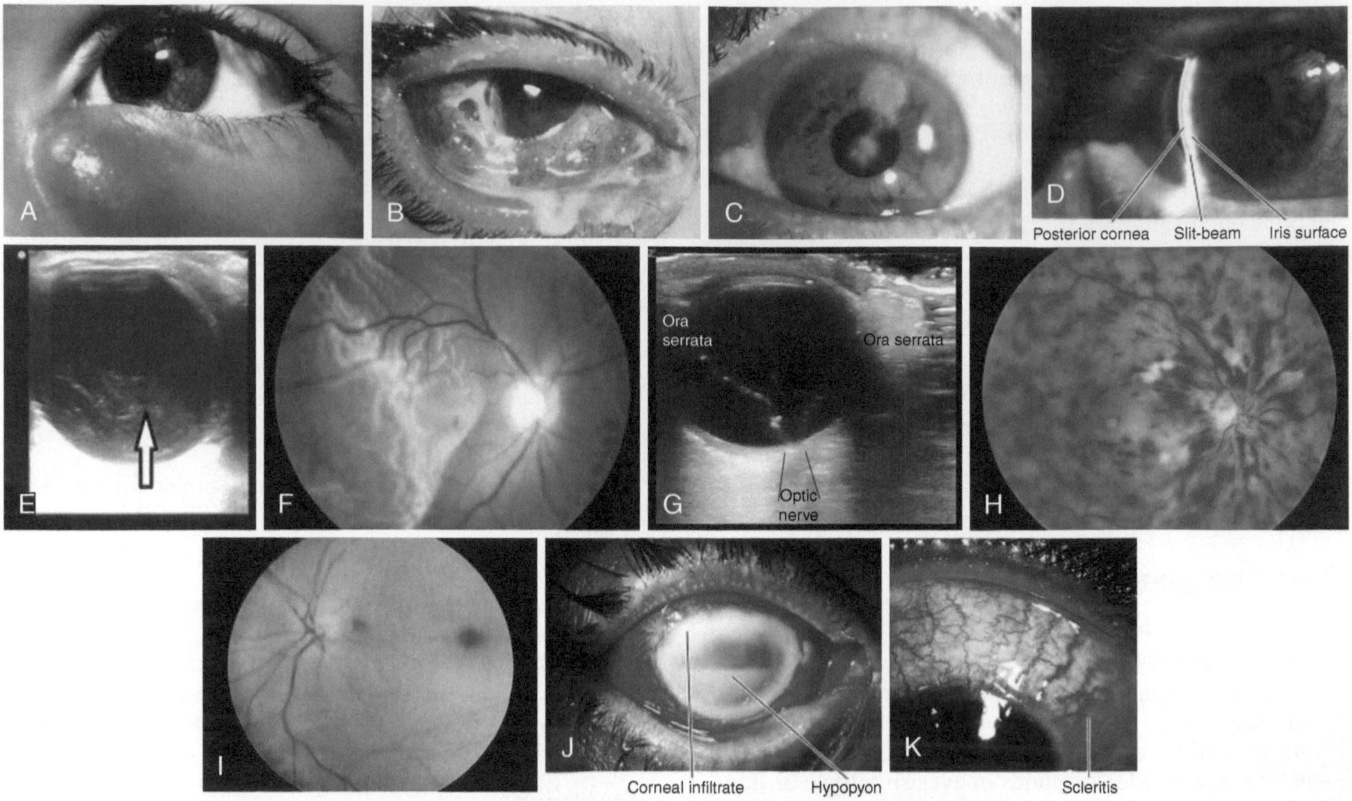

FIG. 43.3 **A**, Dacrocystitis. (Courtesy Jeffrey Lee, MD, University of California San Diego.) **B**, Bacterial conjunctivitis. (From Goldman, L., & Schaefer, A. I. (Eds.) (2012). *Goldman-Cecil medicine* (24th ed.). Saunders.) **C**, Herpes simplex keratitis. (Courtesy www.tedmontgomery.com). Elsevier.) **D**, Angle closure glaucoma. (From P. Kaiser, N. Friedman, & R. Pineda II. (2014). *The Massachusetts Eye and Ear Infirmary illustrated manual of ophthalmology* (4th ed., Fig. 6.1). Elsevier.) **E**, Vitreous hemorrhage. (Courtesy Douglas Brunette, MD.) **F**, Retinal detachment. (Courtesy www.tedmontgomery.com) **G**, Retinal detachment. (Figure 1 from Mohebbi, M. R., Bernard, R. L., & Stickles, S. P. (2017). 60 year old man with loss of vision in one eye. *Visual Journal of Emergency Medicine, 7*, 26–27.) **H**, Central retinal vein occlusion. (Courtesy www.tedmontgomery.com) **I**, Central retinal artery occlusion. (From R. M. Walls, R. S. Hockberger, & M. Gausche-Hill (Eds.). (2018). *Rosen's emergency medicine: Concepts and clinical practice* (9th ed., p. 813, Fig. 61.28A). Elsevier.) **J**, Endophthalmitis. (From P. Kaiser, N. Friedman, & R. Pineda II. (2014). *The Massachusetts Eye and Ear Infirmary illustrated manual of ophthalmology* (4th ed., p. 245, Fig. 6.10). Elsevier.) **K**, Scleritis. (From P. Kaiser, N. Friedman, & R. Pineda II. (2014). *The Massachusetts Eye and Ear Infirmary illustrated manual of ophthalmology* (4th ed., p. 168, Fig. 4.62). Elsevier.)

Diagnosis and Evaluation

- Clinical examination: must differentiate from keratitis, iritis, or angle closure glaucoma

Treatment

- **Bacterial:** broad-spectrum topical antibiotics (e.g., polymyxin B plus trimethoprim). If contact lens wearer, cover for *Pseudomonas aeruginosa* with a fluoroquinolone or aminoglycoside and advise cessation of contact lens use until infection resolves. If *Neisseria gonorrhoeae* is suspected, treat with ceftriaxone and saline irrigation. Add empiric treatment for *Chlamydia trachomatis*.
- **Viral:** cool compresses and topical lubricating agents
- **Allergic:** educate patients to avoid rubbing their eyes as this can cause mechanical mast cell degranulation. Patients should also decrease contact lens use and limit allergen exposure. Additional treatments include cool compresses and refrigerated artificial tears.

OPHTHALMIA NEONATORUM

General Principles

- Neonatal conjunctivitis that occurs within 30 days from birth; can be allergic, chemical, viral, or bacterial in etiology
- Serious causes include *N. gonorrhoeae*, *C. trachomatis*, and herpes simplex virus (HSV).
- Untreated infections can cause corneal and conjunctival scarring and can lead to visual impairment.
- Suspect in infants of mothers with no prenatal care or maternal history of gonorrhea or chlamydia

Clinical Presentation

- Chemical neonatal conjunctivitis: days 1 to 2 of life
- *N. gonorrhoeae:* days 2 to 5 of life. Profuse, purulent conjunctivitis with swelling of eyelids
- *C. trachomatis:* days 5 to 14 of life. Mild eyelid edema with watery to mucopurulent discharge.
- HSV: weeks 2 to 6 of life. Excessive tearing, conjunctival erythema. Skin demonstrates coalescing vesicles on an erythematous base and lid edema.

Diagnosis and Evaluation

- *N. gonorrhoeae:* Gram stain and cultures of swab of exudates (Thayer-Martin medium)
- *C. trachomatis:* nucleic acid amplification test. Swab everted eyelid, must include conjunctival epithelial cells (exudate not adequate as it is an obligate intracellular organism).
- HSV: slit-lamp examination with fluorescein to identify corneal microdendrites. Swab conjunctiva for HSV viral

culture. Must rule out CNS involvement with cerebrospinal fluid analysis.
- Diagnosis of either gonorrhea or chlamydia should prompt evaluation for the other.

Treatment

- *N. gonorrhoeae:* single-dose ceftriaxone
- *C. trachomatis:* oral erythromycin
- HSV: topical trifluridine and IV acyclovir until CNS and disseminated disease is ruled out. Hospitalization to observe response to therapy. When CNS involvement is excluded, transition to oral acyclovir and continue topical antivirals.

RADIATION (ULTRAVIOLET) KERATITIS

General Principles

- Excessive exposure to UV light leads to superficial burns of the cornea
- Common causes include welder's arc burns and "snow blindness"

Clinical Presentation

- Bilateral eye pain, photophobia, conjunctival erythema 6 to 12 hours after the exposure
- History of exposure and examination with tearing, injection, and edema of bulbar conjunctiva, sparing tarsal conjunctiva
- Hazy cornea, fluorescein examination with multiple superficial punctate staining
- Decreased visual acuity

Diagnosis and Evaluation

- Clinical examination

Treatment

- Oral analgesics for 1 to 2 days
- Lubricant antibiotic ointment, such as erythromycin or polymyxin-bacitracin (prophylaxis against bacterial superinfection)

HERPES KERATITIS

General Principles

- Herpes simplex keratitis: corneal infection and inflammation caused by herpes simplex virus
- Herpes zoster ophthalmicus: reactivation of latent varicella zoster virus in the ophthalmic branch of the fifth cranial nerve (V_1)

Clinical Presentation

- Herpes simplex virus
  - Eye pain, visual changes, watery discharge
  - Ciliary flush (conjunctival injection near limbus)
  - Dendritic lesions of the cornea on fluorescein staining (Fig. 43.3C)
  - Decreased corneal sensation
- Herpes zoster ophthalmicus (HZO)
  - Prodrome of headache, malaise, fever followed by a painful, unilateral dermatomal maculopapular skin eruption leading to vesicular ulceration and crusting
  - Hyperemic conjunctivitis, uveitis, episcleritis, or keratitis may occur with onset of rash.
  - **Vesicular lesions on the tip or side of the nose (Hutchinson sign)** indicate involvement of nasociliary nerve and are highly associated with ocular involvement.
  - Pseudodendrites (coarse, heaped-up, epithelial plaques without terminal bulbs) on fluorescein staining of cornea

Diagnosis and Evaluation

- Clinical diagnosis
- Slit-lamp findings pathognomonic in HSV

Treatment

- Ophthalmologic consult to characterize the extent of disease
- HSV
  - Most common form is epithelia keratitis, which can be treated with topical antivirals (trifluridine) and oral acyclovir
  - **Avoid steroids.**
- HZO
  - Oral antivirals (e.g., valacyclovir, famciclovir, acyclovir)
  - Topical antibiotics (e.g., erythromycin) to prevent secondary infection
  - Topical steroids
  - Immunocompromised patient or sight-threatening disease requires IV acyclovir and admission.

PTERYGIUM

General Principles

- Chronic fibrovascular growth caused by UV light exposure
- Higher incidence in outdoor jobs, patients who do not wear sunglasses, male sex

Clinical Presentation

- Triangular, thickened conjunctiva on the nasal side that **may encroach onto the cornea** and threaten vision

Diagnosis and Evaluation

- Clinical examination

Treatment

- Artificial tears for symptom relief
- Referral for surgical excision if visual acuity or visual axis is affected

Anterior Segment

ACUTE ANGLE-CLOSURE GLAUCOMA

General Principles

- Aqueous humor normally fills the anterior segment and drains through the anterior chamber angle. When this pathway is narrowed, build-up of aqueous humor causes increased intraocular pressure (IOP) and damage to the optic nerve.

Clinical Presentation

- Severe eye pain, headaches, decreased vision, nausea and vomiting, halos around lights

- Conjunctival redness
- **"Cloudy" or "steamy" cornea**
- Shallow anterior chamber
- Mid-dilated pupil that reacts poorly to light
- **Increased IOP greater than 30 mm Hg**
- Often precipitated by pupil dilation (evening, entering a movie theater, iatrogenic)

Diagnosis and Evaluation

- Clinical examination including visual acuity, IOP, slit-lamp examination of anterior segment (will reveal shallow chamber: Fig. 43.3D), and nondilated fundus examination

Treatment

- Emergent ophthalmologic consult
- Topical medication to decrease IOP
  - Topical β-blockers (e.g., timolol maleate) to decrease aqueous humor production
  - Topical α_2 agonist (e.g., apraclonidine) to decrease aqueous humor production
  - Parasympathomimetic (e.g., pilocarpine) to contract the iris sphincter muscle, facilitating the outflow of aqueous humor
- Acetazolamide (systemic carbonic anhydrase inhibitor). Avoid in sickle cell disease.
- Repeat IOP 30 to 60 minutes after medication administration. Redose if IOP is greater than 40 mm Hg.

UVEITIS

General Principles

- Inflammation of the three structures that make up the uvea, which include the (1) iris, (2) ciliary body, and (3) choroid. Most commonly associated with systemic autoimmune disease, such as **ankylosing spondylitis** or infections (HSV, cytomegalovirus, toxoplasmosis).

Clinical Presentation

- Painful red eye, photophobia, and often a decrease in visual acuity
- Ciliary flush, "cell and flare" in anterior chamber (white cells and protein)

Diagnosis and Evaluation

- Clinical examination, including slit-lamp examination and dilated fundoscopy

Treatment

- Ophthalmologic consult to confirm diagnosis, treat underlying cause

Posterior Segment/Retina

VITREOUS HEMORRHAGE

General Principles

- Blood in the vitreous space
- Diabetes, retinal tear, vitreous detachment, and trauma are common causes.

Clinical Presentation

- Sudden onset of floaters and decreased vision
- Ophthalmoscopy with poor or no view of fundus, red reflex diminished or absent
- Ultrasound with echogenic debris in the vitreous humor (Fig. 43.3E)

Diagnosis and Evaluation

- Clinical examination
- Ocular ultrasound

Treatment

- Ophthalmologic consult to evaluate for retinal detachment (requires emergent treatment)
- Limit activity.
- Avoid anticoagulation.
- Elevate head of bed to allow blood to settle to optimize visualization of the retina on repeat examinations.

RETINAL DETACHMENT

General Principles

- Results from accumulation of fluid between the neurosensory retina and the underlying retinal pigment epithelium
- Can be categorized by those that initially involve macula ("macula off") and those that do not ("macula on")

Clinical Presentation

- **Painless** flashes of light and floaters
- Cloudy or classically "**curtain-like**" visual loss
- "Mac-on": central vision preserved, minimal change in visual acuity
- "Mac-off": visual acuity between 20/40 and counting fingers
- In large retinal detachments, a bullous detachment with retinal folds can be seen on fundoscopy (Fig. 43.3F).

Diagnosis and Evaluation

- Ultrasound with a discrete hyperechoic line in the posterior chamber that **does not** cross (is instead tethered to) the optic nerve. This finding can help differentiate retinal detachment from vitreous detachment (detachment of vitreous from the retina) or vitreous hemorrhage, in which the hyperechoic material does cross (Fig. 43.3G) the optic nerve.

Treatment

- Macula **on:** emergent ophthalmologic consult for surgical repair within 24 hours. Most symptomatic retinal detachments will progress to involve the macula if not treated.
- Macula **off:** urgent ophthalmologic referral

CENTRAL RETINAL VEIN OCCLUSION

General Principles

- Thrombus formation in the retinal vein leads to increased venous pressure, which causes retinal ischemia and subsequent vision loss.
- Causes include mechanical compression, poor circulation, vasculitis, and hypercoagulability.

Clinical Presentation

- Monocular, sudden-onset, painless blurred vision or vision loss
  - Nonischemic: mild, no afferent pupillary defect (APD), retina with perfusion
  - Ischemic: visual acuity less than 20/100, **APD present**, causes decreased arterial flow to the retina
- Retinal hemorrhages give a classic "blood and thunder" appearance on funduscopic examination (Fig. 43.3H).
- Dilated and tortuous retinal veins with macular and optic disc edema in affected eye

Diagnosis and Evaluation

- Clinical examination

Treatment

- Ophthalmologic consult for intravitreal antivascular endothelial growth factor injection, intravitreal triamcinolone injection, and possible laser photocoagulation
- Workup and treatment of underlying hypercoagulability

CENTRAL RETINAL ARTERY OCCLUSION

General Principles

- Caused by embolic occlusion, most commonly by plaque material originating from the ipsilateral carotid artery

Clinical Presentation

- Monocular, **painless** vision loss that may be preceded by transient blindness or have a stuttering course
- Retinal examination with "cherry red" macula (Fig. 43.3I), "boxcar" segmentation of blood in retinal veins and ischemic retinal whitening. **APD is present.**

Diagnosis and Evaluation

- Clinical examination
- An ophthalmologist may confirm unclear cases with fluorescein angiography.
- Erythrocyte sedimentation rate and C-reactive protein to evaluate for giant cell arteritis if patient is more than 50 years of age and without visible retinal emboli

Treatment

- Intraarterial thrombolytic therapy is controversial.
- Anterior chamber paracentesis may be performed by an ophthalmologist if the patient is not a thrombolysis candidate and symptoms are less than 24 hours.
- Measures to include: dislodge the embolus by manipulating the IOP, including ocular massage, systemic medications (IV acetazolamide, mannitol), and topical medications
- Vasodilator medication (pentoxifylline, nitroglycerin, isosorbide dinitrate)
- Occlusions of more than 4 hours duration are usually not amenable to therapy.

Optic Nerve

OPTIC NEURITIS

General Principles

- Inflammatory demyelination of the optic nerve
- Most cases occur in women and in patients between 20 and 40 years of age.
- Presenting feature in 15%–20% of all cases of **multiple sclerosis (MS)**

Clinical Presentation

- Monocular, **painful** vision loss that peaks at 1 to 2 weeks; pain worsened by eye movement
- Flashes of lights
- **Loss of color vision** out of proportion to loss of visual acuity
- Afferent pupillary defect
- Swelling and hyperemia of the optic disc, blurred disc margins on fundoscopy

Diagnosis and Evaluation

- Magnetic resonance image of the brain and orbits, with and without gadolinium, to confirm diagnosis and assess for MS

Treatment

- Benefits of steroids are controversial, but IV methylprednisolone may reduce the risk of conversion to MS and improve the speed of visual recovery.

Globe

ENDOPHTHALMITIS

General Principles

- Bacterial or fungal infection within the eye involving the vitreous and/or aqueous humor. Most common bacterial pathogen is coagulase-negative *Staphylococci*.
- Most commonly caused by exogenous inoculation of organisms after trauma or surgery
- Less commonly due to hematogenous spread

Clinical Presentation

- Typically presents **within 1 week of surgery or injury**, with a decrease in visual acuity and eye pain that worsens over 12 to 24 hours
- Examination may reveal chemosis, hyperemia of conjunctiva, or **hypopyon** (Fig. 43.3J).

Diagnosis and Evaluation

- Clinical examination
- Confirmed by positive culture of aqueous or vitreous aspirate

Treatment

- Broad-spectrum IV antibiotics to cover gram-positive bacteria, gram-negative bacteria, and anaerobes
- Emergent ophthalmologic consult for intravitreal antibiotics
- Severe or refractory cases may require vitrectomy.

SCLERITIS

General Principles

- 50% associated underlying systemic illness, including **rheumatoid arthritis** and granulomatosis with polyangiitis (previously called Wegener granulomatosis)
- High risk for vision loss

Clinical Presentation

- Severe, constant, boring pain that is worse at night or early morning and radiates to the face and periorbital region; commonly worsened by eye movement
- Scleral edema, violaceous discoloration of the globe (Fig. 43.3K)
- Tenderness (test by exerting pressure over closed eyelid)

Diagnosis and Evaluation

- Clinical examination

Treatment

- Ophthalmologic consult for guidance on nonsteroidal antiinflammatory drugs (NSAIDs), glucocorticoids, and/or systemic immunosuppressants

EPISCLERITIS

General Principles

- Inflammation of the episcleral layer; unlike scleritis, does **not threaten vision**

Clinical Presentation

- Acute onset of redness, irritation, and watering of the eye without vision changes
- Bright red episcleral discoloration (vs. deeper purple color of scleritis)

Diagnosis and Evaluation

- Clinical examination
- Introduction of topical phenylephrine eye drops should produce rapid, transient improvement in episcleral erythema, allowing better evaluation of underlying sclera.

Treatment

- Successive therapy with topical lubricants, topical NSAIDs, topical glucocorticoids, and oral NSAIDs

SUGGESTED READINGS

Guluma, K., & Lee, J. E. (2018). Ophthalmology. In R. M. Walls, R. S. Hockberger, & M. Gausche-Hill (Eds.), *Rosen's emergency medicine: Concepts and clinical practice* (9th ed., pp. 790–819). Elsevier Saunders.

Kaiser, P., Friedman, N., & Pineda, R., II. (2014). *The Massachusetts Eye and Ear Infirmary illustrated manual of ophthalmology* (4th ed.). Elsevier Saunders.

Dental Emergencies

KATHLEEN YIP, MD, and RYAN PEDIGO, MD, MHPE

Dental emergencies are classified as either traumatic or atraumatic. They may range from simple, requiring just pain control, to life-threatening, requiring intubation and intravenous antibiotics. Additionally, a broad differential must be considered, because many conditions may mimic dental pain but are actually nonodontogenic in origin.

Anatomy

Basic Information

- Twenty deciduous (primary) teeth are eventually replaced by 32 permanent (secondary) teeth (Fig. 44.1)
  - Primary teeth begin erupting at approximately 6 months of age.
  - Permanent teeth begin replacing primary teeth at age 5 or 6 years.
  - Teeth are labeled from top right to top left, then bottom left to bottom right, with primary teeth represented by letters (A through T) and permanent teeth represented by numbers (1 through 32).
- The crown of tooth includes (from outside to in) enamel, dentin, and pulp.
- The root of tooth has cementum instead of enamel, which attaches to the alveolar bone with the help of the periodontal ligament (Fig. 44.2).
  - Periodontal ligament viability is crucial to successful reimplantation.

Dentoalveolar Trauma

Clinical Presentation

- Concussion: dental pain with percussion and no mobility of the tooth
- Subluxation: mobility of the tooth is present, but remains in correct anatomic position
- Luxation: there is mobility of the tooth and it is not in anatomic position (e.g., partially out of socket, forced into the socket, inward or outward) (Fig. 44.3).
- Avulsion: complete extrusion of the tooth
- Alveolar ridge fracture: entire segment of teeth is displaced
- Tooth fractures are classified using the Ellis classification system (Fig. 44.4).
  - Ellis I: involvement of the enamel only
  - Ellis II: involvement of the enamel and dentin
  - Ellis III: involvement of all three layers (enamel, dentin and pulp)

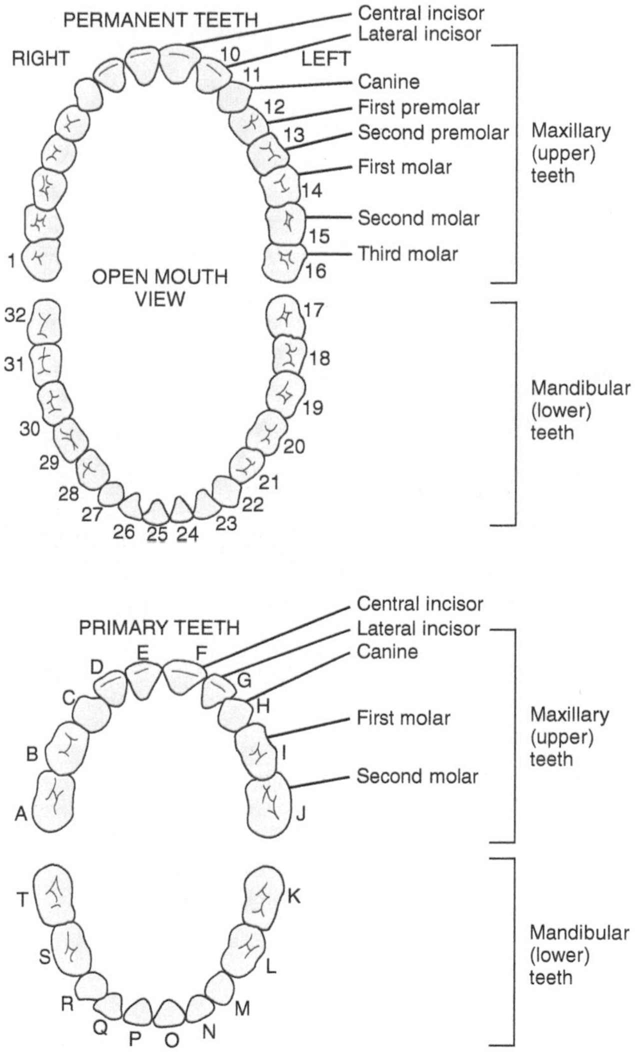

FIG. 44.1 Identification of teeth. (Modified from Roberts, J. (2014). *Roberts & Hedges' clinical procedures in emergency medicine*, (6th ed., Fig. 64.2, p 1344.). Elsevier.

Disorders of the Tooth, Gingiva, and Periodontium

Clinical Presentation

- Pulpitis: demineralization of the enamel and exposure of the dentin facilitates infection to the pulp; condition is usually caused by untreated caries. Can be reversible (pain with stimulus, such as cold) or irreversible (pain without stimulus).

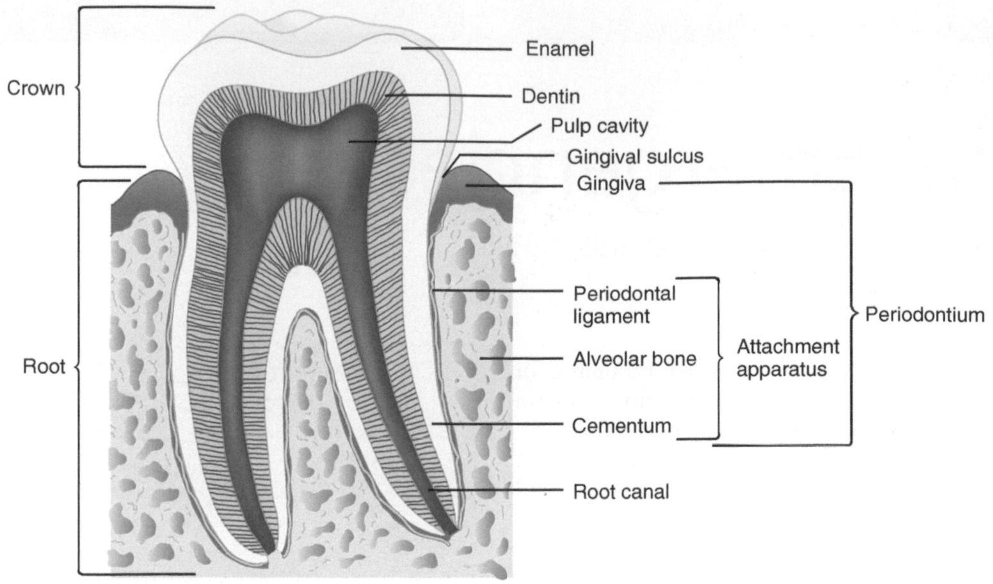

FIG. 44.2 Anatomy of the tooth. (From Pedigo, R. A., & Amsterdam, J. T. Oral medicine. (2018). In R. M. Walls, R. S. Hockberger, & M. Gausche-Hill (Eds.), *Rosen's emergency medicine: Concepts and clinical practice*, (9th ed., Fig. 60.1). Elsevier.)

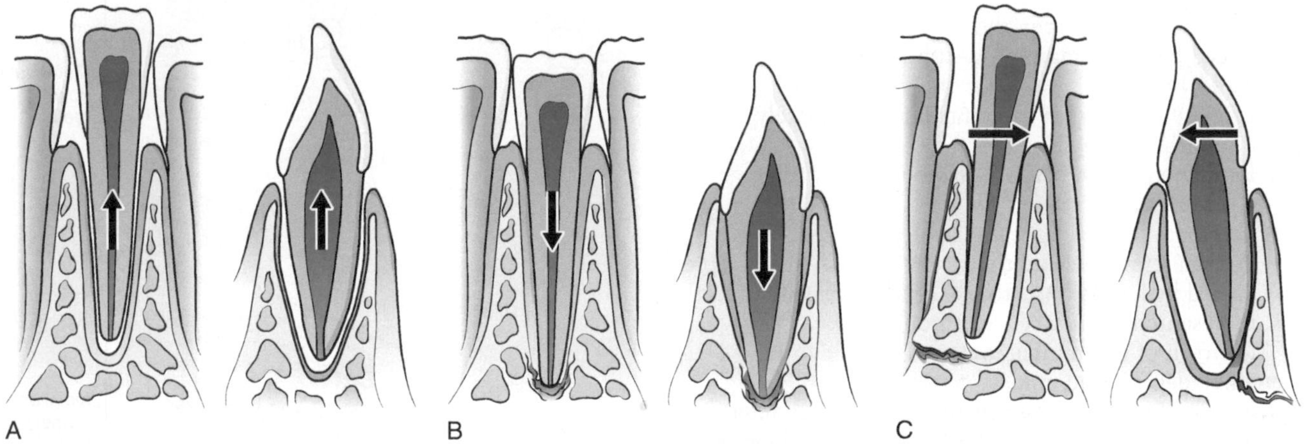

FIG. 44.3 Luxation of teeth. (From Roberts, J. (2014). Roberts and Hedges' clinical procedures in emergency medicine (6th ed., Fig. 64.9). Elsevier.

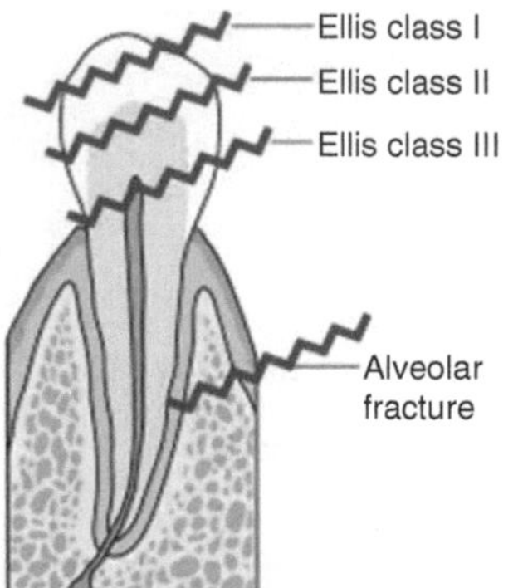

FIG. 44.4 Ellis classification of tooth fractures. (Fowler, G. C. (2011). Management of dental injuries. In J. L. Pfenninger & G. C. Fowler (Eds.), Pfenninger and Fowler's procedures for primary care (pp. 511–515, Fig. 81.2). Elsevier/Mosby.

- Gingivitis: inflammation of the gingiva only
- Periodontitis: inflammation of the periodontium (gingiva, periodontal ligament, alveolar bone, and cementum), leading to loosening or loss of teeth over time
- Acute necrotizing ulcerative gingivitis (ANUG, or trench mouth): bacterial invasion of the periodontium and gingiva
  - Seen in immunocompromised individuals, such as those with human immunodeficiency virus (HIV) or diabetes
  - Usually polymicrobial (especially *Fusobacterium* species and spirochetes)
- Gingival hyperplasia: ranges from enlargement of the interdental papillae up to gingiva; often owing to long-term phenytoin, cyclosporine, or calcium channel blocker use
- Pericoronitis: inflammation as a result of food and bacteria that are trapped within a flap of gingiva (operculum), which can occur when teeth are erupting through the gingiva
  - Most commonly occurs at the third molar (wisdom tooth)
- Alveolar osteitis (dry socket): dislodgement of the clot after a tooth extraction, usually 3 to 4 days after extraction, leading to pain from localized osteomyelitis

Odontogenic Abscesses and Deep Neck Infections

Clinical Presentation

- Major risk factors include diabetes and HIV.
- In children, they are caused by sequelae of oropharyngeal infections (e.g., tonsillitis leading to a peritonsillar abscess or retropharyngeal lymphadenopathy leading to a retropharyngeal abscess).
- In adults, they are more commonly caused by dental infections.
- In immunocompetent individuals, an irreversible pulpitis can lead to the formation of a periapical abscess, which may be localized and drained in the emergency department.
- In immunocompromised patients or with aggressive organisms, an odontogenic infection can commonly spread into the fascial planes.
- Maxillary odontogenic infections usually involve the canine space or the buccal space, leading to swelling along the cheek.
  - Spread may occur into the infraorbital space and cavernous sinus, leading to cavernous sinus thrombosis.
- Mandibular odontogenic infections may involve the submental, sublingual, and/or submandibular space.
  - If one or two of these spaces are affected, there will be focal midline or unilateral swelling.
  - Ludwig angina occurs when all three mandibular spaces are affected bilaterally.
    - Other less-common causes of Ludwig angina include a fractured mandible, traumatic intubation, or laceration at the floor of the mouth.
    - Signs and symptoms include dysphagia, a "hot potato" voice, tongue swelling, and sore throat.
    - Physical findings may include bilateral submandibular swelling, elevation of the floor of the mouth, a "woody" consistency of the floor of the mouth, trismus, and tenderness to palpation of the neck.
    - Ludwig angina is a clinical diagnosis, although a computed tomography (CT) scan may be helpful to visualize the extent of the spread and identify a drainable collection.

Diagnosis and Evaluation

- All teeth must be accounted for in the setting of trauma.
  - Teeth can be aspirated, swallowed, or embedded in a laceration. A significant intrusive luxation can also mimic a tooth avulsion.
  - Radiographs may be helpful in locating the missing tooth.
  - CT maxillofacial scan may be useful for identifying mandible and subtle alveolar ridge fractures.
- When considering a deep space neck infection, physical examination may be unreliable in determining the extent of the infection.
  - A complete blood count may or may not show leukocytosis.
  - CT scan with contrast should be considered.
- Not all dental pain is odontogenic in origin so a broad differential should be considered (Box 44.1).

BOX 44.1 *Differential Diagnosis of Orofacial Pain*

ODONTOGENIC CAUSES	**PERIODONTAL CAUSES**
Dental caries	Gingivitis
Pulpitis (reversible or irreversible)	Periodontal disease
Periapical abscess	Acute necrotizing ulcerative gingivitis
Tooth eruption	**TRAUMATIC CAUSES**
Pericoronitis	Dental fractures
Alveolar osteitis	Concussion
Bruxism	Subluxation
OTHER INFECTIOUS CAUSES	Luxation (intrusive, extrusive, or lateral)
Oral candidiasis	Avulsion
Herpes simplex virus	Facial fractures
Varicella zoster	Alveolar ridge fractures
Herpangina	Soft-tissue injuries
Hand, foot, and mouth disease	**OTHER CAUSES**
Sexually transmitted infections	Angina pectoris
Parotitis (e.g., mumps)	Cranial neuralgias (e.g., trigeminal neuralgia)
ONCOLOGIC CAUSES	Stomatitis
Squamous cell carcinoma	Mucositis (owing to nutritional deficiencies, aphthous ulcers, and so forth)
Kaposi sarcoma	Erythema migrans
Lymphoma	Pyogenic granuloma
Leukemia	Atypical odontalgia
Graft versus host disease	Ulcerative diseases (e.g., Crohn disease, Behçet syndrome, lichen planus)
Melanoma	Temporal arteritis
	Gingival hyperplasia

Pedigo, R. A. (2017). Dental emergencies: Management strategies that improve outcomes. Emergency Medicine Practice, 19(6), 1–24. EB Medicine. www.ebmedicine.net Used with permission.

Treatment

- Airway
  - Airway compromise is the leading cause of death from Ludwig angina.
  - Flexible endoscopically guided intubation under sedation is preferred.
  - Trismus and displacement of the tongue owing to swelling and infection may make direct laryngoscopy difficult; neuromuscular blockade will not relieve the trismus.
- Analgesia
  - Nonsteroidal anti inflammatory drugs (NSAIDs) are superior to acetaminophen and opioids owing to their anti inflammatory properties.
  - Orofacial nerve blocks can be considered if dental pain or a laceration is localized to a single nerve distribution.

- Supraperiosteal: provides analgesia to a single tooth (more effective for maxillary teeth than mandibular teeth, owing to thinner bone).
- Mental: provides analgesia to the ipsilateral lower lip and chin; no significant dental analgesia.
- Inferior alveolar: provides analgesia to the entire ipsilateral mandible and mandibular teeth. Also includes lower lip and chin (the inferior alveolar nerve becomes the mental nerve as it exits the mental foramen).
- Infraorbital: provides analgesia to the ipsilateral midface and upper lip.

- With alveolar osteitis, treatment is primarily analgesia, as well as packing with a "dry socket paste" or eugenol and referral back to the dentist who performed the extraction.

- Traumatic injuries
  - Storage and handling
    - Teeth should only be handled by the crown, because the periodontal ligament cells present on the root of the tooth are easily damaged.
    - Storage should occur in Hanks balanced salt solution, oral rehydration solution, or milk to preserve periodontal ligament viability.
  - Reimplantation
    - Teeth can be gently rinsed with saline prior to reimplantation.
    - Only permanent teeth should be considered for reimplantation.
      - Reimplantation of primary teeth may interfere with eruption of permanent teeth.
    - After placing the tooth in anatomic position, splint the tooth using dental splinting material.
    - Doxycycline is the first-line post-reimplantation antibiotic prophylaxis; penicillin VK can be prescribed for children or for patients with tetracycline allergies.
    - Chlorhexidine rinses, gentle brushing, a soft diet, and dental follow-up are also indicated.
  - Tooth fractures
    - Ellis I: Nonurgent dental referral
    - Ellis II: Cover exposed dentin with calcium hydroxide paste as a temporary fix to prevent spread of bacteria to the pulp: this requires 24- to 48-hour follow-up with a dentist for further treatment.
    - Ellis III: Treat as an Ellis II fracture, but requires dental referral within 24 hours. Do not perform a pulpectomy owing to a high risk of infection.
    - Alveolar ridge fracture: consultation of a dentist, if possible, for rigid splinting; urgent follow-up with dentist within 24 hours
  - Soft-tissue injuries
    - Buccal lacerations do not need to be closed unless the laceration is large enough where food may become embedded.
    - Gingival lacerations are complex and may require specialty consultation.
    - Frenulum lacerations are generally not repaired, but in children should raise concern for abuse.
    - Tongue lacerations do not usually require repair unless they are gaping, expose muscle, or do not achieve hemostasis otherwise.
- Antibiotics
  - Necrotizing periodontal disease: oral antibiotics and chlorhexidine rinses
  - Pericoronitis: chlorhexidine rinses. Do not debride the operculum.
  - Periapical abscess: antibiotics are only indicated in patients with systemic symptoms or in an immunocompromised state.
  - Acceptable oral antibiotics include penicillin VK and amoxicillin/clavulanate; in penicillin-allergic patients, clindamycin or metronidazole may be used (Table 44.1).
  - Ludwig angina: aggressive intravenous antibiotics and airway management decreases mortality to less than 10%.
    - Antibiotics must cover *Streptococcus* spp., *Staphylococcus* spp., and anaerobes such as *Bacteroides fragilis*.
    - Immunocompetent patients will require ampicillin/sulbactam plus vancomycin OR clindamycin monotherapy.
    - Immunocompromised patients will require extended spectrum beta lactam antibiotics (e.g., piperacillin/tazobactam, meropenem) and the addition of vancomycin (with methicillin-resistant *Staphylococcus aureus* risk factors).

TABLE 44.1 *Recommended Antibiotics for Severe Periodontal Disease, Severe Pericoronitis, and Simple Odontogenic Infections*

Antibiotic	Dose	Duration	Notes
Penicillin VK	500 mg PO four times a day	10 days	None
Amoxicillin/ clavulanate	500 mg/125 mg PO q8hrs or 875/125 mg PO BID	10 days	None
Clindamycin	300 mg PO four times a day	10 days	If allergic to penicillin
Metronidazole	500 mg PO BID	10 days	If allergic to penicillin

Abbreviations: PO, by mouth; q8hrs, every 8 hours; BID, two times per day.
Adapted from Pedigo, R. A., & Amsterdam, J. T. (2018). Oral medicine. In R. M. Walls, R. S. Hockberger, T. M. Gausche-Hill (Eds.), *Rosen's emergency medicine: Concepts and clinical practice*, (9th ed., Table 60.2). Elsevier.

SUGGESTED READINGS

Pedigo, R. A. (2017). Dental emergencies: Management strategies that improve outcomes. *Emergency Medicine Practice*, *19*(6), 1–22.

Pedigo, R. A., & Amsterdam, J. T. (2018). Oral medicine. In R. M. Walls, R. S. Hockberger, & M. Gausche-Hill (Eds.), *Rosen's emergency medicine: Concepts and clinical practice* (9th ed., pp. 770–790). Elsevier.

CHAPTER 45

BOARD REVIEW

Oropharyngeal Emergencies

KELSEY WILHELM, MD, BS, and RYAN PEDIGO, MD, MHPE

Oropharyngeal complaints in the emergency department range from common and benign presentations to the rare and life-threatening. Emergency medicine physicians should maintain a high index of suspicion for underlying immune compromise, and pursue additional work-up, as necessary. Disease processes involving the oropharynx are often associated with the risk of rapid decompensation and airway compromise. Following is an overview of a variety of common, nontraumatic oropharyngeal complaints seen in the emergency department.

Oral Cavity

APHTHOUS STOMATITIS

General Principles

- Commonly referred to as "canker sore," this ulcerative disease has an incidence of 20%–40% and a higher prevalence in professionals, nonsmokers, and those with higher socioeconomic status.
- Although the etiology and pathogenesis are unclear, aphthous stomatitis is often triggered by psychological stress, hormonal changes, or certain foods. Recurrent oral ulcerations could be manifestations of other conditions, including, but not limited to, infections, medication side effects, and systemic diseases, such as autoimmune disease, inflammatory bowel disease, celiac disease, Behçet syndrome, or human immunodeficiency virus (HIV) infection.

Clinical Presentation

- Involves the nonkeratinized epithelium, especially labial and buccal mucosa. The vermillion border is a commonly affected area.
- Begins as an erythematous macule that ulcerates and forms a yellowish-white, central, fibropurulent eschar usually measuring 2–3 mm in diameter
- Two other systemic conditions, Sweet syndrome and PFAPA (*p*eriodic *f*ever, *a*phthous ulcers, *p*haryngitis, and *a*denitis), also manifest aphthous ulcers as part of the disease process.

Diagnosis and Evaluation

- Aphthous ulcers are a clinical diagnosis.

Treatment

- In mild cases, no treatment is necessary, and spontaneous resolution occurs within 10 to 14 days. Consider symptomatic treatment with over-the-counter medications.
  - Analgesics
  - Amlexanox paste
  - Chlorhexidine gluconate mouthwash
  - Topical corticosteroids, such as triamcinolone acetonide oral paste

HERPES GINGIVOSTOMATITIS

General Principles

- Primary oral infection with the HSV, commonly referred to as a "cold sore," affects 60%–90% of the population in the United States. This disease occurs at two peak ages: children (6 months to 5 years) and young adults (early 20s).
- Frequency varies from 1 to 12 or more recurrences per year, but both frequency and severity of outbreaks generally decrease over time. Outbreaks can occur in response to stress, UV exposure, fever, trauma, pregnancy, or menstruation. Herpes simplex virus-1 is more common in oral, facial, and ocular lesions.

Clinical Presentation

- Primary herpetic infection is commonly associated with lymphadenopathy, fever, and malaise. Recurrent herpetic infections can be elicited by history. Patients usually experince classic phases of herpes simplex virus (Table 45.1).
- Lesions heal within 2 to 3 weeks. However, the herpes virus remains dormant in the facial and trigeminal ganglions, which periodically reactivates, resulting in recurrent sores in the same area.

TABLE 45.1 *Classic Phases of Herpes Simplex Virus*

Prodromal (day 0–1)	Tingling, itching, and reddening of the skin around the infected site
Inflammation (day 1)	Swelling and redness
Pre-sore (day 2–3)	Tiny, hard, inflamed papules and vesicles that may be pruritic or painful
Open lesion (day 4)	Vesicles break open and coalesce to create one open, weeping ulcer. May develop a fever and lymphadenopathy
Crusting (day 5–8)	A honey- or golden-colored crust starts to form from the syrupy exudate.
Healing (day 9–14)	New skin begins to form underneath the scab. A series of scabs will form over the sore (called a Meier complex).
Postscab (12–14 days)	A reddish area may linger at the site of infection.

Diagnosis and Evaluation

- Herpes gingivostomatitis is a clinical diagnosis. Available laboratory studies, although not required for diagnosis, include:
  - Viral culture (gold standard) and/or polymerase chain reaction
  - Direct immunofluorescence
  - Tzanck smear

Treatment

- Analgesia (e.g., acetaminophen, ibuprofen, or viscous lidocaine) is recommended to ensure adequate oral intake. In younger patients, local anesthetic systemic toxicity has been described with viscous lidocaine and should be avoided.
- Antiviral therapy
  - Immunocompetent host: oral antivirals (e.g., acyclovir, valacyclovir)
  - Immunocompromised host: intravenous antivirals
    - Treatment does not affect the dormant virus in nerve ganglions.

ORAL CANDIDIASIS (ORAL THRUSH)

General Principles

- Oral candidiasis is an opportunistic infection that can occur when normal host immunity or host flora are disrupted, allowing for overgrowth of *Candida albicans*. Infection may manifest as three clinical syndromes: acute candidiasis (pseudomembranous or erythematous candidiasis), chronic candidiasis (denture-related, hyperplastic, or medial rhomboid glossitis), or angular cheilitis.
- Risk factors include extremes of age, recent antibiotic use, smoking history, steroid use, xerostomia, denture use, and immunocompromise.

Clinical Presentation

- Pseudomembranous: adherent, white, curd-like plaques that may be wiped off and leave an erythematous base. Patients may describe a "cotton-like" sensation in the mouth, which is sometimes associated with loss of taste.
- Erythematous: red, macular lesions, often accompanied by a burning sensation.
- Perlèche (angular cheilitis): erythematous, scaling fissures at the corners of the mouth. Superinfection with *Staphylococcus* species is possible.

Diagnosis and Evaluation

- Most cases are diagnosed clinically. Providers should consider performing a KOH preparation of the scrapings if there is clinical uncertainty. Consider HIV testing if no other etiology is determined or if risk factors are present.
  - Treatment is targeted against *Candida* species with antifungals. Topical agents are appropriate for patients with their first presentation of mild thrush. Oral azole therapy is reserved for patients with moderate to severe oropharyngeal candidiasis, recurrent disease, or HIV with CD4 count less than 100 cells/μL, which is a risk for developing esophageal candidiasis.
    - Nystatin oral suspension
    - Clotrimazole
    - Fluconazole: reserved for moderate to severe disease
    - Voriconazole: reserved for *Candida* species that are resistant to fluconazole
  - Adults with dentures should be reminded to clean and disinfect dentures frequently. If the patient is being breastfed, the mother should treat her nipples before and after feeding.

Salivary Gland

SIALADENITIS

General Principles

- Sialadenitis is inflammation of the salivary glands. Sialolithiasis is the formation of calculi in the ductal system of the salivary glands. It is the most common cause of sialadenitis.
- The submandibular gland is most commonly affected because 80%–90% of stones develop in the submandibular (Wharton) duct, 10%–20% of calculi form in the parotid (Stensen) duct, and 1% form in the sublingual duct.

Clinical Presentation

- Painful, tender submandibular gland, associated with halitosis
- Symptoms are worse with eating.

Diagnosis and Evaluation

- Clinical diagnosis
- Ultrasound may be useful if there is clinical uncertainty.

Treatment

- Many stones will pass spontaneously.
- Start sialogogues (e.g., sour lozenges, lemon juice), which stimulate salivary secretions and help expel the stone. Local heat and hydration are also effective.
- Palpable stones may also be "milked" from the duct by stroking in a posterior-to-anterior direction.

SUPPURATIVE PAROTITIS

General Principles

- Serious bacterial infection of the parotid gland often occurs in patients with decreased salivary flow and is caused by retrograde migration of oral bacteria into the salivary ducts and parenchyma.
- This infection is usually caused by anaerobes, and *Streptococcus* and *Staphylococcus* species.
- Risk factors include dehydration, extremes of age, xerostomia, medications leading to dehydration, or decreased salivary flow (diuretics, beta-blockers, anticholinergic medications), and chronic illnesses (anorexia/bulimia nervosa, cystic fibrosis, HIV, Sjögren syndrome).

Clinical Presentation

- Rapid onset, erythematous skin overlying unilateral parotid gland, fever, trismus, and purulent drainage from the parotid duct

Diagnosis and Evaluation

- Clinical evaluation considering other differential diagnoses of facial swelling

Treatment

- Supportive care
  - Hydrate the volume-depleted patient.
  - Massage and apply heat to the affected gland.
  - Stimulate salivation using sialagogues, such as lemon drops.
- Antibiotics (for staphylococcal, streptococcal, and gram-negative coverage)
  - Amoxicillin/clavulanate OR clindamycin

VIRAL PAROTITIS

General Principles

- Viral parotitis is an acute nonsuppurative sialadenitis most often caused by paramyxoviruses (e.g., mumps).
- Less common causes include influenza, parainfluenza, coxsackie, echovirus, and HIV.
- This disease is most common in children younger than 15 years. Patients are contagious for up to 9 days after onset of parotid swelling.

Clinical Presentation

- Prodrome of fever, malaise, headache, myalgias, and arthralgias
- Unilateral or bilateral (75%) parotid swelling associated with otalgia, trismus, and dysphagia, all worse with chewing/eating. Displacement of the pinna can be seen.
- Complications of mumps virus include unilateral orchitis (20%–30% of male patients), aseptic meningitis, pancreatitis, nephritis, and sensorineural hearing loss.

Diagnosis and Evaluation

- Diagnosis is clinical, but the health department may want specific laboratory testing: buccal swab, immunoglobulin M, polymerase chain reaction, and so forth.

Treatment

- Supportive care with heat and analgesia
- Dietary modification to minimize secretory activity

Pharynx and Tonsils

INFECTIOUS PHARYNGITIS

General Principles

- In adults, infectious pharyngitis is caused by a bacterial infection 5%–10% of the time, in comparison with 30%–40% in children younger than 15 years. The remainder of infections appears to be viral in etiology.
- In adults, group A β-hemolytic *Streptococcus pyogenes* (GABHS) is the most common pathogen responsible for bacterial infections in adults. Less commonly, groups B, C, and G *Streptococcus*, *Fusobacterium necrophorum*, *Neisseria gonorrhoeae*, *Corynebacterium diphtheriae*, *Mycoplasma pneumoniae*, and several chlamydial species have been isolated.
- Providers should consider other etiologies of pharyngitis including early HIV, Epstein-Barr virus, and tuberculosis.

Clinical Presentation

- Local tissue inflammation, including palatine tonsils, uvula, soft palate, and posterior pharyngeal wall. Symptoms appear rapidly and can include fever, chills, malaise, odynophagia, cervical lymphadenopathy, hoarseness, trismus, headache, and rhinorrhea.
- The pharynx typically has erythema and gray-white symmetric exudates on swollen tonsils. Petechiae may be present on the soft palate and foul breath is common.
- Transmission is direct person-to-person through saliva or nasal secretions.
- If the patient has scarlatiniform rash, consider scarlet fever.

Diagnosis and Evaluation

- Owing to the significant overlap in findings with other causes of pharyngitis, GABHS tonsillopharyngitis is difficult to accurately diagnose clinically.
- Rapid streptococcal tests (RSTs) have a reported specificity and sensitivity of up to 95% when used in correct, high-risk groups.
- Scoring systems, such as the Modified Centor Criteria (Table 45.2), stratify patients into high-, intermediate-, and low-risk groups.
- A negative RST result in a child should be followed by a confirmatory culture. Adults with negative RST results do not require confirmatory cultures because of the lower incidence of group A *Streptococcus* infection and extremely low risk for complications.
  - Throat culture sensitivity is 90%–95%.

Treatment

- Can be delayed up to 9 days and prevent major sequelae. The therapeutic goals of antibiotic treatment for GABHS pharyngotonsillitis are:
  - To shorten the acute illness (antibiotics shorten course by approximately 16 hours)
  - To prevent nonsuppurative complications (e.g., acute rheumatic fever, acute glomerulonephritis)
  - To prevent suppurative complications (e.g., peritonsillar abscess, retropharyngeal abscess, Lemierre syndrome)

TABLE 45.2 ***Centor Criteria Scoring for Determining Testing and Treatment for Group A Beta-Hemolytic Streptococcal Pharyngitis***

- Tonsillar exudates
- Tender anterior lymphadenopathy or lymphadenitis
- Absence of cough
- History of fever

Centor Score	Testing and Treatment
0 or 1	None
2 or 3	Treatment based on results of rapid streptococcal test results
4	Treat without testing

(Adapted from Melio, F. (2018). Upper respiratory tract infections. In R. M. Walls, R. S. Hockberger, & M. Gausche-Hill (Eds.), *Rosen's emergency medicine: Concepts and clinical practice* (9th ed., pp. 857–870, Box 65.1 and Table 65.2). Elsevier.)

- First-line antibiotics
  - 10-day oral course of penicillin V or single intramuscular injection of benzathine penicillin
  - If mild penicillin allergy: cefuroxime
  - If severe penicillin allergy: azithromycin or clindamycin
- Steroids
  - Multiple studies have shown that steroids are effective at reducing the clinical symptoms and shortening the course of the illness in severe cases. Should be reserved for patients with severe swelling or odynophagia.
  - Often a single dose of dexamethasone 10 mg PO/IV (or equivalent dosing of alternative corticosteroid) is effective.

PERITONSILLAR ABSCESS

General Principles

- Peritonsillar abscess (PTA) and tonsillitis are the most common neck infections in adolescents and young adults, with PTA accounting for one-third of all soft-tissue abscesses of the head and neck. This polymicrobial abscess grows between the tonsillar capsule and the superior constrictor and palatopharyngeus muscles.
- Common pathogens include *Streptococcus* and *Staphylococcus* species, anaerobes, *Eikenella*, *Haemophilus influenzae*, and *Fusobacterium necrophorum*.
- Serious complications that may arise include airway obstruction, ruptured abscess, retropharyngeal abscess, mediastinitis, septic thrombophlebitis of the internal jugular vein (Lemierre syndrome), and erosion into the carotid sheath. Of patients affected, 10%–15% experience a recurrence, sometimes requiring subsequent tonsillectomy (Quinsy tonsillectomy).

Clinical Presentation

- Symptoms include severe unilateral sore throat, dysphagia, and otalgia.
- Signs include fever, tender cervical lymphadenopathy, trismus, muffled "hot potato voice," pharyngotonsillar exudates, soft palate fullness, and contralateral deflection of edematous uvula.

Diagnosis and Evaluation

- Imaging is not routinely performed when the diagnosis is clinically apparent.
- If the patient's examination is limited secondary to trismus, a deep space infection is suspected, or there is diagnostic uncertainty, a computed tomography (CT) scan of the neck with contrast is indicated.

Treatment

- Treatment usually involves intravenous fluid hydration, antibiotics, pain control, and steroids (dexamethasone 10 mg IV/PO) prior to drainage of the abscess. In 50% of pediatric patients, symptoms resolve with medical management alone.
- Abscess drainage for source control or if no improvement on medical management.
  - Needle aspiration procedure
    - Spray topical anesthetic, then inject 1 to 2 mL of lidocaine with 1:100,000 epinephrine into the mucosal of the lateral soft palate.
    - Aspirate with 18-g needle lateral to tonsil, at the area of fluctuance. First, aspirate at the superior pole. If unsuccessful, aspirate at the middle and inferior poles (Fig. 45.1).

Peritonsillar Abscess: Incision and Drainage

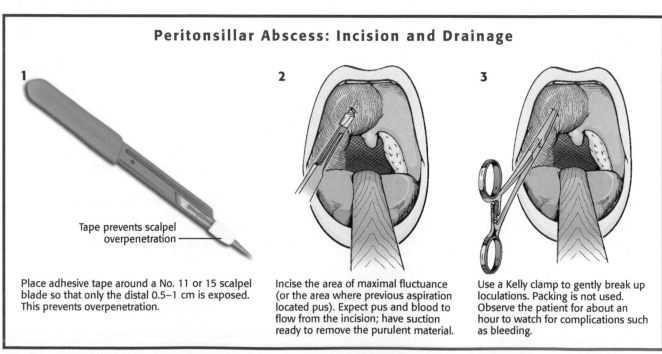

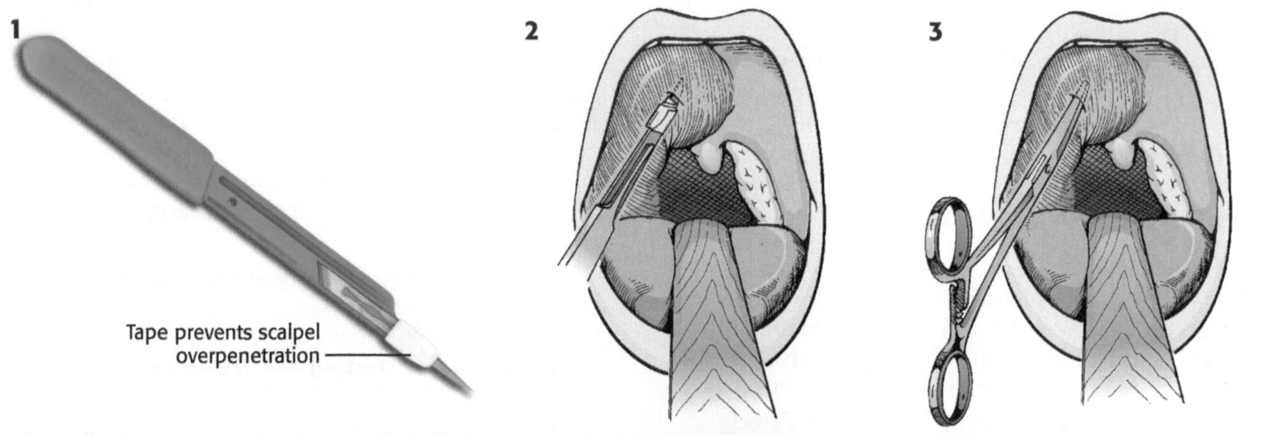

1. Place adhesive tape around a No. 11 or 15 scalpel blade so that only the distal 0.5–1 cm is exposed. This prevents overpenetration.
2. Incise the area of maximal fluctuance (or the area where previous aspiration located pus). Expect pus and blood to flow from the incision; have suction ready to remove the purulent material.
3. Use a Kelly clamp to gently break up loculations. Packing is not used. Observe the patient for about an hour to watch for complications such as bleeding.

FIG. 45.1 Peritonsillar abscess: incision and drainage. (From Riviello, R. (2019). Otolaryngologic procedures. In J. R. Roberts, C. B. Custalow, & T. W. Thomsen (Eds.), *Roberts and Hedges' clinical procedures in emergency medicine and acute care* (7th ed., pp.1338–1383.e2, Fig. 63.13). Elsevier.)

- If unsuccessful, consider expert consult or proceed with incision and drainage of the abscess.
  - Use a #11 or #15 blade. Do not insert the blade more than 1 cm deep and only advance posteriorly. The carotid artery is 2.5 cm behind and lateral to tonsil.
- Antibiotic coverage for *Streptococcus* species, anaerobes, *Eikenella*, *H. influenzae*, and *S. aureus*
  - Outpatient options: oral clindamycin or amoxicillin/clavulanate
  - Inpatient options: ampicillin/sulbactam, piperacillin/tazobactam, or IV clindamycin

POST-TONSILLECTOMY HEMORRHAGE

General Principles

- The incidence of post-tonsillectomy hemorrhage is approximately 3.9% in adults and 1.6% in children. The highest incidence is in 21- to 30-year-old persons.

Clinical Presentation

- Hemoptysis
- Recent tonsillectomy
  - Primary post-tonsillectomy hemorrhage (0–24 hours)
  - Secondary post-tonsillectomy hemorrhage (more than 24 hours)
    - Second peak of bleeding in between 7 and 10 days when scabs slough off

Diagnosis and Evaluation

- Examine posterior oropharynx, and do not disturb clot if bleeding is controlled.
- Type and screen, hemoglobin and hematocrit

Treatment

- Airway management (anticipate difficulty, surgical backup)
- IV, O_2, monitor, nothing by mouth, and maintain upright position
- Otolaryngology consult recommended as rebleeding is common. Discuss patient age, level of cooperation, visible clot, hematemesis, and bleeding diathesis.

Minor Bleeding

- Benzocaine spray or rinse with cold water
- Direct pressure with tonsillar pack or gauze infused with tranexamic acid (TXA) or lidocaine with epinephrine on a long clamp or Magill forceps

Uncontrolled Bleeding

- Nebulized TXA 250 mg for patients less than 25 kg and 500 mg for patients more than 25 kg
- Nebulized racemic epinephrine 0.05 mL/kg (max 0.5 mL) of 2.25% solution quantity sufficent to be diluted with normal saline to make total volume of 3 mL.
- If the above fails, intubate patient and tightly pack the oropharynx to tamponade bleeding, and emergency otolaryngology consultation is indicated for uncontrolled post-operative bleeding.

Deep Space Neck Infections

RETROPHARYNGEAL ABSCESS

General Principles

- This polymicrobial abscess develops in the retropharyngeal space between the posterior pharyngeal wall and the prevertebral fascia, usually occurring lateral to the midline. Posterior to the retropharyngeal space is the "danger space" and prevertebral space, both of which communicate with the mediastinum, allowing for the rapid spread of infection and life-threatening complications (Fig. 45.2).

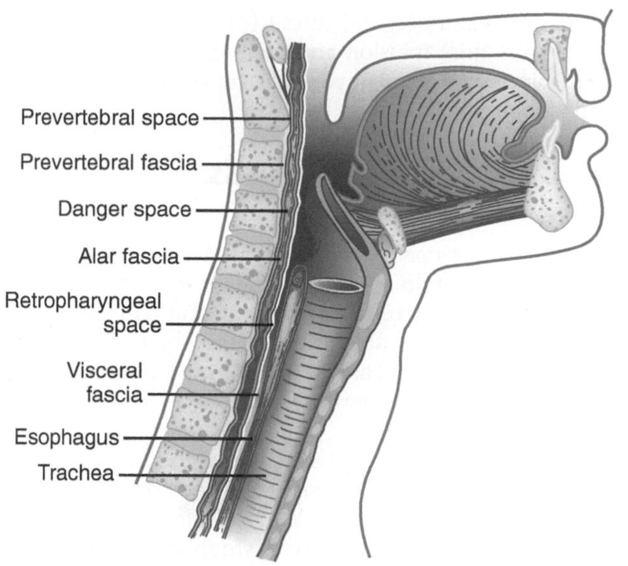

FIG. 45.2 Lateral view of the neck showing the relationship of fascia to the prevertebral danger area and retropharyngeal and submandibular spaces. (From Melio, F. (2018). Upper respiratory tract infections. In R. M. Walls, R. S. Hockberger, & M. Gausche-Hill (Eds.), *Rosen's emergency medicine: Concepts and clinical practice* (9th ed., pp. 857–870, Fig. 65.7). Elsevier.)

- This disease process is most common in children (96% occur in those under the age of 6 years), because suppurative lymphadenitis is the primary source of infection. Additionally, this can develop after direct inoculation from trauma (e.g., child falling with a stick/toothbrush in the mouth or fishbone).

Clinical Presentation

- Initial symptoms: odynophagia, fever, dysphagia, and torticollis
- Late symptoms: stridor, respiratory distress, and chest pain (mediastinitis)
- Patient may prefer to keep head in extension and lay supine to prevent posterior abscess and edematous posterior wall to collapse into the airway.
  - Tenderness on moving the larynx and trachea side to side (tracheal rock sign) is commonly present.

Diagnosis and Evaluation

- Lateral x-ray can demonstrate prevertebral soft-tissue swelling.
  - Prevertebral space should be less than 7 mm at C2, 14 mm at C6 in children, and less than 22 mm at C6 in adults.
- Gold standard: CT of the neck with IV contrast

Treatment

- Secure airway. Take care to avoid disruption of abscess—risk of rupture is significant. Tracheostomy or fiberoptic intubation may be necessary.

- Emergent ear, nose, and throat (otolaryngology) consult, as most require incision and drainage.
- Antibiotics: IV clindamycin OR cefoxitin OR ampicillin/sulbactam.

PARAPHARYNGEAL ABSCESS

General Principles

- The parapharyngeal space is divided into two compartments by the styloid process. The anterior compartment contains connective tissue, muscle, and lymph nodes. The posterior compartment contains the carotid sheath, which contains the carotid artery, internal jugular vein, vagus nerve, cranial nerves IX through XII, and sympathetic chain.
- Parapharyngeal abscesses are usually polymicrobial, originating from an odontogenic source or contiguous spread from other deep neck space infections (e.g., PTA, parotitis, sinusitis, suppurative lymphadenitis).

Clinical Presentation

- Symptoms usually include odynophagia, swelling of the neck, and occasionally torticollis. History may elicit prior pharyngitis or odontogenic infection.
    - Signs of involvement of the anterior compartment include medial tonsillar displacement, posterolateral pharyngeal wall bulging, fever, trismus, edema, and swelling at the angle of the mandible.
    - Signs of involvement of the posterior compartment include many of the same signs mentioned above. However, if the anterior compartment is spared, there may be little to no trismus, retropharyngeal swelling, and posterior displacement of the tonsillar pillar.
- Complications include airway obstruction, abscess rupture, spread to surrounding spaces (necrotizing mediastinitis), pericarditis, myocardial abscess, empyema, osteomyelitis of the mandible, cavernous sinus thrombosis, meningitis, ipsilateral Horner syndrome, cranial nerve neuropathies, carotid artery erosion or aneurysm, and Lemierre syndrome.

Diagnosis and Evaluation

- Ultrasonography, CT, and magnetic resonance imaging are more useful than lateral radiography in diagnosing parapharyngeal abscess and its complications.
- Angiography, Doppler flow studies, and magnetic resonance angiography may also be helpful in evaluating vascular complications.

Treatment

- Intravenous antibiotics: clindamycin OR cefoxitin OR ampicillin/sulbactam
- Surgical consultation with otolaryngology is necessary.

SEPTIC THROMBOPHLEBITIS OF THE INTERNAL JUGULAR VEIN (LEMIERRE SYNDROME)

General Principles

- This rare disease is characterized by disseminated abscesses and thrombophlebitis of the internal jugular vein as a sequela of an oropharyngeal infection.
- The predominant pathogen is a gram-negative anaerobic bacillus, *Fusobacterium necrophorum*. These bacteria penetrate the nearby jugular vein causing thrombophlebitis, bacteremia, and septic emboli.

Clinical Presentation

- Usually affects young, healthy adults who developed a PTA
- Persistent odynophagia, fever, fatigue, and lymphadenopathy are common.
- Sequela can include pneumonia, septic arthritis, meningitis, sepsis, and intracranial complications.

Diagnosis and Evaluation

- CT angiography is considered the gold standard.
- Point-of-care ultrasound may reveal thrombus within internal jugular vein.
- Blood cultures (primarily growth of *F. necrophorum*, but *S. aureus* is common in drug users.)

Treatment

- Intravenous antibiotics, such as piperacillin/tazobactam or a carbapenem
- Surgical drainage of abscess with jugular vein ligation and resection required for uncontrolled sepsis and respiratory failure from septic emboli
- No evidence for or against anticoagulation

DESCENDING NECROTIZING MEDIASTINITIS (CERVICOTHORACIC NECROTIZING FASCIITIS)

General Principles

- This is a rare but serious complication of a common periodontal or oropharyngeal infection with a reported mortality rate of 25%–40%. The infection spreads inferiorly into the mediastinum through the deep cervical fascia by way of the "danger" space or carotid space. The infection results from polymicrobial organisms from oral flora.
- The high rate of mortality is related to the nonspecific and subtle clinical findings. Immunocompromised patients are at higher risk.

Clinical Presentation

- Prior odontogenic or oropharyngeal infection that is not improving despite antibiotics
- Worsening edema, inability to tolerate sections, or other signs of sepsis and deep space neck infections
- Physician should have a high index of suspicion because presentations can be subtle initially and decompensate rapidly.

Diagnosis and Evaluation

- If suspicion is high for deep space infection on examination, resuscitate and ensure ability to maintain airway while lying flat for a contrast-enhanced CT of the neck and chest.
- Plain radiographs can demonstrate subcutaneous air but have lower sensitivity than CT.

Treatment

- Intravenous antibiotics, airway management, and surgical drainage by surgical specialist

Larynx/Trachea

EPIGLOTTITIS

General Principles

- Epiglottitis continues to be a life-threatening cellulitis of the supraglottic structures; it leads to obstruction of the upper airway in both children and adults. Despite the great success of the *Haemophilus influenzae* type B (HIB) vaccine, which has limited the incidence of this disease, the high morbidity and mortality of this disease remains.
- As the epiglottis enlarges, it curls posteriorly and inferiorly to obstruct the airway.
- Most cases can be attributed to the lack of immunization with HIB, failure of antibody production, or immunocompromised status.

Clinical Presentation

- Rapid and progressive symptoms in toxic patient with drooling, fever, respiratory distress, inspiratory stridor, and tripod posture

Diagnosis and Evaluation

- Diagnosis of epiglottis is made with direct visualization of the larynx, which usually occurs in the operating room.
- In children who are mildly symptomatic and a broader differential is considered, cervical radiographs may be helpful.
  - Edema of the epiglottis and bulging of the aryepiglottic folds on lateral films may be present (thumbprint sign).

Treatment

- Patient should be allowed to sit in a position of comfort.
  - Avoid interventions causing pain, anxiety, or crying.
- Emergent ENT consult and coordinate with anesthesia regarding airway management
- Intubation in a controlled setting (e.g., the operating room) or an awake tracheotomy is usually appropriate.

LARYNGITIS

General Principles

- Acute laryngitis is commonly a self-limited inflammatory condition lasting less than 3 weeks. It is associated with either an upper respiratory tract infection or acute vocal strain.

Clinical Presentation

- Hoarseness resulting from an upper respiratory infection
- Usually associated with rhinorrhea, cough, and odynophagia

Diagnosis and Evaluation

- Consider differential diagnosis: acute vocal fold pathology (screaming, protracted coughing), malignancy, and vocal cord paralysis.

Treatment

- Symptomatic care (hot tea with honey, voice rest)

BACTERIAL TRACHEITIS

General Principles

- This rare but potentially life-threatening disease can occur in isolation or as a secondary infection of a viral croup.
- Common pathogens include *S. aureus*, *Moraxella catarrhalis*, *S. pneumoniae*, *H. influenzae*, and anaerobes.
- This infection causes an inflammatory process that involves the subglottis and trachea with edema, ulceration, and pseudomembrane formation followed by copious exudative sloughing contributing to airway obstruction.

Clinical Presentation

- Peak age is 3- to 5-years-old, usually beginning with viral prodrome.
- Progression to severe inspiratory stridor, respiratory distress, and copious purulent secretions
  - Similar symptoms to croup and epiglottitis may be seen, but severe decompensation, high fever, and purulent secretion aid in differentiation.
  - Classically, a child may have been treated with racemic epinephrine and steroids for croup, with no clinical improvement.

Diagnosis and Evaluation

- Diagnosis is clinical, but radiographs of the neck may show subglottic narrowing (steeple sign) with ragged tracheal epithelium or concomitant pneumonia.

Treatment

- Emergent intubation is usually necessary; bronchoscopy can confirm diagnosis and aid therapeutically. Use a smaller tube, if appropriate, to prevent future airway scarring.
- Antibiotics: third-generation cephalosporin (cefotaxime or clindamycin) + methicillin-resistant *S. aureus* coverage (clindamycin or vancomycin)

TRACHEOSTOMY COMPLICATIONS

General Principles

- Many tracheostomy complications can present to the emergency department, including bleeding, infection, obstruction, and dislodgement.
- Indications for tracheostomy are variable, and it is important to confirm some basic information, including date of placement, size of the tracheostomy tube (cuffed or uncuffed), and if the patient had a laryngectomy (if so, only able to ventilate through stoma and cannot orally intubate).

Clinical Presentation

- Bleeding tracheostomy site. Local oozing or brisk bleeding may be noted.
- Increased respiratory distress, fever, erythema, and purulent secretions may all be present in the case of tracheostomy site infections.
- Hypoxia, respiratory distress, severe coughing/gagging may be signs of obstruction.

Diagnosis and Evaluation

- Tracheostomy bleeding may be present, but minor, in the first few days after placement owing to a lack of hemostasis, raw mucosa, suctioning, and other manipulations.
  - If brisk bleeding noted, consider tracheoinnominate fistula.
- Infected appearing tracheostomy site
  - Foul-smelling discharge, fever, or erythema of the site may be noted.
- Obstructed tracheostomy tube
  - Consider other causes of respiratory distress before assuming obstruction. Attempt suctioning and assess patency.
- Dislodged tracheostomy tube
  - Determine whether tube is dislodged from the trachea and obtain date of placement.
  - Evaluate with fiberoptic scope to verify tube placement.

Treatment

- For the bleeding tracheostomy site, assess severity of the bleed.
  - Treat local bleeding with silver nitrate if bleeding source is identified.
  - Treat brisk bleeding as a tracheoinnominate fistula until proven otherwise. Most patients present within the first 3 weeks (but may present later) after tracheostomy. The mortality rate is very high.
    - Obtain emergent surgical assistance.
    - Hyperinflate the cuff (85% successful), to tamponade bleeding.
    - If the above fails, withdraw tube while placing pressure against the anterior trachea. Apply digital pressure of the innominate artery against the manubrium from inside the tracheostomy tract and proceed to the operating room.
    - Correct coagulopathies and administer blood products, as needed.
- Suspect tracheostomy infection.
  - Initiate broad-spectrum antibiotics to cover *Staphylococcus*, *Pseudomonas*, and *Candida* species.
  - Supportive care, suctioning, oxygenation
- Suspected tracheostomy obstruction
  - Preoxygenate and place sterile saline solution into trachea and then suction.
  - If this fails, inner cannula of tube can be removed and cleaned.
- Tracheostomy tube dislodgement
  - If fresh tracheostomy, may be able to pull at stay sutures to bring the trachea closer to the stoma
  - Bag-valve-mask (BVM) and look for bubbling at tracheostomy site
  - Take care when replacing not to create a false tract.

AIRWAY FOREIGN BODY

General Principles

- Airway foreign body is a potentially life-threatening situation requiring prompt evaluation and usually operative intervention.
- It is most common in young children (1–3 years of age), but consider in any child with respiratory symptoms.
- The object can be lodged in upper airway (20% of cases) or bronchi (80%).

Clinical Presentation

- History of eating or playing with a small object (or unsupervised) followed by sudden coughing, gagging, dyspnea, dysphonia, tachypnea, respiratory distress, or color change
  - Symptoms can be delayed more than 24 hours.
  - Consider aspiration event in sudden collapse or cardiac arrest.
  - If lodged in the larynx/trachea, stridor or dysphonia may be present.
- Persistent wheezing that is not responsive to bronchodilators and decreased breath sounds may represent lower airway obstruction.

Diagnosis and Evaluation

- Diagnosis may be clinical, but a chest radiographs may be useful in the diagnosis, although does not rule out a foreign body.
  - Radiographs are negative in more than 50% tracheal foreign bodies, 25% bronchial foreign bodies, and may be missed if very small and/or radiolucent.
  - Inspiratory/expiratory films may show relative hyperinflation proximal to obstruction on end-expiration. Consider lateral decubitus films.
- Button battery aspiration warrants urgent ENT consult and prompt operative removal to avoid necrosis, perforation, and potential airway strictures.

Treatment

- Complete airway obstruction
  - If conscious: Heimlich maneuver, chest thrusts (obese or pregnant patients), back-blow/chest thrust (infants)
  - If object is visible, remove manually (avoid pushing the object further into the airway).
  - Consider laryngoscopy to view object and remove with Magill forceps.
  - If unsuccessful, bag-valve mask or intubate (may dislodge object and improve situation to partial or more distal obstruction).
  - If unable to intubate or ventilate, consider emergent cricothyrotomy. If obstruction distal to cricothyroid, this procedure will not help. Consider other transtracheal ventilation or intubation while pushing the foreign body distally.
- Partial airway obstruction
  - Place patient on monitor, administer supplemental oxygen, and allow a position of comfort.
  - Consider urgent ENT and anesthesia consultation.
  - May need rigid bronchoscopy to remove obstruction. Avoid blind finger sweep.

ANGIOEDEMA

General Principles

- Angioedema is a paroxysmal self-limited localized swelling of the skin or mucosal tissues resulting from inflammatory mediators acting on the vasculature causing extravasation of fluid into the interstitium.
- Patients typically present with nondependent and asymmetric edema. Angioedema can occur with urticaria, as a component of anaphylaxis, or in isolation. The known causes of angioedema can be subdivided into

mast cell-mediated etiologies (associated with urticaria), bradykinin-mediated etiologies, and idiopathic angioedema. Isolated uvular angioedema, or Quincke disease, is a relatively rare presentation of angioedema of the upper airway.

Clinical Presentation

- Mast cell-mediated etiologies of angioedema are associated with urticaria and/or pruritus.
  - Caused by mast cell release of inflammatory mediators, including histamine, leukotriene C4, and prostaglandin D2, increasing capillary permeability and causing edema
  - If angioedema occurs in the setting of anaphylaxis, other signs and symptoms may be present, including flushing, throat tightness, bronchospasm, hypotension, and gastrointestinal symptoms.
  - Allergic angioedema is an IgE-mediated type 1 hypersensitivity reaction.
- Bradykinin-mediated etiologies occur as a result of bradykinin overproduction or inhibition of bradykinin degradation.
  - Angiotensin-converting enzyme (ACE) inhibitor-induced angioedema results from excessive bradykinin.
  - Incidence is highest within the first month of the initial dose; however, it may occur at any time.
    - 40% present months to years after initial dose with overall incidence of 0.1%–2.2% (more common in African-American populations).
  - Hereditary angioedema
    - Congenital (autosomal-dominant) or acquired loss of C1 esterase inhibitor leads to unregulated activity of vasoactive mediators (bradykinin) associated with complement pathway.
    - Edema of face, extremities, bowel wall
  - Idiopathic angioedema occurs with uncertain etiology of symptoms.

Diagnosis and Evaluation

- Mast cell-mediated angioedema
  - Clinical diagnosis in the setting of allergic presentation, with or without anaphylaxis
- Hereditary angioedema
  - Suspect in patients with a history of recurrent peripheral angioedema and abdominal pain
  - 75% experience onset of symptoms before age 15 years
  - C4 level screens may be low, with decreased levels of C1 and C4 esterase inhibitors, confirming the diagnosis
- ACE inhibitor-induced angioedema
  - Patient recently may have been started on an ACE-I or have taken it at some point in the past

Treatment

- In general, consider definitive airway management if voice change, hoarseness, stridor, or dyspnea is present. Always prepare for a difficulty airway, which can include the need for fiberoptic assistance, ENT/anesthesia consult, surgical airway, or transfer to the operating room.
- If allergic component is present:
  - Consider epinephrine 0.3 mg intramuscular.
  - Consider glucagon 1 to 5 mg IV if patient is on beta-blockers and not responding to epinephrine.
- Hereditary angioedema
  - Patients often communicate a history of hereditary angioedema or have a medical bracelet or ID.
    - Consider 2 units of fresh frozen plasma for possible etiology related to bradykinin or C1-esterase deficiency.
  - First-line therapies
    - C1 esterase inhibitor (C1-INH)
    - Ecallantide (kallikrein inhibitor for angioedema)
    - Icatibant (bradykinin receptor antagonist)
- ACE inhibitor-induced angioedema
  - Typical anaphylaxis medications do not affect bradykinin levels, but consider them.
    - Epinephrine 0.3 mg intramuscular
    - Diphenhydramine 50 mg IV
    - Methylprednisolone 125 mg IV
  - Consider ecallantide.

SECTION SEVEN

BOARD REVIEW

Hematologic/ Oncologic

Blood Transfusion

KIERON K. BARKATAKI, DO, and ALEX HUANG, MD

- Transfusion therapy involves giving blood that has been separated into individual components for storage.
- Before transfusion, the donor and recipient blood must be tested for compatibility.
- Indications for transfusion include significant anemia, thrombocytopenia, coagulopathy, or acute blood loss.
- Complications can occur and vary in severity and management.

Preparation and Storage

- Packed red blood cells (PRBCs) are prepared by removal of plasma and platelets from whole blood.
- A preservative is added to provide PRBCs a shelf life of 42 days.

Type and Screen/Crossmatch

- Transfusion of PRBCs requires matching the donor and recipient blood type and checking the recipient's plasma for antibodies.
- Order a type and screen (ABO group, Rh type, antibody screen for non-ABO Rh antibodies) when there is a possibility for transfusion. A type and crossmatch should occur before blood transfusion; this involves mixing the recipient's serum with donor red blood cells (RBCs) and checking for agglutination.
- In emergency situations, when there is no time for crossmatching, type O Rh-negative blood, or "universal donor" blood, is used because it contains no antigens.
- Type O Rh-positive blood may be used for male patients, but it should be avoided in women of childbearing potential.
- Rh-negative females can develop RhD antibodies when exposed to Rh-positive PRBCs, which leads to risk of hemolytic disease of the newborn during subsequent pregnancies.
- Patients with blood type AB are considered "universal recipients."

Indications for Packed Red Blood Cells

- PRBC transfusion is indicated for the purpose of increasing oxygen-carrying capacity in patients with acute blood loss or significant anemia.
- In patients with active bleeding (e.g., trauma or massive gastrointestinal bleed), the fall in hemoglobin/hematocrit level may lag behind.
- Decision to transfuse should be based on clinical signs and symptoms, such as hemodynamic instability, despite fluid resuscitation, inability to stop bleeding, and possibility of further blood loss.
- In patients with chronic anemia, transfusion should be considered at hemoglobin concentrations <7 g/dL.
- However, in patients with active cardiac disease (e.g., ongoing acute coronary syndrome), the transfusion threshold is suggested to be increased to 8–9 g/dL.
- One unit of PRBC (250 mL) raises the hemoglobin by 1 g/dL in adults.
- Generally transfused over 1–2 hours, but can be done more rapidly in unstable patients.

Indications for Platelets

- Platelet transfusion is indicated in patients with platelet count <5,000–10,000/mm^3, <50,000/mm^3 in patients with active bleeding or scheduled to undergo invasive procedures, and <100,000/mm^3 in patients undergoing high-risk procedures such as neurologic or cardiac surgery.
- Platelets are also used in conjunction with PRBCs and plasma as part of a massive transfusion protocol.
- One apheresis-collected platelet unit (concentrate pooled from six donor units) increases the platelet count by up to 50,000/mm^3.
- Platelet levels should be checked after transfusion to ensure adequate response and to assess for possible platelet destruction from processes such as autoimmune destruction, splenic sequestration, and thrombosis.

Indications for Fresh Frozen Plasma

- Fresh frozen plasma (FFP), which contains fibrinogen and all coagulation factors, is indicated for replacement of coagulation factors in massive transfusion protocols (MTPs) and in cases of disseminated intravascular coagulation, severe liver dysfunction, and for reversal of warfarin-induced coagulopathy.
- FFP can also be used for bleeding secondary to an individual factor deficiency if the specific factor replacement is not available.
- Initial dose of FFP is 3 to 5 units in an adult (10–15 mL/kg), which can raise each coagulation factor level by up to 20%.

Indications for Cryoprecipitate

- Cryoprecipitate is derived from FFP and contains fibrinogen, factor VIII, and smaller amounts of von Willebrand factor, factor XIII, and fibronectin.
- Cryoprecipitate is sometimes given as part of an MTP, but the main indication is fibrinogen level <100 mg/dL, usually secondary to disseminated intravascular coagulation or severe liver dysfunction.
- Standard dose for cryoprecipitate is 10 U for an adult.

Contraindications

Patient's beliefs/value system prohibit receiving blood products (e.g., Jehovah's Witnesses).

Equipment and Supplies

- PRBCs are given through a large-bore intravenous line with normal saline.
- Lactated Ringer solution should be avoided with PRBCs because it can lead to clotting owing to its calcium content.
- If a rapid rate of transfusion is indicated, a pressure bag may be used to increase the infusion rate.
- A Level 1 rapid transfuser, which is capable of warming fluids and blood products to body temperature, may be used to transfuse as rapidly as 1 L/min.

Complications of Blood Transfusion

- Resulting from ABO incompatability when the recipients' antibodies cause hemolysis of donor RBCs, *hemolytic transfusion reactions* are usually due to clerical errors in patient identification (Table 46.1).
  - Symptoms include fever, tachycardia, dyspnea, hematuria, syncope, shock, and disseminated intravascular coagulopathy.
  - Management consists of immediately stopping the transfusion, aggressive intravenous fluid hydration, and initiating vasopressors if patient remains hypotensive.
- A type and crossmatch and a Coombs test should be performed; a positive Coombs test result, post transfusion, confirms the diagnosis.

TABLE 46.1 *Complications of Blood Transfusions*

Acute Complications	Delayed Complications
Hemolytic reactions	Infectious transmissions
Febrile reactions	
Allergic reactions	
Transfusion-related acute lung injury	
Electrolyte disturbances	

TABLE 46.2 *Risk of Viral Transmission From Transfusion*

Virus	Infection Risk for Number of Units Transfused
HIV	1 per 1.5 million
Hepatitis B	1 per 300,000
Hepatitis C	1 per 1 million
Parvovirus B19	1 per 10,000
CMV	Rare; use leukocyte-reduced blood to decrease risk of CMV transmission

CMV, cytomegalovirus; *HIV,* human immunodeficiency virus.

- *Febrile transfusion reactions* consist of fever and chills during or shortly after a transfusion.
  - Management includes stopping the transfusion, administering antipyretics, and initiating the workup for a hemolytic reaction.
  - Transfusion may be restarted if the workup is negative for a hemolytic reaction and the patient responds to antipyretics.
- *Allergic transfusion reactions* are characterized by urticaria and pruritus during transfusion and, in severe cases, patients can have bronchospasm, hypotension, and anaphylaxis.
  - Management includes stopping the transfusion and administering antihistamines. In mild cases the transfusion can be resumed if symptoms resolve with antihistamines.
  - In severe anaphylaxis, patients require more aggressive treatment such as volume resuscitation, epinephrine, steroids, and bronchodilators.
  - More common in patients with immunoglobulin A deficiency, allergic transfusion reactions can be mitigated by transfusing washed PRBCs (from plasma).
- *Transfusion-related acute lung injury* is a rare complication believed to be caused by a reaction between transfused antibodies and recipient leukocytes.
  - It presents with respiratory distress with hypoxia and bilateral pulmonary infiltrates.
  - Management includes stopping the transfusion and providing respiratory support, with intubation and mechanical ventilation, if necessary.
- Hypocalcemia can result after a transfusion due to citrate, a blood preservative, which binds calcium.
- Because citrate is metabolized by the liver, this effect is usually insignificant in patients with healthy hepatic function.
- Recent improvements in blood donor screening have significantly reduced the risk of infection transmission from transfusions. However, a small risk of viral transmission remains (Table 46.2).

Massive Transfusion Protocol

- With massive or uncontrolled hemorrhage, a patient may require greater than 50% replacement of patient's total blood volume within 24 hours.
- In such cases, an institution-specific MTP must be initiated to guide the process.

- The goal of MTP is to increase cardiac output, maintain oxygen delivery, and achieve hemostasis.
- "Massive transfusion" is generally defined as more than 10 U of PRBCs within 24 hours (e.g., replacement of entire blood volume) or more than 4 U of blood products within 1 hour.
- Cases requiring MTP are commonly related to trauma but can also involve ruptured aortic aneurysms, gastrointestinal bleeding, or obstetric complications.
- Indications may include immediate inability to achieve hemostasis, positive focused assessment with sonography in trauma, systolic blood pressure less than 90 mm Hg without sustained response to 1 L of crystalloid solution, and signs of class IV hemorrhagic shock.
- Advanced trauma life support guidelines support using low ratios (1:1:1) of PRBCs to plasma and platelets, although the exact ratio is controversial.
- Complications that can be avoided, monitored for, and corrected include coagulopathy, hypothermia, acidosis, hyperkalemia, and volume overload.
- In addition to blood products, tranexamic acid, an antifibrinolytic, and calcium supplementation may be indicated.
- Tranexamic acid may aid in reversing coagulopathy and decrease mortality.
- Calcium administration combats the citrate-induced hypocalcemia.

SUGGESTED READINGS

Coil, C. J., & Santen, S. A. (2016). Transfusion therapy. In J. E. Tintinalli, J. S. Stapczynski, O. J. Ma, D. M. Yealy, G. D. Meckler, & D. M. Cline (Eds.), *Tintinalli's emergency medicine: A comprehensive study guide* (8th ed., pp. 1518–1524). McGraw-Hill Education.

Emory, M. (2018). Blood and blood components. In R. M. Walls, R. S. Hockberger, & M. Gausche-Hill (Eds.), *Rosen's emergency medicine: Concepts and clinical practice* (9th ed., pp. 1455–1462). Elsevier.

Hemostatic Disorders

DANIEL QUESADA, MD

- Characterized by defects in hemostasis, bleeding disorders increase one's susceptibility to ongoing blood loss.
- In the emergency department, most bleeding is a result of some traumatic event, often occurring in patients with normal hemostasis.
- However, there are also patients who may have inherited or acquired coagulation defects resulting in a hemorrhagic diathesis.
- With careful attention to the history and physical examination, patients with pathologic bleeding can usually be identified.
- The process of hemostasis (i.e., clot formation) is an orchestrated response involving platelets, the clotting cascade, blood vessel endothelium, and fibrinolysis.

Basic Information/Categories of Hemostasis

- Disorders of primary hemostasis
  - Platelet disorders (general)
  - Quantitative thrombocytopenia
    - Immunologic thrombocytopenic purpura (ITP)
    - Thrombotic thrombocytopenic purpura (TTP)
    - Hemolytic uremic syndrome (HUS)
    - Disseminated intravascular coagulopathy (DIC)
  - Qualitative thrombocytopenia
    - Congenital (Von Willebrand disease)
    - Acquired (disease and drugs)
    - Disorders of secondary hemostasis
  - Overview of intrinsic/extrinsic pathway
  - Inherited disorders
  - Acquired disorders
  - Vitamin K-associated disorders
  - Drug-induced

General Principles

- Normal hemostasis occurs as a response to internal/external bleeding via a mechanism that involves an orchestrated series of checks and balances working in conjunction with each other.
- The goal of hemostasis is to limit blood loss.
- Primary hemostasis involves the formation of a platelet plug and is the initial physiologic sequence triggered by blood loss.
- The formation of cross-linked fibrin to strengthen the platelet plug accounts for the end point of secondary hemostasis.
- Primary and secondary hemostasis is counter-regulated by the fibrinolytic system.

Primary Hemostasis

- Triggered by damage to the vascular endothelial surface
- Results in the interaction of exposed normal vascular endothelium (collagen) and platelets, as well as the release of Von Willebrand Factor (VwF) and fibrinogen, resulting in a complex cross-linked aggregate termed a platelet plug or hemostatic plug (Fig. 47.1)

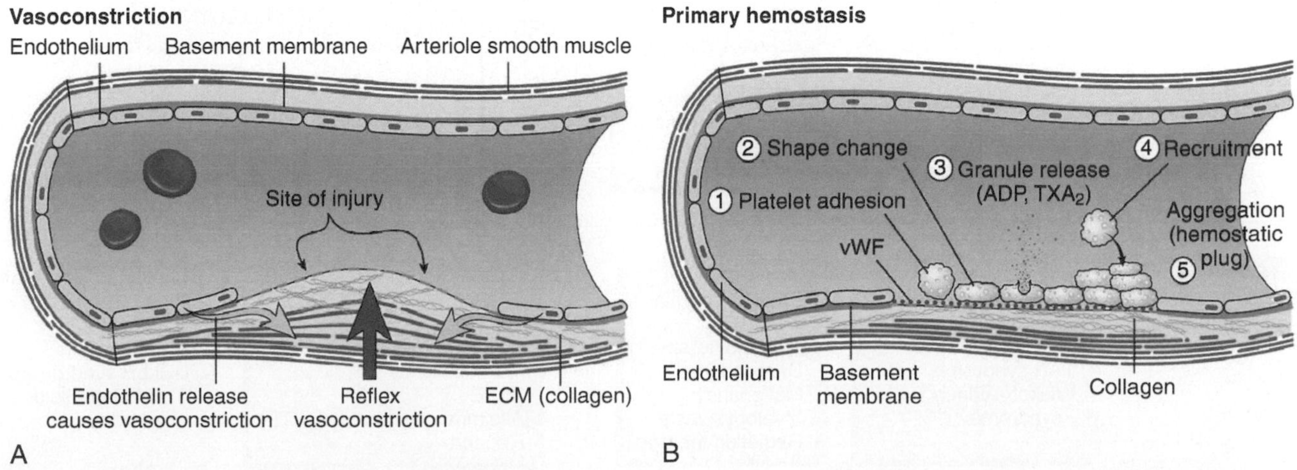

FIG. 47.1 Initial blood clotting process of primary hemostasis. (From Salvatore Cito, S., Mazzeo, M, & Badimon, L. (2019). *Thrombosis Research.* Elsevier Ltd.) *ECM* = Extracellular Matrix, *vWF* = Von Willebrand Factor, *ADP* = Adenosine diphosphate, *TXA2* = Thromboxane A2

PLATELET DISORDERS

Overview

- Acquired platelet (PLT) disorders can be quantitative (thrombocytopenic) or qualitative.
- Quantitative defects can be caused by decreased production, increased destruction, increased splenic sequestration, or a combination of the three (Fig. 47.2).

Clinical Presentation

- Manifest as nonpalpable petechiae are most prominent in the lower extremities, areas of poor blood flow, and/or gravity-dependent areas.
- Other findings include purpura, mucosal bleeding, hemoptysis, hematuria, and hematochezia.
- Risk factors for bleeding include age, comorbid conditions, (i.e., renal disease, liver disease), alcoholism, connective tissue disease, hypertension (HTN), peptic ulcer disease, and patients susceptible to falls, certain lifestyles, and medications.
- Platelet count less than 10,000/µL increases the risk of spontaneous bleeding, particularly intracranial bleeding.

Diagnosis and Evaluation

- Initial evaluation of a patient who exhibits signs/symptoms of hemorrhage should be aimed at stabilizing the circulatory system.
- History and physical focusing on chief complaint, family history, recent illness, and medications
- Determine early on the potential need for blood products.
- Laboratory work: complete blood count (CBC) with peripheral blood smear to evaluate for thrombocytopenia/anemia and red blood cell (RBC) morphology, respectively.

Treatment

- Always treat any underlying condition and control symptoms.
- Consider prophylactic platelet transfusion if count is less than 10,000/µL, given the high risk for spontaneous bleeding.
- **NO** transfusion needed if more than 50,000/µL.
- If platelet count is 10,000 to 50,000/µL, transfuse if the patient is at risk of bleeding with trauma or an invasive procedure.
- Transfuse for spontaneous bleeding or if excessive bleeding occurs after a procedure.
- One pack of platelets (single donor unit) increases PLT count by 50,000 to 60,000/µL in a 70-kg male.
- Some conditions (e.g., DIC, TTP) may be refractory or unresponsive to transfusions and may even worsen the condition by generating thrombi.

Quantitative Platelet Disorders

IMMUNOLOGIC THROMBOCYTOPENIC PURPURA

- Thrombocytopenia secondary to increased destruction can be a result of medications, infections, or autoimmune diseases.
- ITP is an acquired autoimmune disease that results in the rapid destruction of platelets mediated by the production of auto-antibodies that attach to circulating platelets and are then removed by the reticuloendothelial system.
- ITP may present at all ages.
- May have an acute or chronic course
- Acute ITP is more common in young children, equal male-to-female ratio, and typically resolves in 1 to 2 months.
- Chronic ITP lasts more than 3 months; there is a higher incidence in adults, with a higher female predilection, and it is more commonly associated with other autoimmune disorders.
- Rarely remits spontaneously or with treatment.

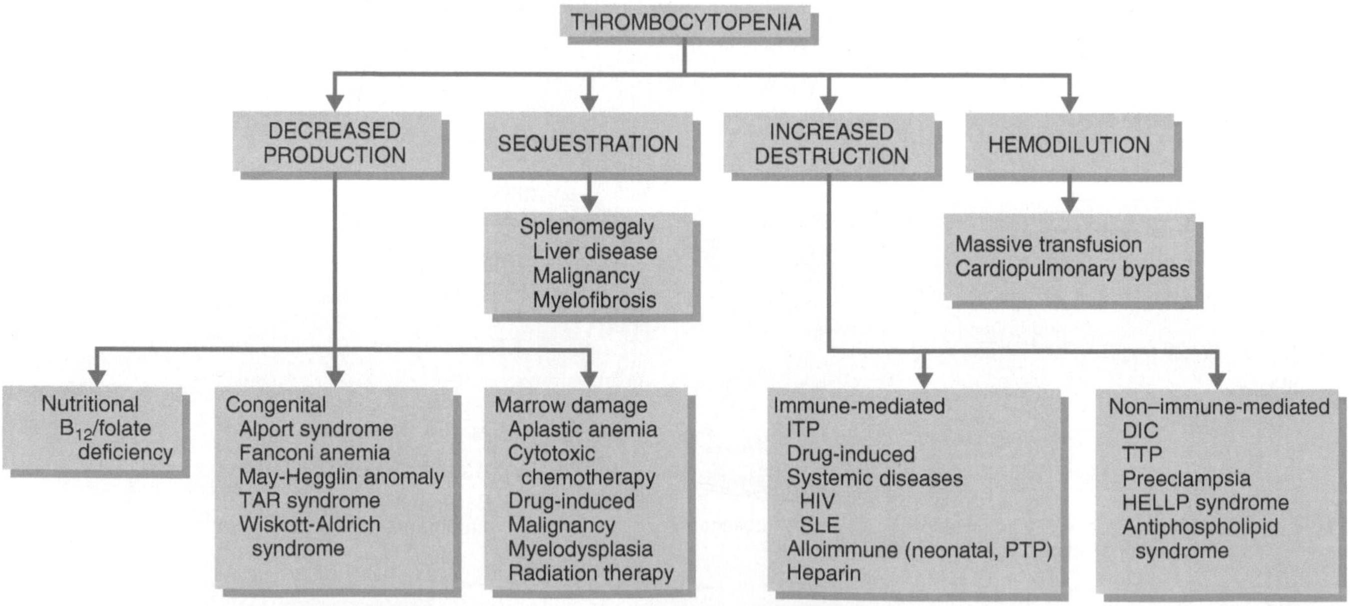

FIG. 47.2 Disorders of hemostasis: Bleeding. (From Tormey, C., A, & Rinder, H. (2016). Disorders of hemostasis: Bleeding. In I. J. Benjamin, R. C. Griggs, E. J. Wing, & J. G. Fitz (Eds.), *Andreoli and Carpenter's Cecil essentials of medicine* (9th ed., pp. 544–563). Elsevier Saunders.)

Clinical Presentation

- Most common sign involves the development of petechiae.
- Mild epistaxis, gingival bleeding, and menorrhagia in females of childbearing age
- Other than petechiae, the physical examination is generally unremarkable.
- Presence of lymphadenopathy, hepatosplenomegaly, pallor, or hyperbilirubinemia suggests an alternative diagnosis.

Diagnosis and Evaluation

- Clinical diagnosis is based on history and physical examination.
- Physical examination is remarkable for the presence petechiae/purpura.
- Thrombocytopenia on CBC
- Peripheral smear may show large, well-granulated platelets, fewer in number.
- Normal bone marrow biopsy and no other identifiable cause of thrombocytopenia

Treatment

- Minimize bleeding risk by avoiding antiplatelet medications (i.e., aspirin and nonsteroidal antiinflammatory drugs [NSAIDs]).
- Avoid unnecessary procedures.
- Asymptomatic, otherwise healthy, with platelet count less than 50,000/µL requires NO treatment.
- Platelet count less than 50,000/µL + bleeding or significant risk factors for bleeding requires treatment.
- Platelet count less than 30,000/µL requires treatment.
- Initial treatment in adults: a short course of high-dose oral dexamethasone (pulse dexamethasone of 40 mg/day without a taper)
  - Alternative: prednisone 60 to 100 mg/day and tapered after platelet count reaches normal levels
- ITP refractory to steroids may require splenectomy as an alternative treatment.
- Life-threatening bleeds require high-dose steroids (i.e., methylprednisolone 1 to 2 g intravenously (IV) × 2 to 3 days + IV immunoglobulin (IVIG).
- Platelets may be transfused with active acute bleeding after administration of the first dose of steroids or IVIG.
- Admit patients who have ITP-related bleeds.
- Hospitalization is not required for asymptomatic patients with platelet count greater than 20,000 to 30,000/µL.

47

THROMBOTIC THROMBOCYTOPENIC PURPURA

- A consumptive thrombocytopenia owing to a mutation in ADAMTS13 gene (VwF cleaving protease)
- Absence of ADAMTS13 results in circulating large VwF multimers leading to clumping of platelets and thrombus formation (Fig. 47.3). A hyaline thrombi complex may occlude small vessels in the pancreas, adrenals, heart, lungs, and kidneys.
- Risk factors for TTP include flu-like illnesses (with gastrointestinal [GI] component), pregnancy, oral contraceptive use, human immunodeficiency virus, and medications (e.g., cyclosporine, ticlopidine, penicillin, and metronidazole).
- Up to 80% mortality if untreated (down to 10% with plasma exchange)

Clinical Presentation

- Most common in females 30 to 50 years of age, African-Americans, and obese patients.
- Pregnancy is most common precipitating event for TTP (second trimester, most common).

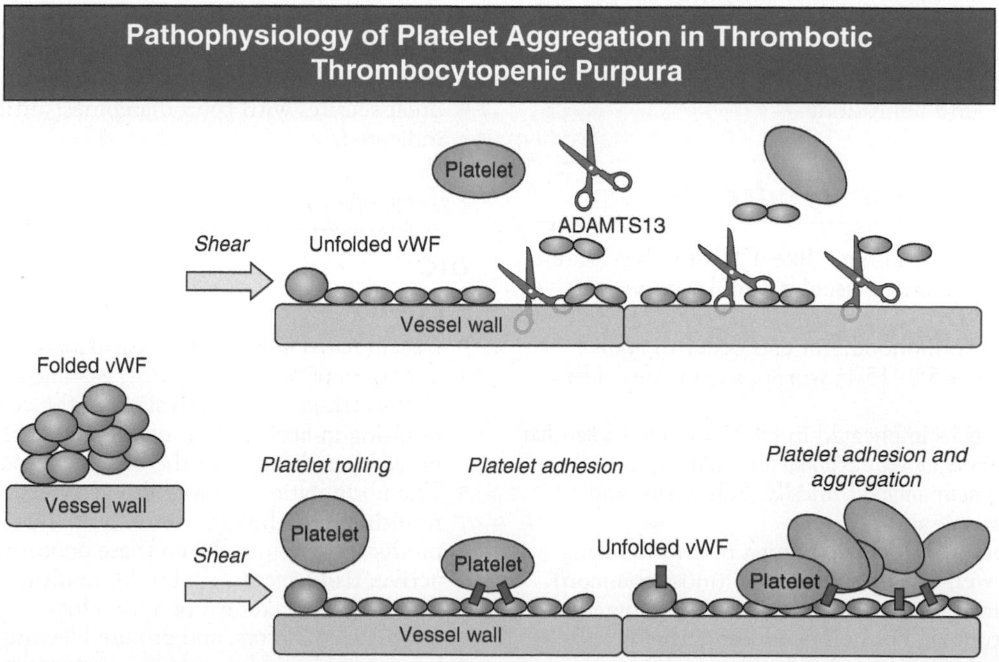

FIG. 47.3 Pathophysiology of platelet aggregation in thrombotic thrombocytopenic purpura. *vWF,* Von Willebrand factor. (From Norris, M., Ruggenenti, P. L., & Remuzzi, G. (2019). Thrombotic microangiopathies, including hemolytic uremic syndrome. In J. Feehally, J. Floege, M. Tonelli, & R. J. Johnson (Eds.), *Comprehensive clinical nephrology* (6th ed., pp. 343–356). Elsevier Inc.)

- Presents with evidence of microangiopathic hemolytic anemia, bleeding manifestations, renal disease, thrombocytopenia, fever, and NEUROLOGIC deficits (i.e., altered mental status, cephalgia, seizure, cerebrovascular accident [CVA], aphasia, and so forth).
- Patients commonly complain of fatigue and dyspnea on exertion (often from anemia).
- Physical examination may demonstrate pallor, jaundice, and scleral icterus (from hemolysis).
- Oliguria, myocardial infarction, cardiac conduction disorders, and HTN indicate end-organ damage.

Diagnosis and Evaluation

- Mostly a clinical diagnosis, because ADAMTS13 levels are usually not immediately available.
- CBC with peripheral smear will show evidence of thrombocytopenia and fragmented RBCs on smear, respectively.
- Increased reticulocyte count.
- Increased lactate dehydrogenase and indirect bilirubin, with decreased haptoglobin suggestive of RBC hemolysis.
- International normalized ratio (INR) less than 1.5 (if greater than 1.5, more suggestive of disseminated intravascular coagulation [DIC]).

ELEVATED CREATININE IS INDICATIVE OF ACUTE KIDNEY INJURY

Treatment

- Plasma exchange is essential treatment for TTP, and it is superior to plasma infusion alone.
- Glucocorticoids (dose is based on risk stratification).
- Rituximab is used as part of the initial therapy based on emerging evidence that exacerbations and relapses are reduced.
- Caplacizumab for high-risk patients.
- Avoid platelet transfusion unless uncontrolled hemorrhage.
- Splenectomy, if refractory to treatment or relapsing.
- Relapse occurs in 40% of patients.
- Intensive care unit admission.

Hemolytic Uremic Syndrome

- Hemolytic uremic syndrome, like TTP, involves platelet aggregation in the microvascular circulation via the mediation of VwF.
- Disease of early childhood, but can occur in adults.
- Overall mortality 5%–15%; worse prognosis in older children/adults.
- Multiple organisms implicated in HUS include *Escherichia coli*, *Shigella*, *Yersinia*, *Campylobacter*, *Salmonella*, *Streptococcus pneumoniae*, *Varicella*, Echovirus, and Coxsackie virus A and B.
  - *E. coli* serotype 0157:H7 or Shiga toxin producing *E. coli* is a well-known precipitant (most common).
  - *E. coli* toxins bind to receptors found on glomerular and renal tubular, epithelial, and endothelial cells.
- Results in renal microvascular damage and formation of platelet thrombi; mediated by VwF (as in TTP).
- Toxin also potentiates release of large VwF multimers.

Clinical Presentation

- Often follows a prodromal illness (children typically have prodromal illness with abdominal pain, vomiting, and diarrhea).
- Onset of HUS typically occurs 5 to 10 days after diarrhea develops.
- *E. coli* 0157:H7 produces bloody diarrhea in up to 40% of patients.
- Urine will commonly contain protein and blood, although it may be normal.

Diagnosis and Evaluation

- History and physical examination may vary.
- Symptoms can include abdominal pain, nausea, vomiting, fever, lethargy, and seizures.
- Physical examination findings and signs can include petechiae, anemia, hypertension, and altered mental status.
- Microangiopathic hemolytic anemia: hemoglobin usually less than 8 g/dL.
- Platelet count less than 60,000.
- Peripheral smear: fragmented RBCs.
- Urinalysis: hematuria, protein, leukocytes.
- Blood urea nitrogen/creatinine elevated, sometimes associated with oliguria.
- Lactate dehydrogenase and bilirubin are high and haptoglobin is low.
- Coomb's tests and coagulation panel are normal.

Treatment

- Supportive: airway, breathing, and circulation (ABCs), IV access, monitor, correct electrolyte disturbances, and return the patient to an euvolemic state.
- Mild HUS with fewer than 24 hours of urinary symptoms requires only fluid and electrolyte correction.
- Hemodialysis is first-line therapy in the setting of renal failure.
- Antimotility drugs are not indicated.
- Transfuse plateletst if less than 50,000 and actively bleeding.
- Transfuse RBCs if patient is symptomatic and Hb is less than 7 g/dL.
- Treat seizures with benzodiazepines; antibiotics are not indicated.

Fibrinolytic Disorders

DIC

Overview

- Disseminated intravascular coagulation (DIC), also known as consumption coagulopathy, is an acquired syndrome characterized by the activation of the coagulation system resulting in fibrin formation leading to the formation of blood clots throughout the body's microcirculation.
- The fibrinolytic system is also activated during DIC, resulting in pathologic fibrinolysis and split/degradation product formation. When these opposing pathways are active, tissue factor is released, resulting in thrombin formation, breakdown of fibrin clots, consumption of coagulation factors, and profuse bleeding (Fig. 47.4).
- The various conditions/diseases that can trigger DIC are diverse (Table 47.1); however, the deregulated formation of thrombin is central to its pathogenesis.

Pathogenesis of disseminated intravascular coagulation

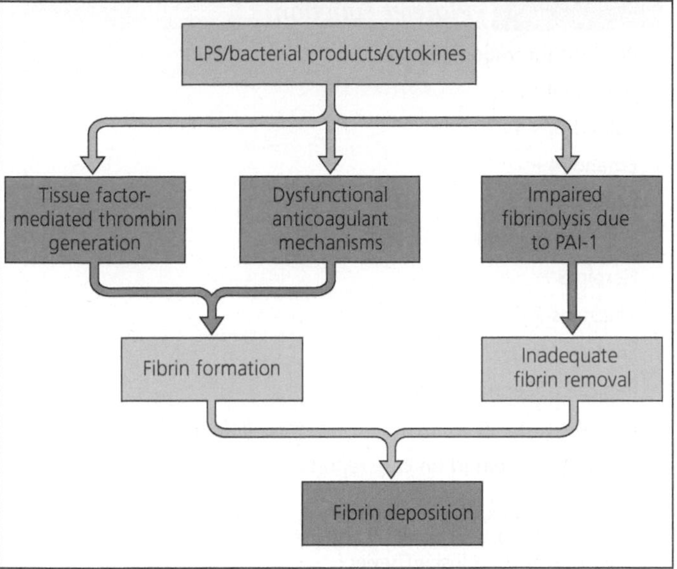

FIG. 47.4 Pathogenesis of disseminated intravascular coagulation. (From Cohen, J., Powderly, W., & Opal, S. (2017). *Infectious disease* (4th ed., p. 423). Elsevier.)

TABLE 47.1 ***Precipitating Etiologies of Disseminated Intravascular Coagulation***

Conditions	Examples	Clinical Impact
Severe infectious diseases	Gram ± sepsis	May lead to end-organ failure
Malignancy	Solid tumors	Solid tumor: hemorrhagic
	Leukemia	Leukemia: hemorrhagic
Trauma	Multitrauma	Acute bleeding, followed by pro-thrombotic state
	Brain injury	
	Burns	
Obstetric complications	Abruptio placentae	Combination of bleeding/thrombosis
	Amniotic fluid embolism	
Vascular malformations	Aortic aneurysm	Primarily hemorrhagic + severe thrombocytopenia
	Large hemangiomas	
Immunologic reactions	Transfusion reactions, toxins, and snake bites	
Heat stroke		Thrombosis > bleeding
Post cardiopulmonary resuscitation		Thrombosis > bleeding

From Marx, J. A., Hockberger, R. S., Walls, R. M., Adams, J., & Rosen, P. (2010). *Rosen's emergency medicine: Concepts and clinical practice* (7th ed.). Mosby/Elsevier.

- Thrombin generation results in the formation of small fibrin clots being deposited in the microcirculation, eventually leading to widespread thrombotic occlusion of the vasculature and end-organ dysfunction.

Clinical Presentation

- Clinical features of DIC depend on the underlying precipitating illness/condition.
- Despite simultaneous hemorrhage and thrombus formation, bleeding usually predominates and is the most common manifestation of DIC.
- Signs of bleeding can range from ecchymosis to widespread bleeding from the gastrointestinal tract, genitourinary tract, surgical wounds, subcutaneous sites, and venipuncture sites.

Diagnosis and Evaluation

- Patients may manifest signs and symptoms of bleeding with evidence of multiorgan failure (i.e., renal, hepatic, pulmonary, and neurologic dysfunction) secondary to ischemia, and vital sign instability.
- The degree of DIC correlates with the extent of organ dysfunction.
- Laboratory findings (Table 47.2) suggest simultaneous bleeding and thrombotic diathesis.
- Imaging is indicated per physician discretion to identify the underlying precipitating condition.

Treatment

- Supportive care in the form of ABCs, IV fluids, and cardiopulmonary monitoring
- The key is to identify the underlying cause (e.g., sepsis, cancer) and initiate appropriate treatment, directed at the specific cause.

QUALITATIVE/FUNCTIONAL PLATELET ABNORMALITIES

Overview

- Platelets are often dysfunctional, even with elevated/normal PLT count.
- A wide variety of acquired medical conditions can account for abnormal platelet function (Table 47.3).

TABLE 47.2 ***Laboratory Findings in Acute Disseminated Intravascular Coagulation***

Platelet count	DECREASED
Fibrinogen	DECREASED
PT (INR)	INCREASED
PTT	INCREASED
D-dimer	INCREASED
Peripheral smear	Schistocytes and Helmet cells

Adapted from Marx, J. A., Hockberger, R. S., Walls, R. M., Adams, J., & Rosen, P. (2010). *Rosen's emergency medicine: Concepts and clinical practice* (7th ed.). Mosby/Elsevier.

PT, prothrombin time; *PTT*, partial thromboplastin time; *INR*, international normalization ratio.

TABLE 47.3 Medical Conditions Associated with Qualitative Platelet Abnormalities

Uremia
Liver disease
DIC
Antiplatelet antibody (ITP, SLE)
Myeloproliferative disorders (PCV, CML)
Preleukemias (AML, ALL)
Multiple myeloma

Adapted from Marx, J. A., Hockberger, R. S., Walls, R. M., Adams, J., & Rosen, P. (2010). *Rosen's emergency medicine: Concepts and clinical practice* (7th ed.). Mosby/Elsevier.

ALL, acute lymphocytic leukemia; *AML*, acute myelogenous leukemia; *CML*, chronic myelogenous leukemia; *ITP*, idiopathic thrombocytopenic purpura; *PCV*, polycythemia vera; *SLE*, systemic lupus erythematous; *DIC*, disseminated intravascular coagulation.

TABLE 47.4 Common Anticoagulation Medications Encountered in Emergency Room and Effects on Platelet Function

Drug	Onset	Duration of Action
Aspirin	1 hr	Life span of platelet
NSAIDS	1 hr	1 day
Clopidogrel	1–2 days	4–10 days

Adapted from Marx, J. A., Hockberger, R. S., Walls, R. M., Adams, J., & Rosen, P. (2010). *Rosen's emergency medicine: Concepts and clinical practice* (7th ed.). Mosby/Elsevier.

hr, hour; *NSAIDs*, nonsteroidal antiinflammatory drugs.

- Many commonly used drugs can also alter platelet function (Table 47.4).
- Other drugs can decrease platelet production (Table 47.5).

Clinical Presentation

- Can manifest petechiae or more substantial bleeding, such as purpura, mucosal bleeding, gastrointestinal bleeding, or genitourinary bleeding.
- Abnormal function with thrombocytosis can lead to a thromboembolic event (i.e., deep venous thrombosis, mesenteric thrombosis, splenic vein thrombosis, cerebrovascular accident, myocardial infarction).

Diagnosis and Evaluation

- Stabilize patient and assess early on potential need for transfusion.
- History and physical: concentrate on chief complaint, medical history, and medications.
- CBC will have normal to elevated platelet count.
- Prolonged bleeding time may be present.

Treatment

- Treat underlying condition.
- Discontinue medications associated with an increased risk of bleeding.
- If patient is also thrombocytopenic, then consider transfusion to raise count to 50,000/μL.

TABLE 47.5 Drugs That Produce Thrombocytopenia or Impair Platelet Function

Produce thrombocytopenia
Heparin 4+
Sulfa drugs 4+
Ethanol 4+
Aspirin 3+
Indomethacin 3+
Heroin 3+
Thiazides 2+
Furosemide 2+
Penicillins/Cephalosporins 1+
Note: 4+ to 1+ indicates relative incidence, from more frequent to less frequent, based on case reports

Adapted from Marx, J. A., Hockberger, R. S., Walls, R. M., Adams, J., & Rosen, P. (2010). *Rosen's emergency medicine: Concepts and clinical practice* (7th ed.). Mosby/Elsevier.

- In macroglobulinemia and related disorders, elevated levels of viscous proteins interfere with function and many require plasmapheresis.

CONGENITAL (VON WILLEBRAND DISEASE)

Overview

- Most common congenital bleeding disorder (1% of population).
- Three types:
  - Partial quantitative (most common).
  - Qualitative (abnormal function).
  - Near complete deficiency (autosomal recessive).
- Von Willebrand factor functions in normal hemostasis:
  - Cofactor for platelet adhesion.
  - Carrier protein for factor VIII.

Clinical Presentation

- Skin and mucosal bleeding is common in people with Von Willebrand disease (particularly in children and adolescents).
- Recurrent epistaxis, gingival bleeding, unusual bruising, gastrointestinal (GI) bleeding, and menorrhagia.

Diagnosis and Evaluation

- History, physical examination, and family history (autosomal-dominant inheritance).
- Diagnostic testing includes bleeding time, activated partial thromboplastin time (aPTT), factor VIII, coagulant activity, Von Willebrand factor-antigen, and Von Willebrand factor activity.
- Common laboratory results include increased bleeding time, decreased Von Willebrand factor antigen, decreased Von Willebrand factor activity, increased aPTT (owing to decreased factor VIII), and NORMAL PT.
- Blood type affects the VwF (ex: type O has 30% reduction in Von Willebrand factor levels).
- Any adrenergic stimulus, such as acute illness or stress, can result in an increase in Von Willebrand

TABLE 47.6 Mechanism of Action of Common Oral Anticoagulation Drugs

Drugs	Mechanism	Uses
Aspirin	Permanently inhibits COX-1 and COX-2	CAD, CVA-TIA
NSAIDs	Reversibly inhibits COX-1	Limited
Dipyridamole	Inhibits PDE; increases cAMP	TIAs
Ticlopidine Clopidogrel	Inhibits ADP, PlatAg; active metabolite	TIAs-CVA CAD, PVD

Adapted from Marx, J. A., Hockberger, R. S., Walls, R. M., Adams, J., & Rosen, P. (2010). *Rosen's emergency medicine: Concepts and clinical practice* (7th ed.). Mosby/Elsevier.

CAD, Coronary artery disease; *CVA*, cerebrovascular accident; *TIA*, transient ischemic attack; *COX*, cyclooxygenase; *PDE*, phosphodiesterase; *cAMP*, cyclic adenosine monophosphate; *ADP*, adenosine diphosphate; *PlatAg*, platelet aggregation; *PVD*, peripheral vascular disease; *NSAIDs*, nonsteroidal antiinflammatory drugs.

factor levels and lead to a missed diagnosis. High levels of estrogen during pregnancy can also lead to elevated Von Willebrand factor levels.

Treatment

- Avoid antiplatelet medications (Table 47.6).
- DDAVP (desmopressin) (0.3 μg/kg to a maximum of 20 μg intravenously) and/or cryoprecipitate, depending on type of Von Willebrand Disease.
- Route of administration of DDAVP can be intravenous, subcutaneous, or intranasal.
- Recombinant human factor VIIa or factor VIII bypassing agents if severe (type 3) disease or in those who develop inhibitors to replacement VwF.

ACQUIRED (RENAL DISEASE)

Background

- Renal disease can lead to qualitative platelet and clotting factor abnormalities.
- Uremic toxins cause inhibition of platelet aggregation and platelet-vessel wall adhesion.
- Preventative measures include optimizing nutrition: folate, vitamin B12, and iron repletion.
- Anemia often accompanies renal failure secondary to decreased RBC production.

Clinical Presentation, Diagnosis, and Evaluation

- Manifestations include fatigue, pallor, light-headedness.
- Prolonged bleeding time.
- Metabolic manifestations of uremia include metabolic acidosis (Kussmaul breathing), elevated potassium, phosphorous, and magnesium, and decreased calcium.
- Platelet count may be slightly decreased, but is often normal.
- Bleeding occurs at mucosal sites, puncture sites, and from GI sources.

Treatment

- Aimed at prevention and directed at treatment of acute bleeding.
- Treatment of acute bleeding includes dialysis, RBCs, desmopressin, conjugated estrogens, cryoprecipitate, and, rarely, platelets.
- Cryoprecipitate and platelets are only indicated in life-threatening bleeds.

ACQUIRED (ASPIRIN-INDUCED)

Background

- Multiple drugs can cause a qualitative platelet thrombocytopenia disorder.
- Aspirin is commonly used for primary prevention of transient ischemic attack, cerebrovascular accident, and myocardial infarction.
- Irreversibly inhibits cyclooxygenase (COX-1), which in turn inhibits the synthesis of thromboxane A2, leading to vascular dilation and increased bleeding.
- Inhibition is irreversible and effective for the life span of circulating platelets (7 to 10 days).

Clinical Presentation, Diagnosis, and Evaluation

- History of easy bruising.
- GI bleeding (upper and/or lower source).
- Prolonged bleeding time.
- Acid–base respiratory and metabolic disorder may be present with significant ingestion.

Treatment

- Intravenous access, monitor, and fluid resuscitation plus or minus packed RBC if hemodynamic instability is present.
- Discontinue medication.
- Direct mechanical pressure to bleeding site, if accessible.
- Reverse any coprescribed anticoagulants.
- Platelet transfusion in life-threatening bleeds.

Secondary Hemostasis

OVERVIEW (FIG. 47.5)

- Reaction of plasma coagulation proteins by a tightly regulated mechanism composed of an "intrinsic" and "extrinsic" pathway.
- Final product is cross-linked fibrin, which strengthens the platelet plug formed by primary hemostasis.
- Counter-regulated by the fibrinolytic system.
- Physiologic inhibitors of hemostasis include protein C, S, and anti-thrombin III.
- Deficiencies in these proteins results in a hypercoagulable state.

Inherited Disorders

HEMOPHILIA

Overview

- A disorder of coagulation caused primarily by a deficiency or defect in one of two circulating plasma proteins.
- Hemophilia A (classic hemophilia) is caused by a deficiency in factor VIII and is the most common cause of hemophilia in the United States.
- Hemophilia B (Christmas disease) is caused by deficiency in factor IX.
- Hemophilia A and B are clinically indistinguishable from each other.
- Severity of disease/bleeding reflects the percent of factor levels (degree of deficiency).

47

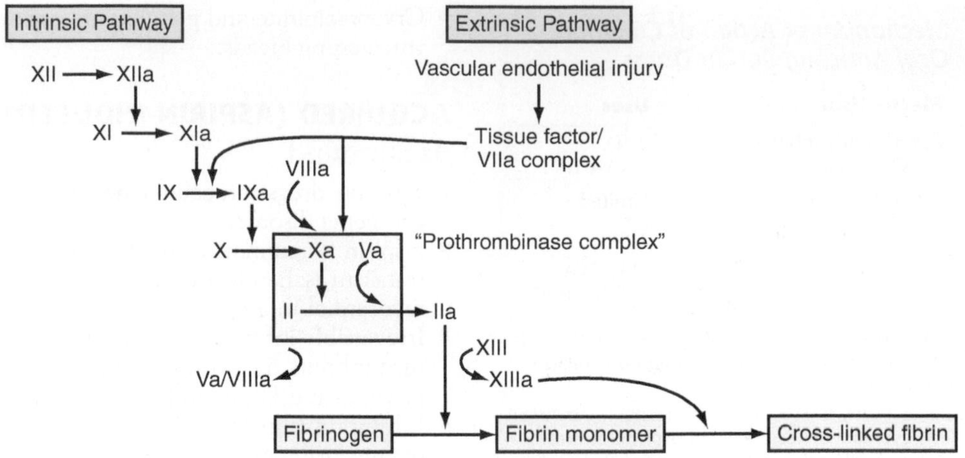

FIG. 47.5 Coagulation cascade incorporating extrinsic and intrinsic pathways of coagulation. (From Estafanous, F. G., Barasch, P. G., & Reves, J. G. (2001). *Cardiac anesthesia: Principles and clinical practice* (2nd ed., p. 320). Lippincott Williams & Wilkins.)

Clinical Presentation

- Degree of bleeding depends on severity of disease.
- Joints and muscles are the most common areas into which bleeding occurs.
- Bleeding can also occur in the abdomen, retroperitoneum, or central nervous system.
- Any trauma or surgical procedure can also result in difficulty in controlling bleeding.

Diagnosis and Evaluation

- ABCs, IV access, monitor.
- Consider early and complete factor replacement simultaneously with other resuscitative and diagnostic maneuvers.

Treatment

- Two treatment options:
  - Recombinant factor replacement.
  - Plasma-derived factor.
- Recombinant factor is the purer and safer (i.e., lower likelihood for viral transmission) of the two options, but the more costly one.
- Dosing is based on clotting factor volume of distribution, half-life, and hemostatic level of factor required to control bleeding (Box 47.1).
- Early airway management is appropriate. Consider risk of bleeding into neck, tongue, retropharynx, or pharynx.
- Known hemophilia with new onset headache or localizing neurologic symptom or blunt head injury should receive immediate factor replacement followed by emergent head computed tomography.
- Hemarthrosis is one of the most common manifestations of hemophilia.
- No central line placement without initial factor replacement.

BOX 47.1 *Recombinant factor dosing*

Factor VIII required = weight (kg) × 0.5 × (% change in factor activity needed)
Factor IX required = weight (kg) × 1.0 × (% change in factor activity needed)

From Marx, J. A., Hockberger, R. S., Walls, R. M., Adams, J., & Rosen, P. (2010). *Rosen's emergency medicine: Concepts and clinical practice*. (7th ed). Mosby/Elsevier.
kg, kilogram.

- No intramuscular injections.
- No aspirin or NSAIDs.

Acquired Disorders

Overview and Clinical Presentation

- Liver-associated coagulopathies are often seen in association with certain medications (i.e., sulfa drugs and penicillin), malignancies, autoimmune disorders, viral infections, intravenous drug abuse (IVDA), or alcohol abuse.
- The liver synthesizes almost all proteins involved in hemostasis, with the exception of factor VIII. Thus, the extrinsic pathway is largely affected, as compared with the intrinsic pathway (i.e., PT greater than aPTT) plus or minus platelet dysfunction.
- Portal HTN secondary to cirrhosis increases splenic sequestration of platelets and increases fibrinolysis.

Diagnosis and Evaluation

- PT is a sensitive indicator of hepatic synthetic function.
- Significant liver disease can lead to prolonged PT, aPTT, and bleeding time.
- Decreased fibrinogen levels (less than 100 mg/dL) may also be seen with significant disease.
- GI (upper and lower) bleeding in the form of melena/hematochezia/hematemesis.
- May present with physical examination findings consistent with liver disease, such as abdominal distension, extremity edema, jaundice, tremors, ecchymosis, as well as altered mental status.

Treatment

- No treatment is required if the patient has no active bleeding despite laboratory abnormalities.
- Treat coagulopathy if clinically significant bleeding or patient pending invasive procedure/surgery.
- Transfuse RBCs to maintain adequate hemoglobin levels and maintain hemodynamic stability.
- Administer oral or IV vitamin K for all patients with liver disease and active bleeding.
- If pending procedures or have active bleeding in the setting of prolonged PT and aPTT, fresh frozen plasma

(FFP) can be used to replace coagulation factors temporarily.
- Administer cryoprecipitate in patients with active bleeding and fibrinogen levels below 100 mg/dL.
- Consider platelets and DDAVP may be considered if patient is thrombocytopenic.

VITAMIN K-ASSOCIATED DISORDERS

Overview and Clinical Presentation

- Vitamin K is required for carboxylation of clotting factors II, VII, IX, and X.
- Vitamin K is fat-soluble and therefore can be affected by malabsorption, which can be caused by impaired bile acid metabolism (i.e., primary biliary cirrhosis), cholestasis, treatment with bile acid binders, and poor nutrition.

Clinical Presentation, Diagnosis, and Evaluation

- GI loss (i.e., mouth, upper, and lower GI tract), epistaxis, intracerebral hemorrhage, and ecchymosis.
- Prolonged PT.

Treatment

- Administer Vitamin K orally, subcutaneously, intramuscularly, or parenterally, depending on the situation.
- 4-Factor prothrombin complex concentrate (4F-PCC) is first-line treatment in serious life-threatening bleeds, regardless of INR levels.
- Fresh frozen plasma is a second-line treatment if 4F-PCC is not available.
- Transfuse PRBCs to maintain adequate hemoglobin levels and hemodynamic stability.

DRUG-INDUCED DISORDERS OF SECONDARY HEMOSTASIS

Overview and Clinical Presentation

- Anticoagulants have various targets in the clotting cascade.
- Multiple types of anticoagulation medications exist that may be used, depending on patient diagnosis and disposition.
- Direct oral anticoagulants can be categorized as direct thrombin (IIa) inhibitors or direct factor Xa inhibitors.
- Direct thrombin inhibitors, such as dabigatran, exert their effects by direct, selective, and reversible binding to the active site of thrombin.
- Idarucizumab has been approved for reversal of dabigatran.
- Factor Xa inhibitors, such as rivaroxaban, apixaban, and edoxaban, selectively and reversibly block the activity of clotting factor Xa.
- Andexanet alfa has been approved for reversal of factor Xa inhibitors.

Clinical Presentation, Evaluation, and Diagnosis

- History focusing on chief complaint, current medications, dosing, and reason for anticoagulation.
- Evaluate for signs and symptoms of hemorrhage/bleeding, such as vital sign instability, altered mental status, and/or headache suspicious for intracranial bleed, positive-guaiac test, or ecchymosis/petechiae.
- Laboratory work should consist of complete blood count, renal function, coagulation panel, and fibrinogen.
- Imaging should be considered if evidence of trauma or patient has an altered sensorium.
- INR ≥ 5, recent surgery, thrombocytopenia, antiplatelet medication, and GI disease (i.e., ulcer and inflammatory bowel disease) are all risk factors for bleeding.

Treatment

- ABCs, IV access, oxygen and monitor.
- Consider activated charcoal if acute intoxication and no evidence of altered sensorium.
- Do not induce emesis.
- Monitor PT/INR.
- Type and cross if severe bleeding present.
- Treatment of warfarin-induced bleeding will depend on INR value and severity of bleeding (Fig. 47.6).
- Treatment of other anticoagulated-related bleeding will depend on INR value, severity of bleeding, and the type of anticoagulant taken (Table 47.7).

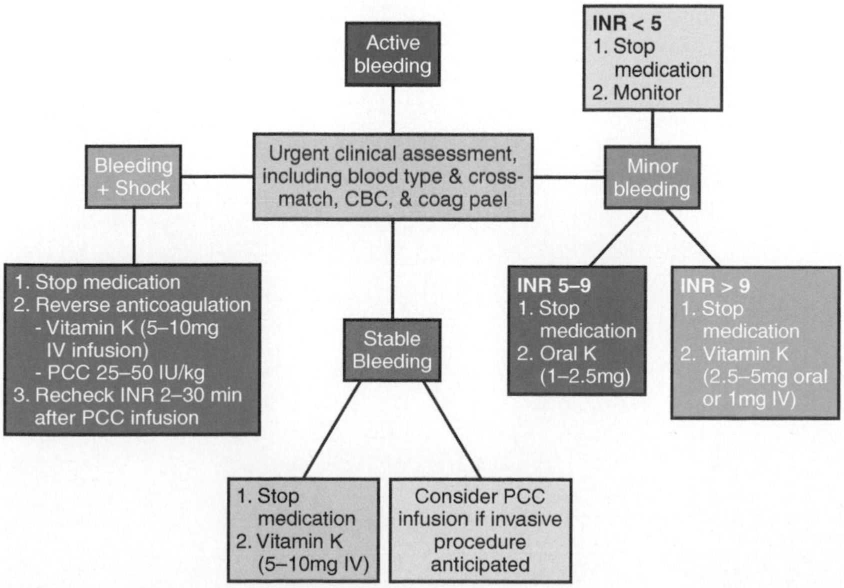

FIG. 47.6 Medical approach to warfarin-induced bleeding. *PCC,* prothrombin complex concentrates; *CBC,* complete blood count; *IV,* intravenous; *INR,* international normalization ratio. (Adapted from Marx, J. A., Hockberger, R. S., Walls, R. M., Adams, J., & Rosen, P. (2010). *Rosen's emergency medicine: Concepts and clinical practice* (7th ed.). Mosby/Elsevier.)

47

TABLE 47.7 *Mechanism of Action and Antidotes of Common Anticoagulation Medications*

Agent	Mechanism of Action	Dose/Route Administration	Antidote
LMWHs (enoxaparin)	Activate antithrombin III and inhibit thrombin	Subcutaneous	Protamine sulfate
Warfarin	Blocks synthesis of vitamin K (factors 2,7,9,10)	Oral	Vitamin K, FFP, PCC
Fondaparinux	Xa inhibitor	Subcutaneous	Consider rFVII
Dabigatran	Direct IIa inhibitor	Oral	Idarucizumab
Rivaroxaban	Xa inhibitor	Oral	Adexanet Alfa
Apixaban	Xa inhibitor	Oral	Adexanet Alfa
Edoxaban	Xa inhibitor	Oral	Adexanet Alfa

Adapted from Marx, J. A., Hockberger, R. S., Walls, R. M., Adams, J., & Rosen, P. (2010). *Rosen's emergency medicine: Concepts and clinical practice* (7th ed.). Mosby/Elsevier.

LMWH, low-molecular-weight heparin; *FFP*, fresh frozen plasma; *PCC*, prothrombin complex concentrates; *rFVII*, recombinant factor VII.

SUGGESTED READING

Dupre, A. A., & Janz, T. G. (2018). Disorders of hemostasis. In R. M. Walls, R. S. Hockberger, & M. Gausche-Hill (Eds.). *Rosen's emergency medicine: Concepts and clinical practice* (9th ed.). Elsevier.

CHAPTER **48** BOARD REVIEW

Lymphomas

LEV LIBET, MD

Lymphomas account for a diverse group of malignancies that arise from lymphocytes. The two major categories of lymphoma are Hodgkin and non-Hodgkin lymphoma. The incidence of Hodgkin and non-Hodgkin lymphoma in North America is approximately 2.7 cases and 20 cases per 100,000, respectively.

General Principles

- Lymphoma is a hematologic malignancy of the lymphocyte lineage and is primarily found in the lymphatic system, in contradistinction to leukemia, where the malignant cells are primarily found in the bone marrow and blood stream.
- The progenitors for various lymphomas are B lymphocytes, T lymphocytes, and natural killer cells.
- The two broad categories of Hodgkin and non-Hodgkin lymphoma are further subdivided into numerous distinct lymphoma types.

Hodgkin Lymphoma (HL)

CATEGORIES OF HL

- Hodgkin lymphoma (HL) is defined by the presence of Reed Sternberg cells or Reed Sternberg variants, CD 30, and/or CD 15 antigens (CD stands for cluster of differentiation). This is further subcategorized into classic Hodgkin lymphomas (CHL), which make up 95% of HL, and nodular lymphocyte predominant (NLP), which makes up the remaining 5%. NLP is characterized by the absence of CD 30 antigen.
- Classic Hodgkin lymphoma
  - Nodular sclerosis: 70% of CHL
  - Mixed cellularity: 20%–25% of CHL
  - Lymphocyte-depleted
  - Lymphocyte-rich
- Nodular lymphocyte predominant: 5% of HL. Characterized by popcorn cells and absence of CD 30 antigen.

Basic Information

- Risk factors for HL include first-degree relative with HL, immunocompromise, Epstein-Barr virus, and human immunodeficiency virus (HIV). In fact, HL is an AIDS-defining illness.
- There is a bimodal distribution of disease, with the first peak between ages 15 and 40, and a second peak in those older than 55.
- Spread of lymphoma is generally to proximal lymph nodes.

Clinical Presentation

- Lymphadenopathy, a central component to the presentation, occurs in the cervical, axillary, supraclavicular, or inguinal regions.
- With progression, there is the development of B symptoms: fevers, weight loss, and/or night sweats.
- Dyspnea, chest pain, fatigue, and sensitivity to alcohol may also be present. The sensitivity to alcohol presents as either pruritus or chest pain shortly after ingestion in those with a mediastinal mass.

Diagnosis and Evaluation

- Involves laboratory evaluation, imaging, and pathologic evaluation
  - Laboratory evaluation: complete blood count with differential, renal function, and liver function may be unremarkable. Erythrocyte sedimentation rate, lactate dehydrogenase (LDH), and uric acid may be elevated.
  - Imaging: computed tomography scan, positron emission tomography scan, and magnetic resonance imaging for staging purposes
  - Biopsy of lymph node: fine needle aspiration (FNA), needle core biopsy, excisional biopsy. FNA does not provide any architectural information, whereas an excisional biopsy does and therefore is the most comprehensive option.
  - Immunophenotyping: immunohistochemistry, flow cytometry

Treatment

- Prior to the commencement of treatment, imaging is used to stage the disease. Classically, the Ann Arbor classification system is used (Fig. 48.1); however, there is also the more recent Lugano classification. The letter A indicates the absence of B symptoms, whereas the letter B indicates their presence. Prognosis is generally good for early-stage HL with 5-year survival being 90% or greater. There are various treatment modalities.
- Drug therapy
  - Chemotherapy: multiple regimens
  - Immunotherapy: a variety of biological agents that either attack the malignant cells directly or stimulate the immune system to more effectively target malignant cells. Examples include monoclonal antibodies, cytokines, checkpoint inhibitors, and adoptive cell transfer.
- Radiation therapy
- Stem cell transplant: autologous vs. allogeneic

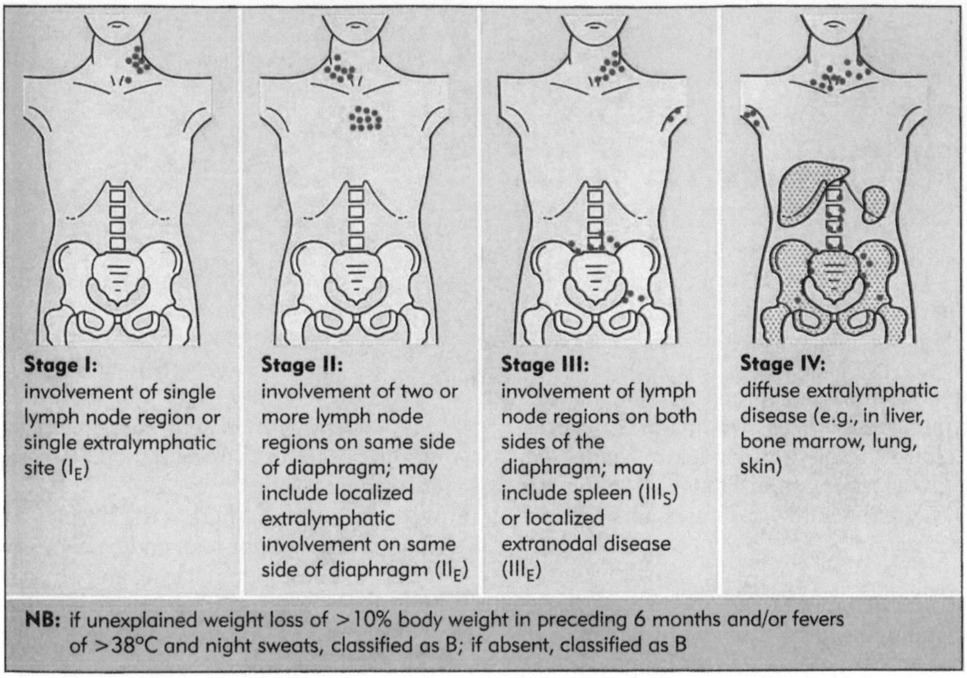

Stage I:
involvement of single lymph node region or single extralymphatic site (I_E)
Stage II:
involvement of two or more lymph node regions on same side of diaphragm; may include localized extralymphatic involvement on same side of diaphragm (II_E)
Stage III:
involvement of lymph node regions on both sides of the diaphragm; may include spleen (III_S) or localized extranodal disease (III_E)
Stage IV:
diffuse extralymphatic disease (e.g., in liver, bone marrow, lung, skin)
NB: if unexplained weight loss of >10% body weight in preceding 6 months and/or fevers of >38°C and night sweats, classified as B; if absent, classified as B

FIG. 48.1 Ann Arbor staging system for Hodgkin lymphoma. (From Hoffbrand, A. V., & Pettit, J. E. (2010). *Color atlas of clinical hematology* (4th ed.). Mosby. Originally modified from Hoffbrand, A. V., & Pettit, J. E. (1993). *Essential haematology* (3rd ed.). Blackwell Science Publications.)

Non-Hodgkin Lymphoma

- There are more than 80 types of NHL, according to the World Health Organization (WHO).
- Fig. 48.2 shows various types and their relative prevalence. B-cell lymphomas make up the vast majority of NHL (85%). The remaining 15% is shared by natural killer and T-cell lymphomas.
- NHL is also classified as either indolent or aggressive where indolent refers to slow growing and aggressive refers to fast growing. Indolent NHL can progress to aggressive NHL. The goal of treatment is to achieve remission; cure is not possible.

CATEGORIES OF NHL

Indolent B-cell Lymphomas

- Small lymphocytic lymphoma/chronic lymphocytic leukemia: believed to be the same entity, but is classified based on the predominant location of the abnormal cells. Up to 50% of patients may be asymptomatic. Chronic lymphocytic leukemia may progress to diffuse large B-cell lymphoma (DLBCL), which is the aggressive form. This progression is called Richter's transformation.
- Follicular lymphoma: may also transform into an aggressive type.
- Waldenstrom macroglobulinemia: high levels of monoclonal protein (paraprotein) in the form of immunoglobulin M
- Marginal zone lymphoma (MZL)
  - Extranodal marginal zone lymphoma, also known as mucosal-associated lymphoid tissue
  - Nodal marginal zone lymphoma
  - Splenic marginal zone lymphoma

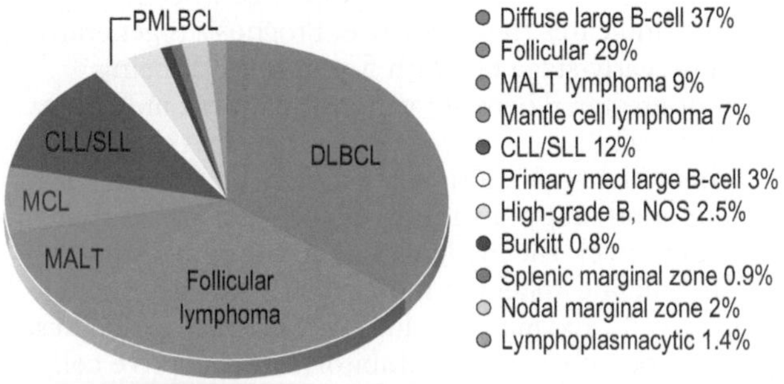

FIG. 48.2 Malignant disease. (From Gallagher, C. J. (2017). *Kumar and Clark's clinical medicine, 2017* (pp. 583–644). Elsevier Ltd. All rights reserved.)

Indolent T-cell Lymphomas

- Cutaneous T-cell lymphoma (mycosis fungoides): presents with patches, plaques, or ulcerations.

Aggressive Types of B-cell lymphomas

- Diffuse large B-cell lymphoma: most common type of lymphoma, accounting for 25% of NHL; however, it is a category that encompasses several heterogeneous entities.
- Burkitt lymphoma: mostly found in Africa
- Double- lymphoma
- Mantle cell lymphoma

Aggressive Types of T-cell Lymphomas

- Lymphoblastic lymphoma/leukemia: it is suggested that acute lymphocytic leukemia is the same entity.

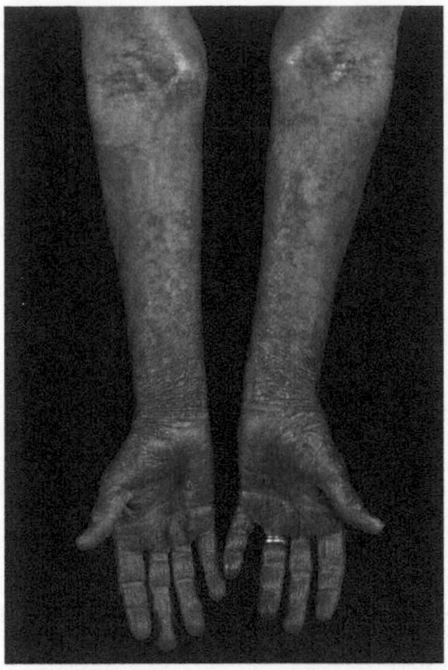

FIG. 48.3 Sézary syndrome. (From Kubica, A. W. & Pittelkow, M. R. (2014, April). Sézary syndrome. *Surgical Pathology Clinics*, 7(2), 191–202.)

- Sézary syndrome (Fig. 48.3): a form of cutaneous lymphoma. Large patches of erythroderma are present as well as palmoplantar keratoderma.
- Peripheral T-cell lymphoma: a hodgepodge of various types of lymphomas
- Anaplastic large cell lymphoma: systemic type

Clinical Presentation

- The clinical presentation is variable and depends on the specific type of NHL. Patients will often have painless lymphadenopathy; however, in a significant percentage, the disease will arise from extranodal, extramedullary tissues.
- Patients may note the presence of B symptoms. Additionally, they may note fatigue, dyspnea, easy bruising, and frequent infections.

Diagnosis and Evaluation

- Involves laboratory evaluation, imaging, and pathologic evaluation.
  - Complete blood count, chemistry, liver tests, LDH, human immunodeficiency virus, hepatitis panel
  - Fine needle aspiration (FNA), core needle biopsy, excisional biopsy
  - Computed tomography/positron emission tomography scan/magnetic resonance imaging for staging purposes
  - Immunophenotyping: immunohistochemistry and/or flow cytometry

Treatment

- Poor prognostic indicators are age more than 60 years, requiring assistance with daily activities, elevated LDH, stages III and IV. There are various treatment modalities which depend on the NHL type, stage, and patient factors.
- Active surveillance: for those with indolent type lymphomas.
- Drug therapy
  - Chemotherapy: multiple regimens
  - Immunotherapy
    - Radioimmunotherapy
    - CAR (chimeric antigen receptor) T-cell therapy depicted in Fig. 48.4. This is a type of adoptive cell transfer. The patient's T-cells are genetically modified to produce chimeric antigen receptors. They are multiplied and then delivered back to the patient. The major complication of this intervention is cytokine release syndrome, which induces a systemic inflammatory response that can vary in

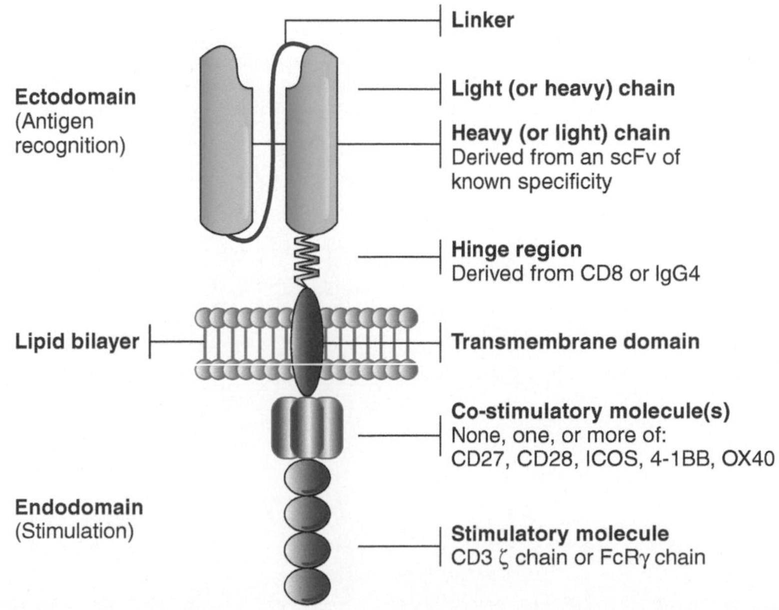

FIG. 48.4 Anatomy of a chimeric antigen receptor (CAR). All the indicated components (with the exception of the lipid bilayer, which is an integral part of the host cell membrane) are typically produced as a single polypeptide encoded by one plasmid. (From Gill, S., Maus, M. V., & Porter, D. L. (2016). Chimeric antigen receptor T cell therapy: 25 years in the making. *Blood Reviews*, 30(3), 157–167.)

severity but may include hemodynamic instability and death.
- Targeted therapy: drugs that target molecules that help control the growth and survival of lymphoma cells
- Radiation therapy
- Stem cell transplant: autologous vs. allogeneic

Complications of Treatment

- The most important iatrogenic complication is acute tumor lysis syndrome. It is most commonly seen in high-grade lymphomas and acute leukemias. It is seen hours to days after chemotherapy and results in various metabolic derangements, which are the result of extensive cell death. The cellular byproducts overwhelm renal excretion capabilities. Additionally, the precipitation of uric acid crystals and calcium phosphate crystals further hinders renal excretion. Laboratory derangements include hyperuricemia, hyperkalemia, hyperphosphatemia, and hypocalcemia. Symptoms are unreliable and laboratory evaluation must be undertaken. This may be a life-threatening entity because of the combination of hyperkalemia and hypocalcemia, which may result in malignant arrhythmias. Approach to treatment:
  - Address the hyperkalemia: This requires an early electrocardiogram and myocyte membrane stabilization with calcium, if necessary. Early hemodialysis may be required.
  - Hydration: This is vital for the dilution of extracellular fluid and providing sufficient volume for renal perfusion.
  - Allopurinol: A xanthine oxidase inhibitor that prevents further conversion of byproducts into uric acid. This will not reduce uric acid levels acutely.
  - Rasburicase: A recombinant urate oxidase that can acutely reduce uric acid levels by converting uric acid into a more soluble entity, allantoin.

SUGGESTED READINGS

Armitage, J. O. (2010). Early-stage Hodgkin's lymphoma. *New England Journal of Medicine, 363*, 653–662.

Aster, J. C., & Posdnyakova, O. (2018, June 11). *Epidemiology, Pathologic Features and Diagnosis of Classic Hodgkin Lymphoma.* UpToDate.com.

Belcher, C., & Rogers, R. (2016). *Tumor Lysis Syndrome – Diagnosis and Treatment.* emDocs.net.

Bryant, A. J., & Newman, J. H. (2013). Alcohol intolerance associated with Hodgkin lymphoma. *CMAJ: Canadian Medical Association Journal*, 185, E353. Retrieved from https://www.cancer.org/cancer/lymphoma.html

Long, B. (2018). *CAR T-Cell Therapy – What do you Need to Know for the ED?* emDocs.net.

Salama, M., & Hoffman, R. (2018). Progress in the classification of hematopoietic and lymphoid neoplasms: Clinical implications. In Hoffman, R., Benz, E. J., Jr., Silberstein L. E., Heslop, H. E., Weitz, J. I, Anastasi, J., ... Abutalib, S. A. (Eds.), *Hematology: Basic principles and practice* (7th ed.) Elsevier.

Smith, A., Crouch, S., Lax, S., Li, J., Painter, D., Howell, D., et al. (2015). Lymphoma incidence, survival and prevalence 2004-2014: sub-type analysis from the UK's haematological malignancy research network. *British Journal of Cancer*, 112, 1575–1584.

Ugras-Rey, S. (2014). Selected oncologic emergencies. In J. A. Marx, R. S. Hockberger, & R. M. Walls (Eds.), *Rosen's emergency medicine: Concepts and clinical practice* (8th ed.). Elsevier Saunders.

Pancytopenia

JAMES ROSBRUGH, MD

Pancytopenia is a description of a condition more so than a final diagnosis in and of itself. The presenting symptoms are widely varied based on the underlying cause and on the cell lines most significantly involved. Likewise, the management options are numerous and depend on many factors.

General Principles

Definition

- All three of the blood cell lines (*erythroid, myeloid, megakaryocytic*) are below normal reference ranges.
  - Red blood cells (RBCs): hemoglobin (Hb) <12 g/dL (nonpregnant women), <13 g/dL (men)
  - White blood cells (WBCs): absolute neutrophil count (ANC) <1800/μL (some sources define as <1500/μL)
  - Platelets: <150,000/μL

Mechanism

- Can occur individually or in combination
  - Replacement/infiltration of bone marrow (crowds out stem cells)
    - Hematologic malignancies
    - Myelofibrosis
    - Metastatic cancers
    - Various infections
  - Bone marrow aplasia (slows or stops cell production)
    - Medications or toxins
    - Nutritional deficiencies
    - Immune-mediated destruction
    - Radiation
    - Infections
    - See "Aplastic anemia" below.
  - Blood cell destruction/sequestration (destroys/traps cells already made)
    - Destruction
      - Disseminated intravascular coagulopathy
      - Thrombotic thrombocytopenic purpura (TTP)
      - Megaloblastic disorders
      - Myelodysplasia
    - Sequestration
      - Splenomegaly

Categories of Pancytopenias

- Acquired (up to 80% of cases)
  - Most causes listed above
  - Aplastic anemia—specific form of pancytopenia
    - Hypocellular bone marrow with no abnormal cells, fibrosis, or other abnormal infiltrate
    - Depression of at least two hematopoietic cell lines
    - Most common cause: autoimmune damage to hematopoietic stem cells
  - Commonly associated causes
    - Drugs
      - Anticonvulsants: carbamazepine, phenytoin (Dilantin), valproic acid, felbamate
      - Antibiotics: sulfonamides, chloramphenicol, nitrofurantoin
      - Immunosuppressants: mycophenolic acid, azathioprine, cyclosporine
      - Chemotherapy agents
      - Antiinflammatory: gold, indomethacin
    - Toxins: benzene, glue, organic solvents
    - Radiation
    - Viral infections: Epstein-Barr virus, human immunodeficiency virus, hepatitis, some herpes
- Congenital
  - Fanconi anemia—most common form of inherited pancytopenia
    - Autosomal recessive inheritance pattern
    - Multiple physical deformities include:
      - Microcephaly
      - Short stature
      - Developmental delays
      - Abnormal skin pigmentations, café au lait spots
      - Thumb and/or radii deformities
    - Prone to various cancers, including acute myeloid leukemia
    - Usually develop pancytopenia by adulthood
  - Dyskeratosis congenital (Zinsser-Engman-Cole syndrome)
    - Rare, X-linked recessive
    - Most have characteristic triad
      - Reticulated skin hyperpigmentation
      - Dystrophy of the nails
      - Oral leukoplakia
    - Seventy percent die of bone marrow failure complications (usually opportunistic infections or bleeding) with mean age of 16 years.
  - Various other rare congenital conditions can develop some form of bone marrow suppression. Refer to Suggested Readings for more information.

Commonly Associated Emergencies

- Concomitant hematologic emergencies (examples)
  - Hemolytic uremic syndrome
  - Disseminated intravascular coagulopathy
  - TTP
  - Hemophagocytic lymphohistiocytosis
- Metabolic emergencies from the underlying cause
  - Acute renal failure (due to tumor lysis, multiple myeloma, etc.)
  - Hypercalcemia (due to leukemia, metastatic cancers, etc.)

Clinical Presentation

Varies based upon the degree that different cell lines are affected. Examples:

- Anemia
  - Easy fatigability
  - Chest pain or dyspnea on exertion
  - Claudication
  - Pallor
- Neutropenia
  - Fevers
  - Severe infections
  - Opportunistic infections (e.g., thrush)
- Thrombocytopenia
  - Petechiae
  - Easy bleeding (epistaxis, bleeding gingiva, hematuria, blood per rectum, etc.)

Diagnosis and Evaluation

- Complete blood count (include WBC differential and RBC indices)
- Peripheral blood smear
- Reticulocyte count
- Chemistry panels (electrolytes, serum urea nitrogen, creatinine, liver function tests, calcium, lactate dehydrogenase, uric acid)
- Coagulation (prothrombin time, partial thromboplastin time)
- Blood type and screen
- Specialized studies (not emergent, usually after hematology department referral)
  - Bone marrow biopsy
  - Immune-mediated studies (antinuclear antibody and DNA titer, Coombs test, rheumatoid factor)
  - Viral studies (HIV, Epstein-Barr virus, parvovirus, hepatitis A, B, and C, etc.)
  - Vitamin levels (B_{12}, folate)

Treatment

- Minor pancytopenia, asymptomatic (See reference ranges in "General Principles: Definition" above.)
  - Does not require emergency intervention
  - Prompt hematology department consultation recommended within days to weeks
- Moderate, severe, or symptomatic—may need emergent treatment
  - Anemia
    - Asymptomatic patients: consider transfusion of packed RBCs if Hb < 6–7 g/dL.
    - Symptomatic patients
      - Confirm that symptoms are not a result of a separate condition (e.g., pulmonary embolism).
      - May need packed RBC transfusion even if Hb ≥7.0, up to 10 g/dL, to control symptoms
      - Patients with preexisting coronary artery disease may require transfusion at slightly higher Hb levels.
  - Neutropenia
    - New-onset moderate (ANC <1000/µL) or severe (ANC <500/µL)
      - Immediate hematology department consultation and/or
      - Hospitalization
    - Neutropenic fever
      - ANC <1000/µL with either
        - Fever (temperature ≥38°C/100.4°F) or ≥38.3°C/101.0°F on one measurement)
        - Other evidence of infection
      - Initiate treatment
        - Blood cultures
        - Broad-spectrum antibiotics within 60 minutes of presentation
        - Immediate hematology department consultation
  - Thrombocytopenia
    - Consider platelet transfusion and immediate hematology department consultation if:
      - Severe (platelets <10,000/µL) due to high risk of bleeding
      - Moderate (platelets <50,000/µL) with concerning bleeding, or a condition in which bleeding is anticipated, such as:
        - Pregnancy
        - Clinical condition that will require prompt invasive procedure (e.g., surgery)
    - Other conditions may require specific treatment (eg., plasma exchange may be necessary to treat TTP, immunologic thrombocytopenic purpura might require immunoglobulin G, etc.).

SUGGESTED READINGS

Al Jefri, A. (2019). Marrow failure syndromes. *Medscape*. Retrieved October 17, 2019 from https://www.emedicine.medscape.com/article/993616-overview.

Bakhshi, S. (2019). Aplastic anemia. *Medscape*. Retrieved October 17, 2019, from https://www.emedicine.medscape.com/article/198759-overview.

Berliner, N. (2019). Approach to the patient with pancytopenia. *UpToDate*. Retreived October 17, 2019, from https://www.uptodate.com/contents/approach-to-the-adult-with-pancytopenia.

Carson, J., & Kleinman, S. (2020). Indications and hemoglobin thresholds for red blood cell transfusion in the adult. *UpToDate*. Retreived October 17, 2019, from https://www.uptodate.com/contents/indications-and-hemoglobin-thresholds-for-red-blood-celltransfusion-in-the-adult.

CHAPTER **50**

BOARD REVIEW

Red Blood Cell Disorders

JOSHUA TOBIAS, MD

Red blood cell disorders cover a group of diseases that affect the number of red blood cells (RBCs) in circulation resulting in either too few (anemia), too many (polycythemia), or disruption of the oxygen-carrying protein, hemoglobin. The function of the RBC is to deliver oxygen from the lungs to the tissues and carbon dioxide from the tissues to the lungs. RBC disorders affect the oxygen delivery system, causing organ tissue injury throughout the body.

Categories of Red Blood Cell Disorders

- Anemia: blood loss, increased destruction, or decreased production of red blood cells.
- Polycythemia: overproduction of blood cells from malignant change of the bone marrow or in response to an underlying condition.
- Methemoglobinemia: congenital or acquired elevation of methemoglobin levels.

General Principles for Approach and Treatment of RBC Disorders

- Correct any reversible causes (blood loss, hypoxia, dehydration, medications).
- Assess the need for emergent transfusion or phlebotomy.

Anemias

- Anemia is the absolute decrease in the number of circulating RBCs. The diagnosis is based upon laboratory measurements of RBC indices that are below the accepted normal values (Table 50.1). Anemia is the most common hematologic disorder and affects about 25% of the world's population. It is more prevalent in children, pregnant women, and the elderly. This decrease in RBCs may result from blood loss, increased destruction, or decreased production. In the emergency department (ED), acute hemorrhage is the most common etiology for anemia.

APLASTIC ANEMIA

General Principles

- Aplastic anemia is a rare disorder characterized by suppression of bone marrow function that results in progressive pancytopenia with a hypocellular bone marrow. Aplastic anemia may be acquired (>80%) or inherited. Acquired cases may be idiopathic or secondary to infection, exposure to toxins or drugs, or nutritional deficiencies.

Clinical Presentation

- The presentation relates to the decreased production of cells across all blood lines.
  - Anemia: pallor, headaches, palpitations, dyspnea, or fatigue.
  - Thrombocytopenia: mucosal bleeding, gingival bleeding, petechial rash.
  - Neutropenia: opportunistic infections, recurrent infections, oral infections.

Diagnosis and Evaluation

- Diagnosed with blood testing and bone marrow evaluation.
- Complete blood count (CBC) testing reveals pancytopenia often with normochromic anemia.
- Bone marrow biopsy reveals hypocellular bone marrow.
- Magnetic resonance imaging may be used to assess cellularity of axial skeleton.

Treatment

- Supportive, including transfusions and treatment of infections.
  - Infections are a major cause of mortality.
  - Broad-spectrum antibiotics should be initiated to cover *Pseudomonas* and *Staphylococcus* infections along with antifungal treatment, especially for *Aspergillus* infections.
- Immunosuppression
- Hematopoietic stem cell transplantation

HEMOGLOBINOPATHIES

General Principles

- Hemoglobinopathies may be secondary to structural defects in the hemoglobin molecules (e.g., sickle cell disease) or from diminished production of one of the subunits (α or β). This diminished production can result in abnormal association of normal subunits due to the decreased number of other subunits (e.g., thalassemias). Genetic defects result in the abnormal production of one of the globin chains of the hemoglobin molecule and cause anemia. Common in those of African, Indian, Asian, and Mediterranean descent, the most clinically significant hemoglobin gene defects occur on the beta hemoglobin chain.

TABLE 50.1 Adult Reference Ranges for Red Blood Cells[a]

Measurement (Units)	Men	Women
Hemoglobin (g/dL)	13.6–17.2	12.0–15.0
Hematocrit (%)	39–49	33–43
Red cell count ($\times 10^6/\mu L$)	4.3–5.9	3.5–5.0
Reticulocyte count (%)	0.5–1.5	
Mean cell volume (fL)	82–96	
Mean cell hemoglobin (pg)	27–33	
Mean cell hemoglobin concentration (g/dL)	33–37	
Red cell distribution width	11.5–14.5	

[a]Reference ranges vary among laboratories. The reference ranges for the laboratory providing the result should always be used in interpreting test results.

From Kumar V., Abbas, A. K, & Aster, J. C. (2015). Red blood cell and bleeding disorders. In V. Kumar, A. K. Abbas, & J. C. Aster (Eds.), *Robbins and Cotran pathologic basis of disease* (9th ed., pp. 629–667). Elsevier.

Clinical Presentation

- Often related to the anemia, but the patient can present with jaundice, splenomegaly, iron overload, and vasoocclusive crisis.

Diagnosis

- Often diagnosed in childhood. Incidental findings of mild microcytic anemia may warrant investigation of at-risk populations. Hemoglobin electrophoresis is the diagnostic test of choice.

Evaluation and Treatment

- Blood transfusion in extreme cases; folate supplementation, antibiotic prophylaxis for asplenic patients.

SICKLE CELL DISEASE

General Principles

- Genetic disorder due to the mutation in the hemoglobin beta gene found on chromosome 11. This defect results in hemoglobin S and sickle-shaped RBCs. These sickle-shaped cells can block blood vessels and damage tissue and organs. Sickle cell anemia is the most common inherited blood disorder in the United States and is screened in all newborns. It is most prevalent in African Americans; about 1 in 400 are born with sickle cell anemia and 1 in 12 carry the gene. About one in 1400 Hispanic Americans of Caribbean ancestry also have the disease.

Clinical Presentation

- The disease is present at birth but symptoms do not arise until 5–6 months of age because of the presence of hemoglobin F. Symptoms can range from mild to severe. Early findings include anemia, jaundice, swelling of the hands and feet, and delayed growth.
  - Vasoocclusive or acute pain crisis.
    - Caused by sickled cells occluding blood flow and oxygen delivery to tissues.
    - Pain can be anywhere, but most commonly presents in abdomen, arms, chest, low back, and legs.
    - Can be triggered by high altitude, dehydration, illness, stress, and ambient temperature changes.
  - Severe anemia
    - Aplastic crisis usually caused by parvovirus B19 infection.
    - Splenic sequestration with trapping of RBCs leading to splenomegaly and a weakened or nonfunctioning spleen (autosplenectomy).
  - Infectious
    - Asplenic individuals are at risk for infection, especially owing to encapsulated bacteria such as *Streptococcus pneumoniae*, *Haemophilus influenzae*, and *Neisseria meningitides*.
  - Acute chest syndrome (ACS)
    - Caused most commonly by infection but can be due to sickling in the blood vessels of the lungs.
    - Damages areas of the lungs and impairs oxygen exchange.
    - Usually starts a few days after a vasoocclusive crisis begins (often during in-patient hospitalization).
    - Symptoms include chest pain, cough, fever, and dyspnea.
  - Cerebrovascular accident
    - Can be found in as many as 24% of people by age 45.
    - Often large vessels such as the internal carotid or middle cerebral are affected with devastating consequences.
    - Dysarthria, motor weakness, facial droop.
    - Recurrence rate of 50% within 2 years.
  - Sickle cell retinopathy
    - More common in sickle cell trait.
    - Present with flashes or floaters.
  - Other presentations: cardiomegaly, pulmonary hypertension, kidney disease, priapism, gallstones, liver disease, leg ulcers, and avascular necrosis (Table 50.2).

Pregnant patients have increased episodes of pain crisis, hypertension, infections, and blood clots with higher risk for miscarriage, premature births, and babies that are small for gestational age.

Diagnosis and Evaluation

- Newborns in the United States are tested for sickle cell disease as part of newborn screening. This testing also determines whether the newborn has sickle cell trait. Evaluation of the patient in the ED is based on the presenting concern.
- Anemia: baseline CBC
  - Hemoglobin: 5–9 g/dL
  - Hematocrit: 17–29%
  - Reticulocyte count: elevated, depending on bone marrow function. A depressed count is concerning for aplastic crisis.
  - Peripheral blood smear: target cells, elongated cells, and sickle cells. Asplenic patients have Howell-Jolly bodies.
- Vasoocclusive crisis
  - Occurs in about 50% of all patients with hemoglobin S.
  - Variable occurrence from rare to monthly in some patients.
  - Sudden onset and may last hours to days.

TABLE 50.2 *Organ Damage Seen in Sickle Cell Disease*

Organ or System	Injury
Skin	Stasis ulcer
Central nervous system	Cerebrovascular accident
Eye	Retinal hemorrhage, retinopathy
Cardiac	Congestive heart failure
Pulmonary	Intrapulmonary shunting, embolism, infarct, infection
Vascular	Occlusive phenomenon at any site
Liver	Hepatic infarct, hepatitis resulting from transfusion, hepatic sequestration, intrahepatic cholestasis
Gallbladder	Increased incidence of bilirubin gallstones caused by hemolysis
Spleen	Acute sequestration
Urinary	Hyposthenuria, hematuria
Genital	Decreased fertility, impotence, priapism
Skeletal	Bone infarcts, osteomyelitis, aseptic necrosis
Placenta	Insufficiency with fetal wastage
Leukocytes	Relative immunodeficiency
Erythrocytes	Chronic hemolysis

From Marx, J. A., Hockberger, R. S., & Walls, R. M. (2010). *Rosen's emergency medicine: Concepts and clinical practice* (7th ed.). Mosby.

  - Often no trigger is found, but look for cause: hypoxemia, dehydration, infection, or body temperature changes from environment.
  - Can affect any body part.
  - May be seen in hands and feet of infants up to 18 months of age (dactylitis).
- Infection
  - Asplenic patients at high risk for encapsulated bacterial infection.
  - Consider osteomyelitis (staphylococcal and salmonella) with persistent pain and fever.
- ACS
  - Leading cause of death. The diagnosis of ACS requires both (1) a new infiltrate on chest radiograph (CXR), and (2) one or more of the following: chest pain, temperature >38.5°C, respiratory symptoms (tachypnea, wheeze, cough), or hypoxia.
  - Pediatrics: usually secondary to infection. Chest pain, fever, cough, tachypnea, leukocytosis. CXR may reveal infiltrates in the upper lobes.
  - Adults: dyspnea and severe chest pain. CXR may reveal multilobar disease. Higher mortality in adults secondary to higher proportion caused by bone marrow and fat emboli.
- Cerebrovascular accident (CVA)
  - Usually ischemic in children and hemorrhagic in adults.
  - Hemiparesis is the usual presentation.
  - Other deficits depend on the location of the infarction.
  - May only see decrease in cognitive function.
  - Computed tomography reveals large or established infarcts.
  - Magnetic resonance angiography reveals small or acute infarcts and may reveal previous silent infarcts.
- Sickle cell retinopathy
  - Localized vascular occlusion with associated proliferative retinopathy, vitreous hemorrhage, and retinal detachment.
  - May have floaters, flashes, or blurry vision.
  - Can affect vision with occlusion of perifoveal capillaries.
  - Visual acuity, intraocular pressure, and retinal examination should be performed.
  - May see peripheral neovascularization on funduscopic examination.

Treatment

- Anemia
  - Transfusion is not required for usual anemia or pain crisis.
  - Simple or exchange transfusion required for severe anemia due to:
    - Acute splenic sequestration
    - Parvovirus B19 infection resulting in aplastic crisis
    - Severe ACS and hemoglobin 1 g below baseline
    - Acute ischemic stroke
    - Multisystem organ failure
    - Hepatic sequestration
    - Priapism refractory to usual therapy
  - Preoperative transfusion to a hemoglobin of 10 g/dL may decrease complications from hypoxia, dehydration, and/or hypothermia.
  - Exchange transfusion recommended for severe ACS, which includes oxygen saturations <90% despite supplemental oxygen.
- Vasoocclusive crisis
  - Hydration to maintain euvolemia; overhydration may increase risk of atelectasis and ACS. Avoid normal saline because it can lead to hyperchloremic metabolic acidosis and predispose to further sickling.
  - Analgesic: initiate analgesic therapy within 30 minutes of triage and 60 minutes of presentation.
  - Mild to moderate pain: nonsteroidal antiinflammatory drugs (NSAIDs) unless contraindicated.
  - Severe pain: parenteral opioids. Give subcutaneously if intravenous access not obtainable.
  - Reassess pain every 15–30 minutes until the patient reports the pain is under control.
  - Avoid meperidine.
  - Patient-controlled analgesia better than as-needed basis.
  - Use NSAIDs as an adjuvant analgesic unless contraindicated.
  - Oral anti-histamine for patients with pruritis from opioids.
- Infection (fever)
  - Temperature >38.5°C requires workup for sepsis.
  - Cover for streptococcal pneumonia and gram-negative enteric organisms.
  - Consider hospitalization for temperature >39.5°C or ill-appearing.
  - Investigate for ACS with immediate CXR in those with fever, shortness of breath, tachypnea, cough, and/or rales.

- Consider osteomyelitis in febrile patients with bony tenderness accompanied by erythema and swelling.
- ACS
  - Hospitalize
  - Broad-spectrum antibiotics, supplemental oxygen, and bronchodilators as needed.
  - Closely monitor for bronchospasm, acute anemia, and hypoxemia.
  - Transfuse when hemoglobin is >1 g/dL below baseline and below 9 g/dL.
  - Exchange transfusion for severe ACS (pulse oximetry <90% despite supplemental oxygen), increasing respiratory distress, progressive pulmonary infiltrates, and/or decline in hemoglobin concentrations despite RBC transfusion.
  - Incentive spirometer while awake.
- Acute CVA
  - Confirm with neuroimaging.
  - For ischemic CVA, initiate exchange transfusion in consultation with a sickle cell disease expert; exchange transfusion preferred over simple transfusion.
  - Neurology department consult for both ischemic and hemorrhagic CVA.
  - Neurosurgery department consult for hemorrhagic CVA.
  - Hydroxyurea if unable to implement exchange transfusion.
- Retinopathy
  - Check for hyphema in trauma.
  - Ophthalmology department referral; management may involve laser photocoagulation.

THALASSEMIAS

General Principles

- The thalassemias are a group of disorders in which one or more of the globin chains has a defect that disrupts the normal ratio of α-globin to β-globin production.
  - Disruption of the normal ratio causes precipitation of the unpaired globin chains and the destruction of RBC precursors in the bone marrow (ineffective erythropoiesis) and circulation (hemolysis).
  - Affected people have variable degrees of anemia and extramedullary hematopoiesis, which leads to bone changes, impaired growth, and iron overload.
- The two most common thalassemias are α and β. α-Thalassemia is caused by a gene deletion of one or more of the four α-globin genes.
  - α-Thalassemia is prevalent in southern China, Malaysia, and Thailand.
  - β-Thalassemia is highly prevalent in Africa and is caused by mutations to one or both of the β-globin genes. The mutations cause reduced expression or complete absence of the β-globin.

Clinical Presentation

- In α-thalassemia, severity of the disease correlates to the amount of normal globin production.
  - Loss of all four α chains results in either death in utero or soon after birth owing to severe anemia and hydrops fetalis.
  - Loss of three α-chain genes leads to hemoglobin H disease. The clinical severity varies from an asymptomatic state to severe transfusion-dependent anemia. Most patients require episodic transfusions and develop some degree of iron overload by adulthood.
  - Loss of two α-chain genes results in mild anemia, hypochromia, and microcytosis, with no obvious clinical manifestations.
  - Loss of a single α-chain gene leads to a silent carrier state.
- β-Thalassemia is due to gene mutation of one or both β-globin genes, and the severity of disease correlates to the amount of normal globin production. Newborns are asymptomatic because of the presence of hemoglobin F, and the diseases of thalassemia (major, intermedia, and minor) manifest at around 4–6 months of age.
  - β-Thalassemia major patients have severe and lifelong transfusion-dependent anemia. Presentation may include pallor, jaundice, and dark urine from hemolysis and abdominal swelling from hepatosplenomegaly. The severe anemia may lead to high-output heart failure, failure to thrive, and infection. Extramedullary hematopoiesis causes skeletal abnormalities of the face and long bones. Iron overload is seen later and this may affect the heart, liver, and endocrine organs.
  - β-Thalassemia intermedia is also known as non–transfusion-dependent thalassemia. Patients tend to have anemia and the typical age of presentation is 2–4 years. They may have mild to moderate anemia or become transfusion-dependent by the third or fourth decade with presentations ranging from symptoms of anemia to some degree of iron overload.
  - β-Thalassemia minor is a carrier state and is often asymptomatic. Mild anemia may be found.

Diagnosis and Evaluation

- Often there is a known family history of thalassemia or it may be suspected in a neonate, infant, or child with symptomatic anemia.
  - If the family history is positive and the type of thalassemia is known, this information will help guide the workup.
  - A negative family history does not eliminate the disease from diagnosis, because both parents may be carriers.
- Initial laboratory testing should include a CBC, blood smear, and iron studies. Bone marrow evaluation is not required but genetic testing and/or hemoglobin analysis confirms the diagnosis.
  - CBC reveals a microcytic, hypochromic anemia. RBC count is increased and reticulocyte counts are surprisingly low for the severity of anemia.
  - Iron studies help differentiate thalassemia from iron deficiency anemia (ferritin is low in iron deficiency) and to determine whether iron overload is present in those who are diagnosed with thalassemia.
- Other laboratory findings may include an elevated lactate dehydrogenase and indirect bilirubin from hemolysis.

Treatment

- RBC transfusion is needed for symptomatic anemia. Many patients with major or intermedia thalassemia are on a chronic transfusion regimen with transfusions being initiated at pretransfusion values of 9–10 g/dL. This higher pretransfusion indicator is used to prevent extramedullary hematopoiesis and the posttransfusion goal is 12–13 g/dL.

- Folic acid is given to patients on chronic transfusion regimens to compensate for the increased folate requirements due to the increased RBC turnover. The typical dose is 1–2 mg/d.
- Iron overload is seen in patients with β-thalassemia major or intermedia. Iron chelation is initiated with chronic transfusion therapy, serum ferritin levels greater than 1000 ng/mL, liver iron concentration that exceeds 3 mg of iron per gram of dry weight, or after the transfusion of 20–25 U of RBCs. Iron chelation and chronic transfusion therapy have allowed long-term survival in many patients.
  - Other considerations include luspatercept (a subcutaneous agent that improves RBC maturation), splenectomy, and allogeneic hematopoietic cell transplantation.

HEMOLYTIC ANEMIA

General Principles

- The typical lifespan of a RBC is 110–120 days. Age-dependent destruction occurs at a rate of about 1% of RBCs daily. Hemolysis increases the rate of premature destruction, and may be caused by intrinsic or extrinsic abnormalities to the RBC, inherited or acquired conditions, and immune versus nonimmune mechanisms.

Clinical Presentation

- Symptoms similar to those for anemia: fatigue, weakness, shortness of breath, pallor, etc.
- Patient may have jaundice.
- Severity of anemia depends on rapidity of the onset of the hemolysis.

Diagnosis and Evaluation

- Rapidly identify those patients with potentially life-threatening conditions that may require immediate intervention such as transfusion, plasmapheresis for thrombotic thrombocytopenic purpura, or hydration and diuresis for transfusion reactions.
- Once stabilized and the diagnosis of hemolytic anemia is made, obtain a thorough history and perform a physical examination to look for potential causes of hemolysis. Obtain CBC, peripheral smear, reticulocyte count, direct antiglobulin (Coombs) test. May add lactate dehydrogenase, bilirubin, and haptoglobin to help diagnose hemolysis.

Treatment

- Depends on the type of hemolysis.
- Corticosteroids 1–1.5 mg/kg initiated in the ED if due to autoimmune disease; may take 1–3 weeks to see effects.
- Transfusion for severe anemia in consultation with hematologist because transfusion may worsen the hemolytic process.
- Discontinue or avoid any causative drug or toxin.

HYPOCHROMIC ANEMIA/IRON DEFICIENCY ANEMIA

General Principals

- Iron deficiency anemia (IDA) is a frequent cause of chronic anemia seen in the ED, especially in women of childbearing age.
- The major causes of iron deficiency are decreased dietary intake, reduced absorption, and blood loss.
- In resource-rich countries, blood loss is the major cause.
- Reduced absorption can occur in celiac disease, *Helicobacter pylori* infection, and bariatric surgery.

Clinical Presentation

- Similar to other causes of anemia with fatigue, weakness, dyspnea, etc.
- Patients may have a history of pica, especially pagophagia (pica for ice).
- Red urine may be found in patients who have ingested beets (beeturia). This is found in about 10% of healthy people and 50% of IDA patients.

Diagnosis and Evaluation

- Patients may have tachycardia, pallor, and dyspnea.
- May see glossitis, cheilosis, and dry, rough skin.
- CBC may show low RBC count, low hemoglobin and hematocrit, low absolute reticulocyte count, and low mean corpuscular volume.
- Reduced or absent iron stores are characteristic, but a low serum iron level cannot be used to diagnose iron deficiency (anemia of chronic disease is also often characterized by low iron levels).
- In those without comorbidities, serum ferritin <15 mg/mL is considered the criterion standard for the diagnosis of IDA.
- Serum ferritin levels <41 mg/mL in patients with comorbidities (chronic inflammation increases ferritin levels) and transferrin saturation <16% also suggests IDA.
- Note that the anemia should also resolve with iron administration in IDA.

Treatment

- Iron administration
  - Oral iron (325 mg of ferrous sulfate three times daily) given between meals.
  - Parenteral iron if more rapid repletion required, oral iron is not tolerated, or patient is unlikely to be effectively treated with oral iron (severe anemia, ongoing blood loss, nonresponder in the past).

MEGALOBLASTIC ANEMIA

General Principles

- Megaloblastic anemia is a form of macrocytic anemia in which nucleic acid metabolism is impaired, leading to reduced efficiency of cell division and nuclear cytoplasmic dyssynchrony. Causes include deficiency of vitamin B_{12}, folate, or copper, or it can be caused by medications that interfere with purine or pyrimidine metabolism.

50

Clinical Presentation

- Usually asymptomatic from the anemia unless it is severe, which may result in the typical presentation of fatigue, weakness, dyspnea, etc.

Diagnosis and Evaluation

- Mean corpuscular volume greater than 100 fL or by observing larger-than-normal RBCs on peripheral smear.
- Search for causes of vitamin B_{12} or folate deficiency such as alcoholism, liver disease, hypothyroidism, gastric bypass, and medications that interfere with deoxyribonucleic acid synthesis or liver disease.

Treatment

- Oral replacement of vitamin B_{12} unless absorption is poor, as in pernicious anemia or intestinal blind loop.
- Folic acid can be replaced orally or parenterally.
- Stop any offending medication.

Polycythemia

General Principles

- Increased hemoglobin and/or hematocrit in peripheral blood. Hemoglobin >18.5 g/dL in males or >16.5 g/dL in females is considered elevated and hematocrit levels greater than 49% and 48%, respectively. Polycythemia can be relative, in which the elevated level is due to a decrease in plasma volume as seen in diuresis or dehydration.
- Absolute polycythemia is an increase of RBC mass and can be divided into primary and secondary polycythemia. Primary polycythemia is an increase in RBC mass caused by autonomous production of RBCs (polycythemia vera). Secondary polycythemia is an increase in RBC mass caused by an elevated serum erythropoietin (tissue hypoxia).

Clinical Presentation

- Polycythemia is often found as an incidental finding on a CBC.
- Patients may present with complaints of thrombosis (CVA, myocardial infarction, deep venous thrombosis, pulmonary embolism), hypertension, pruritus, or hemorrhage.

Diagnosis and Evaluation

- Diagnosis is made by a CBC with an elevated hemoglobin and/or hematocrit.
- Evaluation is based upon the presenting complaint.
- Patients with signs of thrombosis, hemorrhage, or other emergent findings require prompt evaluation.

Treatment

- Patients presenting with emergent conditions such as thrombosis require immediate treatment such as hydration or phlebotomy.
- Goal is a hematocrit <45%, which has been shown to decrease the incidence of thrombosis.
- Low-dose aspirin may be prescribed.

Methemoglobinemia

General Principles

- Methemoglobinemia occurs when the ferrous (Fe^{2+}) irons of heme are oxidized to the ferric (Fe^{3+}) state and are unable to reversibly bind oxygen, resulting in impaired oxygen delivery to the tissues.
- Methemoglobinemia can be congenital or acquired. Owing to a deficiency in cytochrome b5 reductase, patients with congenital disease typically have cyanosis but may be asymptomatic.
- The acquired form is more common and results from ingestion of drugs or toxins that cause an increase in methemoglobin and can be severe and even fatal.
  - The most common drugs are dapsone, topical anesthetics, and inhaled nitrous oxide, whereas the chemicals include aniline dyes, benzene derivatives, antifreeze, and chlorates.

Clinical Presentation

- Early symptoms of acquired methemoglobinemia include cyanosis with pale or blue skin and lips, tachycardia, headache, dyspnea, and lethargy.
- At higher levels, respiratory depression, coma, seizures, and death may occur.
- Methemoglobin levels of 8%–12% (1.5 g/dL) result in clinically detectable cyanosis. Symptoms typically occur when levels rise to more than 10%.
- When methemoglobin levels are >30%–40%, severe symptoms of hypoxia and even death could occur (Table 50.3).

Diagnosis and Evaluation

- Maintain a high index of suspicion when the patient presents with sudden onset of cyanosis, especially after

TABLE 50.3 ***Signs and Symptoms Associated with Methemoglobin Blood Concentrations***

Methemoglobin Concentration (g/dL)	% of Total Hemoglobin	Symptoms
<1.5	<10	None
1.5–3.0	10–20	Cyanotic skin discoloration
3.0–4.5	20–30	Anxiety, lightheadedness, headache, tachycardia
4.5–7.5	30–50	Fatigue, confusion, dizziness, tachypnea, increased tachycardia
7.5–10.5	50–70	Coma, seizures, arrhythmias, acidosis
>10.5	>70	Death

From Cortazzo, J. A., & Lichtman, A. D. (2014). Methemoglobinemia: A review and recommendations for management. *Journal of Cardiothoracic and Vascular Anesthesia, 28*(4), 1043–1047.

ingestion or use of a known agent that can cause methemoglobinemia.

- Hypoxia does not improve with oxygen administration.
- Blood is dark red, chocolate, or brown when drawn.
- Normal partial pressure of oxygen in the alveoli when there is clinical cyanosis.
- The preferred method for detecting the presence of methemoglobin is direct analysis of the blood on the absorption spectrum. Methemoglobin has a peak absorbance at 631 nm on the cooximeter.
- Pulse oximetry and arterial blood gas determination are not accurate methods for analysis.

Treatment

- Discontinue the offending agent.
- Levels less than 20% and asymptomatic patients often do not require any treatment.
- If symptomatic or with severe levels of methemoglobinemia, stabilization of airway, breathing, and circulation may be required.
- Methylene blue (MB) is the treatment of choice. Administer 1–2 mg/kg of MB intravenously over 5 minutes and the typical result is a decrease in methemoglobin to levels of less than 10% within 1 hour. Dose may be repeated at 1 hour if levels remain greater than 20%, but this is unusual.
- Ascorbic acid has also been used when MB was unavailable but requires multiple infusions and may take 24 hours or longer to decrease levels below 10%.
- If MB is unavailable or contraindicated (glucose-6-phosphate dehydrogenase deficiency), blood transfusion, exchange transfusion, or hyperbaric oxygen therapy can be performed.

SUGGESTED READINGS

Auerbach, M. (2019). Causes and diagnosis of iron deficiency and iron deficiency anemia in adults. *UpToDate*. Retrieved December 13, 2019, from https://www.uptodate.com/contents/causes-and-diagnosis-of-iron-deficiency-and-iron-deficiency-anemia-in-adults

Denshaw-Burke, M. Methemoglobinemia. Medscape (eMedicine). https://emedicine.medscape.com/article/204178-overview

National Heart, Lung and Blood Institute. (2014). *Evidence-based management of sickle cell disease: Expert panel report 2014*. Clinical Practice Guidelines. https://www.nhlbi.nih.gov/health-topics/evidence-based-management-sickle-cell-disease

Tefferi, A. (2019). Prognosis and treatment of polycythemia vera. *UpToDate*. Retrieved December 13, 2019, from https://www.uptodate.com/contents/prognosis-and-treatment-of-polycythemia-vera

CHAPTER 51

BOARD REVIEW

White Blood Cell Disorders

LEV LIBET, MD

The complete blood count, the most commonly ordered test in the emergency department, contains a wealth of information. This chapter focuses specifically on the white blood cell count. The two general immune cell lines are granulocytes, which are the phagocytic cells (neutrophils, monocytes, basophils, and eosinophils), and lymphocytes. These cell lines make up the two broad categories of leukemia. In this chapter, we discuss various leukemias, multiple myeloma, and leukopenia.

Leukemia

General Principles

- Leukemias make up nearly a third of all hematopoietic cancers. Fig. 51.1 shows the broad breakdown of hematopoietic cancers in North America. Resulting from a disruption in hematopoiesis, with leukemia, the progenitor cell fails to differentiate properly and proliferates uncontrollably. As opposed to lymphoma, the predominant location of the abnormal cell line in leukemia is in the peripheral circulation or bone marrow, rather than in the lymphatic system.
- If the progenitor cell is myeloid (granulocyte), then myeloid leukemia results, whereas lymphocytic leukemias result from lymphoid progenitors.
- Leukemias are categorized by their progenitor cells and further described as either acute or chronic: acute lymphocytic leukemia (ALL), chronic lymphocytic leukemia (CLL), acute myeloid leukemia (AML), and chronic myeloid leukemia (CML) (see Fig. 51.1).

ACUTE LYMPHOCYTIC LEUKEMIA (ALL)

General Principles

- ALL is the most common form of leukemia in the pediatric population, accounting for 75%; overall, it is the most common malignancy in children.
- Comprising approximately 13% of leukemias in adults, ALL arises from a B-cell progenitor 75% of the time and from a T-cell progenitor in the remainder.

Clinical Presentation

- Presenting symptoms are often vague; they include fatigue, lethargy, dizziness, and dyspnea. These symptoms are at least partly related to the resulting anemia. Patients will often have lymphadenopathy, abdominal discomfort, and easy bruising/bleeding. B symptoms, which are fever, night sweats, and weight loss, may be present.
- Signs that may be noted on examination include pallor, petechiae, ecchymoses, lymphadenopathy, and hepatosplenomegaly.

Diagnosis and Evaluation

- The complete blood count and differential are imperative in making the diagnosis. In general, the white blood cell (WBC) count is significantly elevated, although a normal leukocyte count or leukopenia may also be seen. The WBC differential may demonstrate the presence of blasts. Most patients will also be anemic and mildly thrombocytopenic, but only a minority will have profound thrombocytopenia.

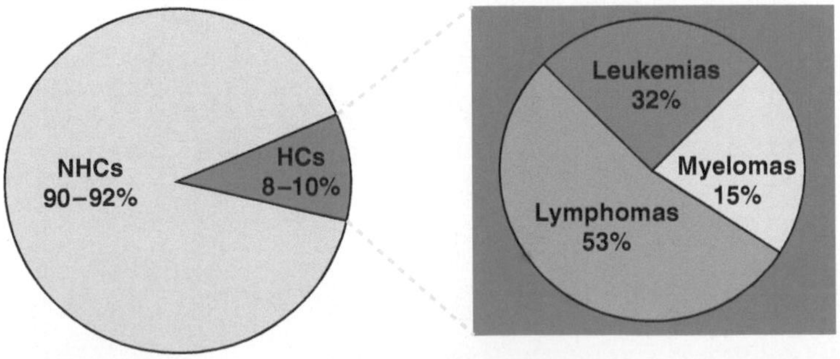

FIG. 51.1 Hematopoietic cancers. (With data from Howlader, N., Noone, A.M., Krapcho, M. et al., (Eds). SEER Cancer Statistics Review, 1975–2009 (Vintage 2009 Populations), National Cancer Institute. Bethesda, MD, *http://seer.cancer.gov/csr/1975_2009_pops09/*, based on November 2011 SEER data submission, posted to the SEER website, April 2012.) [From Mak, T. W. (2014). *Primer to the immune response*, ed 2. 2014, Chapter 20, pp. 553–585). Elsevier Inc.]. NHCs, nonhematopoietic cancers; HCs, hematopoietic cancers.

- The definitive diagnosis is made by bone marrow aspiration and biopsy. The bone marrow cells are analyzed by flow cytometry and immunophenotyping.
- Other laboratory abnormalities may include hyperphosphatemia, hyperkalemia, hyperuricemia, and elevated lactate dehydrogenase, owing to rapid cell turnover.
- Chromosomal assessment is performed using fluorescent in situ hybridization and polymerase chain reaction.

Treatment

- A testament to advances in cancer treatment, the survival rate has increased from 10% in 1960 to 90% in 2009. Response to treatment is the single most powerful prognostic factor.
- Prognosis declines with age: 5-year survival rate for adolescents, those aged 40 to 60, and those older than 60 are, respectively, 42%–63%, 24%, and 18%. Prognosis is worse in those less than 1 year of age at the time of diagnosis and in those with higher WBC counts on presentation.
- Treatment occurs in three phases.
  - Phase I: Induction therapy (4 to 6 weeks). If the Philadelphia chromosome is present, then a tyrosine kinase inhibitor is used.
  - Phase II: Consolidation or an intensive combination chemotherapy (6 to 8 months). Intrathecal chemotherapy may be used. In this phase, allogenic stem cell transplant is considered, if the patient is a candidate.
  - Phase III: Maintenance phase (2 to 3 years)
- In the emergency department, treatment for potential complications, such as neutropenic fever, tumor lysis with associate electrolyte abnormalities, and hyperviscosity should be prioritized.

CHRONIC LYMPHOCYTIC LEUKEMIA (CLL)

- CLL is also discussed under the heading of non-Hodgkin lymphoma, because it is classified as a small lymphocytic lymphoma when the disorder predominantly presents in the lymphatics.

General Principles

- A B-cell disorder generally afflicting patients older than 50, CLL is a low-grade lymphoproliferative disorder.
- In 2% to 10% of patients, CLL may undergo a transformation to an aggressive diffuse large B-cell lymphoma, a process called Richter's syndrome.

Clinical Presentation

- B symptoms are present in only approximately 10% of patients and, thus, most patients are asymptomatic at the time of diagnosis.
- Fatigue, easy bruising, and lymphadenopathy may be present and 20% to 50% of patients will have hepatosplenomegaly.

Diagnosis and Evaluation

- The absolute clonal lymphocyte count is generally greater than 5000/µL. The cells are then further categorized using flow cytometry and immunophenotyping. Cells are evaluated for the expression of CD19, CD20, CD5, and CD23 antigens (CD stands for cluster of differentiation).
- Imaging is not necessary until the patient is symptomatic.

Treatment

- Treatment is not necessary until the patient is symptomatic.
- Once symptomatic, purine analogues and chemoimmunotherapy are used.

ACUTE MYELOID LEUKEMIA (AML)

General Principles

- This type of leukemia is defined by the proportion of blasts in circulation and/or bone marrow. The clonal expansion of myeloid cells interferes with normal blood cell production, resulting in anemia and thrombocytopenia. Increasing incidence with age, AML may be primary or secondary.
- Secondary AML may arise after the use of alkylating agents, in association with certain genetic diseases, such as Fanconi's anemia, or if CML or myelodysplastic syndrome converts to AML.

Clinical Presentation

- The median age at presentation is 65. Similar to other leukemias, vague symptoms, such as anorexia, fatigue, and weight loss, predominate. Symptomatic anemia, such as dizziness and dyspnea on exertion, is often present.
- Assess for easy bruising and bleeding owing to thrombocytopenia (Fig. 51.2).
- Patients may display signs of leukemic infiltration, such as hepatosplenomegaly, bone pain, gingival infiltration, and leukemia cutis. Patients are also susceptible to infection.
- Some patients may develop hyperleukocytosis to a degree that cell counts exceed 100,000/µL, which may precipitate hyperviscosity syndrome. The clinical presentation depends on where the vascular sludging is most prominent. Patients may present with dyspnea, visual disturbances, mucosal bleeding, and a variety of neurologic complaints, including dizziness, focal weakness, headache, and seizures. Fig. 51.3 shows engorged retinal veins and deep retinal hemorrhages resulting from hyperviscosity syndrome.

51

Diagnosis and Evaluation

- Presence of 20% or more blasts in the peripheral smear and/or on bone marrow biopsy. There are nine subtypes

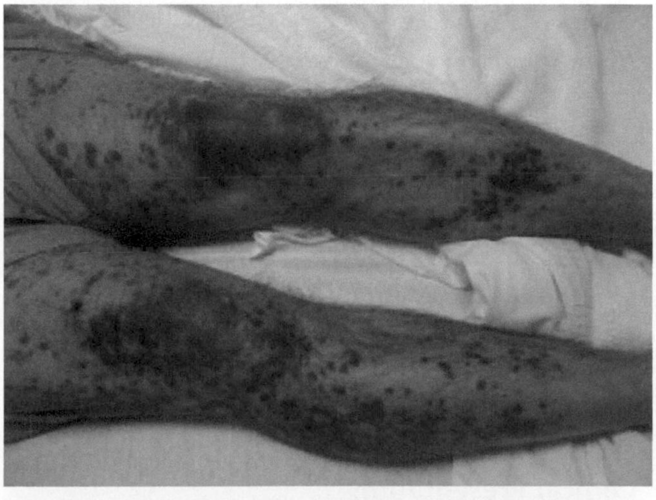

FIG. 51.2 Acute myelogenous leukemia. El Tal, A. K., Zeina T., (2008). Cutaneous vascular disorders associated with internal malignancy. *Dermatologic Clinics* 26(1).

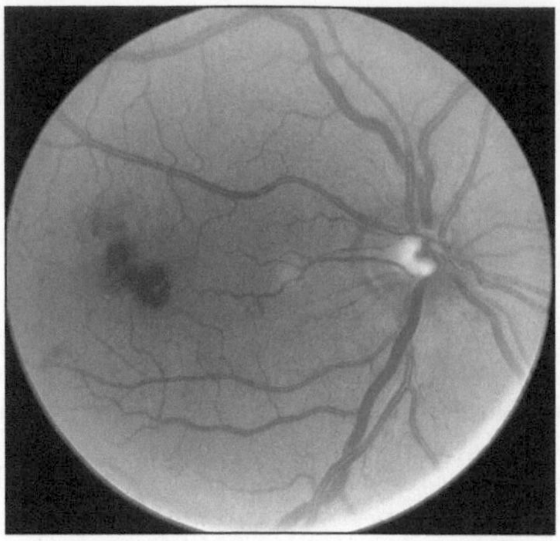

FIG. 51.3 Chronic myeloid (myelogenous) leukemias and myelodysplastic/myeloproliferative neoplasms. (From Hoffbrand, A. V. (2010). *Color atlas of clinical hematology* (Chapter 13, (pp. 233–246), Fig. 13.5). Elsevier)

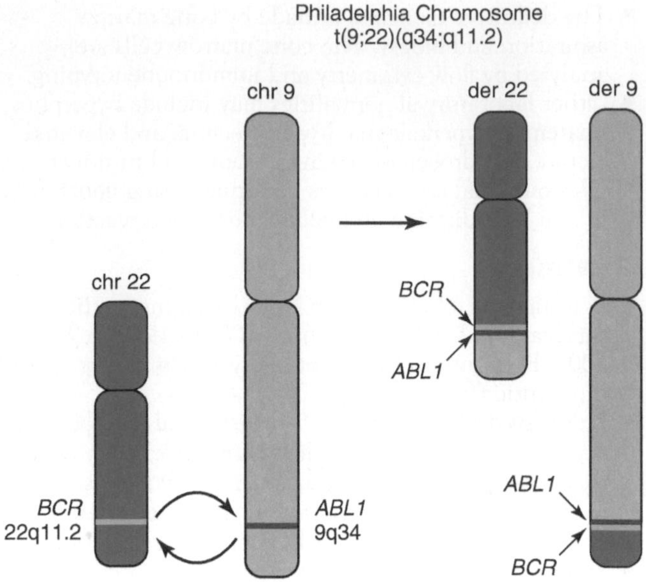

FIG. 51.4 Chronic myelogenous leukemia. (From Rathore, R. (2019). *Ferri's clinical advisor 2019* (pp. 329–330.e1, Fig. 188.1). Elsevier.)

and the diagnosis may be difficult to differentiate from other entities, such as leukemoid reaction or myelodysplastic syndrome.

Treatment

- The goal of treatment is to induce remission, which is defined as less than 5% blast cells. Induction therapy is then followed by allogenic bone marrow transplantation, autologous bone marrow transplantation, or chemotherapy alone.
- An important complication of treatment is tumor lysis syndrome, which is discussed in Chapter 48, Lymphomas.
- Hyperviscosity syndrome requires aggressive treatment. This involves supportive care and rehydration in the emergency department. Definitive treatment is emergent leukapheresis, and the postprocedure target WBC is fewer than 100,000. If the patient is comatose secondary to hyperviscosity, an emergent two-unit phlebotomy is indicated, followed by crystalloid replacement.

CHRONIC MYELOID LEUKEMIA (CML)

General Principles

- The third most common form of leukemia, CML comprises 15% of all leukemias and is defined by the presence of premature peripheral and bone marrow myeloid cells. This entity is caused by the presence of the Philadelphia chromosome, which is a fusion of the *BCR* gene on chromosome 22 and the *ABL* gene on chromosome 9 (Fig. 51.4).
- Myeloid leukemia exists on a spectrum that is described by the percent of blast cells present. In the initial phase of CML, there are less than 10% blasts. Without treatment, CML will progress to the accelerated phase in which there are 10%–19% blasts and eventually into the blast phase, defined by the presence of 20% blasts in the periphery or bone marrow.

Clinical Presentation

- Symptoms are generally indolent and progress over a course of 3 to 5 years.
- Patients will present with fatigue, malaise, mild weight loss, and perhaps night sweats. In contrast, patients with a blast crisis may manifest more prominent symptoms of fever, arthralgia, abdominal distention, anorexia, early satiety, petechiae, and/or purpura and spontaneous bleeding. Lymphadenopathy is uncommon, however.

Diagnosis and Evaluation

- The presence of more than 20% myelocytes and/or metamyelocytes in the peripheral circulation or in the bone marrow is diagnostic of CML.
- The cells are then further categorized using flow cytometry and immunophenotyping.

Treatment

- The advent of tyrosine kinase inhibitors revolutionized the treatment of myeloid leukemia. They are most effective in the chronic phase of disease, but are used in all stages. Interferon alpha may be used as second-line treatment. Chemotherapy followed by allogenic stem cell transplant is considered in those who are otherwise healthy.
- Poor prognostic indicators are age greater than 60, elevated white blood cell count, elevated platelet count, and poor response to tyrosine kinase inhibitors.

Multiple Myeloma (MM)

General Principles

- MM is a plasma cell neoplasm that is defined as clonal proliferation of plasma cells, the presence of a monoclonal protein, and associated organ dysfunction.
- It is believed to be on a spectrum of disease with monoclonal gammopathy of undetermined significance (MGUS) at the benign end. MGUS is thought to progress to smoldering myeloma and eventually symptomatic multiple myeloma.

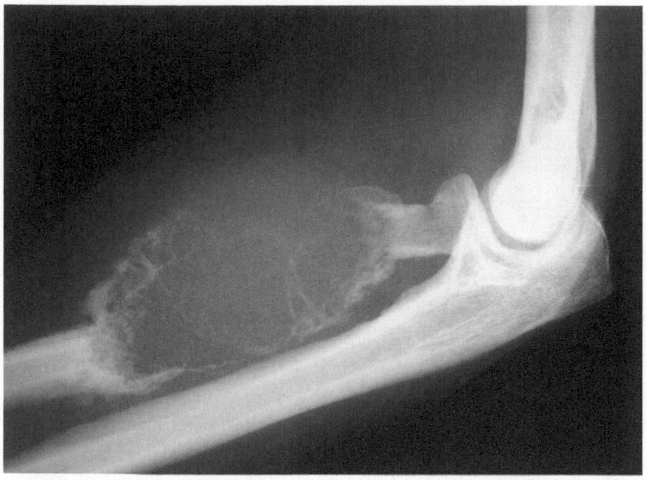

FIG. 51.5 Hematopoietic tumors. (From McCarthy, E. F. (2010). *Bone and Soft Tissue Pathology* (Chapter 18, (pp. 379–388, Fig. 18.3). Saunders, an imprint of Elsevier, Inc.)

Clinical Presentation

- The median age at presentation is 50 years. Most patients will present with anemia owing to bone marrow infiltration.
- Thus, 80% of patients will have bone involvement, and 58% of patients will have bone pain. Fig. 51.5 shows an example of a large lesion causing bone destruction. Some will present with pathologic fractures, including vertebral body compression fractures. 20%–40% of patients will have renal dysfunction.
- Hypercalcemia, secondary to osteoclastic activity, is the other contributor to symptoms and the adage "stones, bones, groans, and psychiatric overtones" is a reminder of signs and symptoms of which to be aware. Hypercalcemia may display the electrocardiographic changes of shortened QT-interval, prolonged PR-segment, widened QRS-wave, and atrioventricular blocks.

Diagnosis and Evaluation

- Complete blood count will often demonstrate a decline in the other cell lines. The creatinine and calcium level are crucial.
- Serum protein electrophoresis and urine protein electrophoresis assess for monoclonal protein (M-protein) and will likely provide the diagnosis. Table 51.1 displays the relative incidence of paraprotein types.

TABLE 51.1 *Incidence of Paraprotein Types.*

Protein	Incidence (%)
IgG	52
IgA	21
IgD	1.5
IgM (predominantly Waldenstrom Macroblobulinemia)	12
Bence Jones only	11

(From Marshall, W. J. (2017). *Clinical Chemistry* (Chapter 16, (pp. 275–291). Elsevier Ltd.)

- Bone marrow aspiration will demonstrate 10% clonal plasma cells; Fig. 51.6 provides a summary of the pathologic findings seen in MM.

Treatment

- The treatment for MGUS and smoldering myeloma is observation.
- For MM, a two- to three-agent induction protocol is used, followed by maintenance treatment. Depending on baseline health status, patients may be eligible for allogeneic bone marrow transplant.
- Treatment of hypercalcemia depends on the level, with the caveat that if symptomatic, urgent treatment is required. Severe hypercalcemia is defined as more than 14 mg/dL and, at this level, all patients require hydration with crystalloids, intravenous bisphosphonates (zoledronic acid, pamidronate, ibandronate), and calcitonin. Glucocorticoids can be considered and in those patients refractory to intravenous bisphosphonates or who have a contraindication to bisphosphonates, denosumab can be considered. As the treatment of hypercalcemia requires time, these patients need to be admitted. Once the calcium level is 18 mg/dL or greater, or if there is resulting neurologic compromise, dialysis is recommended.

Leukopenia

General Principles

- Etiologies for leukopenia may be congenital or acquired.
  - Congenital
    - Severe congenital neutropenia
    - Cyclic neutropenia
    - DiGeorge Syndrome
    - Others
  - Acquired
    - Infection
      - Sepsis
      - Human immunodeficiency virus
      - Other viruses: parvovirus, cytomegalovirus, influenza, hepatitis A, hepatitis B, Epstein-Barr virus
    - Drug-induced
      - Antineoplastic agents
      - Immunosuppressive agents
      - Clozapine
      - Methimazole, propylthiouracil
      - Sulfasalazine
      - Levamisole
      - Radiation
    - Metastatic infiltration/myelodysplastic syndrome
    - Immune
      - Primary autoimmune neutropenia
      - Secondary autoimmune neutropenia: hyperthyroidism, systemic lupus erythematosus, rheumatoid arthritis (RA), granulomatosis with polyangiitis
      - Large granular lymphocyte syndrome: often seen with RA
    - Nutritional deficiencies: Vitamin B_{12}, folate, and copper are specifically associated with neutropenia.
    - Chronic idiopathic neutropenia

51

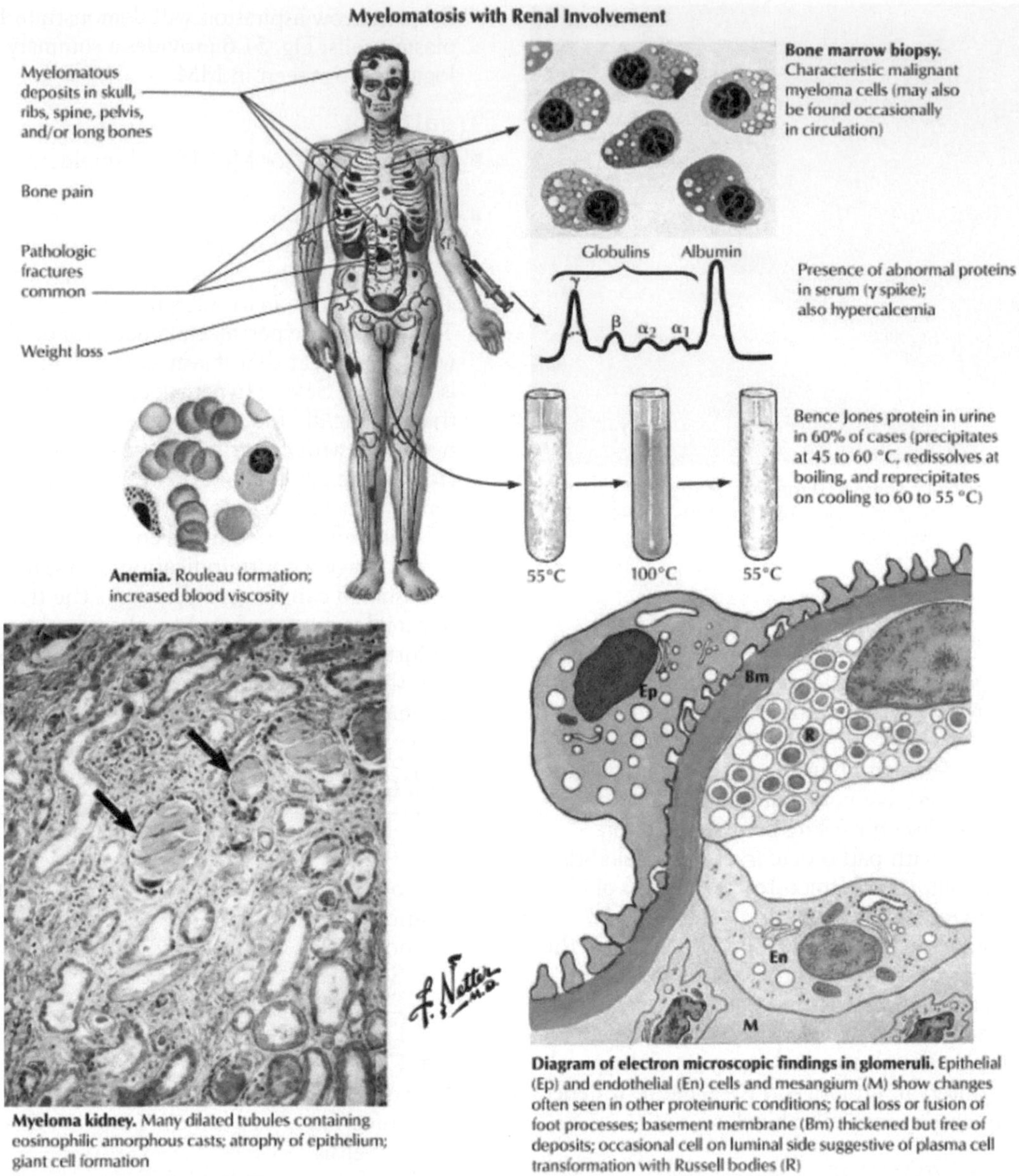
Myelomatosis with Renal Involvement
Myelomatous deposits in skull, ribs, spine, pelvis, and/or long bones
Bone pain
Pathologic fractures common
Weight loss
Bone marrow biopsy. Characteristic malignant myeloma cells (may also be found occasionally in circulation)
Globulins
Albumin
γ
β
α2
α1
Presence of abnormal proteins in serum (γ spike); also hypercalcemia
Bence Jones protein in urine in 60% of cases (precipitates at 45 to 60 °C, redissolves at boiling, and reprecipitates on cooling to 60 to 55 °C)
55°C
100°C
55°C
Anemia. Rouleau formation; increased blood viscosity
Ep
Bm
R
En
M
F. Netter M.D.
Myeloma kidney. Many dilated tubules containing eosinophilic amorphous casts; atrophy of epithelium; giant cell formation
Diagram of electron microscopic findings in glomeruli. Epithelial (Ep) and endothelial (En) cells and mesangium (M) show changes often seen in other proteinuric conditions; focal loss or fusion of foot processes; basement membrane (Bm) thickened but free of deposits; occasional cell on luminal side suggestive of plasma cell transformation with Russell bodies (R)

FIG. 51.6 From Buja, L. M., & Krueger, G. (2014). Netter's illustrated human pathology (2nd ed., Chapter 6: Kidneys, ureters, and urinary bladder). Saunders Elsevier. (Netter illustration used with permission of Elsevier Inc. All rights reserved. www.netterimages.com.)

Clinical Presentation

- Leukopenia, in and of itself, does not confer any symptoms. However, as the white blood cell count decreases, the risk of infection increases. Fewer immune cells are available to participate in an immune and inflammatory response, which leads to diminished or atypical symptomatology and signs of illness.

Diagnosis and Evaluation

- Based on the absolute neutrophil count, neutropenia is stratified into mild (1000 to 1500/μL), moderate (500 to 1000/μL), and severe (less than 500/μL).

Treatment

- Treatment depends on the underlying cause of leukopenia.

RECOMMENDED READINGS

Emerson, G., & Kaide, C. G. (August, 2018). Rapid fire: acute blast crisis/hyperviscosity syndrome. *Emergency Medicine Clinics of North America*, 36, 603–608.

Kolitz, J. E. (September, 2017). *Overview of Acute Myeloid Leukemia in Adults*. UpToDate.com.

Nabhan, C., & Rosen, S. T. (2014). Chronic lymphocytic leukemia: A clinical overview. *Journal of the American Medical Association*, 312, 2265–2276.

Palumbo, A., & Anderson, K. (2017). Multiple myeloma. *New England Journal of Medicine*, 364, 1046–1060.

Ugras-Rey, S. (2013). Selected oncologic emergencies. In J. A. Marx, R. S. Hockberger, & R. M. Walls (Eds.), *Rosen's emergency medicine: concepts and clinical practice* (8th ed.). Elsevier Saunders.

CHAPTER 52

BOARD REVIEW

Oncologic and Hematologic Emergencies

SEAN HEAVEY, MD, and RICK McPHEETERS, DO

Patients with cancer, cancer-related complaints, or complications from treatment of their cancer represent approximately 4% of all emergency department (ED) visits. The ED serves as the gateway for all hospital admissions, and emergency providers need to be aware of potential medical and surgical emergencies that are specific to patients with cancer and those undergoing treatment.

Local Tumor Effects

MALIGNANT AIRWAY OBSTRUCTION

Background

- Primary or metastatic lung cancer (breast, colorectal, and renal cancers are most common lung metastases) or malignancies adjacent to the airway (esophageal cancer, thyroid cancer, mediastinal tumors) may cause mechanical airway obstruction.
- Mechanism of airway obstruction (Fig. 52.1)
  - External compression of airway or direct tumor growth into the airway

Clinical Presentation

- Variable: spectrum from mild cough and exertional dyspnea to hemoptysis, asphyxiation, postobstructive infections
  - If no prior cancer diagnosis, patients may present multiple times and receive treatment for common causes of dyspnea (e.g., bronchitis) or be misdiagnosed with asthma or chronic obstructive pulmonary disease (COPD).
  - Presentation will depend on chest wall compliance, muscle strength, acuity of onset, rapidity of tumor growth, and severity of underlying comorbid diseases.

Diagnosis and Evaluation

- Initial evaluation should focus on assessing airway and breathing.
- Radiographic studies
  - Radiography: chest radiograph (CXR) may not be helpful unless underlying tumor is large enough to cause significant airway distortion; assessment of airways is limited by overlying bones and mediastinal structures.
  - Computed tomography (CT): can provide a good view of the anatomy within and surrounding the airway
- Pulmonary function testing
  - Generally speaking, peak flow before and after bronchodilator treatment will not change with a fixed obstruction (e.g., tumor). However, there may be some improvement if there is underlying reactive airway disease.

Management

- Advanced airway management: bag-valve-mask ventilation, endotracheal intubation, emergent surgical airway (cricothyrotomy or tracheostomy). Consider emergent ear nose and throat surgery consult for upper airway obstruction.
  - Extracorporeal membrane oxygenation can be used as a temporizing and life-saving measure in patients with complete airway obstruction until definitive airway management is performed with stenting or surgery to bypass or remove the obstruction.

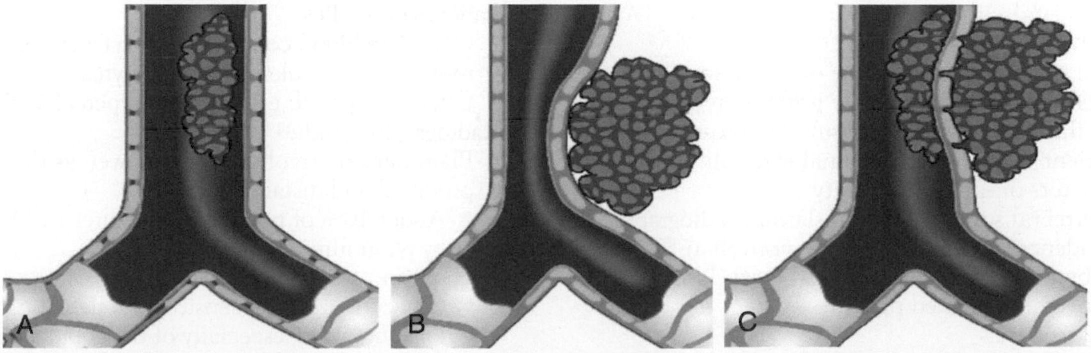

FIG. 52.1 Mechanisms of malignant airway obstruction in oncologic patients (Chua, A.-P., Santacruz, J. F., & Gildea, T. R. (2011). Pulmonary complications of cancer therapy and central airway obstruction. In *Supportive Oncology* (pp. 309–325). Elsevier. https://doi.org/10.1016/B978-1-4377-1015-1.00029-1)

- Emergent referral to specialists (otolaryngology, pulmonology, cardiothoracic surgery) for definitive management

MALIGNANT SPINAL CORD COMPRESSION

Background

- Tumor invasion of the epidural space with compression of the thecal sac
- Suspect in all patients with known cancer and back pain; 70% will be in a thoracic location
  - Spinal metastases are present in 3% to 5% of all patients dying from cancer.

Clinical Presentation

- Back pain: may be worse when supine; often the initial presenting symptom
  - May be worse at night and progress to radicular pain
- Motor weakness
  - Preferentially affects lower extremity flexors; hyperreflexia below the level of the lesion
- Sensory changes: tingling, ascending numbness and paresthesias
  - In cases of complete compression, a spinal sensory level that is one to five levels below the disease may be present.
- Urinary retention, overflow incontinence, bowel dysfunction

Diagnosis and Evaluation

- Complete and thorough physical and neurologic examinations. Postvoid residual or postvoid bladder ultrasound may also be helpful if urinary retention is suspected.
- Imaging
  - Magnetic resonance imaging (MRI) with intravenous (IV) contrast: preferred modality for initial evaluation of suspected epidural spinal cord compression; preferentially within 24 hours of presentation
  - CT myelography is an acceptable alternative if patients cannot undergo MRI, although use and availability may be institution-dependent.
    - This procedure involves direct injection of contrast into the thecal sac by lumbar puncture and can cause complications requiring urgent surgical spinal decompression. Neurosurgery should be consulted prior to the procedure and be available to address any complications.

Management

- Determine if mechanically stable or unstable spine
  - Patients who are mechanically unstable require surgical stabilization of spine. Consult a neurosurgeon for any patient with suspected spinal instability.
    - Predictors of spinal instability
      - Vertebral subluxation/translation, radiographic evidence of bone deformity, more than 50% vertebral body collapse, bilateral facet destruction, movement-related pain
- Symptomatic care
  - Glucocorticoids: reduction of inflammation and pain
    - Suggested regimen: 10 mg dexamethasone IV, then 4 mg orally every 6 hours, daily
  - Pain control: begin with nonopioid analgesics and escalate to mild-moderate opioids, as needed. Many models for escalating analgesia (such as the World Health Organization Pain Ladder) exist.
    - Referral to a pain specialist may be required.
  - Foley catheterization for urinary retention
- Definitive management: in consultation with primary oncologist/oncology team (radiation oncology, neurosurgery, and so forth). May be useful to consult patient's primary oncologist for recommendations regarding inpatient vs. outpatient treatment.
  - Surgical fixation or vertebroplasty for spinal instability, surgical decompression, conventional external beam radiation therapy

PATHOLOGIC FRACTURES

Background

- Bone metastases are common in solid tumors: lung, breast, prostate, kidney, and thyroid cancers; also common with multiple myeloma.
  - Bone is the third most common organ affected by metastatic disease; most commonly to the skull, axial skeleton, pelvis, and proximal femur.
- Pathologic fracture is a fracture through an area of bony pathology.
  - Fractures can be imminent (extensive bony destruction, but not through and through fracture).
  - Most common in lytic bone disease (e.g., multiple myeloma); also can occur with blastic metastases

Clinical Presentation

- Location-dependent: sudden onset of pain, deformity, or inability to bear weight or ambulate
  - Fractures occur with minimal trauma.
- Spine: pain on axial loading (sitting, standing)
- Neurologic symptoms
  - Caused by tumor compression of the spinal cord rather than the fracture itself, but can also occur if the fracture impinges on adjacent nerves

Diagnosis and Evaluation

- Physical examination: evidence of bony tenderness, decreased range of motion, saddle anesthesia, decreased anal sphincter tone. A complete neurologic examination is paramount.
- Laboratory studies
  - Complete blood count (CBC) to examine for concurrent anemias, leukopenia/leukocytosis
  - Chemistry panel: evaluate for hypercalcemia.
- Radiographic studies
  - Plain films of involved bone, as well as the joint proximal and distal to it
    - About 10% of pathologic fractures will be missed by plain films.
  - CT scan
    - CT scans are more sensitive for detecting pathologic fractures, especially of the shoulder, spine, and pelvis owing to their complex anatomy. Further, CT imaging is more useful for examination of the bone cortex vs. plain films.

- MRI
  - More sensitive and specific for detection of underlying tumor in spinal cord, soft tissues, and marrow
  - Not necessarily needed emergently

Management

- Pain control
  - Opioid therapy is first line for moderate to severe cancer pain.
- Consult primary oncologist and/or orthopedic surgeon to determine surgical vs. nonsurgical management options.
- Nonsurgical therapy
  - Bracing
  - Osteoclast inhibiting agents (bisphosphonates)
  - Systemic therapies: chemotherapy, hormonal therapy, immunotherapy
- Surgical management
  - Durable fixation or excision of bone and endoprosthetic reconstruction
- Radiation therapy
  - Recommended for most patients after fixation; provides pain relief, promotes mineralization, and improves functional status

MALIGNANT PERICARDIAL EFFUSION AND CARDIAC TAMPONADE

Background

- Most commonly associated with lung and breast cancers
- May also be related to chemotherapy or radiation
- Malignant pericardial effusions can lead to cardiac tamponade with impaired ventricular filling and decreased cardiac output.

Clinical Presentation

- Effusion without tamponade
  - Symptoms may be vague, related to underlying cause.
    - Dyspnea, tachycardia
- Effusion with subacute tamponade
  - Dyspnea, chest discomfort or fullness, easy fatigability
  - Hypotension with narrow pulse pressure
- Effusion with acute cardiac tamponade
  - Chest pain, dyspnea, hemodynamic instability
  - Pulseless electrical activity

Diagnosis and Evaluation

- Physical examination, with focus on airway, breathing, and circulation
  - Friction rub, pulsus paradoxus
    - Beck triad: hypotension, muffled heart sounds, jugular venous distention
- Electrocardiogram (ECG): decreased QRS complex voltage, electrical alternans
- CXR: enlarged cardiac silhouette with clear lung fields; detection of concomitant pleural effusions
- Cardiac ultrasound
  - Point-of-care ultrasound is quick, reliable, and accessible, even in patients in extremis

Management

- Initial assessment of airway, breathing, and circulation
- Acute pericardial effusion, with evidence of tamponade
  - Emergent ultrasound-guided percutaneous pericardiocentesis
- Prevention of fluid accumulation: up to 60% of patients have reaccumulation
  - Consult cardiothoracic surgery or interventional cardiology. Options include prolonged catheter drainage, pericardial window, balloon pericardiotomy, or pericardial sclerosis.

SUPERIOR VENA CAVA (SVC) SYNDROME

Background

- Majority of cases caused by external compression by mass rather than SVC thrombus
  - Compression and thrombus can coexist.
  - Compression by tumor, enlarged lymph node, or direct tumor invasion
- Often a gradual process, allowing for good collateral circulation to develop; however, rapid tumor growth may not allow time for good collaterals to develop.

Clinical Presentation

- Facial swelling or plethora, chest pain, stridor, cough, hoarseness, shortness of breath owing to pleural effusion
- Increased intracranial pressure with altered mental status (AMS), laryngeal edema causing hoarseness, syncope or near-syncope from SVC compression, and decreased cardiac output
- Physical examination
  - Distention of neck veins and chest wall veins, arm edema, cyanosis, facial plethora
  - Pemberton sign: plethora with raised arms (Fig. 52.2)

Diagnosis and Evaluation

- Imaging
  - Plain radiographs: most patients will have radiographic abnormality, such as mediastinal widening, pleural effusion, etc.
  - CT scan: venography can provide a detailed view of the anatomy.
  - Traditional venography: allows for visualization and direct intervention with endovascular recanalization in the event of a blockage
- Laboratory studies
  - CBC and coagulation studies

Management

- Evaluate for any airway compromise owing to tumor effect or edema causing compression of the airway; evaluate for respiratory distress and impending respiratory collapse.
- Presence of severe symptoms presents a medical emergency requiring either immediate endovascular recanalization with SVC stent placement or transfer to a facility with these capabilities.
- Systemic anticoagulation: if thrombus is present and causing SVC symptoms
  - Limits thrombus extension, does not speed up breakdown of existing clot
  - Remove indwelling catheters associated with thrombus.

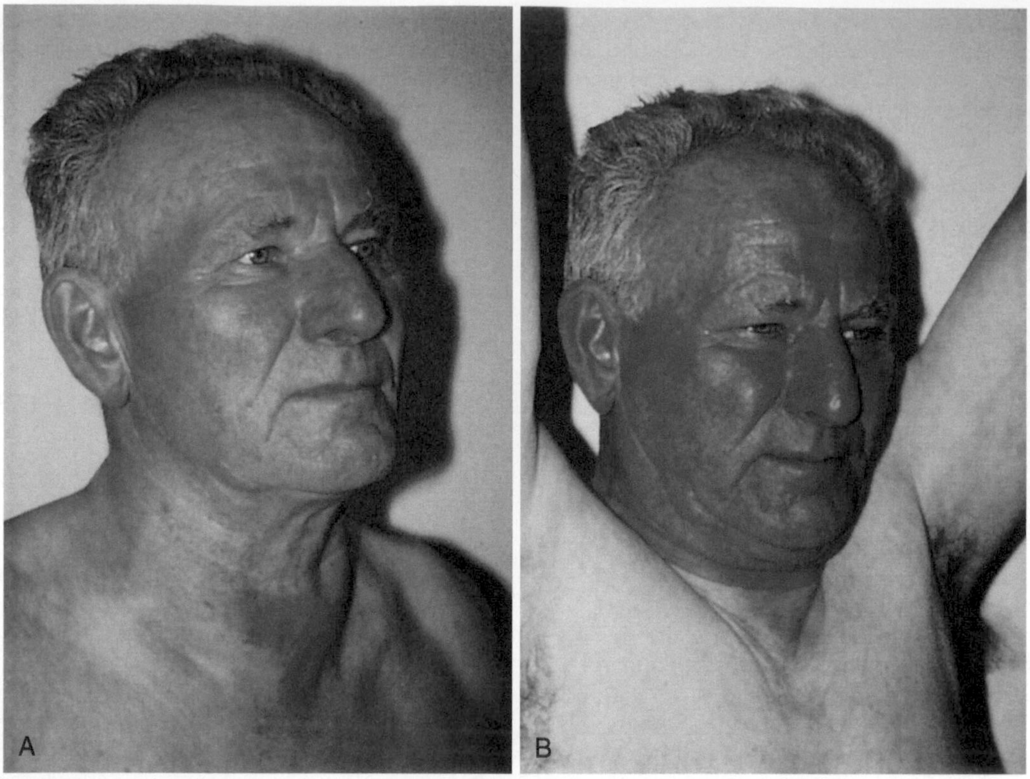

FIG. 52.2 Pemberton's sign in superior vena cava syndrome. **A**, Normal. **B**, Increased plethora of the face when arms are raised above the head for 30 seconds, consistent with compression of the superior vena cava. (Swartz, M. H. (2014). The head and neck. In M. H. Swartz (Ed.), *Textbook of physical diagnosis* (7th ed., pp. 145–160.e1, Fig. 6.14.). Saunders.)

- Glucocorticoids
  - Patients with severe airway compromise who are not candidates for stenting and who are going to receive immediate radiation treatment
  - Patients with SVC symptoms owing to a known steroid-sensitive malignancy
- Radiation therapy
  - Patients will need referral and evaluation by radiation oncologist for radiotherapy.

Metabolic Derangements

TUMOR LYSIS SYNDROME (TLS)

Background

- Associated with leukemia and lymphoma, specifically acute lymphocytic leukemia, Burkitt lymphoma, and non-Hodgkin's lymphoma
  - Rare in solid tumor malignancies, but case reports exist
- Owing to rapid turnover of tumor cells (occurring spontaneously with rapid tumor growth, or after treatment)
  - Risk factors: high proliferation rate, large tumor burden, tumor infiltration of the kidney, or extensive bone marrow involvement
  - Physiology: cell lysis with release of intracellular contents, including potassium and phosphate (which binds calcium and causes hypocalcemia), and uric acid
- Cairo-Bishop definition (Table 52.1)
  - Encompasses both laboratory and clinical definitions of TLS

TABLE 52.1 *Cairo-Bishop Definition of Tumor Lysis Syndrome*

Laboratory Tumor Lysis Syndrome (LTLS)	
Requires 2 or more laboratory abnormalities within 3 days before or 7 days after cytotoxic therapy	
Potassium	≥ 6 mEq/L or 25% increase from baseline
Uric acid	≥ 8 mg/dL or 25% increase from baseline
Phosphorus	≥ 6.5 mg/dL (children), ≥ 4.5 mg/dL (adults), or 25% increase from baseline
Calcium	≤ 7mg/dL or 25% decrease from baseline
Clinical Tumor Lysis Syndrome	
Requires presence of LTLS plus one of more of the following	
Renal involvement	Creatinine ≥ 1.5 × ULN
Cardiac involvement	Arrhythmia/sudden death
Neurologic involvement	Seizure

mEq/L, milliequivalents per liter; *mg/d*, milligrams per deciliter; *ULN*, upper limit of normal.

(Wagner, J., & Arora, S. (2014). Oncologic emergencies. *Emergency Medicine Clinics of North America, 32*(3), 509–525.)

Clinical Presentation

- Symptoms based on electrolyte abnormalities
  - Hyperkalemia (most-immediate/life-threatening): dysrhythmias

- Hypocalcemia: abdominal pain, cramping, AMS, tetany, seizures
- Hyperphosphatemia: may result in acute kidney injury (AKI) owing to precipitation of calcium phosphate crystals
- Hyperuricemia: renal failure, nausea, vomiting
- Acute renal failure
  - Uremic symptoms: nausea, vomiting, confusion
  - Uric acid precipitation causing crystal induced nephropathy: flank pain, hematuria

Diagnosis and Evaluation

- Laboratory evaluation: CBC, chemistries, uric acid, lactate dehydrogenase, urinalysis (UA)
- ECG: looking for dysrhythmias owing to electrolyte abnormalities

Management

- Aggressive fluid hydration with a urine goal output of more than 2 mL/kg/hr (between 2 and 5 liters per 24 hours for most adults)
- Management of electrolyte abnormalities
  - Hyperkalemia: only give calcium gluconate for cardiovascular instability to avoid worsening calcium phosphate deposition.
  - Hypocalcemia: treat with calcium gluconate only if symptomatic to avoid worsening calcium phosphate precipitation.
  - Hyperphosphatemia: normal saline and acetazolamide, if normal renal function. Consider dialysis if refractory.
  - Hyperuricemia
    - Rasburicase (urate oxidase): can be used for both prevention and treatment
    - Allopurinol: only helpful for prevention of further uric acid formation

HYPERCALCEMIA OF MALIGNANCY

Background

- Multiple mechanisms
  - Parathyroid hormone-related protein release: squamous cell carcinomas, breast cancer, renal cell carcinoma, endometrial cancers
  - Local osteolysis: primarily owing to bone metastasis from multiple myeloma, lung cancers, and breast cancers
  - Production of vitamin D analogs: Hodgkin's lymphoma

Clinical Presentation

- Symptomatic hypercalcemia: "Stones, Bones, Moans, Groans"
  - Renal calculi and renal failure
  - Bony pain and or pathologic fractures
  - Abdominal pain, nausea, vomiting
  - Lethargy, AMS, depression

Diagnosis and Evaluation

- Laboratory studies: CBC, chemistries, liver function tests, albumin
- 12-lead ECG

Management

- Calcium less than 12 mg/dL or asymptomatic
  - No treatment
  - Avoid thiazides, lithium, dehydration (all exacerbate hypercalcemia)
- Calcium greater than 14 mg/dL or severe symptoms
  - Intravenous rehydration with isotonic fluids
    - Infusion rate of 200 to 300 mL/hr with urine output goal of 1 to 2 mL/kg/hr
  - Calcitonin (4 units/kg IV or subcutaneous): lowers calcium within 2 to 4 hours
    - Tolerance: diminishing effect with repeat dosing
  - Bisphosphonates: lowers calcium within 12 to 48 hours
    - Good in cases of hypercalcemia caused by excessive bone resorption
  - Replete electrolytes
  - Diuretics are not routinely recommended, although furosemide is appropriate in patients with renal insufficiency, or heart failure with clinical volume overload.
  - Dialysis
    - Indications: renal failure, calcium greater than 18 mg/dL, severe hypervolemia

HYPONATREMIA AND SYNDROME OF INAPPROPRIATE ANTIDIURETIC HORMONE SECRETION

Background

- Cancers associated with ectopic antidiuretic hormone (ADH) secretion: lung, mesothelioma, duodenal, pancreatic, renal, adrenal, urothelial, cervical, ovarian, prostate, brain, carcinoid

Clinical Presentation

- Symptoms of hyponatremia: severity of symptoms is related to both the degree of hyponatremia (serum sodium less than 120 mEq/L indicates severe hyponatremia) and the chronicity of hyponatremia. Patients with an acute change in serum sodium are likely to have more severe symptoms than those with chronic hyponatremia.
  - Mild: abnormal gait, confusion, cognitive deficits
  - Moderate: nausea, headache, confusion
  - Severe: seizures, coma, vomiting

52

Diagnosis and Evaluation

- Evaluation
  - CBC, chemistries panel, serum osmolality, UA, urine osmolality, urine sodium
- Diagnostic criteria
  - Serum osmolality less than 275 mOsm/kg
  - Urine osmolality greater than 100 mOsm/kg
  - Urine sodium greater than 30 mmol/L

Management

- Severe symptoms
  - 100 to 150 mL bolus of 3% hypertonic saline over 20 minutes; may repeat bolus twice if patient remains acutely symptomatic (i.e., seizing)
  - After bolus, may infuse 3% hypertonic saline at 20 to 100 mL/hr with goal correction rate of 0.5 to 1 mEq/hr; maximum correction of 12-mEq/L change per 24 hours

- Moderate symptoms
  - 100 to 150 mL bolus of 3% saline over 20 minutes, then normal saline infusion to maintain volume. Goal rate of correction is no more than 10 mEq/L in the first 24 hours, and no more than 8 mEq/L each subsequent 24-hour period.
- Asymptomatic or mild: water restriction

ADRENAL INSUFFICIENCY

Background

- Owing to decreased hormone production secondary to exogenous corticosteroid use suppressing endogenous adrenal function or tumor invasion of the adrenal glands
  - Mineralocorticoid deficiency leads to hyponatremia, hyperkalemia, and acidosis
  - Glucocorticoid deficiency leads to hypoglycemia and hypotension
- Precipitated by sudden withdrawal of exogenous corticosteroids OR increased physiologic stressors (infection, myocardial infarction, surgery, or trauma)

Clinical Presentation

- Weakness, nausea, vomiting, refractory hypotension
- Abdominal tenderness, dehydration
- Confusion, AMS, lethargy

Diagnosis and Evaluation

- Laboratory findings: hypoglycemia, hyponatremia, hyperkalemia, low bicarbonate

Management

- Obtain cortisol levels, adrenocorticotropin hormone level, and serum renin, but do NOT delay treatment for results.
- Stress-dose steroids
  - Hydrocortisone 2 mg/kg up to 100 mg IV bolus
  - Dexamethasone 4 mg IV
  - Isotonic crystalloids
  - Supportive care

CARCINOID SYNDROME

Background

- Carcinoid tumors are typically neuroendocrine malignancies arising from the gastrointestinal system, lungs, kidneys, or ovaries. Carcinoids may be malignant or benign.
  - Symptoms of carcinoid syndrome result from tumor production of serotonin, histamine, bradykinin, and/or prostaglandins.

Clinical Presentation

- Flushing, hypotension and shock (owing to vasodilatory effects of kinin and prostaglandin), diarrhea, bronchospasm
- Tricuspid or pulmonary valvular lesions: owing to serotonin-induced fibrogenesis

Diagnosis and Evaluation

- Elevated urinary 5-hydroxyindoleacetic acid
- Imaging for tumor workup/staging, including CT, MRI, or radionucleotide imaging; may be performed in the outpatient setting
- Echocardiography (to look for valvular manifestations)

Management

- Treat shock and right-sided heart failure
- Symptomatic management
  - Octreotide to relieve flushing
  - Antihistamines
  - Loperamide for diarrhea
- If tumor is restricted to a specific area, surgical removal may be curative.

Hematologic and Immunologic Derangements

THROMBOEMBOLISM

Background

- Increased risk of thromboembolic events in patients with malignancy
  - Neoplastic cells and chemotherapies can both promote hypercoagulable state; tumor compression of vasculature can cause stasis.
- High mortality: second leading cause of death in cancer patients

Clinical Presentation

- Deep vein thrombosis: isolated limb swelling and pain
- Pulmonary embolism: shortness of breath, tachycardia, chest pain, syncope, and cardiovascular collapse (if saddle embolism)

Diagnosis and Evaluation

- CT pulmonary angiogram
- Lower extremity duplex ultrasound
- Coagulation studies, CBC, chemistries

Management

- Anticoagulation with enoxaparin, heparin, or direct-acting oral anticoagulants
  - Low molecular weight heparin, such as enoxaparin, preferred over unfractionated heparin based on American Society of Clinical Oncology guidelines
  - Warfarin is associated with higher rates of serious bleeding and venous thromboembolism recurrence when compared with low molecular weight heparin and is not recommended.
- Inferior vena cava filter placement is indicated for patients with recurrent venous thromboembolism despite adequate anticoagulation or patients in whom systemic anticoagulation is contraindicated.

NEUTROPENIC FEVER

Background

- Although dependent on a specific chemotherapy regimen, neutrophil nadir is typically 5 to 10 days after chemotherapy, with neutrophil counts rebounding 5 days after the nadir.

- Definition: temperature greater than 38 degrees Celsius (°C) for 1 hour or single temperature greater than 38.3 °C with absolute neutrophil count less than 1000 cells/mm^3. Severe neutropenia is defined as absolute neutrophil count less than 500.

Clinical Presentation

- Owing to attenuated immune response, there is absence of typical signs and symptoms to localize infectious source.
  - A careful physical examination is warranted, including an examination of all indwelling catheter sites. Defer rectal examination to prevent seeding bacteremia.

Diagnosis and Evaluation

- Laboratory studies: CBC with differential, blood cultures (including cultures drawn from all indwelling catheters), UA, urine culture, chemistries, LFTs
- Imaging: CXR
  - May appear normal in patients with neutropenia because neutrophils are required for infiltrates to appear
- Additional studies based on presenting symptoms: stool studies, lumbar puncture, CT

Management

- Multinational Association of Supportive Care in Cancer (MASCC) Risk Index Score for Febrile Neutropenia can be used to risk stratify patients and predict complications.
  - MASCC Risk Index Score stratifies patients into those who are low risk for complications owing to febrile neutropenia and those who are not low risk based on the following criteria: (1) burden of illness, (2) presence of hypotension with systolic blood pressure less than 90 mm Hg, (3) underlying COPD, (4) cancer type (solid vs. hematologic), (5) level of dehydration, (6) inpatient vs. outpatient status at onset of fever, and (7) age greater than 60 years.
    - Higher scores are associated with a lower risk for complications.
- Empiric antibiotics (Table 52.2)
  - Broad spectrum empiric coverage with anti-pseudomonal cephalosporin or extended spectrum penicillin. Add vancomycin for mucositis, catheter site infection, hypotension, or high risk for methicillin resistant *Staphylococcus aureus* (MRSA).
- Admit in conjunction with treating oncologist.

HYPERVISCOSITY SYNDROME

Background

- Impaired blood flow caused by high levels of paraproteins or blood cells
  - Causes sludging and stasis; impairs microcirculation and leads to tissue hypoperfusion.
- Most common in acute leukemia, polycythemia, and myeloma

Clinical Presentation

- Vague initial symptoms: fatigue, abdominal pain, headache, blurry vision, dyspnea, fever, AMS.
- Thrombosis or bleeding are also possible presentations.

TABLE 52.2 ***Empiric Antibiotics for Neutropenic Fever***

First-line therapy	Cefepime Carbapenem (meropenem or imipenem-cilastatin) Piperacillin-tazobactam
Severe penicillin allergy or complication (hypotension or pneumonia)	Aminoglycoside Fluoroquinolone
Suspected catheter-related infection, skin and soft-tissue infection, health care-associated infection, or hemodynamic instability, add extended gram-positive coverage	Vancomycin Linezolid Daptomycin

(From White, L., & Ybarra, M. (2014). Neutropenic fever. *Emergency Medicine Clinics of North America, 32*(3), 549–561.)

- Symptoms are worse with dehydration.

Diagnosis and Evaluation

- Laboratory studies: CBC, chemistries
  - White blood cell (WBC) greater than 100,000
  - Hematocrit greater than 60%
  - Peripheral smear with rouleaux formation
  - Abnormal protein electrophoresis

Management

- Hydration with isotonic fluids
- Hematology consult for plasmapheresis or leukapheresis if hyperviscosity is caused by leukostasis
  - If plasmapheresis is unavailable, phlebotomy of 2 to 3 units of blood, then infusion of 2 to 3 liters of IV fluids as a temporizing measure

LEUKOSTASIS AND HYPERLEUKOCYTOSIS

Background

- Hyperleukocytosis is defined as WBC greater than 50,000 to 100,000.
- Leukostasis is *symptomatic* hyperleukocytosis.
  - Medical emergency with 20% to 40% mortality within 1 week
  - Most commonly associated with blast crisis in acute myeloid leukemia or chronic myeloid leukemia; brain and lungs primarily affected

Clinical Presentation

- Fevers are common and associated with concurrent infection.
- Neurologic: range from headache to coma, stupor, and death
- Respiratory: respiratory distress, respiratory failure

Diagnosis and Evaluation

- CBC with WBC greater than 50,000 to 100,000
- Platelets, prothrombin time, d-dimer, fibrinogen (up to 40% of patients are found to have disseminated intravascular coagulation)
- CXR may show pulmonary interstitial infiltrates.

TABLE 52.3 *Drug-Specific Side Effects of Chemotherapy*

Side Effect	Chemotherapy Agent/Class
Cardiotoxicity	Anthracyclines (doxorubicin)
Progressive pulmonary fibrosis	Bleomycin Busulfan
Neurotoxicity (neuropathy)	Cisplatinum Vinka Alkaloids (Vinblastine, Vincristine)
Nephrotoxicity	Cisplatinum Tyrosine Kinase Inhibitors (Imatinib)
Skin (plantar-palmar dermatitis)	5-fluorouracil
Reproductive sterility	Anthracyclines (doxorubicin) Alkylating Agents (cyclophosphamide) Docetaxel
Secondary malignancy	Alkylating agents (cyclophosphamide)

(Gallagher, C. J., Smith, M., & Shamash, J. (2017). Malignant disease. In P. Kumar & M. Clark (Eds.), *Kumar and Clark's Clinical Medicine* (9th ed., pp. 583–644). Elsevier.)

Management

- Asymptomatic hyperleukocytosis: hydroxyurea
- Leukostasis
  - IV fluids since dehydration can worsen symptoms
  - Hydroxyurea and plasmapheresis are temporizing.
  - Chemotherapy is the only therapy shown to improve survival.
- ICU admission

Treatment-Related Complications

COMMON SYSTEMIC TOXICITIES OF CHEMOTHERAPEUTIC AGENTS

- Nausea, vomiting, hair loss, myelosuppression, mucositis, and fatigue are most common.
- Specific chemotherapy agents and their toxicities (Table 52.3)

Chemotherapy-Induced Nausea and Vomiting

BACKGROUND

- Chemotherapy can be emetogenic, working centrally on noxious chemoreceptors in the chemoreceptor trigger zone in the medulla.

Clinical Presentation

- History of recent chemotherapy with persistent nausea and vomiting
- Clinical signs of dehydration/malnutrition

Diagnosis and Evaluation

- Rule out infection, brain metastasis, and edema as causes of nausea and vomiting.

TABLE 52.4 *Antiemetic Drugs for Chemotherapy-Related Nausea and Vomiting*

Dopamine receptor antagonists	Metoclopramide Promethazine*
Serotonin receptor antagonist	Ondansetron
Corticosteroids	Dexamethasone
Benzodiazepines	Lorazepam
Histamine receptor antagonists	Diphenhydramine

*Not currently approved by the Food and Drug Administration for treatment of chemotherapy-related nausea and vomiting.

Management

- Rehydration with IV fluids
- Correct electrolyte abnormalities.
- Antiemetic agents (Table 52.4)

STEM CELL TRANSPLANT COMPLICATIONS

Background

- High lifetime risk of complications in patients after transplant

Clinical Presentation

- Gastrointestinal complications: diarrhea (graft-versus-host disease [GVHD], neutropenic enterocolitis, viral enteritis), odynophagia and dysphagia (acute GVHD mucositis, infectious mucositis, chronic GVHD with stricture), abdominal pain (acute GVHD, viral hepatitis, biliary disease, vasoocclusive disease)
- Pulmonary complications: radiation pneumonitis, pulmonary edema, pleural effusions (increased hydrostatic pressure and increased capillary permeability), bronchiolitis obliterans, diffuse alveolar hemorrhage, GVHD
- Infectious complications: viral (cytomegalovirus pneumonitis is most fatal), bacterial (pneumonia, endocarditis, urinary tract infection, colitis, meningitis), fungal (candida, pneumocystis, aspergillus)
- Skin complications: GVHD rash, dermatitis

Management

- Definitive management requires specialty care
- In the ED, focus on supportive care: supplemental oxygen, noninvasive positive-pressure ventilation, intubation, bronchodilators, corticosteroids, broad-spectrum antibiotics if infection is suspected.

COMPLICATIONS ASSOCIATED WITH BIOLOGICS AND SMALL MOLECULE INHIBITORS

Background

- Many new targeted therapies for cancer, including small molecule inhibitors and biologic therapies with targeted antibodies
  - Unique side effects caused by interactions with immune system

Clinical Presentation

- Patients on small molecule inhibitors or biologic agents presenting with immune-related complaints
  - Diarrhea, colitis, pneumonitis, dermatitis, vasculitis

Diagnosis and Evaluation

- Clinical diagnosis: maintain high clinical suspicion
- Basic laboratory studies: CBC, chemistries

Management

- Consult with treating oncologist
- Systemic glucocorticoids indicated for neurologic, pulmonary, or cardiac toxicity

SUGGESTED READINGS

Barquín-García, A., Molina-Cerrillo, J., Garrido, P., Garcia-Palos, D., Carrato, A., & Alonso-Gordoa, T. (2019). New oncologic emergencies: What is there to know about immunotherapy and its potential side effects? *European Journal of Internal Medicine*, 66, 1–8.

Khan, U. A., Shanholtz, C. B., & Mccurdy, M. T. (2014). Oncologic mechanical emergencies. *Emergency Medicine Clinics of North America*, *32*(3), 495–508.

McCurdy, M. T., & Shanholtz, C. B. (2012). Oncologic emergencies. *Critical Care Medicine*, *40*(7), 2212–2222.

Wagner, J., & Arora, S. (2014). Oncologic metabolic emergencies. *Emergency Medicine Clinics of North America*, *32*(3), 509–525.

SECTION EIGHT

BOARD REVIEW

Immune system

Systemic Rheumatic Disease

JAGDIPAK S. HEER, MD, and SARAH GRACIE GONZALEZ, MD

Formerly referred to as collagen vascular disorders, systemic rheumatic diseases are a group of autoimmune disorders that can range from a focal presentation of a specific organ system to systemic manifestations.

Raynaud Phenomenon

General Principles

- Raynaud phenomenon (RP) is characterized by vasoconstriction of the distal digits induced by cold temperatures or emotional stress.
- More common in women, and can be associated with migraines, livedo reticularis, and fibromyalgia.
- Considered a primary condition if it occurs without an underlying cause.
- RP is secondary when it is part of another systemic rheumatic disease or a hematologic abnormality (e.g., systemic lupus erythematosus [SLE]) or cryoglobulinemia, respectively.

Clinical Presentation

- Typically begins in a single digit, and spreads to other digits, but usually spares the thumb. Can also affect the toes.
- Has a sharp demarcation of white coloration owing to vasoconstriction, followed by cyanosis owing to tissue hypoxia, and eventually erythema when reperfusion occurs
- Presents as white and blue finger skin pallor (Fig. 53.1)
- Nailfold capillary microscopy can help distinguish between primary and secondary RP.
- Predisposing factors include hypothyroidism, prior occupational trauma, and frostbite.

Diagnosis and Evaluation

- Diagnosis is made by history and physical examination findings.
- Can be isolated or a symptom of a systemic autoimmune disorder (e.g., SLE, scleroderma, mixed connective tissue disease, Sjogren's syndrome, and dermatomyositis/polymyositis).
- Differential diagnosis includes peripheral neuropathy, acrocyanosis, and complex regional pain syndrome.
- Obtain antinuclear antibody (ANA) and other specific antibody tests if an underlying autoimmune disorder is suspected.

Treatment

- Treatment includes nonpharmacologic therapies, such as keeping digits warm and avoiding cold temperatures.
- Calcium channel blockers, such as amlodipine, are the mainstay of pharmacologic therapy.

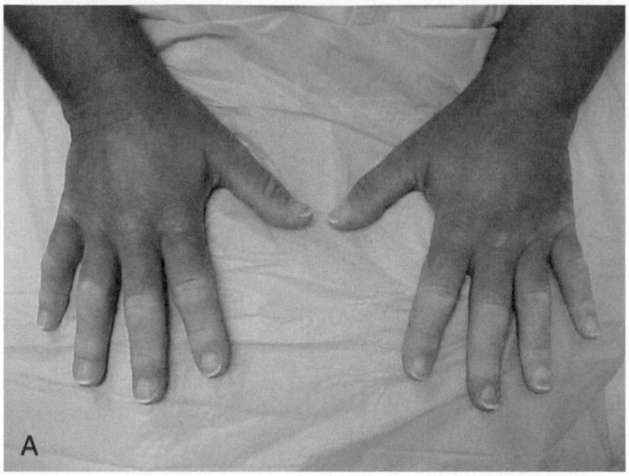

FIG. 53.1 Raynaud phenomenon. (From Fuhlbrigge, R. (2016). Raynaud phenomenon and vasomotor syndromes. In R. E. Petty, R. M. Laxer, C. B. Lindsley, & L. Wedderburn (Eds.), *Textbook of pediatric rheumatology* (7th ed., pp. 436–447.e3, Fig. 311). Elsevier.)

Reactive Arthritis (Formerly Reiter's Syndrome)

General Principles

- Form of spondyloarthritis that occurs following a recent extraarticular infection, caused by certain enteric and genitourinary pathogens.
- Classic triad of "can't pee, can't see, can't climb a tree;" which represents urethritis, conjunctivitis, and arthritis.

Clinical Presentation

- Presents as an acute asymmetric oligoarthritis 1–4 weeks following an inciting infection, such as urethritis or gastroenteritis.
- Usually associated with enteric bacteria, such as *Salmonella*, *Shigella*, *Yersinia*, *Campylobacter*, and *Clostridium difficile*.
- Most common genital pathogen is *Chlamydia trachomatis*.
- Symptoms include arthritis, dactylitis, and back pain.
- Common extraarticular symptoms include conjunctivitis, uveitis, oral lesions, and cutaneous and nail changes.

Diagnosis and Evaluation

- Patients will have elevated acute phase reactants, erythrocyte sedimentation rate (ESR), and C-reactive protein (CRP).
- There is a genetic predisposition with human leukocyte antigen-B27.

- Plain radiographs can be done to exclude other underlying causes of symptoms, but there is no specific finding on a plain radiograph that can establish the diagnosis.
- Arthrocentesis should be performed on patients presenting with a joint effusion to exclude septic arthritis. Synovial fluid should be examined for cell count and differential, crystals, gram stain, and culture.
- Pathogens typically cannot be cultured from the joints in reactive arthritis.

Treatment

- Treatment of the underlying active infection, if indicated (e.g., chlamydia); otherwise, symptomatic treatment of the arthritis with nonsteroidal antiinflammatory drugs (NSAIDs).
- Good prognosis with spontaneous remission in 6–12 months. However, a few will develop pain or evolve to a chronic spondylarthropathy.

Rheumatoid Arthritis

General Principles

- Rheumatoid arthritis is a chronic systemic inflammatory disease that involves the synovial joints. Uncontrolled rheumatoid arthritis (RA) leads to erosion of cartilage and bone, resulting in joint deformities.

Clinical Presentation

- Insidious onset of synovial joint inflammation and pain in a symmetric presentation. Disease course can fluctuate with exacerbations and reductions of disease activity.
- Commonly involves the metacarpal joints, proximal interphalangeal joints, wrists, and metatarsophalangeal joints; can have symptoms in other synovial joints, such as elbows, shoulders, ankles, and knees.
- Presents with morning stiffness that improves with movement.
- Can lead to swan neck deformity and boutonniere deformity (Figs. 53.2 and 53.3) when erosion to the cartilage and bone occurs.
- Extraarticular features of anemia, scleritis, muscle weakness, and skin ulcers are a few of the many features that can occur.
- Cricoarytenoid joint involvement can cause hoarseness and inspiratory stridor.
- Cervical subluxation owing to longstanding joint instability can lead to subluxation, causing cord compression, and can present with hyperreflexia and Babinski reflex.
- Juvenile Inflammatory arthritis (previously juvenile rhumatoid arthritis) has a number of manifestations including arthritis with evanescent salmon-colored rash and fever spikes 1-2 times per day.

Diagnosis and Evaluation

- The 2010 American College of Rheumatology (ACR)/ European League Against Rheumatism (EULAR) classification criteria for RA is based on synovitis in the joints and serologic abnormalities to make the diagnosis.
  - Serologic tests include rheumatoid factor, anticitrullinated peptide/protein antibody, ESR, and CRP.
  - Plain radiographs may demonstrate joint space narrowing, periarticular osteopenia, and bony erosions.

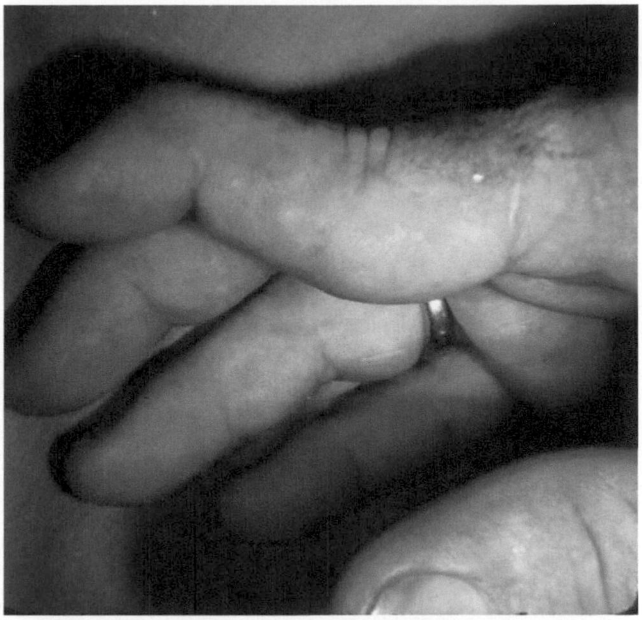

FIG. 53.2 Swan neck deformity. (From Waldman, S. D. (2016). Physical diagnosis of pain: An atlas of signs and symptoms (3rd ed., p. 195), Fig. 123.2). Elsevier.)

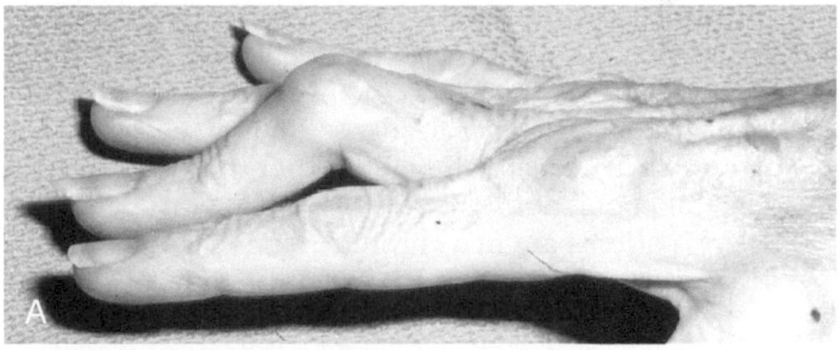

FIG. 53.3 Boutonniere deformity. (From Williams, K., & Terrono, A. L. (2011). Treatment of boutonniere finger deformity in rheumatoid arthritis. *Journal of Hand Surgery,* 36(8), 1388–1393.)

Treatment

- Treatment can involve a combination of antiinflammatory therapy (e.g., NSAIDs and steroids), disease-modifying antirheumatic drugs, and biologic agents.
- Physical and occupational therapy also help with mobility and function.
- Treatments can also have their own set of complications; thus, it is important to perform appropriate screenings and laboratory work prior to the initiation of therapy.

53

Systemic Lupus Erythematosus

General Principles

- Systemic lupus erythematosus is a systemic autoimmune disorder that can affect multiple organ systems and can range from mild to life-threatening symptoms.

Clinical Presentation

- Systemic lupus erythematosus can present with a broad range of symptoms. Table 53.1 lists the common clinical presentations based on organ system. The difficulty in treating patients with systemic autoimmune disorders stems from

TABLE 53.1 Common Systemic Lupus Erythematosus (SLE) Presentations

Organ System	Common Presentations
Constitutional	Fatigue, fever, weight loss, lymphadenopathy
Pulmonary	Pleural effusion, pleurisy, pneumonia, pulmonary embolism
Cardiac	Pericarditis, myocarditis, pericardial effusion
Renal	Nephritis
Nervous system	Seizures, psychosis, autonomic dysfunction, neuropathy
Dermatologic	Malar rash, discoid rash, hair loss, photosensitivity
Musculoskeletal	Myositis, arthritis/arthralgias
Vascular	Vasculitis, Raynaud's phenomenon
Ophthalmologic	Uveitis
Hematologic	Leukopenia, thrombocytopenia, anemia

the fact that any organ can be affected, and single or multiple organ systems can be affected during a disease flare.

- Clinical course is variable, with some patients having a benign course with remissions and few exacerbations, whereas others have a rapidly progressive fulminant course leading to death.
- Mortality is two to five times greater than in the general population.
- Many patients are in a chronic immunocompromised state owing to immunosuppressant therapy.
- Treating patients with SLE and differentiating the underlying etiology based on the clinical presentation can be difficult. There are a few important pearls to remember when evaluating patients with lupus:
  - Patients can have accelerated atherosclerosis and can present with acute coronary syndrome at a young age.
  - Patients who are positive for anticardiolipin antibody present with recurrent miscarriages and venous thromboembolism.
  - It is also important to consider side effects from immunosuppressant medications (e.g., infection and avascular necrosis).
- Patients can also have overlapping autoimmune disorders and have mixed connective tissue disease.

Diagnosis and Evaluation

- There are two longstanding classifications systems for the diagnosis of SLE:
  - The American College of Rheumatology 1997 criteria, which uses 4 of 11 criteria to meet the diagnosis of SLE
  - Systemic Lupus International Collaborating Clinics 2012 classification criteria, in which patients must meet 4 of 17 criteria
- In 2019 the EULAR and ACR developed a new classification system with more sensitivity and specificity.
  - It uses the ANA titer as the entry criterion, and then has additive criteria that have a weighted point system.
  - The additive criteria are grouped into clinical and immunology domains, as shown in Table 53.2.
- On average, it takes patients with lupus 6 years from onset of symptoms to a diagnosis of SLE, making it very unlikely to diagnose a patient in one encounter. It is important to take a thorough history and perform a physical examination and to consider the possibility of drug-induced lupus.
- Laboratory studies should include complete blood cell count, complete metabolic panel, urinalysis, and urine pregnancy.
- In the acute setting, an ESR and CRP can be useful when it is difficult to differentiate the underlying cause of symptoms. Although not definitive, if the ESR rise is greater than the rise in the CRP, the symptoms more likely may be owing to lupus. Conversely, if the CRP rise is greater than the ESR rise, the cause may not be an exacerbation of lupus but could be caused by an underlying infection.
- Specific antibody tests, such as ANA and anti-dsDNA, may be helpful for the outpatient provider following the patient, but are not helpful in the acute care setting owing to processing time for antibody tests.

Treatment

- Treatment can involve a combination of anti-inflammatory therapies. Disease-modifying anti-rheumatic drugs (e.g., azathioprine, methotrexate), immunosuppressants (e.g., mycophenolate), and biologic agents (e.g., rituximab) are all used commonly off label for the treatment of SLE. The only U.S. Food and Drug Administration-approved medications for SLE are hydroxychloroquine, steroids and, in more recent years, the biologic agent, belimumab.

Vasculitis

General Principles

- Vasculitides comprise a group of disorders defined by the presence of inflammatory leukocytes in vessel walls, which causes bleeding and compromise of the lumen, resulting in ischemia and necrosis. Classification is by the size of the vessel predominately involved as shown in Fig. 53.4. Other classifications include those associated with an etiology of another underlying disease (e.g., SLE, RA, or cryoglobinemia vasculitis caused by hepatitis C).
  - Large vessel: Takayasu and giant cell
  - Medium vessel: polyarteritis nodosa and Kawasaki
  - Small vessel: microscopic polyangiitis, Behcet's, granulomatosis with polyangiitis and Henoch-Shonlein purpura.

Clinical Presentation

- Presentation is based on each type of vasculitis; however, some commonalities are seen among the different syndromes. Patients will usually have systemic symptoms of fever, fatigue, weight loss, and arthralgias. A detailed history, including drug use, infectious disease exposure, and medications, will help in delineating if a vasculitis is the underlying cause.

TABLE 53.2 *2019 Classification Criteria for Systemic Lupus Erythematosus (SLE)**

Entry Criterion: Antinuclear antibody (ANA) at a titer ≥1:80 on Hep-2 cells or an equivalent test (ever)

Clinical Domains and Criteria	Weight	Immunology Domains and Criteria	Weight
Constitutional Fever	2	Antiphospholipid antibodies Anticardiolipin antibodies OR Anti-β2GP1 antibodies ORLupus anticoagulant	2
Hematologic Leukopenia Thrombocytopenia Autoimmune hemolysis	3 4 4	Complement Proteins Low C3 OR low C4 Low C3 AND low C4	3 4
Neuropsychiatric Delirium Psychosis Seizure	2 3 5	SLE-specific antibodies Anti-dsDNA antibody OR Anti-Smith antibody	6
Mucocutaneous Nonscarring alopecia Oral ulcers Subacute cutaneous OR Discoid lupus Acute cutaneous lupus	2 2 4 6		
Serosal Pleural or pericardial effusion Acute pericarditis	5 6		
Musculoskeletal Joint involvement	6		
Renal Proteinuria > 0.5g/24 h Renal biopsy class II or V lupus nephritis Renal biopsy class III or IV lupus nephritis	4 8 10		
Total of highest score in each domain. Classify as SLE with entry criterion fulfilled AND a score of 10 or more of additive criteria.			

*American College of Rheumatology (ACR)/European League Against Rheumatism.

Note: If an entry criterion is absent, do not classify as SLE. Do not count a criterion if a more likely explanation than SLE. Criterion needs to occur at least once. Criteria do not need to count simultaneously.

(From Aringer, M., Costenbader, K., Daikh, D., et al. 2019. European League Against Rheumatism/American College of Rheumatology classification criteria for systemic lupus erythematosus. *Arthritis & Rheumatism* 71(9), 1400–1412. Epub 2019 August 6.)

- A child with 5 days of fever accompanied by oral changes, rash, non-purulent conjunctivitis, extremity changes and cervical lymphadenopathy >1.5 cm likely has Kawasaki Disease.
- A child under 10 years with symmetric palpable purpura on legs and buttocks, arthritis, and abdominal pain may have HSP.

Diagnosis and Evaluation

- Physical examination findings can be subtle and include sensory and/or motor neuropathy, palpable purpura, and an abnormal vascular examination. Absent or diminished pulses or tender superficial arteries, along with bruits or blood pressure discrepancies can help in identifying a vasculitis, especially a large-vessel vasculitis. Testing should include a complete blood cell count, complete metabolic panel, ESR, CRP, viral hepatitis serologies, serum cryoglobulins, urinalysis with urine sediment, and blood cultures to rule out infection.
- More specific testing includes an ANA, complement levels and antineutrophil cytoplasmic antibody. Symptoms will guide further testing (e.g., chest radiograph) if respiratory symptoms present. Biopsy of the involved tissue is critical for diagnosis, but not always possible. It is important to rule out mimics of vasculitis (e.g., endocarditis, drug exposure).

Treatment

- Treatment is based on the specific vasculitis and the extent of the disease. In general, treatments entail immunosuppressive therapy and antiinflammatory medications (e.g., NSAIDs and prednisone).

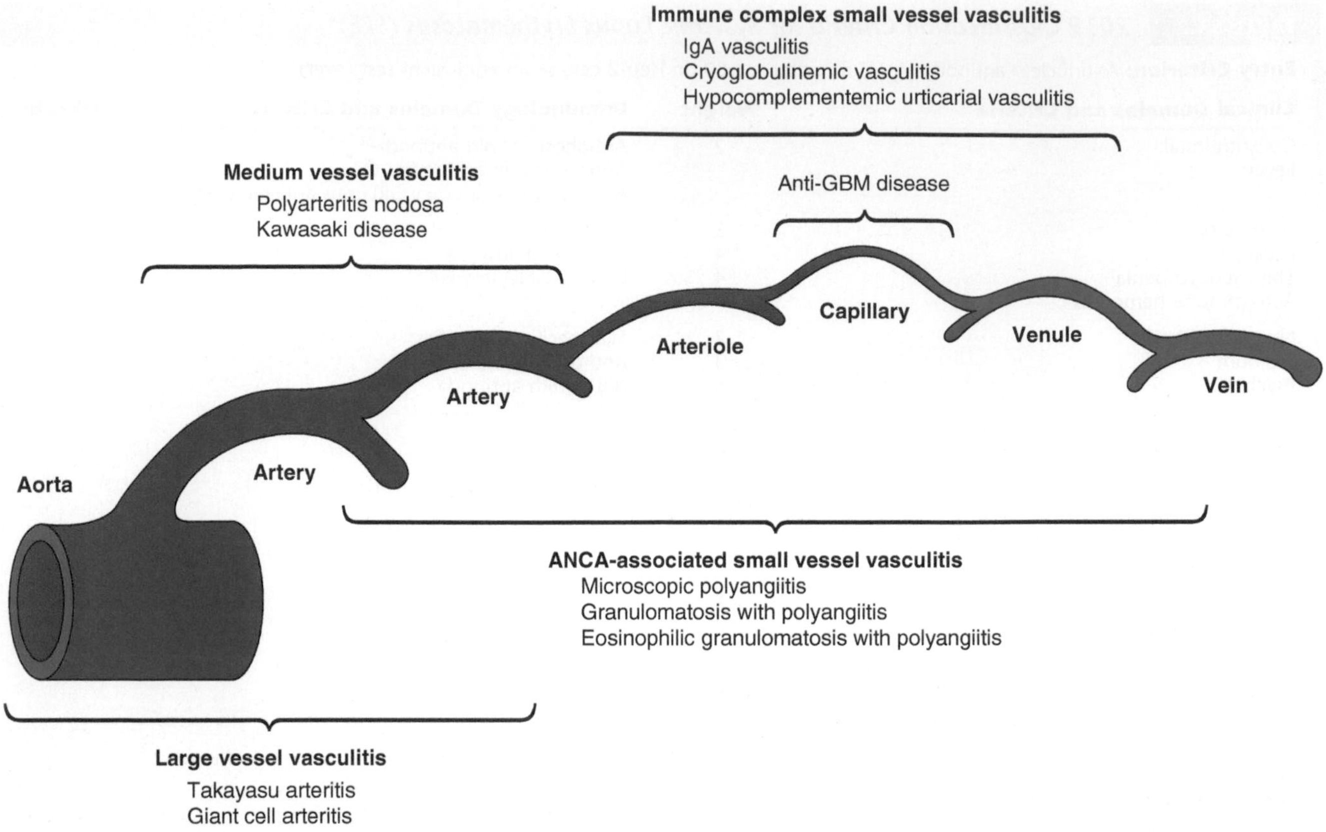

FIG. 53.4. Classification of vasculitis based on vessel size. (From Jennette, J. C., Weimer, E. T., & Kidd, J. (2017). Vasculitis. In R. A. McPherson & M. R. Pincus (Eds.), *Henry's Clinical Diagnosis and Management by Laboratory Methods* (23rd ed., pp. 1016–1031.e2, Fig. 53.1). Elsevier [Modified from Jennette, J. C., Falk, R. J., Bacon, P. A., et al. (2013). 2012 revised International Chapel Hill Consensus Conference Nomenclature of Vasculitides. *Arthritis & Rheumatism, 65*(1), 1–11.])

SUGGESTED READINGS

Lupus is a Cruel Mystery We Must all Solve Together. Available at: https://www.lupus.org/understanding-lupus August 10, 2019.

Merkel, P. A. *Overview of An Approach to the Vasculitides and Adults*. UpToDate. Available at: https://www.uptodate.com/contents/overview-of-and-approach-to-the-vasculitides-in-adults?search=vasculitis&source=search_result&selectedTitle=1~150&usage_type=default&display_rank=1 August 11, 2019.

Merkel, P. A. *Overview of the Management of Vasculitis in Adults*. UpToDate. Available at: https://www.uptodate.com/contents/overview-of-the-management-of-vasculitis-in-adults?search=vasculidites%20treatment&source=search_result&selectedTitle=1~150&usage_type=default&display_rank=1#H172114463 August 11, 2019.

Venables, P. J. W. *Clinical Manifestations of Rheumatoid Arthritis*. UpToDate. Available at: https://www.uptodate.com/contents/clinical-manifestations-of-rheumatoid-arthritis?search=RA&source=search_result&selectedTitle=4~150&usage_type=default&display_rank=4#H1597589 August 14, 2019.

Yu, D. T., & van Tubergen, A. *Reactive Arthritis*. UpToDate. Available at: https://www.uptodate.com/contents/reactive-arthritis?search=reiters%20syndrome&source=search_result&selectedTitle=1~129&usage_type=default&display_rank=1 August 12, 2019.

CHAPTER 54

Hypersensitivity

ISAAC GRABIEL, DO, and RICK McPHEETERS, DO

- Hypersensitivity is an inappropriate immune response to generally harmless antigens.
- There are four classes of hypersensitivity reactions.
  - Type I (also known as immediate or anaphylactic) is an immunoglobulin E (IgE)-mediated degranulation of mast cells and/or basophils and occurs immediately after a patient's second exposure to the antigen.
  - Type II (cytotoxic) occurs when IgG or IgM antibodies react to cell antigens, resulting in complement activation.
  - Type III (immune complex) results in immune complex deposition and complement activation.
  - Occurring 24–48 hours after antigen exposure, type IV (also known as cell mediated or delayed) involves the response of activated T cells to cell surface–bound antigens.
- Patients may present with a wide range of symptoms, with varying degrees of severity, including urticaria, pruritus, angioedema, abdominal pain, vomiting, diarrhea, bronchospasm, tachycardia, hypotension, or cardiovascular collapse.
- Diagnosis and evaluation are based on the type of hypersensitivity, although it is largely a clinical diagnosis.
- Workup should include the consideration of other diagnoses while stabilizing the patient.

Allergic Reaction

General Principles

- An allergic reaction occurs when the immune system overreacts to a harmless substance (allergen). Although some cases of allergic reactions are idiopathic, common exposures include medications, insect toxins, and foods.

Clinical Presentation

- May present with urticaria, angioedema, abdominal pain, vomiting, diarrhea, wheezing, stridor, conjunctivitis, or allergic rhinitis. IgE-mediated anaphylaxis is the most severe presentation.

Diagnosis and Evaluation

- This is a clinical diagnosis. Attempt to identify exposure, ensure stabilization of patient, all while considering alternative diagnoses.

Treatment

- Identification, removal, and avoidance of inciting exposure.
- Treatment depends on severity of disease and body system(s) involved; however, antihistamines are a mainstay of treatment.

Anaphylaxis

General Principles

- Life-threatening and rapid in onset, anaphylaxis is the most severe form of allergic reaction. Approximately half of fatalities occur within the first hour and usually result from asphyxiation.
- Most common cause in children is foods, whereas insect stings and medications are more common in adults.

Clinical Presentation

- May present with signs of allergic reaction with concomitant respiratory or cardiovascular compromise (distributive shock).
- Skin and mucosal involvement (hives, lips-tongue-uvula swelling) occurs in up to 90% of episodes.
- Respiratory involvement (stridor, wheezing) occurs in up to 70%.
- Gastrointestinal and cardiovascular signs and symptoms (vomiting, diarrhea, syncope, dizziness, tachycardia, and hypotension) each occur in up to 45%.

Diagnosis and Evaluation

- Diagnosis is clinical. Consider anaphylaxis when there is involvement of two or more body systems with or without hypotension or airway compromise (Box 54.1).

Treatment

- Eliminate exposure. First-line therapy is epinephrine (Table 54.1).
- Steroids, histamine-1 receptor blocker (H_1) and H_2 antihistamines, intravenous (IV) fluids in setting of hypotension, nebulized albuterol in cases of bronchospasm, glucagon for patients on β-blockers with refractory hypotension.

Angioedema

General Principles

- Self-limited, localized swelling of cutaneous and subcutaneous tissue secondary to capillary dilation.
- Classified by mechanism: (1) activation of mast cells (allergic), often associated with urticaria and/or pruritus, (2) generation of bradykinin (hereditary, angiotensin-converting enzyme inhibitor induced), not associated with urticaria and/or pruritus, and (3) unknown pathophysiology (idiopathic, infection).

BOX 54.1 Clinical Criteria for Anaphylaxis

Anaphylaxis is highly likely when any one of the following three criteria are fulfilled.

1. Acute onset of an illness (minutes to several hours) with involvement of the skin, mucosal tissue, or both (generalized hives, pruritis or flushing, swollen lips-tongue-uvula) AND AT LEAST ONE OF THE FOLLOWING:
   a. Respiratory compromise (e.g., dyspnea, wheeze-bronchospasm, stridor, reduced PEF, hypoxemia)
   b. Reduced BP or associated symptoms of end-organ dysfunction (e.g., hypotonia [collapse], syncope, incontinence)
2. Two or more of the following that occur rapidly after exposure to a *likely* allergen for that patient (minutes to several hours):
   a. Involvement of the skin/mucosal tissue (e.g., generalized hives, itch-flush, swollen lips-tongue-uvula)
   b. Respiratory compromise (e.g., dyspnea, wheeze-bronchospasm, stridor, reduced PEF, hypoxemia)
   c. Reduced BP or associated symptoms (e.g., hypotonia [collapse], syncope, incontinence)
3. Reduced BP after exposure to *known* allergen for that patient (minutes to several hours)
   a. Infants and children: low systolic BP (age specific) or greater than 30% decrease in systolic BP
   b. Adults: systolic BP of less than 90 mm Hg or greater than 30% decrease from that person's baseline

BP, blood pressure; *PEF*, peak expiratory flow.

From Lee, S., Bashore, C., Lohse, C. M., Bellolio, M. F., Chamberlain, A., Yuki, K., Hess, E. P., & Campbell, R. L. (2016). Rate of recurrent anaphylaxis and associated risk factors among Olmsted County, Minnesota, residents: A population-based study. *Annals of Allergy, Asthma & Immunology, 117*(6), 655–660.e2.

TABLE 54.1 Epinephrine Dosing in Hypersensitivity

Anaphylaxis	Epinephrine Dosing
Initial therapy	Epinephrine: 0.3–0.5 mg (1:1,000 dilution) IM (pediatric, 0.01 mg/kg, maximum 0.5 mg)
Nonresponsive to IM injections and volume resuscitation	IM (preferred) or SC every 5–15 minutes as needed
Cardiovascular collapse or impending cardiovascular collapse, nonresponsive to IM injections and infusion not available	Epinephrine infusion of 0.1 µg/kg/min (pediatric, 0.1–1 µg/kg/min) titrated to effect Epinephrine: 0.5–1 mL of 0.1 mg/mL (1:10,000) epinephrine slow IV push over 1–10 minutes for adults and adolescents (not recommended in infants and children). Use with extreme caution.

IM, intramuscular; *IV*, intravenous; *SC*, subcutaneous.

Clinical Presentation

- Although presentation depends on underlying mechanism, there may be edema of face, lips, mouth, throat, larynx, uvula, extremities, genitalia, and gastrointestinal tract. There is potential for airway obstruction.
- Angiotensin-converting enzyme inhibitors account for approximately 30% of all angioedema cases presenting to emergency departments.

Diagnosis and Evaluation

- Although usually a clinical diagnosis, serum C1 esterase inhibitor levels may be ordered by the primary care provider to screen for hereditary angioedema (this can be done as an outpatient).
- Determining likely underlying mechanism allows for directed therapy.

Treatment

- Primarily supportive; protecting the airway when necessary.
- Allergic angioedema is treated with antihistamines and glucocorticoids with epinephrine added in severe cases.
- Acute hereditary angioedema treatment options include purified C1 inhibitor concentrate, ecallantide, icatibant, or fresh frozen plasma (contains C1 inhibitor) when other therapies are unavailable.

Drug Allergies

General Principles

- Drug allergies are adverse reactions caused by an immunologic reaction elicited by a drug.
- May be IgE-mediated (anaphylaxis, angioedema, urticaria), cytotoxic (hemolytic anemia), immune-complex-mediated (serum sickness), or cell-mediated (Stevens-Johnson syndrome).
- Drug allergies may also present as toxic epidermal necrolysis (TEN), drug rash with eosinophilia, and systemic symptoms syndrome.

Clinical Presentation

- Depending upon underlying pathophysiology, the presentation may range from an urticarial rash to anaphylaxis or TEN.

Diagnosis and Evaluation

- Diagnosis is clinical. Evaluate for airway compromise, end-organ damage, and signs of shock.

Treatment

- Identify and withdraw offending agent.
- Treatment is supportive with oral or parenteral antihistamines and corticosteroids.
- For severe cases such as Stevens-Johnson syndrome or TEN, admission to the intensive care unit setting is warranted (preferably a burn unit).

SUGGESTED READINGS

Mitchell, M. S. (2013). Anaphylaxis, acute allergic reactions, and angioedema. In Cline, D. M., Ma, O. J., Cydulka, R. K., Meckler, G. D., Handel, D. A., & Thomas, S. H. (Eds.), *Tintinalli's emergency medicine: Just the facts* (3rd ed., p. 34). McGraw-Hill Education.

Rowe, B. H., & Gaeta, T. J. (2016). Anaphylaxis, acute allergic reactions, and angioedema. In Tintinalli, J. E., Stapczynski, J. S., Ma, O. J., Yealy, D. M, Meckler, G. D. & Cline D. M. (Eds.), *Tintinalli's emergency medicine: A comprehensive study guide* (8th ed., pp. 74–79). McGraw-Hill Education.

Zuraw, B. (2019). An overview of angioedema: Clinical features, diagnosis, and management. *UpToDate*. Retrieved September 25, 2019, from https://www.uptodate.com/contents/an-overview-of-angioedema-clinical-features-diagnosis-and-management

CHAPTER 55

BOARD REVIEW

Transplant-Related Problems

ELIZABETH SIACUNCO, MD, and RACHEL O'DONNELL, MD

- To diminish an immune response to the graft, the transplant patient needs to be receiving immunosuppressive therapy.
- Most patients need a level of chronic immunosuppression to prevent rejection and loss of a graft.
- This ongoing immunosuppression predisposes the patient to infections.
- Other transplant-related complications include disorders of the transplanted organ/altered physiology, rejection, graft-versus-host disease, or medication side effects.
- These patients can present to the emergency department with life-threatening emergencies.

Immunosuppression

General Principles

- As a result of immunosuppression, transplant patients are at high risk for infection.
- Various strategies utilized to prevent infection include extensive pretransplant screening and evaluation in addition to universal, targeted, and preemptive prophylaxis with medications and vaccinations. Despite such measures, infection is common after transplant.
- The type of infection to which the patient is most susceptible to varies based on the time frame after surgery (Fig. 55.1).
  - First month after a transplant: patient is not clinically immunosuppressed yet. Thus they are most susceptible to nosocomial infections, including postoperative wound infections, catheter-related infections, and aspiration or other infections from antimicrobial-resistant species. Rarely, the patient can also develop an infection that was present in the donor blood or organ.
  - Between 1 and 6 months post transplant: patient undergoes the most intensive immunosuppression and is thereby most susceptible to opportunistic infections.
  - After 6 months: opportunistic infections are still common, depending on the net state of immune suppression. As immune suppression is weaned over time, community-acquired infections rather than opportunistic infections become more likely.

Clinical Presentation

Initial presentation varies because these patients may have few clinical findings (e.g., may not manifest peritoneal signs) owing to an impaired inflammatory response.

Diagnosis and Evaluation

- Complete blood count
- Inflammatory markers (lactate, C-reactive protein, procalcitonin)
- Baseline function tests of transplanted organ (kidney, liver, etc.)
- Blood and urine cultures (if indicated)
- Low threshold for chest radiograph and other imaging
- Image the transplanted organ liberally (if indicated)

Treatment

- Posttransplant infections may be difficult to treat. Given the patient's already complex medication regimen, more attention must be given to drug toxicities, drug interactions, and increased resistance to antibiotics.
- The treatment should always be discussed with the transplant team. Should the patient need urgent antimicrobial intervention, consider initiating the following medication recommendations in the emergency department:
  - Skin wound: broad-spectrum antibiotic (carbapenem or piperacillin/tazobactam) + methicillin-resistant *Staphylococcus aureus* (MRSA) coverage (vancomycin or linezolid)
  - Pneumonia: may be community-acquired, hospital-acquired, atypical, or opportunistic
    - Carbapenem OR
    - Cefotaxime + gentamycin OR
    - Piperacillin/tazobactam
    - Add MRSA coverage or fungal therapy if suspected.
    - Suspected *Pneumocystis jirovecii*: prednisone + trimethoprim/sulfamethoxazole
  - Intraabdominal infection: metronidazole + (carbapenem or piperacillin/tazobactam)
  - Meningitis: frequently due to *Listeria*, cefotaxime + vancomycin
  - Gastrointestinal/genitourinary infections: treat with usual antimicrobial agents
  - Suspected fungal disease: fluconazole (amphotericin has higher toxicity)
  - Suspected cytomegalovirus (CMV): ganciclovir
  - Suspected varicella/herpes simplex virus: acyclovir
  - Suspected Epstein-Barr virus: reduction of immunosuppression regimen
  - Suspected toxoplasmosis: pyrimethamine + sulfadiazine + folinic acid

Rejection

General Principles

- Rejection is defined as a decline of graft function associated with pathologic changes in graft tissue. There are four types of rejection:
  - Hyperacute rejection: occurs within minutes to hours of transplantation. Preformed antibodies in the donor

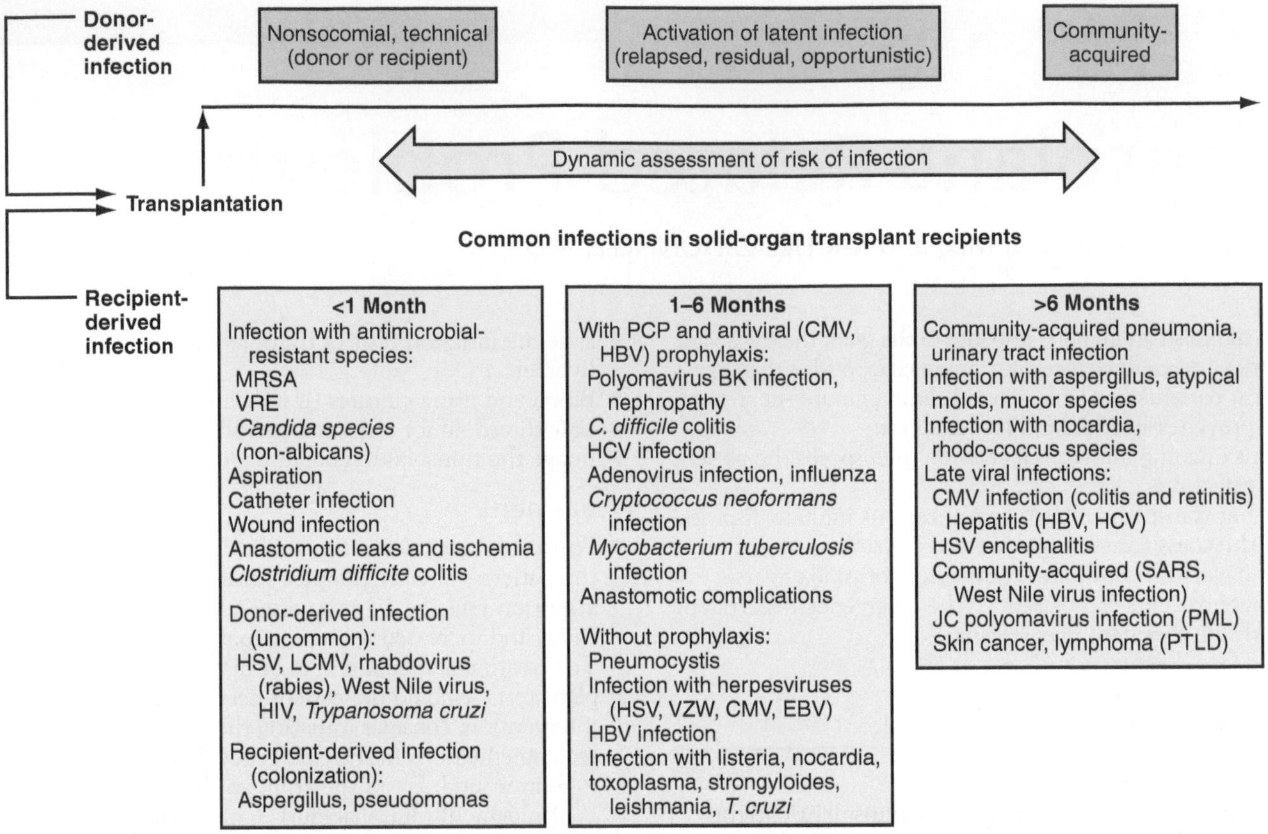

FIG. 55.1 Timeline of common infections in the immunocompromised host. *CMV*, cytomegalovirus; *EBV*, Epstein-Barr virus; *HBV*, hepatitis B virus; *HCV*, hepatitis C virus; *HIV*, human immunodeficiency virus; *HSV*, herpes simplex virus; *LCMV*, lymphocytic choriomeningitis virus; *MRSA*, methicillin-resistant *Staphylococcus aureus*; *PCP*, *Pneumocystis carinii* pneumonia; *PML*, progressive multifocal leukoencephalopathy; *PTLD*, posttransplantation lymphoproliferative disorder; *SARS*, severe acute respiratory syndrome; *VRE*, vancomycin-resistant *Enterococcus faecalis*; *VZV*, varicella-zoster virus. (From Fishman, J. A. (2007). Infection in solid-organ transplant recipients. *New England Journal of Medicine, 357*, 2601–2614.)

attack the graft, activating a response that destroys the graft's vascularization.
  - Acute rejection: occurs between 1 week to several months after transplantation. Acute rejection is categorized into T-cell–mediated (cellular) rejection and antibody-mediated (humoral) rejection. This manifests as a decline in function of the transplanted organ and is confirmed by histologic changes in the tissue.
  - Chronic rejection: occurs months to years after transplant. It results in scarring and fibrosis of the transplanted organ.
  - Graft-versus-host disease: occurs when immune cells from the donor (graft) attack the cells of the recipient, activating an immune response, which manifests as disease in the recipient
- Long-term use of immunosuppressive medications is aimed at preventing rejection.
- Rejection can occur at any time, and because it usually presents with nonspecific symptoms, one must maintain a high index of suspicion.

CARDIAC TRANSPLANT

Clinical Presentation

- Typically asymptomatic (most commonly detected on surveillance biopsy)
- No angina or pain, owing to denervation of heart after transplant (can have silent ischemia or infarction)
- Congestive heart failure symptoms: dyspnea, orthopnea, palpitations, syncope or near-syncope, hepatic congestion
- Dysrhythmias

Diagnosis and Evaluation

- Electrocardiogram: both recipient and donor sinus nodes are present, resulting in two P waves on electrocardiogram; only the donor P wave correlates with the QRS.
- Serial cardiac enzymes
- Echocardiogram: worsening systolic and/or diastolic function
- Confirmed with endomyocardial biopsy

Treatment

- Always consult transplant team; treatment without confirmation by biopsy is contraindicated unless patient is unstable.
- Rejection: high-dose glucocorticoids (methylprednisolone 500–1000 mg intravenously (IV)
- Bradydysrhythmia: isoproterenol (atropine has no effect on the denervated heart)
- Hypotension: inotropic agents such as dopamine or dobutamine

LUNG TRANSPLANT

Clinical Presentation

- Typically asymptomatic (most commonly detected on surveillance biopsy)
- Fever, nonproductive cough, dyspnea on exertion
- New hypoxia
- Chronic rejection/late complications: obliterative bronchiolitis and posttransplant lymphoproliferative disease

Diagnosis and Evaluation

- Pulse oximetry
- Arterial blood gas, complete blood cell count, electrolytes, appropriate drug levels
- Consider concomitant infection: blood cultures, sputum cultures, bronchoalveolar lavage samples, CMV viral load
- Spirometry: worsening pulmonary function tests
- Chest x-ray, computed tomography of chest
- Pleural fluid analysis
- Confirmed by transbronchial biopsy

Treatment

- Always consult transplant team
- High-dose glucocorticoids (methylprednisolone 500–1000 mg IV)
- Must rule out infection because steroids can precipitate and exacerbate opportunistic infections

LIVER TRANSPLANT

Clinical Presentation

- Nonspecific: fever, malaise
- Abdominal pain, hepatomegaly, increasing ascites

Diagnosis and Evaluation

- Rise in some or all of the liver function tests: aminotransferases, alkaline phosphatases, γ-glutamyl transpeptidase, bilirubin
- Must rule out surgical complications: biliary obstruction/leakage, hepatic artery thrombosis, or recurrence of preexisting liver disease
- Abdominal ultrasound can help rule out other etiologies.
- Confirmed by liver biopsy

Treatment

- Always consult transplant team
- High-dose glucocorticoids (methylprednisolone 500–1000 mg IV)

KIDNEY TRANSPLANT

Clinical Presentation

- Most are asymptomatic.
- Occasionally present with fever, oliguria, graft pain and/or tenderness, weight gain (fluid retention), generalized malaise
- Worsening hypertension

Diagnosis and Evaluation

- Acute rise in serum creatinine: >25% from patient's baseline
- Urinalysis: pyuria or worsening proteinuria
- Elevated plasma levels of donor-derived cell-free DNA
- Immunosuppressive drug levels, if available: rejection usually occurs when patient is noncompliant with medications or when patient's medication regimen has been aggressively reduced.
- Renal ultrasonography
- Confirmed by renal allograft biopsy

Treatment

- Always consult transplant team.
- High-dose glucocorticoids (methylprednisolone 250 mg IV q6)

GRAFT-VERSUS-HOST DISEASE

Clinical Presentation

- Targeted organs are typically the skin, gastrointestinal tract, and liver.
  - Skin: maculopapular skin rash (pruritic or painful) with scaling
  - Gastrointestinal: typically diarrhea, but may also have anorexia, nausea, vomiting, abdominal pain
  - Liver: abnormalities in liver function tests

Diagnosis and Evaluation

- A clinical diagnosis if the patient presents with a classic maculopapular rash, diarrhea, and rising serum bilirubin within 2–3 weeks of the hematopoietic cell transplantation
- Liver function tests: an increase in alkaline phosphatase and transaminases, with rising serum bilirubin within first 100 days of hematopoietic cell transplantation
- Electrolyte abnormalities may be seen, depending on the severity of diarrhea.

Treatment

- Depends on the organs involved, severity of symptoms, prophylactic regimen used
- Systemic steroids (typically prednisone or methylprednisolone) daily until clinical improvement
- If gastrointestinal graft-versus-host disease, then supplemental nutrition may also be indicated.

SUGGESTED READINGS

Brennan, D. C., Alhamad, T., & Malone, A. (2020). Clinical features and diagnosis of acute renal allograft rejection. *UpToDate*. https://www.uptodate.com/contents/kidney-transplantation-in-adults-clinical-features-and-diagnosis-of-acute-renal-allograft-rejection?search=diagnosis%20renal%20allograft%20rejection&source=search_result&selectedTitle=1~150&usage_type=default&display_rank=1.

Cline, D. M., Ma, O. J., Cydulka, R. K., Meckler, G. D., Handel, D. A., & Thomas, S. H. (2012). *Tintinalli's emergency medicine manual* (7th ed.). McGraw-Hill Medical.

Eisen, H. J. (2020). Acute cardiac allograft rejection: Diagnosis. *UpToDate*. https://www.uptodate.com/contents/heart-transplantation-in-adults-diagnosis-of-acute-allograft-rejection?search=cardiac%20allograft%20rejection&source=search_result&selectedTitle=1~150&usage_type=default&display_rank=1.

Pilewski, J. (2018). Evaluation and treatment of acute lung transplant rejection. *UpToDate*. https://www.uptodate.com/contents/evaluation-and-treatment-of-acute-lung-transplant-rejection?search=treatment%20lung%20transplant%20rejection&source=search_result&selectedTitle=1~150&usage_type=default&display_rank=1.

Reddy, K. R. (2021). Liver transplantation: Diagnosis of acute cellular rejection. *UpToDate*. https://www.uptodate.com/contents/liver-transplantation-in-adults-clinical-manifestations-and-diagnosis-of-acute-t-cell-mediatedcellular-rejection-of-the-liver-allograft?search=diagnosis%20liver%20transplant%20rejection&source=search_result&selectedTitle=1~150&usage_type=default&display_rank=1.

Immune Complex Disorders

MANISH AMIN, DO, and ISAAC GRABIEL, DO

- Immune complex disorders encompass a group of inflammatory conditions mediated by antigenantibody interactions and complement activation.
- Immune complex formation and complement activation trigger inflammatory mediators resulting in organ and tissue injury.
- In general, many organ systems can be involved, and thus patients often present with multiple constitutional symptoms and nonspecific signs, often making a diagnosis difficult.
- Diagnosis and treatment are based on the organ system(s) involved.
- Common entities are mucocutaneous lymph node syndrome (Kawasaki syndrome), rheumatic fever, sarcoidosis, and poststreptococcal glomerulonephritis.

BOX 56.1 *Diagnostic Criteria for Kawasaki Disease*

Unexplained fever of at least 5 days' duration associated with four of these criteria:
- Cervical lymphadenopathy where at least one lymph node is >1.5 cm in diameter
- Mucositis (strawberry tongue; cracked, red lips)
- Polymorphous rash
- Bilateral nonexudative conjunctivitis
- Extremity changes: indurated edema to the dorsum of the hands and feet, diffuse erythema of the palms and soles

Incomplete Kawasaki disease presents with fever of at least 5 days' duration associated with fewer than four of the five criteria cited above.

Mucocutaneous Lymph Node Syndrome (Kawasaki Syndrome)

General Principles

- Owing to inflammation of muscular arteries, Kawasaki syndrome is one of the most common childhood vasculitides.

Clinical Presentation

- Patients present with evidence of systemic inflammation associated with signs of mucocutaneous inflammation.

Diagnosis and Evaluation

- Arthritis and cardiovascular findings are not part of the diagnostic criteria (Box 56.1) but do support the diagnosis. No laboratory studies are diagnostic.

Treatment

- The disease process is self-limited and treatment is supportive.
- Nevertheless, intravenous immunoglobulin reduces the feared complication of coronary artery aneurysms, which can also result from incomplete Kawasaki disease.

Rheumatic Fever

General Principles

- Acute rheumatic fever occurs 2–4 weeks after group A *Streptococcus* (GAS) pharyngitis. It can also occur after streptococcal pyoderma in patients from tropical regions.

Clinical Presentation

- Depending on the organ system involved, patients present with arthritis, carditis, chorea, erythema marginatum, and subcutaneous nodules.
- Most commonly, patients present with an acute febrile illness associated with arthritis and carditis.
- Less commonly, patients present with neurologic or behavioral disorders associated with Sydenham chorea.

Diagnosis and Evaluation

- Based on the revised Jones criteria for the diagnosis of acute rheumatic fever (modified in 2015), patients need either two major criteria, or one major and two minor criteria, plus laboratory evidence of a preceding group A streptococcal infection.
  - Major criteria for diagnosis
    - Polyarthritis
    - Cardiac inflammation (carditis, pericarditis, or heart valve disease)
    - Subcutaneous nodules
    - Chorea
    - Erythema marginatum
    - Polyarthralgia or monoarthritis (major criteria for high-risk patients only)
  - Minor criteria for diagnosis
    - Fever
    - Elevated erythrocyte sedimentation rate or C-reactive protein
    - Polyarthralgia
    - Prolonged PR interval on electrocardiogram
    - Monoarthralgia (minor criteria for high-risk patients only)

Treatment

- Eradication of the bacteria to stop any further immunologic response.
- Treatment does not change the course of the rheumatic fever once the immunologic response has begun. Symptomatic treatment includes high-dose aspirin for arthritis, steroids for carditis, and antipsychotic medications for chorea.
- The most feared complication is due to progressive damage to the cardiac valves, resulting in heart failure.

Sarcoidosis

General Principles

- A multisystem granulomatous disorder, sarcoidosis is characterized pathologically by noncaseating granulomas in involved organs.
- The disease typically affects young adults.
- The etiology is unknown, but the incidence varies among geographic regions and race, most commonly afflicting Blacks.

Clinical Presentation

- Patients most frequently present with cough, dyspnea, and chest pain.
- The pulmonary symptoms are often accompanied by nonspecific constitutional symptoms such as fatigue, malaise, fever and weight loss.
- Extrapulmonary manifestations may include visual changes, dry eyes or mouth, parotid swelling, palpitations, syncope, and muscle weakness.
- Physical examination may also demonstrate wheezing or crackles, skin changes (erythema nodosum), lymphadenopathy, splenomegaly, or uveitis.

Diagnosis and Evaluation

- Diagnosis requires three elements: (1) compatible clinical and radiographic manifestations, (2) exclusion of other diseases that may present similarly, and (3) histopathologic detection of noncaseating granulomas.
- Evaluation may reveal bilateral hilar lymphadenopathy on chest radiograph, elevated serum angiotensin-converting enzyme, hypercalciuria, or hypercalcemia.

Treatment

Corticosteroids are the primary treatment modality, although spontaneous resolution is common.

Poststreptococcal Glomerulonephritis

General Principles

- A sequela of group A streptococcal infection (typically after GAS pharyngitis or skin infections), poststreptococcal glomerulonephritis is caused by deposition of circulating immune complexes, with streptococcal antigenic components, in the kidneys.

Clinical Presentation

- Most frequently occurring in children 5–7 years of age, the presentation may range from asymptomatic, microscopic hematuria to acute nephritic syndrome (red to brown urine), with proteinuria, generalized edema, hypertension, and elevated serum creatinine.
- The latency period post-GAS pharyngitis is 1–3 weeks, whereas the latency period post-GAS skin infection is 3–6 weeks.

Diagnosis and Evaluation

- Urinalysis may show hematuria, pyuria, and proteinuria. Antistreptolysin O titer and immunoglobulin G levels are elevated.
- Complement levels (C3 in particular) are significantly depressed.

Treatment

- There is no specific therapy for poststreptococcal glomerulonephritis, and the treatment is largely supportive and focused on treating clinical manifestations of disease, such as volume overload or hypertension.
- General measures include sodium and water restriction and loop diuretics.
- Antibiotics have a role only if there is still currently a GAS infection.

SUGGESTED READINGS

King, T. (2017). Clinical manifestations and diagnosis of pulmonary sarcoidosis. *UpToDate*. Retrieved 9/17/2019 from https://www.uptodate.com/contents/clinical-manifestations-and-diagnosis-of-pulmonary-sarcoidosis

Niaudet, P. (2018). Poststreptococcal glomerulonephritis. *UpToDate*. Retrieved 9/1/2019 from https://www.uptodate.com/contents/poststreptococcal-glomerulonephritis

Perlstein, D., & Mersch, J. (2018). Rheumatic fever. *MedicineNet*. Retrieved 9/3/2019 from https://www.medicinenet.com/rheumatic_fever/article.htm#rheumatic_fever_acute_rheumatic_fever_or_arf_facts

Steer, A., & Gibofsky, A. (2018). Acute rheumatic fever: Clinical manifestations and diagnosis. *UpToDate*. Retrieved 8/16/2019 from https://www.uptodate.com/contents/acute-rheumatic-fever-clinical-manifestations-and-diagnosis

Sundel, R. (2018). Kawasaki disease: Clinical features and diagnosis. *UpToDate*. Retrieved 8/7/19 from https://www.uptodate.com/contents/kawasaki-disease-clinical-features-and-diagnosis

Szczygielska, I., Hernik, E. Kołodziejczyk, B., Gazda, A., Maślińska, M., & Gietka, P. (2018). Rheumatic fever–new diagnostic criteria. *Reumatologia*, 56(1), 37–41. doi:10.5114/reum.2018.74748

Warren, J., & Ward, P. (2017). Immune complex diseases. Wiley Online Library. doi:10.1002/9780470015902.a0002164.pub3

Medication-Induced Immunosuppression

JAGDIPAK S. HEER, MD, and VIKRAM SHANKAR, MD

General Principles

- Immunosuppressants are medications that inhibit the immune system in various ways and may be used to induce an immunosuppressed state for organ transplant recipients or reduce the frequency of autoimmune/inflammatory disease flares.
- Immunosuppressive drugs act by modifying critical pathways in the inflammatory process.
- Choice of medication depends on disease severity, disease progression rate, organ involvement, and degree of immunosuppressive effect required.
- Diseases treated by immunosuppressive drugs are often autoimmune in etiology and include rheumatoid arthritis, systemic lupus erythematosus, scleroderma, inflammatory bowel disease, multiple sclerosis, psoriasis, and vasculitides.
- Immunosuppressive agents may be used to prevent organ and tissue transplantation rejection.

Clinical Presentation

- Patients receiving immunosuppressive therapy are at increased risk of infection secondary to immunodeficiency.
- Risk factors for infection include duration of use, concomitant use of other immunomodulators, baseline functional status, nature of disease, age, and the degree of exposure to health-care settings.
- Patient may present with leukopenia, fever, rash, arthritis, nausea/vomiting, sepsis and septic shock, and/or adverse reactions in any organ system (Table 57.1).
- Immunosuppressed host may not manifest "classic" signs and symptoms of disease because of altered physiology e.g., patient may not mount a fever, develop leukocytosis, nor develop an abscess fluid collection because they are neutropenic.

Diagnosis and Evaluation

- Evaluation should be based on the patient's specific history, physical examination, and therapeutic regimen.
- Leukopenia may point to a bacterial infection and lymphocytosis may represent a viral etiology such as cytomegalovirus.
- Each immunosuppressive agent may present with a range of specific adverse reactions (Table 57.2), and evaluation should aim to differentiate between the medication side effect and a more sinister underlying disease process.

Treatment

Glucocorticoids

- Glucocorticoids are antiinflammatory and immunosuppressive drugs that include prednisone, dexamethasone, and hydrocortisone.
- These drugs work by inhibiting molecules associated with inflammation, including arachidonic acid metabolites, cytokines, and chemokines.
- Glucocorticoids are used for induction and maintenance of immunosuppression, acute cellular rejection, and antibody-mediated rejection.
- Adverse effects include hyperglycemia, high blood pressure, truncal obesity, osteoporosis, and adrenal cortical atrophy.

Cytostatics

- Cytostatics work by inhibiting cell division and include alkylating agents, antimetabolites, azathioprine, and methotrexate.
- Azathioprine is a purine analog that inhibits DNA synthesis and suppresses proliferation of activated T-cell lymphocytes.
- Methotrexate is a folic acid analog commonly used to treat such autoimmune diseases as rheumatoid arthritis.

Antibodies

- Antibodies, including polyclonal antibodies, monoclonal antibodies, T-cell receptor-directed antibodies, and interleukin-2 receptor-directed antibodies, may be used to treat malignancies and autoimmune disorders, and prevent acute rejection. They include the following:
  - Antithymocyte globulin, equine
  - Antithymocyte globulin, rabbit
  - Rituximab
  - Basiliximab
  - Belatacept
  - Bortezomib
  - Eculizumab

Drugs Acting on Immunophilins

- Drugs acting on immunophilins include cyclosporine, tacrolimus, and sirolimus.
- Cyclosporine inhibits calcineurin by binding to cyclophilin, blocking several cytokines and inhibiting T-lymphocyte activation and proliferation.
- Tacrolimus works by inhibiting calcineurin with the same effects as cyclosporine, but with 50–100 times greater potency.

TABLE 57.1 *Side Effects of Immunosuppressive Therapies by System*

System	Side Effects
Constitutional	Anorexia, fevers, dizziness, malaise, generalized weakness
Eyes	Blurry vision, loss of sight, conjunctivitis, cataracts
Ears/mouth	Tinnitus, decreased hearing, gingival hyperplasia, stomatitis
Pulmonary	Cough, dyspnea, pneumonitis, pleural effusion, interstitial lung disease
Cardiovascular	Hypertension, tachy-/bradycardia, CHF, hypotension, syncope
Gastrointestinal	Nausea and vomiting, diarrhea, gastritis, pancreatitis, constipation, ascites
Musculoskeletal	Myopathy, muscle atrophy, osteoporosis, osteopenia, avascular necrosis, tendon rupture
Hematologic	Thrombocytopenia, neutropenia, lymphopenia, anemia, thrombosis
Metabolic	Abnormal K, Na, Ca, Mg, Phos, hyper-/hypoglycemia, hyperlipidemia
Integumentary	Skin thickening/thinning, edema, hirsutism, hair loss
Neurologic	Vertigo, tremors, neuropathy, cerebral edema, confusion, agitation, paresthesias
Endocrine	Adrenal suppression, thyroiditis and thyroid storm, diabetes
Immune	Infections, anaphylaxis, other allergic reactions
Renal	Renal failure, nephrotoxicity, dysuria

CHF, congestive heart failure; *K,* potassium; *Na,* sodium; *Ca,* calcium; *Mg,* magnesium; *Phos,* phosphorus.

TABLE 57.2 *Side Effects and Mechanism of Action of Select Immunosuppressive Therapies*

Medication	Mechanism of Action	Adverse Reaction
Prednisolone	Binds to glucocorticoid receptors interacting with DNA to inhibit inflammatory genes	Muscle wasting, impaired wound healing, adrenal suppression, gastric ulceration, weight gain, skin thinning, nausea, bone loss, avascular necrosis
Azathioprine	Inhibits purine metabolism	Nausea, vomiting, myelosuppression, hepatotoxicity, acute pancreatitis
Cyclosporine	Inhibits calcineurin phosphatase and T-cell activation	Nephrotoxicity, hepatotoxicity, cardiotoxicity, neurotoxicity, gingival hyperplasia, hypomagnesemia, gastrointestinal upset; heavily metabolized by CYP3A4
Mycophenolate	Inhibits guanosine monophosphate metabolism	Diarrhea, abdominal pain, nausea, neutropenia, neurotoxicity
Tacrolimus	Inhibits calcineurin phosphatase and T-cell activation	Nephrotoxicity, hepatotoxicity, cardiotoxicity, neurotoxicity, posttransplantation diabetes mellitus. CYP3A inducers may decrease tacrolimus blood concentration. There are many interactions with food (e.g., grapefruit juice increases serum tacrolimus levels).
Sirolimus	Inhibits target of rapamycin and T-cell proliferation	Delayed wound healing, thrombocytopenia, hyperlipidemia, increased toxicity of calcineurin inhibitors. CYP3A4 and P-gp inducers may decrease sirolimus blood concentration.

CYP34A, cytochrome P450 3A4; *P-gp,* P-glycoprotein.

- Sirolimus inhibits transduction of signals to the mammalian target of rapamycin complex, causing immunosuppression and antiproliferation.

SUGGESTED READINGS

Calvert, J. H. (2016). The transplant patient. In Tintinalli, J. E., Stapczynski, J .S., Ma, O. J., Yealy, D. M., Meckler, G. D., & Cline, D. M. (Eds.), *Tintinalli's emergency medicine: A comprehensive study guide* (8th ed., pp. 2002–2010). McGraw-Hill Education.

Chao, N. (2019). Overview of immunosuppressive agents used for prevention and treatment of graft-versus-host disease. *UpToDate.* Retrieved May 31, 2019, https://www.uptodate.com/contents/overview-of-immunosuppressive-agents-used-for-prevention-and-treatment-of-graft-versus-host-disease?search=overview%20of%20immunosuppressive%20agents%20used%20for%20prevention&source=search_result&selectedTitle=1~150&usage_type=default&display_rank=1

Cline, D. M. (2013). The transplant patient. In Cline, D. M., Ma, O. J., Cydulka, R. K., Thomas, S. H., Handel, D. A., & Meckler, G. D. (Eds.), *Tintinalli's emergency medicine: Just the facts* (3rd ed., pp. 357–362). McGraw-Hill Education.

Systemic Infectious Diseases

CHAPTER **58**

BOARD REVIEW

Sepsis, Septic Shock, and Toxic Shock Syndrome

CAMERON W. HARRISON, MD, and ALLISON FERREIRA, MD

Sepsis is characterized by an exaggerated and often dysregulated response to an infectious insult. The phenotype of the response varies based on individual host factors, but sepsis implies a life-threatening condition with secondary damage to multiple organ systems. The incidence of sepsis appears to be increasing. This may be driven by population aging, a greater number of immunosuppressed patients, the emergence of multidrug-resistant bacteria, and/or an increased focus on early recognition of sepsis.

Definitions and Clinical Criteria

- There is no gold standard test for the diagnosis of sepsis; the clinical criteria to diagnose sepsis have evolved over the years.
- The latest guidelines, Sepsis-3 developed in 2016, focus on the dysregulated host response to infection and operationalize the definition of sepsis using the sequential organ failure assessment (SOFA) score.
  - SOFA score involves multiple physiologic and laboratory measures of end-organ dysfunction, many of which are impractical for emergency department use. A score >2 represents organ dysfunction and correlates with a greater than 10% risk of in-hospital mortality.
  - The quick SOFA score was developed by the Sepsis-3 group as a bedside clinical tool for the identification of septic patients.
    - The score is positive if two of the following three criteria are met: respiratory rate ≥22, altered mentation, and systolic blood pressure ≤100 mm Hg.
    - If the quick SOFA score is positive in someone without a known infection, prompt consideration of an occult infection is indicated.
  - A pediatric SOFA (pSOFA) score has been developed and predictive up to age 21 years.

Application of Definitions and Clinical Criteria

Sepsis

- Life-threatening organ dysfunction caused by a dysregulated host response to infection.
- A documented or suspected infection and an acute increase of ≥2 SOFA points.

Septic Shock

- A subset of sepsis in which underlying circulatory and cellular metabolism abnormalities are profound enough to cause hemodynamic instability and substantially increase mortality.
- Sepsis criteria met as above plus vasopressors are required to elevate mean arterial pressure (MAP) ≥65 mm Hg and lactate >2 mmol/L (or 18 mg/dL) despite adequate fluid resuscitation.

Clinical Presentation

- The clinical presentation of sepsis can vary from minimally symptomatic to comatose and hypotensive.
- Patients may be febrile (temperature ≥38°C) or hypothermic (≤36°C; associated with poorer prognosis).
- History and a thorough physical examination are critical, particularly to determine source.
  - Cough, sputum production, dyspnea may indicate a pulmonary source.
  - Dysuria, frequency, hematuria, or back pain may indicate a urinary source.
  - Presence of a central venous catheter with fevers may indicate a line infection.
  - Examine the patient's back, sacrum, genitals for evidence of skin source (including necrotizing soft tissue infections).
  - Jaundice could indicate a biliary source.

Diagnosis and Evaluation

- Consider broadening workup as clinically indicated.
  - Complete blood count with differential
    - May see leukocytosis or leukopenia (defined as >12,000 or <4,000 white blood cells/μL, respectively). Leukopenia is associated with poorer prognosis.
    - May see neutrophilic predominance and immature neutrophils (bands).
    - May see thrombocytopenia.
  - Comprehensive metabolic panel
    - May identify hepatic dysfunction.
    - Creatinine increased by 0.3 from baseline indicates acute kidney injury.
    - Hyperglycemia (plasma glucose >140 mg/dL) may be present in the absence of diabetes.
    - Electrolyte disturbances consistent with adrenal insufficiency (e.g., hyponatremia, hyperkalemia) may be seen.
  - Prothrombin time/international normalized ratio may be elevated (international normalized ratio >1.5) in hepatic dysfunction or disseminated intravascular coagulation.
  - Lactate elevated (>2 mmol/L).
  - Arterial blood gas (venous blood gas may be substituted under most conditions).

- Blood cultures, two sets (unless endocarditis is suspected, in which case three sets of blood cultures are recommended)
  - Culture any indwelling lines.
  - If possible, blood cultures should be drawn before antibiotics unless this would cause a significant delay in time to antibiotics.
  - Positive blood cultures are found only about 50% of the time.
- Urinalysis and urine culture
- Consider site-specific cultures: sputum, wound, stool, etc.
- Chest radiograph.
- Advanced imaging with computed tomography or ultrasound should be considered on a case by case basis depending on the history and physical exam to identify an intra-abdominal source, or deep space infection.

Treatment

- Resuscitation strategy has been controversial, although there are some general guidelines with which most experts would agree. The 2016 Surviving Sepsis Campaign International Guidelines for Management of Sepsis and Septic Shock include the following points:
  - Intravenous antibiotics for sepsis and septic shock.
    - Initiation of broad-spectrum antibiotics.
    - Antibiotics should be narrowed once pathogen has been identified.
    - Every hour delay is associated with increased mortality and end-organ dysfunction.
      - Current guidelines recommend appropriate antibiotics be administered within 1 hour.
      - Antibiotics guided based on likely source and local antibiograms.
  - Fluid resuscitation with normal saline or lactated Ringer solution at 30 mL/kg.
    - The fluid tolerance and volume status of the patient should be considered before, during, and after administering this amount of fluid. For example, aggressive fluid resuscitation is likely to be detrimental to a patient who has cardiogenic shock.
    - We are increasingly aware of the incidence of sepsis-induced cardiomyopathy in patients without history of heart failure who may not tolerate the standard 30 mL/kg fluid.
    - Point of care ultrasonography can be useful in determining both volume status and fluid tolerance.
      - May also use passive leg raise test to determine fluid responsiveness, equivalent to a temporary bolus of 500 mL of fluid
    - Guidelines currently recommend that fluid bolus be completed within 3 hours.
  - Norepinephrine as first-line vasopressor
    - Initiated as soon as possible if patient has inadequate perfusion after appropriate fluid resuscitation.
    - Epinephrine or vasopressin as second-line vasopressor.
      - Epinephrine may be more useful for patients requiring more inotropy and/or chronotropy.
  - Source control.
    - Removing of indwelling lines, kidney stone, or gallstone that may be obstructed, drainage of abscesses, and debridement of necrotic tissue.
  - For pediatric sepsis, 10-20 mL/kg boluses should be given with reassessment and epinephrine (for cold shock) and norepinephrine (for warm shock) are recommended vasopressors.
  - Stress-dose steroids (hydrocortisone or dexamethasone) if history of or risk factors for adrenal insufficiency or has vasopressor-refractory shock.
  - Goal MAP of 65 mm Hg.
    - Goal MAP varies between patients; must determine adequate perfusion based on improvement in lactate, urine output, mental status, or other organ dysfunction.

Toxic Shock Syndrome

58

General Principles

Toxic shock syndrome (TSS) is a clinical syndrome caused by superantigens released by toxin-producing bacteria (*Staphylococcus aureus* and *Streptococcus*) that cause a sudden onset of fever, rash, hypotension, and multisystem organ damage. In the early 1980s, the incidence of TSS rose in the setting of tampon use by menstruating women. This improved with removal of certain brands and types of tampons from the market along with increased awareness of the disease. Now only half of cases are associated with feminine hygiene products. Other causes of TSS include an assortment of conditions that may introduce or harbor *S. aureus* (or *Streptococcus* in some cases) including mastitis, sinusitis, osteomyelitis, open skin wounds, necrotizing fasciitis, burns, respiratory infections, nasal or other types of packing, and surgical or postpartum wounds, among others. A high index of clinical suspicion is necessary because it has been reported that up to 45% of TSS due to *Streptococcus* did not have an identified portal of entry.

Pathophysiology and Mechanisms

- May involve *S. aureus* (methicillin-sensitive or methicillin-resistant *S. aureus* [MRSA]) or *Streptococcus*.
  - *Streptococcus* toxic shock usually presents without the characteristic rash.
- Multiple types of exotoxins are released in TSS, many of which cause intense immune system responses.

Clinical Presentation and Evaluation

- Should be suspected in individuals who are otherwise healthy who present with rapid onset of symptoms including fever, rash, and hypotension along with symptoms present in multiple organ systems. Gastrointestinal symptoms, especially diarrhea, are usually prominent.
- Diagnosed clinically with laboratory testing along with cultures.
- Probable case meets the laboratory criteria plus four of the following five clinical criteria, while a confirmed case meets all five of the criteria:
  - Centers for Disease Control and Prevention clinical criteria:
    - Fever
    - Rash
      - Rash is usually diffuse, red, and macular.
      - Usually involves palms and soles.
      - Rash can be transient.
    - Desquamation
      - Usually 1–3 weeks after initial illness.
    - Hypotension

- Three or more of the following systems affected:
  - Gastrointestinal: vomiting, diarrhea
  - Muscular: myalgias, creatine kinase elevation twice the upper limit of normal
  - Mucous membranes: vaginal, oropharyngeal, conjunctival hyperemia
  - Renal: serum urea nitrogen or creatinine more than twice the upper limit of normal, pyuria
  - Hepatic: bilirubin or transaminases more than twice the upper limit of normal
  - Hematologic: platelets <100,000/μL
  - Central nervous system: confusion, altered mental status without focal neurologic findings when fever and hypotension are absent.
- Laboratory criteria
  - Blood or cerebrospinal fluid cultures often negative in the case of *Staphylococcus*-related TSS but more likely to be positive if *Streptococcus* is the causative organism.
  - Microbial identification not required for confirmation of the diagnosis.

Treatment

- Involves early and aggressive resuscitation
  - Patients can have extensive capillary leak requiring a lot of volume resuscitation.
  - Vasopressors usually needed to maintain adequate perfusion.
- Early removal of the infection source
  - Important to perform a vaginal examination with removal of a possibly contaminated tampon.
  - Evaluate for nasal packing
  - Surgical debridement
    - Including incision and drainage for any possible abscesses.
- Antibiotics
  - Need coverage for methicillin-sensitive S. *aureus* and MRSA as well as *Streptococcus*
    - Clindamycin, vancomycin, and piperacillin/tazobactam (or a carbapenem) are good first-line agents.
    - Clindamycin is the drug of choice for inhibiting toxin synthesis.
    - Vancomycin to cover MRSA.
    - Piperacillin/tazobactam to cover other organisms that could cause a similar clinical picture.
- Intravenous immunoglobulin used in severe cases
  - Literature is limited on this treatment.
- No evidence for steroid use in TSS
  - Can be considered if patient is believed to have adrenal insufficiency

Disposition

- Patient should be admitted to the intensive care unit for appropriate monitoring and treatment.
- Surgical consult should strongly be considered for wounds and debridement of source.

SUGGESTED READINGS

Puskarich, M. A., & Jones, A. E. (2016). Sepsis. In Tintinalli, J. E., Stapczynski, J. S., Ma, O. J., Yealy, D. M. Meckler, & G. D., Cline, D. M. (Eds.), Tintinalli's emergency medicine: A comprehensive study guide (8th ed.). McGraw-Hill Education.

Shapiro, N. L. (2015). Bacteremia, sepsis, and septic shock. *Harwood-Nuss' clinical practice of emergency medicine*. In Wolfson, A. B., Cloutier, R. L., Hendey, G. W., Ling, L. J., Rosen, C. L., & Schaider, J. J. (Eds.) (6th ed.). Lippincott Williams & Wilkins.

Singer, M., Deutschman, C. S., Seymour, C. W., Shankar-Hari, M., Annane, D., Bauer, M., … Angus, D. C. (2016). The third international consensus definitions for sepsis and septic shock (Sepsis-3). *Journal of the American Medical Association, 315*(8), 801–810. doi:10.1001/jama.2016.0287

CHAPTER **59** BOARD REVIEW

Systemic Bacterial Infections

ALEXANDER DAGUANNO, MD, BS, and KELLY PAINTER, MD, FACEP

Meningococcemia (Neisseria meningitidis)

Basic Information

- Encapsulated gram-negative diplococci infection transmitted by inhalation of aerosolized particles and colonization of the nasopharynx.
- Life-threatening disease predominantly of the young, with 50% of cases occurring in the first year of life and a second peak in young adults 15 to 25 years of age.
- High rate of mortality and morbidity if treatment is delayed.
- High-risk populations include college students, premature infants, and patients with complement deficiency (congenital or medication-induced), asplenia, or human immunodeficiency virus.

Clinical Presentation

- Most frequently manifests as one of four syndromes: meningitis (covered in chapter 78 Disorders Presenting with Headache and Associated Symptoms), meningitis with meningococcemia, meningococcemia without clinical evidence of meningitis, or pharyngitis but can rapidly progress.
  - Early symptoms (hours): fever, nausea/vomiting, headache, sore throat, coryza, myalgias.
  - Later symptoms (typically within first 24 hours): purpuric/hemorrhagic rash, meningismus, altered mental status.
- Clinical signs may involve multiple systems:
  - Neurologic: altered mentation, meningismus; focal deficits and seizures uncommon.
  - Dermatologic: petechial rash most commonly affecting trunk, lower body, palms and soles, often involving mucus membranes; may not be present on initial presentation. Lesions may coalesce into large purpuric/ecchymotic lesions (Fig. 59.1) owing to disseminated intravascular coagulation. Purpuric lesions may develop a gray necrotic center, which is pathognomonic for meningococcal infection.
  - Cardiovascular: hypotension, tachycardia, myocarditis with heart failure and pulmonary edema, poor perfusion and capillary refill 2 seconds is an early finding especially in children.
  - Adrenal: Waterhouse-Friedrichsen syndrome (adrenal hemorrhage causing adrenal insufficiency); consider this if hypotension is unresponsive to fluids and vasopressors.

Diagnosis and Evaluation

- Laboratory signs of infection are nonspecific, including elevated white blood cell count with bandemia, lactic acidosis, thrombocytopenia, hyponatremia.
- Cerebral spinal fluid (CSF) studies are consistent with bacterial meningitis and gram stain demonstrates gram-negative diplococci.
- Gold standard for diagnosis is the isolation of *Neisseria meningitidis* by culture from blood or CSF. Blood cultures are positive in 40%–75% of patients and CSF positive in 90%. Lumbar puncture is contraindicated if signs of increased intracranial pressure are present and in patients with septicemia and shock if positioning will compromise their condition.
- Polymerase chain reaction on whole blood or urine antigen can be used for diagnosis.
- Skin biopsy or scrapings may be used, but typically are not indicated.

Treatment

- Broad-spectrum antibiotics and fluid resuscitation should be initiated immediately after clinical suspicion of diagnosis. Patients should be placed in isolation, with droplet precautions.
- Do NOT delay giving antibiotics until after lumbar puncture.

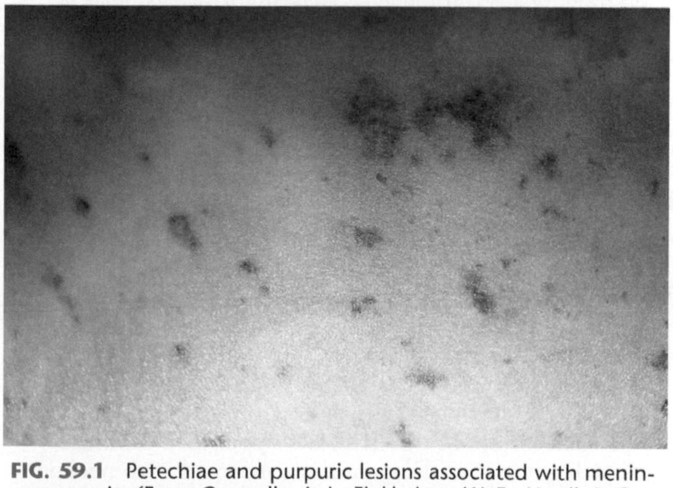

FIG. 59.1 Petechiae and purpuric lesions associated with meningococcemia. (From Connolly, A. J., Finkbeiner, W. E., Ursell, P. C., & Davis, R. L. (2016). Atlas of gross autopsy pathology. In A. J. Connolly, W. E. Finkbeiner, P. C. Ursell, & R. L. Davis (Eds.), *Autopsy pathology: A manual and atlas* (3rd ed., pp. 186–319, Fig. 16.13). Elsevier.)

- Given that microbiologic diagnosis is often unavailable in the emergency department (ED), empiric antibiotic therapy should include a third-generation cephalosporin (ceftriaxone 100 mg/kg (max 2 grams) in pediatrics and 2 grams in adults q12 hours) plus age-appropriate coverage for other causes of bacterial meningitis (see chapter 78 Disorders Presenting with Headache and Associated Symptoms).
- Start vasopressors if hypotension unresponsive to fluids (see Chapter 58. Sepsis, Septic Shock, and Toxic Shock Syndrome).
- The Centers for Disease Control and Prevention recommends that high-risk groups receive both the meningococcal conjugate vaccine (MenACWY) and the serogroup B meningococcal vaccine (MenB).
- Close contacts should receive prophylactic ciprofloxacin or rifampin, regardless of prior immunization status. Individuals who have a contraindication for fluoroquinolones can receive intramuscular ceftriaxone.

Mycobacterium tuberculosis (TB)

Basic Information

- Slow-growing, acid-fast aerobic rod; transmitted via respiratory droplets; primarily affects the lungs. Risk factors include travel to endemic area, crowded living conditions, immunocompromised status, and homelessness.
  - Primary TB: granulomatous infection of lung or extrapulmonary tissues.
  - Latent TB: primary infection becomes dormant and patients are asymptomatic and develop a positive purified protein derivative (PPD).
  - Reactivation TB: host becomes immunocompromised and latent disease becomes active and symptomatic.

Clinical Presentation

- Primary TB: usually asymptomatic, but may resemble pneumonia.
- Latent TB: asymptomatic with +PPD 1 to 2 months after exposure.
- Reactivation TB: variable clinical presentation to include pulmonary TB (prolonged cough, night sweats, fever, weight loss, hemoptysis) or extrapulmonary TB (Pott disease, osteomyelitis, pericarditis/pericardial effusion, arthritis, sterile pyuria with urinary symptoms, exudative pleural effusions, meningitis with lymphocyte predominance, cervical lymphadenitis or "scrofula").

Diagnosis and Evaluation

- Chest x-ray (CXR) study is a crucial component of diagnosis at all stages.
  - Primary TB: CXR can be normal or show nonspecific infiltrate, often with regional lymphadenopathy, termed "Ghon complex."
  - Latent TB: CXR does not show any signs of TB; use +PPD to diagnose latent infection.
  - Reactivation TB: CXR shows upper lobe infiltrate with cavitation. Diagnosis is confirmed with nucleic acid amplification test of the sputum, which is more sensitive than an acid-fast bacillus smear and also can determine antibiotic susceptibility. Cultures of sputum, blood, and tissue are gold standard for diagnosis of active infection, but can take up to 6 weeks to result.

Treatment

- Latent TB (+PPD) is treated with 6 to 9 months of isoniazid (INH) or 3 months of INH and rifampin.
- Reactivation TB requires a four-drug regimen with rifampin, isoniazid, pyrazinamide, and ethambutol (RIPE). Baseline laboratory tests (LFTs) should be obtained before starting RIPE. Meningitis and pericarditis are treated with RIPE plus corticosteroids.

Nontuberculous Mycobacterium

Basic Information

- Nontuberculous mycobacteria (NTM) can cause four clinical syndromes in humans: pulmonary disease, disseminated disease, superficial lymphadenitis, and skin and soft tissue infections.

NONTUBERCULOUS MYCOBACTERIAL PULMONARY DISEASE

- Most often from Mycobacterium avium complex (MAC); encompasses many genetically similar species acquired from the environment (e.g., municipal water sources). It is not spread by human or animal contact and most often is seen in the setting of underlying lung disease (chronic obstructive pulmonary disease, bronchiectasis, pneumoconiosis, cystic fibrosis, or previous TB infection).

Clinical Presentation

- Similar to TB with cough, fatigue, dyspnea, chest discomfort, or hemoptysis. Fever and weight loss are less common than in TB.

Diagnosis and Evaluation

- Diagnosis requires microbiologic confirmation from sputum cultures and/or bronchial-alveolar lavage. Radiographic findings include reticular or reticulonodular infiltrates, cavitary disease (upper lobe predominant), pulmonary nodules, and multifocal bronchiectasis.

Treatment

- Treatment is prolonged and requires multiple medications. First-line treatment is macrolide with ethambutol and rifampin. If close follow-up is possible, macrolide therapy can be started in the ED. Ethambutol and rifampin have significant side effects that require monitoring and should be delayed for outpatient management.

DISSEMINATED NONTUBERCULOUS MYCOBACTERIAL DISEASE

- Occurs primarily in severely immunocompromised patients (e.g., acquired immunodeficiency syndrome, leukemia, chronic immunosuppressive medication use); most commonly from MAC.

Clinical Presentation

- Fever, night sweats, weight loss, fatigue, malaise, anorexia. Organ-specific signs and symptoms reflect major sites of involvement and include cough, lymphadenopathy, hepatosplenomegaly, diarrhea, and abdominal pain.

Diagnosis and Evaluation

- Clinical diagnosis in the ED as confirmation requires positive blood or tissue culture for mycobacteria. Transaminitis, anemia, neutropenia, or pulmonary infiltrates may be seen.

Treatment

- In general, requires inpatient admission for intravenous (IV) antibiotics (macrolide along with ethambutol and rifampin) and infectious disease consultation.

NONTUBERCULOUS MYCOBACTERIAL LYMPHADENITIS

- Common form of lymphadenitis in children, most often owing to MAC.

Clinical Presentation

- Unilateral, nontender cervicofacial lymphadenitis that slowly enlarges over weeks and does not respond to antibiotics directed toward *Staphylococcus* and *Streptococcus*. Initially is pink and progresses to purple in color.

Diagnosis and Evaluation

- Diagnosis can be presumed based on clinical characteristics and a positive acid-fast bacillus stain.

Treatment

- Surgical excision without antibiotic therapy is first-line treatment. Patients should be referred to general surgery for outpatient management. **Incision and drainage of lymph nodes are contraindicated** owing to a high probability of developing a sinus tract.

NONTUBERCULOUS MYCOBACTERIAL SKIN AND SOFT TISSUE INFECTIONS

- Can be caused by multiple species of nontuberculous mycobacteria. Infection is transmitted through environmental sources (e.g., swimming pools and natural bodies of water) after cutaneous trauma.

Clinical Presentation

- Variable, but includes ulcers, folliculitis, erythematous papules and nodules. Starts as painless, slowly growing indurated areas that begin to ulcerate after weeks, most often without systemic signs or lymphadenopathy.

Diagnosis and Evaluation

- Consider diagnosis if history of water exposure with cutaneous injury and lack of response to anti-*Staphylococcal/Streptococcal* antibiotics. A +PPD can support the diagnosis in patients without risk factors for TB. Definitive diagnosis is made by isolation of nontuberculous mycobacteria in wound culture or biopsy.

Treatment

- Empiric treatment with macrolide and fluoroquinolone, doxycycline, or trimethoprim-sulfamethoxazole may be initiated from the ED. If abscess is present, incision and drainage in the ED are indicated.

Necrotizing Fasciitis

Basic Information

- Rare, rapidly progressive infection of skin/soft tissue associated with high mortality; may be polymicrobial (type I) or monomicrobial (type II).
- Type I infections are most often caused by mixed aerobic and anaerobic bacteria and usually occur in older adults or diabetics and immunocompromised patients with underlying comorbid conditions.
- Type II infections are typically caused by group A *Streptococcus* or *Staphylococcus aureus* and can occur in healthy persons of any age.
- Risk factors include penetrating trauma, blunt trauma, skin/mucosal breach, recent surgery, and immunosuppression.

59

Clinical Presentation

- Early on, skin will be relatively normal appearing. The patient will present with **pain out of proportion to the examination;** must have a high index of suspicion to diagnose this early or it will progress rapidly over hours to include signs of cellulitis (erythema, warmth, pain, edema, tenderness) and formation of bullae or crepitus, often with systemic signs and sepsis (fever, tachycardia, hypotension).

Diagnosis and Evaluation

- Laboratory findings are nonspecific and include leukocytosis, hyponatremia, lactic acidosis, elevated creatinine, and elevated inflammatory markers such as C-reactive protein and erythrocyte sedimentation rate.
- Hyponatremia (Na^+ less than 135 mEq/L) is associated with increased mortality and may be an early prognostic indicator.
- Laboratory risk indicator for necrotizing fasciitis score based on white blood cell count, hemoglobin, sodium, glucose, creatinine, and C-reactive protein has limited sensitivity and should not be used to rule out the diagnosis.
- Imaging is sometimes helpful. Plain radiographs and bedside ultrasound may show air in soft tissues. Computed tomography or magnetic resonance imaging may show air, inflammation, or purulence within tissue planes.
- Surgical exploration is definitive diagnosis.

Treatment

- Emergent surgical consult for rapid surgical debridement is essential. Treatment for shock, including aggressive fluid resuscitation, should be initiated immediately. Empiric broad-spectrum antibiotics to cover polymicrobial infection are indicated. Vancomycin plus a third-generation cephalosporin are necessary to cover methicillin-resistant *Staphylococcus aureus*, *Streptococcus*, and gram-negative organisms. Clindamycin should be added to cover anaerobes and to treat toxin-elaborating strains of streptococci and staphylococci.

Clostridial Infections

Basic Information

- *Clostridium* species are widespread in nature owing to their ability to form endospores.
- Gas-producing, anaerobic gram-variable rods that can cause cellulitis (local along fascial planes) or myonecrosis/gas gangrene (invades healthy muscle tissue).
- Traumatic gas gangrene, predominantly caused by *C. perfringens*, results from deep penetrating or crush injury.
- Spontaneous gas gangrene, usually caused by *C. septicum*, occurs via hematogenous seeding from a gastrointestinal (GI) portal of entry. Risk factors include colon cancer, irritable bowel disease, diverticulitis, recent GI surgery, chemotherapy, radiation therapy, acquired immunodeficiency syndrome, necrotizing enterocolitis, and leukemia.

Clinical Presentation

- Anaerobic cellulitis: pain, erythema, edema at site of wound infection.
- Traumatic gas gangrene: skin initially appears pale then rapidly develops a bronze appearance, followed by red/purple discoloration. Skin becomes exquisitely tender and may develop bullae. Systemic signs develop rapidly, including fever and tachycardia, followed by shock, intravascular hemolysis, and multiorgan failure.
- Spontaneous gas gangrene: abrupt onset of severe muscle pain with rapid development of edema and bullae surrounded by skin with violaceous hue; may progress to septic shock.

Diagnosis and Evaluation

- Diagnosis is clinical. Imaging with computed tomography or magnetic resonance imaging may be useful to detect gas in deep tissues. Blood cultures (aerobic and anaerobic) should be obtained and may be positive. Definitive diagnosis requires demonstration of gram-variable rods at the site of entry. Drainage from surgical procedures shows presence of organisms, but absence of neutrophils.

Treatment

- Emergent surgical debridement in the operating room in addition to fluid resuscitation and broad-spectrum antibiotics to cover *Clostridium* species (clindamycin and piperacillin/tazobactam).

Clostridium tetani (Tetanus)

Basic Information

- Tetanus is caused by the exotoxin tetanospasmin produced by the spore-forming bacteria *Clostridium tetani*, which is ubiquitous in soil. Infection occurs following a break in the skin from a wound, rusty nail, or dirty needle used for IV drug use. Exotoxin causes blockage of the release of inhibitory neurotransmitters γ-aminobutyric acid and glycine, inducing spastic paralysis and tetany.

Clinical Presentation

- Incubation period is 3 to 21 days, typically shorter in neonatal tetanus.
- Local tetanus: muscle spasm near the site of injury; usually self-limited, but may progress to generalized tetanus.
- Generalized tetanus (most common): diffuse muscle rigidity and periodic spasms that result in trismus (lockjaw), risus sardonicus (sardonic smile), opisthotonus (severe muscle spasm causing arching of the back), respiratory failure.
- Neonatal tetanus: uncommon in the United States owing to sterilization of instruments used to cut umbilical cord and passive immunity from vaccinated mothers; irritability and poor feeding in the first week of life.
- Cephalic tetanus: occurs after facial trauma or otitis media, leading to cranial nerve dysfunction, which can mimic Bell palsy.

Diagnosis and Evaluation

- Diagnosis is clinical; no useful laboratory tests and cultures are often negative. "Spatula Test" = brushing of the posterior pharynx with a tongue depressor causes the patient to uncontrollably bite down on the tongue depressor. Sensitivity and specificity is more than 90% for tetanus infection.

Treatment

- Supportive care, including benzodiazepines for muscle spasm and magnesium or beta-blockers for sympathetic hyperactivity; immediate treatment with human tetanus immunoglobulin (TIG), followed by aggressive wound debridement (after the tetanus immunoglobulin to avoid release of more exotoxin); tetanus immunization at the opposite site of immunoglobulin. Metronidazole can be given after immunoglobulin and immunization.

Treponema pallidum (Syphilis)

Basic Information

- Bacterial spirochete responsible for the sexually transmitted infection syphilis
- Reportable to the public health department

Clinical Presentation

- Primary syphilis: painless genital ulcer with indurated border (chancre) that heals spontaneously over 2 to 6 weeks (Fig. 59.2A).
- Secondary syphilis: occurs 4 to 8 weeks after healing of a chancre, presenting with flu-like illness; may see nonpruritic maculopapular rash that spreads from trunk to extremities (Fig. 59.2B) and often involves the palms and soles; may be pustular and/or involve mucous membranes; can also see condyloma lata, which are wart-like lesions on genitals. Renal involvement may include nephrotic syndrome and/or acute renal failure. Symptoms resolve spontaneously.
- Latent syphilis: asymptomatic period with positive rapid plasma reagin or VDRL test, commonly lasting 3 to 4 years.

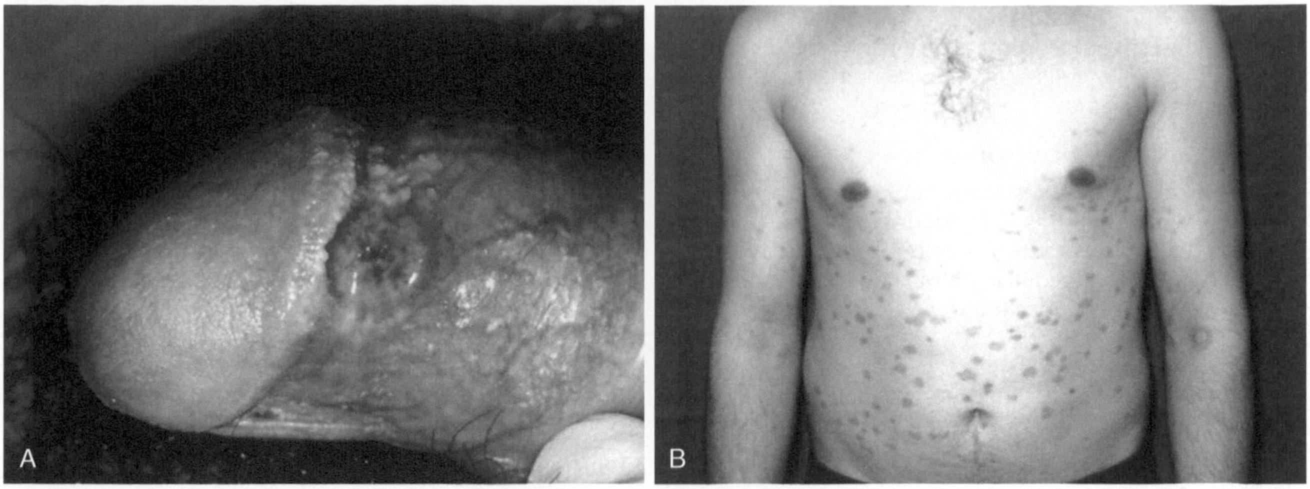

FIG. 59.2 **A,** Painless penile chancre seen in primary syphilis. **B,** Secondary syphilis rash. (From Sukthankar, A. (2014). Syphilis. *Medicine, 42*(7), 394–398, Figs. 3 and 4.)

- Tertiary syphilis: cardiovascular syphilis results in ascending aortic aneurysm and aortic valve regurgitation; typically occurs 15 to 30 years after an initial infection. Gummas present as ulcers or granulomatous nodules, which can occur anywhere, including skin, mucous membranes, bones, and internal organs.
- Neurosyphilis: can occur at any stage of infection; may present with meningitis, central nervous system vasculitis with ischemic stroke, ocular syphilis with uveitis, progressive dementia and personality changes, or tabes dorsalis, which is a disease of the dorsal columns of the spinal cord that causes sensory ataxia, lancinating pain, and the Argyll-Robertson pupil (normal accommodation, impaired reactivity to light); typically presents more than 20 years after a primary syphilis infection.

Diagnosis and Evaluation

- Screening tests are the rapid plasma reagin (RPR) or VDRL; these are nonspecific, positive more than 2 weeks after the first chancre, but false positives do occur. The confirmatory test is the fluorescent treponemal antibody absorption test. CSF studies, including VDRL, can be used to diagnose neurosyphilis in patients whose fluorescent treponemal antibody absorption test is positive.

Treatment

- Primary and secondary syphilis: benzathine penicillin 2.4 million units intramuscular (alternative: doxycycline orally for 14 days).
- Latent and tertiary syphilis: benzathine penicillin 2.4 million units weekly for 3 weeks (alternative: doxycycline orally for 28 days).
- Neurosyphilis: penicillin G 3 to 4 million units IV every 4 hours for 10 to 14 days.

JARISCH-HERXHEIMER REACTION

- A self-limited syndrome of acute fever, headache, malaise, myalgias, and sweating within 24 hours of initiating an antibiotic against spirochetes.

Corynebacterium diphtheriae (Diphtheria)

Basic Information

- Gram-positive rod, which may produce respiratory disease, cutaneous disease, or an asymptomatic carrier state.

Clinical Presentation

- Respiratory diphtheria (caused by toxin-producing strains): symptoms include sore throat, malaise, low-grade fever; can see cervical lymphadenopathy, erythema of pharynx, spots of gray and white exudates on the tonsils, and development of "pseudomembrane," which bleeds when scraped (Fig. 59.3). The membrane then spreads throughout the respiratory tract, causing nasal discharge, cough, hoarseness, and respiratory failure. Systemic manifestations caused by dissemination of diphtheria toxin include myocarditis, cranial neuropathy (palatal paralysis), peripheral neuropathy, and renal failure.

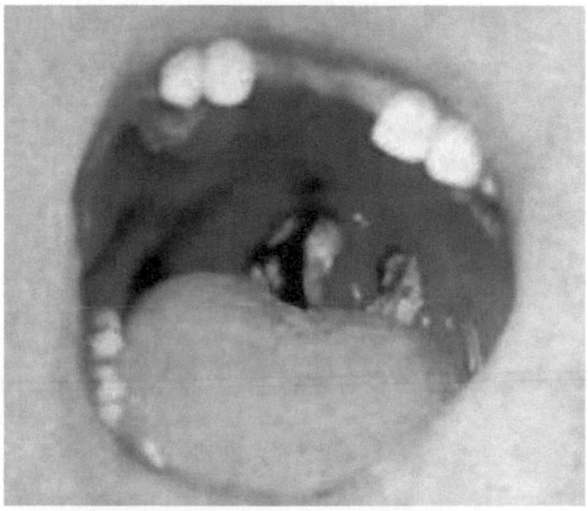

FIG. 59.3 Gray pseudomembrane in patient with diphtheria pharyngitis. (From Pham, L. L., Bourayou, R., Maghraoui-Slim, V., & Koné-Paut, I. (2017). Laryngitis, epiglottitis and pharyngitis. In J. Cohen, W. G. Powderly, & S. M. Opal (Eds.), *Infectious diseases* (4th ed., pp. 229–235.e1, Fig. 25.7). Elsevier.)

- Cutaneous diphtheria: caused by toxigenic and nontoxigenic strains; chronic, nonhealing sores or shallow ulcers with a dirty gray membrane; often seen after trauma in the homeless or intravenous drug users.

Diagnosis and Evaluation

- Based on clinical manifestations and risk factors. Presumptive diagnosis is made by identifying gram-positive rods in "Chinese character" distribution on Gram stain. Definitive diagnosis requires culture from respiratory tract secretion or skin lesion.

Treatment

- If signs of airway obstruction occur, prepare for a difficult intubation and consider consultation with anesthesia, if available. Supportive care includes respiratory droplet and contact precautions, and IV erythromycin or penicillin G. Antitoxin available from the Centers for Disease Control and Prevention is recommended in severe cases.

SUGGESTED READINGS

French, P. (2007). Syphilis. *BMJ*, *334*(7585), 143–147. doi:10.1136/bmj.39085.518148.BE.

Goh, T., Goh, L. G., Ang, C. H., & Wong, C. H. (2013). Early diagnosis of necrotizing fasciitis. *British Journal of Surgery, 101*(1), e119–e125. doi:10.1002/bjs.9371.

Heckenberg, S. G. B., de Gans, J., Brouwer, M. C., Weisfelt, M., Piet, J. R., Spanjaard, L., van der Ende, A., & van de Beek, D. (2008). Clinical features, outcome, and meningococcal genotype in 258 adults with meningococcal meningitis. *Medicine*, *87*(4), 185–192. doi:10.1097/md.0b013e318180a6b4.

Biological Warfare Agents

JESSA BAKER, MD, and GREGORY J. MORAN, MD

General Principles

A variety of microorganisms have potential to be used as biological warfare agents. The ideal agent would be capable of producing illness in a large proportion of those exposed, be disseminated easily to expose large numbers of people, remain stable and infectious despite environmental exposure, and be available to terrorists. Fortunately, few microorganisms have all these characteristics. The Centers for Disease Control and Prevention (CDC) has identified the organisms believed to have the greatest potential for use in bioterrorism (https://emergency.cdc.gov/bioterrorism/). Category A agents have the top priority for public health preparedness given their suitability for weaponization and lethality. Categories B and C are lower priority, but are recognized as potential agents.

As the front line of clinical medicine, emergency departments will be key to effective recognition, management, and surveillance of a natural or intentional outbreak. In addition to the challenge of treating illnesses, emergency clinicians will be faced with serious logistical problems. Personnel, medications, and other resources are likely to be insufficient; the federal government has stores of antibiotics, but rapid distribution will be difficult and demand for treatment and prophylaxis will exceed supply. Isolation of victims may also be necessary, which will be another hospital challenge. Lastly, preparing for the panic and chaos that a bioterrorism attack would cause is also necessary; thousands of people, ill or healthy, could descend on emergency departments and clinics, seeking evaluation and treatment.

Category A Agents

These agents are easy to disseminate, cause high morbidity and mortality, and require specific enhancements of the CDC's diagnostic capacity and enhanced disease surveillance.

ANTHRAX (*BACILLUS ANTHRACIS*)

- Natural source: zoonotic disease of persons who handle contaminated animal products (hair or hides); forms spores that are stable over long periods and can withstand exposure to air, sunlight, and some disinfectants.

Clinical Presentation

- Three distinct clinical syndromes in humans: cutaneous, inhalation, and gastrointestinal
  - Cutaneous anthrax
    - Most common, usually spread through contact with infected animals (cows, sheep, and horses, or their products); could present after contact with spores mailed in envelope, etc.
    - Typically produces large black eschars on the skin, lymphadenopathy, fever, malaise, and nausea.
    - Mortality rate of less than 1% if treated, can occasionally become systemic with mortality rates up to 20%.
  - Gastrointestinal anthrax
    - Rare in humans, acquired by ingesting inadequately cooked meat from infected animal; could result from intentional food contamination.
    - Oral or esophageal or lower gastrointestinal lesions may develop, causing abdominal pain, fever, and diarrhea that progresses to a sepsis with high mortality.
  - Inhalational anthrax
    - Rarely seen but could be spread by aerosolization with intentional attack, rapidly fatal.
    - Early symptoms similar to influenza: malaise, dry cough, and mild fever, progressing to chills, sweats, nausea, and vomiting, with chest pain and respiratory distress.
    - Almost all patients have chest radiograph or computed tomography scan abnormality, including infiltrates, pleural effusion, or mediastinal widening.
    - Illness often progresses to septic shock and death approximately 24–36 hours after onset of respiratory distress.

Diagnosis

- Mainly clinical diagnosis in order to ensure prompt treatment.
- *B. anthracis* is detectable through gram stain of the blood and blood culture on routine media.
- May also be identified in cerebrospinal fluid (CSF); approximately 50% of cases have hemorrhagic meningitis.
- Chest films may show a widened mediastinum and pleural effusions (late findings).

Infection Control Precautions

- Not spread person-to-person.
- Standard precautions recommended.
- Spores may be present after recent exposure; bathe with soap and water and store contaminated items in a sealed plastic bag.

Treatment and Prophylaxis

- Penicillin is the preferred treatment; however, penicillin-resistant strains exist.
- **Empiric** treatment with ciprofloxacin or another fluoroquinolone is recommended until susceptibility is known (penicillin not recommended as *empiric* treatment).

- *B. anthracis* is also susceptible to tetracyclines, erythromycin, chloramphenicol, and gentamicin.
- Exposure prophylaxis is recommended for those with suspected or confirmed exposure: ciprofloxacin or doxycycline in addition to vaccination (three-dose series).
- Spores can be dormant for a long time; a 60-day course of antibiotics is recommended for prophylaxis after exposure.

PLAGUE (*YERSINIA PESTIS*)

- Natural source: rodents via fleas.

Clinical Presentation

- Painful adenopathy several days after the infected fleabite.
- Illness progresses within several days to septicemia without treatment.
- 5%–15% of patients will develop a secondary pneumonia after 2–3 days that can progress to septicemia with ecchymoses and extremity necrosis.
- Aerosol dispersal with resulting pneumonic plague would be more likely in a bioterrorism attack.

Diagnosis

- Identify *Y. pestis* in Gram, Wayson, or Wright-Giemsa stain of blood, sputum, or lymph node aspirate.
- Definitive diagnosis with cultures; colonies of *Y. pestis* are usually 1–3 mm in diameter and have been described as having a "beaten copper" or "hammered metal" appearance.

Infection Control Precautions

- Strict respiratory isolation until treated for at least 3 days.

Treatment and Prophylaxis

- Streptomycin is the traditional preferred agent.
- Doxycycline, gentamicin, ceftriaxone, chloramphenicol, and fluoroquinolones should also be effective.
- Antibiotic course for minimum of 10 days or for 4 days after clinical recovery.
- Postexposure prophylaxis: doxycycline or a fluoroquinolone for 6 days.

SMALLPOX (VARIOLA)

- Source: no nonhuman sources; now only exists in secure laboratory stores.

Clinical Presentation

- Incubation period is approximately 12 days.
- Febrile prodrome with chills, body aches, nausea, vomiting, and abdominal pain.
- Characteristic rash develops on extremities and spreads centrally; skin lesions evolve slowly from macules to papules to vesicles to pustules, each stage lasting 1–2 days, all at the same stage of development (unlike varicella); may become umbilicated or confluent.
- Mortality is approximately 30% among unvaccinated persons (data from populations without modern medical care); death occurs late in the first week or during the second week.

Diagnosis

- Electron microscopy or gel diffusion on vesicular scrapings.
- Smallpox specimens should be handled under biosafety level 4 conditions.
- Vesicular eruption in which varicella cannot be identified should alert clinicians to possible smallpox.

Infection Control Precautions

- Transmitted person-to-person through respiratory droplets.
- **Identification of even a single case of smallpox would signal an infectious disease emergency of worldwide significance.**
- **If smallpox is suspected: immediately contact local health department and hospital infection control officer.**
- **Containment of any subsequent outbreak is of highest importance; strict quarantine with respiratory isolation for anyone exposed with respiratory isolation for 17 days.**
- Virions can also remain viable on fomites for up to 1 week; all laundry should be autoclaved or washed in hot water with bleach, standard hospital antiviral surface cleaners are adequate for disinfecting surfaces.

Treatment and Prophylaxis

- Supportive
- No known effective treatment exists against smallpox.
- Cidofovir (used for cytomegalovirus) may be active, but no data currently show efficacy in humans.
- Vaccine based on the vaccinia virus is effective up to several days after exposure; potential for secondary transmission following administration of live vaccine exists but is uncommon.

HEMORRHAGIC FEVERS

The hemorrhagic fevers are Ebola hemorrhagic fever, Marburg hemorrhagic fever, Lassa fever, Bolivian hemorrhagic fever, Congo-Crimean hemorrhagic fever, and Rift Valley fever.

- See Chapter 65. Emerging Infections: Pandemic Viruses.

Treatment and Prophylaxis

- Lassa fever, Bolivian hemorrhagic fever, Congo-Crimean hemorrhagic fever, or Rift Valley fever may benefit from ribavirin.

BOTULISM

- Natural source: neurotoxins produced by the bacillus *Clostridium botulinum*; most cases result from the ingestion of improperly prepared or canned foods.

Clinical Presentation

- Fairly characteristic presentation and can usually be diagnosed with clinical signs and symptoms alone.
- Clinical syndrome is similar whether toxins are ingested or inhaled.
- Toxins block the cholinergic synapses and thereby interfere with neurotransmission.
- After incubation period of 1–5 days, patients generally present with neurologic manifestations: bulbar palsies (diplopia and mydriasis), dysarthria and dysphagia, progressive weakness followed by skeletal muscle paralysis; cause of death is usually respiratory failure.

Diagnosis

- Clinical and epidemiologic grounds.
- Laboratory testing not helpful.

Infection Control Precautions

- Standard
- Bathe thoroughly with soap and water and discard contaminated clothes after skin or aerosol exposure.

Treatment and Prophylaxis

- Hemodynamic and ventilatory support.
- Full recovery may take weeks to months.
- Trivalent equine antitoxin available from CDC; effective only at preventing further deterioration.

TULAREMIA

- See Chapter 63. Tick-Borne Illnesses.

Category B Agents

Category B agents are somewhat easy to disseminate. They cause moderate morbidity and low mortality and require specific enhancements of the CDC's diagnostic capacity and enhanced disease surveillance.

COXIELLA BURNETII (Q FEVER)

- Natural source: rickettsial organism *C. burnetii* carried by infected livestock (sheep, cattle, goats), humans infected by inhaled/aerosolized spores, which last weeks to months in environment.

Clinical Presentation

- Nonspecific; most common are fever, chills, and headache.
- Incubation period can vary considerably from approximately 10 days up to several weeks.
- Most have self-limited febrile illness that resolves within 1 or 2 weeks.
- Mortality is low: 2.4%.
- May manifest as pneumonia: many patients have radiographic evidence of pneumonia but no cough; multiple rounded opacities (often pleural-based) are a suggestive pattern.
- Various chronic manifestations: culture-negative endocarditis, intravascular infection, acute hepatitis, liver granulomas, and osteomyelitis.

Diagnosis

- Serologic testing through complement fixation, indirect fluorescent antibody, or enzyme-linked immunosorbent assay.
- Titers may not be elevated until 2–3 weeks into the illness.

Infection Control Precautions

- No person-to-person spread.

Treatment and Prophylaxis

- Tetracyclines are most commonly used for treatment.
- Other drugs that have been used include macrolides, quinolones, chloramphenicol, rifampin, and trimethoprim-sulfamethoxazole.
- Optimal duration of therapy is unclear; generally given for 5–7 days.

BRUCELLA SPECIES (BRUCELLOSIS)

- Natural source: zoonotic infection spread via direct contact with animal secretions through breaks in the skin, infected aerosols, or ingestion of unpasteurized dairy products.

Clinical Presentation

- Varied and nonspecific, viral-like prodrome.
- Symptoms begin 2–4 weeks after exposure, followed by relapsing and remitting symptoms.
- Infection tends to localize in tissues with large numbers of macrophages, such as lung, spleen, liver, central nervous system, bone marrow, and synovium.
- Rarely fatal.
- Liver involvement is common; hepatic granulomas are characteristic of some species, such as *B. abortus*.
- Skeletal complications: osteomyelitis, and tenosynovitis of large weight-bearing joints (e.g., sacroiliac, hips, knees, ankles).
- Hematologic findings: anemia, leukopenia, and thrombocytopenia.
- Serious complications: endocarditis (2%) and central nervous system infection (<5%).

Diagnosis

- Serology
- Slow growing; laboratory should hold cultures for 4 weeks.
- Presumptive diagnosis can be made on the basis of high or rising antibody titers; most have titers higher than 1:160.

Infection Control Precautions

- Human-to-human transmission seems to be rare; isolation is not necessary.
- Organisms are highly infectious through aerosol, and culture specimens may pose a threat to laboratory workers.
- Contact isolation should be used for those with open, draining lesions.

Treatment and Prophylaxis

- Antibiotics reduce the severity and duration of illness.
- Combination treatment is most effective: doxycycline plus rifampin for 6 weeks.
- Gentamicin or streptomycin is sometimes included in the regimen for more severe infections such as endocarditis.
- Postexposure prophylaxis would likely be effective and cost-effective in a bioterrorism setting.

BURKHOLDERIA MALLEI (GLANDERS)

- Natural source: carried by horses, mules, or donkeys; spread via broken skin or nasal mucosa or aerosol form.

Clinical Presentation

- Tender nodule with local lymphangitis.
- Inoculation of the eyes, nose, and mouth can result in mucopurulent discharge with ulcerating granulomas.
- Systemic invasion: incubation period after infection through inhalation (most likely in a bioterrorism event) is 10–14 days, followed by generalized papular or pustular eruption, fever, myalgias, headache, pleuritic chest

pain, lymphadenopathy and splenomegaly; fatal within 7–10 days.

Diagnosis

- Blood cultures usually negative, except in the terminal stages of septicemia.
- Serologic tests usually show rise in titers by second week of illness.
- Complement fixation titers are more specific but less sensitive.
- Polymerase chain reaction testing can differentiate *B. mallei* and *B. pseudomallei.*

Infection Control Precautions

- Standard and airborne isolation precautions.
- Culture specimens pose a threat to laboratory personnel: biosafety level 3 precautions are indicated.

Treatment and Prophylaxis

- No studies, given paucity of cases.
- Sulfadiazine has been effective in experimental animal infections and humans.
- Agents known to be effective for human melioidosis include tetracyclines, trimethoprim-sulfamethoxazole, amoxicillin-clavulanate, and chloramphenicol.

ALPHAVIRUSES

The alphaviruses include Venezuelan equine encephalomyelitis, eastern equine encephalomyelitis, and western equine encephalomyelitis.

- Natural source: mosquito-borne.

Clinical Presentation

- Nonspecific viral prodrome: fever, headache, and myalgia, a fraction will progress to frank encephalitis.
- Ill horses in the vicinity should suggest an equine encephalitis virus.
- Eastern equine encephalomyelitis is the most severe, with high mortality rates and high rates of neurologic sequelae; western equine encephalomyelitis and Venezuelan equine encephalomyelitis have lower rates of progression to neurologic symptoms.
- Infants and elderly most prone to developing encephalitis; initial viral prodrome is followed by confusion, somnolence, and potentially coma.
- Laboratory test results: leukopenia in the early stages, which can progress to leukocytosis, CSF protein is elevated, and lymphocytic pleocytosis is usually present.

Diagnosis

- Can sometimes be isolated from blood during the early stages of illness; viremia has usually resolved by the time encephalitis symptoms develop.
- Can sometimes be isolated from CSF or postmortem brain tissue.
- Serologic testing of the CSF or serum.
- Virus-specific immunoglobulin M antibodies can be detected with enzyme-linked immunosorbent assay.

Infection Control Precautions

- Isolation not necessary.
- No person-to-person transmission.

Treatment and Prophylaxis

- Supportive
- Inactivated vaccines are available for eastern equine encephalomyelitis, western equine encephalomyelitis, and Venezuelan equine encephalomyelitis, but none are widely used.

RICIN TOXIN FROM *RICINUS COMMUNIS* PLANT

- Natural source: castor bean.

Clinical Presentation

- Ricin toxin inhibits protein synthesis.
- As inhaled aerosol, the toxin can produce symptoms within 4–8 hours.
- Typical symptoms include fever, chest tightness, cough, dyspnea, nausea, arthralgias, and profuse sweating.
- Symptoms should improve within several hours with sublethal dose.
- Lethal doses produced necrosis of the respiratory tract and alveolar filling in 36–72 hours after exposure in animal studies.
- Ingested toxin causes gastrointestinal symptoms: nausea, vomiting, and diarrhea.
- Large toxin exposures associated with gastrointestinal hemorrhage and hepatic, splenic, and renal necrosis.
- Death can occur from hypovolemic shock, disseminated intravascular coagulation, microcirculatory failure, and multiple organ failure.

Diagnosis

- Clinical and epidemiologic.

Infection Control Precautions

- No person-to-person transmission.

Treatment and Prophylaxis

- Supportive, including ventilatory.
- Gastric decontamination with charcoal may be beneficial.

EPSILON TOXIN OF *CLOSTRIDIUM PERFRINGENS*

- See Chapter 59. Systemic Bacterial Infections.

STAPHYLOCOCCAL ENTEROTOXIN B

- See GI (see Chapter 4 Large Bowel).

FOOD-BORNE OR WATER-BORNE AGENTS

Food- or water-borne agents include *Salmonella* species, *Shigella dysenteriae*, Shiga toxin-producing *Escherichia coli*, *Vibrio cholerae*, and *Cryptosporidium parvum*.

- See GI (see Chapter 4. Large Bowel).

Category C Agents

Category C agents are emerging pathogens that could be engineered for mass dissemination in the future because of availability, ease of production and dissemination, and potential for high morbidity and mortality and major health impact.

NIPAH VIRUS

- Natural source: pigs, primarily in south Asia.

Clinical Presentation

- Fever, headache, and myalgias, and eventually develop signs of meningitis or encephalitis.
- Respiratory symptoms less common.

Diagnosis

- Specialized testing in a reference laboratory, such as the CDC or U.S. Army Medical Research Institute of Infectious Diseases (USAMRIID).
- Immunoglobulin M antibodies can be detected in blood and CSF.

Infection Control Precautions

- Virus has been isolated from respiratory secretions and urine of patients infected; however, person-to-person spread not identified.

Treatment and Prophylaxis

- Supportive
- Reduction in mortality with ribavirin.

HANTAVIRUSES

- See Chapter 65. Emerging Infections: Pandemic Viruses.

OTHER VIRUSES TO CONSIDER

- Tick-borne hemorrhagic fever viruses (see Chapter 65. Emerging Infections: Pandemic Viruses)
- Tick-borne encephalitis viruses (see Chapter 65. Emerging Infections: Pandemic Viruses)
- Yellow fever
- Multidrug-resistant tuberculosis (see Chapter 66. Drug Resistance)

SUGGESTED READINGS

Centers for Disease Control and Prevention. (2000). Biological and chemical terrorism: Strategic plan for preparedness and response. Recommendations of the CDC Strategic Planning Workgroup. *Morbidity and Mortality Weekly Report. Recommendations and Reports*, 49(RR04), 1–14. https://www.cdc.gov/mmwr/preview/mmwrhtml/rr4904a1.htm.

Moran, G. J., Talan, D. A., & Abrahamian, F. M. (2008). Biological terrorism. *Infectious Disease Clinics of North America, 22*, 145–187.

Schultz, C. H., & Koenig, K. L. (2018). Weapons of mass destruction. In R. M. Walls, R. S. Hockberger, & M. Gausche-Hill (Eds.), *Rosen's emergency medicine: Concepts and clinical practice* (9th ed., pp. 2418–2428). Elsevier.

Fungal Infections

ASHLEY VUONG, MD, MA, and FREDRICK M. ABRAHAMIAN, DO, FIDSA, FACEP

Systemic fungal infections are commonly encountered in immunocompromised populations and can affect all organ systems.

Aspergillosis

General Principles

- Caused by *Aspergillus*.
- Often occurs in immunocompromised people.
- Infection can range from a hypersensitivity reaction to invasive infections.
- Often spread through inhalation and presents as a lung infection.

ALLERGIC BRONCHOPULMONARY ASPERGILLOSIS

- Occurs almost exclusively in patients with asthma or cystic fibrosis.

Clinical Presentation

- Presents as recurrent asthma exacerbations.

Diagnosis and Evaluation

- Obligatory criteria: *Aspergillus* skin test positivity or elevated serum immunoglobulin (>1,000 IU/mL) against *A. fumigatus*.
- Two or more other criteria
  - Serum antibodies against *A. fumigatus*.
  - Radiographic evidence of pulmonary opacities consistent with allergic bronchopulmonary aspergillosis.
    - Chest x-ray (CXR) may show mucus plugging, consolidations in upper or middle lobes, or central bronchiectasis.
  - Total eosinophil count >500 cells/μL (glucocorticoid-naive).

Treatment

- Systemic glucocorticoids and antifungal therapy with itraconazole or voriconazole.

ASPERGILLOMA (FUNGUS BALL)

- Arises in preexisting pulmonary cavities in immunocompetent hosts.

Clinical Presentation

- Simple aspergillomas may be asymptomatic.
- Chronic pulmonary aspergillosis.
  - Weight loss, chronic productive cough, hemoptysis, shortness of breath.

Diagnosis and Evaluation

- CXR: intracavitary mass surrounded by crescent of air.
- *Aspergillus* immunoglobulin A-positive.

Treatment

- Azole antifungals (itraconazole or voriconazole).

INVASIVE ASPERGILLOSIS

- Occurs in patients with immunosuppression (e.g., neutropenia).

Clinical Presentation

- Can present as pulmonary aspergillosis, tracheobronchitis, rhinosinusitis, central nervous system (CNS) infection, endophthalmitis, endocarditis, cutaneous aspergillosis, gastrointestinal (GI) aspergillosis, or disseminated infection.
- Most common presentation is pulmonary aspergillosis.
  - Classic triad in neutropenic patients: fever, pleuritic chest pain, and hemoptysis.

Diagnosis and Evaluation

- Single or multiple nodules with surrounding ground-glass infiltrates (the halo sign) on computed tomography (CT) scan.
- Diagnosis based on biopsy showing hyphal elements invading tissue.

Treatment

- Voriconazole with or without the addition of an echinocandin.
- Adjunctive treatments may include surgery and reduction of immunosuppression.

Systemic Candidiasis

General Principles

- Can present as urinary tract infection, meningitis, endocarditis, empyema, mediastinitis, pericarditis.
- Risk factors.
  - Immunosuppression, invasive lines, microbiota composition changes.

HEPATOSPLENIC OR CHRONIC DISSEMINATED CANDIDIASIS

Clinical Presentation

- Persistent fever, right upper quadrant pain, nausea, vomiting, anorexia.

Diagnosis and Evaluation

- Elevated serum alkaline phosphatase.
- Characteristic lesions in the liver, spleen, and kidneys on ultrasonography, magnetic resonance imaging, and CT.
- May be present even if blood cultures are negative.

URINARY TRACT INFECTION

- May present as colonization or infection.
- Infection generally occurs in patients with diabetes or anatomic abnormalities.

Clinical Presentation

- Typical symptoms of urinary tract infection (dysuria, frequency, suprapubic discomfort).
- Typical symptoms of pyelonephritis (flank pain, costovertebral angle tenderness, abdominal tenderness).

Diagnosis and Evaluation

- Fungal casts, which signify kidney involvement, can help diagnose infection.
- Abdominal CT and ultrasonography may show hydronephrosis, fungal balls, or perinephric abscesses.

OSTEOARTICULAR INFECTION

- Occurs in the setting of hematogenous spread or direct inoculation.
- Adults are most likely to have vertebral involvement.
- Children are more likely to have infections in the long bones of the extremities.

Clinical Presentation

- Most common symptoms include pain and decreased range of motion.

Diagnosis and Evaluation

- Diagnosis requires visualization of *Candida* on culture of the involved site.

MENINGITIS

- Occurs in the setting of disseminated candidiasis in premature neonates or direct inoculation from ventricular drainage devices.

Clinical Presentation

- Presents as fever, nuchal rigidity, altered mental status, headache.
- May also present as sepsis or organ failure in neonates.

Diagnosis and Evaluation

- Diagnosed through positive cerebrospinal fluid (CSF) culture.

ENDOCARDITIS

- Most common cause is fungal endocarditis.
- Occurs in patients with prolonged candidemia who have prosthetic heart valves or central venous catheters, or are intravenous drug users.

Clinical Presentation

- Presents similarly to bacterial endocarditis: fever, new heart murmur, new-onset heart failure.

Diagnosis and Evaluation

- Positive blood cultures.
- Vegetations on echocardiography.

PERITONITIS AND INTRAABDOMINAL INFECTIONS

- Usually part of a polymicrobial infection after intraabdominal injury or a complication of peritoneal dialysis.
- May also cause pancreatic abscess, gangrenous cholecystitis, fungal ball, common bile duct obstruction.

Clinical Presentation

- Presents with the same symptoms as bacterial peritonitis: fever, chills, abdominal pain.

Treatment

- Local infections: topical or oral nystatin or azole drugs.
- Invasive candidiasis: intravenous echinocandins (e.g., caspofungin, micafungin).

Blastomycosis

General Principles

- Caused by the fungus *Blastomyces dermatitidis*.
- Most frequent clinical manifestation is asymptomatic infection (50%) or chronic pneumonia.
- Risk factors
  - Associated with moist soil and wood.
  - Distributed in the southeast and midwest parts of the United States (the Mississippi and Ohio River valleys).

61

Clinical Presentation

- Common symptoms: productive cough, fever, chest pain, shortness of breath, B symptoms (fever, weight loss, night sweats).

Diagnosis and Evaluation

- CXR demonstrates alveolar infiltrates, a mass lesion, or a miliary or reticulonodular pattern.
- Chest CT can show nodules, consolidations with or without cavitation, and "tree-in-bud" opacities without hilar adenopathy (unlike histoplasmosis).
- Broad-based yeast buds.
- Definitive diagnosis requires growth of *Blastomyces*.

Treatment

- Non-CNS mild to moderate disease: itraconazole.
- Severe disease: lipid formulation amphotericin B and then itraconazole (non-CNS) or voriconazole (CNS) for step-down therapy.

Coccidioidomycosis

General Principles

- Also known as Valley fever.
- Caused by the fungus *Coccidioides immitis*.
- Generally distributed in the southwestern region of the United States.

- Transmitted through inhalation of airborne spores.
- Exposure more common in dry periods after a rainy season.
- Common in immunocompetent hosts (unlike other systemic fungal infections).
- Risk factors:
  - Immunosuppression, pregnancy, diabetes.
  - Black or Filipino heritage.

Clinical Presentation

- More than half of infections are asymptomatic.
- May present with typical signs and symptoms of respiratory infection.
  - Fever, malaise, cough, pleuritic chest pain, sore throat.
- Severe cases can present with arthralgias and cutaneous manifestations such as erythema nodosum and erythema multiforme.
- Disseminated disease presents with constitutional symptoms (severe night sweats, weight loss, fever) and dyspnea at rest.
  - Typically presents in immunocompromised or Black or Filipino individuals.
- Meningeal coccidioidomycosis presents as headache, nausea, vomiting, altered mental status, blurry vision.

Diagnosis and Evaluation

- Suspect coccidioidomycosis in patients who:
  - Live in or have recently traveled to endemic areas.
  - Have a prolonged course (>1 week) of a respiratory illness.
  - Have cutaneous symptoms (erythema nodosum or erythema multiforme).
- Diagnosis confirmed through serologic testing or isolation of *Coccidioides* in culture.
- Features of severe disease:
  - Weight loss >10% of body weight.
  - Night sweats >3 weeks.
  - Symptoms >2 months.
  - Infiltrates in more than half of one lung or in both lungs.
  - Anticoccidioidal complement fixing antibody concentrations >1:16.

Treatment

- No treatment is necessary in immunocompetent patients with mild disease.
- In severe disease, including coccidioidomycosis meningitis:
  - Fluconazole or itraconazole for nonpregnant patients.
  - Amphotericin B in the most severe cases or during first-trimester pregnancy (due to the risk of teratogenicity with azoles).

Histoplasmosis

General Principles

- Caused by the fungus *Histoplasma capsulatum*.
- Endemic to the Ohio, Missouri, and Mississippi River valleys.
- Found in soil, bird, and bat droppings.
- Risk factors
  - Disruption of soil leads to aerosolization of the fungus that can be inhaled
  - Associated with high-risk activities including spelunking, excavation, and building demolition.

Clinical Presentation

- May infect both immunocompetent and immunocompromised patients.
- Presentation of disease will differ greatly based on a person's ability to contain the infection.
- Can present as acute pulmonary histoplasmosis, chronic pulmonary histoplasmosis, disseminated disease, or mediastinitis.

ACUTE PULMONARY HISTOPLASMOSIS

- Most cases are asymptomatic or self-limited.
- Symptoms occur 1–4 weeks after exposure.
- Presents with flu-like symptoms: fever, chills, headache, myalgia, cough, substernal chest pain (coryza and sore throat are not typical symptoms).
- CXR may show hilar or mediastinal lymphadenopathy.

CHRONIC PULMONARY HISTOPLASMOSIS

- Typically occurs in those with underlying lung disease.
- Presents with symptoms like re-activation tuberculosis: productive cough, dyspnea, chest pain, fevers, fatigue, night sweats, cavitary, fibrotic apical infiltrates on radiography.

DISSEMINATED HISTOPLASMOSIS

- Occurs in immunocompromised patients who cannot form granulomas to contain the infection.
- Disseminated infection can be acute or chronic.
  - Acute infection can present as fever, fatigue, hepatosplenomegaly, pancytopenia, or shock and multiorgan failure.
  - Chronic infection presentation differs based on the organ system involved.
    - Hematologic: pancytopenia.
    - Liver/spleen: hepatosplenomegaly.
    - GI and oropharynx: mucosal or intestinal ulceration.
    - Adrenal glands: adrenal insufficiency.
    - Cardiac: pericarditis.
    - CNS: focal brain lesions or meningitis.

MEDIASTINITIS

- Dissemination of *Histoplasma* to the mediastinal lymph nodes
- Mediastinal granulomas or fibrosing mediastinitis may be asymptomatic or can cause mass-effect disease.
  - May lead to superior vena cava syndrome, esophageal compression, or airway obstruction.

Diagnosis and Evaluation

- CXR may be normal or show pneumonitis with adenopathy, focal pulmonary infiltrates, or diffuse infiltrates.
- Laboratory testing may show mild anemia, elevated alkaline phosphatase (in chronic or disseminated disease), or elevated lactate dehydrogenase (in AIDS patients).
- Definitive diagnosis: sputum cultures, blood cultures, antibody testing, or serum/urine antigen testing.

Treatment

- Acute pulmonary disease:
  - <4 weeks or asymptomatic: usually self-limited, no treatment.
  - >4 weeks: itraconazole; severe: amphotericin B with methylprednisolone.

- Chronic cavitary pulmonary disease: itraconazole.
- Mediastinal granuloma: itraconazole.

Pneumocystis Pneumonia

General Principles

- Also known as PCP/PJP.
- Caused by yeast-like fungus *Pneumocystis jiroveci (carinii)*.
- Most common opportunistic infection and most commonly identified cause of death in AIDS patients.
- Risk factors
  - Immunosuppression (especially CD4 count <200), severe malnutrition.

Clinical Presentation

- Dyspnea, dry cough, fever, fulminant respiratory failure with hypoxemia.

Diagnosis and Evaluation

- CXR: diffuse, bilateral interstitial infiltrates ("bat-wing" appearance).
- CT scan: ground glass opacities or cystic lesions in the lungs.
- Definitive diagnosis: isolation of the *Pneumocystis jiroveci* in sputum via tinctorial staining, fluorescent antibody staining, or PCR assay.

Treatment

- Trimethoprim/sulfamethoxazole.
- Alternative regimens: trimethoprim-dapsone or clindamycin-primaquine.
- Adjunctive corticosteroids in moderate to severe disease (A-a O2 gradient ≥35 and/or a partial pressure of arterial oxygen <70 mm Hg).

Cryptococcus Neoformans

General Principles

- Encapsulated yeast found worldwide.
- Spreads through inhalation.
- Risk factors
  - Immunocompromised, liver disease, sarcoidosis.

Clinical Presentation

- Most commonly presents as indolent meningoencephalitis.
- Common presenting symptoms include fever, headache, nausea, altered mental status, focal neurologic deficits (only one-fourth to one-third of patients present with stiff neck, photophobia, or vomiting).
- Can also present as pulmonary cryptococcosis (symptoms include cough and dyspnea) and rarely as disseminated disease.

Diagnosis and Evaluation

- Neuroimaging result is typically normal.
- CSF studies are the key to diagnosis.
  - CSF studies usually consistent with fungal meningitis:
    - Color: clear
    - Opening pressure: normal to elevated
    - White blood cell count: <500 cells/μL
    - Protein: >200 mg/dL
    - Glucose: low to normal
  - CSF can be normal in extreme immunocompromise.
  - CSF positive for *Cryptococcus* antigen has 100% sensitivity and specificity.
  - Other important CSF studies include *Cryptococcus* culture and India ink capsule stains.

Treatment

- Pulmonary:
  - Non–AIDS associated: fluconazole, itraconazole, or voriconazole
  - AIDS associated: fluconazole
- Meningitis:
  - Non–AIDS associated: amphotericin B with or without flucytosine followed by fluconazole.
  - AIDS associated: amphotericin B with flucytosine followed by fluconazole.
    - Highly active antiretroviral therapy 2–10 weeks *after* the start of treatment for *Cryptococcus* to reduce risk of immune reconstitution syndrome.

Mucormycosis

General Principles

- Caused by the *Mucor* mold.
- Spread through inhalation.
- Risk factors include uncontrolled diabetes mellitus, glucocorticoid therapy, hematologic malignancy, hematopoietic cell or organ transplantation, iron treatment or iron overload, HIV/AIDS, intravenous drug use, trauma/burns, malnutrition.

Clinical Presentation

Varies based on the location of the infection.

- Rhino-orbital-cerebral
  - The most common site of *Mucor* infection.
  - Initially presents similarly to acute bacterial sinusitis (fever, headache, swelling and pain around the sinuses).
  - May rapidly invade contiguous structures over the course of a few days.
    - Invasion causes tissue necrosis and eschar formation on the palate, mucosa, or overlying skin.
      - May present with nasal ulceration, periorbital swelling, vision loss, ophthalmoplegia, altered mental status.
- Pulmonary
  - Inhalation of *Mucor* causes a necrotic pneumonia.
  - Presents with fever and hemoptysis.
- Gastrointestinal
  - Ingestion of spores may cause necrotic ulceration of the GI tract.
  - May result in bowel infarction and hemorrhagic shock.
- Cutaneous
  - Spore inoculation through wounds.
  - Forms painful ecthyma-like lesion.
  - May develop into progressive tissue necrosis.
- Disseminated
  - Typically occurs in cases of severe immunocompromise.
  - Often spreads from primary pulmonary or cerebral infections.
  - High mortality rate (96%).

Diagnosis and Evaluation

- CT useful for surgical intervention.
- Definitive diagnosis requires visualization of nonseptate hyphae, right-angle branching *Mucor* on histopathology.

Treatment

- Aggressive and emergent treatment is vital.
- Requires a combination of surgical debridement and treatment with amphotericin B.

SUGGESTED READINGS

Enoch, D. A., Ludlam, H. A., & Brown, N. M. (2006). Invasive fungal infections: A review of epidemiology and management options. *Journal of Medical Microbiology, 55*(pt. 7), 809–818.

Garber, G. (2001). An overview of fungal infections. *Drugs, 61*(Suppl. 1), 1–12.

Shoham, S., & Marr, K. A. (2012). Invasive fungal infections in solid organ transplant recipients. *Future Microbiology, 7*(5), 639–655.

Protozoa and Parasites

ALEXANDRA McLEROY-WALLACE, MD, and MATTHEW WAXMAN, MD, DTM&H

Protozoal and parasitic infections represent a large number of species that may be both locally acquired in the country of origin and encountered in returning travelers. Protozoa species and parasites have varied presentations, depending on the organ system that they invade and host immune status. An understanding of the organism's life cycle, exposure to endemic areas, diagnostic tests, and treatment in the acute setting are summarized below. Many of the diagnostic tests for parasites and protozoa are not readily available in the emergency department, nor will the results be available in a timely manner to the emergency medicine provider. A high index of suspicion to the possibility of one of these infections and obtaining specialty consultation or referral is a key feature in managing such diseases in emergency medicine.

Protozoa

MALARIA

General Principles

- Organism: *Plasmodium* species (*P. falciparum*, *P. vivax*, *P. ovale*, *P. malariae*).
- *P. falciparum* causes the most severe infection.
- *P. vivax* and *P. ovale* can reside in the host hepatocytes in a dormant state causing symptoms months to years after initial infection.
- Vector: Anopheles mosquito.
- Endemic areas: Africa, Asia, Central America, South America.
- Life cycle: sporozoites transmitted through mosquito saliva migrate to the liver, following rounds of division resulting in cell lysis and release of merozoites which in turn invade erythrocytes and become trophozoites. Cyclic red blood cell (RBC) lysis releases merozoites to infect other erythrocytes.

Clinical Presentation

- Malaise, anemia, abdominal pain, headache, upper respiratory complaints (cough). Although fever is the prominent clinical clue, cyclical fevers (occurs from lysis of RBCs) with predictable patterns are rarely encountered clinically.
  - *P. falciparum*: infected RBCs become adherent to microvasculature and result in ischemia in arterioles and capillaries leading to encephalopathy (cerebral malaria), metabolic acidosis, renal failure, noncardiogenic pulmonary edema, and disseminated intravascular coagulation.

Diagnosis and Evaluation

- Any returning traveler with fever from an area endemic for malaria should undergo testing in the emergency department.
- Anemia, hypoglycemia, acute renal failure, hemolysis, and hyperbilirubinemia may be present in severe disease.
- Thick peripheral blood smears identify the presence of blood parasites and should be sent from the ED, and can often be reviewed by a hospital microbiologist or pathology.
- Thin smears speciate the blood parasite and require light microscopy skills (Fig. 62.1 A-B). In endemic areas, light microscopy is often not performed when rapid diagnostic tests are available.
- Admit those with severe disease (sepsis, end organ damage) and those who cannot take medication orally.

Treatment

- All patients with high suspicion for malaria should receive specialty consultation because treatment depends on organism and resistance patterns.
- *P. falciparum*:
  - Quinine plus doxycycline OR quinine plus clindamycin OR mefloquine.
  - Proguanil-atovaquone for cerebral malaria and multiorgan involvement.
  - Intravenous (IV) quinine is currently not available in the United States.
  - IV artesunate for severe malaria is only available in the United States through the Centers for Disease Control and Prevention (CDC) malaria hotline at 770-488-7788.
- *P. vivax*, *P. ovale*, and *P. malariae*:
  - Chloroquine only in areas of Latin America without substantial resistance (Haiti, Dominican Republic, Central America).
  - Primaquine: for hepatic phase of *P. ovale* and *P. vivax*.
    - Induces hemolysis in patients with G6PD deficiency.
  - Artemether/lumefantrine: an oral agent for uncomplicated malaria.

AMERICAN TRYPANOSOMIASIS (CHAGAS DISEASE)

General Principles

- Organism: *Trypanosoma cruzi*.
- Vector/host: reduviid bug ("kissing bug"); excretes feces containing trypomastigotes that enter through a bite wound.
- Life cycle: amastigotes invade the cardiac muscle and conduction system, as well as smooth and autonomic muscle in the esophagus and colon.
- Endemic areas: Central and South America.

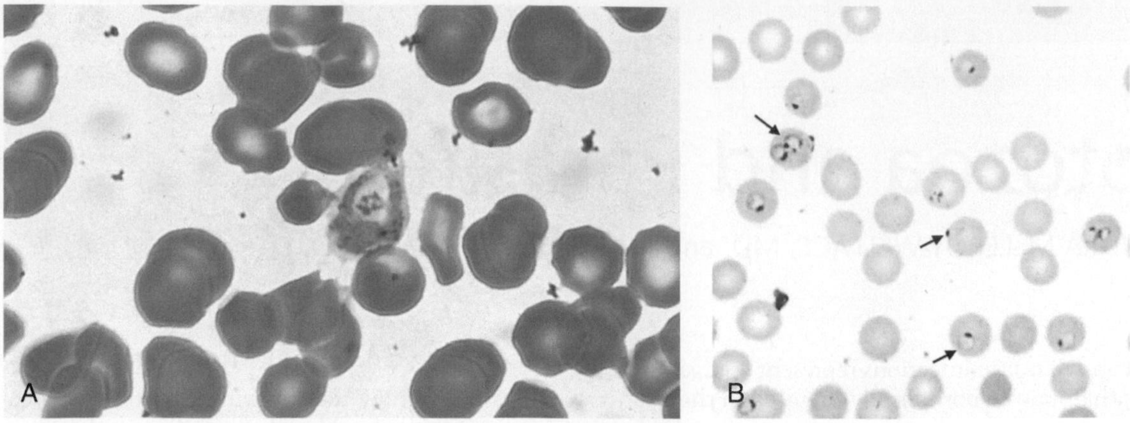

FIG. 62.1 Thick (**A**) and thin (**B**) smear peripheral blood smears demonstrating *P. falciparum* infection. (**A**, From Zitelli, B. J., McIntire, S., & Nowalk, A. J. (2018). *Zitelli and Davis' atlas of pediatric physical diagnosis* (7th ed., pp. 419–454, Fig. 12.21). Elsevier; **B**, From Kafai, N. M., & Odom John, A. R. (2017). Malaria in children. *Infectious Disease Clinics of North America, 32*(1), 189–200, Fig. 1.)

Clinical Presentation

- Infected bite site (chagoma): often around eyes, causing painless unilateral periorbital edema.
- Fever, malaise, pedal edema, hepatosplenomegaly: generally lasts 1 to 2 months.
- "Indeterminate" (dormant) phase: only 25% of those infected with the infection progress.
- Invasion of the myocardium, smooth and autonomic muscle of the esophagus and colon: typically becomes clinically significant decades after exposure.
  - Myocarditis, dilated cardiomyopathy, dysrhythmias, conduction blocks, congestive heart failure.
  - Gastrointestinal (GI) symptoms: achalasia, megacolon, hepatosplenomegaly, and elevated aminotransferases.

Diagnosis and Evaluation

- Serology (e.g., enzyme-linked immunosorbent assay [ELISA] and immunofluorescent antibody test [IFA]). Trypomastigotes are rarely visualized on peripheral blood smear in acute disease. Cerebrospinal fluid, lymph node, or cardiac biopsy required in chronic disease.
  - Delayed diagnosis of heart failure with preserved ejection fraction and right bundle branch block (RBBB) on electrocardiogram may be seen in immigrants from endemic areas.

Treatment

- Nifurtimox or benznidazole: less than 50% cure rate and not effective in advanced disease.
- Symptomatic treatment of GI and cardiac complications, such as automatic implantable cardioverter defibrillator (AICD) placement, antiarrhythmics, congestive heart failure treatment, cardiac transplantation (although disease can recur in the transplanted heart).

AMEBIASIS

General Principles

- Organism: *Entamoeba histolytica.*
- Vector: ingestion of amebic cysts.
  - Associated with poor sanitation and hygiene.
  - Recent outbreaks in men who have sex with men (*E. histolytica*).
- Life cycle: colonizes the large bowel wall and can seed the brain and/or lungs; transmission via the fecal-oral route.
- Endemic areas: worldwide, especially in developing areas with poor sanitation.

Clinical Presentation

- High fevers, right upper quadrant pain from liver abscess, dysentery.
- Invasive inflammatory diarrhea mixed with mucus and blood, associated with tenesmus, colitis, and even bowel perforation.
- Can seed the lungs, presenting as pulmonary lesions and/or effusions.

Diagnosis and Evaluation

- Stool ova and parasite.
- Ultrasound or computed tomography (CT) visualization of liver abscess.

Treatment

- Metronidazole or tinidazole.
- Most liver abscesses resolve with medication, but interventional radiology (IR) drainage may be required for biliary obstruction.

GIARDIASIS

General Principles

- Organism: *Giardia lamblia.*
- Acquired by ingestion of cysts in unfiltered spring water, typically seen in campers and daycare center outbreaks.
- Life cycle: colonizes the duodenum and jejunum.
- Endemic area: United States (most common intestinal parasite in this country).

Clinical Presentation

- Diarrhea, steatorrhea
- Flatulence
- Abdominal cramping, bloating
- Weight loss owing to malabsorption

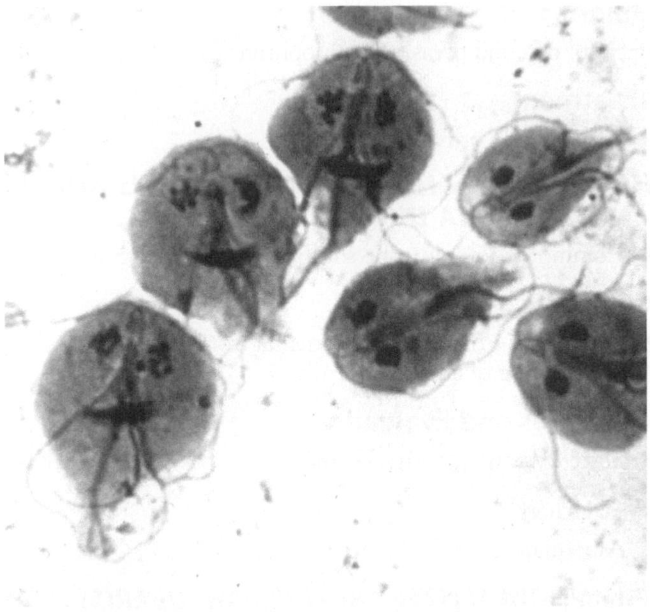

FIG. 62.2 Giardia in culture. (From Adachi, J. A., Backer, H. D., & DuPont, H. L. (2017). Infectious diarrhea from wilderness and foreign travel. In P. S. Auerbach, T. A. Cushing, & N. S. Harris (Eds.), *Auerbach's wilderness medicine* (7th ed., pp. 1859–1874, Fig. 82.2). Elsevier.)

Diagnosis and Evaluation

- Multiple stool ova and parasite collections may be needed for diagnosis (Fig. 62.2).
- Fecal immunoassays may be needed for definitive diagnosis.

Treatment

- Metronidazole (or tinidazole or nitazoxanide).

TOXOPLASMOSIS

General Principles

- Organism: *Toxoplasma gondii.*
- Typically occurs in patients with AIDS with CD4 less than 100 cells/mm^3 or other immunocompromised hosts.

Clinical Presentation

- Headache, fever
- Altered mental status
- Seizures
- Focal neurologic deficits
- Can cause retinal hemorrhages and optic neuritis

Diagnosis and Evaluation

- Multiple subcortical ring-enhancing lesions on CT of the brain in an immunocompromised patient.
- Antitoxoplasma IgG can be sent, but the result will not be back while the patient is in the emergency department.
  - In rare cases, antibodies may be negative and a biopsy may be necessary for diagnosis.
- Lumbar puncture is not needed to confirm the diagnosis, but it should be considered to evaluate for other central nervous system (CNS) pathology with similar clinical presentation, such as CNS abscess, cytomegalovirus, herpes simplex virus, mycobacterium, lymphoma, tuberculosis, fungal infection, or Kaposi sarcoma.

Treatment

- Pyrimethamine plus sulfadiazine and folic acid.
- Prophylaxis for immunocompromise with CD4 les than 100 cells/mm^3: trimethoprim/sulfamethoxazole daily.
- Steroids can reduce the mass effect from CNS lesions.
- Seizure prophylaxis for patients with CNS involvement.

CRYPTOSPORIDIUM

General Principles

- Organism: *Cryptosporidium parvum*
- A common cause of diarrhea in immunocompromised patients, but can also occur in immunocompetent hosts.
- Vector: cysts transmitted by fecal-oral contamination of food and water sources.
  - Cysts are extremely hardy and can survive long periods of time outside of a host and are resistant to chlorine-based disinfectants.

Clinical Presentation

- Watery diarrhea typically presenting in an immunocompromised host.

Diagnosis and Evaluation

- Stool ova and parasite with acid-fast stain, or ELISA or polymerase chain reaction.

Treatment

- Most immunocompetent patients recover spontaneously with supportive care.
- Nitazoxanide can decrease stool frequency.
- Patients with HIV should be treated with highly active antiretroviral therapy to reconstitute the immune system.
- Confirmed cases should be reported to the local public health department.

LEISHMANIASIS

General Principles

- Organism: *Leishmania mexicana* and *L. tropica* (cutaneous), *L. braziliensis* (mucosal).
- Vector: sandfly bite.
- Endemic areas: Middle East, India, East Africa, Mediterranean coast, Brazil; typically presents in the United States in soldiers or others returning from endemic areas.

Clinical Presentation

- In the United States, typically presents in soldiers, immigrants, or others returning from long-duration stay in endemic areas with cutaneous lesions.
  - Cutaneous: painless chronic ulcerating skin lesions that can be singular or diffuse, resembling lepromatous leprosy.
  - Mucosal: attacks and erodes the mucocutaneous skin borders of the nose and mouth, and can involve the trachea and larynx.

- Visceral: fever in immunocompetent hosts, hepatosplenomegaly, neutropenia, weight loss.

Diagnosis and Evaluation

- Light microscopy of biopsied lesions or serum polymerase chain reaction for diagnosis of visceral leishmaniasis.

Treatment

- Cutaneous manifestations are often self-limited, requiring only symptomatic treatment.
- Amphotericin B or oral miltefosine for visceral or resistant disease.

Nematodes (Roundworms)

- This class of parasite has the following characteristics:
  - Vector: contaminated soil with organisms that penetrate directly through skin.
  - Colonizes the intestines and can often mimic other abdominal pathology, including appendicitis, colitis, and bowel obstruction.
  - Pulmonary involvement resulting in *Loeffler syndrome*: dry cough, eosinophilia, and dyspnea caused by pulmonary infiltration.
  - Endemic areas: tropics and subtropical climates such as Latin America and Southeast Asia.

Diagnosis and Evaluation

- Stool ova and parasite, eosinophilia, ELISA.

Treatment

- Albendazole or ivermectin.

STRONGYLOIDES (*STRONGYLOIDES STERCORALIS*)

- Clinically significant infection in the immunocompromised patient such as individuals with HIV, but also seen in immunocompetent and elderly individuals in tropical and subtropical areas worldwide.

Clinical Presentation

- Serpiginous, pruritic dermatitis at the entry site.
- Persistent diarrhea, weight loss, and abdominal pain.
- Pulmonary involvement with cough, dyspnea, and even respiratory failure.

Diagnosis and Evaluation

- Stool ova and parasite may not show eggs for more than 1 month while organisms migrate through the lungs and then to the GI tract.

Treatment

- Thiabendazole, albendazole, or ivermectin.

WHIPWORM (*TRICHURIS TRICHIURA*)

Clinical Presentation

- Bloody diarrhea, iron-deficiency anemia, abdominal pain, fever.

Diagnosis and Evaluation

- Stool ova and parasite, eosinophilia.

Treatment

- Albendazole or ivermectin.

HOOKWORM (*NECATOR AMERICANUS AND ANCYLOSTOMA DUODENALE*)

- Commonly found in the southeastern United States.

Clinical Presentation

- Significant iron-deficiency anemia from GI blood loss; major cause of anemia globally.

Diagnosis and Evaluation

- Stool ova and parasite, eosinophilia.

Treatment

- Albendazole, or pyrantel pamoate.

PINWORM (*ENTEROBIUS VERMICULARIS*)

- Life cycle involves migration of the female worm to the rectum at night to deposit eggs.
- Commonly seen in children with anal pruritus.

Clinical Presentation

- Anal itching, particularly at night.

Diagnosis and Evaluation

- "Scotch tape test"; eggs seen on microcopy.

Treatment

- Albendazole or pyrantel pamoate.

ASCARIASIS (*ASCARIS LUMBRICOIDES*)

- Migrates through the intestines to primarily affect the lungs.

Clinical Presentation

- Loeffler syndrome: pulmonary infiltration with dry cough, wheezing, infiltrative disease.
- GI involvement: abdominal pain, cramping. High worm load can cause bowel obstruction.

Diagnosis and Evaluation

- Stool ova and parasite, eosinophilia.

Treatment

- Albendazole or ivermectin.

Cestodes (Tapeworms)

- This class of parasite is acquired by ingestion of the larval (cyst) stage of the associated organism, which resides in the intestines, but is notable for involvement of other organ systems.

CYSTICERCOSIS

General Principles

- Organism: *Taenia solium* (pork tapeworm).
- Vector: undercooked pork.

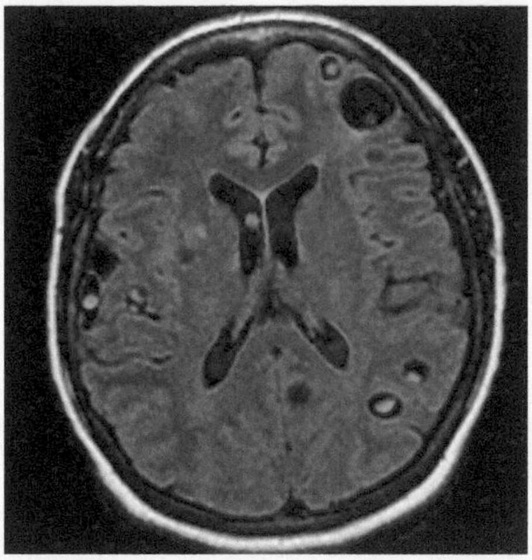

FIG. 62.3 MRI findings of cysticercosis. (From Garcia, H. H., & Gilman, R. H. (2020). Larval cestode infections (cysticercosis). In E. T. Ryan, D. R. Hill, T. Solomon, N. E. Aronson, & T. P. Endy (Eds.), *Hunter's tropical medicine and emerging infectious diseases* (10th ed., pp. 941–945). Elsevier Courtesy, Dr. T. Nash, NIAID, NIH)

Clinical Presentation

- Often asymptomatic, but active CNS lesions cause seizure and encephalopathy secondary to enlarging cysts producing an intense immunologic response, inflammation, fibrosis, and calcification.
- Liver involvement can cause cirrhosis decades later.

Diagnosis and Evaluation

- Stool ova and parasite.
- CT scan with ring-enhancing lesions (Fig. 62.3).
- Cysticerci may occur in more than one anatomic region at the same time, and/or may be present at different stages (e.g., viable cysts, enhancing cysts, and some older calcified cysts) at the same time.
- Serologic testing (enzyme-linked immunoelectro-transfer blot available from the CDC) can be performed in patients with suspected disease and neuroimaging is not diagnostic.

Treatment

- Praziquantel or albendazole.
- Corticosteroids and antiepileptics for symptom control.
- Neurosurgical consult if CT of the brain shows signs of obstructive hydrocephalus.

FISH TAPEWORM

- Organism: *Diphyllobothrium latum.*
- Vector: raw fish.

Clinical Presentation

- Vitamin B_{12} deficiency: organisms compete with the human host for absorption of vitamin B_{12}.

Diagnosis and Evaluation

- Stool ova and parasite.
- CBC showing macrocytic anemia.

Treatment

- Praziquantel.

ECHINOCOCCOSIS

- Organism: *Echinococcus granulosus*, *E. multicaris.*
- Vector: definitive host = canine; transient host = sheep and cattle.
  - Spread by fecal-oral contamination and exposure to dogs and/or livestock.

Clinical Presentation

- Hydatic cysts (cysts containing larvae and scolices) in the liver, brain, and lungs that cause symptoms according to the organ affected.
- Echinococcal disease can cause anaphylaxis if cyst ruptures.

Diagnosis and Evaluation

- CT scan and ultrasonography show cysts.

Treatment

- Albendazole.
- Surgical resection in specific cases (with caution so as not to promote seeding and anaphylactoid reaction).

Trematodes (Flatworms/Flukes)

SCHISTOSOMIASIS

General Principles

- Organism: *Schistosoma haematobium*, *S. japonicum*, *S. mansoni.*
- Life cycle: intermediate host = freshwater snails; permanent host = humans. Cercariae penetrate skin and reside in the venous system, migrating to the intestine (*S. mansoni*), bladder (*S. haematobium*), or CNS (*S. japonicum*).
- Endemic areas: worldwide includes lakes and rivers of North Africa (especially Nile River Valley), Sub-Saharan Africa, Brazil, Venezuela, Caribbean, rural Southeast Asia.

Clinical Presentation

- Common clinical scenario is "swimmer's itch" and rash after swimming in endemic area: Africa, Middle East, Asia.
- Pulmonary: Katayama fever syndrome of fever, cough, and diffuse pulmonary nodules.
- GI: hepatosplenomegaly, cirrhosis, and liver failure due to worm pairs ensnared in the liver that cause periportal fibrosis and portal hypertension.
- Genitourinary: hematuria and hydroureter, primarily caused by *S. haematobium.*

Diagnosis and Evaluation

- Stool ova and parasite.

Treatment

- Praziquantel.

SUGGESTED READINGS

Centers for Disease Control and Prevention. (April 24, 2019). Parasites. Available at: https://www.cdc.gov/parasites/.

Marx, J. A., Hockberger, R. S., & Walls, R. M. (2014). *Rosen's emergency medicine: Concepts and clinical practice* (8th ed., pp. 1768–1784). Elsevier.

Ryan, E. T., Hill, D. R., Solomon, T., Aronson, N. E., & Endy, T. P. (2019). *Hunter's tropical medicine and emerging infectious diseases e-book* (10th ed.). Elsevier.

CHAPTER 63

BOARD REVIEW

Tick-Borne Illnesses

GREGORY J. MORAN, MD, and ELIZABETH TANG FERREIRA, MD

A vector-borne illness, initial identification of the tick and removal is key to initial emergency department (ED) management. Most presentations are vague, with skin manifestations and occasionally some component of a neurologic deficit. For most of the following diseases, doxycycline is often the first-line agent, with some exceptions in children and pregnancy.

Lyme Disease (LD)

General Principles

- The most common vector-borne illness in North America and Europe.
- Caused by the spirochete *Borrelia burgdorferi*.
- Transmitted by saliva from the bite of the Ixodes tick.
- Most reported cases are observed in the northeastern, mid-Atlantic, and north-central states during the summer months (May to August) when human outdoor activities are at their peak and Ixodes nymphal activity is most prominent.
- Ticks require approximately 36 hours of feeding for successful *B. burgdorferi* transmission, at which time the ticks are notably engorged.

Clinical Presentation

Early Localized Infection

- Presents 1 to 2 weeks and up to 30 days after a tick bite; bites are commonly found in crevices, such as base of neck, axilla, groin, popliteal fossa.
- The most common presentation is a rash known as erythema migrans:
  - Classically a solitary expanding smooth red target lesion with a ring of clearing around the original site of tick attachment (Fig. 63.1);
  - Size ranges from 5 cm to 60 cm; rarely presents with central necrosis, crusting, or induration;
  - Usually not pruritic or painful.
- Constitutional symptoms resembling a viral syndrome including fatigue, malaise, low-grade fever, anorexia, headache. May also endorse photophobia, nausea, neck stiffness with normal neurologic and cerebrospinal fluid (CSF) findings.
- Musculoskeletal symptoms include asymmetric migratory arthralgia and myalgias.

Early Disseminated Infection

- Occurs after latent period, weeks to months after infection and involves the skin, eyes, nervous system, and heart.

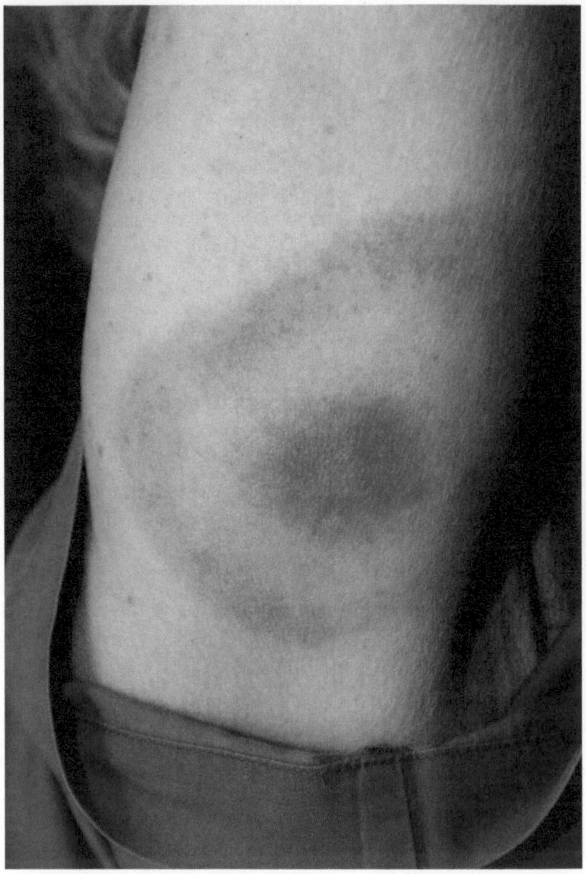

FIG. 63.1 Erythema migrans. (From Centers for Disease Control and Prevention Public Health Image Library. Image number 9875.)

- Neurologic manifestations affect approximately 15% of patients who have progressed from early localized infection and include:
  - Lymphocytic meningitis
    - Constellation of headache, nausea, lethargy, and irritability.
    - CSF shows lymphocytic pleocytosis and antibodies to *B. burgdorferi*.
    - Brain imaging is normal.
  - Cranial nerve palsies, unilateral or bilateral
    - Facial nerve is most commonly affected.
    - One of few diseases causing bilateral cranial nerve palsy.
  - Lyme encephalitis
    - May have notable papilledema, especially in children.
    - Peripheral neuropathies are common with motor or sensory radiculopathies and mononeuritis.

- Cardiac manifestations (Lyme carditis) affect 4% to 10% of untreated Lyme disease and are often transient. Nonspecific constellation of light-headedness, syncope, chest pain, palpitations, and dyspnea.
- Most commonly presents with atrioventricular conduction block, affecting 90% of patients with Lyme carditis. Rarely will the conduction block be complete and require pacemaker placement.
- Ocular manifestations present with keratitis, conjunctivitis, chorioretinitis, retinal detachment, optic neuritis, and blindness.

Late Disseminated Infection

- Presents months to years after initial infection and includes neurologic and arthritic symptoms.
- Arthritis: involving large joints (e.g., knees, hips, shoulders, elbows), may be intermittent or persistent, can have a painless joint effusion, may progress to chronic synovitis.
- Neurologic manifestations are vague, with wide variety in clinical presentations.
  - Lyme encephalopathy (changes in memory, mood, cognition, sleep).
  - Central and peripheral nerve pathology is typical and includes radicular pain, numbness in stocking glove distribution, in addition to cranial nerves, spinal roots, and peripheral plexus.

Diagnosis and Evaluation

- No testing necessary for patients with evidence of erythema migrans (pathognomonic for LD), or with history of tick bite and living in an endemic area.
- Indications for serologic testing include:
  - Recent travel to endemic area of LD, risk factor for tick exposure, and symptoms consistent with early disseminated or late LD.
  - Two-step testing is recommended, starting with enzyme immunoassay (EIA). If EIA is negative, no further testing is recommended. If EIA is positive or indeterminate, an immunoblot test ("Western blot") is done. Results are considered positive only if the EIA and the immunoblot are both positive.
- Do not perform serologic testing for screening in asymptomatic patients or in those with nonspecific symptoms, because there is a high rate of positive serology in people without LD.

Management

- Treatment varies, depending on staging and patient presentation.
  - Early localized (i.e., erythema migrans) or early disseminated treatment includes:
    - Doxycycline 100 mg twice daily for 10 days in adults, and 2.2 mg/kg twice daily for 10 days in children greater than 8 years of age.
    - Amoxicillin is preferred in pregnant or lactating women, and children younger than 8 years of age, with dosing of 500 mg three times daily for 14 days in adults and 50 mg/kg divided into 3 daily doses for 14 days in children less than 8 years of age.
- Neurologic disease
  - Oral antibiotics as above are appropriate if CSF findings are unremarkable.
  - If evidence of meningitis, encephalitis, or cranial neuropathies, parenteral antibiotic therapy is indicated, which includes ceftriaxone 2 g intravenous (IV) daily for 14–28 days in adults, and ceftriaxone 75 mg/kg IV for 14-28 days in children.
- Cardiac disease
  - Oral antibiotics are appropriate if PR-interval is less than 0.30 on ECG or first-degree atrioventricular (AV) block.
  - High-degree AV block requires parenteral antibiotics.
- Arthritis
  - Oral doxycycline or amoxicillin for a 1-month course or longer.
- Prophylaxis-begins within 72 hours of tick removal and is indicated in patients with the following:
  - Attached tick is identified as *I. scapularis* and has been attached 36 or more hours.
  - Local infection rate with *B. burgdorferi* 20% or more.
  - Doxycycline is not contraindicated. Doxycycline prophylactic dosing is a single 200 mg oral dose in adults, and a single 4 mg/kg oral dose in children over 8 years of age.

Spotted Fever Rickettsiosis (SFR)

General Principles

- Previously "Rocky Mountain Spotted Fever".
- Systemic vasculitis caused by the obligate intracellular bacterium *Rickettsia rickettsii*.
- More common in the Midwest and southeastern United States than in the Rocky Mountains.
- Affects any organ system and commonly begins as a viral syndrome with fever during the SFR season from April to September.
- In the western United States it is carried by the vector *Dermacentor andersoni*, a wood tick; in the eastern United States it is carried by the America dog tick *Dermacentor variabilis*.

Clinical Presentation

- Skin: rash spreads centripetally, beginning on the hands/wrists, and soles/ankles. Begins macular and progresses to a petechial and maculopapular rash (Fig. 63.2). Develops commonly on the third day of illness. Approximately 10% of patients do not present with a rash. If severe, purpura, skin sloughing, ulceration, and gangrene may manifest. Rarely the tick bite may also have an eschar.
- Central nervous system (CNS)
  - Headache is the predominant complaint. May be severe, and can lead to meningeal inflammation and cerebral vasculitis.
  - Rickettsial encephalitis (severe headache, confusion, stupor, coma, and seizures).
- Other CNS symptoms include Guillain-Barre syndrome, focal neurologic deficits, deafness, sensory neuropathy, tardive dyskinesia
- Cardiovascular
  - Myocarditis and myocardial vasculitis.
  - Atrioventricular block, dysrhythmias (atrial and ventricular tachycardia, atrial fibrillation).
  - Left ventricular dysfunction.

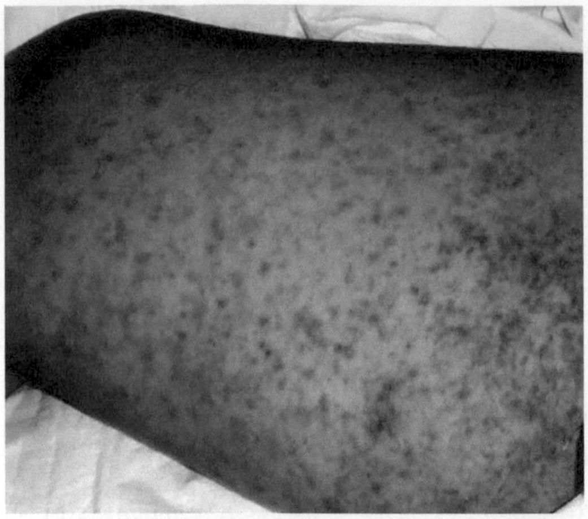

FIG. 63.2 Rocky Mountain Spotted Fever Rash (Spotted Fever Rickettsiosis) (From Biggs, H. M., Behravesh, C. B., Bradley, K. K., Dahlgren, F. S., Drexler, N. A., Dumler, J. S., Folk, S. M., Kato, C. Y., Lash, R. R., Levin, M. L., Massung, R. F., Nadelman, R. B., Nicholson, W. L., Paddock, C. D., Pritt, B. S., & Traeger, M. S. (2016). Diagnosis and management of tickborne rickettsial diseases: Rocky Mountain spotted fever and other spotted fever group rickettsioses, ehrlichioses, and anaplasmosis—United States. *Morbidity and Mortality Weekly Report: Recommendations and Reports*, 65(2), 1–44, Fig. 21.)

- Pulmonary: Rickettsial pneumonitis from microvascular injury, fluid leakage into interstitium and alveolar airspace; life-threatening.
- Gastrointestinal: symptoms present early in illness and include nausea, vomiting, diarrhea, and abdominal pain.

Diagnosis and Evaluation

- No rapid test to confirm SFR; treatment should be initiated immediately if clinical diagnosis is suspected.
  - History of camping or outdoor activity between April and September in endemic area.
  - Viral syndrome with rash and fever.
  - Laboratory studies: nonspecific.
  - Lumbar puncture is indicated in patients with headache, fever, and evidence of meningeal irritation (also to rule out meningococcemia, which has a similar presentation). CSF will show elevated protein and pleocytosis, with either lymphocytic or polymorphonuclear leukocyte (PMN) predominance.
  - Serum serologic testing via immunofluorescence antibody is the gold standard, with sensitivity 94% to 100% after 14 days, but much lower at onset of symptoms. Enzyme-linked immunosorbent assay is increasing in use. Neither diagnostic tool is a rapid test.
  - Skin biopsy may be helpful in the acute setting, only when rash is present.

Management

- Doxycycline is the general drug of choice (usually oral, but IV in severe cases).
- In pregnancy, chloramphenicol is the drug of choice.
- In severe cases, resuscitation efforts will be focused on wide-spread systemic vasculitis leading to hypotension, renal failure, disseminated intravascular coagulation (DIC), acute respiratory distress syndrome (ARDS), and shock. Small serial boluses of isotonic saline recommended; vasopressors may be added if patient is unresponsive to IV fluids.

Anaplasmosis (Ehrlichiosis)

General Principles

- *Ehrlichia chafeensis*, *Ehrlichia ewingii*, and *Anaplasma phagocytophilum* are gram-negative intracellular coccobacilli that cause ehrlichiosis and anaplasmosis, respectively.
- Although separate causes, they present similarly and are managed in identical fashions.
- *E. chafeensis* causes human monocytic ehrlichiosis (HME), *E. ewingii* causes human ewingii ehrlichiosis (HEE), and *A. phagocytophilum* cases human granulocytic anaplasmosis (HGA).
- HME and HEE are transmitted mainly via the Lone Star tick (*Amblyomma americanum*), whereas HGA is transmitted via *I. scapularis* in the eastern United States and *I. pacificus* in the western United States.

Clinical Presentation

- Presents after incubation period of 5 to 14 days, with fevers, headache, myalgia, nausea, vomiting, and with or without diarrhea.
- Severity of illness varies; most recover uneventfully with outpatient antibiotics, but some require hospitalization for severe illness.
- Nervous system
  - Ehrlichiosis presents with meningitis, encephalitis, seizures, and possibly coma.
  - Anaplasmosis presents with peripheral nerve palsies predominantly.
- Skin: nonpruritic, nontender erythematous maculopapular or petechial rash appears at 5 to 7 days of illness on trunk and extremities, seen in most ehrlichiosis cases and 10% of anaplasmosis cases.
- Complications include meningoencephalitis, seizures, thrombocytopenia and life-threatening hemorrhage, DIC, ARDS, myocarditis, and renal failure.

Evaluation and Management

- Physical examination may show rash; if peripheral nerve palsies, suspect anaplasmosis and if meningismus or acute encephalopathy, suspect ehrlichiosis.
- Laboratory studies: nonspecific; may show anemia, thrombocytopenia, leukopenia, hyponatremia, elevated aspartate aminotransferase and alanine aminotransferase.
- Polymerase chain reaction (PCR) is the test of choice in ED. Peripheral blood smears may be helpful.
- Cotesting for Lyme disease indicated because of sharing the same vector.
- Preferred treatment is doxycycline.
- Failure to improve after 24 to 48 hours indicates a diagnosis other than HME, HEE, HGA.

Tularemia

- Caused by the gram-negative coccobacillus *Francisella tularensis*.
- Transmitted via Lone Star tick (*A. americanum*), Rocky Mountain wood tick (*Dermacentor andersonii)*, and dog tick (*D. variabilis*).

- May also be transmitted occasionally by aerosols from activities such as running a lawnmower over an infected carcass, or movement of infected hay.

Clinical Presentation

- Presents with two syndromes that begin after an incubation period of 2 to 21 days.
- Patients first develop abrupt onset of constitutional symptoms, including fever, chills, headache and myalgias.
- May be an associated nonspecific maculopapular, papulovesicular rash.
- Symptoms may last 1 to 4 weeks.
- Tularemia complications are similar to other tick-borne infections and include septic shock, meningitis, ARDS, peri- or endocarditis, hepatic failure, rhabdomyolysis, renal failure, osteomyelitis, peritonitis.

Ulceroglandular Tularemia

- Constitutional symptoms (abrupt fever, chills headache, myalgias).
- Solitary ulcerative skin lesion at site of bite about 0.5 cm to 3 cm in diameter, with undermined borders and with flat black or red base (Fig. 63.3).
- Regional lymphadenopathy is common and may be necrotic or suppurative.

Typhoidal (Systemic) Tularemia

- Systemic febrile illness without prominent regional adenopathy or other localizing signs of other major forms of tularemic disease. Lower prevalence than ulceroglandular tularemia, but has a higher mortality rate.
- Constitutional symptoms as above, but can rapidly progress to sepsis.

Tularemic pneumonia

- Presents as dry cough, pleuritic chest pain, and dyspnea.

Evaluation and Management

- Physical examination
  - Pathognomonic ulcer with regional lymphadenopathy, which may be present in up to 70% of patients.
  - Ocular manifestations of conjunctivitis and corneal ulcers (urgent ophthalmologic consult is warranted).

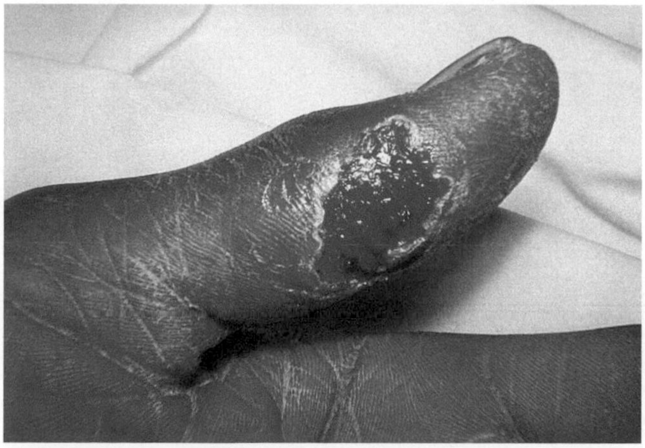

FIG. 63.3 Ulceroglandular tularemia. Ulcer caused by Francisella tularensis. (Reproduced from CDC, courtesy Emory U./Dr. Sellers. Reprinted from Tyring, S. K., Burnett, M., & Mwesigye, F. (2017). Anthrax, *plague, diphtheria, trachoma, and miscellaneous bacteria.* In S. K. Tyring, O. Lupi, & U. R. Hengge (Eds.), *Tropical dermatology* (2nd ed.), Fig. 28.24. Elsevier.)

  - A yellow-white pseudomembrane may be seen in the oropharynx.
  - Typhoidal tularemia may have pulse-temperature dissociation, which presents with a bradycardia relative to the height of fever.
- Laboratory studies: nonspecific and may have mildly elevated transaminases.
- Imaging: chest x-ray may have classic tularemic triad of hilar adenopathy, ovoid opacities, and pleural effusions; may also show multiple cavitary infiltrates.
- PCR and serology confirm the diagnosis.
- Treatment
  - Streptomycin or gentamicin.
- Disposition: most require admission for parenteral antibiotics.

Babesiosis

- Disease of red blood cell hemolysis caused by the intraerythrocytic protozoan *Babesia microti.*
- Transmitted via the tick vectors *I. scapularis and I. pacificus.*

Clinical Presentation

- Manifests on a spectrum from mild flu-like illness to fulminant sepsis.
- Occurs 1 to 6 weeks after tick attachment.
- Symptoms include high fevers, significant diaphoresis, fatigue, headache, and myalgias.
- May be jaundiced if severe intravascular hemolysis has transpired.
- Major risk factors include patients who are immunosuppressed and asplenic, neonates, and the elderly.
- Can be cotransmitted with Lyme disease.
- Complications are similar to those of other tick-borne illnesses and include DIC, ARDS, renal failure.

Evaluation and Management

- Physical examination will show high fever, with or without hepatosplenomegaly, and a small percentage of patients will have jaundice.
- Laboratory studies demonstrate intravascular hemolysis.
- PCR is most sensitive; peripheral smears may show the organism in red blood cells and is more quickly available.
- Treatment
  - Atovaquone plus azithromycin.
- If no improvement in 48 hours with evidence of massive hemolysis (Hgb <10 g/dL) and organ failure, consider exchange transfusion.

63

Tick-Borne Relapsing Fever

- Disease caused by spirochetes in the *Borrelia* genus and transmitted via soft ticks (*Ornithodoros*).
- Most prevalent in California, Rocky Mountains, and central Texas.

Clinical Presentation

- 4 to 18 day incubation period
- Presents with the constellation of fever, headache, myalgias, arthralgias, diarrhea, vomiting, nonspecific

maculopapular rash, meningismus, and cranial nerve palsies.
- Symptoms come and go in an episodic fashion lasting approximately 3 days and resolving for 1 week only to return later.
- Complications are similar to those of previously discussed tick-borne illnesses.

EVALUATION AND MANAGEMENT

- Laboratory studies show thrombocytopenia, elevated transminases, hematuria.
- PCR for diagnosis; peripheral blood smear may show spirochetes, but is insensitive.
- Treatment
  - Doxycycline.
- Disposition: observation of patients for 12 hours after initiating antibiotics because a Jarisch-Herxheimer reaction may develop, leading to fatal cardiovascular collapse.

Tick Paralysis

- Symptoms develop after approximately 4 to 7 days of feeding by ticks *Dermacentor andersoni* (the Rocky Mountain wood tick) and *Dermacentor variabilis* (the American dog tick).
- Symptoms begin with a sense of weakness, fatigue, and paresthesias, despite a normal sensory examination.
- Rarely patients develop an unsteady gait that progresses to an ascending complete paralysis, and is the cause of mortality, similar to that of Guillain-Barre syndrome.
- Presentation is variable and may be isolated to the bulbar muscles or single extremities.
- Paralysis typically abates on discovery and removal of the tick, but it is not immediate.

Tick Removal and Disposal

- Using fine-tipped tweezers, grasp the tick as close to the skin's surface as possible and pull upward with even and steady pressure.
- Avoid twisting or jerking so as not to detach the body from the mouth; if the mouth remains in skin, remove it with tweezers.
- After tick removal, thoroughly clean the bite area and your hands with rubbing alcohol or soap and water.
- Never crush a tick with your fingers.
- Dispose of a live tick by putting it in alcohol, placing it in a sealed bag/container, wrapping it tightly in tape, or flushing it down the toilet.

SUGGESTED READING

Biggs, H. M., Behravesh, C. B., Bradley, K. K., Dahlgren, F. S., Drexler, N. A., Dumler, J. S., Traeger, M. S. (2016). Diagnosis and management of tick-borne rickettsial diseases: Rocky Mountain spotted fever and other spotted fever group Rickettsioses, Ehrlichioses, and Anaplasmosis — United States. MMWR. *Recommendations and Reports*, 65(No. RR-2), 1–44.

Centers for Disease Control and Prevention. (2018). *Tickborne Diseases of the United States: A Reference Manual for Health Care Providers* (5th ed.). Available at: https://www.cdc.gov/ticks/tickbornediseases/TickborneDiseases-P.pdf.

Centers for Disease Control and Prevention. *Tick Removal* | Ticks |. Centers for Disease Control and Prevention. Available at: https://www.cdc.gov/ticks/removing_a_tick.html. Accessed August 20, 2019.

Shapiro, E. D. (2014). Lyme disease. *New England Journal of Medicine*, *370*, 1724–1731.

Viral Infections

STEVEN BOLGER, MD, and GREGORY J. MORAN, MD

Viral infections are one of the most commonly encountered illnesses in the emergency department. Although many viral infections are self-limited, certain viral illnesses have the potential for morbidity and mortality that require prompt diagnosis and treatment.

Influenza

- Influenza is caused by a single-stranded RNA virus from the orthomyxovirus family. The two most common types of influenza that cause infections in humans are influenza A and B; influenza A is more likely to cause serious infections. Influenza is transmitted via respiratory secretions, most commonly through sneezing and coughing and then direct contact.

Clinical Presentation

- Patients with influenza present with fever accompanied by body aches and respiratory symptoms, most commonly in late November through March.
- Most cases are self-limited in healthy patients. The elderly, young children, and those with comorbid conditions are more likely to develop complications, such as respiratory failure.
- Influenza can cause exacerbations of chronic conditions, such as congestive heart failure or chronic obstructive pulmonary disease, and bacterial superinfection, such as *Staphylococcus aureus* pneumonia.

Diagnosis and Evaluation

- Diagnosis of influenza is usually clinical with fever and respiratory symptoms in a community with known cases of influenza.
- Laboratory confirmation is not typically necessary, but it can be useful in patients at higher risk for complications and in hospitalized patients.
- Rapid antigen assays identify surface proteins in influenza A and B.
  - They have low sensitivity of 50%–70% and specificity greater than 98%.
- Reverse-transcriptase polymerase chain reaction (RT-PCR) yields results in about an hour; it has a sensitivity of approximately 92%–95% and a specificity of greater than 98%.

Treatment

- Most patients will have self-limited illness requiring symptomatic care only.
- Early treatment with antivirals can shorten the duration of the illness and may reduce the risk of some complications, such as otitis media, pneumonia, and respiratory failure.
  - Early treatment of hospitalized adult patients with influenza has been associated with a decreased mortality.
  - In hospitalized children, early treatment has been shown to shorten the duration of hospitalization.
- Centers for Disease Control and Prevention guidelines recommend antiviral treatment as early as possible for any patient with confirmed or suspected influenza who meets any of the following criteria:
  - Is hospitalized
  - Has severe, complicated, or progressive illness
  - Is at higher risk for influenza complications (Box 64.1).
- Antiviral treatment can be considered for healthy patients if initiated within 48 hours of illness onset.
- Oseltamivir (75 mg oral twice daily for adults) is the recommended antiviral.
  - Baloxavir is an alternate option that is given as a single dose of 40 mg for patients who are 40 to 80 kg or 80 mg for patients greater than 80 kg.

BOX 64.1 *Patients at Higher Risk for Influenza Complications Who Should Receive Antiviral Treatment*

- Children younger than 2 years of age
- Adults 65 years of age and older
- Patients with chronic pulmonary (including asthma), cardiovascular (except hypertension alone), renal, hepatic, hematologic (including sickle cell disease), and metabolic disorders (including diabetes mellitus), or neurologic and neurodevelopment conditions (including disorders of the brain, spinal cord, peripheral nerve, and muscle, such as cerebral palsy, epilepsy, stroke, intellectual disability, moderate to severe developmental delay, muscular dystrophy, or spinal cord injury)
- Patients with immunosuppression, including human immunodeficiency virus (HIV) infection and medications
- Patients who are pregnant or postpartum (within 2 weeks of delivery)
- Patients younger than 19 years of age who are receiving long-term aspirin- or salicylate-containing medications
- American Indians/Alaska Natives
- Obese patients with body-mass index (BMI) 40 or greater
- Residents who are in nursing homes and other chronic care facilities

(From Fiore, A. E., Fry, A., Shay, D., Gubareva, L., Bresee, J. S., & Uyeki, T. M. (2011). Antiviral agents for the treatment and chemoprophylaxis of influenza: Recommendations of the Advisory Committee on Immunization Practices. *Morbidity and Mortality Weekly Report*, 60(RR-01), 1–24. https://www.cdc.gov/mmwr/preview/mmwrhtml/rr6001a1.htm)

Herpes Simplex Virus

- Herpes simplex virus type 1 (HSV-1) and herpes simplex virus type 2 (HSV-2) are double-stranded DNA viruses that cause oral and genital infections and, rarely, central nervous system (CNS) infections.
  - Although HSV-1 is commonly acquired through nonsexual contact in childhood, HSV-2 is typically acquired through sexual activity.
    - Transmission occurs via direct mucosal contact with ulcers or through exchange of saliva, vesicle fluid, semen, or cervical fluid.
  - HSV-1, one of the most common causes of viral encephalitis, occurs most commonly in patients younger than 20 years of age and those more than 50 years of age.
    - The mortality rate for untreated HSV encephalitis in more than 70%; many survivors have neurologic sequelae.
  - HSV-2, one of the most common causes of viral encephalitis in neonates, is typically acquired from the maternal genital tract at the time of delivery.
  - HSV-1/2 remain latent in sensory ganglia following transmission and cause localized vesicular eruptions when reactivated.

Clinical Presentation

- The clinical presentation of HSV-1/2 varies, depending on the body site affected and primary versus recurrent infection. Most HSV infections are subclinical.
  - Primary HSV-1 infections result in more extensive lesions involving mucosal and extramucosal sites accompanied by fever and malaise.
    - Gingivostomatitis and pharyngitis are typical manifestations of primary HSV-1 infection (Fig. 64.1).
    - Less common manifestations include herpetic whitlow, herpes gladiatorum, eczema herpeticum, and herpes keratitis.

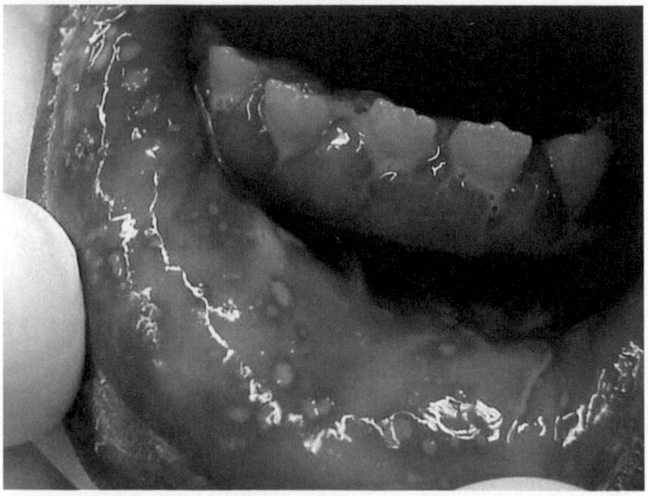

FIG. 64.1 Gingivostomatitis caused by primary HSV-1 infection. (From Fatahzadeh, M, & Schwartz, R. A. (2007). Human herpes simplex virus infections: Epidemiology, pathogenesis, symptomatology, diagnosis, and management. *Journal of the American Academy of Dermatology, 57*(5), 737–763.)

  - Primary HSV-2 infection commonly results in genital lesions (Fig. 64.2). About one-third of women with primary HSV-2 infection develop a viral meningitis syndrome.
  - Recurrent HSV infections typically cause localized painful vesicular lesions that are either orolabial or genital.
  - Bell palsy and herpes zoster ophthalmicus may occur with HSV-1 reactivation in the facial nerve or ophthalmic branch of the trigeminal nerve, respectively.
  - HSV encephalitis presents with acute-onset fever with neurologic symptoms, including focal seizures, ataxia, hemiparesis, cranial nerve deficits, and altered mental status.
  - HSV infections in immunocompromised hosts can cause widespread dissemination, including pneumonia, esophagitis, hepatitis, and colitis.
  - Neonates can present with three manifestations, typically within the first month of life:
    - lesions of the skin, eye or mouth.
    - disseminated sepsis-like syndrome.
    - meningitis. The latter two have high morbidity/mortality.

Diagnosis and Evaluation

- Most mucocutaneous HSV diagnoses do not require laboratory confirmation. If needed, confirmation is done by swabbing fluid from an unroofed vesicle for viral culture, polymerase chain reaction (PCR), or direct fluorescent antibody testing.
- PCR testing of cerebrospinal fluid (CSF) for HSV-1/2 is the preferred diagnostic method for HSV meningitis or encephalitis.
  - Viral DNA can be detected within the first 24 hours and remains positive for a week or longer.
  - Identification of temporal lobe lesions on CT or magnetic resonance imaging is suggestive of HSV encephalitis.
  - Electroencephalogram will show typical intermittent, high-amplitude slow waves localized to temporal lobes.

Treatment

- Treatment depends on disease severity and the immune status of the patient.
  - Patients who are immunocompetent with primary HSV-1 or HSV-2 can be treated with oral acyclovir, valacyclovir, or famciclovir for 7 to 10 days.
    - Recurrent orolabial infections usually do not require treatment.
  - Patients with HSV encephalitis or disseminated disease or patients who are immunocompromised with severe mucocutaneous disease should be given intravenous (IV) acyclovir.
    - Acyclovir should be given IV empirically when HSV encephalitis is suspected.
    - Similarly, empiric acyclovir should be given to neonates with suspected HSV.

Epstein-Barr Virus

- Epstein-Barr virus (EBV), the most common cause of infectious mononucleosis, is associated with multiple malignancies, including B-cell lymphoma, Hodgkin lymphoma, Burkitt lymphoma, and nasopharyngeal carcinoma. EBV

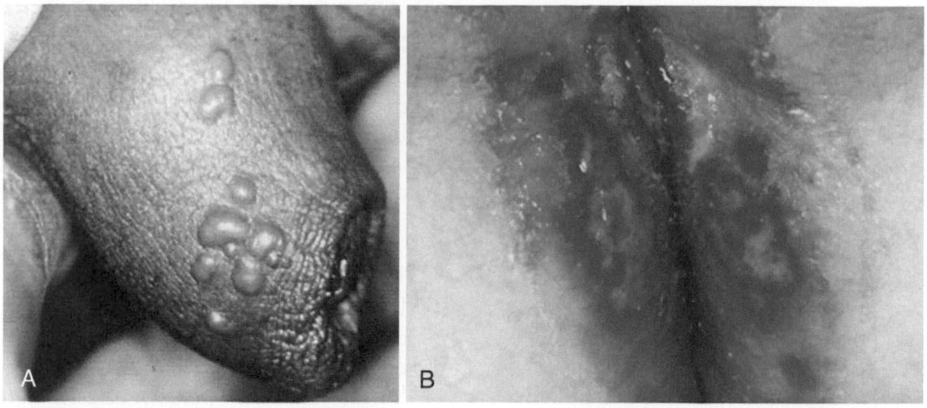

FIG. 64.2 Genital lesions on penis (**A**) and vagina (**B**) owing to primary HSV-2 infection. (From Genital herpes infection. (2019). In *Elsevier Point of Care*. Elsevier.) A: From Johnston C et al: Genital herpes. In: Morse SA et al, eds: Atlas of Sexually Transmitted Diseases and AIDS. 4th ed. London, England: Saunders; 2010:169–85, Figure 10.13; B: From Hudson MJ et al: Medical conditions with genital/anal findings that can be confused with sexual abuse. In: Jenny C, ed: Child Abuse and Neglect: Diagnosis, Treatment and Evidence. St Louis, MO: Saunders; 2011:93–105, Figure 12–20

is transmitted via salivary secretions and infects B lymphocytes, which results in enlargement in lymphoid tissue.

Clinical Presentation

- Manifestations depend on the patient's age and immune status.
  - Infections in infants and young children are often asymptomatic or cause mild pharyngitis.
  - Teenagers and young adults can develop infectious mononucleosis, which presents with fever, lymphadenopathy, and pharyngitis.
    - Tonsillar exudates are common (Fig. 64.3); splenomegaly occurs in a majority of patients with infectious mononucleosis.
    - The duration of symptoms is typically 2 to 3 weeks, although fatigue can last for months.

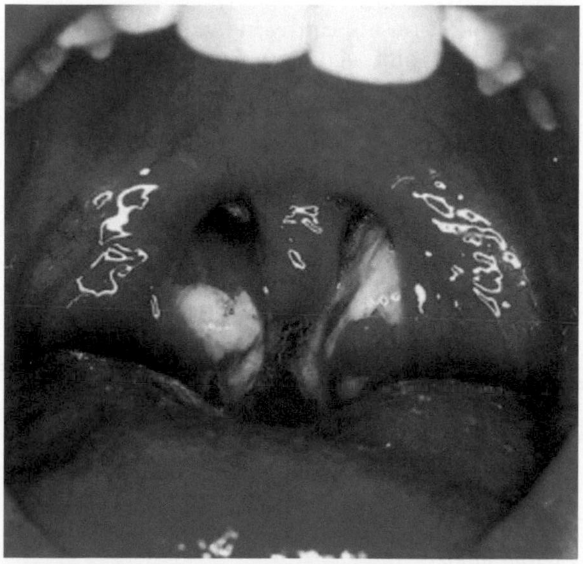

FIG. 64.3 White tonsillar exudates owing to Epstein-Barr virus (EBV) infection. (From Epstein-Barr virus infection. (2019). In *Elsevier Point of Care*. Elsevier.) From Michaels MG et al: Infectious disease. In: Zitelli BJ et al, eds: Zitelli and Davis' Atlas of Pediatric Physical Diagnosis. 6th ed. Saunders; 2012:469–529, Figure 12–10B

  - Patients with infectious mononucleosis who are treated with ampicillin or amoxicillin for suspected streptococcal pharyngitis often develop a morbilliform rash.
  - EBV can cause multiorgan system involvement, including encephalitis, meningitis, hepatitis, myocarditis, and hematologic disorders.

Diagnosis and Evaluation

- Complete blood cell count and mononucleosis spot (monospot) test can confirm the diagnosis of infectious mononucleosis, but is not typically required.
  - Complete blood cell count will show lymphocytosis with more than 50% lymphocytes with atypical lymphocytes on peripheral smear.
  - The monospot test identifies a heterophile antibody produced in response to EBV infection; a positive result is considered diagnostic in the appropriate clinical context.
  - The monospot test may be negative early in the course of the disease, so a second test may be required with a high clinical suspicion for EBV infection.

Treatment

- Most cases of EBV infection are self-limited and require only supportive care, including rest and analgesia.
- The patient should be instructed to avoid all contact sports for a minimum of 3 weeks after illness onset owing to a risk of splenic rupture.
- Corticosteroids are recommended only for those patients with severe disease, such as upper airway obstruction, neurologic disease, or hemolytic anemia.
  - Corticosteroid use has not been shown to be effective in controlling symptoms.

Varicella-Zoster Virus

VARICELLA

- Varicella-zoster virus (VZV) is the causative organism for both varicella (chickenpox) and herpes zoster (shingles). Varicella, which is more common in the winter and spring months, is spread via aerosolized droplets of respiratory secretions from individuals with varicella. Vaccination against varicella is generally administered in childhood and has significantly reduced the disease burden over the past several decades.

Clinical Presentation

- Patients with varicella present with fever and rash accompanied by nonspecific symptoms, such as headache, malaise, and loss of appetite.
- The rash consists of lesions at varying stages including papules, vesicles, and crusted lesions that are more concentrated on the torso and face.

Diagnosis and Evaluation

- Varicella is a clinical diagnosis and does not require any diagnostic testing.

Treatment

- Healthy patients with varicella require supportive care only.
- Antiviral agents, such as acyclovir, can decrease the number of lesions and shorten the duration of illness if started within 24 hours of onset of rash, although they are not routinely recommended in healthy patients.
- Antiviral agents can be considered in patients at risk for complications, including those patients with chronic skin or pulmonary disorders and those who are immunocompromised.
- Varicella is highly contagious, so airborne precautions should be initiated as soon as possible.

HERPES ZOSTER

- Herpes zoster occurs in patients previously infected with VZV once the immune response against the virus wanes, usually with advancing age. VZV remains latent in the dorsal root ganglion following initial infection and can later reactivate, resulting in herpes zoster. Iatrogenic immune suppression, human immunodeficiency virus (HIV) infection, organ transplantation, and lymphoproliferative disorders increase the risk of herpes zoster. Varicella virus can be transmitted to nonimmune individuals via direct contact with vesicle fluid before the vesicles crust over.

Clinical Presentation

- Patients with herpes zoster initially present with pain, pruritus, and paresthesias that occur in one or more adjacent dermatomes and are accompanied by malaise, headache, and photophobia.
- These symptoms are followed by a maculopapular rash that becomes vesicular and most commonly affects the chest and face and does not cross the midline.
- Reactivation of VZV along the ophthalmic distribution of the trigeminal nerve, which is called herpes zoster ophthalmicus, can lead to corneal damage.
- Reactivation of VZV along the seventh cranial nerve can cause facial nerve paralysis and lesions along the auditory canal and is called herpes zoster oticus.
- Dissemination of VZV consists of herpes zoster involving more than three dermatomes and more often occurs in patients who are immunocompromised.

Diagnosis and Evaluation

- Diagnosis of herpes zoster is clinical; it is based on clusters of vesicles and papules present in a dermatomal distribution.
- Laboratory testing can be performed for patients with atypical illness or severe disease and consists of viral culture, antigen testing, or PCR testing of fluid from a freshly unroofed vesicle.

Treatment

- Patients with herpes zoster who present within 72 hours of clinical symptoms should be treated with antiviral therapy consisting of acyclovir, valacyclovir, or famciclovir.
- For patients who present after 72 hours, antiviral therapy should be given only if new lesions are appearing at the time of presentation. There is minimal benefit of antiviral therapy in patients with lesions that have crusted.
- Patients who are immunocompromised should be treated with antiviral therapy regardless of the time since the onset of the rash.
- Patients with disseminated herpes zoster or CNS involvement or those severely immunosuppressed with herpes zoster require admission for IV acyclovir.
- Antiviral therapy promotes rapid healing of skin lesions, decreases the severity and duration of acute pain, and reduces viral shedding.

CYTOMEGALOVIRUS

- Cytomegalovirus (CMV) is a herpesvirus that causes a wide variety of diseases, ranging from asymptomatic infections in healthy patients to life-threatening pneumonia in those who are immunosuppressed. CMV is not highly contagious and is spread via sexual contact, saliva, breastfeeding, transplantation, and blood transfusion and through the placenta from mother to child.

Clinical Presentation

- Primary infection in healthy individuals is usually asymptomatic, although some patients may develop a heterophile-negative infectious mononucleosis syndrome consisting of fever, myalgias, and atypical lymphocytosis.
- Congenital and neonatal infections can carry a high mortality rate and present with jaundice, hepatosplenomegaly, petechiae, growth retardation, and microcephaly.
- Infections in patients who are immunocompromised can be severe and involve any organ system.
  - Patients with HIV and a CD4 count less than 50 cells/mm^3 can develop CMV retinitis, which presents with painless vision loss.

Diagnosis and Evaluation

- Diagnostic testing for CMV includes PCR testing, antibody testing, histologic analysis, and viral culture from body fluid, such as urine, blood, semen, tears, saliva, and vaginal fluid.

Treatment

- Infection in healthy patients is usually self-limited and requires only supportive care.

- Systemic antivirals, such as ganciclovir, valganciclovir, foscarnet, and cidofovir, can be used for severe CMV infection in consultation with an infectious disease specialist.

Human Immunodeficiency Virus

- HIV infection is a leading cause of infectious disease-related mortality worldwide, with approximately 36 million deaths caused by HIV-related illnesses in 2013. The vast majority of new infections occur in the developing world, with almost 5% of adults in sub-Saharan Africa positive for HIV. Although the number of new cases of HIV annually is decreasing, there are approximately 50,000 new cases of HIV each year in the United States.
  - The main risk factors for HIV infection are found in men who have sex with men and in injection drug use.
  - The HIV virus selectively targets CD4+ T cells after infection.
  - Transmission of HIV occurs via semen, vaginal secretions, blood or blood products, breast milk, and from mother to child through the placenta.

Clinical Presentation

- Patients with acute HIV infection present with fever, pharyngitis, fatigue, rash, headache, and lymphadenopathy.
  - The diagnosis of acute HIV infection is often missed because symptoms appear similar to common viral illnesses.
  - Symptoms develop 2 to 4 weeks after exposure and may last 2 to 10 weeks.
- Seroconversion usually occurs 3 to 8 weeks after HIV infection.
- Viral load and CD4+ T-cell count are most predictive of disease burden in patients with HIV.
- The Centers for Disease Control and Prevention defines acquired immunodeficiency syndrome (AIDS) as either a CD4 count less than 200 cells/mm^3 or occurrence of HIV-related opportunistic infection or cancer.

Diagnosis and Evaluation

- The most common method for diagnosis of HIV infection is detection of antibodies to the virus; most currently available tests also detect p24 antigen, which is positive during acute HIV infection symptoms prior to seroconversion.

Clinical Presentation

- Infections are the most common cause of hospitalizations in persons who are HIV-positive. We will limit our discussion to the most common infectious complications of HIV and aspects of treatment that are important for the emergency physician.
  - HIV-positive patients with a CD4 count greater than 500 cells/mm^3 have infection risk similar to immunocompetent patients.
  - HIV-positive patients with a CD4 count between 200 and 500 cells/mm^3 have some increased risk of bacterial respiratory infections and tuberculosis.
  - HIV patients with a CD4 count less than 200 cells/mm^3 are at risk of *Pneumocystis jirovecii* pneumonia, and CNS infections, including cryptococcal meningitis and toxoplasmosis; those with counts less than 50 are at risk of infection with *Mycobacterium avium* complex and cytomegalovirus.

Pulmonary Complications in HIV-Positive Patients

- The most common cause of pneumonia in HIV-positive patients in the United States is *Streptococcus pneumoniae.*
- *Pneumocystis jirovecii* pneumonia (PCP) is the most common opportunistic infection among patients with AIDS. This fungal infection is discussed in Chapter 61.

Neurologic Complications in HIV-Positive Patients

- Computed tomography with IV contrast and lumbar puncture (LP) should be considered for patients who are HIV-infected with a CD4 count below 200 and symptoms, such as fever and headache.
  - Toxoplasmosis causes focal encephalitis.
    - Patients present with headache, focal neurologic deficits, fever, seizures, and altered mental status.
    - Patients require treatment with IV pyrimethamine plus sulfadiazine and leucovorin or trimethoprim-sulfamethoxazole; steroids may be indicated for edema with mass effect.
  - Cryptococcal meningitis presents most commonly with fever and headache, either with or without altered mental status.
    - The presentation is often subtle with no meningismus, and the diagnosis generally requires lumbar puncture with CSF cryptococcal antigen testing or staining with India ink.
    - Elevated opening pressure greater than 25 mm Hg is common.
    - Initiate treatment with IV amphotericin B and oral flucytosine for 14 days followed by fluconazole for 8 weeks. Some mild cases may be treated primarily with oral fluconazole in consultation with infectious disease.

Gastrointestinal Complications in HIV-Positive Patients

- Oral candidiasis is characterized by plaques with an erythematous base that are present on the tongue and buccal mucosa and are easily scraped off.
  - Development of oral candidiasis is a poor prognostic sign and predictive of progression to AIDS.
  - Clotrimazole or nystatin suspension or troches are first-line treatment for oral candidiasis, and oral fluconazole can be used for refractory or recurrent disease.
- Dysphagia and odynophagia indicate esophagitis, which is most common in patients who are HIV-positive with a CD4 count less than 100 cells/mm^3, and it can be caused by *Candida*, herpes simplex virus, or cytomegalovirus.
  - Patients are treated presumptively with oral fluconazole or ketoconazole for 2 to 3 weeks with endoscopy; biopsy is reserved for patients who fail to respond to appropriate therapy.

Dermatologic Complications in HIV-Positive Patients

- Kaposi sarcoma consists of painless, raised, brown or purple papules that do not blanch and are most common on the face, chest, genitals, and oral cavity. (Details are given in Chapter 21.)

Ophthalmic Complications in HIV-Positive Patients

- Cytomegalovirus retinitis, the most frequent and serious ocular opportunistic infection, is the leading cause of blindness in patients with AIDS. Treatment requires IV ganciclovir.

Treatment

- Decisions regarding initiation of HIV antiretroviral therapy or any changes in therapy should be made in consultation with an infectious disease specialist.
- Initial treatment regimens typically consist of three drugs, including two nucleoside reverse transcriptase inhibitors and a nonnucleoside reverse transcriptase inhibitor, protease inhibitor, or integrase strand transfer inhibitor.
- Immune reconstitution inflammatory syndrome is a paradoxical worsening of preexisting infectious processes that occurs weeks or months following initiation of antiretroviral therapy. It is most common in patients with opportunistic infections, such as Cryptococcus or *Mycobacterium avium* complex, at the time antiretroviral treatment is initiated.
  - Treatment consists of nonsteroidal antiinflammatory agents for mild to moderate symptoms, and corticosteroids for severe cases.
  - Antiretroviral therapy should be continued during the episode of immune reconstitution inflammatory syndrome.

Rabies

- Human rabies infection is rare in the United States. Infection is invariably fatal, although infection can be prevented by rabies postexposure prophylaxis for high-risk animal exposures. Rabies infection is caused by the Lyssavirus, which is transmitted to humans from rabid animals, most commonly through bites.

Clinical Presentation

- Early symptoms are a prodrome of nonspecific flu-like symptoms, including fever, malaise, sore throat, headache, and nausea. Neurologic symptoms can include paresthesia, pain, and pruritis starting in the nerve distribution of the infecting bite.
- Patients then develop an acute neurologic syndrome consisting of fluctuating consciousness, hyperactivity, hypersalivation, persistent fever, painful pharyngeal spasms ("hydrophobia"), and seizures.

Diagnosis and Evaluation

- Rabies is usually a clinical diagnosis in developing countries when nonimmunized patients present after a bite by a rabid animal.
- The diagnosis is often delayed in developed countries owing to unrecognized exposure.
- Diagnosis can be confirmed by isolation of the virus from saliva, detection of antirabies antibodies in serum or CSF, and virus-specific immunofluorescent staining of a skin biopsy specimen.

Treatment

- There is no effective treatment for rabies, although the infection can be effectively prevented through postexposure prophylaxis.
- The decision to initiate rabies postexposure prophylaxis is based on type of exposure, circumstances regarding the exposure, vaccination history of the animal, local rabies epidemiology in animals, and availability of animal observation or rabies testing.
- Postexposure prophylaxis should be considered in cases of any potential exposure between a human and a bat, including patients in a room with a bat even without known physical contact if the person may not have been aware of contact (e.g., sleeping infant or intoxicated adult).
- Raccoons, skunks, and foxes are more likely to be infected with rabies, whereas squirrels, rats, and rabbits are unlikely to be infected with rabies in the United States.
- Immunocompetent patients who have not been previously vaccinated against rabies should receive the rabies vaccine on the day of exposure (day 0) followed by repeat vaccinations on days 3, 7, and 14.
  - Patients who are immunocompromised should receive a fifth dose of the rabies vaccination on day 28.
- Rabies immune globulin should be administered at the site of the bite on the day of exposure (day 0) in patients who have not previously received a rabies vaccination series.

SUGGESTED READINGS

Fiore, A. E., Fry, A., Shay, D., Gubareva, L., Bresee, J. S., & Uyeki, T. M. (2011). Antiviral agents for the treatment and chemoprophylaxis of influenza—Recommendations of the Advisory Committee on Immunization Practices. *Morbidity and Mortality Weekly Report, 60*(1), 1–24.

Maartens, G., Celum, C., & Lewin, S. R. (2014). HIV infection: Epidemiology, pathogenesis, treatment, and prevention. *Lancet, 384*(9939), 258–271.

Manning, S. E., Rupprecht, C. E., Fishbein, D., Hanlon, C. A., Lumlertdacha, B., Guerra, M., Meltzer, M. I., Dhankhar, P., Vaidya, S. A., Jenkins, S. R., Sun, B., & Hull, H. F. (2008). Human rabies prevention—United States, 2008: Recommendations of the Advisory Committee on Immunization Practices. *Morbidity and Mortality Weekly Report, 57*(RR-3), 1–28.

Emerging Infections: Pandemic Viruses

HAIG AINTABLIAN, MD, MS, and MATTHEW WAXMAN, MD, DTM&H

At the time of this writing, severe acute respiratory syndrome coronavirus 2, or SARS-CoV-2, is a novel RNA coronavirus that emerged from Wuhan, China, in December 2019. SARS-CoV-2 causes coronavirus disease 19, or COVID-19 and has spread in a global pandemic. Given the uncertainty of current knowledge about the life cycle of the virus and of the diagnosis and treatment of COVID-19, the authors have decided not to include an extensive discussion of this important virus.

The emergency physician is required to recognize the presentation of infections once confined to remote parts of the globe. Because emergency physicians are on the front line of health care, we need to be aware of outbreaks of emerging infections and familiar with their clinical presentations. Emerging and newsworthy infections such as Ebola, H1N1 influenza virus, severe acute respiratory syndrome (SARS), Middle East respiratory syndrome (MERS), and Zika virus have been predominantly viral, as opposed to bacterial, in etiology. Specialized testing for many emerging viral infections are not readily available in the emergency department, and supportive care and infection control are the mainstays of treatment. When there is clinical suspicion for an emerging viral infection, public health authorities should be notified immediately to help provide guidance on diagnostic testing and to institute public health efforts.

General Principles

List of Emerging Infectious Viruses

- Emerging viral infections most relevant to the emergency physician include filoviruses, such as Ebola and Marburg virus, which share route of transmission, intermediate hosts, and symptomatology, Hantaviruses, Lassa virus, H1N1 influenza virus (swine flu), H5N1 influenza virus (avian flu), SARS, MERS, Chikungunya, and Zika virus.

Common Preventive Measures

- Preventive measures for viruses include isolation, barrier methods, and respiratory precautions when encountering patients with a suspected infection.
- Personal protective equipment may include mask, gown, shoe covers, gloves, and respiratory precautions such as an N95 mask based on the specific virus and route of transmission.
- Quarantine may be required by public health authorities to contain outbreaks of some of these pandemic viruses such as Ebola virus.
- Vaccination exists for influenza virus and Ebola virus.

The Importance of Tropism

- Tropism, or a biologic organism's specificity toward infecting a subtype of host cells, is important in understanding a specific virus's symptoms. For example, many of the viruses that cause hemorrhagic complications have a tropism for endothelial cell lines, causing cell lysis of endothelium during their replication cycles. This, although not important for board memorization, aids in understanding the specific symptoms caused by these viruses. An excellent example of tropism and its effects on symptomatology is seen in chikungunya, a virus that has a predilection for musculoskeletal tissue and joints.

Crimean-Congo Hemorrhagic Fever Virus

General Principles

- Spread via the ixodid ticks, especially *Hyalomma*. These ticks are reservoirs and vectors for the Crimean-Congo hemorrhagic fever virus. Amplifying hosts for the virus include livestock such as cattle, goats, sheep, and hares. Transmission to humans occurs through contact with infected ticks or animal blood, and from human to human with infected blood or other body fluid.
- Located predominantly in Eastern Europe, the Mediterranean, northwestern China, central Asia, southern Europe, Africa, the Middle East and the Indian subcontinent.
- Has a diffuse tropism with multiple human cell lines affected.

Clinical Presentation

- Viral incubation after a tick bite (or bodily exposure to virus) is about 1–3 days followed by a flu-like prodrome of myalgia, headache, and nausea.
- About 5–6 days after the initial exposure, altered mental status develops slowly; intraoral petechiae, nosebleeds, gradually worsening hemorrhagic vomiting, and dark stools increase, ultimately leading to hepatic failure and bleeding into the skin.
- Those who survive (about 60% of those infected) may recover within 2 weeks of symptom onset.

Diagnosis and Evaluation

- In the emergency department (ED), diagnosis is mostly clinical, using a history or physical examination suggestive of tick bite followed by viral prodrome and ultimately hemorrhagic conversion.

- Laboratory tests, including complete blood count, comprehensive metabolic panel, urinary analysis and so forth, are useful in assessing the degree of anemia, hepatic involvement, renal failure, and dehydration.
- Definitive testing includes many options from enzyme-linked immunosorbent assay (ELISA), real time polymerase chain reaction (RT-PCR), antigen detection, or viral isolation on cell culture.
  - Early on in the course of infection, antibody production and therefore detection is limited, so antibody-specific tests may not be accurate.

Treatment

- Supportive. Ribavirin may have potential benefit.
  - *Prevention:* tick prevention and avoidance of infected body fluid or livestock.

Filoviruses: Ebola Virus Disease and Marburg Virus

General Principles

- Intermediate hosts and reservoirs include fruit bat species throughout sub-Saharan Africa with the terminal hosts being humans and great apes infected via bats. The exact mechanism of transmission of Ebola virus disease (EVD) to humans has not been established. Spread by contact, especially with corpses during funeral rites (EVD).
- Located predominantly in West and Central Africa.
- Diffuse tropism with multiple cell lines affected, including liver, spleen, intestinal linings, testes, and eyes.

Clinical Presentation

- Wide variation in symptoms and disease course.
- Rapid death is commonly from dehydration due to gastrointestinal losses early in disease.
- Early symptoms include fever, nausea, vomiting, malaise, and muscle aches. Nonspecific early symptoms may mimic malaria or other endemic diseases such as dengue or Marburg virus disease.
- Metabolic acidosis, dehydration, and renal failure with resultant tachypnea are common in critically ill patients.
- Although hemorrhagic complications such as conjunctival suffusion, bloody diarrhea, and bleeding diathesis are associated with EVD, they have been relatively rare in recent epidemics.
- EVD has a high mortality rate (about 70% of those infected) and a relatively low infectivity rate (about 10% of household contacts).

Evaluation and Diagnosis

- Unless during an outbreak, where clinical suspicion is high, Ebola and Marburg can be difficult to diagnose because early symptoms mimic those of other pathogens such as malaria or typhoid.
- In the ED, the diagnosis is clinical (high index of suspicion for travel to a region with ongoing outbreak), with confirmatory tests (PCR) done inpatient.
- As for other hemorrhagic viruses, complete blood count, comprehensive metabolic panel, and urinary analysis are useful in assessing the degree of anemia, presence of acidosis, and renal failure.

Treatment

- Supportive care including aggressive electrolyte repletion and intravenous hydration.
  - *Prevention:* avoidance of all infected body fluids. Vaccine for EVD is available only during outbreaks. Encapsulated viruses are killed by sodium hypochlorite (bleach).

Hantaviruses

General Principles

- Spread by contact with aerosolized rodent urine, feces, or saliva. Risk factors include camping.
- Located in all continents but Australia; outbreaks in the Four Corners region of the southwestern United States.
- Specific tropism for blood vessel and pulmonary cell lines.
- Multiple strains exist, and present as two major forms of hantavirus – hemorrhagic fever with renal syndrome (HFRS), and hantavirus cardiopulmonary syndrome (called HCPS or HPS). In the US, Andes and South America predominantly see HCPS.

Clinical Presentation

- Flu-like symptoms including fever, myalgia, headache, then rapidly decompensating pulmonary edema, shock, coagulopathy, arrhythmias in Hantavirus cardiopulmonary syndrome found in North America.
- Classic hemorrhagic fever with renal syndrome (HFRS) presents with fever, hemorrhage, hypotension, and AKI, but the course can be extremely variable. This is more common with the strains in Europe and eastern Asia.

Diagnosis and Evaluation

- Diagnosis requires a high clinical suspicion in a patient with risk factors such as rodent exposure, camping in an endemic area, presenting with pulmonary edema.
- Confirmatory testing involves serologic assays including ELISA, PCR, and antigen detection.
- ED workup should focus on cause of pulmonary edema with chest x-ray, B-type natriuretic peptide and infectious disease workup. Early in the course of illness (in the prodromal phase), patients may have a rapid drop in platelet count, elevated hepatocellular enzymes, lactate and LDH. Marked leukocytosis and immunoblasts are seen in the serum in severe illness.

Treatment

- Supportive care may require airway management and critical care in patients with Hantavirus pulmonary syndrome. Ribavirin should be considered.
  - *Prevention:* minimize contact with rodents when engaging in outdoor activities in affected areas.

H1N1 Influenza

General Principles

- Known as "swine flu," H1N1 is a zoonotic infection because it is acquired from pigs or infected humans. Spread is via inhalation or contact with virus.
- Worldwide presence.

- Predominantly infects the respiratory tract, including respiratory mucosa.

Clinical Presentation

- Common flu-like symptoms such as fever, chills, pharyngitis, myalgia, headache, and generalized fatigue begin early in the course of H1N1.
- In patients with severe disease who are hospitalized, pulmonary complications including secondary bacterial infection and acute respiratory distress syndrome (ARDS) are common.
- Systemic complications may occur in younger, healthy people disproportionately *more* than unhealthy people (as compared with typical influenza); about 60% of those who died from swine flu had no prior medical comorbidities.

Diagnosis and Evaluation

- Cannot be clinically distinguished from seasonal influenza virus. Diagnosis requires epidemiologic exposure to pigs or indirect exposure by contact with farm, slaughterhouse, or animal fair within 1 week of symptom onset.
- Rapid diagnostic tests for influenza may or may not be sensitive for H1N1 strains. In the proper clinical setting, a nasopharyngeal swab should be collected for diagnostic testing in conjunction with local health authorities.

Treatment

- Supportive care. Oseltamivir or zanamivir is of limited benefit unless given within first few days of infection.
  - *Prevention:* vaccination, hand hygiene, and contact precautions.

H5N1 Avian Flu

General Principles

- Spread via direct contact with infected birds. Direct human-to-human spread is uncommon.
- Mostly concentrated in Asia, but reported worldwide.

Clinical Presentation

- Symptoms begin with a typical flu-like illness including fever, cough, pharyngitis, and myalgia.
- Early in the disease course, patients may develop systemic complications including pneumonia, ARDS, and cytokine storm.

Diagnosis and Evaluation

- Clinically similar to H1N1. Commercially available rapid diagnostic influenza tests do not identify subtype and may be misleading.
- In the clinical scenario of influenza symptoms with travel to Asia and avian exposure, consider PCR testing in conjunction with public health authorities.

Treatment

- Supportive care. Oseltamivir or zanamivir are of limited benefit unless given early in infection.
  - *Prevention:* vaccination, hand hygiene, and contact precautions; avoidance of poultry farms and birds during epidemics in Asia.

Lassa Virus

General Principles

- *Mastomys* family of rodent is the vector. Virus is shed in rodent urine. Ingestion of food contaminated with rodent urine and inhalation are routes of transmission. Human-to-human contact can occur via body fluid.
- Located predominantly in West Africa.

Clinical Presentation

- Flu-like symptoms including fever, myalgia, and headache, followed by hemorrhagic symptoms including pulmonary hemorrhage and hematemesis.
- Clinical presentation may be indistinguishable from Ebola, which can lead to misdiagnosis during times of Ebola virus outbreaks.

Diagnosis and Evaluation

- Diagnosis is guided by nonspecific viral symptoms, travel to West Africa, and rodent exposure.
- Definitive testing should be done in conjunction with local public health authorities and includes PCR.
- Laboratory testing such as complete blood count and basic metabolic panel may be helpful to guide treatment of anemia, dehydration, and acidosis.

Treatment

- Supportive care and ribavirin.
  - *Prevention:* avoiding rodents during outbreaks.

SARS Coronavirus

General Principles

- Emergence of severe viral respiratory illness in Asia (China and Hong Kong) in 2003–2004. No cases have been reported since 2004.
- Bats may have been involved in the emergence of SARS.

Clinical Presentation

- Severe illness initially with muscle pain, headaches, and high fever.
- May progress after 2–14 days to cough, dyspnea, pneumonia, respiratory failure, and ARDS.

Diagnosis and Evaluation

- Clinical suspicion should be guided by concern for the reemergence of SARS with multiple cases of severe viral pneumonia coming from Asia.
- Definitive diagnosis with PCR or other molecular testing in conjunction with public health authorities.

Treatment

- Supportive care focusing on ARDS. Steroids may decrease inflammatory contribution to ARDS.
  - *Prevention:* quarantining of infected individuals with respiratory precautions during outbreaks.

MERS Coronavirus

General Principles

- Severe viral respiratory illness recently recognized in humans in 2012 after an outbreak in the Middle East.
- All patients either have traveled to the Arabian Peninsula or have had close contact with persons who traveled there.
- Route of transmission unclear but involves respiratory secretions and human-to-human contact. Some cases involve exposure to camels.

Clinical Presentation

- Cough, fever, and shortness of breath often progress to severe illness with high mortality.
- Variable incubation period of 2–14 days.
- Comorbid conditions such as diabetes or chronic lung disease may be a risk factor for severe illness.

Diagnosis and Evaluation

- Diagnosis is guided by respiratory symptoms and history of travel or exposure to persons from the Arabian Peninsula.
- PCR diagnostic testing in conjunction with local health department.

Treatment

- Supportive care. Patients with comorbid conditions should avoid camel exposure.

Chikungunya

General Principles

- Spread by *Aedes* mosquito species.
- Traditionally found in Asia and Africa, but since 2000 endemic in Central and South America.

Clinical Presentation

- Symptoms begin 4–7 days after mosquito bite and include fever, headaches, and a maculopapular rash.
- Severe arthralgias including joint pain and swelling of lower back, knees, wrists, and phalanges are characteristic of the virus.
- Symptoms resolve by 2 weeks, but some patients experience chronic musculoskeletal pain and disability.

Diagnosis and Evaluation

- Clinical suspicion raised by a history of mosquito bites, travel to endemic regions, and symptoms of severe joint pain. There is significant overlap between dengue fever and chikungunya, with the latter having more prominent joint involvement.
- Testing includes PCR early in presentation and ELISA in chronic disease.

Treatment

- Supportive. No vaccination or medication is proven to be effective.
  - *Prevention:* mosquito control.

Tick-Borne Encephalitis Viruses

General Principles

- *Ixodides* tick acts as both vector and reservoir. Rodents are definitive hosts; humans act as accidental hosts. Infection is also possible by consuming raw (unpasteurized) milk.
- Located worldwide, notably in Siberia, Russia, Saudi Arabia, and India.
- Neurotropic, preferentially targeting large neurons of the anterior horn of spinal cord.

Clinical Presentation

- Incubation period is 1–2 weeks, with mild flu-like symptoms including fever and myalgia.
- After a brief remission of 1 week, new symptoms develop in a large proportion of those infected, leading to meningismus and encephalitic symptoms causing the largest morbidities associated with the virus.

Diagnosis and Evaluation

- History and physical examination may include tick exposure (with a tick still attached to the patient).
- Leukopenia, thrombocytopenia, and elevated results from liver function tests are common diagnostic findings early on in the infection.
- Lumbar puncture will likely show pleomorphic leukocytosis.
- Definitive testing involves cerebrospinal fluid and serologic studies for viral culture, IgM, and/or IgG.

Treatment

- Supportive care with medications, including steroids, to address cerebral edema.
  - Aggressive search for and removal of tick are required.
  - *Prevention:* avoidance of tick exposure.

Zika Virus

General Principles

- Spread via the *Aedes* mosquito vector. Blood-borne and sexual human-to-human transmission has been documented. Vertical transmission or intrauterine infection causes significant fetal morbidity and mortality.
- Located predominantly in Central and South America.
- Broad tropism including neural progenitor cells, optic epithelium, placental endothelial cells, Leydig and Sertoli cells, vaginal epithelium, and exocrine tissue.

Clinical Presentation

- Most patients are asymptomatic or have mild symptoms and do not seek medical care.
- Symptoms include a maculopapular rash, conjunctivitis, and fever.
- Clinical importance of Zika virus is the effects in utero including microcephaly and fetal demise.

Diagnosis and Evaluation

- Diagnosis in the ED should be considered for patients with fever and constitutional symptoms with recent mosquito exposure from an endemic area. Pregnant patients with symptoms from an endemic area require referral to obstetrics for prenatal screening and evaluation.

- Nucleic acid amplification testing is the diagnostic test of choice. Testing should only be ordered in conjunction with local public health authorities.

Treatment

- Supportive care including nonsteroidal antiinflammatory agents.
  - *Prevention:* avoidance of mosquitos. Pregnant women should consider avoiding travel to affected areas to prevent birth defects.

SUGGESTED READINGS

Centers for Disease Control and Prevention. *Viral hemorrhagic fevers (VHFs)*. Centers for Disease Control and Prevention. Retrieved from: http://www.cdc.gov/vhf/index.html.

McMichael, A. J. (2004). Environmental and social influences on emerging infectious diseases: Past, present and future. *Philosophical Transactions of the Royal Society of London*, 359(1447), 1049–1058. doi:10.1098/rstb.2004.1480.

CHAPTER 66

BOARD REVIEW

Drug Resistance

DAVID HAASE, MD, and FREDRICK M. ABRAHAMIAN, DO, FIDSA, FACEP

Excessive use of antibiotics can result in the development of antibiotic-resistant bacteria. Antibiotic stewardship programs ensure appropriate antibiotic use and provide guidance to health-care providers in selecting antibiotics.

General Principles

- Examine local resistance patterns using antibiograms. Antibiograms consist of antimicrobial susceptibility data of various bacteria to selected antibiotics that are created using culture data from inpatient and outpatient services.
- The shortest duration of antibiotic therapy should be selected to minimize adverse side effects.
- Risk factors for harboring resistant organisms can include history of recent antibiotic use, nursing home stay, or recent hospitalization.
- Institute appropriate precautions (e.g., contact precautions) to minimize the spread of the pathogen.

Methicillin-Resistant *Staphylococcus aureus*

- Resistant to oxacillin and most other β-lactams, including most cephalosporins.
- Community-associated methicillin-resistant *Staphylococcus aureus* (MRSA) often manifests as skin and soft tissue infections that frequently are treated with trimethoprim/sulfamethoxazole, doxycycline, or clindamycin.
- MRSA can also be encountered with endocarditis, pneumonia, and osteomyelitis.
- Vancomycin and daptomycin are commonly used intravenous anti-MRSA agents; however, daptomycin is not used for pneumonia because of its poor respiratory tract concentrations.
- Linezolid is often used in the setting of vancomycin allergy, but its use is limited by its myelosuppression properties and potential serotonergic interactions.

Drug-Resistant Tuberculosis, Mycobacterium tuberculosis

- Tuberculosis (TB) usually requires multidrug therapy owing to varied resistance, often empirically with isoniazid, rifampin, pyrazinamide, and ethambutol.
- Drug-resistant tuberculosis refers to an isolate of tuberculosis that has resistance against isoniazid, rifampin, pyrazinamide, ethambutol, or streptomycin.
- Multidrug-resistant TB refers to an isolate of TB that is resistant to at least both isoniazid and rifampin.
- Extensively drug-resistant TB refers to a type of multidrug-resistant TB that is resistant to isoniazid and rifampin, plus any fluoroquinolone and at least one of three injectable second-line drugs such as amikacin, kanamycin, or capreomycin.
- Predictors of resistance include prior episodes of tuberculosis, worsening tuberculosis while receiving therapy, travel to endemic areas of known resistance, or contact with a person with known resistant TB.
- Treatment of drug-resistant TB is complicated, involves using expanded regimens, and should be managed by experts in the disease.

Extended-Spectrum β-Lactamase Bacteria

- Extended-spectrum β-lactamases (ESBLs) refers to enzymes produced by *Enterobacteriaceae*, often *Klebsiella pneumoniae* or *Escherichia coli*, that break down β-lactams (e.g., cephalosporins) except carbapenems.
- Usually, resistance to ceftriaxone is indicative of ESBL resistance.
- Typically found in infections common for *E. coli* or *K. pneumoniae*, such as urinary tract infections (UTIs), bacteremia, and nosocomial pneumonia.
- Often found in hospitalized patients; however, there is a rising trend of community-acquired ESBL infections, including UTIs.
- Treatment is generally with a carbapenem.

Vancomycin-Resistant Enterococci

- Most vancomycin-resistant enterococci organisms are *Enterococcus faecium*, which colonize the gastrointestinal tract and can be spread via hand-to-hand transmission.
- Associated with health-care infections.
- Can be seen in immunocompromised people, including those with bacteremia, subacute endocarditis, UTIs, or intraabdominal infections.
- With increasing resistance to β-lactams and aminoglycosides, treatment can consist of linezolid or daptomycin.

Carbapenem-Resistant Enterobacteriaceae (CRE)

- Commonly being *Klebsiella pneumoniae or Escherichia coli*, these organisms are resistant to most β-lactam antibiotics, including carbapenems, and most infections are from inpatient facilities.
- Infections range from bacteremia, pneumonia, to UTIs, often with high mortality rates.
- Risk factors include exposure to health-care settings like hospitals and long-term care facilities and recent exposure to carbapenems or cephalosporins.
- Treatment depends on the susceptibility profiles, with expert consultation.

Gonococcal Resistance, Neisseria gonorrhoeae

- Resistance initially developed to penicillins and has spread to fluoroquinolones.
- Increasing reports of decreased susceptibility to oral cephalosporins as well as azithromycin.
- Current recommended therapy for confirmed gonococcal urogenital infection is a single dose of intramuscular ceftriaxone. Presumptive additional treatment with doxycycline is recommended if chlamydia coinfection has not been ruled out.

SUGGESTED READINGS

Cyr, S. S., Barbee, L., Workowski, K. A., Bachmann, L. H., Pham, C., Schlanger, K., Torrone, E., Weinstock, H., Kersh, E. N., & Thorpe, P. (2020). Update to CDC's treatment guidelines for gonococcal infection, 2020. *Morbidity and Mortality Weekly Report*, 69(50), 1911.

Stevens, D. L., Bisno, A. L., Chambers, H. F., Dellinger, E. P., Goldstein, E. J., Gorbach, S. L., Hirschmann, J. V., Kaplan, S. L., Montoya, J. G., & Wade, J. C. (2014). Practice guidelines for the diagnosis and management of skin and soft tissue infections: 2014 update by the infectious diseases society of America. *Clinical Infectious Diseases*, 59(2), e10–e52.

SECTION TEN

BOARD REVIEW

Musculoskeletal

Bone and Joint Infections

ADEDAMOLA OGUNNIYI, MD

Basic Information

Anatomy

- Bone tissue has two types:
  - Compact: Bone is dense without cavities; forms the shaft of long bones and the outer edge of all bones.
  - Spongy: Bone is also referred to as medullary or cancellous bone; found at the ends of long bones and in irregular bones. It is metabolically active and is composed of trabeculae (a bony lattice), containing marrow.
- Long bones are divided into the following sections (Fig. 67.1):
  - Diaphysis, the bone shaft, is composed of the medullary canal (with marrow), overlying compact bone, and periosteum.
  - Metaphysis connects the diaphysis and the epiphysis.
  - Epiphysis, found at the ends of long bones and covered by a layer of cartilage, is the area of bone involved in joint articulation.
- Joints are formed by the articulation of two bones. They are covered by a fibrous synovial capsule, which is lined by synovial cells that produce fluid that keeps the space lubricated.

General Principles

- Bone and joint infections often result from hematogenous spread, but can also result from direct inoculation from trauma, operative procedures, or puncture wounds (including animal and human bites). Contiguous spread from adjacent infections is another means through which bones or joints become infected.
- Classified as acute (lasting less than 2 weeks), subacute (lasting 2 to 6 weeks), and chronic (infections lasting over 6 weeks), the acuity of bone and joint

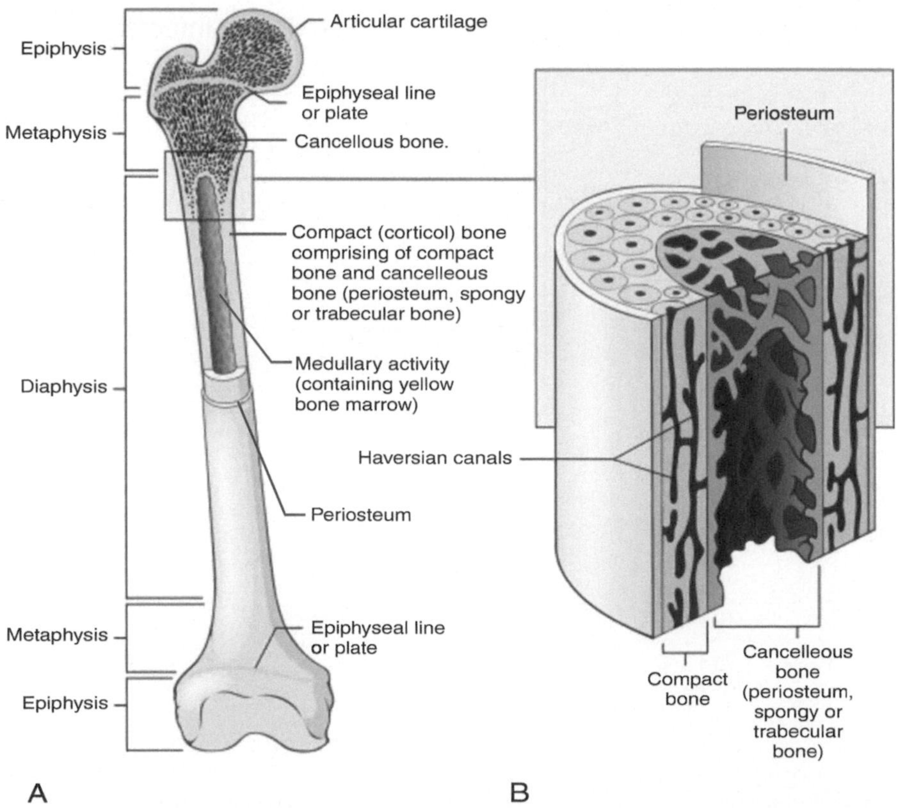

FIG. 67.1 Diagram of bone marked with an inset showing an enlarged view of compact cortical bone. (From Chabner, D.-E. (2021). *The language of medicine* (12th ed., pp. 543–612, Fig. 15.1). Elsevier.)

infections may alter treatment options and duration of therapy.

- Conditions that increase the risk of bone and joint infections include diabetes mellitus, immunosuppression (e.g., acquired immune deficiency syndrome [AIDS] and chronic steroid use), sickle cell disease, concurrent joint disease (e.g., rheumatoid arthritis or gout), and those with prosthetic implants.
- In general, bone and joint infections are monomicrobial and *Staphylococcus aureus* is the most common cause in all age groups, aside from neonates (in whom group B streptococci, *Escherichia coli*/gram-negative coliforms, and *Staphylococcus epidermidis* are the most common pathogens).
  - Box 67.1 provides a list of the common bacterial pathogens involved in the pathophysiology of bone and joint infections.
- Certain types of infection are more likely to be polymicrobial; these include posttraumatic osteomyelitis, diabetic foot osteomyelitis, and chronic infections.
- Although most bone and joint infections are bacterial, other pathogens (viruses, fungi, or parasites) can also affect these areas, particularly in patients infected with the human immunodeficiency virus (HIV) or in patients with AIDS.

Osteomyelitis

- Osteomyelitis is an infection of the bone and medullary cavity (marrow). Bone is resistant to infection unless there is direct trauma to the area, an impairment/compromise in blood flow, a foreign body, and/or seeding of the tissue (either hematogenously or from an external source). Chronic osteomyelitis is difficult to treat with antibiotics alone for the following reasons:
  - Necrotic infected bone (referred to an involucrum) has a limited blood supply, making it difficult for antibiotics to penetrate the area.
  - Infecting bacteria form a biofilm with most organisms existing in a dormant state.
- In children, osteomyelitis tends to be more acute and acquired hematogenously. In contrast, bone infections in adults occur more commonly from contiguous spread or direct inoculation.
  - The exception is in vertebral osteomyelitis, which occurs secondary to bacteremia in patients with indwelling lines, intravenous access devices (such as ports), or a history of intravenous (IV) drug use.
- Complications include bacteremia, local extension into nearby tissues (leading to conditions like pneumonia, spinal cord compression, epidural abscesses, and meningitis) and pathologic fractures.

BOX 67.1 *Bacterial Pathogens in Bone and Joint Infections*

Staphylococcus aureus (methicillin-sensitive and methicillin-resistant)
Streptococci (group A and B)
Staphylococcus epidermidis (including methicillin-resistant strains)
Enterobacteriaceae
Hemophilus influenzae (less common in the postvaccination era)
Escherichia coli
Streptococcus pneumoniae (in septic arthritis)
Anaerobes (in chronic osteomyelitis and diabetic foot infections)
Pseudomonas aeruginosa (in intravenous drug use, infected prostheses, and puncture wounds)
Eikenella corrodens (in human bites)
Pasteurella multocida (in animal bites)
Salmonella sp. (in patients with sickle cell disease)
Kingella kingae
Mycobacterium tuberculosis

(Adapted from Raukar, N. P., & Zink, B. J. (2018). Bone and joint infections. In R. M. Walls, R. S. Hockberger, & M. Gausche-Hill (Eds.), *Rosen's emergency medicine: Concepts and clinical practice* (9th ed., pp. 1693–1709). Elsevier.)

Clinical Presentation

- Patients may complain of fevers and chills, although this is not always present (for instance, as often occurs with postsurgical osteomyelitis).
- Other symptoms include pain in the affected bone, swelling, and warmth.
  - Children may present with a limp, difficulty bearing weight, or a decreased range of motion in the affected extremity.
  - Patients with vertebral osteomyelitis may complain of back pain or neurologic symptoms (if the infection extends into the epidural space or results in nerve compression).
- Examination findings include tenderness to palpation of the affected bone, erythema, warmth, and soft-tissue edema.
  - Sinus tracts may be present with chronic disease.

Diagnosis

- Definitive diagnosis is made by a microbiologic identification of the infective organism in the affected bone (which is obtained either by resection or needle aspiration).
  - This also guides the choice of antibiotics.
- Laboratory studies are not specific for osteomyelitis; however, patients may have elevated erythrocyte sedimentation rate (ESR) and C-reactive protein levels.
  - An ESR greater than 70 mm/hr (83%–92% sensitivity) may predict an underlying bone infection in a person with a diabetic foot infection.
  - Be aware that other infections (such as cellulitis) may also result in an elevated ESR, so values should be interpreted based on the clinical context.
- Cultures (blood, urine, and so forth) may be helpful in patients with hematogenous spread.
  - Blood cultures are positive in about 60% of pediatric patients with acute hematogenous osteomyelitis.
  - Anaerobic or fungal cultures may be useful in suspected polymicrobial infections in those with risk factors.

- Imaging
  - X-ray abnormalities may lag behind symptoms by 7 to 10 days.
    - Findings on x-ray include cortical lucencies (representing areas of bone destruction), periosteal elevation, soft-tissue edema, and sclerotic bone in advanced disease.
  - Computerized tomography (CT) may be useful for identifying infections in areas that are difficult to visualize on x-ray (such as the pelvis or sternum).
    - Findings include areas of lucency or gas (if abscesses are present).
  - Magnetic resonance imaging (MRI) is superior to x-rays in the detection of areas of osteomyelitis, especially at an earlier disease stage.
    - Gadolinium can help differentiate between soft-tissue infections and osteomyelitis.
- The differential diagnosis for osteomyelitis includes bone tumors, metastases, occult fractures, and bone infarcts (in patients with sickle cell disease).

Treatment

- Obtain a thorough past medical history because a patient's underlying risk factors may alter the type of bacteria involved, and therefore influence treatment.
- Treatment usually involves a combination of surgical debridement and antibiotic therapy.
  - Generally, antibiotics are not started until a bone biopsy is obtained to guide antibiotic therapy (exception is if the patient is septic).
  - Antibiotics should cover for *S. aureus*, but the treatment regimen should also take into consideration patient risk factors and the potential for concurrent infections.
    - Table 67.1 provides a summary of the recommended empiric antibiotic treatment regimens for suspected osteomyelitis.
    - Standard treatment regimen involves 4 to 6 weeks of IV antibiotics followed by a course of oral antibiotics.
    - Treatment involves input from both the surgical team and the infectious disease specialists to guide appropriate therapy.
- Vertebral osteomyelitis can be treated with IV antibiotics alone, but surgery may be required if complications (e.g., an unstable spine) are present or for diagnostic purposes.
- Diabetic foot osteomyelitis, often managed by amputation, if there is failure of antibiotic treatment.

Septic Arthritis

- Septic arthritis is an orthopedic emergency, because these infections result in damage to articular cartilage (owing to a release of lysosomal enzymes as part of the inflammatory response), which can ultimately lead to chronic arthritis (or avascular necrosis in children).
  - Extension into the developing bone tissue in children may also lead to decreased growth and a limb-length discrepancy.
- Incidence is increased in patients with rheumatic arthritis.
  - Patients with underlying crystal arthropathies (such as gout and pseudogout) are also at increased risk for this condition.
- Infections are either spread hematogenously or occur owing to direct inoculation of the joint (iatrogenically, from an infected foreign body or secondary to direct penetrating trauma).
- Septic arthritis is more common in children than in adults, where *S. aureus* is the most common pathogen.
  - Frequent sites of infection include the knee and hip in children and the knee, hip, and shoulder in adults.

TABLE 67.1 Empiric Treatment Regimens in Osteomyelitis

Age Group/Risk Factor	Common Pathogens	Recommended Antibiotics
Neonates to 3 months	*S. aureus*, group B streptococci, Enterobacteriaceae, gram-negative rods	Third generation cephalosporin; penicillinase-resistant penicillin + gentamicin (or vancomycin for methicillin-resistant *S. aureus*)
3 months to 14 years	*S. aureus*, group A streptococci, *H. influenzae*	Third generation cephalosporin + penicillinase-resistant penicillin (or vancomycin + a third generation cephalosporin)
14 years to adults	*S. aureus*	Penicillinase-resistant penicillin (or vancomycin)
Diabetic foot infections, chronic osteomyelitis	*S. aureus*, Enterobacteriaceae, anaerobes	Penicillinase-resistant penicillin + a fluoroquinolone + metronidazole (or a penicillinase-resistant penicillin + third generation cephalosporin + clindamycin)
Prosthetic joints	*S. aureus*, *S. epidermidis*, *P. aeruginosa*	Vancomycin + a fluoroquinolone (or imipenem)
Intravenous drug use	*S. aureus*, *P. aeruginosa*, Enterobacteriaceae	Third generation cephalosporin ± an aminoglycoside
Mammalian bites	*E. corrodens*, *P. multocida*	Penicillin; third generation cephalosporin; trimethoprim-sulfamethoxazole
Plantar puncture wounds	*P. aeruginosa*	Third generation cephalosporin; a fluoroquinolone
Sickle cell disease	*S. aureus*, *Salmonella* sp.	Third generation cephalosporin, + penicillinase-resistant penicillin (or a fluoroquinolone)

(Adapted from Raukar, N. P., & Zink, B. J. (2018). Bone and joint infections. In R. M. Walls, R. S. Hockberger, & M. Gausche-Hill (Eds.), *Rosen's emergency medicine: Concepts and clinical practice* (9th ed., pp. 1693–1709). Elsevier.)

- The most common type of septic arthritis in sexually active patients is gonococcal arthritis.
  - This occurs following a disseminated gonococcal infection (in about 40% of patients).
  - Gonococcal arthritis is typically monoarticular, but may be polyarticular.

Clinical Presentation

- Patients may present with acute joint pain and swelling, with a decrease in the range of motion (as movement exacerbates pain).
  - Systemic symptoms include fevers, chills, and malaise.
  - Children may present with an inability or refusal to bear weight on the affected extremity.
- Examination may reveal tenderness, warmth, edema, and erythema of the joint, with significant pain when manipulated.
  - The joint may also be held in the position of comfort, which is usually in a slightly flexed position.
- Patients' underlying risk factors may alter the presentation.
  - Immunocompromised patients may present with minimal pain and few systemic symptoms.
- Consider Lyme arthritis in endemic areas.
  - Often presents in the later stage of the disease (i.e., months after exposure).
  - It initially presents with migratory polyarthralgias that then affect one joint.

Diagnosis

- Laboratory studies (particularly the white blood cell [WBC] count) are often not specific or sensitive enough for a definitive diagnosis of septic arthritis and are interpreted based on the clinical context.
  - ESR is elevated in approximately 90% of cases, so it may be a useful marker (along with the C-reactive protein).
  - The Kocher criteria (i.e., a temperature above 38°C, inability to bear weight on the joint, ESR greater than 40 mm/hr, and a WBC count greater than 12,000 cells/mm^3) may be helpful in differentiating between septic arthritis and transient synovitis in children.
- A synovial fluid analysis, including a gram stain, culture, WBC count and differential, and crystal analysis should be performed on fluid aspirated from the joint (in a sterile fashion).
  - WBC counts greater than 50,000 with a neutrophilic predominance were previously thought to be definitive for the condition, but it is important to note that patients may still have septic arthritis with lower synovial WBC counts.
    - In patients with suspected periprosthetic infections, the orthopedic team should be contacted to obtain synovial fluid under sterile conditions. Note that the threshold synovial WBC count for diagnosing a periprosthetic infection is lower.
- The definitive diagnostic test for septic arthritis is the synovial fluid culture.
  - In patients where gonococcal infection is suspected, the fluid should be cultured on prewarmed chocolate agar.
- Blood cultures may also be useful.
  - Cultures of potential infected areas, such as throat, urine, rectum, or genitourinary area, are helpful in gonococcal arthritis.
  - Western blot or enzyme-linked immunosorbent assay testing may also be useful in patients with suspected Lyme disease/arthritis.
- Imaging
  - X-rays cannot diagnose septic arthritis, but may help rule out other conditions (such as osteomyelitis or abscesses).
  - Ultrasound imaging may help identify joint effusions and guide aspiration.
  - CT and MRI do not have a large role in the diagnosis of septic arthritis, but again can help identify other conditions (such as osteomyelitis or a psoas abscess).
- Differential diagnosis for septic arthritis is broad and includes transient synovitis (in children), osteomyelitis, Legg-Calve-Perthes disease, slipped capital femoral epiphysis, juvenile rheumatoid arthritis, crystalline arthropathies, reactive arthritis, and osteoarthritis.

Treatment

- Prompt diagnosis is important because this is an orthopedic emergency.
- Treatment involves both surgical intervention and antibiotic treatment.
  - Antibiotics should cover for *S. aureus*, but the treatment regimen should also take into consideration patient risk factors.
    - Therapy should also include treatment for chlamydia in sexually active adults and adolescents.
  - Table 67.2 provides a summary of the recommended empiric antibiotic treatment regimens for septic arthritis.
- Empiric antibiotics should be started as soon as synovial fluid is obtained.

SUGGESTED READING

Raukar, N. P., & Zink, B. J. (2018). Bone and joint infections. In R. M. Walls, R. S. Hockberger, & M. Gausche-Hill (Eds.), *Rosen's emergency medicine: Concepts and clinical practice* (9th ed., pp. 1693–1709). Elsevier.

TABLE 67.2 *Empiric Treatment Regimens for Septic Arthritis*

Age Group/Risk Factor	Common Pathogens	Recommended Antibiotics
Neonates to 3 months	*S. aureus*, group B streptococci, Enterobacteriaceae	Third generation cephalosporin + a penicillinase-resistant penicillin (or vancomycin for methicillin-resistant *S. aureus* + gentamycin)
3 months to 14 years	*S. aureus*, group A streptococci, *S. pneumoniae, H. influenzae*	Third generation cephalosporin + a penicillinase-resistant penicillin (or vancomycin + a third generation cephalosporin)
14 years to adults	*S. aureus*, streptococci, Enterobacteriaceae, *N. gonorrhoeae* (in sexually active patients)	Third generation cephalosporin or a penicillinase-resistant penicillin (or vancomycin + a third generation cephalosporin; penicillin + an aminoglycoside; or a third generation cephalosporin)
Prosthetic joints	*S. aureus, S. epidermidis, P. aeruginosa*	Vancomycin + a fluoroquinolone (or a penicillinase-resistant penicillin + antipseudomonal aminoglycoside)
Intravenous drug use	*P. aeruginosa, S. aureus*, Enterobacteriaceae	Penicillinase-resistant penicillin + an antipseudomonal aminoglycoside or a fluoroquinolone (or vancomycin and a fluoroquinolone)
Mammalian bites	*E. corrodens, P. multocida*	Penicillin; third generation cephalosporin; trimethoprim-sulfamethoxazole

(Adapted from Raukar, N. P., & Zink, B. J. (2018). Bone and joint infections. In R. M. Walls, R. S. Hockberger, & M. Gausche-Hill (Eds.), *Rosen's emergency medicine: Concepts and clinical practice* (9th ed., pp. 1693–1709). Elsevier.)

Bone Tumors

MICHAEL T. JORDAN, MD, and MANPREET SINGH, MD, MBE

Although metastatic bone malignancy is 25 times more common than primary bone malignancy, it is important to think about primary bone neoplasms when evaluating patients presenting with bone pain or a soft tissue mass because the morbidity and mortality can be high. About half of all primary bone malignancies will result in death.

Multiple Myeloma

Basic Principles

- Malignant proliferation of plasma cells that leads to overproduction of a monoclonal immunoglobulin
- Accounts for 1%–2% of all cancers; mostly seen in the elderly (median age at diagnosis is 66 years)
- Most common primary bone malignancy
- Causes skeletal destruction by forming osteolytic lesions and causing osteopenia, both of which may lead to pathologic fractures
- Osteoclasts are activated through the receptor activator of nuclear factor κ B (RANK) pathway by plasma cells.
- More often seen in African-Americans and males
- Infection is the most common cause of death in multiple myeloma because monoclonal antibodies lack antigenic diversity.

Clinical Presentation

- May present with a wide spectrum of complaints: bone pain (chest and/or back), fatigue, weight loss, and radiculopathy
- Patients may also present in acute renal failure secondary to light chain infiltration of the kidneys causing light chain cast nephropathy or renal failure owing to hypercalcemia.
- Less commonly, patients can present with spinal cord compression from an extramedullary plasmacytoma or pathologic fracture of the spinal column.
- Infection is a common presentation, as multiple myeloma is an immunodeficiency.
- May present with cryoglobulinemic vasculitis secondary to the increased viscosity of blood, which can lead to altered mental status, syncope, and stroke
- Laboratory abnormalities that may be present include a normochromic, normocytic anemia, elevated creatinine, hypercalcemia, and increased serum total protein. Coagulopathy can also occur owing to dysfibrinogenemia.

Diagnosis and Evaluation (Box 68.1; Fig. 68.1)

- Plain radiographs will often show multiple lytic lesions.
- Whole body computed tomography (CT), whole body magnetic resonance imaging (MRI), or whole-body positron emission tomography scan is preferred for detection of bone involvement compared to plain radiographs.
- Serum protein electrophoresis and/or 24-hour urine protein electrophoresis will detect elevated monoclonal proteins with a single spike on a densitometer tracing.
- The most common monoclonal proteins in order are as follows: IgG, IgA, kappa, or lambda light chains.
- Urinalysis will show large, waxy, laminated casts owing to monoclonal proteins known as Bence Jones proteinuria; urine dipstick will be negative for protein because it detects albumin rather than monoclonal proteins.

BOX 68.1 *Diagnostic Criteria for Multiple Myeloma*

Bone marrow plasma cells 10% or more OR biopsy-proven plasmacytoma
AND one of the two following:
Presence of end-organ damage (i.e., CRAB [hypercalcemia, renal insufficiency, anemia, bone pain]) **OR**
Presence of biomarker associated with likely end-organ damage (e.g., serum M protein, free light chain).

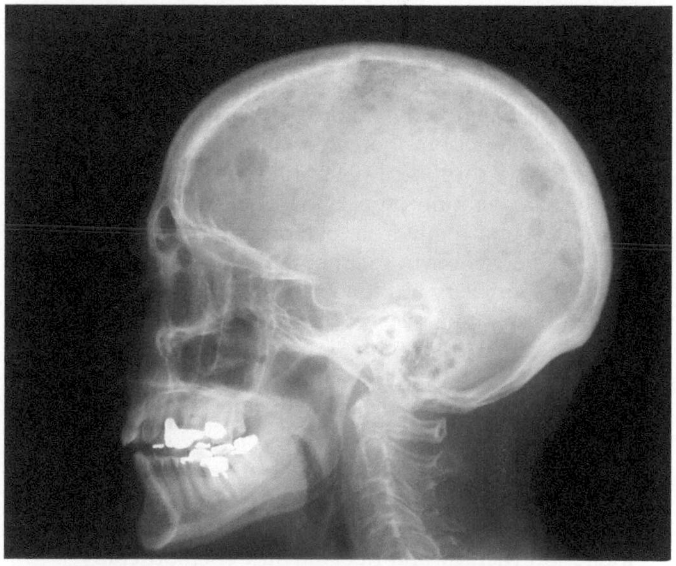

FIG. 68.1 Osteolytic lesions in the skull of a patient with multiple myeloma. (From Rajkumar, S. V., & Dispenzieri, A. (2020). Multiple myeloma and related disorders. In J. E. Niederhuber, J. O. Armitage, J. H. Doroshow, M. B. Kastan, & J. E. Tepper (Eds.), *Abeloff's clinical oncology e-book* (6th ed., p. 1890, Fig. 101.2). Elsevier Health Sciences.)

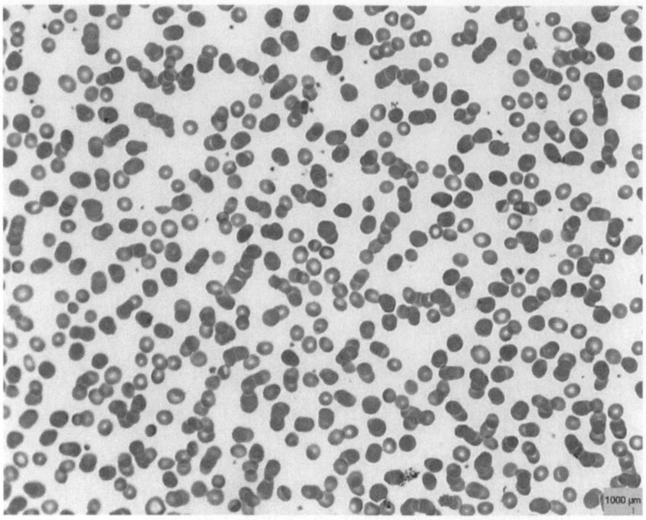

FIG. 68.2 Rouleaux are stacked red cells resulting from the presence of high levels of circulating acute-phase proteins. Rouleaux are commonly seen in patients with myeloma, other paraproteinemia, autoimmune disorders and chronic inflammation. (Courtesy Creative Commons CC0 1.0 Universal Public Domain Dedication.)

- Tubulointerstitial renal disease from the monoclonal proteins is diagnosed by biopsy.
- Hypercalcemia from increased bone turnover may be reflected as a shortened QTc on electrocardiogram.
- Rouleaux formation on peripheral smear (Fig. 68.2)
- Pseudohyponatremia from paraproteinemia
- Increased erythrocyte sedimentation rate secondary to increased viscosity in blood
- Hyperphosphatemia
- High IL-6 may be present in the blood because it stimulates proliferation of plasma cells.
- Bone marrow biopsy for definitive diagnosis. Refer to Box 68.1 for diagnostic criteria.

Treatment

- If eligible, hematopoietic cell transplantation after induction therapy and neoadjuvant chemotherapy
- Chemotherapy if ineligible for hematopoietic cell transplantation
- Treat acute hypercalcemia, renal failure, and symptomatic anemia appropriately.

Osteosarcoma

Basic Principles

- Most common primary pediatric bone tumor; 3% of all childhood cancers
- Around two-thirds of those diagnosed with nonmetastatic disease under the age of 40 will be long-term survivors or cured of the disease with appropriate treatment.
- Survival is less than 20% with metastatic disease.
- It is bimodal because it peaks in early adolescence and over the age of 65.
- Overproduction of osteoid and immature bone by malignant osteoblasts

Clinical Presentation

- Often an adolescent during a growth spurt
- Bone pain for several months that worsens with activity and is more painful at night
- Absence of constitutional symptoms (e.g., fevers, weight loss, night sweats, and decreased appetite are typically absent)
- Large soft-tissue mass on examination that is tender to palpation
- Occurs at metaphysis of long bones; most commonly at the distal femur followed by the proximal tibia
- One-fifth will have metastases at presentation; most common metastatic site is the lung followed by bone.
- Less frequently presents as a pathologic fracture
- Risk factors include prior cancer treatment, Paget disease of bone, benign bone disease, hereditary retinoblastoma, or Li-Fraumeni syndrome.

Diagnosis and Evaluation (Fig. 68.3)

- Classic radiographic finding is a "sunburst" pattern.
- The "sunburst" pattern describes a lytic lesion with a periosteal reaction and cortical disruption at or near the metaphysis.
- Can also see Codman triangle: new, subperiosteal bone formed when periosteum is raised away from the bone
- Laboratory abnormalities frequently present include an elevated alkaline phosphatase, lactate dehydrogenase (LDH), and erythrocyte sedimentation rate (ESR).
- High LDH is associated with poor outcomes.
- MRI and biopsy for definitive diagnosis

Treatment

- Surgery: limb-sparing surgery or amputation, if needed (depends on location and extent of the primary tumor)
- Neoadjuvant chemotherapy; response is a major prognostic factor.
- MAP therapy (methotrexate, doxorubicin, cisplatin) is often the regimen of choice for nonmetastatic disease; no standard approach if metastatic.
- Typically, radiation-resistant; however, if involving base of skull or sacrum, can consider intensity-modulated radiation therapy

Chondrosarcoma

Basic Principles

- Third most common primary bone malignancy after multiple myeloma and osteosarcoma
- Caused by overproduction of chondroid matrix in the medullary cavity
- Around 90% of chondrosarcomas are of low metastatic potential.
- Osteochondromas and enchondromas can be precursor lesions.

Clinical Presentation

- Occurs commonly in the pelvis and central skeleton
- Occurs in patients over 40 years of age, with a male predominance

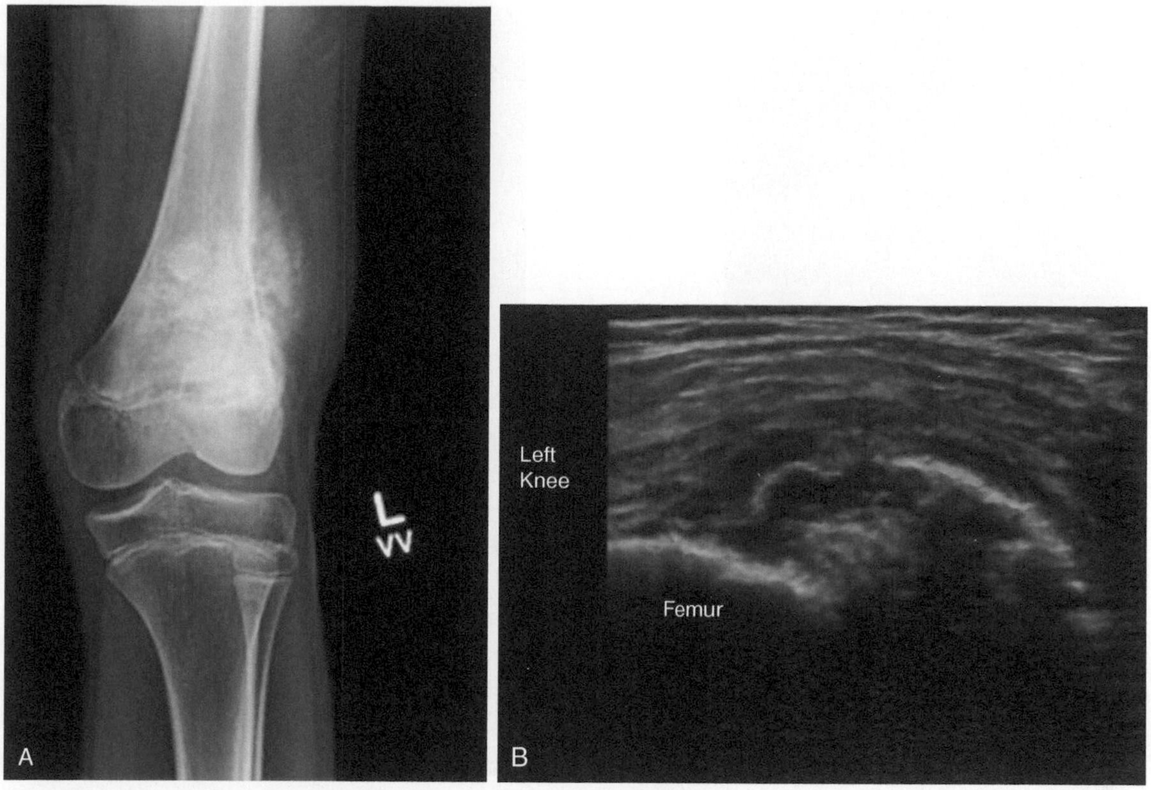

FIG. 68.3 **A**, Sunburst appearance of suspected osteosarcoma. **B**, Ultrasound of the same patient showing cortical destruction and bony mass. (Courtesy M. Jordan, M. Singh, & K. Preston-Suni, Harbor-UCLA Medical Center, 2019.)

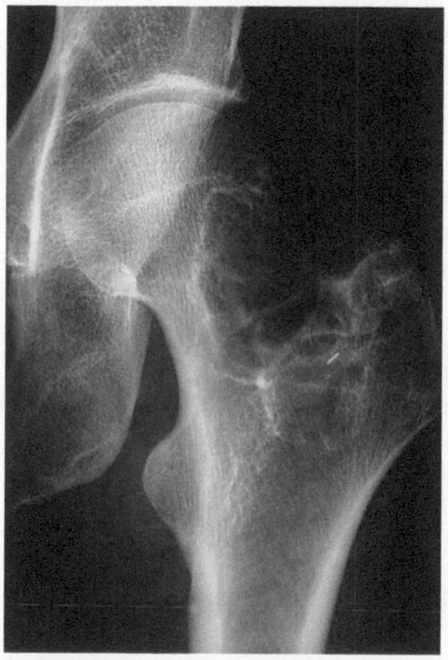

FIG. 68.4 **Chondrosarcoma with cortical bone destruction.** (From Anderson, M. E., DuBois, S. G., & Gebhardt, M. C. (2020). Sarcomas of bone. In J. E. Niederhuber, J. O. Armitage, J. H. Doroshow, M. B. Kastan, & J. E. Tepper (Eds.), *Abeloff's clinical oncology e-book* (6th ed., p. 1636/e1, eFig. 89.4A). Elsevier Health Sciences.)

- Often will present with local swelling and pain or a pathologic fracture; very slow-growing tumors

Diagnosis and Evaluation (Fig. 68.4)

- Plain radiographs reveal punctate calcifications and cortical bone destruction.
- CT or MRI to assess extent of bone involvement
- Bone biopsy for definitive diagnosis

Treatment

- Surgery is the definitive treatment.
- Radiation and chemotherapy are ineffective because the tumor is very slow-growing.

Ewing Sarcoma

Basic Principles

- Highly aggressive malignant bone or soft-tissue tumor arising from cells of the neuroectoderm
- One-fourth of patients will have metastasis at the time of presentation; it is assumed that almost all patients have subclinical metastasis.
- Presence and location of metastasis are the major prognostic factors for survival.
- Metastasis is most frequently seen in bone (spine most common) and lungs.
- Around 70%–80% survival in those with nonmetastatic disease
- More common in males

Clinical Presentation

- Constant pain for months over site of malignancy; worse with exercise and at night
- Site will be edematous and tender to palpation; mass can sometimes be appreciated.

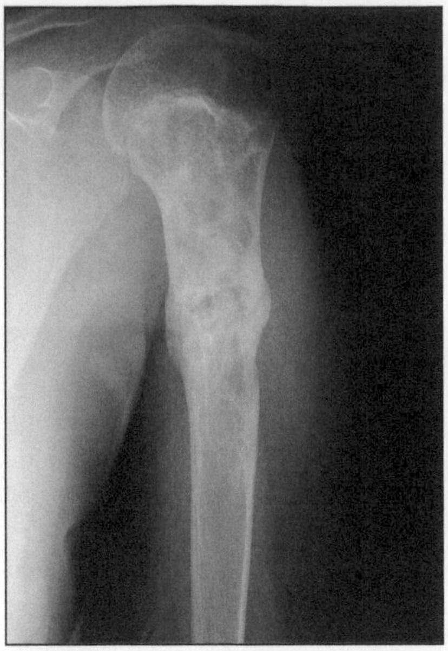

FIG. 68.5 Ewing sarcoma and associated pathologic fracture. Significant periosteal reaction seen on x-ray. (From Anderson, M. E., DuBois, S. G., & Gebhardt, M. C. (2020). Sarcomas of bone. In J. E. Niederhuber, J. O. Armitage, J. H. Doroshow, M. B. Kastan, & J. E. Tepper (Eds.), *Abeloff's clinical oncology e-book* (6th ed., pp. 1604–1654, eFig. 89.5A). Elsevier Health Sciences.)

- Most often found in pelvis, axial skeleton, or diaphysis of femur with a small minority arising in soft tissues
- Pelvic tumors are more regularly associated with metastatic disease.
- Fever, weight loss, fatigue, night sweats occur in less than 20% of patients.
- Pathologic fractures can occur.

Diagnosis and Evaluation (Fig. 68.5)

- Appearance on plain radiographs often is described as "onion peel" or "moth-eaten" appearance referring to the respective periosteal bone formation and osseous destruction.
- LDH is a prognostic factor with elevated levels conferring lower overall survivability.
- Definitive diagnosis is made with biopsy; workup often includes positron emission tomography scan to investigate presence of metastatic disease.
- t(11;22) translocation is often seen.

Treatment

- Neoadjuvant and adjuvant chemotherapy
- Surgery and/or radiation therapy for local control of disease

Giant Cell Tumor

Basic Principles

- Benign tumor that is locally aggressive causing osteolytic destruction
- Although classified as benign lesions, metastasis does occur in a small percentage of patients, typically to the lungs. However, these are known as benign pulmonary implants because they do not carry the same poor prognostic implication as lung metastasis from other malignancies.

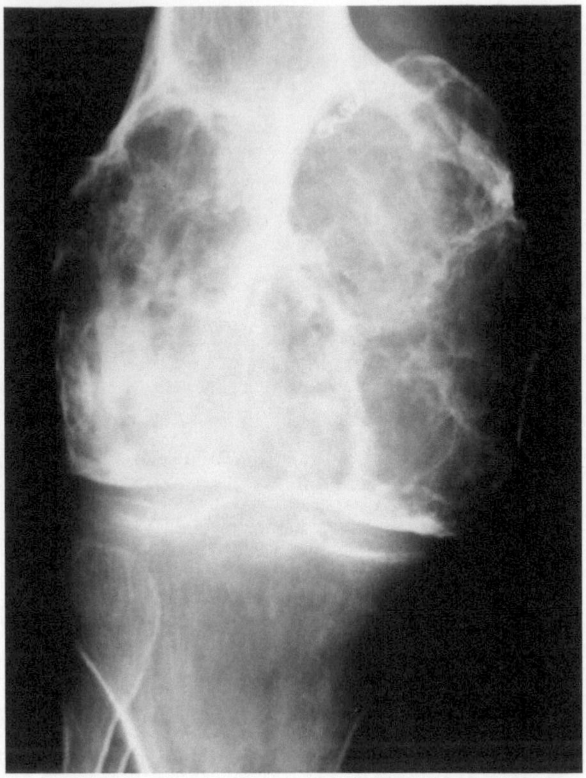

FIG. 68.6 Giant cell tumor at the epiphysis, which appears as a lytic lesion. (From Czerniak, B. (2016). *Dorfman and Czerniak's bone tumors* (2nd ed., p. 737, Fig. 10.38A). Elsevier Health Sciences.

- Of all primary bone tumors, 3%–5%; around 20% in the Chinese population
- Increased incidence in patients who have been diagnosed with Paget disease of the bone

Clinical Presentation

- Pain and edema over a joint near a long bone (usually around the knee) in a young female adult
- Can present as a pathologic fracture
- Nearly all present with just a single tumor site.

Diagnosis and Evaluation (Fig. 68.6)

- Plain radiograph showing a large lytic mass with soap bubble appearance
- Obtain chest plain film to look for pulmonary metastasis.
- CT and MRI for more accurate assessment of tumor
- Biopsy for definitive diagnosis

Treatment

- Surgery is the treatment of choice.
- RANKL inhibitors (Denosumab) for unresectable metastatic disease
- Can recur locally after curettage

Other Malignant Bone Tumors (Table 68.1; Fig. 68.7)

- The more common malignant primary bone tumors have been discussed above.
- Table 68.1 describes other rare malignant bone tumors.

TABLE 68.1 *Less-Common Primary Malignant Bone Tumors*

Name	Presentation	Radiograph Findings	Clinical Importance
Adamantinoma	Bone pain over anterior tibia in adolescent or young adult	Soap bubble osteolytic appearance on plain radiograph	Metastasis to lungs May need amputation
Chordoma	Constant pain if in sacrum Neurologic deficits if at base of skull, most commonly in cranial nerves to the eye	Plain radiograph will show a destructive bone lesion, often with an associated soft tissue mass	Slow-growing, but locally aggressive Metastasis is uncommon; local recurrence is much more likely
Fibrosarcoma and undifferentiated pleomorphic sarcoma	Similar to osteosarcoma, except malignant fibroblasts but less common	Most common in distal femur and proximal tibia	Similar outcome to osteosarcoma
Primary bone lymphoma	Adult over 40 years of age with bone pain or pathologic fracture	Bone destruction Soft-tissue mass	5-year survival is greater than 50% with radiation and chemotherapy

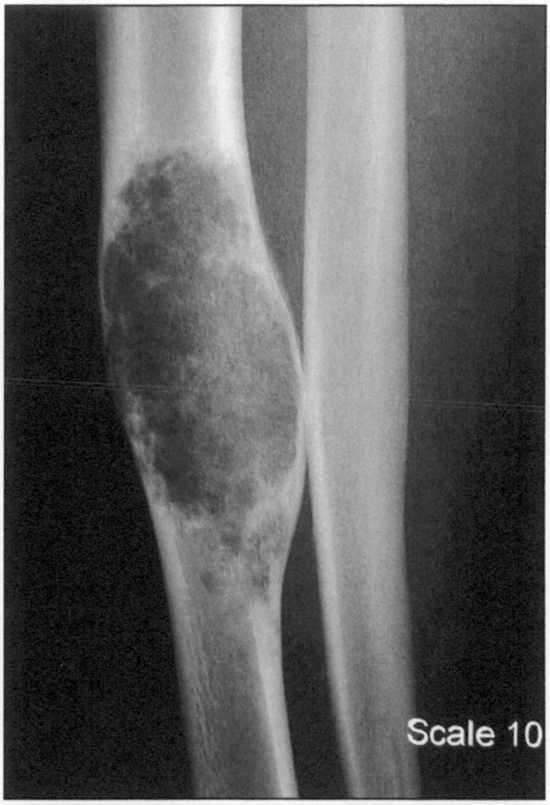

FIG. 68.7 Soap bubble appearance on x-ray. This patient had biopsy proven adamantinoma of anterior tibia. (From Anderson, M. E., DuBois, S. G., & Gebhardt, M. C. (2020). Sarcomas of bone. In J. E. Niederhuber, J. O. Armitage, J. H. Doroshow, M. B. Kastan, & J. E. Tepper (Eds.), *Abeloff's clinical oncology e-book* (6th ed., p. 1890, Fig. 89.17A). Elsevier Health Sciences.)

Benign Bone Tumors (Table 68.2; Figs. 68.8 and 68.9)

- Benign bone tumors are about 100 times more common than primary bone malignancy.
- The true incidence is unknown because most are an incidental finding on imaging.
- Table 68.2 describes some of the more common benign bone tumors.

SUGGESTED READINGS

Czerniak, B. (2016). Benign osteoblastic tumors. In B. Czerniak (Ed.), *Dorfman and Czerniak's bone tumors* (2nd ed., pp. 144–199). Elsevier Health Sciences.

Niederhuber, J. E., Armitage, J. O., Doroshow, J. H., Kastan, M. B., & Tepper, J. E. (2020). Sarcomas. *Abeloff's clinical oncology e-book* (pp. 1604–1654.e8). Elsevier Health Sciences.

TABLE 68.2 *Benign Bone Tumors*

Name	Presentation	Radiograph Findings/Location	Clinical Importance
Chondroblastoma	Bone or joint pain in adolescent	Epiphysis of long bones; may cross growth plate	Growth disturbance Arthritis
Enchondroma	Soft-tissue mass in hands or feet of adolescent Seen in Ollier disease or Mafucci syndrome	Metaphysis of long bones in hand or feet Oval lesion with sclerotic edges and central lucency	Malignant transformation to chondrosarcoma if multiple lesions present
Langerhans cell histiocytosis of bone	Painful swelling of skull in children, typically frontal bone, or long bones	Lytic, punched-out lesion	Lesion of skull can be associated with diabetes insipidus or other CNS disease Pathologic fracture of long bone
Osteoblastoma	Adolescent male with chronic pain in spine; most often seen in posterior column	Similar to osteoid osteoma, but typically more than 2 cm	May appear like osteoid osteoma on plain film, but DOES NOT respond to aspirin/NSAIDs
Osteochondroma	Adolescent male with painless mass over distal femur	Osseous spur that arises from cortex pointing away from joint	Observation without treatment Small risk of transformation to chondrosarcoma
Osteoid osteoma	Adolescent male with bone pain over femur Pain worse at night and unrelated to activity	Radiolucent nidus with sclerotic edges most often seen in proximal femur	Nidus produces prostaglandins, aspirin/NSAIDs can relieve pain Most resolve

CNS, central nervous system; *NSAIDs*, nonsteroidal antiinflammatory drugs.

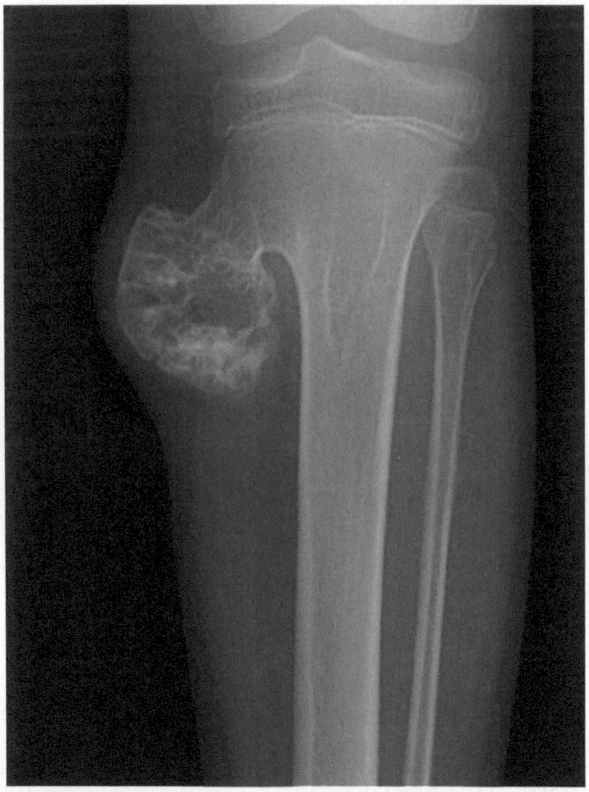

FIG. 68.8 Osteochondroma of the proximal tibial metaphysis. Czerniak, B. (2016). *Dorfman and Czerniak's bone tumors* (2nd ed., p. 443, Fig. 6.75A). Elsevier Health Sciences.)

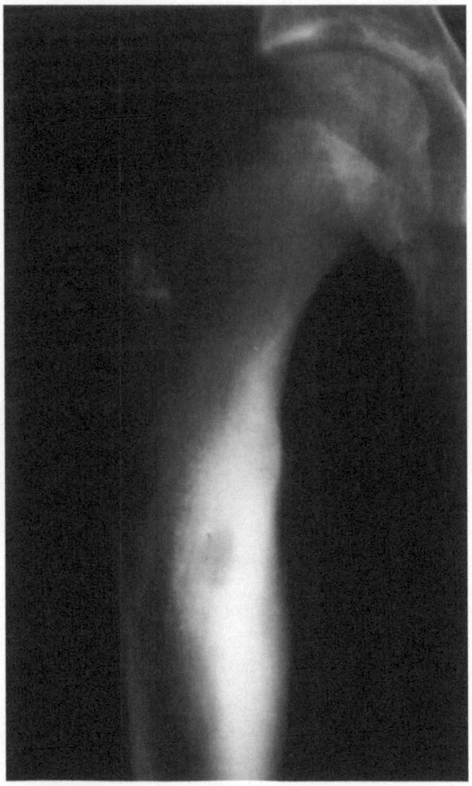

FIG. 68.9 Osteoid osteoma with radiolucent nidus and surrounding sclerosis. Czerniak, B. (2016). *Dorfman and Czerniak's bone tumors* (2nd ed., p. 148, Fig. 4.4A). Elsevier Health Sciences.)

CHAPTER **69** BOARD REVIEW

Pathologic Fractures

ALEXANDRA GROSSMAN, MD, and MANPREET SINGH, MD, MBE

Osteoporosis

General Principles

- A clinical condition characterized by reduced bone mass (osteopenia) and skeletal fragility that results in an increased risk of fractures.
- A significant public health problem, resulting in over 1.5 million fractures per year in the United States with substantial associated morbidity and mortality. For example, in individuals who have sustained a hip fracture, one in five will die within the first year and less than one-third will regain their baseline functional status.
- Low bone mass in osteoporosis results from an imbalance between bone resorption and formation and is defined by a bone mineral density (BMD) score more than 2.5 standard deviations below the young adult mean.
- There are two types: primary and secondary osteoporosis. Primary osteoporosis is related to normal aging and estrogen deficiency states (i.e., postmenopause), whereas secondary osteoporosis results from chronic conditions that accelerate bone loss. Table 69.1 highlights risk factors for osteoporosis.

Clinical Presentation

- Patients with osteoporosis may present with a "fragility fracture," defined as a fracture that occurs with minimal trauma (i.e., ground-level fall) or no identifiable trauma at all.
- The most common locations for these fractures include vertebral, proximal femur, distal forearm, and proximal humerus.

TABLE 69.1 *Risk Factors for Osteoporosis*

Modifiable	Nonmodifiable
Smoking	Age
Alcohol	Ethnicity (white/Asian race)
Nutritional deficiencies (Ca, Vit D)	Gender
Sedentary lifestyle / immobilization	Chronic glucocorticoid therapy
Low body mass index (BMI)	Personal history of fractures
Excessive alcohol intake	Low BMI (less than 21 kg/m^2)
Poor nutritional status	Medical history (renal/metabolic/endocrine/rheumatological)

- Vertebral body compression fractures are the most common manifestation of osteoporosis and they most commonly affect the thoracic spine. Patients may present with mid or upper back pain that is typically worsened by activity and relieved by rest. However, these fractures are also commonly asymptomatic and found incidentally on imaging.
- Consequences of vertebral fractures include chronic pain and spinal deformity (kyphosis), the latter of which can impair pulmonary function and result in restrictive lung disease.
- Distal forearm fractures are one of the most common symptomatic "first" fragility fractures.

Diagnosis and Evaluation

- History should include assessment of risk factors for fragility fractures, including a history of falls, prior fractures, comorbid medical problems, tobacco use, chronic medications, alcohol consumption, and low physical activity levels.
- Physical examination should include appropriate evaluation of the specifically injured body part. Additionally, patients should be examined for signs of underlying systemic disease that may contribute to secondary osteoporosis. A few examples of such physical manifestations include lid lag and goiter (thyroid disease), moon facies or truncal obesity (Cushing's disease), and cachexia (malignancy, eating disorder).
- In the emergency department (ED), laboratory tests should include a complete metabolic panel to evaluate for renal dysfunction, hepatic disease, and disorders of calcium or phosphorus homeostasis. Specifically, hypocalcemia and hypophosphatemia may indicate malabsorption, vitamin D deficiency, or osteomalacia. Workup for secondary causes of osteoporosis may include thyroid function tests, 24-hour cortisol excretion, testosterone/estrogen levels, parathyroid hormone levels, although these are typically done on an outpatient basis.
- X-rays should be obtained to evaluate for fractures. Note that plain radiographic studies as obtained in the ED are not sufficiently sensitive to diagnose early osteoporosis because they will only show changes after more than 30% of bone mineral density has been lost.
- Vertebral compression fractures (Fig. 69.1) are typically diagnosed on lateral radiography of the vertebral column by a decrease in vertebral body height of at least 20% or a 4-mm reduction from baseline height.

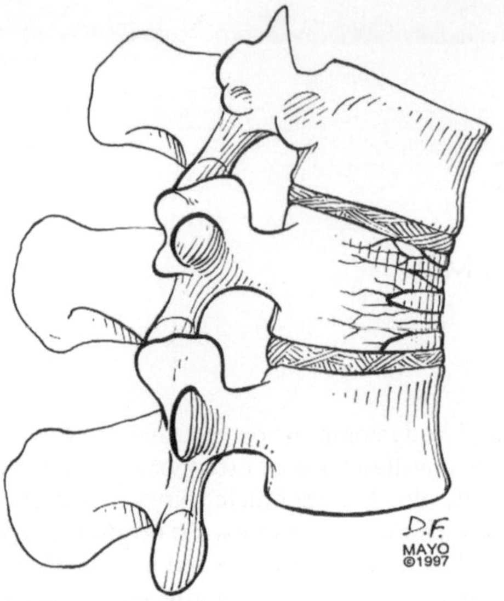

FIG. 69.1 Thoracic compression fracture with reduction in anterior vertebral height and wedging of the vertebrae. (From Hanson, T. (2019). Thoracic compression fracture. In W. R. Frontera, J. K. Silver, & T. D. Rizzo, Jr. (Eds.), *Essentials of physical medicine and rehabilitation: Musculoskeletal disorders, pain, and rehabilitation* (4th ed., pp. 228–233, Fig. 42.1). Elsevier.)

- Patients with concern for osteoporotic fracture should be referred for an outpatient BMD test (Box 69.1).

Management

- ED patients with suspected fragility fracture should be counseled on their risk for osteoporosis and referred for outpatient testing and treatment.
- Pharmacologic options for osteoporosis treatment work by inhibiting osteoclast-mediated bone resorption or stimulating osteoblastic bone formation. Bisphosphonates, which inhibit bone remodeling, are the most commonly prescribed class of medications. Other options include hormone replacement therapy (estrogens and selective estrogen-receptor modulators), denosumab (biologic agent), and the anabolic agent teriparatide. These medications should be initiated in the outpatient setting.
- Patients should be educated on preventive measures, including adequate dietary calcium and vitamin D intake, regular weight-bearing and muscle strengthening exercises, fall safety, and avoidance of smoking and alcohol consumption.
- Spinal compression fractures should be treated with analgesia, early mobilization, physical therapy, and referral for initiation of testing and treatment measures, as above. Thoracolumbar bracing may be prescribed for 6 to 8 weeks, although this is controversial and supported by limited evidence. Bracing carries a risk of pressure ulcerations, impaired pulmonary function, and muscle weakness and should be initiated with caution.

BOX 69.1 *Who Should Get a Baseline Bone Density Test?*

Recommendations from the National Osteoporosis Foundation

- Women aged 65 years or older or men 70 years or older
- Postmenopausal women younger than 65 with one or more additional risk factors
- Men aged 50–69 with one or more risk factors
- Anyone with a fracture after age 50

Tumor-Related

General Principles

- Pathologic fractures can occur secondary to primary bone tumor or metastatic disease, the latter being the most common type of bone malignancy.
- Bone is the third most common site of malignant metastatic spread, following liver and lungs. Cancers of the prostate and breast are most strongly associated with bone metastases, with one autopsy study demonstrating a prevalence of 70% of these patients. Other malignancies that commonly spread to bone include thyroid, renal, and lung carcinomas. Although less frequent, sarcomas, lymphomas, melanomas, gastrointestinal malignancies as well as bladder carcinomas are all also capable of bony spread.
- Hematologic malignancies can also affect bone, particularly multiple myeloma. Skeletal lytic lesions are present in 60% of affected patients at the time of diagnosis.
- Primary bone tumors can be both benign (most common) or malignant. Benign tumors include endochondromas, osteochondromas, osteoid osteomas, and giant cell tumors. Malignant tumors include osteosarcoma, Ewing sarcoma, and chondrosarcoma and can affect both pediatrics and adults.

Clinical Presentation

- Metastatic bone lesions predominantly involve areas of red marrow, such as the axial skeleton (vertebrae, ribs, sternum), pelvis, and skull. The vertebral column is the most frequent site of bony metastasis (50%–70%), specifically the thoracic spine (T4-T7).
- Fractures from bone metastasis often occur with no or minimal trauma. In patients with known malignancy, all patients with bone fracture in the absence of significant trauma should be considered to have metastases.
- Although bony metastases are often asymptomatic, pain is the most common clinical presenting symptom. Pain is classically described as progressive, dull, and nonmechanical. A history of pain preceding the fracture is an important historical clue that should alert the clinician to the possibility of a metastatic lesion; one study found that pain preceded the fracture in 85% of patients with pathologic fractures from bone metastasis.
- Spinal metastases can cause compression of the nerve roots or spinal cord resulting in radiculopathy as well as motor, sensory, bladder, or bowel dysfunction. Up to 20% of patients with malignant spinal cord compression may have no known history of cancer.
- Hypercalcemia occurs in 10% of patients with bone metastases; if symptomatic, it may present with fatigue, altered mental status, abdominal pain, and vomiting.

Diagnosis and Evaluation

- All patients with fracture following minimal or no trauma should be evaluated for the possibility of pathologic fracture, particularly in the setting of known active or prior malignancy.

- Patients should be asked about any history of prior radiation therapy to the affected area, associated symptoms concerning for metastatic disease (weight loss, fevers, and so forth), or spinal cord involvement.
- Physical examination should be tailored to the specific complaint. Any concern for vertebral involvement warrants a thorough neurologic examination to evaluate for spinal cord compromise.
- Radiography is often the first-line imaging test (Fig. 69.2). Features suggesting underlying malignancy include marked lysis or high density of the matrix, cortical breaks, periosteal reaction, spread to adjacent soft tissues, or multifocal lesions (suggestive of metastatic disease).
- Computed tomography (CT) or magnetic resonance imaging (MRI) may be used to help confirm the diagnosis of a pathologic fracture, differentiate primary bone tumor from metastatic lesion, and determine the extent of disease. CT is excellent for visualizing the bone cortex, although MRI is more sensitive for underlying bone marrow abnormalities and soft-tissue lesions. MRI may be necessary to distinguish between insufficiency and pathologic fractures when the diagnosis is unclear. Considered the "gold standard" for assessing spinal metastatic disease, MRI should be obtained emergently with any concern for spinal cord compression.
- Laboratory tests should include a complete blood cell count, metabolic panel, and hepatic function tests. Anemia in combination with renal failure or elevated protein may point toward a diagnosis of multiple myeloma. Hypercalcemia is another finding frequently associated with malignancy and metastatic bone lesions. Note, however, that osteoblastic metastases, such as can occur with prostate cancer, may result in severe hypocalcemia. Additional laboratory tests, such as markers of inflammation (erythrocyte sedimentation rate or C-reactive protein) or tumor markers may be sent when indicated.

Management

- In the ED, treatment efforts should focus on providing adequate analgesia. Opioids tend to be first-line for cancer-related pain, although several studies have shown nonsteroidal antiinflammatory drugs to be particularly effective for short-term relief of metastatic bone pain.
- Adjuvants for treatment of metastatic bone disease include steroids and bisphosphonates. Certain types of malignancies may also respond to targeted hormonal and biological drug therapies, such as tamoxifen for breast cancer, antiandrogens for prostate cancer, and sunitinib in renal cell carcinoma. These medications should be initiated by a specialist.
- Used to provide symptomatic relief for bone metastases, palliative radiotherapy is the standard treatment for uncomplicated, painful bone metastases not associated with a pathologic fracture.
- Impending or complete pathologic fracture may require operative repair or reconstruction to stabilize the lesion. Pathologic long bone fractures may be stabilized by fixation with an intermedullary nail and bone cement or excised and reconstructed with a prosthesis. Vertebroplasty or kyphoplasty may be indicated for management of vertebral compression fractures.

Pediatrics

General Principles

- Pathologic fractures in children can be caused by a wide range of disorders that cause abnormal bone structure, including genetic disease, metabolic abnormalities, infection, neuromuscular disorders, and tumors.
- In children, most pathologic fractures are owing to benign tumors, although malignancy must be ruled out. Osteosarcoma is the most common primary bone malignancy, although systemic hematologic malignancies, such as leukemia, can also affect the bone. Pathologic fracture was reported as the initial presenting symptom

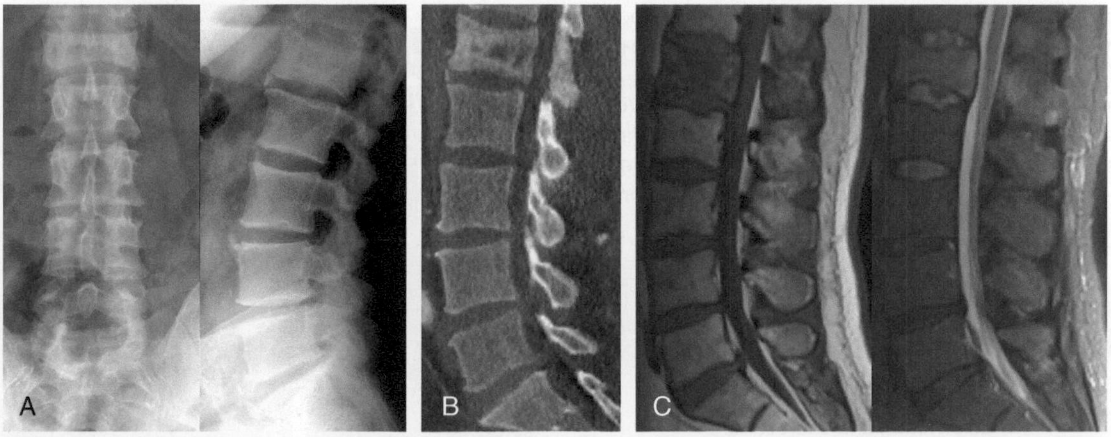

FIG. 69.2 Patient status post road traffic accident with concern for pathologic fracture on plain radiograph. A, Anteroposterior and lateral radiographs demonstrating a biconcave wedge of L1 with sclerotic appearances, lucent center, and thickened cortices suggestive of pagetic change. **B,** Computed tomography reconstruction better demonstrates these characteristic appearances. **C,** T1 (*left*) and Short-TI Inversion Recovery (STIR) (*right*) sagittal images are less specific for the bone pathology, but demonstrate retained marrow fat and acute edema changes further reassuring against a marrow infiltration pathology. (From Woo, T., Tyrrell, P. N. M., Leone, A., Cafarelli, F. P., Guglielmi, G., & Cassar-Pullicino, V. (2019). Radiographic/MR imaging correlation of spinal bony outlines. *Magnetic Resonance Imaging Clinics of North America, 27*(4), 625–640, Fig. 1.)

in 5%–12% of all patients with childhood acute lymphoblastic leukemia.

- Abnormal bone mineralization resulting in an increased risk of fracture in the skeletally immature, Rickets may occur due to congenital and acquired metabolic disorders that cause deficiency or impaired function or vitamin D, calcium, and/or phosphate.
- Neuromuscular diseases, such as cerebral palsy, are associated with an increased fracture risk owing to low bone density subsequent to chronic immobilization.
- As pathologic fractures typically present to the ED and may the first sign of serious underlying disease, appropriate recognition is critical.

Clinical Presentation

Disorders of Bone Mineralization

- Osteogenesis imperfecta (OI) is a heterogenous group of disorders characterized by abnormal collagen synthesis resulting in "brittle bones" with an increased risk of fracture. There are now eight recognized subtypes that vary in inheritance, severity, and clinical features (Table 69.2).
- Fibrous dysplasia (FD) is a benign disease in which normal bone is replaced by fibrous tissue. It can be focal (monostotic) or diffuse (polystotic) and can occur in isolation or as part of a syndrome. In McCune-Albright syndrome, for example, FD occurs with endocrine abnormalities. Clinical manifestations can vary. Radiographically, FD results in a well-circumscribed area of radiolucency surrounded by reactive bone, described as a "ground glass opacity."
- Rickets, which causes defective bone mineralization and increases the risk of fracture most prominetly affects areas of rapid growth, such as the distal femur, proximal tibia, distal radius and ulna, proximal humerus, and anterior ribs (Box 69.2).
- Radiographically, rickets is characterized by widening and bowing of the growth plate, frayed or fractured metaphysis, and beading at the costochondral junction ("rachictic rosary"). Common causes include:
  - Nutritional rickets can result from deficiencies of vitamin D, calcium, or phosphorus from either poor dietary intake, inadequate sun exposure, or malabsorption. Although more common in developing countries, it can occur in infants who are exclusively breast-fed without vitamin D supplementation. Dark skin is a risk factor because larger concentrations of the pigment melanin impair the skin's ability to produce vitamin D from sunlight. Laboratory studies will show low to normal serum calcium, low phosphorus, increased parathyroid hormone, and low vitamin D levels.
  - Familial hypophosphatemic rickets (also known as vitamin D–resistant rickets), an X-linked disorder, is the most common cause of heritable rickets. A mutation in the phosphate-regulating gene results in renal wasting of phosphorus and subsequent hypophosphatemia.
  - Hereditary vitamin D–dependent rickets is caused by a mutation resulting in an inability to convert vitamin D to its active form or a defect in the vitamin D intracellular receptor (type I and II, respectively).

TABLE 69.2 Clinical Features of Osteogenesis Imperfecta

Skeletal	Numerous and atypical fractures during childhood, long bone and vertebral deformities, and short stature
Extraskeletal	Hearing loss, abnormal dentition, joint hypermobility and recurrent dislocations
Cardiovascular	Aortic root dilation, mitral valve prolapse
Neurologic	Macrocephaly, hydrocephalus, basilar invagination

BOX 69.2 Clinical Features of Rickets

- Short stature
- Long-bone deformity (bowing)
- Skeletal kyphosis
- Frontal bossing
- Open anterior fontanelle
- Developmental delay

Note: Infants less than 6 months may present with hypocalcemic tetany or seizures.

Benign Bone Lesions

- Unicameral bone cysts, a benign osteolytic lesion centered in the metaphysis and diaphysis of long bones, are the most common cause of pathologic fracture in children (Fig. 69.3). Fractures most commonly occur in the proximal humerus followed by the proximal femur.
- Aneurysmal bone cysts are responsible for one-third of pathologic fractures and are typically found in the femur, tibia, fibula, humerus, and spine (Fig. 69.4). They can mimic malignant lesion because they are locally aggressive and result in periosteal destruction.

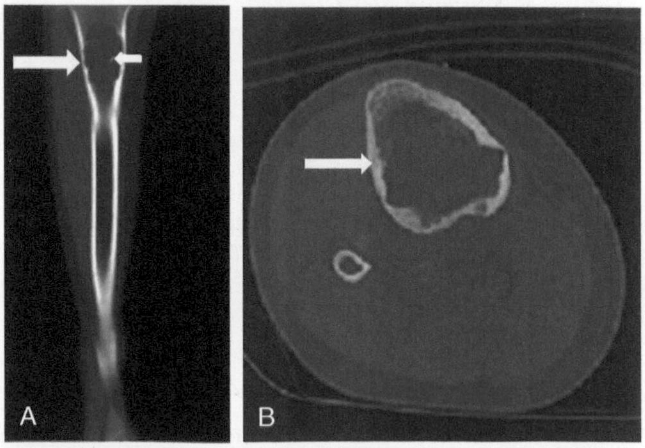

FIG. 69.3 A 12-year-old girl with unicameral bone cyst of tibia. Coronal (**A**) and axial (**B**) computed tomography images show expansile lytic lesion (*long arrow*) containing septa (*small arrow*). (From Noordin, S., Allana, S., Umer, M., Jamil, M., Hilal, K., & Uddin, N. (2018). Unicameral bone cysts: Current concepts. *Annals of Medicine and Surgery, 34*, 43–49, Fig. 2.)

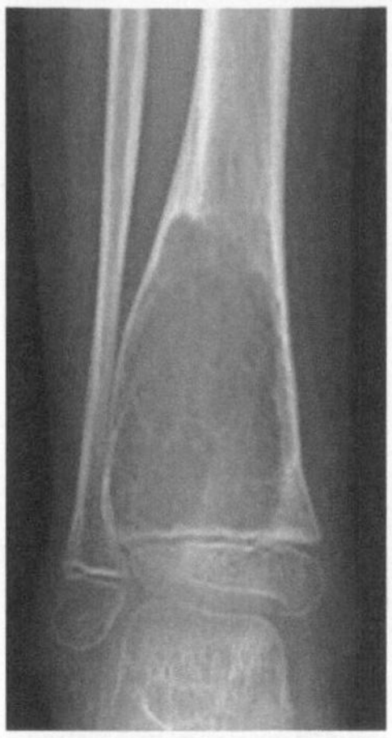

FIG. 69.4 Radiograph of aneurysmal bone cyst. (From Rosenberg, A. E., Nielsen, G. P., Krishnasetty, V., & Rosenthal, D. I. (2007). Disorders of the skeletal system including tumors. In E. Gilbert-Barness (Ed.), *Potter's pathology of the fetus, infant and child* (2nd ed., pp. 1797–1835, Fig. 34.1.4). Mosby.)

- Nonossifying fibromas are common, benign focal lesions that are typically asymptomatic. Although most often discovered by chance, they can be associated with a pathologic fracture. It is characterized by an osteolytic, lobular lesion in the metaphysis of long bones, most commonly the distal femur (Fig. 69.5).

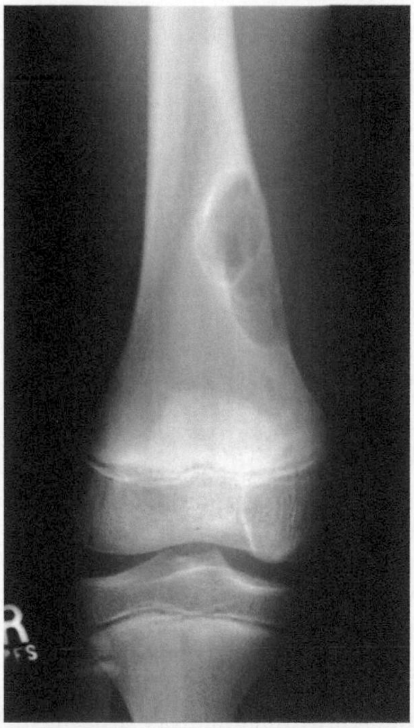

FIG. 69.5 Anteroposterior and lateral radiograph of nonossifying fibroma, consisting of a metaphyseal, circumscribed radiolucency with a sclerotic rim. The lesion is eccentric and ovoid with a long axis parallel to the long axis of the bone. (From Horvai, A., & Link, T. Nonossifying fibroma. High-yield bone and soft tissue pathology. In *Elsevier Point of Care*. 2012. 147–148, Fig. 1.)

Diagnosis and Evaluation

- A thorough history should be obtained. Key historical elements to obtain include events surrounding the fracture (i.e., trauma) as well as any history of preceding pain, associated systemic symptoms, or prior fractures. Family history of relevant disease should be elucidated and the child's nutrition and feeding practices assessed.
- On physical examination, in addition to examination of the fracture site itself, one should look for physical signs that may indicate an underlying chronic genetic or metabolic/nutritional disorder. Such signs include skeletal and limb deformities, short stature, joint hypermobility, blue or gray sclera (OI), abnormal dentition, and forehead bossing. Skin should be examined for pallor, bruising, or petechiae, which may indicate underlying hematologic abnormality.
- Laboratory evaluation should include a complete metabolic panel, with specific attention paid to calcium and phosphorus levels. Other tests to evaluate for metabolic bone disease, such as urinary calcium, vitamin D levels, or parathyroid hormone levels, can be done as an outpatient. A complete blood count should be performed to evaluate for evidence of infection or hematologic malignancy.
- X-rays are typically the first-line imaging test performed in the ED. Advanced imaging, including CT scan and MRI, may be indicated, depending on the fracture lesion.

Treatment

- Treatment should be centered on analgesia, appropriate management of the fracture, and reversal of the underlying cause.
- Fractures should be managed with casting or surgical fixation, depending on the specific fracture.
- Underlying nutritional or metabolic disorders must be corrected to ensure optimal bone healing and to prevent additional fractures. This can most commonly be accomplished by supplementation of vitamin D, calcium, and/or phosphorus.

SUGGESTED READINGS

Canavese, F., Samba, A., & Rousset, M. (2016). Pathological fractures in children: Diagnosis and treatment options. *Orthopaedics & Traumatology, Surgery & Research, 102*(1), S149–S159.

Chang, C. Y., Rosenthal, D. I., Mitchell, D. M., Handa, A., Kattapuram, S. V., & Huang, A. J. (2016). Imaging findings of metabolic bone disease. *Radiographics, 36*, 1871–1887.

Dionyssiotis, Y. (2010). Management of osteoporotic vertebral fractures. *International Journal of General Medicine, 3*, 167–171.

McCarthy, J., & Davis, A. (2016). Diagnosis and management of vertebral compression fractures. *American Family Physician, 94*(1), 44–50.

Stankovits, L. M., & Lopyan, A. H. (2019). Genetic and metabolic conditions. *Pediatric Clinics of North America, 67*(1), 23–43.

Disorders of the Spine

OMID ADIBNAZARI, MD, BS, and DAVID TANEN, MD

Disorders of the spine can range from simple pain syndromes requiring minimal intervention to life-threatening infections or conditions requiring emergent surgical intervention. They can be classified based on the portion of the spine affected, whether this is regional or pertaining to specific structures. Because back pain is one of the most common emergency department complaints, and most back pain will improve without intervention within several weeks, attention must be paid to ensure that red flags for emergent causes of spinal pathology are not missed.

Disc Disorders

Basic Information

- Intervertebral discs lie between vertebrae in the spinal column and form fibrocartilaginous joints.
- Discs are composed of an outer fibrous ring, the anulus fibrosus, and an inner gel-like center, the nucleus pulposus.
  - Disc herniation occurs when unbalanced mechanical pressure causes deformation of the anulus fibrosus.
  - Degenerative disc disease occurs over time from loading and from age-related dehydration and decreased load-bearing ability of discs.
- Discitis is infection of an intervertebral disc, most commonly caused by *Staphylococcus aureus* via hematogenous seeding.

Clinical Presentation

- Back pain at level of disc disease, with associated symptoms and signs depending on disorder
  - Positive straight leg raise and crossed straight leg raise may be seen with disc herniation causing sciatica.
  - Cord compression (or cauda equina syndrome) or spinal nerve root compression symptoms may suggest intrusion into the spinal canal or neural foramina from disc herniation.
    - Most sensitive finding is urinary retention (increased postvoid residual)
    - May also have saddle anesthesia, lower extremity paresthesia or weakness, or fecal incontinence
  - History of intravenous drug use, bacteremia, endocarditis, fever, and sepsis may be found in discitis.

Diagnosis and Evaluation

- Disc herniation is generally a clinical diagnosis in the emergency department unless cord compression symptoms or signs are present, when emergent magnetic resonance imaging (MRI) is indicated.
- Discitis may be visualized with good sensitivity on contrast-enhanced computed tomography (CT), or with MRI if available.
  - Elevated erythrocyte sedimentation rate or C-reactive protein may be seen in discitis.

Treatment

- Disc herniation and degenerative disc disease can generally be managed conservatively with pain control, activity modification, and outpatient physical therapy.
  - Disc herniation with cord compression or cauda equina syndrome requires emergent neurosurgery consultation; may consider intravenous glucocorticoids.
- Discitis requires a prolonged antibiotic course and may require surgical intervention if complications arise (e.g., abscess).

Inflammatory Spondylopathies

Basic Information

- Inflammation of the spinal column may be caused by a variety of disorders.
  - Ankylosing spondylitis is the characteristic condition.
    - Associated with HLA-B27 antigen in 90% of patients
  - Can also be caused by postinfectious reactive arthritis, psoriatic arthritis, rheumatoid arthritis, and arthropathy of inflammatory bowel disease

Clinical Presentation

- Generally marked by insidious onset of back pain and stiffness of the vertebral column
  - Ankylosing spondylitis presents classically with morning back stiffness that improves with exercise.

Diagnosis and Evaluation

- Radiographs may show squaring of vertebral bodies; late classic finding is "bamboo spine," with bony bridging between vertebral bodies.
- MRI changes may be seen in the sacroiliac joint early in the disease course.

Treatment

- Nonsteroidal antiinflammatory drugs (NSAIDs), outpatient physical therapy, and rheumatology follow-up
- In consultation with rheumatology, patients may require antirheumatic drugs for severe symptoms.

Spinal Stenosis

Basic Information

- Abnormal narrowing of the spinal canal or neural foramina causing pressure on cord or nerve roots

BOX 70.1 Causes of Spinal Stenosis

Degenerative (Aging)
Spinal ligament thickening
Osteophytic changes
Disc herniation
Degenerative disc disease
Compression fractures
Facet joint breakdown

Arthritis
Osteoarthritis
Rheumatoid arthritis

Miscellaneous
Trauma: burst fractures or spondylolisthesis
Congenital narrowing of spinal canal
Tumors

- Numerous causes (Box 70.1), most commonly caused by degenerative changes of spine

Clinical Presentation

- Neck or back pain, generally worsened with prolonged standing and spinal extension
- Paresthesia and weakness if nerve root compression, generally in upper extremities with cervical spinal stenosis and in lower extremities with lumbar spinal stenosis
  - Pain often improved with spinal flexion (walking uphill, leaning forward) because it increases the diameter of the spinal canal and neural foramina

Diagnosis and Evaluation

- Clinical diagnosis in the emergency department
- Consider MRI if symptoms are more acute and patients have neurologic deficits.

Treatment

- Pain control (NSAIDS, acetaminophen), strengthening exercises, physical therapy
- May require eventual surgical management for severe symptoms

Back and Neck Pain

Basic Information

- Back and neck pain are among the most common emergency department complaints.
- Most common etiology is muscle strain
- Must screen for red flag symptoms and signs (Box 70.2)
- Sacroiliitis, inflammation of the sacroiliac joint, is a commonly overlooked cause of back and buttock pain. Commonly an early finding in ankylosing spondylitis

Clinical Presentation

- Back or neck pain, with additional findings depending on cause
  - Mechanical injury usually associated with movement, lifting, or a prolonged posture
  - Sciatica usually associated with pain, numbness, weakness along the sciatic nerve, with a positive straight leg or crossed straight leg sign

BOX 70.2 Red Flag History and Physical Findings Associated With Back or Neck Pain

CONCERNING FOR INFECTION	CONCERNING FOR CORD COMPRESSION/CES
Fever or evidence of sepsis	Numbness or paresthesia
History of intravenous drug use	Weakness
History of bacteremia or endocarditis	Urinary retention or incontinence (overflow)
Immunocompromised state	Fecal incontinence
Recent gastrointestinal or genitourinary procedure	Malignancy
Weight loss	Severe or rapidly progressive neurologic deficit

CES, cauda equina syndrome.

  - Infectious etiologies such as spinal osteomyelitis, spinal epidural abscess, pyogenic sacroiliitis, and discitis may have associated fever, weight loss, sepsis, and midline spinal tenderness.
  - Spinal cord or nerve compression may have associated urinary or bowel symptoms, or radicular symptoms, such as numbness or weakness at or below the affected level.

Diagnosis and Evaluation

- Mechanical back pain with no red flag features requires no additional emergency department workup.
- Infectious and compressive lesions require additional workup, primarily imaging.
  - Infectious etiologies may have elevations in erythrocyte sedimentation rate or C-reactive protein.
  - Discitis may be seen on contrast-enhanced CT, but other suspected infectious spinal pathologies are best seen with contrast-enhanced MRI.
  - Compressive lesions can be visualized with noncontrast MRI.

Treatment

- Mechanical back pain may be treated with conservative measures, although none have been shown to significantly improve duration of symptoms.
  - NSAIDs, heat therapy, strengthening exercises, physical therapy
- Infectious and compressive etiologies generally require admission for antibiotics and neurosurgical consultation.

SUGGESTED READINGS

Corwell, B. N. (2018). Back pain. In R. M. Walls, R. S. Hockberger, & M. Gausche-Hill (Eds.), *Rosen's emergency medicine: Concepts and clinical practice* (9th ed., pp. 275–284). Elsevier.
Sudhir, A., & Perina, D. (2018). Musculoskeletal back pain. In R. M. Walls, R. S. Hockberger, & M. Gausche-Hill (Eds.), *Rosen's emergency medicine: Concepts and clinical practice* (9th ed., pp. 569–576), Elsevier.

CHAPTER **71**

BOARD REVIEW

Arthropathies

KATHLEEN YIP, MD, and MANPREET SINGH, MD, MBE

Triggered by trauma, infection, or inflammation associated with autoimmune disease, arthritis can develop over hours to years. Tissue destruction can occur through fast-acting catabolic pathways or long-term changes to the composition of the cartilage. Arthritis can be classified as either monoarticular or polyarticular, and acute (less than 6 weeks) or chronic (more than 6 weeks).

Basic Information

Anatomy

- A synovial joint joins the two ends of bone with a fibrous joint capsule lined with a synovial membrane (Fig. 71.1).
- The synovial joint cavity is filled with lubricating synovial fluid, which, along with the articular cartilage, provides nearly frictionless movement.
- The synovium is highly vascular; as a result, infections rapidly spread.

Clinical Presentation

Principles of Arthritis

- True arthritis causes generalized joint pain, warmth, swelling, and tenderness; all parts of the joint are involved.
- Periarticular inflammation (e.g., bursitis, tendinitis) causes focal pain.
- Determining whether the arthritis is monoarticular or polyarticular and acute or chronic is helpful with diagnosis.

Acute Monoarticular Arthritis

- Septic (nongonococcal) arthritis
  - Most common in children younger than 3 and adults over age 55
  - The Kocher criteria demonstrate increasing probability of pediatric septic arthritis with more signs, symptoms, or laboratory abnormalities of the following:
    - Non–weight-bearing on the affected side
    - Erythrocyte sedimentation rate (ESR) more than 40 mm/hr
    - Fever
    - White blood cell (WBC) count greater than 12,000
  - Risk factors include intravenous (IV) drug use, immunocompromise (e.g., chronic alcoholism, human immunodeficiency virus, diabetes), chronic arthritis (e.g., rheumatoid, crystalline or osteoarthritis), and prosthetic implants.
  - Most often occurs through hematogenous spread. However, direct inoculation or contiguous spread from bone or soft tissue is also possible.
  - Most commonly caused by *Staphylococcus aureus* and, increasingly, the methicillin-resistant strains
  - Symptoms include fever, joint pain, and effusion, especially of the knee.
- Gonococcal arthritis
  - More commonly diagnosed in females as most genital gonococcal infections in women are asymptomatic.
  - Usually a localized septic arthritis with modest effusions
  - Disseminated gonococcal infection manifests with bacteremia, migratory arthralgia, tenosynovitis, and characteristic skin lesions (Fig. 71.2).
- Crystal arthropathies
  - Gout
    - Risk factors include obesity, hypertension, diabetes, and thiazide use.
    - Flares are brought on by excess alcohol, stressors, trauma, surgery, and diets containing meat.
    - Acute precipitation of uric acid in the joint from supersaturated extracellular fluid
    - Most commonly occurs in the great toe (metatarsophalangeal joint)
  - Calcium pyrophosphate dihydrate deposition disease (pseudogout)
    - Deposition of calcium complex crystals on articular surfaces
    - Clinical presentation is similar to gout and may mimic septic arthritis.
    - More commonly occurs in the elderly (age more than 65 years) and in the knee

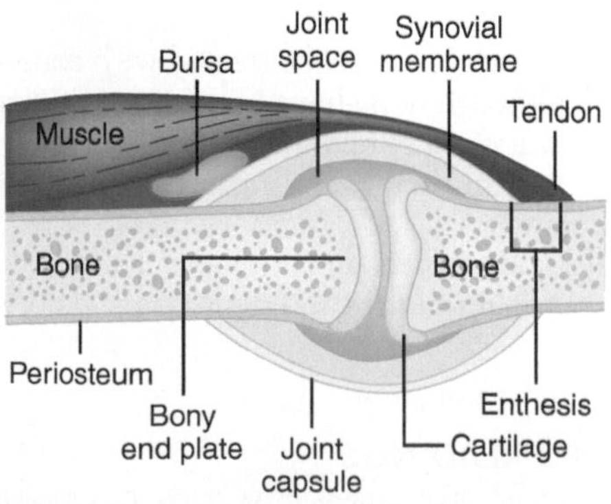

FIG. 71.1 Anatomy of the joint. (Reprinted from Genes, N. (2018). Arthritis. In R. M. Walls, R. S. Hockberger, & M. Gausche-Hill (Eds.), *Rosen's emergency medicine: Concepts and clinical practice* (9th ed., pp. 1375–1391, Fig. 106.1). Elsevier.

Chronic Monoarticular Arthritis: Osteoarthritis (Degenerative Joint Disease)

- Commonly involves the knees in the lower extremities
- In the upper extremities, involvement of the proximal interphalangeal joints and the distal interphalangeal

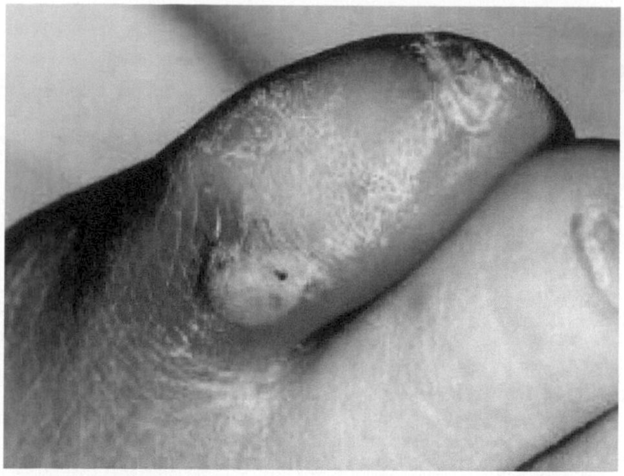

FIG. 71.2 **Pustular skin lesion of disseminated gonorrhea.** (Reprinted from Genes, N. (2018). Arthritis. In R. M. Walls, R. S. Hockberger, & M. Gausche-Hill (Eds.), *Rosen's emergency medicine: Concepts and clinical practice* (9th ed., pp. 1375–1391, Fig. 106.3). Elsevier.

joints of the hands will manifest as Bouchard's and Heberden's nodes, respectively.
- Pain worsens with activity and improves with rest.
- Lacks systemic signs, such as fever
- May display crepitus on active and passive ranging

Slipped Capital Femoral Epiphysis
- Most commonly seen in adolescent boys. Up to half of cases occur bilaterally.
- Presents with discomfort in the groin, ipsilateral thigh, or knee after activity that progresses to pain at rest
- Obtain anteroposterior, lateral, and frog leg views of both hips (Fig. 71.3).

Toxic (Transient) Synovitis
- Nonbacterial inflammatory clinical entity that can cause a limp
- Presents with pain in the hip or knee with an antalgic gait, but minimal systemic symptoms
- Patients are nontoxic appearing.
- Typically presents in boys between 3 and 10 years of age and after resolution of a viral upper respiratory infection
- Must exclude the diagnosis of septic arthritis

Diagnosis and Evaluation
- Blood tests
  - Erythrocyte sedimentation rate, C-reactive protein, WBC count, and serum uric acid are of limited diagnostic value.
  - Blood cultures will be positive in 25%–50% of cases of septic arthritis.
  - Cervical, urethral, rectal, and pharyngeal cultures are positive in 75% of cases of gonococcal arthritis, but blood or synovial cultures are positive in only 10%–50% of cases.
- Radiologic tests
  - Plain radiographs may be helpful in evaluating chronic disease and joint space narrowing, especially in the lower extremities.
  - Ultrasound is useful for evaluating joint effusions and guiding arthrocentesis.
  - Magnetic resonance imaging is more sensitive than plain films for early osteomyelitis.

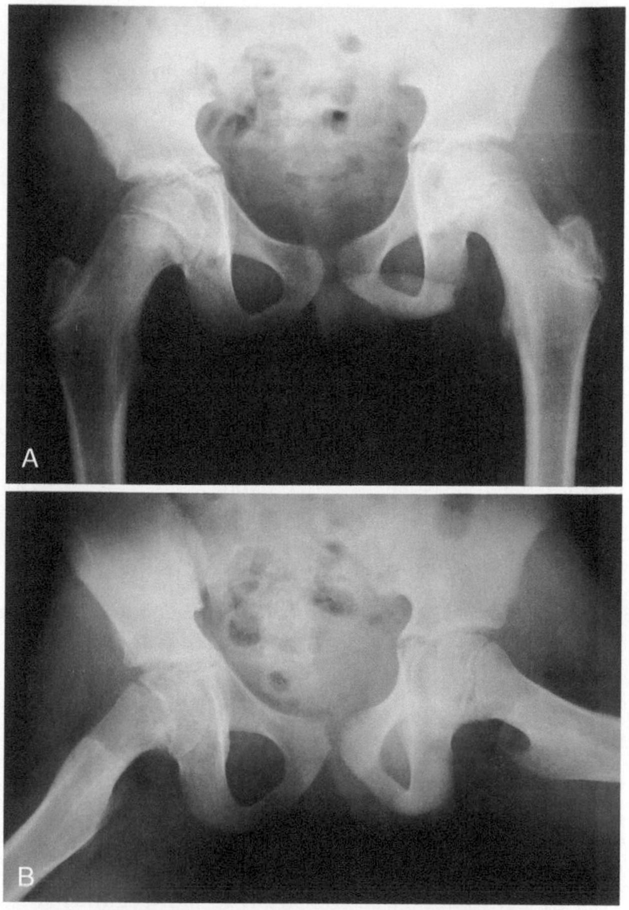

FIG. 71.3 **Radiographic evidence of slipped capital femoral epiphysis.** (Reprinted from McQuillen, K. K. (2018). Musculoskeletal disorders. In R. M. Walls, R. S. Hockberger, & M. Gausche-Hill (Eds.), *Rosen's emergency medicine: Concepts and clinical practice* (9th ed., pp. 2201–2217, Fig. 175.25). Elsevier.)

- Arthrocentesis
  - Synovial fluid analysis is critical in diagnosing septic arthritis versus other causes of joint disease (Table 71.1).
  - Used diagnostically to evaluate joint fluid and traumatic arthrotomy
  - Used as a treatment modality to drain traumatic hemarthroses or instill antiinflammatory agents for analgesia
  - Also recommended in patients with an established diagnosis of arthritis who present with fever and new joint pain or effusion
  - Relatively contraindicated in overlying cellulitis and severe coagulopathy (international normalized ratio above 4.5)
  - An orthopedic surgeon should be consulted before performing a prosthetic joint arthrocentesis.

Treatment
Acute Monoarticular Arthritis
- Septic arthritis
  - Empiric: intravenous antibiotics should be administered if septic arthritis is presumed or if synovial fluid Gram stain is positive.
    - For gram-positive organisms, vancomycin should be administered owing to high rates of methicillin-resistant *Staphylococcus aureus*.

TABLE 71.1 Synovial Fluid Interpretation

Synovium	Normal	Noninflammatory	Inflammatory	Septic
Clarity	Transparent	Transparent	Cloudy	Cloudy, purulent
Color	Clear	Yellow	Yellow	Yellow
Synovial WBC (per mm^3)	< 200	< 200–2000	200–50,000	> 1100 (prosthetic joint) > 25,000; LR=2.9 > 50,000; LR=7.7 > 100,000; LR=28
Synovial PMN	< 25%	< 25%	> 50%	> 64% (prosthetic joint) > 90%
Culture	Negative	Negative	Negative	> 50% positive
Lactate	< 5.6 mmol/L	< 5.6 mmol/L	< 5.6 mmol/L	> 5.6 mmol/L LR > 2.4 to infinity
LDH	< 250 U/L	< 250 U/L	< 250 U/L	> 250 U/L
Crystals	None	None	Gout: needle-shaped with negative birefringence Pseudogout: polymorphic, rhomboid and positively birefringent	None

WBC, white blood cell; *PMN*, polymorphonuclear neutrophils; *LDH*, lactate dehydrogenase; *LR*, likelihood ratio.

    - For gram-negative organisms, a third-generation cephalosporin should be used.
  - Admission is indicated for IV antibiotics and orthopedic washout of the joint.
- Gonococcal arthritis
  - Hospitalization and treatment with intramuscular or IV ceftriaxone and transition to oral cefixime is recommended by the Centers for Disease Control and Prevention.
- Crystal arthropathies (gout and pseudogout)
  - Treatment includes nonsteroidal antiinflammatory drugs (NSAIDs), colchicine, and steroids (either intraarticular steroids once septic arthritis has been ruled out, or oral prednisone).
  - Prophylactic medications, such as allopurinol, febuxostat, and probenecid, should not be stopped or initiated during an acute attack.

Chronic Monoarticular Arthritis (Osteoarthritis)

- Weight loss is one of the mainstays of treatment, especially if the patient is overweight.
- Acetaminophen is considered first-line for pain management; NSAIDs and opioids may be helpful, but have more adverse side effects.

Slipped Capital Femoral Epiphysis

- Patient should be placed on a non–weight-bearing status upon diagnosis.
- Urgent orthopedic surgery consultation
- Admission is required for surgical fixation.
- Complications of delayed diagnosis include avascular necrosis and chondrolysis.

Toxic (Transient) Synovitis

- NSAIDs and return to activity, as tolerated

SUGGESTED READINGS

Genes, N., & Adams, B. D. (2014). Arthritis. In J. A. Marx, R. S. Hockberger, & R. M. Walls (Eds.), *Rosen's emergency medicine: Concepts and clinical practice* (8th ed., pp. 1501–1517). Elsevier.

Genes, N., & Chisolm-Straker, M. (2012). Monoarticular arthritis update: Current evidence for diagnosis and treatment in the emergency department. *Emergency Medicine Practice*, *14*(5), 1–20.

Joint Disorders

SHEETAL KHIYANI, MD

Diseases of the joint can be debilitating, with arthritis being the best known as discussed in the prior chapter. However, many other entities can lead to chronic agonizing pain or a relentless nagging pain that is uncomfortable for the patient.

Legg-Calve-Perthes Disease

Overview

- Rare disorder of childhood, affecting the hip joint
- Blood supply to the femoral head is disrupted, causing avascular necrosis.
- Mostly unilateral presentation, but can be bilateral in 10% of patients
- Boys affected more than girls (4:1), but more severe in girls as compared with boys
- Age of presentation, 4 to 10 years, peak incidence at 5 to 7 years

Pathophysiology

- Continuum of disease process from avascular necrosis of bone to regrowth and reossification
- Etiology is unknown
- Potential risk factors include low birthweight, delayed skeletal maturity, obesity, trauma, adverse social and economic conditions, exposure to tobacco smoke, or a positive family history of the disorder (10% familial).

Clinical Presentation

- Painless, intermittent limp in the initial stages
- Hip pain or referred pain to knee, thigh
- Antalgic gait with limited range of motion, especially internal rotation and abduction

Diagnosis

- Detailed patient history
- Thorough clinical examination: limited internal rotation and abduction
- Imaging: radiographs in anteroposterior (AP) and frog-leg lateral views of pelvis (Fig. 72.1)

Treatment

- Directed toward specific symptoms and depends on patient's age, damage to femoral head, stage of disease at time of diagnosis
- Nonsurgical treatment options
  - Observation: if young at presentation (2 to 6 years) and few changes in femoral head on imaging

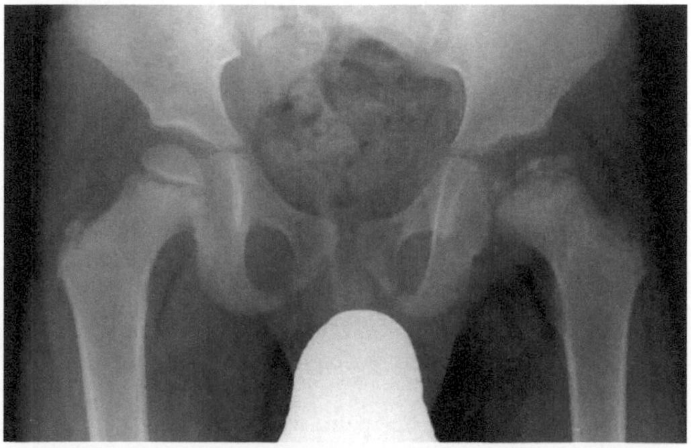

FIG. 72.1 X-ray shows collapsed femoral head (*arrow*) on left side compared with the normal right side. (From Creative Commons: https://en.wikipedia.org/wiki/Legg%E2%80%93Calv%C3%A9%E2%80%93Perthes_disease#/media/File:Roe-perthes.jpg.)

  - Antiinflammatory medications: reduce pain and inflammation
  - Limiting activity: avoid high-impact activities, such as running, jumping. Use crutches or walker to avoid weight bearing on the joint.
  - Physical therapy exercises: focus on hip abduction and internal rotation.
  - Casting and bracing: femoral head deformity may need a cast (Petrie cast) or brace to keep it in its position within the acetabulum.
- Surgery (osteotomy) indicated when child is older (more than 8 years) at presentation; femoral head deformity; or conservative measures have failed.

Prognosis

- Long-term prognosis is good, except in cases of significant femoral head deformity, in which case early development of osteoarthritis is likely.

Slipped Capital Femoral Epiphysis (SCFE)

Overview

- Epiphysis, or head of the femur, slips down and backward off the neck of the femur at the growth plate.
- Presents during periods of rapid growth: in boys, between the ages of 12 and 16; in girls, between the ages of 10 and 14
- Mostly unilateral presentation (left-sided preference), but can be bilateral in 20%–40%, usually within 18 months

Types of SCFE

- **Stable SCFE:** the patient is able to walk or bear weight on the affected hip, either with or without crutches. Most cases of SCFE are stable slips.
- **Unstable SCFE**: a more severe slip; the patient cannot walk or bear weight, even with crutches. Unstable SCFE requires urgent treatment. Complications associated with SCFE are much more common in patients with unstable slips.

Etiology

- Cause is unknown, but certain risk factors increase the likelihood.
  - Overweight (BMI 25–30) or obesity (BMI >30)
  - An endocrine or metabolic disorder, such as hypothyroidism, diabetes, growth hormone deficiency
  - Kidney disease leading to bone disorders
  - Radiation and chemotherapy
  - Medications (such as steroids)
  - Family history of SCFE

Clinical Presentation

- Chronic SCFE in which symptoms are present for weeks to months before diagnosis is the most common presentation.
- Hip, groin, thigh, knee pain: worse after activity, relieved with rest
- Inability to walk or bear weight on the affected limb
- Antalgic gait
- Limb length discrepancy
- External rotation of the affected foot

Diagnosis

- Detailed patient history
- Thorough clinical examination: obligate external rotation (Drehmann sign); internal rotation is painful and limited.

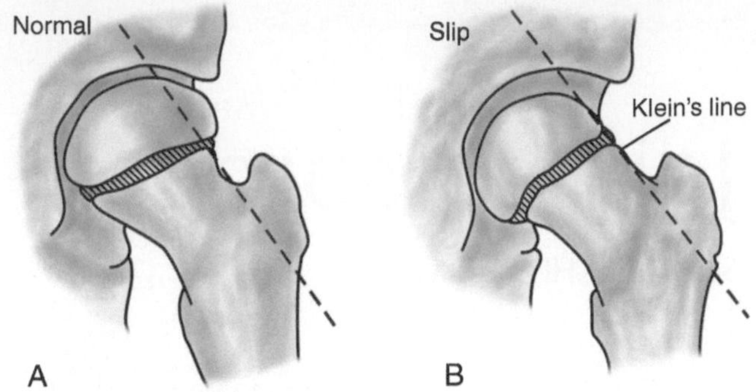

FIG. 72.2 Normal situation of Kline's line in (**A**) compared with (**B**) with a slip when the epiphysis is out of alignment. (From Hubbard, E. W. (2020). School age. In M. D. Miller, J. A. Ahrt, & J. M. MacKnight (Eds.), *Essential orthopaedics* (2nd ed., p. 843, Fig. 213.4). Elsevier.)

- Imaging: anteroposterior and frog-leg lateral views on radiology. Findings on AP view:
  - Klein's line (Figs. 72.2 and 72.3): line drawn along superior border of femoral neck should intersect femoral head; evaluate for asymmetry between two sides.
  - Epiphysiolysis: growth plate widening or lucency
  - Steel sign: a double density at the metaphysis (caused by the posterior lip of the epiphysis being superimposed on the metaphysis).
- Magnetic resonance imaging (MRI) is indicated in preslip condition (MRI will demonstrate widening of the physis with surrounding edema).
- A mild slip involves epiphysis displacement less than one-third of the width of the metaphysis; a moderate slip involves displacement between one-third and one-half of the width; and a severe slip involves displacement greater than one-half of the width.

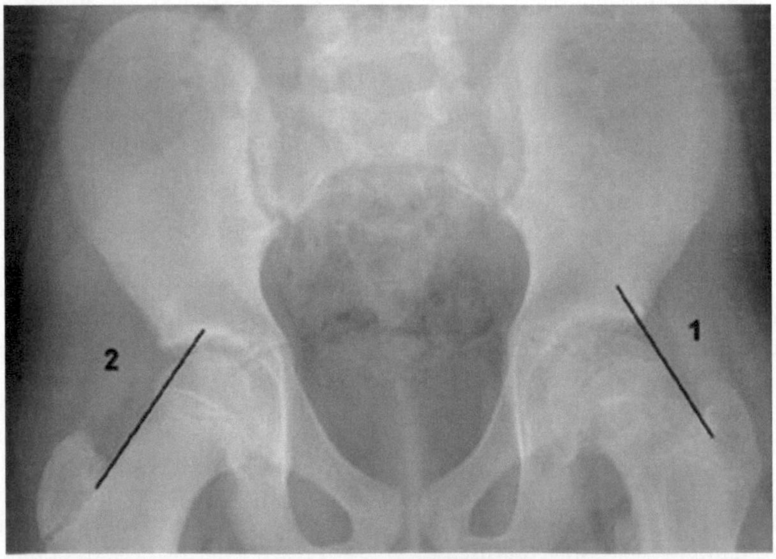

FIG. 72.3 Approximating Klein's line for slipped capital femoral epiphysis on frog-leg x-ray of left SCFE. Klein's line—drawn along the superior aspect of the femoral neck—should intersect a portion of the femoral head as seen on the patient's right hip with *line 2*). *Line 1* on the patient's left hip does not intersect the femoral head and is consistent with SCFE. (From Connolly, B., Krishnamurthy, G., & Manji, A. (2010). Diagnostic imaging and interventional radiology. In A. I. Dipchand, J. N. Friedman, S. Gupta, Z. Bismilla, & C. Lam (Eds.), *The Hospital for Sick Children handbook of pediatrics* (11th ed., Chapter 31, Fig. 14.5). Elsevier.)

Treatment

- Admit patients with acute, unstable slips and consider admission for those with bilateral SCFE.
- After diagnosis, the patient is to be placed in non–weight-bearing crutches or wheel chair and urgently referred to orthopedics.
- Percutaneous *in situ* fixation with screw
- Open reduction and fixation

Prognosis

- Most patients with mild to moderate SCFE who are treated with *in situ* fixation have good to excellent long-term outcomes.
- Unstable SCFE is associated with complications.
  - Avascular necrosis of femoral head
  - Chondrolysis
  - Limb length discrepancy
  - Degenerative arthritis

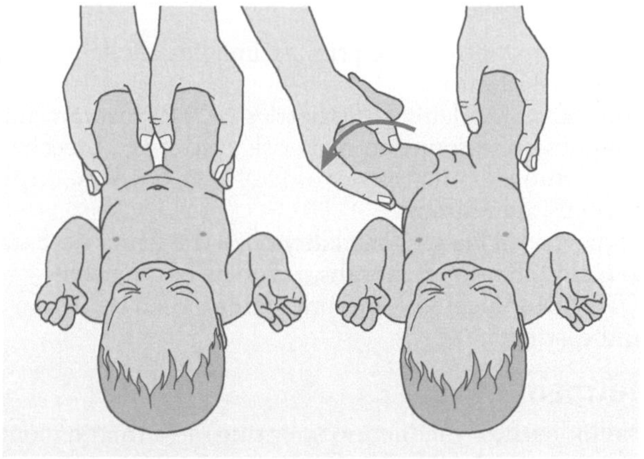

FIG. 72.4 Examination for developmental dysplasia of the hip. (From Stenson, B., & Cunningham, S. (2018). Babies and children. In K. Fairhurst, J. A. Innes, & A. R. Dover (Eds.), *Macleod's clinical examination* (14th ed., p. 297, Fig. 15.14). Elsevier.)

Developmental Dysplasia of the Hip (DDH)

Overview

- Developmental disorder of the hip owing to capsular laxity and mechanical factors
- 1 in 10 infants born with hip instability, but 1 in 500 infants born with a dislocated hip
- Spectrum of abnormal development of hip includes:
  - Subluxation: incomplete contact between the articular surface of the femoral head and the acetabulum
  - Dislocation: complete loss of contact between the articular surface of the femoral head and the acetabulum
  - Instability: ability to subluxate or dislocate the hip with passive manipulation
  - Teratologic dislocation: antenatal dislocation of the hip

Etiology

- Cause is unknown, but certain risk factors increase the likelihood.
  - More common in females (6:1)
  - Native Americans and Laplanders
  - Firstborn children
  - Babies born in the breech position
  - Family history of DDH (parents or siblings)
  - Oligohydramnios

Clinical Presentation

Infant

- DDH is frequently discovered during newborn examination, but sometimes can develop later.
- Hip clicks can be felt on examination, but are nonspecific.
- Because DDH is bilateral in up to 37%, absence of asymmetry does not exclude DDH.
- Barlow test (Fig. 72.4A): dislocates hip by depression and adduction in a flexed femur
- Ortolani test (Fig. 72.4B): reduces a dislocated hip by abduction and elevation in a flexed femur
- Galeazzi sign: patient is supine with hips and knees flexed, and limb length is shorter on side of dislocated hip (Fig. 72.5).

Older Child

- Limb length discrepancy
- Uneven skin folds on the thigh
- Limited abduction
- Limping, toe walking, or a Trendelenburg gait
- Marked swayback (lumbar lordosis)

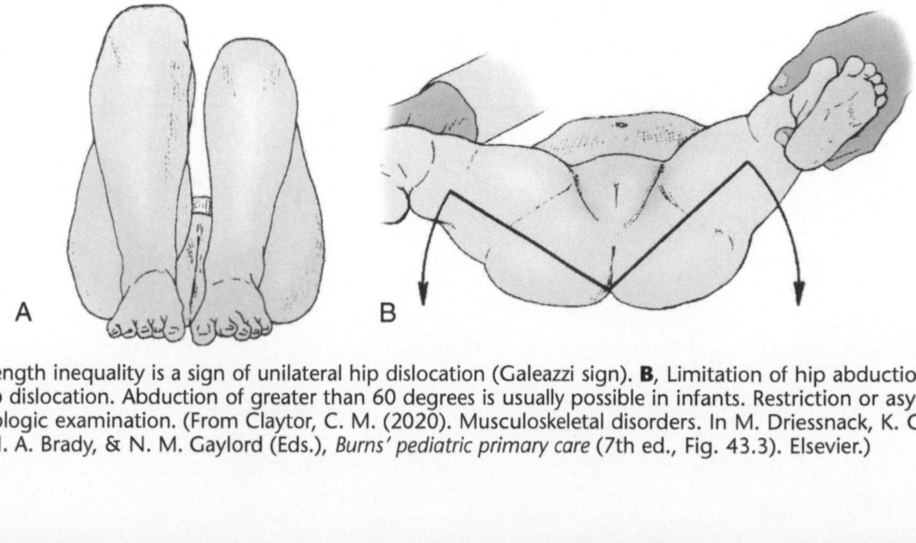

FIG. 72.5 A, Leg-length inequality is a sign of unilateral hip dislocation (Galeazzi sign). **B,** Limitation of hip abduction is often present in older infants with hip dislocation. Abduction of greater than 60 degrees is usually possible in infants. Restriction or asymmetry indicates the need for careful radiologic examination. (From Claytor, C. M. (2020). Musculoskeletal disorders. In M. Driessnack, K. G. Duderstadt, D. L. G. Maaks, N. B. Starr, M. A. Brady, & N. M. Gaylord (Eds.), *Burns' pediatric primary care* (7th ed., Fig. 43.3). Elsevier.)

72

Diagnosis

- Ultrasonography is the primary imaging modality from birth to 4 months.
- American Academy of Pediatrics (AAP) recommends screening ultrasound in high-risk cases (e.g., breech positioning, family history of DDH) at 6 weeks, despite normal examination.
- Radiographs: imaging modality once the femur head starts to ossify after 4 to 6 months, AP view of the pelvis
- CT, MRI indicated sometimes after closed reduction and casting

Treatment

- Pavlik harness (abduction splinting) less than 6 months of age and reducible hip
- Closed reduction and spica cast 6 to 18 months of age and failure of splinting
- Open reduction and osteotomy more than 2 years of age and failure of closed reduction

Prognosis

- Early diagnosis and treatment have good prognosis, whereas delay in diagnosis can lead to complications.

Complications

- Limb length discrepancy
- Delay in walking
- Avascular necrosis of the hip
- Early-onset osteoarthritis

SUGGESTED READINGS

Karkenny, A. J., Tauberg, B. M., & Otsuka, N. Y. (2018). Pediatric hip disorders: Slipped capital femoral epiphysis and Legg-Calvé-Perthes disease. *Pediatrics in Review*, 39(9), 454–463.

Kotlarsky, P., Haber, R., Bialik, V., & Eidelman. M. (2015). Developmental dysplasia of the hip: What has changed in the last 20 years? *World Journal of Orthopedics*, 6(11), 886.

Thawrani, D. P., Feldman, D. S., & Sala, D. A. (2016). Current practice in the management of slipped capital femoral epiphysis. *Journal of Pediatric Orthopedics*, 36(3), e27–e37.

CHAPTER **73**

BOARD REVIEW

Muscle Abnormalities

OMID ADIBNAZARI, MD, BS, and DAVID TANEN, MD

Muscle abnormalities generally manifest as weakness, often associated with muscle pain. These pathologies can be caused by infection, autoimmune reaction, or other insults to muscle cells.

Anatomy

- Skeletal muscle is a form of striated muscle tissue.
  - Made up of multiple bundles of muscle cells called fascicles
- Contents of muscle cells may be released into serum when muscle is damaged.
  - Creatine phosphokinase (CK)
    - Rises in 12 hours after acute injury, peaks at 3 days, normalizes at around 5 days
  - Myoglobin
    - Peaks by 8–12 hours after acute injury and is usually cleared by 24 hours

Clinical Presentation

Inflammatory Myopathies

- Idiopathic inflammatory myopathies with unclear etiologies
- Polymyositis: multisystem disorder with wide clinical manifestations, but characterized by muscle weakness
  - More than 90% of patients present with muscle weakness as the chief complaint.
  - Distribution of muscle weakness is generally symmetric, and affects proximal muscles such as deltoids and hip flexors.
    - Characterized as difficulty climbing stairs, standing up from a seated position, carrying or picking up objects that previously did not feel heavy
  - Generally insidious onset with gradual worsening over months, but occasionally can have acute onset of symptoms
  - Pain is usually mild if present, and stiffness is rare.
  - Can be associated with malignancies
- Dermatomyositis (DM): similar in presentation to polymyositis, but with additional skin findings (Fig. 73.1).
  - Cutaneous findings often precede muscle weakness; weakness is only present in 50%–60% of patients at the time of first evaluation.
  - Gottron papules: erythematous to violaceous papules over extensor surfaces of the hands
  - Gottron sign: Gottron papules affecting extensor surfaces of joints other than the hands
  - Heliotrope eruption: erythematous to violaceous patches of upper eyelids
  - Facial erythema: patients may have photosensitive malar rash similar to that seen in systemic lupus erythematosus, but those with DM frequently have involvement of nasolabial folds.

Pyomyositis

- Purulent infection of skeletal muscle usually arising from a hematogenous source
- *Staphylococcus aureus* is the most common cause of pyomyositis, estimated to cause 70%–90% of cases, followed by *Streptococcus pyogenes*, *Pneumococcus*, *Neisseria*, *Haemophilus*, *Yersinia*, *Pseudomonas*, *Klebsiella*, and *Escherichia coli*.
- Consider in patients with risk factors, such as diabetes mellitus, HIV, intravenous drug use, renal failure, and other immunosuppressive diseases.
- Typically presents with fever and localized muscle pain, usually affecting a single muscle group
  - Multifocal infection may be seen in up to 20% of cases.

Rhabdomyolysis

- Syndrome characterized by muscle cell death and release of intracellular components into the circulation due to various etiologies
- Numerous etiologies (see Table 73.1) that can be broken up into three categories: trauma, nontraumatic exertional, and nontraumatic nonexertional
  - In the emergency setting, consider the diagnosis in patients with crush injury or prolonged down time.
- Classic triad of symptoms is myalgias, red to brown urine due to myoglobinuria, and elevated serum muscle enzymes.
  - More than half of patients may not report any muscle symptoms and present only with changes in urine color or urine output.
- Muscle tenderness and, less commonly, edema may be seen on examination.
- Mental status changes can be present because of urea-induced encephalopathy.

Diagnosis and Evaluation

Polymyositis and Dermatomyositis

- Elevated muscle enzymes, such as CK and lactate dehydrogenase
- Elevated serum and urine myoglobin
- Autoantibodies
  - Antinuclear antibodies in up to 80% of patients
  - Myositis-specific antibodies in 30%–40% of patients, including anti-Jo-1 antibodies, anti-SRP antibodies, and anti-Mi-2 antibodies

Pyomyositis

- Laboratory markers are nonspecific, but may include leukocytosis and elevated inflammatory markers (erythrocyte sedimentation rate and C-reactive protein).

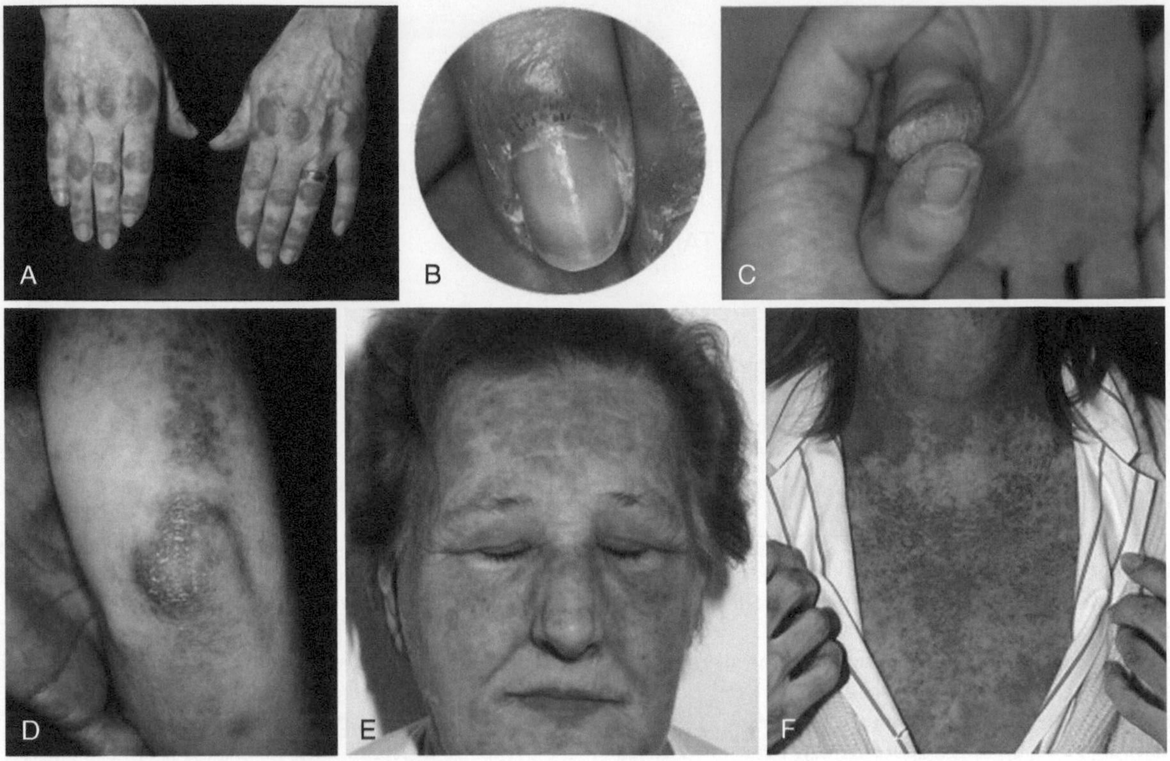

FIG. 73.1 Skin manifestations of dermatomyositis. (A) Gottron papules. (B) Periungual telangiectasia with cuticular hemorrhage and dystrophy. (C) Mechanic's hand. (D) Gottron sign. (E) Heliotrope rash. (F) Poikilodermatomyositis. (From Iaccarino, L., Ghirardello, A., Bettio, S., Zen, M., Gatto, M., Punzi, L., & Doria, A. (2014). The clinical features, diagnosis and classification of dermatomyositis. *Journal of Autoimmunity, 48-49*, 122–127.)

TABLE 73.1 *Causes of Rhabdomyolysis*

Cause	Pathophysiology
Prolonged immobilization	Coma, prolonged general anesthesia
Excessive muscular activity	Seizure, alcohol withdrawal, strenuous exercise, tetanus, dystonia
Muscle ischemia	Thromboembolism, external compression, carbon monoxide poisoning, sickle cell disease
Temperature extremes	Heat stroke, malignant hyperthermia, neuroleptic malignant syndrome, serotonin syndrome, hypothermia/frostbite
Electrolyte abnormalities	Hypokalemia, hypophosphatemia, hyponatremia, hypernatremia
Toxins and recreational drugs	Ethanol, methanol, ethylene glycol, heroin, methadone, barbiturates, cocaine, amphetamine, MDMA (ecstasy), PCP
Trauma	Crush injury, compartment syndrome
Medications	Antihistamines, salicylates, neuroleptics, cyclic antidepressants and selective-serotonin reuptake inhibitors (via serotonin syndrome), anticholinergics, laxatives (likely via electrolyte abnormalities), anesthetics and paralytic agents (especially succinylcholine), quinine, corticosteroids, theophylline, aminocaproic acid, propofol, colchicine, antiretrovirals
Infections	Bacteria: *Escherichia coli*, *Shigella*, *Salmonella*, *Streptococcus pneumoniae*, *Staphylococcus aureus*, group A *Streptococcus*, *Clostridium* Viruses: Influenza A and B, cytomegalovirus, herpes simplex virus, Epstein-Barr virus, HIV, coxsackievirus, West Nile virus, varicella-zoster virus

Used with permission of EB Medicine, publisher of Emergency Medicine Practice. Parekh, R. (2012). Rhabdomyolysis: Advances in diagnosis and treatment. *Emergency Medicine Practice*, *14*(3), 1–16. © 2012 EB Medicine. www.ebmedicine.net

- CK is generally normal to minimally elevated.
- Imaging is the most useful diagnostic tool.
  - Bedside point-of-care ultrasonography can serve as a screening tool, facilitating early diagnosis and treatment.
  - Magnetic resonance imaging is highly sensitive and is considered the gold standard imaging technique, but if unavailable, computed tomography (CT) with intravenous contrast has good test characteristics.

Rhabdomyolysis

- Creatine phosphokinase elevation at least five times the upper limit of normal
  - Usually greater than 5000 IU/L to be considered clinically significant

- May use urinalysis, including dipstick and microscopic analysis, to look for myoglobinuria, which is classic for hematuria without microscopic red blood cells
  - Myoglobinuria lacks sensitivity because it can be absent in up to 50% of patients owing to the rapid clearance of myoglobin.

Treatment

Polymyositis and Dermatomyositis

- Treatment should be in consultation with a rheumatologist, and given the indolent course of these conditions, treatment and consultation may not be indicated in the emergency department.
- Glucocorticoids are first-line initial therapy and recommended in patients with significant muscle weakness.
  - Effective in only about 50% of patients with polymyositis
  - Effective in 80%–90% of patients with DM. However, in one study, more than 90% of patients had symptom flares when steroids were tapered.

Pyomyositis

- Drainage: CT- or ultrasound-guided drainage is an option, but surgical intervention may be required.
- Antibiotics: in mild pyomyositis, antibiotics alone may be appropriate, but most patients present with later-stage disease and require both antibiotics and drainage.
  - Patients typically require weeks of parenteral antibiotics, and treatment may be guided by improvement of clinical and imaging findings.
  - In immunocompetent patients, empiric treatment should consist of staphylococcal coverage, including methicillin-resistant S. *aureus*.
  - For immunocompromised patients, broad-spectrum antibiotics should be started to cover gram-positive, gram-negative, and anaerobic organisms.

Rhabdomyolysis

- Aggressive fluid resuscitation is used to prevent heme-induced acute kidney injury.
  - Optimal fluid type (balanced electrolyte solution vs. normal saline) is not known, but isotonic saline is generally recommended.
  - May start with 1–2 L/hour intravenous fluids, with a urine output goal of 200–300 mL/h (approximately 3 mL/kg per hour)
  - Alkalinization of urine may have benefit in severe rhabdomyolysis.
    - An alkaline solution may be administered when diuresis is established with volume administration.
  - Loop diuretics do not help prevent acute kidney injury, but may help with volume overload from the aggressive fluid administration.

SUGGESTED READINGS

Baddour, L. M., & Keerasuntornpong, A. (2020). Pyomyositis. *UpToDate*. Retrieved May 22, 2019, from https://www.uptodate.com/contents/pyomyositis.

Parekh, R. (2012). Rhabdomyolysis: Advances in diagnosis and treatment. *Emergency Medicine Practice, 14*(3), 1–16.

Parekh, R. (2018). Rhabdomyolysis. In R. M. Walls, R. S. Hockberger, & M. Gausche-Hill (Eds.), *Rosen's emergency medicine: Concepts and clinical practice* (9th ed., pp. 1548–1556). Elsevier.

Shearer, P. (2018). Neuromuscular disorders. In R. M. Walls, R. S. Hockberger, & M. Gausche-Hill (Eds.), *Rosen's emergency medicine: Concepts and clinical practice* (9th ed., p. 1326). Elsevier.

CHAPTER 74

BOARD REVIEW

Overuse Syndromes

OMID ADIBNAZARI, MD, BS, and DAVID TANEN, MD

Overuse syndromes, also known as repetitive strain injuries, comprise a group of injuries to the musculoskeletal and nervous systems that occur because of repetitive movements and mechanical stresses. These injuries can affect any component of the musculoskeletal system, including bones, muscles, and associated soft tissues and nerves.

Bursitis

Basic Information

- A bursa is a closed compartment lined by synovial membrane.
  - Occurs in areas of friction between two layers of tissue
- Inflammation of bursae is termed bursitis.
  - Usually idiopathic, but can have numerous other causes
    - Infection
    - Trauma
    - Rheumatologic disease

Clinical Presentation

- Typically presents as pain over the site of a bursa (Fig. 74.1); usually worsens by putting pressure on the area
  - Olecranon bursitis: pain and swelling over the extensor surface of the elbow
  - Prepatellar bursitis: anterior knee symptoms, often caused by frequent kneeling (gardeners, plumbers, roofers, and so forth)
  - Trochanteric bursitis: lateral hip and thigh symptoms, worse with lying on the hip and walking
  - Ischiogluteal bursitis: "weaver's bottom," pain over the center of the buttock radiating down the back of the leg; worse with sitting on hard surfaces
- May have swelling and fluctuance of the bursa
- Erythema, warmth, and severe tenderness are typical in septic bursitis.
  - Most cases of septic bursitis occur in prepatellar and olecranon bursitis.
- Bursitis should not cause significant limitation in range of motion in most cases.

Diagnosis and Evaluation

- Signs of acute inflammation should prompt aspiration to exclude the presence of crystals or infection.
  - Organisms on Gram stain or culture are diagnostic of infection.
  - White blood cell count greater than 5000/μL^3 suggests infectious etiology, but is nonspecific.

Treatment

- Septic bursitis should be treated with antibiotics with coverage for *Staphylococcus aureus*, including methicillin-resistant *S. aureus*.
  - May consider needle aspiration or surgical intervention with consultant guidance
  - Patients with no underlying medical conditions may be put on a trial of oral antibiotics on an outpatient basis.
- Nonseptic bursitis may be treated conservatively with nonsteroidal antiinflammatory drugs (NSAIDs) and compression.

Muscle Strain

Basic Information

- A strain is a muscle injury that occurs from overstretching, either acutely or from repetitive loading over time.
- Strains commonly result in partial muscle tears as the stress causing them tears muscle fibers.
- Among the most common causes of low back pain

Clinical Presentation

- Typically presents with pain or "tightness" of the affected muscle
- May have associated weakness or functional limitation of the affected muscle
- Contusion often seen with partial muscle tears

Diagnosis and Evaluation

- Clinical diagnosis: localized tenderness over muscle body, functional limitation of affected muscle

Treatment

- Relative rest, ice, compression, elevation
- NSAIDs

Peripheral Nerve Syndrome

Basic Information

- Peripheral nerve syndromes can occur from overuse.
  - Inflammation and swelling of structures surrounding a nerve cause compression.
  - Most common compressive neuropathy is carpal tunnel syndrome (median nerve).
  - Second most common is cubital tunnel syndrome (ulnar nerve).

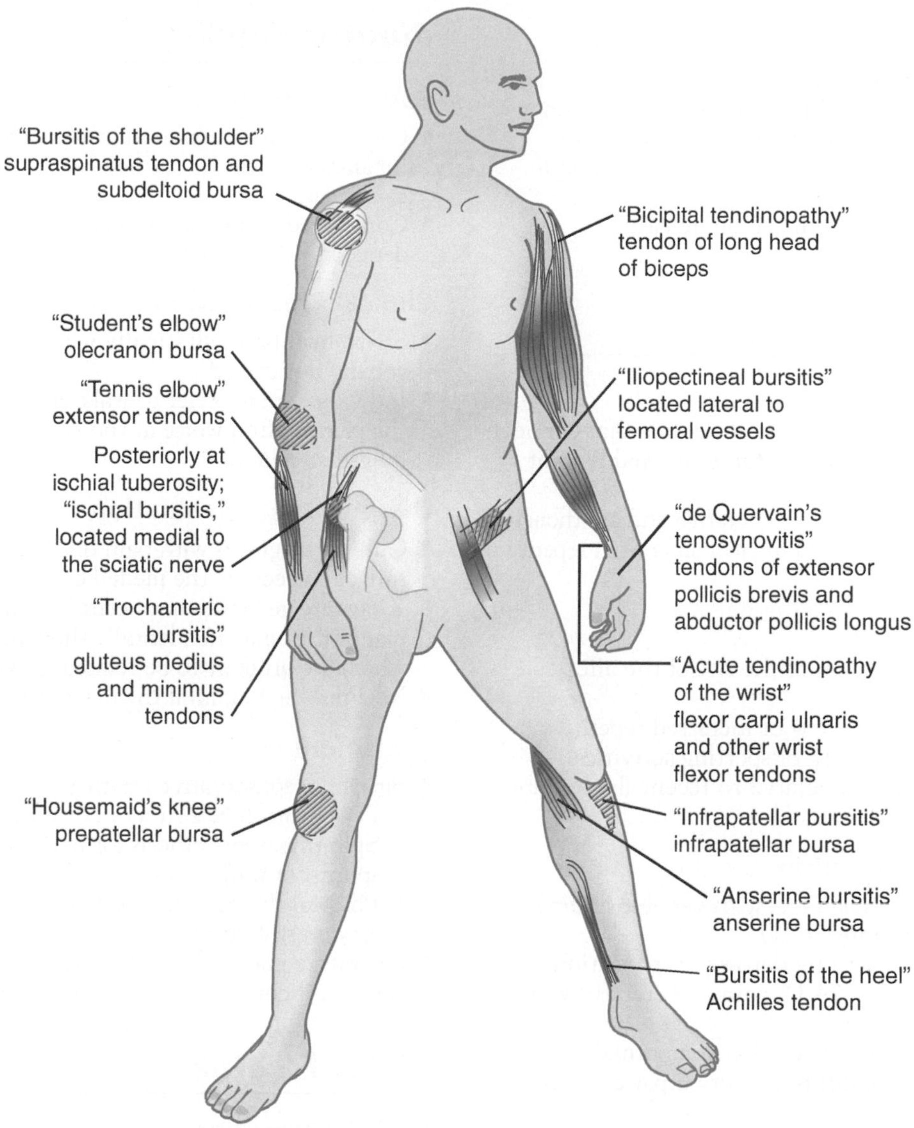

FIG. 74.1 Common sites for tendinopathy or bursitis. (Modified from Branch, W. T. (1987). Office practice of medicine (2nd ed.) W. B. Saunders.)

Clinical Presentation

- Numbness and weakness in distribution of a nerve
  - Carpal tunnel syndrome: numbness of palmar thumb, index finger, middle finger, and radial (toward thumb) aspect of the ring finger; grip weakness and thenar atrophy
    - Tinel sign: pain or paresthesia elicited by tapping over the median nerve at the wrist.
    - Phalen sign (Fig. 74.2): median nerve distribution pain or paresthesia elicited by holding the wrist in full flexion for 60 seconds
- May have pain at the site of impingement and the distribution of the affected nerve

Diagnosis and Evaluation

- Clinical diagnosis in the emergency department
- Outpatients may get magnetic resonance imaging (MRI), ultrasound, and nerve conduction studies.

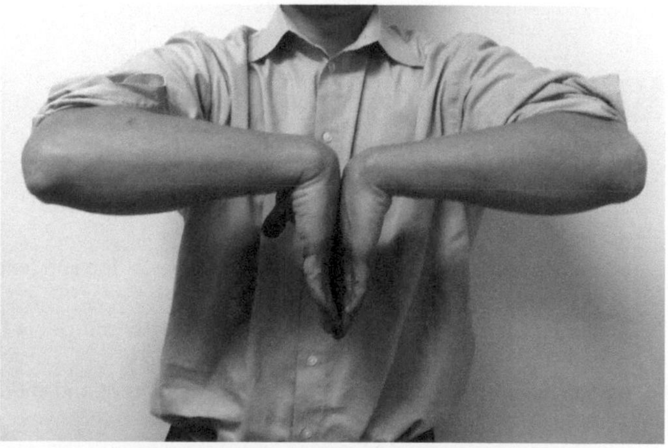

FIG. 74.2 Phalen sign. (From Williams, D. T., & Kim. H. T. (2018). Wrist and forearm. In R. M. Walls, R. S. Hockberger, & M. Gausche-Hill (Eds.), *Rosen's emergency medicine: Concepts and clinical practice* (9th ed., p. 524, Fig. 44.31). Elsevier.)

74

Treatment

- Activity modification, rest
  - Carpal tunnel: wrist splinting in neutral position
- May trial NSAIDs, but little benefit in most cases
- Operative intervention to decrease compression if conservative measures fail
  - Carpal tunnel: flexor retinaculum release

Tendinopathy

Basic Information

- Tendons are dense collagenous structures that connect muscles to bone and transmit forces to enable joint motion.
- Tendinopathies are mostly degenerative and are thought to be caused by accumulated microtrauma from repetitive loading.

Clinical Presentation

- Gradually increasing pain at the site of the affected tendon
- Usually associated with new or increased repetitive stress from change in work or sporting activities
- Tendon rupture may be related to recent fluoroquinolone use.

Diagnosis and Evaluation

- Generally a clinical diagnosis, with variable findings, dependent on site (Table 74.1)
  - Examination showing tenderness over location of the tendon (see Fig. 74.1), pain and crepitus with movement
- May consider x-ray to rule out bony abnormality
- May consider bedside ultrasound or outpatient MRI

Treatment

- Rest, ice, compression, elevation
- NSAIDs

Plantar Fasciitis

Basic Information

- One of the most common causes of foot pain owing to inflammation of the aponeurosis at the origin of the calcaneus
- Considered an overuse injury because it has a high incidence in runners and in those with prolonged walking

Clinical Presentation

- Sharp heel pain, classically with the first step after getting out of bed
- Individuals may prefer to walk on toes (toe-stepping); the pain is often worse at the end of the day after prolonged standing.

Diagnosis and Evaluation

- Clinical diagnosis with pain on palpation on the plantar surface, especially the medial calcaneal tuberosity
- X-rays are generally not necessary; they are often normal or they may incidentally show plantar heel spurs, which are unlikely to be related to symptoms.
- MRI may be helpful if the diagnosis is uncertain.

Treatment

- First-line: conservative treatment
  - Pain control: NSAIDs or cortisone injections
  - Splinting: foot orthosis for heel/arch support, night splints, or walking casts
  - Physical therapy: plantar fascia-specific and Achilles tendon stretching
- Operative management by podiatrist or orthopedic surgeon if conservative management fails

Stress Fracture

Basic Information

- Stress fractures can occur in almost any bone, but it is most common in the lower extremities.

TABLE 74.1 *Common Sites of Tendinopathy and Associated Findings*

Tendinopathy	Involved Muscles/Tendons	Findings
Rotator cuff	Supraspinatus most common; also infraspinatus, teres minor, subscapularis	Positive Jobe sign or empty can test; positive Neer test suggests impingement from decreased subacromial space
Lateral epicondylitis "tennis elbow"	Extensor muscles of forearm (extensor carpi radialis brevis)	Pain with resisted wrist extension and forearm supination
Medial epicondylitis "golfer's elbow"	Flexor and pronator muscles of forearm	Pain with resisted wrist flexion and forearm pronation
De Quervain's tenosynovitis	Extensor pollicis brevis and abductor pollicis longus	Wrist pain with tenderness over radial styloid, exacerbated with Finkelstein test (ulnar wrist deviation while holding the thumb inside a fist)
Patellar tendinopathy	Patellar tendon (connecting patella to tibia)	Tenderness at inferior pole of patella
Achilles tendinopathy	Achilles (calcaneal) tendon	Posterior heel pain, may be edematous and tender

- Occur from repetitive loading
- High-risk stress fractures are often those in bones with vulnerable vascular supply, such as the anterior tibia, medial malleolus, navicular, base of fifth metatarsal.

Clinical Presentation

- Localized pain with insidious onset
- History of change in training regimen in athletes; also may be associated with amenorrhea in female athletes

Diagnosis and Evaluation

- Initial radiographs may be negative; if positive, periosteal reaction, endosteal thickening, or a radiolucent line may be seen.
- May consider bone scan, computed tomography, or MRI as an outpatient

Treatment

- Rest, modification of activity, pain control
- High-risk stress fractures may require immobilization, non–weight-bearing status, and orthopedic or sports medicine consultation.

SUGGESTED READINGS

Hogrefe, C., & Rose, E. M. (2018). Tendinopathy and bursitis. In R. M. Walls, R. S. Hockberger, & M. Gausche-Hill (Eds.), *Rosen's emergency medicine: Concepts and clinical practice* (9th ed., pp. 1392–1401). Elsevier.

Rose, N. G. W., & Green, T. J. (2018). Ankle and foot. In R. M. Walls, R. S. Hockberger, & M. Gausche-Hill (Eds.), *Rosen's emergency medicine: Concepts and clinical practice* (9th ed., pp. 634–658). Elsevier.

Williams, D. T., & Kim, H. T. (2018). Wrist and forearm. In R. M., Walls, R. S. Hockberger, & M. Gausche-Hill (Eds.), *Rosen's emergency medicine: Concepts and clinical practice* (9th ed., pp. 508–529). Elsevier.

CHAPTER 75

BOARD REVIEW

Soft Tissue Infections

MANPREET SINGH, MD, MBE

Soft tissue infections involving the musculoskeletal system are vast and wide. This chapter focuses on limited disease entities, with a special emphasis on hand infections, including felon, paronychia, and flexor tenosynovitis. Please also refer to the cutaneous infection chapter, which covers topics such as cellulitis, abscess, necrotizing fasciitis, and gas gangrene.

Felon

General Principles

- A subcutaneous, pyogenic, slow-growing infection in the pulp space compartment of the distal finger, which typically requires incision and drainage (I&D) to relieve the symptoms
- Epidemiology
  - Commonly accounts for 10%–20% of hand infections, where the thumb or index finger is the predominantly affected digits, because they are more likely to suffer puncture or penetrating trauma wounds.
- Organisms
  - *Staphylococcus aureus* is the most common organism.
  - Consider gram-negative organisms in immunocompromised individuals.
  - *Eikenella corrodens* is seen in diabetics who bite their nails.

Clinical Presentation

- Unilateral digital throbbing pain to the pulp space with erythema is a common presentation, often localized distal to the distal interphalangeal flexion crease. Rarely, the flexor tendon sheath or joint may become involved.
- Pathophysiology
  - Most are caused by a penetrating injury to the area (i.e., needle stick or splinter), but can occur from local spread from a paronychia (to be discussed later).
  - More commonly, 50% of cases have no injury history, making bacterial contamination from nearby eccrine sweat glands a possibility. Intense tissue pressure in the pulp space leads to ischemia from a compartment syndrome of the finger pad.
    - The normal, healthy finger pad is actually composed of 15 to 20 small compartments, separated by septa that extend from the periosteum to the skin.

Diagnosis and Evaluation

- Clinical diagnosis made on examination, with imaging rarely needed, unless concern for fracture or a foreign body.
- Ultrasound, using a high-frequency linear probe with a water bath can be utilized to evaluate for fluid collection in the pulp space, as well as to look for foreign bodies and fractures.
- Complications
  - Fingertip compartment syndrome
  - Flexor tenosynovitis
  - Osteomyelitis
  - Digital tip necrosis

Treatment

- If the felon is early in its presentation (i.e., no drainable abscess), a short course of oral (PO) antibiotics with close observation is recommended. However, most felons require bedside I&D with intravenous (IV) vs. PO antibiotics.
- Antibiotics: definitive drainage is treatment, but you must cover for *S. aureus* (check your local antibiogram for resistance patterns). Some also choose to cover *Streptococcus* with cephalexin, although there is no evidence supporting the need to do so.
  - Trimethoprim-sulfamethoxazole two 160/800 tablets PO every 12 hrs for 7 days
  - Doxycycline 100 mg twice a day for 7 days
  - Clindamycin 450 mg PO every 8 hrs for 7 days
  - Dicloxacillin 250 mg PO every 6 hrs daily for 7 days
- Bedside I&D: digital block prior to performing I&D is crucial for anesthesia. There are two standard approaches (Fig. 75.1):
  - Mid-lateral approach
    - Using a #11 blade, make the incision along the **ulnar aspect** of the index, middle, and ring fingers (digits 2 to 4), and along the **radial aspects** of the thumb and little finger (digit 5), which are the non–pressure-bearing sides of the digits.
      - Start 5 mm distal to flexor DIP crease.
      - Keep the incision distal to flexor DIP crease.
      - Bluntly dissect and explore the wound until the abscess is decompressed.
      - No packing needed, and do not create a "fish-mouth" incision.
  - Volar longitudinal approach
    - Most direct approach with volar incision over the pulp space
  - Novel approach
    - Use an 18-gauge needle to aspirate an abscess and decompress the tiny, engorged compartments. Further compartment release is performed by vigorously massaging the fingertip after the needle decompression to express fluid from the compartments through the needle tracks.

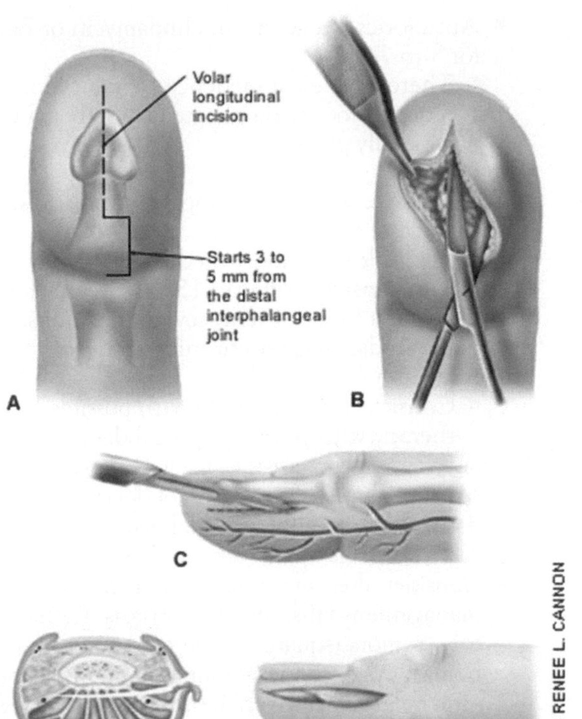

FIG. 75.1 Two approaches for incision and drainage of a felon. A and B, showing direct approach, whereas **C–E** shows lateral approach avoiding the digital arteries. (Courtesy Renee L. Cannon.) (From Clark, D. (2003). Common acute hand infections. *American Family Physician, 68*(11), 2167–2176, Fig. 5.)

- Incisions to avoid (Fig. 75.2)
  - Fish-mouth incision
    - Risk of unstable finger pulp or vascular compromise
  - Double longitudinal or transverse incision
    - Risk of injury to digital nerve and artery
- Debridement: avoid DIP joint and flexor sheath. The main goal is to break up the septa to decompress the infection and prevent compartment syndrome. Gram stain and culture should be sent, and keep the cavity open with gauze wick/drain.
- Disposition
  - Unless the patient is systemically ill or has a complicated infection (i.e., outside the DIP crease), discharge with wound check in 2 days, along with a course of oral antibiotics.
  - Hand surgeon referral is needed if complicated infection or systemically ill-appearing patient. Update the patient's tetanus prior to discharge.

Paronychia

General Principles

- A common soft tissue infection originating at the proximal or lateral nail fold (paronychium)
- Epidemiology
  - Comprises one-third of all hand infections generally occurring in the thumb. It is more common in children with a female propensity (3:11).
- Organisms
  - With acute infections, *S. aureus* dominates in adults, whereas mixed oropharyngeal flora occurs in children and mixed bacterial occurs in diabetics.
  - With chronic infections, *Candida albicans* dominates.

Clinical Presentation

- Pathophysiology
  - Acute paronychia usually results from direct or indirect minor trauma to the area, facilitating bacterial entry, including nail biting, sucking, or getting a manicure.
  - In contrast, chronic paronychia occurs in patients with prolonged exposure to water or chemical irritants (acid/alkali).
  - Thus, paronychia commonly afflicts dishwashers, florists, gardeners, housekeepers, swimmers, and bartenders.
  - Risk factors for chronic infections include diabetes, psoriasis, steroids, and retroviral drugs (indinavir and lamivudine).
- With acute presentation, there is pain, erythema, and swelling to the nail fold with tenderness of usually just one nail. Fluctuance may sometimes be seen, but not always.

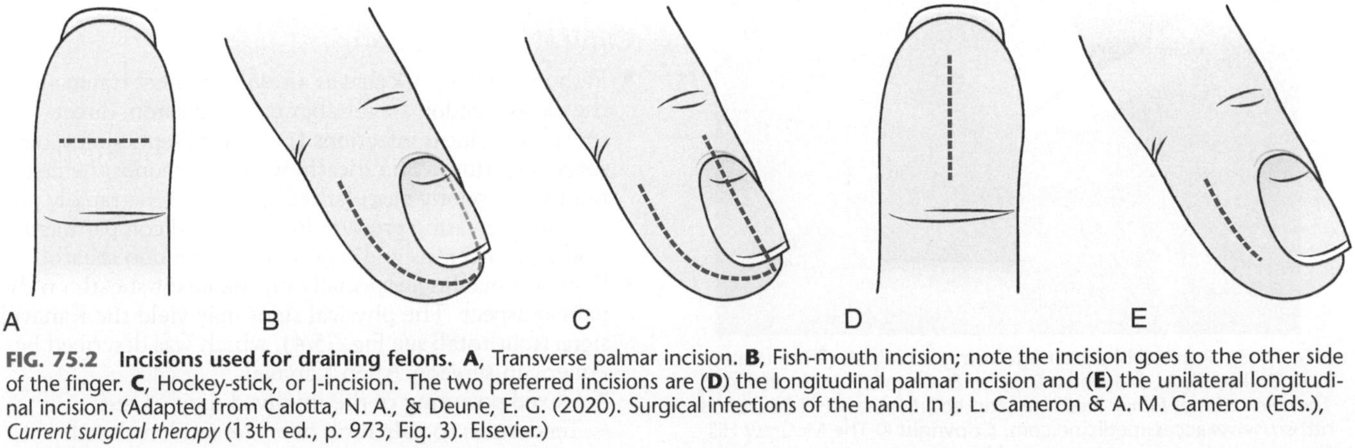

FIG. 75.2 Incisions used for draining felons. A, Transverse palmar incision. **B**, Fish-mouth incision; note the incision goes to the other side of the finger. **C**, Hockey-stick, or J-incision. The two preferred incisions are (**D**) the longitudinal palmar incision and (**E**) the unilateral longitudinal incision. (Adapted from Calotta, N. A., & Deune, E. G. (2020). Surgical infections of the hand. In J. L. Cameron & A. M. Cameron (Eds.), *Current surgical therapy* (13th ed., p. 973, Fig. 3). Elsevier.)

- In contrast, chronic paronychia appears less severe owing to chronic bouts of inflammation, which result in nail plate hypertrophy, nail fold blunting and retraction, and prominent transverse ridges on the nail plate. This can affect multiple nails at a time.

Diagnosis and Evaluation

- Diagnosis relies on clinical presentation with history and physical examination.
- Complications
  - Spread to eponychia
  - Spread to both lateral nail beds (runaround infection)
  - Felon
  - Flexor tenosynovitis
  - Osteomyelitis
  - Subungual abscess ("floating nail")

Treatment

- Both acute and chronic paronychia have noninvasive and invasive treatment approaches, depending on the patient.
  - Acute
    - Noninvasive: warm soaks, topical antibiotics, and avoidance of nail biting
      - Reserved for mild swelling without fluctuance (i.e., abscess)
    - Invasive: I&D (Fig. 75.3) followed by oral antibiotics
      - Anesthesia: digital block
      - Equipment for I&D: Iris scissors, flat tweezers, 18-gauge needle or #11 blade
        - Make an incision into the sulcus between the lateral nail plate and the lateral nail fold.
        - Place material between skin and nail bed to preserve the eponychial fold.
        - Partial or total nail bed removal is an option if infection tracks under the nail plate (rare).
        - Instruct patient to soak finger three times a day in warm water to keep abscess open, or place a wick/gauze if opening is large enough.

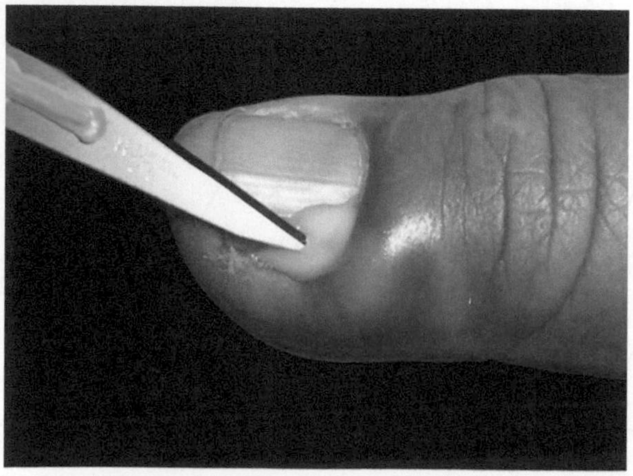

FIG. 75.3 Paronychia drainage using a scalpel. (From Usatine, R. P., Smith, M. A., Mayeaux, E. J., Jr., & Chumley, H. S. (2013). *The color atlas of family medicine* (2nd ed.) McGraw-Hill Education. https://www.accessmedicine.com. Copyright © The McGraw-Hill Companies, Inc. All rights reserved.)

      - Antibiotics: Augmentin, clindamycin or Bactrim for 5 to 7 days
        - There is no clear evidence that antibiotics are required for uncomplicated cases, but they are generally given.
  - Chronic
    - Noninvasive: warm soaks, topical antifungals, and avoidance of finger sucking
      - Miconazole commonly used
        - Can consider Diflucan 150 mg weekly for 4 to 6 weeks for persistent, severe infections.
      - Some studies suggest chronic paronychia to be eczematous.
        - Consider topical steroid with possible systemic therapy with primary medical doctor guidance.
    - Invasive: when conservative, medical management fails
      - Marsupialization by excision of dorsal eponychium down to the level of germinal matrix in severe cases, which is usually left to a hand surgeon
      - Consider alternative diagnoses if conservative management fails, such as psoriasis, Reiter's disease, tumors (squamous cell carcinoma, melanoma), cysts, chancre, human immunodeficiency virus-related paronychia, or herpetic whitlow.
  - Disposition: Discharge home with wound care follow-up with primary medical doctor in 1 to 2 days. Update the patient's tetanus prior to discharge.

Flexor Tenosynovitis

General Principles

- Usually a result of penetrating trauma or direct spread from a nearby infection, flexor tenosynovitis is a true hand emergency. It is an aggressive disease that can lead to debilitating morbidity if not recognized and treated.
- Epidemiology
  - Accounts for 2.5%–9.4% of all hand infections
  - Generally occurs in diabetics, IV drug users, and immunocompromised patients
- Organisms
  - *Staphylococcus aureus* is the most common organism, specifically methicillin-resistant *S. aureus*.
  - However, human bites (*Eikenella*), animal bites (*Pasturella multocida*), and immunocompromised individuals (mixed flora and gram-negative) may be susceptible to other organisms.

Clinical Presentation

- Pathophysiology: Occurs as a result of direct trauma to the closed tendon sheath, but can result from direct spread from local infections (i.e., felon, septic joint, deep space infection). The sheath, which surrounds the flexor tendons, is poorly vascularized; thus, bacteria rapidly proliferate, increasing pressure in this closed compartment, leading to necrosis and rupture of the tendon sheath.
- Pain and swelling, especially on the flexor sheath on the palmar aspect. The physical signs may yield the Kanavel signs (four total; see Fig. 75.4), which was described by American surgeon Allen Kanavel.
  - Flexed posturing of the involved digit at rest
  - Tenderness to palpation over the tendon sheath

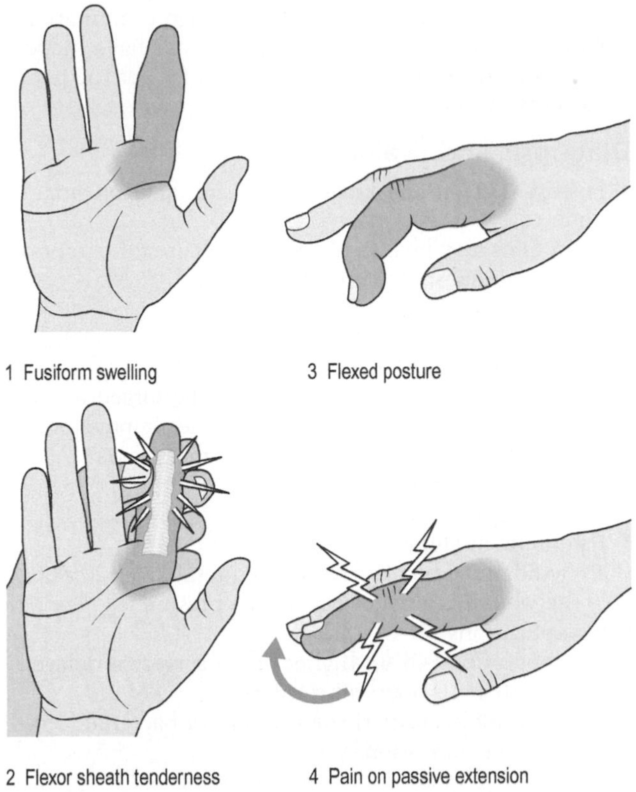

FIG. 75.4 The four Kanavel signs. (From White, T., MacKenzie, S., & Gray, A. (2015). *McRae's orthopaedic trauma and emergency fracture management* (3rd ed., p. 532, Fig. 13.42). Elsevier.)

- Marked pain with passive extension of the digit (generally earliest sign seen)
- Fusiform swelling of the digit (owing to swelling along length of tendon sheath): "sausage digits"
  - The sensitivity, specificity, and interobserver reliability have not been established in the literature (only 54% have all four signs). In addition, they are less reliable in the thumb and small finger, as well as in children.
- Horseshoe abscess: the thumb flexor tendon sheath is in continuity with the radial bursa of the palm, and the small-finger sheath communicates with the ulnar palmar bursa. As a result, infection in one finger can lead to direct infection of the sheath on the opposite side of the hand, resulting in a "horseshoe abscess."

Diagnosis and Evaluation

- Clinical diagnosis based on history and examination; rarely is imaging needed.
  - X-ray may aid in assessing for a foreign body.
  - MRI may be helpful if the diagnosis is uncertain, but cost and availability make it difficult to obtain.
  - An ultrasound using a high-frequency linear probe with a water bath can be utilized to evaluate for a fluid collection between the bone and tendon, as well as to look for foreign bodies.
    - Although ultrasound does not involve ionizing radiation, is noninvasive, and readily available, at this time, no strong evidence exists about its test characteristics (sensitivity and specificity).
- Complications: stiffness owing to adhesions, tendon/pulley necrosis and rupture, infection spread to deep space, soft tissue loss, osteomyelitis

Treatment

- Operative I&D of the flexor tendon (open vs. catheter irrigation method) by hand surgeon
- In the emergency department, antibiotics should be initiated on immediate suspicion of flexor tenosynovitis.
- Rarely, nonoperative measures of splinting for hand mobilization, IV antibiotics, and observation are sought if the diagnosis is uncertain.
- Antibiotics
  - Vancomycin 1 g IV every 12 hrs AND
  - Ampicillin/sulbactam 1.5 g IV every 6 hrs OR cefoxitin 2 g IV every 8 hrs OR Piperacillin/tazobactam 3.375 g IV every 6 hrs
- Disposition: admission to hospital with continued IV antibiotics and hand surgery consultation

Herpetic Whitlow

General Principles

- Distal phalanx infection caused by herpes simplex virus (HSV) through direct inoculation
- Epidemiology
  - Can be found in any age group
    - Children who suck their thumbs
  - HSV-1 (60%) greater than HSV-2 (40%)
  - Often seen among dental and medical personnel, such as respiratory therapists
  - Incidence of 2.4 cases per 100,000 people per year
- Recurrent infections (30%–50%) occur through latent reactivation occurring months to years later following primary infection.

Clinical Presentation

- Pathophysiology
  - Break in epidermal surface of direct introduction of virus into hand through occupation or other type of exposure (i.e., autoinoculation from genital or oral herpes)
- Prodromal pain and tingling to finger before any skin changes
- Vesicular/pustular lesions to pulp and lateral finger edges with abrupt onset of edema, erythema, and localized tenderness to infected finger
  - Can have associated fever, lymphadenitis, and lymphadenopathy (epitrochlear/axillary especially)

75

Diagnosis and Evaluation

- Clinical diagnosis is based on history and physical examination, but it is important to consider in your differential for distal finger infections.
- Laboratory studies available, but not required to make diagnosis
  - Viral culture (gold standard)
  - Polymerase chain reaction or monoclonal antibodies (most sensitive)
  - Serology and direct immunofluorescence (less common)
  - Tzanck smear (poor specificity)

Treatment

- Generally a self-limiting illness, complete resolutions is usually seen within 2 to 4 weeks.
- Apply a dry dressing to prevent disease transmission.
- Incision and drainage should NOT be performed because it is confused with pyogenic bacterial infections (i.e., felon, paronychia).
  - Can lead to concomitant superimposed bacterial infection and viremia (encephalitis in some cases)
- Antivirals: may shorten duration of infection
  - Topical acyclovir 5%
  - Oral acyclovir/valacyclovir
- Disposition: outpatient management

High-Pressure Injection Injuries

General Principles

- Rare surgical emergency with extensive soft tissue damage characterized by a small benign puncture wound from high-pressure equipment, which is often underestimated by both physicians and patients
- Epidemiology
  - Commonly occurs in industrial laborers, through grease, paint, solvent, and fuel guns
  - Injection occurs on upper extremity and nondominant hand.
- Factors affecting injury severity
  - Force of injection
  - Volume injected
  - Time from injury to treatment
  - Material composition (oil-based paint with higher amputation)

Clinical Presentation

- Pathophysiology
  - High-pressure (3000 to 10,000 PSI) force up to 400 mph
  - Dissection along planes of least resistance (i.e., neurovascular bundles)
  - Soft tissue damage owing to impact, vascular ischemia leading to soft tissue necrosis and chemical inflammation, which can lead to compartment syndrome of the hand
- Complaints of severe pain with a benign examination with innocuous punctate wound, but may have hidden soft tissue necrosis depending on how far out the patient presents to the ED

Diagnosis and Evaluation

- History is key in diagnosis. Document duration since onset of events.
- Plain films may be considered to evaluate for extent of radiopaque substance injection.

Treatment

- Splint and elevate injury
- Emergent consult with hand/orthopedic surgeon
  - Early irrigation, debridement, and decompression encouraged to avoid amputation for most cases
- Tetanus prophylaxis
- Prophylactic parenteral antibiotics
- Parenteral analgesia
  - Avoid nerve blocks, including digital blocks, because the wound is already under high pressure.
- Complications
  - Amputation (48%): higher rate if surgery is delayed more than 10 hours after injury.
  - Infection: necrotic tissue is nidus for bacterial growth.
- Disposition: admission

SUGGESTED READINGS

Ahn, L., & Woon, C. (2019, March 26). Felon. Available at: https://www.orthobullets.com/hand/6102/felon.

Cannon, T. A. (2016). High-pressure injection injuries of the hand. *Orthopedic Clinics of North America*, 47(3), 617–624.

May, N. (2018, July 27). Pointing the finger—Paronychia in the emergency department. Available at: http://www.stemlynsblog.org/paronychia/.

Roberts, J. (2019, December). InFocus: Fingertip problems: Felons. Available at: https://journals.lww.com/em-news/fulltext/2010/12000/InFocus__Fingertip_Problems__Felons.4.aspx.

Roberts, J. (2010, November). InFocus: Fingertip problems: Acute paronychia. Available at: https://journals.lww.com/em-news/FullText/2010/11000/InFocus__Fingertip_Problems__Acute_Paronychia.5.aspx.

Rubright, J. H., & Shafritz, A. B. (2011). The herpetic whitlow. *Journal of Hand Surgery*, 36(2), 340–342.

Yoon, R. (2016, October 04). Pyogenic flexor tenosynovitis. Available at: https://www.orthobullets.com/hand/6105/pyogenic-flexor-tenosynovitis.

SECTION ELEVEN

BOARD REVIEW

Nervous System

Cranial Nerve Disorders

REBECCA A. BAVOLEK, MD, and ELIZABETH TANG FERREIRA, MD

Cranial Nerve III: Oculomotor Palsy

General Principles

The third cranial nerve (CN III) innervates four of the six muscles of the globe (superior rectus, medial rectus, inferior rectus, and inferior oblique), the levator palpebrae muscle of the eyelid, and the pupil. CN III is externally surrounded by parasympathetic fibers that control pupillary constriction via the ciliary body and sphincter of the iris. It originates and exits at the level of the midbrain and traverses through the dura, subarachnoid space, and cavernous sinus, traveling alongside the posterior communicating artery before entering the superior orbital fissure to innervate the structures of the eye.

- An approach to a chief concern of diplopia involving CN III should begin with classifying the lesions as neurologically isolated or nonisolated with other neurologic defects or systemic findings. If neurologically isolated, the next step is to determine whether it is pupil-sparing or nonpupil-sparing.

Clinical Presentation

- Complete CN III palsy presents with ptosis, mydriasis with lack of accommodation, and ophthalmoplegia with the eye resting in a "down and out" position where it is abducted, intorted, and slightly depressed. This is due to unopposed superior oblique muscle (CN IV, intorted and depressed) and lateral rectus (CN VI, abducted) activity.
- Partial CN III palsies have a variable spectrum of pupillary response, including normal pupil size and reactivity, a dilated and poorly reactive pupil, or dilated pupil with complete lack of reactivity to light.

Evaluation and Management

- Pupillary function should be evaluated first to initiate an algorithmic approach to the underlying pathology. If the pupil demonstrates dilation and lack of reactivity, consider a space-occupying lesion. If pupillary reactivity is spared, consider ischemic etiology.
- **Complete oculomotor palsy** or isolated pupillary dilation (nonpupil-sparing) should be highly concerning for a space occupying lesion, most likely an aneurysm at the posterior communicating artery causing external compression on the parasympathetic periphery of CN III and warrants investigative imaging with computed tomography (CT) angiogram or magnetic resonance (MR) angiogram. In the context of a traumatic injury, it can signify uncal herniation where the temporal lobe compresses CN III.
  - Management involves neurosurgical consultation if a lesion is identified.
- **Pupil-sparing partial unilateral oculomotor palsy** should signal ischemic causes and is commonly a peripherally isolated diabetic neuropathy, in which case better glucose control is the mainstay of treatment. The microvascular disease affects the inner motor fibers more than the outer parasympathetic fibers, leading to pupil-sparing.
  - Less commonly, it may be due to midbrain infarction, but this should typically present with additional neurologic findings.
- **Mixed findings of incomplete or partial oculomotor palsies** require consideration of multiple causes and warrant advanced imaging with CT or MR imaging (MRI) and potentially additional laboratory studies. Examples include:
  - Trauma causing extraocular muscle entrapment
  - Neuromuscular disease (e.g., myasthenia gravis, Lambert-Eaton syndrome)
  - Demyelinating disease (e.g., multiple sclerosis, Miller Fisher syndrome)
  - Vasculitis (e.g., giant cell arteritis)
  - Thrombosis (e.g., cavernous sinus thrombosis)

Cranial Nerve IV: Trochlear Palsy

General Principles

CN IV (trochlear nerve) innervates the superior oblique muscle of the eye responsible for intorsion and depression of the eye. It exits the brainstem dorsally with a protracted course intracranially, leaving it susceptible to damage in closed head injuries and subarachnoid hemorrhage. This palsy is the most difficult ocular palsy to identify, typically of traumatic, congenital, or microischemic (diabetes mellitus, hypertension) etiology.

Clinical Presentation

CN IV palsy is the most common cause of vertical diplopia and presents with the eye resting in an elevated and extorted position. Patients compensate by tilting the head forward and away from the affected eye to mimic the loss of intorsion and depression.

Evaluation and Management

This is a clinical diagnosis. Isolated peripheral CN IV palsies without other neurologic findings typically do not require advanced imaging, and disposition favors outpatient referral to neurology or ophthalmology for further workup. Yield of CT is low in these cases.

- Fourth-nerve palsy accompanied with signs of brainstem involvement (bilateral palsy, internuclear ophthalmoplegia,

Horner syndrome, or ataxia) signify a central lesion due to infarction or hemorrhage and require imaging to identify the central lesion.

Cranial Nerve VI: Abducens Palsy

General Principles

CN VI (abducens nerve) innervates the lateral rectus muscle of the eye responsible for abduction (lateral movement) of the eye. The nerve travels within the cavernous sinus along the petrous portion of the temporal bone in a tethered fashion, making it susceptible to dysfunction in pathologies with elevated intracranial pressures.

Clinical Presentation

CN VI palsy presents with horizontal binocular diplopia and causes significant visual distortion for the patient. Patients compensate by rotating the head to the affected side or covering the eye.

Evaluation and Management

CN VI palsy is the most common cranial nerve palsy and is considered a non-localizing neurologic finding, given that elevated intracranial pressure from any cause may lead to this condition. As such, it is important to perform fundoscopic examination, looking for papilledema. When imaging is pursued, MRI is preferred over CT because the latter commonly misses most pathologies causing an isolated sixth nerve palsy. In the acute setting, outpatient referral to neurology is the mainstay of management, with follow-up in 3 months. All children under 18 years of age with isolated sixth nerve palsy require MRI because compressive tumors account for approximately 25% of sixth nerve palsies in this demographic group.

Trigeminal Neuralgia (Tic Douloureux)

General Principles

Trigeminal neuralgia is a painful recurring neuropathy of cranial nerve V involving the facial sensory nerves that innervate the cornea, nasal cavity, oral region, and motor nerves, including the muscles of mastication. Current etiologic hypothesis is focused on blood vessel compression of the trigeminal nerve when the nerve root enters the pons as a primary cause.

Clinical Presentation

- Relapsing-remitting disease with paroxysms of excruciating pain that is lancinating, stabbing, or electric shock-like in quality that lasts months to years and progressively increases in frequency
- Commonly generates unilateral spasmodic grimacing or facial contractions
- Most commonly affects the V2 (maxillary branch) along the nerve distribution of V2-V3, but rarely affects V1
- Eventually patients grow averse to shaving, chewing, or touching the face for fear of triggering the pain.

Evaluation and Management

- Patients should have a normal neurological examination result. If a sensory deficit is present, consider compression of the trigeminal nerve due to a central nervous system space-occupying lesion or multiple sclerosis; MRI should be acquired.
- Rule out odontogenic and other local causes of facial pain.
- In the acute setting, pain can be managed with opioid analgesia.
- Carbamazepine is first-line therapy for long term management.
- Oxcarbazepine, lamotrigine, valproic acid, clonazepam, baclofen, and gabapentin have all been shown to have efficacy for long-term management.

Cranial Nerve VII: Facial Palsy

General Principles

Bell palsy is an idiopathic acute peripheral neuropathy involving the facial nerve (CN VII). It is a lower motor neuron deficit characterized by unilateral weakness or paralysis of the muscles used in facial expression. Other identified causes of peripheral CN VII palsy such as Lyme disease or herpes zoster oticus are not termed Bell palsy because Bell palsy refers only to idiopathic facial nerve palsy.

Clinical Presentation

- Unilateral facial weakness or paralysis with lagophthalmos (loss of the nasolabial fold) and drooping of the corner of the mouth.
- Patients are not able to raise their eyebrow on the involved side (vs. in upper motor neuron or central causes of facial nerve palsy wherein raising of the unilateral eyebrow is spared).
- May endorse hyperacusis due to paresis of the stapedius muscle and ageusia of the anterior two-thirds of the tongue.

Evaluation

- Consideration should be given to the causes of new-onset peripheral facial nerve palsy. Differential diagnosis includes:
  - Lyme disease, especially in areas of endemic disease or bilateral palsy
  - Herpes zoster oticus (Ramsay Hunt syndrome): physical examination should include evaluation for vesicles in the external auditory canal, anterior two-thirds of the tongue, and soft palate.
  - Vestibular schwannoma: presents with slowly progressive unilateral hearing loss, tinnitus, vertigo, and disequilibrium
    - A thorough neurologic examination is necessary to ensure that the lesion is not central in origin.

Management

- Oral steroids should be started within 72 hours of symptom onset in patients 16 years or older to prevent long-term complications.

- It is possible that steroids and antivirals are superior to steroids alone in patients with severe facial palsy and should be considered for these cases.
- Recovery usually occurs within 3 months and may take up to 9 months.
- Ophthalmologic care includes lubricating eye drops, wearing glasses, and taping the eye closed at night to prevent corneal injury.

SUGGESTED READINGS

Biousse, V., & Newman, N. J. (2000). Third nerve palsies. *Seminars in Neurology*, *20*, 55.

Rucker, C. W. (1966). The causes of paralysis of the third, fourth and sixth cranial nerves. *American Journal of Ophthalmology*, *61*, 1293.

Rush, J. A., & Younge, B. R. (1981). Paralysis of cranial nerves III, IV, and VI. Cause and prognosis in 1,000 cases. *Archives of Ophthalmology*, 99, 76.

CHAPTER 77

BOARD REVIEW

Demyelinating Disorders

KEVIN WROBLEWSKI, MD, and GREG HENDEY, MD

General Principles

- A demyelinating disease is a disease of the nervous system that damages the myelin sheath of neurons. There are numerous causes of demyelination including inflammatory, infectious, genetic, and granulomatous etiologies, as well as nutritional deficiencies and disease of myelin itself, among others.
- Demyelinating diseases can affect the central nervous system (CNS) and the peripheral nervous system, and therefore have various clinical presentations. This chapter focuses on hallmark demyelinating diseases to provide insight on the typical clinical presentation, diagnosis, and treatment of common demyelinating disorders.

Inflammatory

MULTIPLE SCLEROSIS

Basic Information

- Multiple sclerosis (MS) is the most common autoimmune inflammatory disease of the CNS.
- Exact pathogenesis is unknown. It is widely accepted that a genetic predisposition and unclear environmental factors result in an autoimmune inflammatory response mediated by T cells against myelin.
- Commonly involved CNS regions: periventricular, juxtacortical, cerebellum, and spinal cord; therefore, varied presentations exist depending on the locations of the demyelination.
- Course can be relapsing-remitting (most common), primary or secondary progressive, or progressive-relapsing.
- Greater prevalence among people of northern European descent
- Higher prevalence among women than men, 2:1
- Disease of young adults, typically 18–50 years of age

Clinical Presentation

- Commonly presents as a single, monosymptomatic complaint that develops over days
- Often presents with chief complaint of visual disturbance, due to either optic neuritis (eye pain, vision loss, color vision loss) or internuclear ophthalmoplegia (affected eye does not adduct correctly)
- Common initial symptoms: vision loss, diplopia, paresthesias, weakness, dizziness, bladder/bowel dysfunction, and Lhermitte sign (electrical sensation down the back and limbs when the neck is flexed)

Diagnosis and Evaluation

- Magnetic resonance imaging (MRI) with and without contrast; presence of CNS lesions in both space and time
- Lumbar puncture (LP) (if MRI inconclusive); presence of oligoclonal bands within the cerebrospinal fluid (CSF) that are not seen in serum, or an increased immunoglobulin G index

Treatment

- Intravenous (IV) high-dose methylprednisolone
- Rule out/treat infection (fever or high temperature can cause MS flare [Uhthoff phenomenon]).

GUILLAIN-BARRÉ SYNDROME

Basic Information

- Guillain-Barré Syndrome (GBS) is an acute autoimmune polyneuropathy of the peripheral nervous system that leads to rapidly progressive weakness or paralysis.
- Typically preceded by an infection
  - Most commonly *Campylobacter jejuni*
  - Cytomegalovirus, Epstein-Barr virus, and HIV are other common causes.
  - Molecular mimicry leads to immune-mediated degradation of Schwann cells or myelin.
- Can affect motor, sensory, cranial, and sympathetic nerves
- GBS is a heterogeneous syndrome with multiple forms.
- Acute inflammatory demyelinating polyradiculoneuropathy accounts for 90% of cases in the United States.

Clinical Presentation

- Rapidly progressive (~2 weeks) ascending muscle weakness or paralysis
- Absent or diminished deep tendon reflexes
- Typically symmetric
- ~30% of cases require mechanical ventilation for respiratory muscle weakness.
- ~20% experience severe dysautonomia.

Diagnosis and Evaluation

- LP: shows elevated CSF protein with normal white blood cell count (known as albuminocytologic dissociation)
- Frequent measurement of forced vital capacity and negative inspiratory force is key to predict impending respiratory failure.
- Nerve conduction and electromyography studies help confirm the diagnosis.

Treatment

- IV immunoglobulin or plasma exchange
- Admission to intensive care unit and cardiac monitoring
- Intubation and mechanical ventilation for a forced vital capacity <20 mL/kg, negative inspiratory force <30 cm H_2O, or maximum expiratory pressure <40 cm H_2O in conjunction with clinical findings of impending respiratory failure

Prognosis

- At 1 year post onset and treatment: ~60% have a full recovery, ~14% have severe deficit, and ~5% have died from the disease.

Infectious

NEUROSYPHILIS

Basic Information

- Syphilis is a bacterial infection caused by the spirochete *Treponema pallidum*.
- May be latent for years
- Syphilis has three clinical stages: primary, secondary, and tertiary.
- Neurosyphilis is due to invasion of the CSF.
- Neurosyphilis is common in untreated disease, especially in secondary syphilis.
- Secondary CNS infection involves the CSF, meninges, and vasculature.
  - Can be asymptomatic
- Tertiary infection of the CNS typically involves the brain parenchyma and/or spinal cord.

Clinical Presentation

- Secondary neurosyphilis
  - Headache, confusion, nausea/vomiting, neck stiffness
  - Visual and/or hearing disturbances are common.
  - May or may not have other concomitant signs of syphilis (e.g., rash)
- Tertiary neurosyphilis
  - Paralysis
  - Tabes dorsalis: decreased proprioception and vibration sensation

Diagnosis and Evaluation

- VDRL and fluorescent treponemal antibody absorption (FTA-ABS) tests
- Concomitant HIV testing
- LP
  - + VDRL or FTA-ABS with neurologic, visual, or hearing deficits: require LP
  - + VDRL or FTA-ABS without neurologic, visual, or hearing deficits: no LP
  - + VDRL or FTA-ABS and +HIV: require LP (regardless of neurologic deficits)

Treatment

- Penicillin G 18–24 million U/d intravenously for 10–14 days
- Penicillin allergy: desensitization or ceftriaxone 2 g IV or intramuscularly for 10–14 days
- Monitoring: LP 3–6 months after treatment and every 6 months thereafter until CSF VDRL test is nonreactive and CSF white blood cell count is normal

PROGRESSIVE MULTIFOCAL LEUKOENCEPHALOPATHY

Basic Information

- Progressive multifocal leukoencephalopathy is a demyelinating disease caused by infection of the CNS by JC polyomavirus.
- High morbidity and mortality rates
- Only seen in immunosuppressed individuals, especially HIV/AIDS
- Rarely seen in cancer or transplant patients

Clinical Presentation

- Altered mental status (AMS), visual disturbance, hemiparesis, ataxia
- Seizures

Diagnosis and Evaluation

- CT or MRI: often multifocal areas of white matter demyelination around periventricular and subcortical regions without mass effect or contrast uptake
- CSF polymerase chain reaction for JC polyomavirus
- Gold standard is brain biopsy; however, this is associated with high morbidity and mortality and therefore is indicated only if CSF polymerase chain reaction negative ×2 and other workup is negative.

Treatment

- Restoration of the host's immune system (no direct treatment for JC polyomavirus)
- HIV-positive patients: antiretroviral therapy
- Immunosuppressed patients (e.g., immunomodulators): discontinue offending agent.
- If cerebral edema is present: high-dose glucocorticoid therapy.

Other

OSMOTIC DEMYELINATION SYNDROME

Basic Information

- Formerly known as central pontine myelinolysis
- Results from overly rapid correction of chronic hyponatremia
- The brain adapts to hyponatremia within 48–72 hours; therefore, anything >48 hours is deemed chronic.
- Hyponatremia causes brain edema. In the setting of chronic hyponatremia, this is a low-pressure mechanism with very little risk of herniation.
- Typically occurs at starting [Na^+] of 105 mEq/L or less
- Rare at starting [Na^+] of 120 mEq/L or greater
- Rate of correction should not exceed 6–8 mEq/L in 24 hours

Clinical Presentation

- Clinical manifestations are delayed 2–6 days after overly rapid sodium correction.
- Symptoms may include hypertonia, dysarthria, dysphagia, seizures, paraparesis, quadriplegia, AMS, or coma.
- "Locked-in syndrome": seen in severe cases of osmotic demyelination syndrome; patients are awake, but unable to move or vocalize.

Diagnosis and Evaluation

- MRI findings can lag behind clinical symptoms; concerning symptoms in the appropriate clinical context should raise suspicion of osmotic demyelination syndrome. Typical findings on MRI include demyelination and restricted diffusion of the central pons and basal ganglia.

Treatment

- Symptoms are often irreversible.

- Prevention is key; [Na^+] correction <6–8 mEq/L per 24 hours.
- Close monitoring, [Na^+] every 2–3 hours
- Overly rapid correction, >8 mEq/L per 24 hours, should be treated with dextrose 5% in water or desmopressin.

VITAMIN B_{12} DEFICIENCY

Basic Information

- Vitamin B_{12} (cobalamin) plays an important role in methylation reactions.
- B_{12} is required for DNA synthesis and neuronal myelination.
- The human body cannot synthesize B_{12}; must be obtained from dietary sources.
- B_{12} is found in animal products, like meat, eggs, and dairy products.
- Cereals and breads are commonly fortified with B_{12}; deficiency is uncommon in the United States.
- Vegans and people who have had bariatric surgery or who have pernicious anemia, celiac disease, and inflammatory bowel disease are at risk for deficiency.
- Pernicious anemia results from the lack of intrinsic factor, which is necessary for B_{12} absorption in the ileum.
- B_{12} deficiency leads to a macrocytic anemia, and can cause subacute combined degeneration of the spinal cord, which is degeneration of the posterior and lateral columns of the spinal cord.
- B_9 (folate) deficiency also causes a macrocytic anemia, but does NOT cause neurologic symptoms.

Clinical Presentation

- Vague neuropsychiatric symptoms: fatigue, irritability, depression
- Neuropathic symptoms: decreased proprioception and vibration sensation, balance problems, and paresthesias affecting the legs more severely than the arms
- Glossitis

Diagnosis and Evaluation

- Complete blood count: macrocytic anemia, potentially pancytopenia
- Serum B_{12}: if normal or low-normal levels but clinical picture is consistent, may need to send intermediates in B_{12} and folate metabolism (such as methylmalonic acid and homocysteine, respectively) but this is typically not done in the emergency department.
- Consider checking serum folate (not necessary in those with normal diet and no history of gastrointestinal disease or surgery).

Treatment

- Vitamin B_{12} 1000 μg intramuscularly or subcutaneously (typically weekly until deficiency is corrected, then monthly as maintenance therapy)
- If patient has normal absorption (e.g., dietary deficiency rather than pernicious anemia), oral dosing is effective. For those with impaired absorption, very high oral doses may be effective given that passive diffusion allows for some absorption.

SUGGESTED READINGS

Lew, E. K., & Penney, D. W. (2015). Demyelinating disease. In Wolfson, A. B., Cloutier, R. L., Hendey, G. W., Ling, L. J., Rosen, C. L., & Schaider, J. J. (Eds.), *Harwood-Nuss' clinical practice of emergency medicine* (6th ed., pp. 2065–2069). Wolters Kluwer.

Marra, C. M. (2020, August 12). *Neurosyphilis*. UpToDate. https://www.uptodate.com/contents/neurosyphilis?search=Neurosyphilis&source=search_result&selectedTitle=1~73&usage_type=default&display_rank=1

Olek, M. J., & Howard, J. (2019, October 30). *Evaluation and diagnosis of multiple sclerosis in adults*. UpToDate. https://www.uptodate.com/contents/evaluation-and-diagnosis-of-multiple-sclerosis-in-adults?search=multiple%20sclerosis&source=search_result&selectedTitle=1~150&usage_type=default&display_rank=1

Vriesendorp, F. J. (2018, December 4). *Guillain-Barré syndrome in adults: Clinical features and diagnosis*. UpToDate. https://www.uptodate.com/contents/guillain-barre-syndrome-in-adults-clinical-features-and-diagnosis?search=guillain%20barre&source=search_result&selectedTitle=1~150&usage_type=default&display_rank=1

CHAPTER 78

BOARD REVIEW

Disorders Presenting with Headache and Associated Symptoms

CATHERINE WEAVER, MD, and HANNAH WALLACE, MD, MPH

General Principles

- Headaches account for 3%–5% of all emergency department visits in the United States, making it the fourth most common chief complaint. Although approximately 90% of headache presentations are for benign headaches, the remaining 10% have "can't-miss," potentially life-threatening etiologies. Even benign headaches can cause severe distress to patients; it is crucial for physicians to be proficient in identifying key historical and physical examination findings to evaluate for "red flags" (Table 78.1) that may indicate dangerous etiologies. Any of these findings should prompt physicians to consider further workup to rule out life-threatening etiologies of headaches. Importantly, response to pain medications does *not* exclude life-threatening causes.

Can't-Miss Diagnoses

- Can't-miss headaches are rare, accounting for approximately 10% of headache visits. The differential for headaches, even potentially fatal ones, is broad and encompasses intracranial bleeds, infectious etiologies, vascular pathologies, pressure-related ones, or toxic exposure to carbon monoxide. Consider mass effect from tumor in an older patient with progressively worsening headache over time or in a child with positional headaches and vomiting.

Hemorrhage

- Bleeding in the brain can be spontaneous or traumatic. It can be related to elevated intracranial pressure or coagulopathy owing to anticoagulants, liver disease, and so forth. Most of these presentations are worked up and managed in similar ways, as discussed in the sections below. Remember that airway, breathing, and circulation (ABCs) remain the priority: consider early intubation for patients with declining mental status (and, in the traumatically injured patient, Glasgow Coma Scale [GCS] ≤8). If the patient is intubated, use adequate sedation to allow for ventilator synchrony. Head of bed (HOB) should remain elevated to 30 degrees.

Subarachnoid Hemorrhage

General Principles

- Subarachnoid hemorrhage (SAH) can be traumatic or spontaneous (most common). If spontaneous, it is typically related to rupture of a cerebral artery aneurysm, but arteriovenous malformations and idiopathic etiologies can occur. From 10% to 50% of cases have a sentinel bleed that occurs days to weeks prior to fatal hemorrhage and may present similarly to rupture. Fatality rates up to 50% have been described in cases of missed diagnosis of

TABLE 78.1 *Headache Red Flags*

Patient Characteristics	Signs and Symptoms
Immunocompromise (HIV, malignancy, immunosuppressants)	Altered mental status
No prior headache history or significant change from previous headache	Seizure
Toxic-appearing patient	Sudden or maximal-at-onset pain
Age > 50	Association with exertion (exercise, straining, or orgasm), Valsalva, or posture
Pregnancy or postpartum	Syncope
Anticoagulation use	Recurrent vomiting
Illicit drug use	Neck stiffness or other meningeal signs
Recent chiropractic neck manipulation	Visual disturbances
Trauma	Papilledema found on fundoscopic exam or increased optic nerve sheath diameter via ocular ultrasound
	Acute neurologic deficits

SAH. Risk factors include history of aneurysm or polycystic kidney disease in self or family, severe hypertension, and previous vascular lesions in other areas of the body.

Clinical Presentation

- Sudden, severe ("thunderclap" or "worst of my life") headache, may be exertional or after orgasm; maximal within 1 hour of onset
- Often includes transient alteration of consciousness, neck pain or stiffness, photophobia
- Cranial nerve (CN) III palsy with associated ipsilateral pupillary dilation from a compressive aneurysm
- Severe SAH can present with focal neurologic deficits and coma.

Diagnosis and Evaluation

- Obtain computed tomography (CT) of the head without contrast.
  - If negative and obtained within 6 hours of headache, SAH can be ruled out per 2019 American College of Emergency Physicians (ACEP) clinical policy.
  - If negative and obtained *after* 6 hours of headache, SAH is not yet ruled out, and the patient requires either a lumbar puncture (LP) or computed tomography angiography (CTA). If either test is negative, the diagnosis can be ruled out. If the CTA is positive, it is assumed that the patient has an aneurysmal subarachnoid hemorrhage.
  - If CT of the brain without contrast is positive for subarachnoid hemorrhage, obtain CTA to evaluate for aneurysm location and size.

Treatment

- **Neurosurgery consultation** for surgical clipping or endovascular coiling by interventional radiology (IR).
- Tight blood pressure control. Optimal goal blood pressure is not clear, but American Stroke Association guidelines recommend systolic blood pressure (SBP) less than 160 mm Hg using titratable medication, such as labetalol, esmolol, enalapril, or nicardipine (avoid nitroprusside or nitroglycerin, which can increase intracranial pressure [ICP]).
- Nimodipine (60 mg oral every 4 hours); reduces blood pressure (albeit with lability) and severe neurologic deficit. Exact mechanism is unknown; evidence has *not* shown that it reduces secondary vasospasm.
- Discontinue antithrombotic medications and reverse any anticoagulants.
- Consider seizure prophylaxis (controversial).

Epidural Hematoma

General Principles

Epidural hematomas (EDH) are most commonly caused by trauma that shears the middle meningeal artery, although they can be caused by venous bleeding as well.

Clinical Presentation

- May present with coma or initial loss of consciousness followed by a transient "lucid interval" of normal mentation that rapidly progresses to acute altered mental status (AMS) or somnolence.
- Anisocoria, focal neurologic deficits, evidence of trauma on physical examination, Cushing reflex

Diagnosis and Evaluation

- CT of the brain without contrast demonstrates biconvex hematoma in the middle cranial fossa.

Treatment

- Neurosurgical consultation for surgical evacuation in patients with focal neurologic deficits or symptoms secondary to an acute EDH. Small and asymptomatic EDH may be managed nonsurgically in consultation with neurosurgery.
- Prior to surgical intervention, any coagulopathy must be addressed.
- If evidence of elevated ICP and/or herniation, treat with HOB elevation, hyperventilation, and an osmotic agent (mannitol or hypertonic saline) in consultation with neurosurgery.
- For those with a moderate GCS, consider tranexamic acid (CRASH 3 trial).

Subdural Hematoma

General Principles

Subdural hematomas (SDH), which are caused by shearing of bridging veins, are often, but not always, associated with trauma (acute, subacute, or recurrent minor injuries). Advanced age, history of alcohol dependence, and use of anticoagulants increase risk.

Clinical Presentation

- Gradually increasing headache and confusion; patient may not remember trauma.
- Symptoms typically have a slower onset than EDH and presentation can be delayed.
- If the SDH is large, patient may have signs of increased intracranial pressure or focal neurologic findings. Other symptoms may include altered mental status, irritability, seizures, dizziness, weakness/lethargy, nausea, vomiting, personality changes, and ataxia.

Diagnosis and Evaluation

- CT of the brain without contrast demonstrates crescent-shaped hematoma.

Treatment

- Consult neurosurgery. Treatment depends on size and growth rate. Small SDH can be monitored for reabsorption; others require surgical drainage or craniotomy.
- As with other intracranial hemorrhages, consider reversal of coagulopathies, consider antiepileptic therapy, and address elevated ICP, as needed.
- For those with a moderate GCS, consider tranexamic acid (CRASH 3 trial).

Hemorrhagic Stroke

General Principles

Less common than ischemic strokes, hemorrhagic strokes occur when a blood vessel in the brain ruptures and bleeds into the surrounding tissue. Hemorrhagic strokes can be intracerebral (i.e., intraparenchymal or intraventricular) or subarachnoid. They are more common in patients with preexisting vascular pathology of some kind (such as cerebral amyloid angiopathy, cerebral arteriovenous malformations, or vascular aneurysms) or in patients with severe hypertension.

Clinical Presentation

- Symptoms typically start suddenly; however, unlike in ischemic strokes, hemorrhagic stroke symptoms are more likely to progress as bleeding or edema worsens.
- Symptoms depend on the location of the hemorrhage but typically include headache and focal neurologic deficits, with or without nausea, vomiting, and/or altered mental status.

Diagnosis and Evaluation

- CT of the brain without contrast

Treatment

- Current guidelines recommend a SBP goal of 140 mm Hg using titratable medication, such as labetalol, esmolol, enalapril, or nicardipine (avoid nitroprusside or nitroglycerin as these can increase ICP).
- Discontinue antithrombotic medications and reverse any anticoagulation with appropriate agents. Platelet transfusions should be avoided and may be hazardous.

Pituitary Apoplexy

General Principles

Pituitary apoplexy is very rare but life-threatening and is most commonly caused by a rapidly enlarging, nonfunctioning pituitary macroadenoma that develops hemorrhage and/or infarction. It is most common in men older than age 50 with preexisting adenoma, but it should also be considered in pregnant women owing to massive hyperplasia of lactotrophs causing the pituitary gland to grow significantly, either outgrowing or compressing its blood supply.

Clinical Presentation

- Sometimes sudden, severe headache, with nausea/vomiting, plus or minus meningeal irritation.
- Impaired consciousness, CN palsy, visual disturbances, variable ocular paresis are common.
- Look for hypoadrenalism/adrenal crisis, hypopituitarism (hypotension, hyponatremia).

Diagnosis and Evaluation

- Magnetic resonance imaging (MRI) of the brain with contrast is superior to CT without contrast (sensitivity: 91% vs. 28%).
- Laboratory studies to evaluate pituitary insufficiency in consultation with an endocrinologist

Treatment

- Surgical decompression if persistent visual symptoms, neurologic deficit, or AMS
- Treat secondary adrenal insufficiency with intravenous fluids (IVF), electrolyte replacement, and hydrocortisone.

Infections

MENINGITIS

General Principles

Meningitis, which is the inflammation of the leptomeninges surrounding the brain and spinal cord, can be caused by bacterial, viral, or fungal infections and can be rapidly fatal, even to previously healthy patients. Meningitis is more common in immunocompromised patients, those with general debilitation, extremes of age (very young or very old), accompanying concurrent acute febrile illness, those living in impacted conditions such as military barracks or college dormitories, and patients who are not vaccinated. Patients with recent sinus or ear infection or recent dental, ear nose throat (ENT), or neurosurgical procedure are also at high risk.

Clinical Presentation

- Gradual onset, nonfocal headache with decreased mentation and irritability
- Nuchal rigidity and pain, photophobia; typically fever is present.
- Rare to have focal neurologic findings, but seizures may occur.
- Severely immunocompromised persons may *not* present with fever, nuchal rigidity, or severe headache.
- Infants may just have fever, somnolence, and irritability.
- Look for rash, especially with meningococcal meningitis.
- "Classic" (low-sensitivity) signs:
  - Brudzinski sign: spontaneous flexion of hip with passive flexion of neck
  - Kernig sign: with hips flexed 90 degrees, resistance of full extension of the knees

Diagnosis and Evaluation

- Plus or minus CT of the brain without contrast: always get CT if the patient has evidence of increased ICP (papilledema, focal neurologic deficit, seizures, AMS), history of known central nervous system (CNS) disease, or has any *reason* to have increased ICP (human immunodeficiency virus or acquired immunodeficiency syndrome [HIV/AIDS], history of cancer, recent sinusitis, or other ENT infection or surgery that could lead to abscess)
- Lumbar puncture (see Table 78.2 for typical cerebrospinal fluid [CSF] results)

Treatment

- Most important: do not wait for laboratory, CT, or LP results to treat.
- Give steroids (dexamethasone) before or at same time as antibiotics. Steroids have been shown to decrease hearing loss and neurologic deficits in pneumococcal meningitis.
- Droplet isolation precautions if meningococcemia is being considered.

Treatment by age:

- **Less than 1 month:** ampicillin AND gentamicin OR cefotaxime OR ceftazidime. Consider acyclovir.
- **1 to 23 months:** ampicillin AND vancomycin AND cefotaxime OR ceftriaxone
- **Age 2 to adult:** ceftriaxone OR cefotaxime AND vancomycin ± ampicillin (if more than **50 years of age or immunocompromised,** for listeria)

TABLE 78.2 *Lumbar Puncture Cerebrospinal Fluid Analysis*

	Normal	Viral	Bacterial
Glucose	0.6:1 (CSF:serum) OR 50–80 mg/dL	Normal	< 0.4:1 (CSF:serum) OR < 40 mg/dL ***also consider tuberculosis (TB) or fungal meningitis, neurosyphilis, or some viral infections such as mumps and lymphocytic choriomeningitis (LCMV)
Protein	< 50 mg/dL	50–300 mg/dL ***also consider CNS Lyme disease, neurosyphilis, TB meningitis	100–500 mg/dL
WBC	< 5/mm^3 < 1 PMN/mm^3	< 1000/mm^3 (mostly lymphocytic) ***also consider neurosyphilis or TB meningitis (or very early bacterial meningitis)	>1000/mm^3 (mostly PMN, however early can be lymphocytic) ***also consider TB, mumps, and LCMV

- **Healthcare-associated:** vancomycin AND cefepime OR ceftazidime OR meropenem

Treatment: Other

- Herpes simplex virus (HSV): acyclovir
- Cryptococcus: amphotericin B + flucytosine
- Tuberculosis: isoniazid + rifampin + pyrazinamide + ethambutol
- **Antibiotic prophylaxis** for close contacts of confirmed meningococcal meningitis (household members, day care center contacts, anyone directly exposed to oral secretions):
- Adults: ciprofloxacin 500 mg oral × 1 OR rifampin 600 mg every 12 hours × 2 days.
- Children: oral rifampin OR intramuscular ceftriaxone OR oral azithromycin

Encephalitis

General Principles

Encephalitis and intracranial abscesses share the same risk factors as meningitis. Patients with encephalitis, an infection with inflammation of the brain itself rather than the meninges, generally present with fever, altered mental status, often seizures, and may demonstrate focal neurologic findings; they do not typically develop significant nuchal rigidity or pain. The most common causes of encephalitis are viral infections, but bacterial and noninfectious inflammatory conditions (or postinfectious immune response) can occur as well. The most common causes of viral encephalitis include West Nile virus, herpes simplex virus (HSV), Epstein-Barr virus, varicella zoster, coxsackievirus, influenza, and arthropod-borne viruses. Viruses, such as measles (rubeola), mumps, and German measles (rubella), used to be fairly common causes of encephalitis; there is increasing prevalence relating to a recent decrease in vaccinations. Rabies virus is a rare cause of encephalitis in the United States.

Clinical Presentation

- AMS, fever, seizures; plus or minus headaches, loss of consciousness, vomiting, photophobia, focal neurologic deficits, irritability, plus or minus hallucinations
- HSV encephalitis presents with notable personality changes, temporal lobe changes on CT.
- Rabies encephalitis may present with hydrophobia, aerophobia, pharyngeal spasms, bulbar deficits, hyperactivity subsiding to paralysis and coma.
- Flaccid paralysis: consider West Nile virus encephalitis.
- Grouped vesicles in a dermatomal pattern may suggest varicella zoster virus; but *not* having a rash does not rule this out.

Diagnosis and Evaluation

- See "Meningitis: Diagnosis and Evaluation." Send additional cerebral spinal fluid (CSF) studies, including CSF polymerase chain reaction for HSV-1, HSV-2, and enteroviruses. Consider serology for arboviruses, HIV, and so forth.

Treatment

- See "Meningitis: Treatment" above. Consider steroids and antibiotic therapy. If signs and symptoms concerning for HSV encephalitis, start intravenous (IV) acyclovir early. Other viral encephalitis treatment is primarily supportive.

Brain Abscess

General Principles

Meningitis, encephalitis, and brain abscesses largely share the same risk factors. Patients with abscesses are more likely to demonstrate focal neurologic findings in addition to the AMS, headaches, and fevers that present with meningitis and encephalitis. Brain abscesses especially should be suspected in patients with AIDS and in those who complain of worsening headache, high fevers, and focal neurologic deficits following a sinus infection.

Clinical Presentation

- Headache (often localized to side of abscess), fever, AMS, seizures, and often focal neurologic deficits

correlating with abscess location, plus or minus nuchal rigidity
- Changes in mental status are indicative of severe cerebral edema.
- Vomiting and CN (III and VI) palsies can occur with increased ICP.

Diagnosis and Evaluation

- CT of the brain **with contrast** (or MRI, which is superior but oftentimes more difficult to obtain)
- **Lumbar puncture is contraindicated** in patients with focal neurologic findings.

Treatment

- Antibiotics based on presumptive source of abscess:
  - **Oral, otogenic, or sinus:** metronidazole + either penicillin G for oral source *OR* ceftriaxone or cefotaxime for sinus or otogenic source
  - **Hematogenous spread:** vancomycin for methicillin-resistant *Staphylococcus aureus* coverage plus or minus metronidazole and ceftriaxone OR cefotaxime
  - **Postoperative neurosurgical:** vancomycin + ceftazidime OR cefepime OR meropenem
  - **After penetrating trauma:** vancomycin + ceftriaxone OR cefotaxime + metronidazole if paranasal sinuses are involved
  - **Unknown:** vancomycin + ceftriaxone OR cefotaxime + metronidazole
- Dexamethasone 10 mg IV × 1 then 4 mg IV every 6 hours for mass effect or altered mental status
- **May require needle aspiration or surgical excision:** call neurosurgeon upon diagnosis.

Cavernous Sinus Thrombosis

General Principles

Cavernous sinus thrombosis is an extremely rare complication of common facial infections, such as bacterial sinusitis (typically sphenoidal or ethmoidal), nasal furuncles, or dental infections. These septic thrombi are most often caused by *Staphylococcus aureus* or *Streptococcus* sp., although anaerobes are common when the underlying condition is from a dental or sinus infection. Symptoms and complications of cavernous sinus thrombosis are explained by the location of CN III, IV, VI, as well as the ophthalmic and maxillary branches of CN V that are immediately adjacent to the sinus.

Clinical Presentation

- Severe headache; usually unilateral, in CN V_1 and V_2 dermatomes, retroorbital, frontal
- Proptosis, ophthalmoplegia (especially CN VI palsy), anisocoria, or mydriasis (CN III dysfunction), vision loss, eyelid edema, papilledema, fevers
- Sensation changes localized to the V_1, V_2 dermatomes
- AMS, seizures, and other focal neurologic deficits are signs of CNS spread
- Always consider this diagnosis in patients with orbital cellulitis + CN dysfunction, bilateral eye involvement, or mental status changes.

Diagnosis and Evaluation

- MRI/magnetic resonance venography (MRV) (preferred) or CT/computed tomography venography (CTV). Consider adjunct testing: laboratory studies, cultures, plus or minus LP.

Treatment

- Vancomycin + ceftriaxone OR cefepime + metronidazole, if sinusitis or dental
- May require surgical drainage

Vascular Emergencies

CERVICAL ARTERY DISSECTION

General Principles

Cervical artery dissections, which can be spontaneous or traumatic, can occur in the vertebral or carotid arteries and cause approximately 20% of strokes in adults less than 50 years of age. Disruption of blood vessel intima leads to hematoma formation and eventually thromboembolic stroke.

Clinical Presentation

- Both carotid and vertebral dissections present with neck pain and often headache.
- **Vertebral artery dissections** typically are preceded by recent flexion/extension trauma and present with posterior circulation stroke symptoms (vertigo, dizziness, dyscoordination).
- **Carotid artery dissections** typically present with anterior circulation stroke symptoms, such as hemiplegia, slurred speech, or partial Horner syndrome (ptosis/miosis).

Diagnosis and Evaluation

- CTA (or magnetic resonance angiography [MRA]) of the neck plus or minus the brain

Treatment

- Thrombolysis with tissue-type plasminogen activator (tPA) in setting of acute ischemic stroke.
- **Medical management for stroke prevention:** antiplatelet therapy (aspirin or clopidogrel)

TEMPORAL (GIANT CELL) ARTERITIS

General Principles

Giant cell arteritis (GCA) is a very rare diagnosis, more likely in women and almost exclusively in patients above age 50. Polymyalgia rheumatica and other collagen vascular or inflammatory diseases are present in more than half of patients with this disorder. It is crucial to diagnose GCA early and initiate treatment immediately once highly suspected in order to prevent blindness.

Clinical Presentation

- Localized symptoms: headache with temporal tenderness and jaw claudication
- Consider polymyalgia rheumatica if systemic symptoms: fever, fatigue, nausea/vomiting, myalgias
- Visual symptoms: diplopia, amaurosis fugax, blindness

Diagnosis and Evaluation

- Physical examination with beading and/or tenderness over temporal arteries
- Elevated erythrocyte sedimentation rate (often above 100) plus or minus elevated C-reactive protein, although it may be normal
- Official diagnosis by temporal artery biopsy, but do not delay initiation of steroid therapy

Treatment

- Immediate corticosteroids: high-dose methylprednisolone 500 mg to 1000 mg IV (if vision loss) for 1 to 3 days, then oral prednisone (1 mg/kg/day up to 60 mg). If no vision loss, may begin with prednisone.

CEREBRAL VENOUS THROMBOSIS

General Principles

Cerebral venous thrombosis can be related to infection (such as septic thrombi in the cavernous sinus), trauma, or thrombotic disease from hypercoagulability. It typically presents gradually, but when thrombosed areas of the brain become infarcted, acute stroke-like symptoms can develop. Presentation can therefore vary depending on location and extent of thrombus.

Clinical Presentation

- Gradual-onset headache, may be localized or diffuse
- Plus or minus symptoms of elevated ICP, especially if hemorrhagic transformation (up to one-third)
- May have focal neurologic deficits or seizures; encephalopathy possible

Diagnosis and Evaluation

- MRI/MRV (preferred) or CT/CTV of the brain

Treatment

- Heparin or low molecular weight heparin followed by long-term oral anticoagulation treatment (controversial)
- Plus or minus an antiepileptic, depending on lesion location and seizures on presentation

Pressure-Related and Mass Effect Emergencies

HYPERTENSIVE EMERGENCY WITH ENCEPHALOPATHY

General Principles

Hypertensive emergency with encephalopathy is characterized by significant hypertension in association with severe headache (which may occur before hypertension), vomiting, visual disturbance, seizures, or coma. Hypertensive emergency can be caused by essential hypertension, by secondary causes such as renal, endocrinological, or cardiac disorders, as well as intoxications. Symptoms are thought to be caused by rapidly increasing blood pressure causing vascular injury with ischemia and edema of the brain; meanwhile, high systemic blood pressure induces brain vessel vasoconstriction, increasing permeability and causing worsening edema and sometimes hemorrhage. The distinguishing factor with hypertensive emergency compared with similar syndromes is clinical improvement with reduction of blood pressure.

Clinical Presentation

- Systemic: significant hypertension, nausea, vomiting
- Neurologic: acute-onset headache, altered mental status, seizures, visual disturbances

Diagnosis and Evaluation

- Physical examination, including fundoscopic examination and blood pressure measurements
- Laboratory work to evaluate for end-organ damage, including complete blood cell count (CBC), comprehensive metabolic panel (CMP), troponin, urinalysis (UA)
- Electrocardiogram (ECG) plus or minus electroencephalogram if seizures or significantly impaired consciousness
- CT of the brain without contrast (and/or MRI)

Treatment

- Antihypertensives with goal of mean arterial pressure (MAP) reduction by 10%-20% in first hour, 25% in first day via vasodilation (nicardipine) or beta- or adrenergic-blockade (esmolol, labetalol).

POSTERIOR REVERSIBLE ENCEPHALOPATHY SYNDROME (PRES)

General Principles

A severe form of hypertensive emergency, PRES is generally reversible and often related to medications (especially immunosuppressants), eclampsia, or hypertensive encephalopathy. The pathogenesis of PRES is unclear and thought to be multifactorial.

Clinical Presentation

- Systemic: often significant hypertension, but blood pressure is variable and may be normal
- Neurologic: acute-onset headache, altered mental status, seizures, visual disturbances

Diagnosis and Evaluation

- Noncontrast CT or MRI (more sensitive) of the brain: demonstrates symmetric white matter vasogenic edema, especially in the posterior cerebral hemispheres

Treatment

- Discontinue any causative medications.
- Antihypertensives: consider vasodilators (especially nicardipine) or adrenergic blockers such as labetalol or esmolol. Goal: reduction of MAP by 10%–25% in first hour.

IDIOPATHIC INTRACRANIAL HYPERTENSION (PSEUDOTUMOR CEREBRI)

General Principles

Idiopathic intracranial hypertension is typically associated with young, obese women, with a higher risk in those taking retinoids, tetracyclines, and excessive vitamin A. It is diagnosed in absence of other etiology for intracranial hypertension (mass, abscess, bleeding, or other space-occupying lesion).

Clinical Presentation

- Signs and symptoms of increased ICP: headache, pulsatile tinnitus, papilledema, visual disturbances, but without impaired level of consciousness, no fevers, and generally no other focal neurologic deficits (except CN VI palsy may be seen)

Diagnosis and Evaluation

- MRI/MRV (preferred) or CT of the brain demonstrating no space-occupying lesions or hemorrhage
- LP with elevated opening pressure greater than 200 mm H_2O and normal CSF cells, protein, glucose

Treatment

- LP: diagnostic and therapeutic, although generally temporary
- Weight loss for obese patients plus or minus a low-sodium diet
- Medications: acetazolamide 500 mg oral twice a day (decreases CSF production in the choroid plexus); alternatives: topiramate or furosemide (can also be adjunctive therapy)
- Surgical intervention for refractory cases

TUMOR WITH MASS EFFECT

General Principles

Tumors generally grow slowly with progression of signs and symptoms of increased ICP, focal neurologic findings, and headache. Occasionally more rapid development of vasogenic edema or hemorrhage can cause accelerated decompensation. Without hard neurologic findings or signs of ICP, tumors will be difficult to diagnose and are likely to be missed on initial presentation.

Clinical Presentation

- Progressive, dull, generally nonfocal headache with decreased mentation, vomiting, and eventual focal neurologic deficits or seizures. Wide variability of symptoms, depending on tumor location, growth rate, and any secondary complications.

Diagnosis and Evaluation

- Initial imaging: CT of the brain without contrast; **MRI of the brain** has higher sensitivity/specificity

Treatment

- Tumor treatment varies widely depending on diagnosis.
- Vasogenic edema is generally treated initially by corticosteroids (dexamethasone with dose dependent upon extent of edema and severity of symptoms).
- If intracranial bleeding, any coagulopathy present should be addressed.
- Consult neurosurgery plus or minus neuro-oncology.

PREECLAMPSIA

General Principles

Preeclampsia and eclampsia occur as a spectrum of disease in pregnant and postpartum women. Pathophysiology is poorly understood and thought to be multifactorial. Patients must be more than 20 weeks estimated gestational age (EGA) or fewer than 6 weeks postpartum and normotensive prior to pregnancy. For more information, please refer to Chapter 91, Late Pregnancy Complications.

ACUTE ANGLE CLOSURE GLAUCOMA

General Principles

Acute angle glaucoma typically occurs in patients older than age 40 to 50 (women 4:1 compared with men) with a history of glaucoma. Patients typically report pain increasing in a dark place owing to sudden dilation of pupils, causing outflow obstruction of aqueous humor through the anterior chamber, leading to a rapid increase of the intraocular pressure (IOP).

Clinical Presentation

- Sudden onset of severe, typically unilateral eye pain with blurred vision or vision loss, halos around bright lights, photophobia. Nausea and vomiting are common.
- Physical examination: acute red eye, mid-dilated pupil, poorly reactive, "steamy" cornea, eye may feel firm to palpation

Diagnosis and Evaluation

- Measurement of IOP via tonometer: up to 60 to 80 mm Hg in acute attack (normal: 10 to 21 mm Hg)

Treatment

- Drops: timolol (beta-blocker) + pilocarpine (miotic) + apraclonidine (alpha-2 agonist)
- Intravenous: acetazolamide (contraindicated in sickle cell trait or disease)
- Immediate ophthalmology consultation (consider laser therapy or surgery).

CARBON MONOXIDE POISONING

General Principles

Carbon monoxide poisoning is an important toxicologic cause of morbidity and mortality worldwide. The odorless, colorless gas results from incomplete combustion of carbon-containing substances and causes tissue hypoxia via binding to hemoglobin, which can result in significant neurologic sequelae, reduced life expectancy, and even death. Typical exposures include car exhaust (especially when breathing in enclosed or confined spaces with engine running), poor ventilation of heating equipment such as furnaces, fires, and industrial accidents.

Clinical Presentation

- Multiple household members presenting with similar symptoms.
- Headache, dizziness, weakness, nausea/vomiting, seizure, coma, cardiopulmonary symptoms.
- **Ask about exposures.** Patients often feel better after leaving the exposure site, but have recurrent symptoms when they return.

Diagnosis and Evaluation

- Carboxyhemoglobin (COHb) concentration: severity depends on duration of exposure and the underlying

health of the patient and can be measured via arterial or venous blood gas.
- Does NOT alter standard pulse oximetry; patient will appear to have 100% saturation.
- Assess severity and possible coexistent poisonings (i.e., cyanide). ECG, CBC, basic metabolic panel (BMP), venous blood gas (VBG).

Treatment

- Remove patient from exposure.
- Administer oxygen: 100% via nonrebreather (NRB) or ventilator for at least 6 hours.
- ABCs; consider intubation if consciousness impaired.
- Hyperbaric oxygen therapy may be beneficial for patients with severe carbon monoxide poisoning (prolonged unconsciousness, evidence of end-organ ischemia, such as AMS, ECG changes, chest pain), severe acidosis (pH <7.1), prolonged exposure, COHb >25%, or pregnancy with significant exposure, any severe symptoms, or COHb >20%).

BENIGN DIAGNOSES (SEE TABLE 78.3)

SUGGESTED READINGS

Marx, J. A., Hockberger, R. S., & Walls, R. M. (Eds.). (2014). *Rosen's emergency medicine: Concepts and clinical practice* (8th ed., pp. 170–175). Elsevier/Saunders.

Schoen, J. C., Campbell, R. L., & Sadosty, A. T. (2015). Headache in pregnancy: An approach to emergency department evaluation and management. *Western Journal of Emergency Medicine, 16*(2), 291–301.

Zodda, D., Procopio, G., & Gupta, A. (2019). Evaluation and management of life-threatening headaches in the emergency department. *Emergency Medicine Practice, 21*(2), 1–20.

TABLE 78.3 *Benign Headache Diagnoses*

Disorder/Diagnosis	History + Physical Key Points	Workup?	Treatment
Primary Headaches			
Migraine	Unilateral, throbbing/pulsatile, sometimes auras, n/v, photophobia/phonophobia, worse with activity. More common in women.	Clinical diagnosis	NSAIDs, acetaminophen, antiemetics (i.e., metoclopramide, prochlorperazine), IVF. Intractable: consider dexamethasone, sumatriptan, magnesium, opiate.
Cluster	Unilateral, sudden, cyclical (weeks to months), orbital/supraorbital/temporal with conjunctival injection, lacrimation, facial sweating, rhinorrhea, congestion, miosis, ptosis, eyelid edema. Frequently male.	Clinical diagnosis	**Oxygen**, other above treatments (although antiemetics less successful). Consider intranasal lidocaine or octreotide.
Tension	Bilateral, tight, frequent exacerbations, nonthrobbing, generally does not worsen with normal activity	Clinical diagnosis of exclusion	NSAIDs, acetaminophen, caffeine, antiemetics
Infectious			
Sinusitis	URI, purulent mucus, sinus tenderness, facial or dental pain/pressure	Clinical +/- CT	NSAIDs, nasal glucocorticoids, decongestant, saline irrigation, ± antibiotics
Systemic Illnesses	HA related to PNA, UTI, viral syndrome, or other illness	Work up systemic disease	Treatment of systemic disease + acetaminophen/NSAIDs
Neuropathic			
Occipital Neuralgia	Piercing, throbbing, or shock-like pain in upper neck, back of head, and behind ears. Usually unilateral, sometimes bilateral. Can have dysesthesia at site. Tenderness to palpation at occipital nerve area.	Clinical diagnosis	Trial occipital nerve block (consider bupivacaine ± triamcinolone) into affected area at point of maximal tenderness if someone experienced in procedure is available. NSAIDs, local heat/cold, massage, rest.
Trigeminal Neuralgia	Episodic, severe, shooting/jabbing/electrical pain to trigeminal nerve distribution, typically unilaterally. Often trigged by eating/drinking, touching the face, smiling, speaking, brushing teeth.	Clinical diagnosis ± imaging to rule out other etiology, such as multiple sclerosis, tumor, and so forth	Carbamazepine (first line), oxcarbazepine, lamotrigine, phenytoin, clonazepam, gabapentin. ± baclofen. Eventually may require injections or surgery.
Other			
Post-Lumbar Puncture	Positional (worse with sitting/standing), hours to days after LP	Clinical diagnosis	IVF, caffeine (high dose), blood patch
Analgesia or Caffeine Rebound	Frequent (>3 times / week) analgesic use, daily caffeine use.	Clinical diagnosis	Weaning medication; other symptomatic control while recovering.
TMJ Disease	Clicking or snapping sensation of jaw, decreased mandible ROM, pain with jaw movement. TMJ tenderness, jaw deviation to affected side possible.	Clinical diagnosis	Behavioral modification, trigger avoidance is key. NSAIDs, acetaminophen, tricyclic antidepressants (low dose), muscle relaxants. Oral splints or mouth guards, physical therapy (stretch, strengthen, moist heat, ice).
Dehydration	Mild to severe pain with clear temporal relationship to dehydration. Most similar to tension or migraine HA. Associated thirst + reduced urination.	Clinical diagnosis	Rehydration
Exertional + Post-Coital	Onset with physical or sexual activity. Bilateral, pulsating, self-limiting. More common in hot weather, high altitude.	Clinical diagnosis. **Consider SAH!**	Self-limiting. NSAIDs, sometimes prophylactic, including propranolol.

CT, computed tomography; *HA,* headache; *IVF,* intravenous fluids; *LP,* lumbar puncture; *NSAIDs,* nonsteroidal antiinflammatory drugs; *n/v,* nausea and vomiting; *PNA,* pneumonia; *ROM,* range of motion; *SAH,* subarachnoid hemorrhage; *TMJ,* temporomandibular joint; *URI,* upper respiratory infection; *UTI,* urinary tract infection.

Seizures

DANIEL WEINGROW, DO, and JACQUELINE KURTH, MD

Major Categories of Seizure Types

"Focal aware seizures" roughly correspond to the previous "simple partial seizures" and seizures in which the patient has "focal impaired awareness" correspond to "complex partial seizures" (Fig. 79.1).

General Principals for Approach and Treatment of Seizures

- Check for hypoglycemia and assess and support patient's ABCs (airway, breathing, circulation).
- Consider seizure mimics such as syncope and arrythmia. Seek etiology for seizure, including the possibility of giving vitamin B_6 (pyridoxine) if the patient is taking isoniazid.
- Administer benzodiazepines and antiepileptics if needed to control seizure activity.
- Assess for refractory status epilepticus and nonconvulsive status epilepticus.
- Determine whether a workup of the seizure is indicated.

Status Epilepticus

- Status epilepticus is defined as a seizure lasting more than 5 minutes, or two or more seizures without recovering a normal consciousness between seizures. The overwhelming majority of seizures terminate spontaneously without intervention within 5 minutes. Because of the high rate of non-convulsive seizures, any patient not returning to baseline mental status should raise the concern for sub-clinical status epilepticus.
  - Place the patient on oxygen, and keep the patient's airway patent with jaw thrust, chin lift, or nasopharyngeal airway.
  - Establish intravenous (IV) access, and check bedside glucose for hypoglycemia (typically values <40 mg/dL).
  - First-line therapy is parenteral benzodiazepines.
    - IV lorazepam 0.1 mg/kg (adults 2–4 mg), may repeat 2–4 times
    - IV/intramuscular/intranasal midazolam 0.2 mg/kg (adults 5 mg IV, 10 mg intramuscularly), may repeat two to four times
  - Second-line therapy, administered over 10 minutes, if no response to benzodiazepines, and no concern of secondary causes of seizure (see below)
    - Phenytoin 1 gm IV loading dose
    - Fosphenytoin 20 PE/kg (maximum 1.5 g PE loading dose)
    - Valproic acid 40 mg/kg (maximum 3 g loading dose)
    - Levetiracetam 60 mg/kg (maximum 4.5 g loading dose)
  - If the patient does not respond to second-line therapy, endotracheal intubation is typically required to prevent respiratory failure when titrating high doses of third-line agents, facilitate transport of the patient to imaging or higher level of care, prevention of rhabdomyolysis.
  - All patients intubated require continuous electroencephalography (EEG) monitoring to ensure that the patient is not having non-convulsive status and ensure adequate epileptogenic suppression. If EEG monitoring is not available, transport should be arranged emergently so that this can be facilitated.
  - It is unclear the optimal third-line agent; although high-dose midazolam and propofol drips are commonly used, there is some experience with ketamine, inhaled anesthetic gases, pentobarbital, phenobarbital.
- Consider causes of seizures that are typically refractory to GABA agonists, such as hyponatremia, hypocalcemia, pyridoxine (B_6) deficiency (infantile or secondary to isoniazid), organophosphates, lithium, and eclampsia.

Special Circumstances

HISTORY OF EPILEPSY

- Many seizures in this population are due to a missed dose of anticonvulsants, stressors, or infection.
- If the anticonvulsant levels are subtherapeutic, a loading dose should be given.
- Patients with a history of epilepsy can have breakthrough seizures as an expected course of their seizure disorder.
- Consider performing a workup if there is a deviation from the normal seizure pattern of patients with a history of epilepsy.
- Evaluate for trauma secondary to loss of postural tone in patients with generalized seizures.

FIRST-TIME SEIZURE

- It is important to obtain historical clues to try to distinguish seizure from syncope, when there is doubt then an electroencphalography (EEG) is reasonable to evaluate for syncope.
- There is no indication to admit patients or start antiepileptics for a first-time unprovoked seizure if the patient has returned to their mental baseline.
- Computed tomography of the head should usually be obtained in the emergency department to evaluate for mass or bleeding. However, in a healthy patient who has returned to baseline and has no neurologic deficit and reliable and prompt follow-up, this can be deferred if CT or MRI is obtainable by a primary care doctor within a few days.

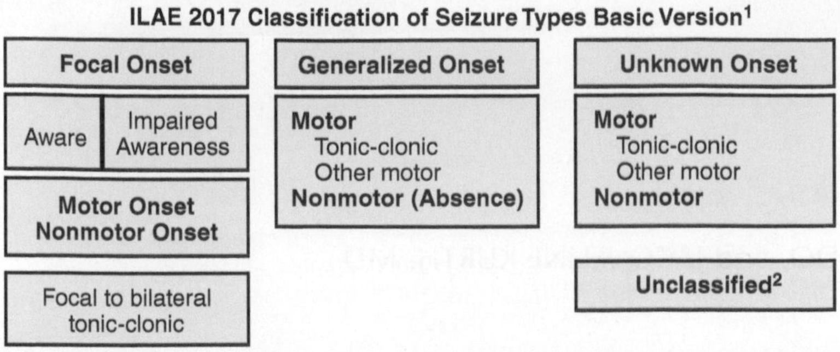

FIG. 79.1 Classification of seizure types. *ILAE*, International League Against Epilepsy. (From Fischer, R. (2017). An overview of the 2017 ILAE operational classification of epilepsy types [Editorial]. *Epilepsy & Behavior, 70*, 271–273.)
[1]Definitions, other seizure types and descriptors are listed in the accompanying paper and glossary of terms.
[2]Due to inadequate information or inability to place in other categories.

- In patients presenting with a provoked seizure, admission should be considered to minimize a recurrent seizure.
- Patients with a first-time seizure who are being discharged need to have specific instructions given to them to avoid dangerous activities, such as swimming, working with hazardous machines, and working at heights.
- A Department of Motor Vehicles form must be filled out in certain states for unexpected lapses in consciousness; reference your local applicable laws. Patients should be instructed not to drive until cleared by a neurologist or primary care physician.

PREGNANCY

- Eclampsia manifests at 20 weeks or more gestation and up to 6 weeks postpartum presenting with seizure, hypertension, edema, and proteinuria.
- High-dose magnesium sulfate 4–8 g IV should be used to treat the seizure, with emergent consultation with obstetrics/gynecology departments, because delivery of the fetus is definitive therapy.

PEDIATRIC FIRST-TIME SEIZURE

- In children who present with a first-time seizure, if they are back to their mental baseline, laboratory tests and neuroimaging from the ED are not routinely recommended. Typically this would be based on history and physical exam, but should be considered in children with focal neurologic findings, young age or developmental delay.
- If the patient does not return to their baseline or any concerning features are present, a workup should be obtained.
- A urine toxicology screen should be obtained if there is concern for ingestion.
- If the child has the appropriate clinical signs, or persistent alteration in mental status, a lumbar puncture should be performed.
- If the child is not high-risk, an outpatient magnetic resonance imaging study of their brain can be considered along with EEG, which can be coordinated with the patient's primary care physician.
- Initiation of anticonvulsants is generally not recommended after a first-time seizure in pediatrics. This allows time for further characterization of the type of seizure. Delay of medication does not increase the risk of epilepsy or worsen the prognosis.

Pediatric Febrile Seizure

SIMPLE FEBRILE SEIZURE

- Febrile seizures are common in the pediatric population and can be divided into simple and complex.
- A simple febrile seizure is a single seizure within a 24-hour period that occurs in a child age 6 months to 5 years. It lasts less than 15 minutes, is generalized at onset, and occurs when there is a fever of 38°C or higher.
- Children who experience a febrile seizure have roughly the same risk of developing epilepsy as the general public.
- No blood testing, neuroimaging, or EEG are necessary for simple pediatric febrile seizures. However, similar to any pediatric fever patient, a thorough examination and appropriate workup should be performed to determine the potential cause of fever.

COMPLEX FEBRILE SEIZURE

- A complex febrile seizure is defined as a seizure in the presence of fever that lasts more than 15 minutes, is localized, or recurs within a 24-hour period.
- In febrile children who appear ill or have prolonged seizure activity, investigation with blood, urine, and potentially cerebrospinal fluid should be performed.

Treatment for Febrile Seizures

- Anticonvulsant therapy is not indicated in febrile seizures. However, in cases of febrile status epilepticus, aggressive antiepileptics should be administered using a similar approach to nonfebrile status epilepticus.
- Antipyretics should be given in children who have a fever; however, there is no evidence that this prevents a recurrent febrile seizure.

SUGGESTED READINGS

Gupta, M. (2007). Mandatory reporting laws and the emergency physician. *Annals of Emergency Medicine*, *49*(3), 369–376.
Tintinalli, J. E., Ma, O. J., Yealy, D. M., Meckler, G. D., Stapczynski, J. S., Cline, D. M., & Thomas, S. H. (2020). *Tintinalli's emergency medicine: A comprehensive study guide* (9th ed.). McGraw Hill Education.
Wijdicks, E. F. M. (2016). *The practice of emergency and critical care neurology*. Oxford University Press.

Delirium

ATILLA UNER, MD, MPH, and CLAUDIE BOLDUC, MD, MPH

General Principles

- Delirium is an under-recognized problem in older patients in the emergency department (ED) that can lead to accelerated functional and cognitive decline, longer hospital stays, undue financial burden on the health-care system, increased rates of institutionalization, and increased morbidity and mortality if not identified and managed early.
- Delirium affects 7%–10% of ED visits for patients aged 65 years or older and is estimated to increase to 25% of visits for this age group by 2030. The emergency physician is uniquely positioned early in the care cycle to identify and intervene on the underlying etiology of delirium to prevent the downstream consequences. Unfortunately, emergency physicians currently overlook delirium as the cause of altered mental status in 75% of cases.

General Principles

Definition

- Delirium is defined as decompensation of cerebral function secondary to a precipitating stressor (e.g., infection) not better accounted for by another preexisting condition, or evolving dementia. Although clinical definitions vary, the *key* defining criteria per the *Diagnostic and statistical manual of mental disorders*, 5th Edition, are summarized as the following:
  - Disturbance in attention (reduced ability to focus) and awareness (reduced orientation)
  - An additional disturbance in cognition (e.g., perception, memory deficit)
  - Rapid onset (hours to days) representing a change from baseline
  - Fluctuations in cognition throughout the day
  - Disturbances not better categorized by a preexisting condition
  - Clinical, laboratory, or imaging evidence that the disturbance is the result of an underlying medical condition
- Additionally, delirium is classically described as being reversible when the underlying process resolves.
- The pathophysiology of delirium is not completely understood and is unlikely to be caused by a single mechanism.

Risk Factors

- Age (>65 years)
- Male sex
- Comorbidity (renal or hepatic disease)
- Dementia
- Polypharmacy

Clinical Presentation

- The chief complaint is often altered mental status for patients with delirium, but not always. Because the earliest manifestation can be subtle and is usually an alteration of consciousness such as inability to focus or deficient attention, the emergency physician should ask pointed questions to the family members to elicit this history. Delirium is categorized into psychomotor subtypes: hypoactive, hyperactive, and mixed. Hypoactive and mixed subtypes are the most prevalent in the ED populations, making up to 96% of cases.
  - Hypoactive: drowsy, lethargic, semi-comatose, appearing depressed
  - Mixed: features of both hypoactive and hyperactive delirium
  - Hyperactive ("agitated"): exhibiting hypervigilance, tachycardia, restlessness; having hallucinations and/or delusions

Delirium Versus Dementia

- Dementia is a well-known predisposing factor for delirium, and delirium is often superimposed on baseline dementia, making it difficult for health care providers to identify a new cognitive impairment. Table 80.1 lists key differentiators between dementia and delirium.
- An exception to these differences is in Lewy body dementia, which presents with rapid onset, fluctuations in consciousness, and parkinsonian motor symptoms.

Diagnosis and Evaluation

Diagnosis

- Several delirium screening tools exist, but many are not realistic for implementation in the ED.
- Inattention as the primary feature of delirium can be quickly ascertained at bedside and has been proposed as a key screening element for delirium.

TABLE 80.1 *Key Differences in Dementia Versus Delirium*

	Dementia	Delirium
Prognosis	Permanent cognitive impairment	Usually reversible
Rate of cognitive decline	Months to years	Hours to days
Consciousness	Attention intact	Fluctuating attention, altered level of consciousness

- Tests include 100 countdown, digit span (recalling and repeating progressively longer sequences of digits), or recitation of the months backwards.
- For patients who cannot speak, the Confusion Assessment Method (CAM) is one of the most widely applied screening tools for delirium. This tool may require history elements from family members at bedside.

Differential Diagnosis of Delirium

- These conditions do not constitute delirium secondary to an acute medical condition and should be ruled out:
  - Dementia
  - Psychiatric condition
  - Acute simple intoxication or withdrawal
  - Subclinical status epilepticus or postictal state
  - Other neurologic syndromes (e.g., Wernicke encephalopathy)

Etiologies/Precipitating Factors for Delirium

- Infection (including central nervous system infections)
- Inflammation (including postoperative)
- Electrolyte abnormality/metabolic causes
- Stroke or intracranial hemorrhage
- Acute coronary syndrome or heart failure
- Hypoxemia or hypercarbia
- Hypertensive encephalopathy
- Shock
- Uncontrolled pain (occult injury/fracture, urinary retention)
- Sleep deprivation
- Iatrogenic (restraints, indwelling urinary catheters)
- Psychoactive medications (anticholinergics, benzodiazepines, narcotics)
- Ingestion/withdrawal

Evaluation

- The evaluation is centered around finding the precipitating factor for the delirium once the diagnosis has been made. Thus the following elements are important in the assessment.

History

- Detailed review of home medications/recent changes
- Recent falls/procedures
- Recent infections/fevers
- History of drug and alcohol abuse

Physical Examination

- Vital signs, point-of-care blood glucose test, and core temperature
- Volume status
- Neurologic examination
- Signs of infection, including a thorough skin examination
- Toxidromes
- Careful examination of joints, extremities for signs of fractures/bruising

Investigations

- Infectious workup: urinalysis, complete blood count, chest x-ray, consider procalcitonin
- Metabolic workup: electrolytes including calcium, liver function tests, ammonia, serum urea nitrogen, creatinine, thyroid-stimulating hormone
- Electrocardiogram
- Computed tomographic scan of the head
- Others based on suspected etiology (troponin, blood gas with co-oximetry, urine drug screen, blood alcohol level, lumbar puncture, electroencephalograph, x-rays of injured limbs)

Treatment and Management

- Nonpharmacologic strategies are the first-line treatments or preventive tactics for all patients with or at risk for delirium. These include frequent re-orientation, quiet rooms, eye contact, cognitive stimulation, sleep protocols (avoiding sedative medications), and addressing sensory impairments (e.g., getting a patient's hearing aids). In addition, restraints should be avoided because they have been shown to prolong delirium when utilized.
  - The environment in most EDs is not conducive to the application of some of these nonpharmacologic strategies.
  - The increasing need to better serve the elderly emergency patient led to the development of the "geriatric ED," which appeared in 2008 and has since become increasingly common. The geriatric ED includes structural and process modifications targeted at improving prognosis in the elderly.
- Ultimately the most successful treatments for delirium are treatments targeted at reversing the precipitating factor.
- Finally, if necessary for patient safety, pharmacotherapies can be employed to manage a patient's symptoms of delirium, such as agitation.
  - Antipsychotics are the preferred agent for the treatment of agitated delirium.
  - Haloperidol and atypical antipsychotics (risperidone, olanzapine, quetiapine) have all been shown to be equally effective.
  - All antipsychotics can result in QT prolongation and have been linked to increased risk of stroke in elderly patients with dementia and thus should be used with caution in this group.
  - Benzodiazepines are not recommended, because they can exacerbate mental status changes or oversedate, especially in the elderly. An exception to this is the treatment of suspected alcohol withdrawal as the precipitating factor.

SUGGESTED READINGS

Han, J. H., Wilson, A., & Ely, E. W. (2010). Delirium in the older emergency department patient—A quiet epidemic. *Emergency Medicine Clinics of North America, 28*(3), 611–631.

Tamune, H., & Yasugi, D. (2017). How can we identify patients with delirium in the emergency department? A review of available screening and diagnostic tools. *American Journal of Emergency Medicine, 35*, 1332–1334.

CHAPTER **81**

BOARD REVIEW

Spinal Cord Disorders

SABRINA M. TOM, MD, and CHELSEA E. ROBINSON, MD

Overview

- Numerous significant pathologies affect the spinal cord. This chapter reviews some of the important nontraumatic causes of spinal cord dysfunction. Traumatic spinal cord injuries, including spinal cord syndromes, and spine disorders are discussed in Chapter 141 (Spine and Neck Trauma).
- Myelopathy is a disease process affecting the neurologic function of the spinal cord. It often results from spinal cord compression, but can also result from pathology intrinsic to the cord itself. In addition to traumatic injuries, common etiologies of myelopathy include autoimmune, infectious, neoplastic, vascular, congenital, and degenerative disorders (Box 81.1).

Extrinsic Spinal Cord Lesions

EPIDURAL COMPRESSION SYNDROMES

- Collective term encompassing spinal cord compression, including conus medullaris and cauda equina syndromes

BOX 81.1 *Differential Diagnosis for Nontraumatic Causes of Myelopathy*

EXTRINSIC LESIONS

Spinal epidural abscess
Spinal epidural hematoma
Neoplasm
Degenerative spine disease
Diskitis, osteomyelitis (e.g., Pott disease)

INTRINSIC LESIONS

Syringomyelia
Transverse myelitis
Multiple sclerosis
Amyotrophic lateral sclerosis
Spinal arteriovenous malformation, subarachnoid hemorrhage
Spinal cord infarction
HIV/AIDS myelopathy
Other viral myelopathies (e.g., polio, coxsackie, West Nile, CMV, EBV, herpes viruses)
Syphilis
Vitamin/mineral deficiencies (e.g., B_{12}, copper)
Environmental (e.g., radiation, electric injury)

Adapted from R. M. Walls, R. S. Hockberger, & M. Gausche-Hill (Eds.) (2018), *Rosen's emergency medicine: Concepts and clinical practice* (9th ed., pp.1298–1306, Box 96-1). Elsevier.

Presentation

- All compression syndromes can cause pain. Motor and sensory findings depend on the level and size of the lesion.
- May have weakness, sensory deficit, and loss of bowel or bladder function.
- Conus medullaris syndrome
  - Terminal end of the spinal cord, approximately L1 in adults
  - Often urinary retention with overflow incontinence, sphincter impairment, or sexual dysfunction
  - May have saddle anesthesia
  - May be distinguished from cauda equina by bilateral or upper motor neuron symptoms, although often difficult to differentiate clinically
- Cauda equina syndrome
  - "The horse's tail," not a true cord syndrome, but affects multiple lumbar and sacral nerve roots simultaneously
  - Urinary retention is the most consistent finding
  - Usually unilateral, radicular pain, paresthesias, asymmetric weakness with loss of distal reflexes
  - Most commonly owing to a metastatic tumor, herniated disc; also by trauma, epidural abscess

Diagnosis and Evaluation

- Magnetic resonance imaging (MRI) is the study of choice for evaluation of spinal cord pathology, including hemorrhage and edema.
- Computed tomography myelography is an inferior alternative if MRI is not available or contraindicated.
- Plain radiographs and computed tomography scans (except CT myelography) are not adequate to evaluate the spinal cord.
- If noncontrast MRI imaging excludes compressive lesions, consider inflammatory or demyelinating disorders. Lumbar puncture (LP) and/or contrast-enhanced MRI may be useful for further diagnosis.

Treatment

- Any compressive spinal cord lesion requires urgent surgical consultation.
- Other adjuncts to treatment depend on etiology of lesion. Infectious etiologies such as spinal epidural abscess, osteomyelitis and diskitis require IV antibiotics targeted at the underlying infectious agent.
- Special considerations for specific diseases that cause spinal cord compression:
  - Epidural abscess
    - Infectious process, pyogenic material in epidural space, often from hematogenous spread of bacteria
    - Most common pathogen is *Staphylococcus aureus*.

- Risk factors include invasive spinal procedure or surgery, diabetes, intravenous (IV) drug use, chronic renal disease, alcohol use, immunosuppression.
- Consider in patients who present with neurologic symptoms and back pain. Typically in thoracic or lumbar spine. May be associated with fever.
- If cauda equina, urinary retention is typically the first neurologic symptom; weakness is a later finding.
- Some may also present with encephalopathy.
- Treatment: IV antibiotics, such as vancomycin plus ceftriaxone (additional coverage if concern for *Pseudomonas aeruginosa*), neurosurgical and infectious disease consultation.

- Neoplasm
  - Spinal cord tumors may cause external compression or intrinsic invasion.
  - Most tumors affecting the spinal cord are metastatic. Lung cancer, breast cancer, and lymphoma are most common.
  - Most common symptom is pain that causes nocturnal awakening, neurologic dysfunction distal to the lesion, progressive difficulty in ambulation; symptoms may begin unilaterally, but progress to bilateral.
  - IV steroids and radiotherapy also considered in addition to acute decompression
- Degenerative spine disease
  - Spinal stenosis is the narrowing of the spinal canal, which can cause compression of the cord. Etiologies include overgrowth of bone or ligaments or a herniated disc.
  - Nonsurgical treatments include physical therapy, analgesic and antiinflammatory medications, and epidural steroid injections.
  - Laminectomy for surgical decompression for progressive neurologic deficits, especially cauda equina syndrome
- Spinal epidural hematoma
  - Typically occurs as a complication of procedures involving spinal dural puncture in patients with bleeding diathesis, such as thrombocytopenia or anticoagulant use, rarely spontaneous.
  - Sudden, severe back pain given vascular etiology, often with radicular component
  - Pain may increase with straining maneuvers that increase intraspinal pressure.
  - Usually a venous bleed that progresses over hours to days
- Pott disease
  - Tuberculosis (TB) spondylitis: infection of the vertebral body from hematogenous spread of TB from other sources, typically the lungs.
  - Causes intervertebral disc collapse, vertebral collapse, and spinal damage.
  - Back pain over the affected vertebra, fever, night sweats, anorexia, and weight loss, followed by secondary compressive myelopathy at the level of the lesion.
  - Typically in thoracic or upper lumbar spine
  - Treatment for TB

Intrinsic Spinal Cord Lesions

- Intrinsic spinal cord lesions can be organized by an anatomic-pathophysiologic classification of dysfunction, depending on the anatomic region affected by the lesion (Fig. 81.1).
- Please refer to Chapter 141 for a more detailed discussion of specific spinal cord syndromes: Anterior, Central, Complete, and Brown-Sequard.

SYRINGOMYELIA

- Fluid-filled cavity within the spinal cord, typically in the cervical or thoracic area
- Commonly associated with Arnold-Chiari I malformations, but can be related to other etiologies, including postinfectious, postinflammatory, neoplastic, and traumatic

Clinical Presentation

- Headache and neck pain are the most common complaints.
- May present as central cord syndrome.
- Most common features on physical examination are lower limb hyperreflexia, weakness and wasting in the hands and arms, "dissociative" sensory loss, and gait disorder.
- Dissociative pattern of sensory deficit is loss of pain and temperature (lateral spinothalamic tract) in the upper extremities with preservation of proprioception and light touch (dorsal columns) in "cape-like" distribution.

Diagnosis

- Magnetic resonance imaging, often nonemergent because the condition is usually slowly progressive.

Treatment

- Refer to neurosurgery for consideration of surgical decompression with fenestration and/or shunt placement.

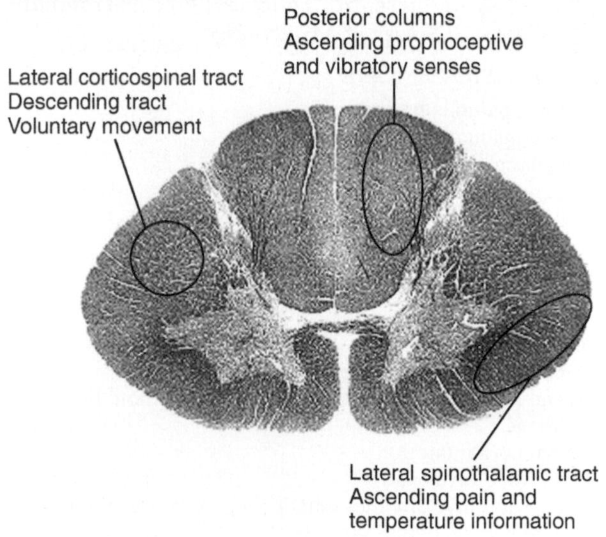

FIG. 81.1 Simplified anatomy and function of spinal cord tracts. (From R. M. Walls, R. S. Hockberger, & M. Gausche-Hill (Eds.) (2018), *Rosen's emergency medicine: Concepts and clinical practice* (9th ed., pp. 1298–1306, Fig. 96.1). Elsevier Photomicrograph courtesy John Sundsten, Digital Anatomist Project, University of Washington.)

TRANSVERSE MYELITIS

- Rare, inflammatory disorder thought to be autoimmune, often in the setting of preceding infection or associated with connective tissue disorders, such as systemic lupus erythematosus, Sjögren syndrome, scleroderma, and rheumatoid arthritis.
- May also be idiopathic.

Clinical Presentation

- Presents with rapid-onset weakness leading to paraplegia, sensory alteration, bowel/bladder dysfunction. Complete cord syndrome or Brown-Sequard syndrome can also be seen.

Diagnosis

- Magnetic resonance imaging with contrast shows signal abnormality over involved segments.
- LP may demonstrate elevated protein and lymphocytosis.

Treatment

- Intravenous steroids often used but limited evidence for their efficacy.

MULTIPLE SCLEROSIS

- See Chapter 77. Demyelinating Disorders.

AMYOTROPHIC LATERAL SCLEROSIS

- Neurodegenerative disorder that produces progressive weakness, with mixed upper and lower motor neuron signs. Usually begins in adults more than 60 years of age.
- Motor neuron degeneration with gliosis replacing lost neurons in the corticospinal tract of the spinal cord and loss of myelinated fibers in motor nerves

Clinical Presentation

- Asymmetric limb weakness with a mixture of upper and lower motor neuron features
- Sensory and sphincter disturbances are usually absent.

Diagnosis and Evaluation

- EMG typically shows denervation in affected muscles. MRI normal.

Treatment

- Refer to neurology. Supportive care; there is no curative treatment.

Spinal Cord Hemorrhage/ Arteriovenous Malformation

- Spinal hemorrhage is rare; it may occur in the same anatomic locations as intracranial hemorrhages: epidural, subdural, subarachnoid, and intramedullary (intraspinal).
- Spinal subarachnoid and intramedullary hemorrhage usually caused by an arteriovenous malformation or trauma.
- Other risks include tumors, cavernous angiomas, and spontaneous bleed from anticoagulation.

Clinical Presentation

- Sudden pain with other symptoms reflecting level and extent of hemorrhage

Diagnosis and Evaluation

- MRI with contrast-enhanced magnetic resonance angiography of the spine

Treatment

- Endovascular occlusion, surgical resection, or both

Spinal Cord Infarction

- Most frequently caused by surgical procedures and pathologies affecting the aorta.
- May be caused by any etiology that can result in brain infarction, including atherosclerosis, embolism, hypercoagulable disorders, and vasculitis.

81

Clinical Presentation

- Anterior spinal cord syndrome is most common: paralysis, loss of bladder function, loss of pain/temperature sensation below the level of the lesion. Dorsal column spared.
- Onset of symptoms is sudden and is frequently associated with back pain.

Diagnosis

- MRI consistent with cord ischemia, but may be normal in the first 24 hours. Diffusion-weighted imaging is more sensitive.

Treatment

- Generally supportive and focused on the underlying aortic pathology and/or secondary stroke prevention

HIV/AIDS Myelopathy

- Human immunodeficiency virus (HIV)/ acquired immunodeficiency syndrome (AIDS) produces vacuolar myelopathy. Pathologic descriptions include demyelination of the dorsal columns and the dorsal half of the lateral columns, with prominent vacuoles within the myelin sheaths.
- Usually in late stages of AIDS

Clinical Presentation

- Progressive, spastic lower extremity weakness, gait disturbance, sphincter dysfunction, accompanied by sensory deficits of vibration and position

Diagnosis

- MRI of the spine is usually normal. Cerebrospinal fluid examination may show nonspecific findings, such as elevated protein.

Treatment

- Directed at antiretroviral therapy, although there is no proven treatment

Syphilis

- Tabes dorsalis, demyelination by tertiary syphilis infection, affecting dorsal columns
- Lancinating (sudden, lightening-like) body pain is an early symptom.
- Progressive loss of vibration and position senses leading to ataxia, followed by weakness, and bladder incontinence

Clinical Presentation

- Characteristic gait is wide and slapping.
- Neurologic examination may demonstrate areflexia, loss of proprioception, vibration, positive Romberg test, Argyll Robertson pupils that accommodate, but do not react to light.

Diagnosis

- Cerebrospinal fluid may be normal or have elevated protein level, lymphocytosis, and reactive VDRL.

Treatment

- IV penicillin for 10 to 14 days

B_{12} Deficiency: Subacute Combined Degeneration of the Spinal Cord

- Affects dorsal and lateral columns, leading to weakness and numbness
- Etiologies include pernicious anemia, vegan diet, decreased absorption from gastrectomy or bariatric surgery, Crohn disease, celiac disease, and medications (e.g., metformin).

Clinical Presentation

- Progressive weakness, sensory ataxia, and paresthesias; ultimately spasticity, paraplegia, and incontinence
- May have neuropsychiatric symptoms, including depression, insomnia, cognitive slowing, and psychosis

Diagnosis

- Examination may demonstrate a positive Romberg sign if the dorsal column is affected.
- Complete blood cell count, vitamin B_{12} level. Not all patients with neurologic abnormalities will have anemia or macrocytosis. MRI may show signal abnormality in dorsal and lateral columns.

Treatment

- B_{12} supplementation and treat the underlying disease causing the deficiency.

SUGGESTED READINGS

Goldman, L., & Schafer, A. I. (2016). *Goldman-Cecil medicine* (25th ed., pp. 2370–2382). Elsevier.

Walls, R. M., Hockberger, R. S., & Gausche-Hill, M. (2018). *Rosen's emergency medicine: Concepts and clinical practice* (9th ed., pp. 1298–1306). Elsevier.

Peripheral Nerve and Neuromuscular Junction Disorders

CHELSEA E. ROBINSON, MD, and SABRINA M. TOM, MD

General Principles

- Individuals presenting with focal weakness should rapidly be evaluated to ensure stabilization of respiratory and circulatory status and to exclude emergent central nervous system disease, including spinal cord disorders. If symptoms of motor and/or sensory deficits appear to be localized to the extremities, consider disorders of the peripheral nerves, neuromuscular junction, or innervated muscles. This chapter reviews some important causes of peripheral weakness, including peripheral nerve disorders and disorders of the neuromuscular junction. Myopathies, or disorders of the muscle, are discussed separately in Chapter 73.

Anatomy *(Fig. 82.1)*

- Anterior and posterior nerve roots exit the spinal cord and converge to form a mixed (motor and sensory) spinal nerve.
  - 31 pairs: 8 cervical, 12 thoracic, 5 lumbar, 5 sacral, 1 coccygeal
  - Posterior ramus innervates the back.
  - Anterior ramus innervates the anterolateral body and supplies all upper extremities through brachial plexus, lower extremities through lumbar plexus.
  - Peripheral autonomic nervous system: sympathetic (thoracolumbar), parasympathetic (craniosacral)

Peripheral Neuropathies

- Disorders involving the axon or myelin sheath of the peripheral nerve.
- Most peripheral neuropathies seen in the emergency department (ED) are subacute or chronic and are associated with long-term morbidity but not mortality.
- Guillan-Barré is an exception, and requires emergent attention.
- Please see Box 82.1 for common causes of acquired peripheral neuropathy.

DEMYELINATING POLYNEUROPATHIES

- Guillan Barré Syndrome and its variants.
- See chapter 77 on Demyelinating Disorders.

DISTAL SYMMETRIC POLYNEUROPATHIES

- The most common type of peripheral neuropathy.
- Common etiologies include diabetes, alcohol use, medications, human immunodeficiency virus (HIV) infection and treatment with antiretrovirals,

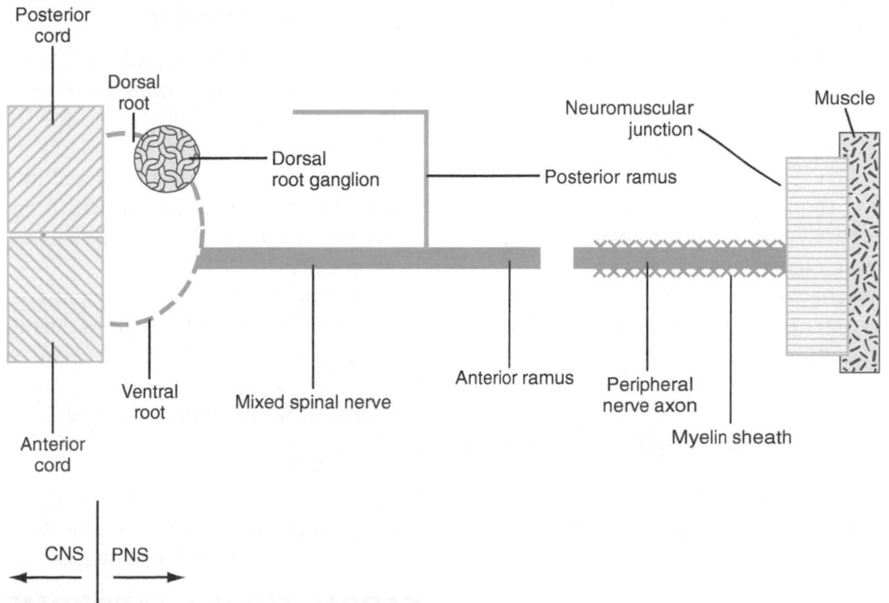

FIG. 82.1 Anatomy of central and peripheral nervous systems with the neuromuscular junction. (From R. M. Walls, R. S. Hockberger, & M. Gausche-Hill (Eds.), *Rosen's emergency medicine: Concepts and clinical practice* (9th ed., Fig. 97.2). Elsevier.)

BOX 82.1 Common Causes of Acquired Peripheral Neuropathy

Metabolic	Diabetes, hypothyroidism, renal failure (uremia), vitamin B_1, B_6, B_{12} deficiency
Malignancy	Direct invasion, compression, paraneoplastic syndromes
Drugs	Isoniazid, phenytoin, amiodarone, antiretrovirals, metronidazole, nitrofurantoin, statins, chemotherapeutic agents
Toxins	Alcohol, heavy metals (lead, arsenic, mercury, thallium), organophosphates
Infections	Lyme disease, human immunodeficiency virus (HIV), diptheria, herpes viruses
Autoimmune/Inflammatory	Guillan-Barré syndrome, connective tissue disorders, vasculitis
Paraproteinemias	Amyloidosis, monoclonal antibody of unknown significance (MGUS), mutliple myeloma
Vascular	Ischemia
Traumatic	Compression, incision

heavy metals, uremia, hypothyroidism and vitamin B deficiencies.
- Box 82.1 lists common causes of peripheral sensorimotor neuropathy.

Clinical Presentation

- Typically characterized by pattern symmetric sensorimotor findings that are worse distally with proximal progression over time.
- Sensory abnormalities (pain, parasthesias, numbness, loss of proprioception) in "stocking-glove" distribution.
- Motor weakness and loss of deep tendon reflexes begin after sensory symptoms. Achilles reflex is the first affected.
- Usually worse in lower than upper extremities.

Diagnosis and Evaluation

- Often clinically suspected based on exam and underlying conditions.
- Diagnosis confirmed with electrophysiologic testing not available in the emergency department: nerve conduction studies and needle electromyography (EMG).
- Electrophysiologic testing can distinguish the anatomic distribution of involvement and the modalities involved (sensory, motor or mixed).

Treatment

- Focus treatment on the underlying condition, if known. For example:
  - If diabetic, tight glycemic control.
  - If from toxin, including alcohol, cessation of exposure.
  - Correct vitamin deficiencies.
- Pain control with gabapentin, other anticonvulants, tricyclic antidepressants, duloxetine. Avoid non-steroidal anti-inflammatory medications (NSAIDs) for long-term use.
- Physical therapy, assistive devices for ambulation, foot care.

RADICULOPATHIES AND PLEXOPATHIES

- Radiculopathy is a condition due to a compressed nerve in the spine. See Chapter X Spine Disorders.
- Plexopathy is a rare disorder involving a network of nerves, either at the brachial or lumbar plexus.

Clinical Presentation

- Brachial plexopathy typically presents with pain in the shoulder or upper arm accompanied by weakness, sensory loss and progressive atrophy in different nerve distributions of the upper extremity. Most commonly due to trauma. Also associated with thoracic outlet syndrome, or injury from radiation therapy.
- Lumbosacral plexopathy typically presents with pain, weakness and sensory deficits in multiple contiguous lumbosacral nerve root distributions. Commonly due to compression from other structures, neoplastic invasion, and diabetic neuropathy.

Diagnosis

- Consider plain films, computed tomography of the chest/abdomen, or magnetic resonance imaging to aid in determining the underlying etiology.
- Definitive diagnosis is made by nerve conduction studies and EMG.

Treatment

- Emergency department management is geared toward fixing reversible causes (joint dislocation/trauma) and pain management.

FOCAL MONONEUROPATHIES

- Mononeuropathy presents as pain, parasthesias, and numbness in the distribution of the affected nerve. They are most often caused by focal nerve compression. See Fig. 82.2 for the neuroanatomy of the upper extremity.

RADIAL NERVE PALSY

Clinical Presentation

- Axillary radial neuropathy occurs from compression of the nerve at the axilla (arm over a chair) and involves weakness of the triceps (inability to extend the elbow).
- Humeral radial neuropathy occurs secondary to compression of the radial nerve as it traverses behind the proximal humerus and results in wrist and finger drop only.
- The majority of radial nerve palsies occur with prolonged improper positioning, such as during deep sleep.

Diagnosis

- Clinical, no imaging indicated

Treatment

- Placing hand in a dynamic splint with the wrist in slight extension will promote healing & restore function
- Expect recovery in 6 to 8 weeks.

CARPAL TUNNEL SYNDROME

- Compression of the median nerve as it travels through the carpal tunnel.
- Most common entrapment mononeuropathy.

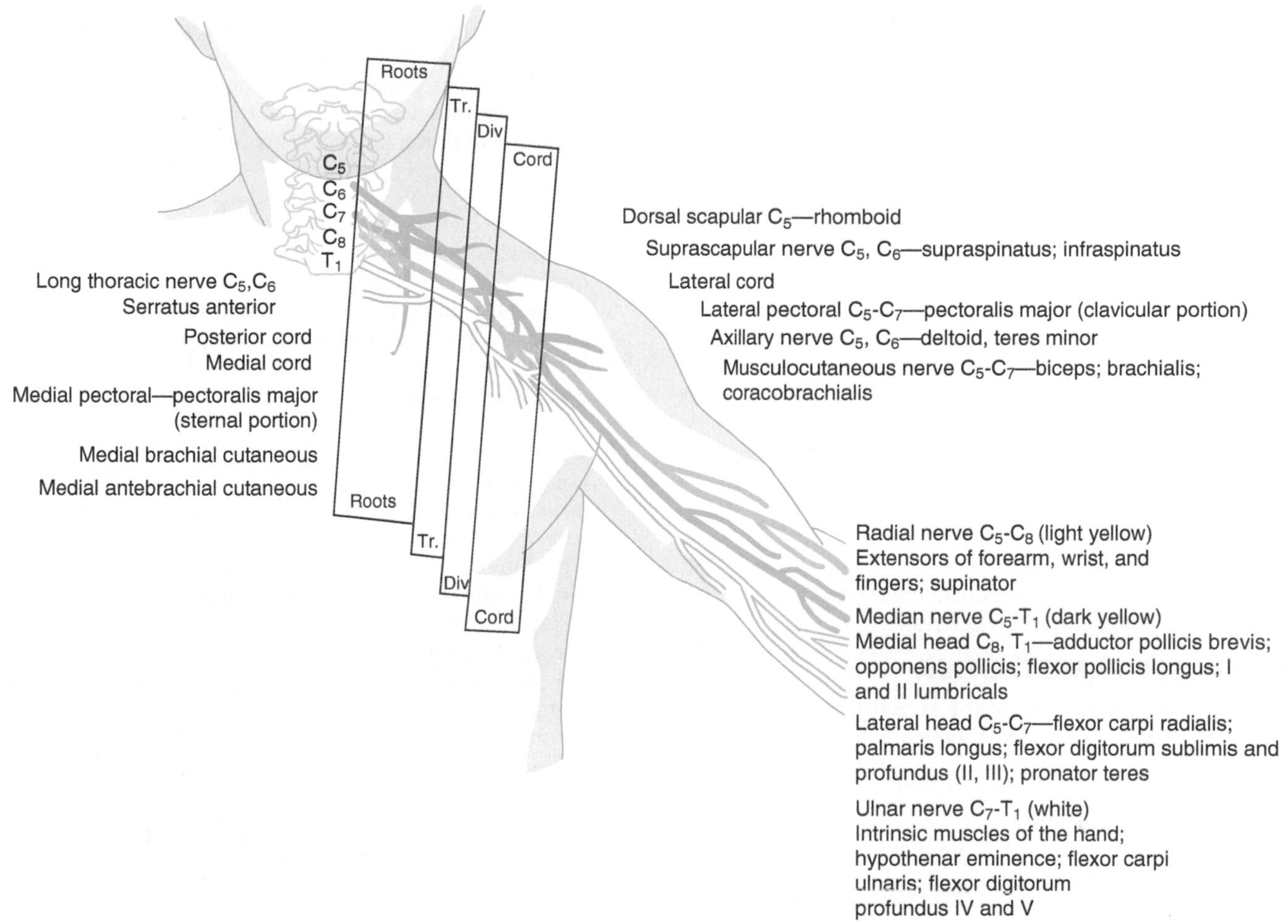

FIG. 82.2 Brachial plexus to nerve branches of shoulder and arm. (From Swaiman, K. F., Ashwal, S., Ferriero, D. M., Schor, N. F., Finkel, R. S., Gropman, A. L., Pearl, P. L., & Shevell, M. (Eds.) (2017), Acquired peripheral neuropathies. *Swaiman's pediatric neurology: Principles and practice* (6th ed., pp. 1081–1085). Elsevier.)

Clinical Presentation

- Pain or paresthesia in the median nerve distribution (first three digits and radial half of the fourth digit). May also see motor deficits.
- Symptoms are usually worse at night and can awaken patients from sleep.
- Predisposing factors are obesity, female gender, diabetes, pregnancy, rheumatoid arthritis, and hypothyroidism.

Diagnosis

- Physical examination: may have a positive Tinel sign (tapping median nerve at the wrist causes electric shock sensation shooting into the hand) or Phalen maneuver (holding wrists in flexion for 1 minute worsens symptoms). Most specific finding is split sensation of the fourth digit's volar aspect (decreased on radial side and normal on ulnar side).
- EMG and nerve conduction studies provide a definitive diagnosis.

Treatment

- Activity modification, nocturnal wrist splinting in a position of comfort
- Glucocorticoid injection
- Surgical referral

ULNAR NEUROPATHY

- Second most common entrapment mononeuropathy after median, arising more often at the elbow followed by wrist.
- Cubital tunnel syndrome if compression is through cubital tunnel at elbow. Other common site of injury at elbow is ulnar condylar groove.

Clinical Presentation

- Elbow: Numbness or parasthesias in ulnar distribution. Variable motor deficits of intrinsic hand muscles, including clawing of 4th and 5th digits. Typically caused by traumatic injury, sustained elbow flexion, or repetitive pronation/supination.
- Wrist: Hand weakness, muscle wasting, and clumsiness. Variable sensory involvement. Caused by repetitive trauma such as frequent tool use or sustained compression from holding handlebars.

Diagnosis

- Physical examination: Sensory testing for splitting of fourth digit with deficits on ulnar side. Motor testing of intrinsic hand muscles (e.g., interossei or pinch to test thumb adduction). Provacative testing with percussion at elbow (Tinel's) or Guyon's canal at wrist.
- Nerve conduction studies and EMG confirm the diagnosis.

Treatment

- Activity modification, nocturnal splinting of elbow in extension. Most resolve with conservative treatment.
- Surgical referral for decompression if needed.

PERONEAL NERVE ENTRAPMENT

- Caused by injury to the peroneal nerve just below the knee as it wraps around the lateral aspect of the fibula. Injury is usually due to compression from prolonged lying, crossing legs, proximal fibular fractures, and casts.

Clinical Presentation

- Acute foot drop (difficulty dorsiflexing foot) and high steppage gait
- Paresthesia and sensory loss over dorsum of the foot and lateral shin

Diagnosis

- Physical examination reveals weakness in foot dorsiflexion and eversion with preserved reflexes.
- EMG and nerve conduction studies for definitive diagnosis.

Treatment

- Remove pressure on the nerve.
- Ankle splint to keep foot dorsiflexed until recovered
- Consider physical therapy referral.

MERALGIA PARESTHETICA

- Caused by compression of the lateral femoral cutaneous nerve (pure sensory nerve), typically as it passes under the inguinal ligament

Clinical Presentation

- Presents with burning pain, paresthesia, and decreased sensation over the upper outer thigh (onset of pain typically subacute).
- Associated with obesity, diabetes, older age, tight belts or garments around the waist, compression from a wallet, and pregnancy

Diagnosis

- Physical examination will show decreased pinprick and light touch over the anterolateral thigh with lower extremity neurologic examination otherwise normal.
- Diagnosis is clinical.

Treatment

- Reduce pressure in the groin area.

Neuromuscular Junction Disorders

MYASTHENIA GRAVIS

- Autoimmune disorder most commonly caused by antibodies against acetylcholine receptors at the neuromuscular junction.
- Associated with thymic tumors and other autoimmune disorders.

Clinical Presentation

- Peak incidence in women in their 20s and men in their 60s
- Hallmark is muscle weakness that worsens with repeated or sustained activity.
- Muscle weakness can be precipitated by infection, pregnancy, medications, or other stressors.
- Ocular muscle weakness (ptosis, diplopia) without pupil involvement is the most common initial manifestation.
- Bulbar muscles (dysarthria, dysphagia), extremity and respiratory muscles may also be involved. Monitor for respiratory failure, known as myasthenic crisis.

Diagnosis

- Physical examination: clinician can perform provocative maneuvers, such as repeated extraocular movements, or having the patient count to 100, and watch for muscle fatigue. It is important to note that in myasthenia gravis, the patient will have normal pupils and reflexes.
- Ice pack test: place an ice pack over the patient's closed eyes for 2 minutes and evaluate for improvement in ptosis.
- Tensilon (edrophonium) test: administer 2 mg intravenous edrophonium (short-acting anticholinesterase inhibitor) and evaluate for improvement in weakness (note: this drug has been discontinued in the U.S.).
- Checking respiratory status: consider intubation when serial readings reveal low forced vital capacity, maximal inspiratory pressures or for worsening clinical status.
- Forced vital capacity
  - Largest volume that the patient can exhale after taking in maximal breath; global assessment of inspiratory and expiratory strength.
  - Consider intubation when less than 15 to 20 mL/kg H_2O.
- Negative inspiratory force
  - Greatest negative inspiratory pressure that the patient can generate.
  - Consider intubation when less negative than 25 to 30 cm H_2O.
- Diagnosis outside the emergency department confirmed with serologic and electrophysiologic testing.

Treatment

- Most important role of the emergency physician is monitoring the patient's respiratory status and ability to handle secretions.
- If intubation is required, If intubation is required, use a non-depolarizing paralytic (rocuronium) at a reduced dose, due to prolonged duration of action. Avoid depolarizing paralytic (succinylcholine), which is likely to be ineffective from decreased acetylcholine receptors on muscle.
- Acetylcholinesterase inhibitors, such as pyridostigmine, are first-line agents.
  - Be aware of possible cholinergic crisis due to excessive treatment causing high levels of acetylcholine. This can mimic a depolarizing paralytic, resulting in muscle weakness and respiratory compromise. Look for muscle fasciulations, nausea/vomiting, diarrhea, salivation, lacrimation, diaphoresis, miosis, or bradycardia.
- Consider steroids, intravenous immunoglobulin, and plasmapheresis in consultation with a neurologist.
- Workup and treatment should be centered around determining the underlying cause of myasthenic crisis (e.g., sepsis, medications).

LAMBERTEATON SYNDROME

- An autoimmune disorder with antibodies against presynaptic voltage-gated calcium channel, usually a paraneoplastic disorder associated with small cell cancer of the lung.

Clinical Presentation

- Typically seen in older men.
- Presents as weakness that improves with repetitive or sustained activity.
- Classic symptoms are weakness in the proximal lower extremities with abnormal gait, hyporeflexia, and autonomic dysfunction manifested as dry mouth.
- Bulbar and ocular symptoms less common.

Diagnosis

- Usually clinical in the emergency department setting: proximal muscle weakness on examination.
- Can check hand grip: will be weak → strong → weak again.
- Diagnosis confirmed with serologic and electrophysiologic testing.

Treatment

- Neurology consult, steroids, intravenous immunoglobulin
- Supportive management and addressing underlying malignancy.

BOTULISM

- See Chapter X on Biological Warfare Agents

TICK PARALYSIS

- See Chapter X on Tick Borne Infections

SUGGESTED READINGS

Shearer, P. (2018). Neuromuscular disorders. In Walls, R. M., Hockberger, R. S., & Gausche-Hill, M. (Eds.), *Rosen's emergency medicine: Concepts and clinical practice* (9th ed., pp. 1321–1327). Elsevier.

Smith, S. A. (2017). Acquired peripheral neuropathies. In K. F. Swaiman, S. Ashwal, D. M. Ferriero, N. F. Schor, R. S. Finkel, A. L. Gropman, P. L. Pearl, & M. Shevell (Eds.), *Swaiman's pediatric neurology: Principles and practice* (6th ed., pp. 2419–2435). Elsevier.

Snow, D. C., & Bunney, E. B. (2018). Peripheral nerve disorders. In R. M. Walls, R. S. Hockberger, & M. Gausche-Hill (Eds.), *Rosen's emergency medicine: Concepts and clinical practice* (9th ed., pp. 1307–1321). Elsevier.

CHAPTER **83**

BOARD REVIEW

Hemorrhagic Stroke

DANIEL WEINGROW, DO, and JACQUELINE KURTH, MD

Subarachnoid Hemorrhage

Basic Information

- Most spontaneous/non-traumatic subarachnoid hemorrhages (SAHs) are secondary to a ruptured aneurysm.
- Other non-aneurysmal causes are arteriovenous malformation (AVM), vasculitis, cerebral artery dissection, coagulation disorders, sympathomimetic drugs, and sickle cell anemia.

Clinical Presentation

- Clinical presentation is on a wide spectrum and is predictive of morbidity, mortality and potential benefits of operative intervention. In obtunded patients or those with diminished mental status, headache is seen in 97% of cases, and typically appears suddenly and is maximal at onset.
  - Neck pain and low back pain may occur from meningismus secondary to nerve root irritation caused by dependent blood.
  - Nausea and vomiting from increased intracranial pressure leading to pressure on the area postrema.
  - Seizures may occur in up to 20% of patients and may be non-convulsive and should be anticipated in any patient presenting with SAH and coma.
  - Vitreous hemorrhage (Terson syndrome) may be seen on fundoscopy in association with SAH and increased intracranial pressure.

Diagnosis

- A non-contrast computed tomography (CT) scan is the initial diagnostic study of choice when evaluating for a subarachnoid hemorrhage. CT may reveal other potential causes of headache and coma. The sensitivity is highest in the first six hours before the hemosiderin is digested by macrophages.
- CT angiography should be performed after the diagnosis of SAH, but should not be performed routinely to screen for aneurysms because 2% of the population will have an incidental cerebral aneurysm.

LUMBAR PUNCTURE AFTER CT

- Owing to the significant morbidity and high lethality of undiagnosed SAH and the potential to intervene and prevent aneurysmal rupture, a very low clinical threshold for performing lumbar puncture should exist in the absence of blood on non-contrast CT done after 6 hours of symptom onset in the appropriate clinical presentation.
  - Lumbar puncture typically reveals non-clotting bloody fluid (more than 100,000 RBCs/mm^3) that does not clear with sequential tubes. No clear cutoff is considered negative for subarachnoid bleeding. False positive results may occur with traumatic taps; however, this blood typically clears in quantity from the first to the last tube evaluated.
  - Xanthochromia is the yellow coloration of cerebrospinal fluid (CSF) produced by red blood cell lysis that is present in nearly 100% of SAH at 12 hours, but may be detectable up to 4 weeks following a sentinel bleed. False–positive findings may occur in jaundice or high protein levels in the CSF.

Treatment

- Admission to the intensive care unit is recommended for close monitoring of neurologic status. Any change may indicate a re-bleed or vasospasm. Patients with SAH and unsecured (unclipped or uncoiled) aneurysms are at highest risk of this complication in the first few days.
- Prognosis of SAH is related to the Hunt and Hess classification of the SAH (Table 83.1).
- Oral/nasogastric nimodipine 60 mg every 4 hours should be administered to all aneurysmal SAH, unless contraindications to beta blockade exist (e.g., hypotension).
- Gentle hydration is encouraged to avoid cerebral salt wasting and hypovolemia.
- Avoidance of hypotension is of paramount importance in preventing ischemia and vasospasm. However,

TABLE 83.1 *Hunt and Hess Classification*

Category	Symptoms	Mortality
Grade 0	Unruptured aneurysm	1.3%
Grade 1	Asymptomatic or mild headache (HA)	1.4%
Grade 2	Moderate to severe HA, nuchal rigidity, cranial nerve palsy	5.4%
Grade 3	Lethargy, confusion, mild focal deficit	18.8%
Grade 4	Stupor, moderate to severe hemiparesis, early decerebrate rigidity	41.9%
Grade 5	Deep coma, decerebrate rigidity, moribund	76.9%

(From Oshiro, E. M., Walter, K. A., Piantadosi, S., Witham, T. F., & Tamargo, R. J. (1997). A new subarachnoid hemorrhage grading system based on the Glasgow Coma Scale: A comparison with the Hunt and Hess and World Federation of Neurological Surgeons Scales in a clinical series. *Neurosurgery, 41*(1), 140–148.)

TABLE 83.2 Anticoagulation Reversal

Anticoagulant	Reversal Agent
Warfarin	Vitamin K 10 mg intravenous (IV) Four-factor prothrombin complex concentrate (PCC) IV based on weight and INR (fresh frozen plasma if PCC unavailable)
Uremic platelet dysfunction	Consider desmopressin (DDAVP) 0.3 mcg/kg IV
Unfractionated heparin	Protamine sulfate (1 mg protamine per 100 units of unfractionated heparin given)
Low molecular weight heparin (LMWH)	If last dose within 8 hours: 1 mg protamine per 1 mg of LMWH If last dose 8 to 12 hours: 0.5 mg protamine per 1 mg of LMWH If last dose more than 12 hours: do not give protamine
Direct thrombin inhibitor or Xa inhibitors	Andexanet alfa for those on factor Xa inhibitors Idarucizumab (Praxbind) may be given to patients taking dabigatran (controversial) Hemodialysis can be considered with dabigatran if Praxbind unavailable Activated charcoal can be considered if apixaban, rivaroxaban, or dabigatran were taken within the last 2 hours

(From Hackmon, J. L., Nelson, A. M., & Ma, O. J. (2016). Spontaneous subarachnoid and intracerebral hemorrhage. In J. E. Tintinalli, J. S. Stapczynski, O. J. Ma, D. M. Yealy, G. D. Meckler, & D. M. Cline (Eds.), *Tintinalli's emergency medicine: A comprehensive study guide* (8th ed., pp.1137–1141). McGraw Hill Education.)

extreme elevations of blood pressure should be avoided owing to the risk of re-bleeding.
- Although there are no formal recommendations, maintaining systolic blood pressure below 160 mm Hg is reasonable. Labetalol and nicardipine are the most commonly used blood pressure medications in SAH.
- Avoiding elevations in intracranial pressure (ICP) with antiemetics (ondansetron preferred as the phenothiazine class may lower seizure threshold), analgesics, and elevating the head of bed to 30° are recommended.
- Antiepileptics are controversial, but levetiracetam and phenytoin are reasonable if used in the short term (particularly if there is concern of non-convulsive seizures in the patients with SAH in a coma).
- Reversal of anticoagulation, which is reviewed in Table 83.2, is recommended to minimize rebleeding.

Intracerebral Hemorrhage

Basic Information

- The majority of intracerebral hemorrhages (ICH) are the result of ruptured penetrating arterial branches deep in the brain (ganglionic) in the striatum (basal ganglia), putamen, lenticular nucleus, internal capsule, globus pallidus, and thalamus and are associated with elevated blood pressure, coagulopathy, and sympathomimetic use.
- These ganglionic bleeds may also occur in the posterior fossa in the brainstem and cerebellum. Lobar hemorrhages occur within 1 cm of the brain surface and are typically associated with structural brain abnormalities, such as an AVM, tumor, aneurysm, or hemorrhagic transformation of ischemic stroke.

Clinical Presentation

- Smooth progression of focal neurologic deficits over the course of minutes to hours (compared with maximal at onset for ischemic stroke) associated with severe headache, vomiting, and deterioration in level of consciousness are characteristic.
- Herniation and compression of the brainstem may produce cranial nerve abnormalities and cardiopulmonary instability.

Diagnosis

- Noncontrast CT is the diagnostic study of choice for detecting bleeding of any type, and it is accurate in estimating location, size, and secondary effect of hemorrhage (edema, mass effect).
- Size of hemorrhage is predictive of mortality and morbidity.
- CT angiography is helpful in determining if the hemorrhage is owing to a structural vascular cause in lobar hemorrhages, in patients with intraventricular hemorrhage (IVH) (high association with AVM), and in younger patients (less than 45 years of age) without a history of hypertension.
- Magnetic resonance imaging is more sensitive for hemorrhage than CT after 12 to 24 hours and more specific than CT in assessing the age of bleeding that is present.

83

Treatment (see Table 83.1)

- Neurosurgical intervention should be emergently considered in patients with cerebellar hemorrhage, in patients with hydrocephalus or IVH, or lobar hemorrhage less than 1 cm from the brain surface.
- Hypertension may contribute to further bleeding; however, the optimal blood pressure management strategy remains undefined after several large multicenter trials. The American Heart Association recommends early and gradual reductions below 140 mm Hg, while avoiding prominent fluctuations using intravenous nicardipine or labetalol.
- Measures to decrease ICP depend on the patient's clinical status. Analgesics, antiemetics, and elevation of the head of bed should be performed in all patients. Those with signs of impending herniation or coma may benefit from mannitol 1 gm/kg and/or the use of continuous hypertonic saline (3%), although the optimal dose and rate are as of yet to be determined through clinical trials.
- If the patient is showing signs of clinical deterioration, neuroprotective intubation is required, and repeat imaging should occur to evaluate for hemorrhagic expansion.
- Anticoagulation reversal is indicated according to Table 83.2.
- Giving platelets to patients who are on antiplatelet agents has been shown to increase mortality in nontraumatic ICH for patients not receiving neurosurgical intervention and is discouraged.
- Desmopressin 0.3 μg/kg may be administered for patients with uremic platelet dysfunction.

- Despite initial enthusiasm showing decreased hematoma expansion, recombinant factor VIIa (rFVIIa) has been associated with increased thromboembolic risk and should be considered with caution in consultation with neurosurgery.

SUGGESTED READINGS

Greenberg, M. S. (2016). *Handbook of neurosurgery*. Thieme.

Tintinalli, J. E., Stapczynski, J. S., Ma, O. J., Yealy, D. M., Meckler, G. D., & Cline, D. M. (2016). *Tintinalli's emergency medicine: A comprehensive study guide* (8th ed.). McGraw Hill Education.

Wijdicks, E. F. M. (2016). *The practice of emergency and critical care neurology*. Oxford University Press.

Ischemic Strokes and Transient Ischemic Attacks (TIAs)

REBECCA A. BAVOLEK, MD, and JACQUELINE KURTH, MD

Basic Information

A stroke can result in devastating neurologic deficits, both temporary, as seen in transient ischemic attacks (TIAs), and permanent, as seen in ischemic strokes. Regardless of the mechanism, the end result of a stroke or TIA is disruption of blood flow to the brain with resulting loss of cellular function.

Definition

- Ischemic stroke: blood flow is disrupted and results in ischemia and infarction of tissue.
- Transient ischemic attack: a transient episode of neurologic dysfunction owing to ischemia *without* infarction of tissue.

Territories

- Anterior cerebral artery infarction
- Middle cerebral artery infarction
- Posterior circulation infarction
- Lacunar infarction

General Principles for Approach and Treatment (Box 84.1)

- Assess and secure the patient's airway, breathing, and circulation (ABCs) as indicated, identify and distinguish true stroke syndrome from stroke mimics, and check a point-of-care (POC) glucose.
- Perform a National Institutes of Health Stroke Scale (NIHSS), obtain a definitive last known well time, and activate the stroke team if available in your institution and within therapeutic windows.
- Obtain imaging to rule out intracranial hemorrhage (ICH) and consider magnetic resonance imaging (MRI), if available.
- Decide on treatment: thrombolysis, thrombectomy, and so forth. Evaluate for inclusion criteria and contraindications.
- Optimize blood pressure, temperature, blood sugar, fluid status, and position the patient with the head of the bed at 30 degrees if the patient is at risk for elevated intracranial pressure or aspiration, and keep the head in neutral position to the rest of the body.

BOX 84.1 *Stroke Mimics*

Seizures (including postictal phase and Todd paralysis)
Syncope
Meningitis/encephalitis
Complex migraine
Brain mass
Epidural/subdural hematoma
Subarachnoid hemorrhage
Hypoglycemia
Hyponatremia
Hypertensive encephalopathy
Hyperosmotic coma
Wernicke encephalopathy
Labyrinthitis
Drug toxicity (lithium, phenytoin, carbamazepine)
Bell palsy
Meniere disease
Demyelinating disease (multiple sclerosis)
Conversion disorder

(From Go, S., & Worman, D. J. (2016). Stroke syndromes. In J. E. Tintinalli, J. S. Stapczynski, O. J. Ma, D. M. Yealy, G. D. Meckler, & D. M. Cline (Eds.), *Tintinalli's emergency medicine: A comprehensive study guide* (8th ed., pp. 1142–1155). McGraw Hill.)

Anterior Cerebral Artery

Basic Information

- Uncommon, accounts for 0.5% to 3% of all strokes.

Clinical Presentation

- Contralateral sensory and motor symptoms; lower extremities are more affected than the upper extremities.
- Right-sided lesions can result in confusion and motor inattention; left-sided lesions are typically associated with akinetic mutism and transcortical motor aphasia.

Middle Cerebral Artery

Basic Information

- The most common vessel involved in a stroke.

Clinical Presentation

- Patients typically present with contralateral upper, greater than lower, extremity sensory and motor loss that also involves the lower (not the upper) face.
- If the dominant hemisphere is involved (usually left hemisphere, regardless of hand dominance), inattention, neglect, and dysarthria without aphasia and confluent apraxia can occur.
- Homonymous hemianopsia and gaze preference to the side of the infarct may be present.

Posterior Circulation

Basic Information

- Posterior circulation strokes are caused by infarction of the vertebrobasilar arterial system.
- Presentations can be subtle and symptoms can be highly variable, so a high degree of suspicion is required to make this diagnosis. Of note, posterior infarction and hemorrhages are not seen well on computed tomography (CT) scans, so an MRI is the test of choice.

Clinical Presentation

- Ataxia, nystagmus, altered mental status, and vertigo.
- Unilateral limb weakness, blurry vision, gait ataxia, cranial nerve VII signs, and sensory deficits may be seen.
- Visual deficits, including contralateral homonymous hemianopsia and unilateral cortical blindness, may be present.

Lacunar Infarction

Basic Information

- These infarcts are most commonly associated with chronic hypertension and increasing age.
- The prognosis is usually considered more favorable than infarcts in other locations.

Clinical Presentation

- Variable, but they can present as pure motor or pure sensory deficits.

Diagnosis

- Identify the stroke with the physical examination and history. Make sure to consider stroke mimics, and ensure the patient's ABCs are stable. Immediately check a POC glucose; an electrocardiogram is helpful to evaluate for arrhythmias, such as atrial fibrillation.
- Once you have identified the patient as potentially having an ischemic stroke within appropriate therapeutic windows, activate your stroke team, if available, at your institution.
- Imaging will be needed and the modality of choice will depend on your facility's capabilities and the history.
  - Noncontrast head CT: consider getting a noncontrast head CT if the history is concerning for an ICH. This imaging test is more rapidly available and it can quickly rule out an ICH if the history is concerning.
  - MRI: most acute ischemic strokes are not seen on a noncontrast CT in the acute phase. Diffusion-weighted MRI is superior to the noncontrast CT for ischemic stroke; however, it can take longer to perform or the patient could have contraindications, such as metal in the body.
  - CT angiography: angiography is used to identify potential endovascular therapies, such as intraarterial thrombolysis and clot retrieval. It is combined with CT perfusion studies to evaluate candidacy for thrombectomy.
  - CT perfusion and MRI perfusion studies show the area of irreversible brain infarct and the area of potentially salvageable ischemic tissue.

Treatment (Box 84.2)

Thrombolysis: Tissue Plasminogen Activator (tPA)

- Intravenous tPA is used within 3 to 4.5 hours after symptom onset, determined from the patient's last known well time.
- Be sure to identify if the patient has any of the exclusion criteria for tPA, and consider the relative contraindications.
- An NIHSS of between 4 and 22 is commonly used as the criterion for administering tPA, although judgment can be used when patients have a lower stroke score with debilitating deficits, such as aphasia.
- Do not give anticoagulants or antiplatelet agents in the initial 24 hours after tPA.

BOX 84.2 ***Inclusion and Exclusion Criteria for Intravenous Alteplase in Acute Ischemic Stroke***

Absolute Exclusion Criteria for tPA Less Than 3 Hours

Neurosurgery, head trauma, or stroke in past 3 months

Any history of intracranial hemorrhage

Clinical presentation suggests subarachnoid hemorrhage or intracranial hemorrhage on computed tomography (CT)

CT shows multilobar infarction (hypodensity greater than one-third cerebral hemisphere)

Uncontrolled hypertension (more than 185 mm Hg systolic blood pressure or more than 110 mm Hg diastolic blood pressure)

Known intracranial arteriovenous malformation, neoplasm, or aneurysm

Active internal bleeding

Arterial puncture at noncompressible site in previous 7 days

Known bleeding diathesis

1. Platelet count less than 100,000
2. Patient has received heparin within 48 hours and has an elevated aPTT (greater than upper limit of normal for laboratory)
3. Current use of oral anticoagulants (ex: warfarin) and INR more than 1.7
4. Current use of direct thrombin inhibitors or direct factor Xa inhibitors

Abnormal blood glucose (less than 50 mg/dL)

Relative Exclusion Criteria for tPA Less Than 3 Hours

Only minor or rapidly improving stroke symptoms

Major surgery or serious non–head trauma in the previous 14 days

History of gastrointestinal or urinary tract hemorrhage within 21 days

Seizure at stroke onset

Post recent myocardial infarction (within 3 months)

Pregnancy

Exclusion Criteria for tPA More Than 3 Hours

Age more than 80 years

History of prior stroke and diabetes

Any active anticoagulant use, regardless of INR

NIHSS greater than 25

aPTT, activated partial thromboplastin time.

(From Demaerschalk, B. M., Kleindorfer, D. O., Adeoye, O. M., Demchuk, A. M., Fugate, J. E., Grotta, J. C., Khalessi, A. A., Levy, E. I., Palesch, Y. Y., Prabhakaran, S., Saposnik, G., Saver, J. L., & Smith, E. E. (2016). Scientific rationale for the inclusion and exclusion criteria for intravenous alteplase in acute ischemic stroke: A statement for healthcare professionals from the American Heart Association/American Stroke Association. *Stroke*, 47(2), 581–641.)

Endovascular Therapies

- Some hospitals have the capacity to perform intra-arterial thrombolysis and clot removal. The decision to proceed with these interventions will be made with your consultants. In general, patients are potential candidates if under 24 hours from last known well time, have a large vessel occlusion, and have a relatively large amount of ischemic penumbra and not as much infarcted tissue (angiography and perfusion imaging required for these determinations).
- Consider discussing these treatments in patients with contraindications to tPA or when their last known well time is unknown.
- In patients who have had a TIA with high-grade internal carotid lesions, carotid endarterectomy should be performed.

Blood Pressure Management

- In patients who are not candidates for reperfusion therapy or thrombolytics, permissive hypertension is advised. No active attempts to lower blood pressure should be made unless the systolic pressure is greater than 220 mm Hg, the diastolic pressure is greater than 120 mm Hg, or if the patient has another medical problem that requires lowering the blood pressure.
- If the patient is to receive tPA, the systolic blood pressure must be less than 185 mm Hg and the diastolic must be less than 110 mm Hg.
- Medications commonly used to lower blood pressure include intravenous labetalol and nicardipine in titration.

Transient Ischemic Attack

Definition

- A transient ischemic attack is defined as a transient episode of neurologic dysfunction without infarction.
- Although symptoms typically last for 1 to 2 hours, there is no defined time course for what determines a TIA.

Management

- If available, MRI with diffusion-weighted imaging is the best imaging modality.
- If MRI is not available, a noncontrast head CT scan can assess for stroke mimics.
- If possible, physicians should obtain cervical vascular imaging with carotid ultrasonography, CT angiography, or magnetic resonance angiography.
- Carotid ultrasonography has accuracy similar to that of magnetic resonance angiography or CT angiography.
- In the past, scoring systems were widely used to help determine which patients are high risk for another stroke in the near future. However, scores such as the $ABCD^2$ have shown not to be reliable.
- The disposition of the patient will depend on the severity of the symptoms, presence of large vessel disease, high degree of stenosis, follow-up, and your suspicion for the high risk for stroke in the future.
- Patients who are being discharged and have known heart disease, or in whom no identifiable cause of their TIA was found, should have an urgent outpatient echocardiogram and possible ambulatory cardiac monitoring.
- Starting aspirin in patients without a cardioembolic source who have had a TIA, and no contraindications, is standard with the addition of a second antiplatelet agent (e.g., clopidogrel) in patients who have high-risk features.
- Anticoagulation is recommended over antiplatelet therapy for patients who have a separate indication for anticoagulation, such as atrial fibrillation and venous thromboembolism.
- Discharged patients should have close follow-up within 48 hours.

SUGGESTED READINGS

Tintinalli, J. E., Stapczynski, J. S., Ma, O. J., Cline, D. M., Cydulka, R., & Meckler, G. D. (2011). *Tintinalli's emergency medicine: A comprehensive study guide* (7th ed., pp. 1142–1155). McGraw Hill.

Wijdicks, E. F. M. (2016). *The practice of emergency and critical care neurology* (pp. 384–437). Oxford University Press.

CHAPTER **85**

BOARD REVIEW

Vertigo

CHELSEA E. ROBINSON, MD, and SABRINA M. TOM, MD

Of patients presenting to the emergency department, 3% do so with dizziness. This chapter focuses on one specific cause of the symptom of dizziness, vertigo.

General Principles

- Vertigo is defined as the perception of movement when none exists.
- Two main categories
  - Peripheral: highly symptomatic, but rarely life-threatening
  - Central: significant morbidity and mortality
- Relevant anatomy (Fig. 85.1)
  - The inner ear contains the cochlea, vestibule, and semicircular canals; it is innervated by CN VIII. CN VIII connects to the brainstem and then to other parts of the cerebellum.
  - The posterior inferior cerebellar artery (branch of vertebral artery) and anterior inferior cerebellar artery (branch of basilar artery) supply the parts of the brainstem and cerebellum that form connections with CN VIII.
- Pathophysiology
  - Benign paroxysmal positional vertigo (BPPV)
    - Most common cause of vertigo
    - Dislodged otolith migrates into the semicircular canal, causing increased excitatory input to vestibular nuclei compared with unaffected ear. Results in sensation of vertigo during head movement.
  - Vestibular neuronitis (VN)
    - Caused by inflammation of the vestibular nerve, usually postviral.
    - Labyrinthitis is defined as inflammation of the vestibular and cochlear nerve. Same clinical presentation as VN, but with hearing loss.
  - Migrainous vertigo
    - The Neuhauser criteria have been developed for diagnosis.
  - Meniere disease
    - Caused by endolymphatic hydrops, or buildup of excess fluid in the endolymphatic system of the inner ear.
  - Posterior circulation insufficiency
    - Defined as insufficient blood flow through the posterior circulation of the brain, which is supplied by the two vertebral arteries which merge to form the basilar artery. The posterior circulation arteries supply the brainstem and cerebellum.

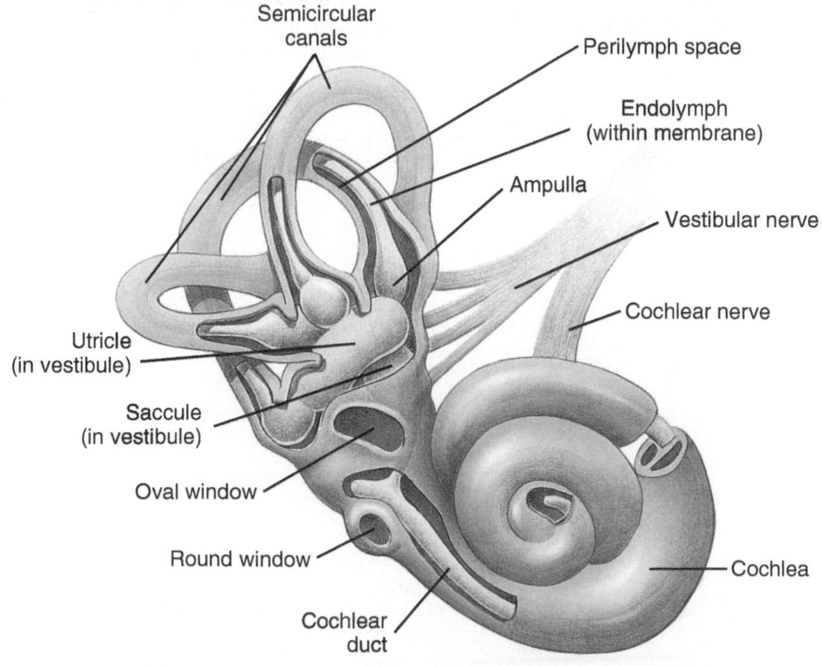

FIG. 85.1 A diagram of the anatomy of the inner ear. (From Patton, K. T., & Thibodeau, G. A. (2013). *Anatomy and physiology* (8th ed., Fig. 26.8, p. 519). Elsevier Mosby).

- Posterior circulation insufficiency can be caused by decreased blood flow from arterial dissection, from atherosclerotic disease in both vertebral arteries or the basilar artery, or by embolic stroke.

Clinical Presentation

- History
  - Attempting to differentiate vertigo from presyncope or disequilibrium may be difficult. Patients with posterior circulation insufficiency can present with vertiginous or nonvertiginous dizziness.
  - History should focus on determining whether symptoms are episodic or constant, duration of symptoms, associated symptoms, and provoking factors.
    - Stroke risk factors, such as previous stroke, diabetes, hypertension, age, atrial fibrillation, and hypercholesterolemia, should also be considered.
  - BPPV is the easiest to differentiate from VN and posterior circulation insufficiency because BPPV presents with sudden onset, short-duration dizziness, and complete resolution of symptoms between episodes.
  - Patients with migrainous vertigo usually have a previous history of migraines with new vestibular symptoms. May not present concurrently with headache.
  - Meniere disease typically presents as progressive hearing loss in the affected ear associated with episodic vertigo. Hearing loss is often associated with the sensation of ipsilateral ear fullness or head pressure. Tinnitus may also be present.
  - Stroke or cerebrovascular accident (CVA) is suggested by a sudden-onset dizziness with persistent, continuous symptoms, often accompanied by other focal neurologic symptoms.

Diagnosis and Evaluation

- Detailed history and physical examination are the most important components in the evaluation of a patient with vertigo.
- See Fig. 85.2 for a broader differential diagnosis of vertigo.
- An algorithm for distinguishing peripheral from central vertigo is outlined in Fig. 85.3.
  - Conduct a full neurologic examination, paying careful attention to hearing; an eye examination looking for pathologic nystagmus, cranial nerves, and ataxia.
    - A normal finger-to-nose test for dysmetria is insufficient to evaluate for cerebellar function.

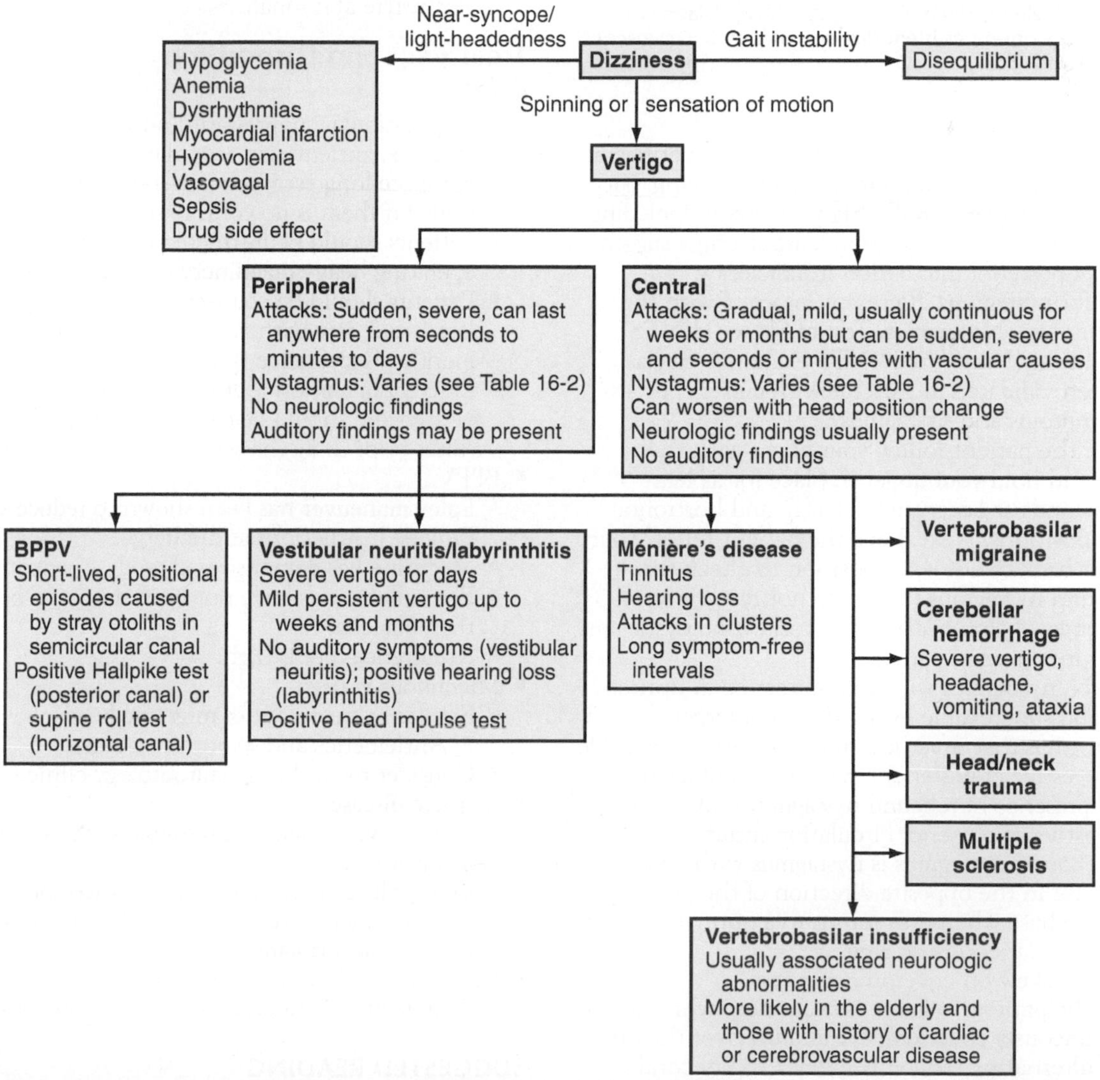

FIG. 85.2 Diagnostic algorithm for dizziness and vertigo. (From Chang, A. K. (2018). Dizziness and vertigo. In R. M. Walls, R. S. Hockberger, & M. Gausche-Hill (Eds.), *Rosen's emergency medicine: Concepts and clinical practice* (9th ed., pp. 145–152, Fig. 16.2). Elsevier.)

85

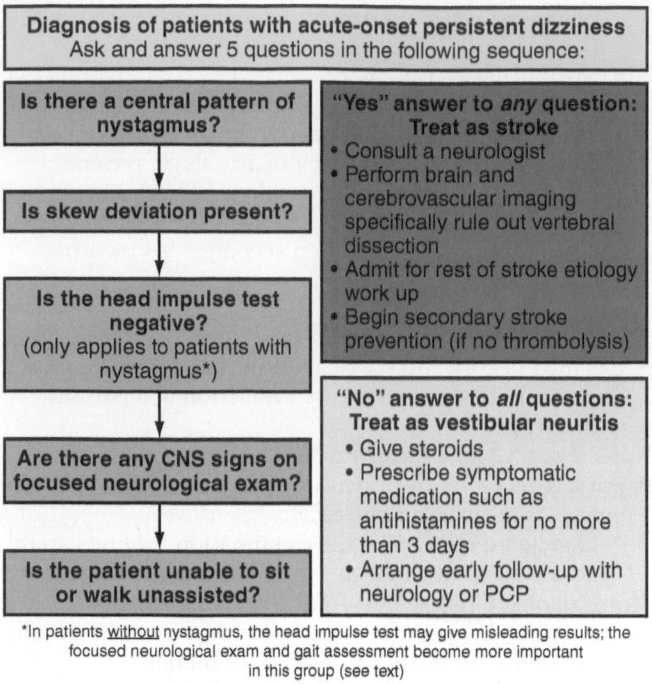

Diagnosis of patients with acute-onset persistent dizziness
Ask and answer 5 questions in the following sequence:
Is there a central pattern of nystagmus?
Is skew deviation present?
Is the head impulse test negative?
(only applies to patients with nystagmus*)
Are there any CNS signs on focused neurological exam?
Is the patient unable to sit or walk unassisted?
"Yes" answer to *any* question:
Treat as stroke
• Consult a neurologist
• Perform brain and cerebrovascular imaging specifically rule out vertebral dissection
• Admit for rest of stroke etiology work up
• Begin secondary stroke prevention (if no thrombolysis)
"No" answer to *all* questions:
Treat as vestibular neuritis
• Give steroids
• Prescribe symptomatic medication such as antihistamines for no more than 3 days
• Arrange early follow-up with neurology or PCP
*In patients without nystagmus, the head impulse test may give misleading results; the focused neurological exam and gait assessment become more important in this group (see text)

FIG. 85.3 Algorithm to help identify central vertigo with acute-onset persistent dizziness. (From Edlow, J. A. (2018). Diagnosing patients with acute-onset persistent dizziness. *Annals of Emergency Medicine, 71*(5), 625–631.)

- Testing of gait is essential. Patients with peripheral disorders may be symptomatic while walking, but will still be able to walk. Signs of ataxia, including inability to walk, sit, or stand, are strongly suggestive of posterior circulation insufficiency.
- Check for nystagmus. If present, proceed with the Head Impulse, Nystagmus, Test of Skew (HINTS) examination (Note: the HINTS examination has only been validated in patients with current, persistent symptoms and nystagmus).
  - Have the patient follow your finger with their eyes and hold your finger in place for at least 10 seconds at eccentric, vertical, and horizontal gaze positions. Next, have the patient follow your finger back to a normal position to check for rebound nystagmus (Note: do not test the very extremes of gaze because this can evoke nystagmus even in a normal patient).
  - In VN, nystagmus will be unidirectional, horizontal, and suppressible by fixating on a target.
  - Nystagmus that is vertical, rotary, or not suppressible is suggestive of posterior circulation insufficiency.
  - The presence of rebound nystagmus is also highly suggestive of posterior circulation insufficiency.
    - Rebound nystagmus is nystagmus with a fast phase in the opposite direction of the previous fast phase when eyes return to a normal position from a far eccentric gaze.
- Check for skew on cover/uncover test
  - Ask the patient to fixate on your nose while you simultaneously cover one eye and uncover the other eye, alternating randomly every 1 to 2 seconds.
  - Vertical movement of the eye to regain fixation on the examiner's nose is highly specific for central vertigo.
- Head impulse test: have the patient fixate on your nose and rapidly turn the patient's head.
  - Positive test: patient's eyes move with the head, then correct in a single saccade, which indicates a peripheral cause of vertigo.
  - Negative test: patient's eyes stay fixated on the target, which is concerning for a central cause of vertigo. Only concerning for central vertigo if the patient has nystagmus.
- Dix-Hallpike and the bow and lean test can be used to diagnose BPPV.
- Imaging
  - Computed tomography of the brain can reveal hemorrhagic stroke, but has very low sensitivity for ischemic stroke, especially in the posterior fossa.
  - Magnetic resonance imaging (MRI) is the standard of care if posterior circulation insufficiency is suspected.
    - If the physical examination suggests posterior circulation insufficiency, neurology should be consulted and the patient should be admitted for stroke evaluation even if the MRI is negative.
- Laboratory testing
  - Limited diagnostic value. Consider evaluating for hypoglycemia, anemia, thyroid dysfunction, and electrolyte abnormalities.

Treatment and Disposition

- VN
  - Use vestibular suppressants: antihistamines, benzodiazepines, antiemetics, scopolamine.
  - For more long-term relief, a short steroid burst can be trialed if there is no contraindication.
  - Patients should be instructed to avoid driving or operating heavy machinery until symptoms resolve.
  - Patients should be counseled that severe symptoms last 1 to 2 days with gradual resolution over weeks to months. Recurrence is rare.
  - Elderly population is at high risk for falls owing to vertigo and should be carefully assessed for functional status prior to discharge.
- BPPV
  - Epley maneuver has been shown to reduce symptoms. Provide instructions at discharge.
  - Meclizine has demonstrated modest benefit.
  - Benzodiazepines have not been shown to be better than placebo.
  - Recurrence rate is high.
- Migrainous vertigo
  - Similar to treatment of migraine headache
    - Antiemetics and serotonin agonists
  - Consider referral to a neurootology clinic.
- Meniere disease
  - May use vestibular suppressants, such as meclizine for acute attacks
  - Limit salt, caffeine, alcohol, and nicotine
  - Can consider diuretic therapy, such as hydrochlorothiazide, acetazolamide, furosemide
- Posterior circulation insufficiency
  - Admission and neurology consultation are indicated.

SUGGESTED READING

Edlow, J. A. (2018). Diagnosing patients with acute-onset persistent dizziness. *Annals of Emergency Medicine, 71*(5), 625–631.

CHAPTER **86**

BOARD REVIEW

Hydrocephalus, Intracranial Hypertension, and Shunt Issues

DANIEL WEINGROW, DO, and THOMAS AKIE, MD, PHD

Basic Principles

- Hydrocephalus, and resultant elevation in intracranial pressure, is the result of derangements of the homeostatic mechanisms of cerebrospinal fluids (CSF). The mainstay of management of hydrocephalus is ventricular shunting and, as many patients coming to the emergency department present subsequent to neurosurgical intervention, understanding the anatomy and function of ventricular shunts is critical to the diagnosis and treatment of these potentially life-threatening disorders.

CSF Physiology

- Cerebrospinal fluid is produced in the choroid plexus in lateral ventricles.
- Flows via the interventricular foramen of Monroe to the third ventricle, then to the area of greatest narrowing, the cerebral aqueduct, then to the fourth ventricle and onward to subarachnoid spaces.
- Absorbed in arachnoid granulations.
- Typical volume is 150 mL, with approximately 450 mL produced daily, therefore maintenance of the homeostatic mechanism is important to prevent accumulation. Infants have less total CSF, but more per kg body weight than adults.

Hydrocephalus

- Hydrocephalus is the accumulation of CSF within the ventricular system.
  - Malabsorptive hydrocephalus: most common, consists of two subtypes:
    - Non-communicating/obstructive: owing to obstruction in the CSF flow proximal to the arachnoid granulations, often caused by cellular obstruction within the ventricular system or mass effect onto the ventricular system.
    - Communicating/non-obstructive: results from decreased absorption at the arachnoid granulations; typically, secondary to particulate material from inflammation/infection or hemorrhage.
  - Hypersecretory hydrocephalus: rare; owing to increased CSF production (e.g., plexus papilloma).
  - Normal pressure hydrocephalus: radiographic appearance of hydrocephalus without an increase in intracranial pressure (ICP), with associated presentation of ataxia, incontinence, and reversible dementia in elderly patients.

Ventricular Shunts

- Ventricular shunts are the primary treatment of hydrocephalus.
  - Most often ventriculoperitoneal (also pleural or atrial shunts)
- Shunt anatomy (Fig. 86.1)
  - Proximal catheter: typically situated in right anterior lateral ventricle, placed via burr hole, drains CSF to shunt device.
  - Shunt device: various types; typically includes valve and reservoir(s); externally palpable.
  - Distal catheter: subcutaneous tubing connects device to site of drainage (most commonly peritoneum).
- Complications: many patients require revision at least once during their lifetime.
  - Undershunting: most common; owing to obstruction of proximal or distal catheter or to shunt device malfunction.
  - Overshunting: can cause "slit ventricles" leading to subdural hematoma or hygroma.
  - Infections: highest risk is 3 to 4 months following placement or revision.

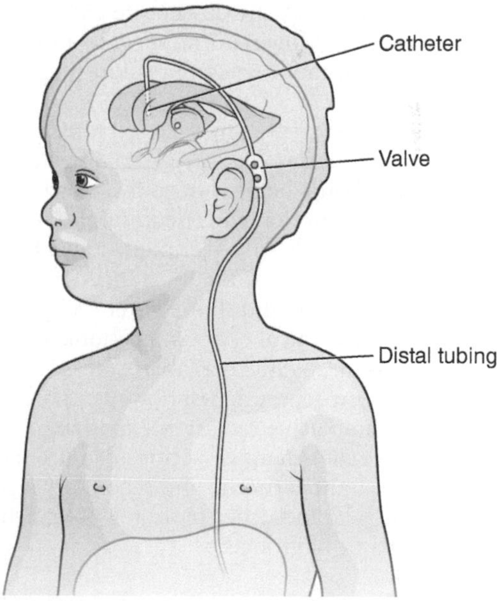

FIG. 86.1 The basic tripartite ventricular shunt system is composed of a ventricular catheter, valve mechanism, and distal tubing. A slit valve may be used in the far end of the distal tubing instead of a more proximally placed valve, as shown. (From Conforto, A., & Wagner, J. G. (2019). Management of increased intracranial pressure and intracranial shunts. In J. R. Roberts, C. B. Custalow, & T. W. Thomsen (Eds.), *Roberts and Hedges' clinical procedures in emergency medicine and acute care* (7th ed., pp. 1243–1257.e2, Fig. 59.12). Elsevier.)

- Distal site complications: bowel injury or obstruction, systemic infections (e.g., endocarditis) from catheter seeding.

Clinical Presentation

- Presenting symptoms of hydrocephalus and shunt malfunctions can range from mild to life-threatening depending on the rapidity of accumulation and resultant change in ICP and mass effect on brain structures.
  - Rapid accumulation can lead to severe altered mental status, coma, and death.
  - Chronic and subacute accumulation is more subtle. Symptoms can mimic systemic illness.
    - Neurologic: headache, cranial nerve palsies, upward gaze deficits, ataxia, hyperreflexia.
    - Cardiovascular: Cushing reflex (bradycardia, hypertension, irregular breathing).
    - Gastrointestinal: nausea, vomiting.
  - In preverbal patients the presentation is typically irritability, lethargy, loss of developmental milestones, diminished level of consciousness, and bulging fontanelle.
  - Parents and caretakers can offer an important perspective into baseline behavior and similarity to prior shunt malfunctions.
  - Important to evaluate for other conditions that may mimic shunt malfunction. Pyelonephritis is a common mimic in patients who are also catheter dependent.

Diagnosis and Evaluation

- In addition to thorough physical examination, neurologic evaluation and careful gait examination, the shunt device itself should be examined.
  - Palpate the distal tubing for kinks, palpable breaks, overlying skin changes, tenderness, inflammation, or CSF accumulation at the device site or burr hole.
  - Palpate reservoir: slow refilling suggests proximal obstruction; resistance to compression suggests distal obstruction.
  - Reservoir may be aseptically accessed for CSF studies using lumbar puncture kit and 23- to 25-gauge butterfly needle (should only be performed by knowledgeable provider in conjunction with neurosurgical consult). Measuring pressure by this technique may also aid in the diagnosis of obstruction.
  - Imaging of the brain and shunt system may be needed when there is a clinical concern of shunt malfunction.
  - CT of the brain: readily available, quick to obtain in most emergency departments; however, potential harm from cumulative radiation exposure.
    - Allows for assessment of ventricular size, positioning of proximal catheter, and secondary signs of increased ICP and other pathology (e.g., subdural hematoma or hygromas).
    - Comparison to prior studies important, because patients may have baseline ventricular enlargement and other neurologic abnormalities.
    - Dilation of ventricles suggests hydrocephalus (expansion of temporal horns of the lateral ventricles is the earliest sign).
  - Magnetic resonance imaging: poor availability in most emergency departments, but no radiation and single axial T2 diffusion-weighted sequences may be performed rapidly.
    - Able to visualize transependymal extravasation of CSF
    - All patients with a programmable shunt undergoing magnetic resonance imaging must have the shunt evaluated by a neurosurgeon, because the magnetic field may modify shunt device settings.
  - Plain film "shunt series": anterior-posterior radiographs of shunt catheter and tubing allowing for radiographic assessment of any potential kinks, breaks, or disconnections.
  - Because approximately one-third of patients with a final diagnosis of shunt malfunction may not have radiographic findings supporting the diagnosis, consultation with neurosurgery may be necessary in patients whose clinical picture could be attributable to the ventricular shunt not functioning correctly.

Treatment

- It is critical to obtain a neurosurgical consult early in the setting of a suspected shunt malfunction and to make management decisions in conjunction with consultant recommendations. Patients with shunt malfunctions may require reprogramming of shunt settings or complete neurosurgical revision of their shunt.
- In patients who are clinically deteriorating owing to herniation, access and drainage of CSF from the shunt reservoir can be a lifesaving temporizing measure while the patient awaits definitive neurosurgical treatment.
- Any patient with concern for a shunt infection requires broad-spectrum antibiotics to cover *Staphylococcus* species as well as gram-negative bacteria and will likely require revision of the shunt by a neurosurgeon.

SUGGESTED READINGS

Madsen, M. A. (1986). Emergency department management of ventriculoperitoneal cerebrospinal fluid shunts. *Annals of Emergency Medicine, 15*(11), 1330–1343.

Osterman, J. L., & Rischall, M. L. (2014). Management of increased intracranial pressure and intracranial shunts. In J. R. Roberts, C. B. Custalow, T. W. Thomsen, & J. R. Hedges (Eds.), *Roberts and Hedges' clinical procedures in emergency medicine* (6th ed.). Elsevier Saunders.

Weingrow, D. W., & Lentz, J. F. (2018). Ventricular shunt evaluation and aspiration. In E. F. Reichman (Ed.), *Reichman's emergency medicine procedures*. McGraw Hill Professional.

SECTION TWELVE

BOARD REVIEW

Obstetrics and Gynecology

CHAPTER **87**

BOARD REVIEW

Adult Gynecology

DANIEL ICHWAN, MD, and PAMELA L. DYNE, MD

Abnormal (or Dysfunctional) Uterine Bleeding (AUB/DUB)

General Principles

- Defined as bleeding that is irregular in volume, frequency, or duration compared with the patient's normal menstrual history
- Most nonpregnant abnormal uterine bleeding (AUB) is not life-threatening, but may be distressing to the patient. Some bleeding (primarily that secondary to fibroids) may require blood transfusion for symptomatic anemia.

Diagnosis and Evaluation

- The differential diagnosis of AUB (and vaginal bleeding) is listed in Table 87.1.
- Presenting symptoms vary significantly and are largely dependent on the severity and etiology of the bleeding. If the bleeding is significant, women may present with symptoms of anemia, including chest pain, shortness of breath, lightheadedness, or syncope.
- Other presenting symptoms may be related to the underlying etiology. It is important to ask targeted questions in an attempt to uncover underlying systemic etiologies manifesting as AUB.
  - Thyroid disease (hypo/hyper): cold/heat intolerance, constipation/diarrhea, changes to hair and skin, and psychomotor symptoms (depression/activation)
  - Polycystic ovarian syndrome (PCOS): can present with symptoms secondary to enlarged ovaries/cysts, including cyst rupture and torsion. May also have acanthosis nigricans.
  - Hyperandrogenism: may present with hirsutism, changes to voice, or acne
  - Hyperprolactinemia: may note breast changes and/or discharge (e.g., galactorrhea). May also present with headache plus or minus homonymous hemianopsia if caused by a primary pituitary tumor.
  - Fibroids: will often present with heavy, irregular, and painful periods. Patient may note an enlarging abdominal mass.
  - Menopause: has an average age of 51 in the United States. Will present with irregular periods, some of which may be heavy, and sometimes with other symptoms of hormonal fluctuation (e.g., "hot flashes," vaginal atrophy).
- History should include the volume and duration of bleeding, menstrual history (last menstrual period [LMP], previous pattern of menstruation [e.g., regular vs, irregular]), obstetric history (gravida, para, infections), history of trauma/vigorous sex, possible retained foreign body, medications (especially contraceptives, assistive reproduction, chemotherapy, anticoagulants, steroids, and antipsychotics), coagulopathy history (von Willebrand disease), endocrine history (PCOS, hypo-/hyperthyroidism, pituitary tumors), and other symptoms, including fever, dysuria, vaginal discharge, abdominal and/or pelvic pain.
- The first step in the physical examination is determining the source of bleeding, if possible (uterine vs. vaginal vs. other including gastrointestinal or urinary). This is especially true in older patients with dementia, when it can be unclear where the bleeding is originating.
- Physical examination should include a pelvic examination with speculum to evaluate for infectious causes, retained foreign bodies, or cervical abnormalities, including cervical malignancy (and to determine the

TABLE 87.1 ***Differential Diagnosis for Common Causes of Uterine and Vaginal Bleeding***

Cause	Notes
Polyps	Causes mid-menstrual cycle bleeding
Adenomyosis	Endometrial glands/stroma within myometrium. Painful, heavy, irregular periods
Leiomyoma (fibroids)	Heavy or irregular bleeding, especially if endometrial-deforming fibroids
Malignancy	Endometrial hyperplasia/cancer. Causes irregular bleeding. Consider especially if age more than 45 years, postmenopausal bleeding or risk factors for endometrial cancer
Coagulopathy	Von Willebrand is the most common
Ovulatory dysfunction	Usually secondary to anovulation, exogenous hormones, or eating disorders. Can also be precipitated by endocrine disorders (PCOS, hyper- or hypothyroidism, pituitary tumors)
Arteriovenous malformations	Can cause life-threatening bleeding.
Infectious	Pelvic inflammatory disease, cervicitis, endometritis
Iatrogenic	Can be seen after any uterine procedure, including uterine biopsies and dilation and curettage (D&C) (both elective and non-elective). If seen after D&C, evaluate for uterine perforation (see Chapter 90. Early Pregnancy Complications)
Vaginal bleeding	Atrophic vaginitis, infections (commonly candida), trauma, foreign bodies

source of bleeding as above). An adnexal or uterine mass or vascular lesions may be identified. Obtain cervical testing for gonorrhea and chlamydia (GC) based on examination or local screening practices. If clinical concern for cervicitis or PID exists, it should be treated (see below).

- After determining the bleeding is in fact uterine and without a clear source on physical examination, the next step is a urine pregnancy test, because this changes the diagnostic algorithm (See Chapter 90. Early Pregnancy Complications).
- Many emergency physicians (EPs) would obtain a complete blood cell count (CBC) to evaluate for anemia, although not strictly necessary in the emergency department (ED) if the patient is hemodynamically stable, with minimal bleeding on examination, and without symptoms of anemia.
- Other testing, such as thyroid-stimulating hormone (TSH) and coagulation studies should be ordered as directed by history and physical examination. Women who are taking warfarin or have an underlying bleeding disorder should have coagulation parameters assessed.
- Pelvic ultrasound is usually not necessary emergently for abnormal uterine bleeding without significant pain (e.g., to evaluate for torsion or other causes of pelvic pain) unless the patient is having severe bleeding requiring transfusion and/or admission. Otherwise this test, although often diagnostic, can usually be deferred to the outpatient setting.
- Those with an increased risk of endometrial hyperplasia or cancer should be referred for outpatient follow-up to obtain an endocervical curettage/endometrial biopsy (ECC/EMB).

Treatment

- If hemodynamically unstable/severe bleeding
  - Stabilize airway/breathing
  - Resuscitate with intravenous (IV) fluids/blood transfusions
  - Correct underlying coagulopathies and reverse anti-coagulants if present
  - Look for trauma or other reversible causes
  - Obstetric/gynecologic (Ob/Gyn) consult/admission with possible operative intervention
  - Consider tranexamic acid
  - Consider intrauterine tamponade with a large Foley or Bakri balloon
  - Consider IV conjugated estrogens
- Determine etiology, if possible (as above, further investigation outside of a physical examination is often only needed for patients with significant bleeding requiring transfusion and/or admission).
- For stable patients, address anemia with transfusion, if needed, guided by symptoms and CBC.
- Iron (plus vitamin C), folate and/or vitamin B_{12} supplementation is recommended for discharged patients.
- Many discharged patients will benefit from hormonal therapy with estrogen-progestin combinations if no contraindications exist (Table 87.2).
  - Medroxyprogesterone 5-30 mg three times a day (TID) for 7 days (especially if concern for endometrial pathology)
  - Oral contraceptive pills (e.g., Ethinyl estradiol 35 μg with 0.25 mg noregestimate TID for 7 days)
- Oral tranexamic acid 1 g three times a day for 5 days may be given with hormonal therapy or alone to help limit bleeding. This is a good option for patients with contraindications to hormonal therapy.
- Patients should be counseled to follow up with Ob/Gyn in 1 to 2 weeks for further evaluation (likely pelvic ultrasound plus or minus ECC/EMB).

TABLE 87.2 Contraindications to Hormonal Therapy for Abnormal Uterine Bleeding

History of venous thromboembolism
Known thrombogenic mutations
35 or more years of age and smoking 15 or more cigarettes/day
Complex migraines
History of hormonal responsive malignancies
Chronic liver disease or liver tumors

Adnexal Masses

- Adnexal masses can be found as either an etiology of a patient's symptoms or incidentally on imaging. In the ED, EPs should focus on life- or organ-threatening complications, including ruptured hemorrhagic cysts and adnexal torsion. Additionally, it is important for EPs to be familiar with follow-up recommendations because many of these masses require outpatient follow-up and are a common incidental finding (Table 87.3). Note that urine or serum pregnancy testing should be performed in all reproductive-age women who present with an adnexal mass.

Hemorrhagic Cysts

General Principles

- Cysts are fluid-filled sacs that develop during the normal menstrual cycle and rupture at ovulation.
- Hemorrhagic cysts occur if a blood vessel in a cyst wall ruptures. Can rupture into the cyst itself or freely into the abdomen causing hemoperitoneum.

Clinical Presentation

- Classic symptoms include sudden unilateral pain mid-menstrual cycle, usually after physical activity or sexual intercourse.
- Can mimic ovarian torsion (see below), although pain tends to abate over time; whereas with torsion, unless intermittent, pain remains constant or worsens with time.

Diagnosis and Evaluation

- After pregnancy has been ruled out, a complete blood count should be drawn, if anemia is suspected secondary to the ruptured hemorrhagic cyst. Serial measurements of hematocrit may be indicated for monitoring.
- Hemodynamic status is a key determinant of whether surgery is indicated.

TABLE 87.3 *Commonly Encountered Ovarian Masses*

Diagnosis	Notes	Follow-Up
Simple cyst	Common, caused by ovulatory cycles.	Does not require follow-up imaging if < 5 cm.*
Hemorrhagic cyst	Caused by bleeding into simple cysts.	Does not require follow-up imaging if < 5 cm.*
Endometrioma	Ectopic endometrial tissue within the ovary. Also called "chocolate cysts." Present with cyclic pelvic pain, dysmenorrhea, and dyspareunia.	Generally, will need follow-up ultrasound in 6–12 weeks.
Dermoid cyst	Usually in 10- 30-year-olds. Ovarian germ cell neoplasm. High risk of torsion.	Needs 1- to 2-week follow-up.
Malignancy	More common with increasing age. Nonspecific symptoms, with bloating, anorexia, constipation, and ascites. Often diagnosed late.	Will need urgent Ob/Gyn follow up.
Tuboovarian abscess (TOA)	Extension of pelvic inflammatory disease into the adnexal structures and fallopian tubes.	Requires intravenous antibiotics and admission for possible operative drainage vs. drainage via interventional radiology.

*Note: These follow-up recommendations are for low-risk patients (e.g., premenopausal healthy young women). For high-risk patients (e.g., older, perimenopausal/menopausal/postmenopausal or with comorbid conditions), follow-up recommendations are more conservative.

- Pelvic examination should be performed in an attempt to localize pain (adnexal vs. abdominal) as well as evaluate for PID or tuboovarian abscesses (TOA) as a cause of unilateral pelvic pain. Ultrasound cannot differentiate a TOA from other complex cystic structures such as hemorrhagic cysts (see below).
- Ultrasound should be obtained for both diagnosis and to rule out torsion because their clinical presentations are similar. Ultrasound will show an ovarian cyst with internal echoes and may show free fluid in the pelvis. A Focused Assessment with Sonography in Trauma (FAST) examination should be completed for hemodynamically unstable women to rule out hemoperitoneum prior to formal ultrasound with radiology.

Treatment

- Provide analgesia usually with nonsteroidal antiinflammatory drugs (NSAIDs) (e.g. ketorolac or ibuprofen)
- Although rare, hemorrhagic cysts can rupture and cause significant hemoperitoneum (hemoperitoneum should be assumed to be a ruptured ectopic in young women until proven otherwise). These patients require resuscitation and an emergent Ob/Gyn consult because they can require operative management.
- Once torsion and hemodynamically significant rupture have been ruled out, patients can be discharged with analgesia and Ob/Gyn or primary care provider follow-up for serial ultrasounds to ensure resolution.
- Can consider oral contraceptive pills (OCPs) to prevent formation of new cysts, in consultation with Ob/Gyn.
- Other types of cysts commonly encountered are simple cysts, dermoid cysts, endometriomas, and malignancies (see Table 87.3 for characterization and recommended follow-up). Of note, concerning adnexal masses tend to be large (> 8 cm), solid, or multi-loculated, and the risk of ovarian torsion increases for ovarian masses ≥ 5 cm.

OVARIAN (ADNEXAL) TORSION

General Principles

- Owing to the partial or complete rotation of the ovary on the infundibulopelvic and uteroovarian ligaments, ovarian torsion initially obstructs venous drainage, eventually leading to decreased arterial blood flow, ischemia, and necrosis of the ovary, with subsequent hemorrhage, peritonitis, and infertility.
- Ovarian enlargement (cyst or masses **usually 5 cm** or greater) increases the risk, but torsion can occur in normal ovaries.
- Usually involves both ovary and fallopian tube (adnexal) torsion
- Usually on the right (70%) owing to increased utero-ovarian ligament length on right and sigmoid colon limiting movement on the left

Clinical Presentation

- Classically presents with sudden, severe, unilateral lower abdominal pain, especially in the setting of exertion, **but** atypical presentations are common with gradual and/or intermittent pain.
- Nausea/vomiting is common (70%).
- May cause fever if ovarian necrosis has developed
- Unilateral lower abdominal/adnexal tenderness on physical examination with or without a palpable adnexal mass

Diagnosis and Evaluation

- Must have a high index of clinical suspicion in women presenting with unilateral lower abdominal/adnexal pain as ultrasound is not always diagnostic
- Laboratory work-up includes a urine pregnancy test (ectopic pregnancies can present similarly) with consideration of a CBC to evaluate for anemia in the event a hemorrhagic cyst is found. If suspicion is very high, may consider preoperative laboratory studies, including a type and screen.
- Diagnostic modality of choice is a transvaginal ultrasound with Doppler.
  - Ovary that is 5 cm or greater owing to cyst/tumor/edema is the most common finding.
  - Normal adnexa (25%)
  - Normal arterial Doppler has poor sensitivity (45%–75%) owing to the dual blood supply of the ovary, but abnormal arterial blood flow has a 100% positive predictive value for torsion.

- As ultrasound is not always diagnostic, definitive diagnosis is only made by direct visualization of a rotated ovary at the time of surgical evaluation.
- If clinical suspicion is high, Gyn should be consulted even if the ultrasound is negative with normal arterial Doppler flow. **Absence of adnexal mass and/or normal arterial blood flow on ultrasound DOES NOT rule out torsion.**

Treatment

- Both ovarian and tubal torsion are gynecologic emergencies and are treated operatively with detorsion and either ovarian conservation or salpingo-oophorectomy.

Cervicitis and Pelvic Inflammatory Disease (PID)

General Principles

- Cervicitis is inflammation or infection of the cervix often caused by sexually transmitted infections (STIs), such as gonorrhea or chlamydia. Other etiologies include irritation from foreign bodies or allergens.
- PID refers to the spectrum of female upper reproductive tract infection including endometritis, tuboovarian abscess and Fitz-Hugh–Curtis syndrome.
- PID is usually associated with ascending lower genital tract infections, especially *Chlamydia trachomatis*, *Neisseria gonorrheae*, and bacterial vaginosis microbes. Can be polymicrobial (including enteric, anaerobic, respiratory microbes) especially in the setting of an intrauterine device (IUD).
- Complications of PID include tuboovarian abscess (TOA), infertility, increased risk of future ectopic pregnancy, and chronic pain.
- Risk factors include a previous history of STIs or PID, younger age, multiple sexual partners and/or lack of barrier protection. IUDs can also increase risk for both STI and non–STI-related PID.

Clinical Presentation

- Cervicitis may be asymptomatic, but, if symptomatic, patients may complain of vaginal discharge, intermenstrual or postcoital bleeding, dyspareunia and/or vaginal irritation.
- PID presents with bilateral lower abdominal pain that worsens with movement. Abnormal uterine bleeding (postcoital or intermenstrual) occurs in up to one-third of patients. Patients may also note abnormal vaginal discharge (75%), dyspareunia, and/or dysuria.
- **Many patients with PID will have systemic symptoms, including fevers, chills, nausea and/or vomiting.**
- Patients with TOAs, a complication of untreated PID, will present with PID symptoms in addition to disproportionate unilateral abdominal and/or pelvic pain.
- Perihepatitis (Fitz-Hugh-Curtis syndrome), which occurs in the setting of PID with inflammation of the liver capsule, will present with right upper quadrant pain in addition to PID symptoms.

Diagnosis and Evaluation

- Cervicitis and PID are clinical diagnoses. No single history, physical, or laboratory finding is sufficiently sensitive or specific.
- A friable cervix with mucopurulent discharge is diagnostic for cervicitis.
- Uterine tenderness is the defining characteristic of PID. There *may* also be cervical motion tenderness although this is not necessary for diagnosis. Cervicitis may also be absent in some cases.
- Presence of an adnexal mass or significant lateralizing adnexal tenderness on examination in the setting of PID suggests the presence of a TOA.
- Right upper quadrant tenderness on examination in concert with PID findings is concerning for Fitz-Hugh-Curtis syndrome.
- Obtain endocervical gonorrhea and chlamydia (GC) swab culture or nucleic acid amplification testing (NAAT).
  - Of note: although the sensitivity and specificity of urine GC testing has been shown to be similar to endocervical testing in the outpatient setting, this has not been validated in the ED. Outpatient urinalyses for GC are generally collected as "dirty" (e.g., first void of the day, first catch of the stream without cleaning before) in comparison with the "clean catch" urines often obtained in the ED. One should likely still obtain endocervical testing when PID is suspected.
- Recommend that the patient receives testing for other STIs, including HIV, hepatitis, and syphilis, generally done through outpatient clinics.
- Laboratory work is generally of low utility unless the patient is getting admitted (see below). Also, Fitz-Hugh-Curtis is inflammation of the hepatic capsule, not an intrinsic hepatitis, so liver function tests are generally normal in this condition and it is a clinical diagnosis.
- Although concurrent pregnancy and PID is extremely unusual, a pregnancy test should be obtained, as it would be an indication for admission and parenteral antibiotics.
- Urinalysis to exclude UTI
- Saline microscopy of vaginal discharge (wet mount) as increased white blood cells are somewhat sensitive (but not specific) for PID. The wet mount can also evaluate for concurrent trichomonas, yeast, or bacterial vaginosis infections.
- Obtain a transvaginal pelvic ultrasound study if concern for TOA, especially if ill-appearing, asymmetric pelvic examination, or failed outpatient PID treatment.

Treatment

- EPs should have a low threshold for empiric treatment of women at risk for STIs with unexplained lower abdominal pain and adnexal/uterine or cervical motion tenderness, regardless of whether cervicitis is found on examination.
- Analgesia, antiemetic, and/or hydration, if necessary
- No evidence to routinely remove an IUD if in place, although not doing so may increase treatment failure rates. This should be discussed with the patient. Note that PID in the setting of an IUD may not be GC-related, but rather, caused by more typical vaginal flora.
- Patient education, partner evaluation (note that many states allow EPs to provide prescriptions for the treatment of male partners without an in-person evaluation), and abstinence until 1 week after treatment and symptom

TABLE 87.4 Recommended Treatment of Cervicitis and Pelvic Inflammatory Disease (PID)

Cervicitis	Ceftriaxone 500 mg intramuscular once (ceftriaxone 1 g for patients ≥ 150 kg) + Doxycycline 100 mg orally, twice daily for 7 days
PID (outpatient)	Ceftriaxone 500 mg intramuscular once (ceftriaxone 1 g for patients ≥ 150 kg) + Doxycycline 100 mg oral, twice daily for 14 days (counsel patients on sun sensitivity) + Metronidazole 500 mg oral, twice daily for 14 days *A recent trial showed that adding metronidazole routinely has significantly lower rates of subsequent pelvic tenderness with similar adverse effects and adherence compared to placebo. Consider metronidazole especially if intrauterine device in place or history/examination concerning for bacterial vaginosis (BV) or trichomonas. Consider Zofran for gastrointestinal side effects. *Azithromycin 1 g orally weekly for 2 weeks if Doxycycline is not tolerated or contraindicated.
PID (inpatient)	Cefotetan 2 g intravenous twice daily or Cefoxitin 2 g intravenous every 6 hours + Doxycycline 100 mg intravenous twice daily. Alternatively, Clindamycin 900 mg intravenous every 8 hours + Gentamycin 3-5 mg/kg intravenous daily or 2 mg/kg intravenous loading, then 1.5 mg/kg intravenous every 8 hours

resolution. Many suggest a test of cure 1 to 2 weeks after completing treatment.

- Treatment of cervicitis and PID is shown in Table 87.4.
- Consider admission if patient is pregnant (although very rare), low probability of adherence, oral intolerance, toxic appearing, TOA, concern for Fitz-Hugh-Curtis, or outpatient treatment failure.
- Outpatient follow-up within 72 hours is recommended.

Vulvovaginitis

General Principles

- There are many causes of vulvovaginitis. They are summarized in Table 87.5.
- Lack of estrogen causes loss of the acidic environment that prevent pathogenic microbes in the vagina. Therefore, pediatric and post-menopausal patients are

TABLE 87.5 Common Causes, Presentations, and Treatment of Vulvovaginitis

	Cause and Presenting Symptoms	Diagnosis	Treatment
Bacterial vaginosis (40%–45%)	Polymicrobial, including *Gardnerella*, *Ureaplasma*, *Mycoplasma*, anaerobes. Presents with thin, gray, homogenous discharge with a fishy odor. Can be recurrent.	"Clue cells" on wet mount (epithelial cells covered with bacteria). pH > 5.	Metronidazole 500 mg oral twice daily for 7 days, Clindamycin cream 2% 1 applicator daily for 7 days, or Metronidazole gel applicator daily for 5 days.
Vulvovaginal candidiasis (20%–25%)	More common in diabetics. Consider blood sugar testing for recurrent, extensive presentations. Also common after antibiotics. Presents as thick, white, "cottage cheese" -like discharge with significant pruritis. Can see other evidence of candida skin infection.	*Candida* species seen with potassium hydroxide (KOH) on wet mount. pH < 5.	Uncomplicated: Azole creams for 1, 3, 7 days. Oral Fluconazole 150 mg once. Complicated: topical azole for 7–14 days or oral Fluconazole 150 mg on day 1 and 3.
Trichomoniasis (15%–20%)	Parasitic sexually transmitted infection. Presents with frothy, green-yellow discharge. Can present with inflammatory changes of the cervix or vulva.	Mobile *Trichomonas* species seen on wet mount. pH > 5.	Metronidazole 2 g oral x 1 dose (recommended by guidelines). Note that trials have suggested Metronidazole 500 mg orally twice daily for 7 days may have higher cure rates with similar adverse effects and adherence.
Pinworms	Intense pruritis, especially at night.	Can visualize worms/eggs under microscopy using cellophane tape to obtain sample.	Treat patient and family with oral Mebendazole 100 mg day 1 and day 7, oral Albendazole 400 mg day 1 and day 14, or oral Pyrantel pamoate 11 mg/kg (max. 1 g) day 1, 14, and 28.
Contact vulvovaginitis	Local swelling, pruritis, and erythema, usually after exposure to a new product.	Clinical	Rule out infectious cause, identify offending agent, cool sitz baths, wet compresses, low potency topical corticosteroids 14 days.
Atrophic vaginitis	Caused by withdrawal of estrogen during/after menopause. Presents with dryness, pruritis, dyspareunia, and vaginal spotting.	Clinical	Topical vaginal estrogen (if no previous GYN malignancy).
Malignancy	More common in elderly patients. Keep on the differential for recurrent, resistant vulvovaginitis, and refer to OB/GYN.	Biopsy	Depends on pathology.

at higher risk (see Chapter 88. Pediatric Gynecologic Emergencies).

Clinical Presentation

- Usually presents with vaginal discomfort (pain or itching), discharge, dyspareunia, vaginal spotting, dysuria, and variable external skin changes
- Other presenting symptoms depend on etiology (see Table 87.5).

Diagnosis, Evaluation, and Treatment

- Depends on etiology. See Table 87.5.

Bartholin Gland Cyst/Abscess

General Principles

- Bartholin glands are located in the labia minora with ducts draining into the posterior vestibule (4 and 8 o'clock positions). Obstruction of the ducts can cause cysts or abscesses. Abscesses may be recurrent.
- Bartholin gland abscesses are usually polymicrobial.

Clinical Presentation

- Presents with pain, induration, and/or difficulty walking, sitting, or with sexual intercourse.
- Cysts may be nontender, but abscesses will generally be tender, warm, and fluctuant (Fig. 87.1).

Diagnosis and Evaluation

- Diagnosis of an abscess is clinical; the physical examination will show a fluctuant mass at the posterior aspect of inferior introitus.
- Evaluate for surrounding cellulitis to help guide management.

Treatment

- It is important to differentiate an uncomplicated cyst from an abscess based on patient presentation and physical examination because they are treated differently.

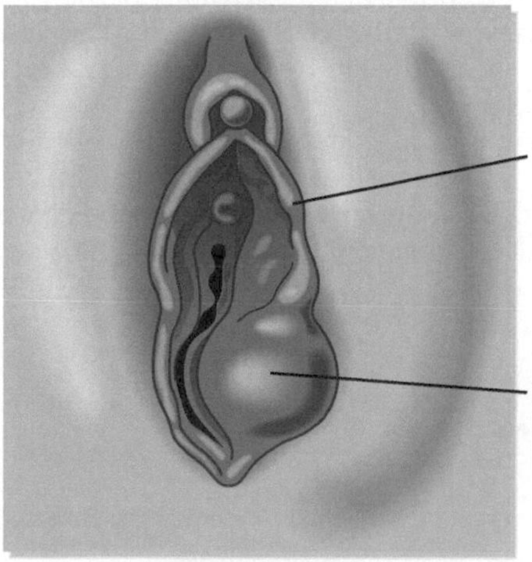

FIG. 87.1 Bartholin gland cyst. (From Adams, J. G., Barton, E. D., Collings, J. L., DeBlieux, P. M. C., Gisondi, M. A., & Nadel, E. S. (2013). *Emergency medicine: Clinical essentials* (2nd ed.). Elsevier Saunders.)

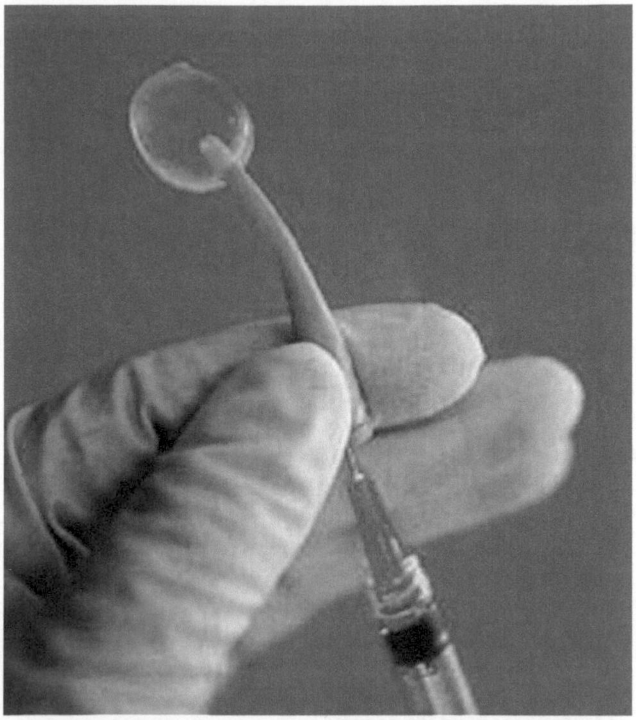

FIG. 87.2 Word catheter. Word catheters are used to develop a fistula from a Bartholin cyst or an abscess to the vestibule. (From Friedrich, E. G. (1983). Vulvar disease (2nd ed.). W. B. Saunders.)

- If a cyst is small (<3 cm) and asymptomatic or minimally symptomatic, they may be managed expectantly with sitz baths and warm compresses.
- Abscesses are usually treated with incision and drainage: local lidocaine, small incision using #11 scalpel on mucosal surface of vestibule, insertion of Word catheter (filled with 2 mL to 4 mL saline). Word catheter may stay in place for 4 to 6 weeks (Fig. 87.2). It is important to insert a Word catheter or the abscess may reaccumulate.
- Analgesia is important because these are painful procedures. May require procedural sedation.
- No antibiotics are needed unless the abscess is recurrent, there are signs of cellulitis, or the patient is immunocompromised (e.g., diabetic).
- Follow-up with OB/GYN in 1 to 2 weeks. Recurrent abscesses often require surgical excision (or marsupialization) and biopsy to rule out an underlying malignancy.

SUGGESTED READINGS

American College of Obstetricians and Gynecologists. Committee Opinion No. 557. Management of acute abnormal uterine bleeding in nonpregnant reproductive-aged women. *Obstetrics and Gynecology, 121*, 891–896, 2013.

Pelvic Inflammatory Disease (PID)—2015 STD Treatment Guidelines. Centers for Disease Control and Prevention. Available at: https://www.cdc.gov/std/tg2015/pid.htm. Accessed March 17, 2019.

Pediatric Gynecologic Emergencies

JAMES JIANG, MD, and NATASHA WHEATON, MD

- Children are susceptible to a variety of specific gynecologic disorders because of their unique anatomy and physiology.
- Performing a gynecologic examination and treating the young female child can be an extremely difficult task for the emergency physician.
- Creating a nonthreatening and soothing environment is critical to facilitating evaluation and treatment.

General Principles

- Normal pediatric gynecologic development
  - Tanner staging (see Table 88.1)
  - Normal puberty onset in girls: 8–13 years old
    - Thelarche: onset of breast development
    - Pubarche: onset of pubic hair development
    - Menarche: onset of menses
- General anatomic features
  - The prepubescent vulva lacks hair or subcutaneous fat and is more susceptible to irritants and trauma.
  - The vestibule is closer to the anus in distance, increasing risk of infection and irritation.
  - The vagina is shorter and lacks distensibility.
  - The hymen is a vascularized membrane separating the vestibule from the vagina, with variability in appearance, shape, and thickness.
- Performing the pediatric gynecologic examination
  - Never physically restrain a child to perform a gynecologic examination. Procedural sedation or examination under anesthesia is preferred to forcibly restraining a child.
  - Allow the parent to remain in the room with the child. Have the parent tell the child that they approve of the examination and explain each step of the examination to the child.
  - To examine the external genitalia, vestibule, or hymen, position the child in the frog-legged position, lying supine on the bed or on the parent's lap. Allow the child's knees to spread apart.
  - To examine the perineum and vaginal vault, position the child in a prone knee-chest position, similar to a crawling baby. Have the child place their elbows and head on the bed.
  - Speculum examination (or any type of internal exam) is rarely indicated in children who are not sexually active, unless required for removal of a foreign body or repair of a traumatic injury, which should be done under sedation or anesthesia.
  - In the prepubescent child, testing for sexually transmitted infections can be done via distal vaginal swab or urine. While some infections (eg, genital warts) can be vertically or accidentally transmitted, the possibility of sexual abuse must be considered when a potentially sexually transmitted infection is identified.

Vulvovaginitis

Clinical Presentation

- Irritation and inflammation of the vulva and outer vaginal vault.
- Children are susceptible due to proximity of the vulva to the anus, lack of protective fat and pubic hair, atrophic vaginal mucosa (due to hypoestrogenic tissue), and thin vulvar skin.
- In young girls it is usually due to inadequate hygiene (poor bathing and urinary/bowel habits). May also be due to local irritants, or infections including group A *Streptococcus*, *Staphylococcus aureus*, *Escherichia coli*, and *Shigella*.

TABLE 88.1 *Tanner Stages*

Tanner Stage	Pubic Hair	Breast Development
1	None	No glandular tissue
2	Sparse, lightly pigmented, straight	Breast bud forms small mound, areola diameter slightly increased
3	Darker pigmentation, slight curling, increased amount	Breast is more elevated, areola continues to widen
4	Coarse, curled, but less than adult	Areola and papilla form mound separate from general breast contour
5	Adult pattern, spreads to medial thigh	Mature, projected nipple, areola follows general breast contour

Candida vaginitis is uncommon in pediatric patients owing to alkaline pH. Sexually transmitted infections, such as gonorrhea, are a rare cause of vulvovaginitis.

Diagnosis and Evaluation

- Clinical diagnosis. Usually presents with pruritis, tenderness, dysuria, erythema, vaginal discharge, and occasionally vaginal bleeding.
- Obtain vaginal cultures if purulent or persistent discharge.

Treatment

- Improve hygiene and avoid local irritants.
- Treat cause, including antibiotics and topical antifungals as indicated (rare).

Vaginal Foreign Body

Clinical Presentation

- Often presents with bloody, purulent, or foul-smelling vaginal discharge due to irritation, which can lead to superimposed infection.
- Discharge is often resistant to treatment and it is not uncommon for foreign bodies to be missed at the index visit.
- Often toilet paper, small toys, coins, or hair accessories.

Diagnosis and Evaluation

- Attempt examination in prone knee-chest position.
- As above, **do not** hold children down to examine them. If unable to visualize, consult with obstetrics/gynecology for an examination under anesthesia or procedural sedation either in the emergency department, in the OR or in clinic at follow-up.

Treatment

- Attempt removal with forceps, swabs, or warm-water irrigation (lavage). Applying a topical anesthetic agent, such as xylocaine jelly before the examination, may be helpful. Most foreign bodies, with the exception of large objects and button batteries, can be successfully removed.
- If unsuccessful, may require sedation or examination under anesthesia.

Premenarchal Vaginal Bleeding

General Principles

- The differential diagnosis is listed in Box 88.1.
- Ensure that the symptoms are due to blood and determine whether the blood is from the genitals, stool, or urine.

BOX 88.1 ***Differential Diagnosis of Premenarchal Vaginal Bleeding***

Onset of menarche, precocious puberty
Vulvovaginitis
Foreign body
Maternal estrogen withdrawal
Urethral prolapse
Trauma or abuse
Neoplasm
Iatrogenic

Diagnosis, Evaluation, and Treatment

- ***Precocious puberty:*** generally considered before 8 years of age or if bleeding occurs out of synchrony with other signs of pubertal development (menarche usually occurs about 2.5 years after the onset of breast development). Characterized by painless bleeding, breast development greater than expected, and estrogenized-appearing vaginal mucosa. Stable patients should have follow-up with pediatric endocrinology.
- ***Maternal estrogen withdrawal:*** neonatal patients. In utero, the fetus is exposed to maternal estrogens. After birth, the neonatal uterine membrane sloughs off, similar to during the menstrual cycle. Occurs typically in the first weeks of life, and lasts only several days. Characterized by painless vaginal bleeding with otherwise normal examination findings. No treatment is needed aside from parental reassurance.
- ***Urethral prolapse:*** usually presents between 2 and 10 years of age with a history of "vaginal bleeding" (although this does not technically involve the vagina), and more commonly in those of African ethnicity. The urethral mucosa extrudes outward through the meatus and appears as a purplish mass between the labia majora. Characterized by painless spotting on underwear, dysuria and difficulty with urination. Can lead to tissue necrosis over time. May be secondary to chronic Valsalva maneuvers, secondary to constipation or chronic cough. Treat with Sitz baths and topical estrogen creams, and treat underlying cause if present.

Imperforate Hymen

General Principles

- Hymenal membrane remains intact, causing vaginal outflow obstruction of menstrual blood.

Clinical Presentation

- In neonates, may present as a bulging introitus.
- At menarche, the patient may present with amenorrhea in a female who has secondary sexual characteristics. Additionally, there may be complaints of cyclic pelvic and lower abdominal pain and/or back pain. Can also present with urinary retention if uterus becomes distended enough with blood products.

Diagnosis and Evaluation

- Tender pelvic or lower abdomen mass
- Accumulation of products causes bulging of the membrane, often presenting as a bluish mass at the vaginal introitus.

Treatment

- Adolescents may require urgent surgical repair, but infants/young girls may have elective repair.

Straddle Injuries

General Principles

- Due to the vagina, perineum, and anus bluntly impacting a hard surface
  - Age 0-4 years: Consider if mechanism offered is a reasonable cause of injury and developmentally

plausible. It can be difficult to differentiate injuries from sexual abuse/ non-accidental trauma from self-inflicted straddle injuries.
  - Age 5–9: most frequently caused by falls and bicycle accidents
- Many straddle injuries result only in superficial abrasions, lacerations, or hematomas.

Clinical Presentation

- Presents with pain and/or bleeding (vaginal, vulvar, or perineal) after a traumatic event
- If presenting without a clear history of traumatic event or in a younger age group, consider nonaccidental trauma.

Diagnosis and Evaluation

- Detailed physical examination is critical. Pay careful attention to the anus, perineum, vulva, urethra, labia, hymen, vagina. Procedural sedation may be necessary.
- Ensure the child is able to urinate.

Treatment

- Minor superficial injuries: supportive care, analgesia. Pain with voiding can be relieved by having the child void in a warm-water bath.
- About 10% of straddle injuries require operative management. Children with significant injuries, expanding hematomas, deep lacerations, urinary retention, persistent vaginal bleeding without identified lesion or rectal bleeding should be evaluated by a pediatric surgeon and/or gynecologist.

Ovarian Torsion

Ovarian torsion, although rare, can occur in pediatric patients and should be considered for any female regardless of age presenting with unilateral pelvic pain. Ovarian torsion involves a previously normal ovary in 25% of pediatric cases.

Clinical Presentation

- Verbal children present similarly to adults with acute-onset lower abdominal/pelvic pain. May be accompanied by vomiting.
- In preverbal or nonverbal children, may present with isolated vomiting. Depending on the age of the child, may or may not be able to communicate accompanying pain.
- Symptoms may be intermittent if there is intermittent ovarian blood flow (e.g., intermittent ovarian torsion).
- Pain is often acute in onset but not always.
- Torsion is most often right-sided (as in adults) and it is commonly mistaken for appendicitis.
- Should be included in the differential diagnosis for an inconsolable female child especially with vomiting and any female child with unilateral pelvic pain.
- Emergency physicians must have a high index of suspicion because this is a difficult diagnosis to make as presenting symptoms vary.

Diagnosis and Evaluation

- Physical examination demonstrates lower abdominal tenderness with or without peritonitis, depending on how long the ovary has been without blood flow.
- Transabdominal ultrasonography is the diagnostic modality of choice. A full bladder can help with ovarian visualization. Just as in adults, flow on ultrasonography does NOT rule out torsion.
- Look for secondary signs of torsion
  - enlarged ovary
  - peripherally displaced follicles
  - a midline ovary
  - free fluid in the pelvis

Treatment

- Prompt obstetrics/gynecology (or pediatric surgery) consult if there is high suspicion (even with flow on ultrasonography).
- As in adults, treatment is operative detorsion of the ovary. Goal is to restore flow within 6–8 hours.

SUGGESTED READINGS

Horeczko, T. (host) (2018, January). Ovarian torsion [audio podcast]. In *Pediatric emergency playbook*. https://pemplaybook.org/podcast/ovarian-torsion/

Stone, C. K., Stephan, M., Humphries, R., & Drigalla, D. (2014). *LANGE current diagnosis and treatment: Pediatric emergency medicine*. McGraw-Hill Education.

Tintinalli, J. E., Stapczynski, J. S., Ma, O. J., Yealy, D. M., Meckler, G. D., & Cline, D. M. (Eds.), (2016). *Tintinalli's emergency medicine: A comprehensive study guide* (8th ed.). McGraw-Hill Education.

CHAPTER 89

BOARD REVIEW

Normal Pregnancy, Labor, and Delivery

ANNA NGUYEN, DO, and PAMELA L. DYNE, MD

Physiologic Changes of Normal Pregnancy

Background Information

- Various physiologic changes occur during pregnancy to accommodate maternal and fetal needs (Table 89.1). It is important to understand and recognize normal changes to identify abnormal findings.

Normal Labor and Delivery

Background Information

- Normal labor progression requires frequent assessment (3 Ps)
  - Power: strength of uterine contractions
  - Passenger: fetal size, lie, presentation and station

TABLE 89.1 *Normal Physiologic and Laboratory Changes Seen in Pregnancy*

System	Physiologic Change	Notes
Cardiovascular	Increased resting heart rate (HR)	Response to increased maternal and fetal metabolic requirements HR is typically NOT more than 95 beats/min (a HR greater than 100 beats/min should be further evaluated)
	Decreased blood pressure (BP)	Owing to decreased systemic vascular resistance from vasodilation and the addition of low-resistance uteroplacental circulation Mean BP 100–105/60
	Increased cardiac output (CO)	Increases by 30%–50% to accommodate flow to fetus Affected by maternal positioning (e.g., compression of the inferior vena cava by the gravid uterus when supine)
	Electrographic changes	Left axis deviation, small Q waves in III/aVF, TWI in III and V1-V3 can be considered normal in pregnancy
Respiratory		
	Respiratory alkalosis	Owing to increased minute ventilation from increased tidal volume Relative decrease in pCO_2 (27–32 mm Hg)
	Shift in oxygen dissociation curve to the right	Relative intolerance to hypoxia
Hematologic	Decreased hematocrit and hemoglobin	Larger increase in plasma volume compared with red blood cell mass (anemia of pregnancy) By third trimester net increase of intravascular volume of 50%
	Leukocytosis or leukopenia	Physiologic neutrophilia occurs in the first trimester and peaks in the third trimester (leukocytosis up to 15 K cells/μL) Any white blood cell count value greater than 20 K or less than 1 K cells/μL is abnormal
	Hypercoagulability	Hormonal changes in pregnancy affect the amount and functionality of clotting factors leading to increased risk of clotting both arterial and venous (e.g., pulmonary embolism/deep vein thrombosis, sinus venous thrombosis and ischemic stroke)
Renal	Decreased BUN/Cr (increased GFR)	Secondary to increased CO and vasodilation increasing BUN/Cr clearance A "normal" Cr of 1.0 mg/dL should be considered abnormal in pregnancy
	Decreased bicarbonate	Metabolic compensation for respiratory alkalosis

BUN, blood urea nitrogen; *Cr*, creatinine; *GFR*, glomerular filtration rate.

  - Pelvis: optimal maternal position to maximize the dimensions of the pelvic inlet upon delivery
- Stages of labor
  - Stage I: onset of regularly occurring contractions to complete cervical dilation, separated by a latent and active phase
    - Latent phase: slow cervical change up to 4 cm
    - Active phase: faster rate of cervical change from 4 cm to complete dilation, usually 1 to 2 cm/hr
  - Stage II: time from complete cervical dilation to delivery of fetus
  - Stage III: time from delivery of fetus to delivery of placenta

Precipitous Delivery in the Emergency Department

Background Information

- Thousands of deliveries in the United States occur precipitously in the emergency department (or prehospital at home/with emergency medical services) each year; thus it is important to review key concepts and procedural points to ensure a safe and successful delivery.

Diagnosis and Evaluation

History

- Essential historical obstetric assessment includes a history of gravidity and parity, evaluation of fetal gestational age, maternal and/or obstetrical medical problems (specifically bleeding diathesis), duration of rupture of membranes, and presence of meconium.
- Women who have had prior vaginal deliveries will often have more rapid labor progression. The emergency physician and team must prepare quickly and anticipate a more rapid delivery in a multiparous patient. This may mean not allowing a multiparous patient who is nearing complete dilation to leave the emergency department and go to labor and delivery because delivery could be imminent and occur before she arrives to the unit.
- Recognition of potential neonatal prematurity helps determine the level of neonatal resuscitation for which the physician and team must be prepared. For unresponsive patients, the gestational age can roughly be determined by measuring the distance in centimeters from the pubic symphysis to the top of the uterine fundus. The number of centimeters estimates the gestational age in weeks.
  - Fewer than 22 weeks: low likelihood of fetal survival
  - 22 to 25 weeks: varies, fetal morbidity/mortality increases with each additional week of prematurity
  - 26 or more weeks: high likelihood of fetal survival
- Assessment of past obstetrical history, such as placenta previa, pre-eclampsia, and prior cesarean sections can help prepare for possible intra- or postpartum emergencies.
  - Do NOT perform a cervical examination if the patient has a known history of placenta previa unless delivery is clearly imminent as it may precipitate life-threatening bleeding.
- Rupture of membranes 18 or more hours before delivery increases the risk of neonatal infections, and this should be appropriately addressed with administration of antibiotics and preparation for neonatal resuscitation.
- Leakage of brown amniotic fluid is concerning for the presence of meconium, and the emergency physician should be prepared for an increased risk of delivering an infant requiring resuscitation.
  - Note that meconium is no longer an indication to perform direct laryngoscopy with suctioning of the airway in a vigorous infant. This should only be performed if the baby is not vigorous.

Physical Examination

- A sterile manual cervical examination is indicated to determine cervical dilation *unless* there is concern for placenta previa or preterm premature rupture of membranes *and* the woman does not appear to be imminently delivering.
- If the woman is voluntarily pushing with her contractions, she is likely in the second phase of labor and will soon deliver.
- If the fetus is crowning from the vagina, delivery is imminent.
- Determine the presenting part, either by ultrasound or examination. Vaginal delivery of a footling breech fetus is contraindicated, and routine breech delivery is not in the usual scope of practice for emergency physicians (see Chapter 92. Complications of Delivery); thus, urgent consultation with obstetric colleagues is essential for all breech presentations.

Treatment

- See Table 89.2 for equipment and supplies recommended for a routine emergency department delivery.
- Steps of a normal vaginal delivery (Fig. 89.1)
  - Presentation of head
    - Protect the perineum: prevent rapid expulsion of fetal head and subsequent tearing of the perineum by applying light pressure on the fetal presenting part with one hand and using the other hand to ease the perineum over the fetal face. Ask the mother to stop pushing, although this is difficult during an unmedicated delivery.
    - Assess for the presence of a nuchal cord and reduce over the head, if possible.
      - If there is resistance to reducing the cord easily over the fetal head, do NOT pull traction owing to the risk of avulsing the cord and precipitating

TABLE 89.2 *Equipment Recommended for an Emergency Department Delivery*

Gauze	Red-top tube to collect fetal blood
Sterile gloves and gowns	Clean towels to dry and swaddle the infant
Two sterile clamps to clamp umbilical cord	Container for placenta
Sterile scissors	Baby warmer (if available)
Bulb suction	Neonatal resuscitative equipment

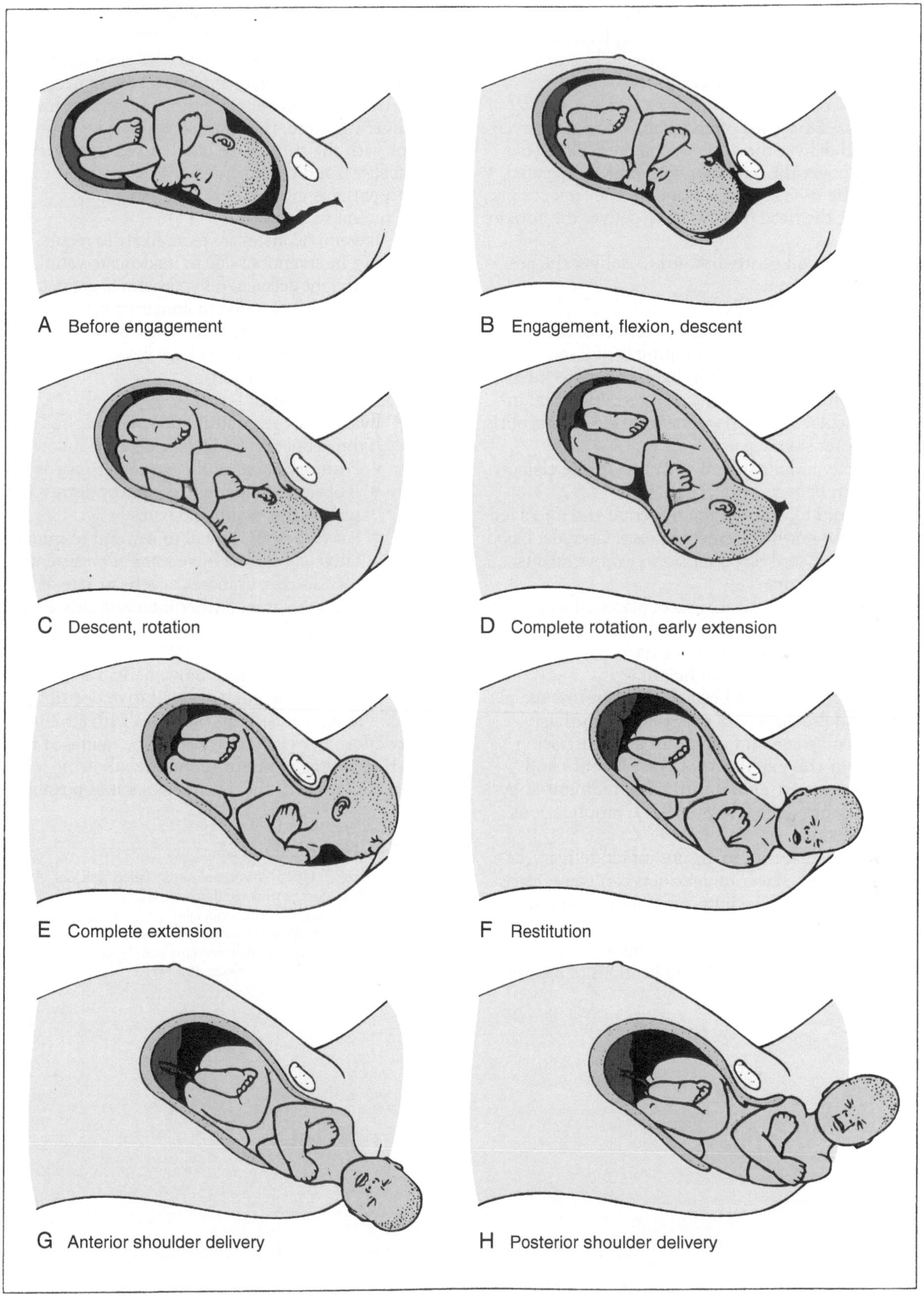

FIG. 89.1 Cardinal movements of labor. (From Kilpatrick, S., & Garrison, E. (2017). Normal labor and delivery. In S. G. Gabbe, J. R. Niebyl, J. L. Simpson, M. B. Landon, H. L. Galan, E. R. M. Jauniaux, D. A. Driscoll, V. Berghella, & W. A. Grobman (Eds.), *Obstetrics: Normal and problem pregnancies* (7th ed., pp. 246–270, Fig. 12.11). Elsevier.)

fetal hemorrhage. In this situation, it is best to allow the fetus to deliver completely and *then* reduce the nuchal cord (see Chapter 92. Complications of Delivery).

- Delivery of body
  - Rotate the fetus (this often occurs without intervention) and deliver the anterior shoulder. Place your left hand over the fetal face with fingers separated around the nose and right hand on the fetal occiput, and guide the head downward to deliver the anterior shoulder.
  - Guide the head gently upward to deliver the posterior shoulder.
  - Deliver the lower body.
- Umbilical cord clamping and collection of cord blood
  - Allow for delayed cord clamping for 60 seconds. Delayed cord clamping has been shown to increase infant iron stores and reduce preterm neonatal intraventricular hemorrhage, necrotizing enterocolitis, and hypotension.
  - Clamp the umbilical cord with two sterile clamps, and cut in between the clamps.
  - Collect cord blood from the placental end into a red-top tube for newborn screening tests. Consider blood gas testing of cord blood for non-vigorous infants.
- Delivery of placenta
  - Look for the three classic signs of placental separation:
    - Lengthening of the umbilical cord
    - Gush of blood from the vagina
    - Elevation of the fundal height
  - Avoid excess traction because this can tear the placenta and precipitate postpartum hemorrhage.
  - Uterine massage and oxytocin administration can aid in the expulsion of the placenta and control postpartum hemorrhage precipitated by uterine atony (see Chapter 92. Complications of Delivery).
  - Inspect the placenta to ensure intact delivery, because retained placental products can cause persistent postpartum bleeding (secondary postpartum hemorrhage).
  - Inspect the perineum for lacerations and repair, as indicated (see Chapter 92. Complications of Delivery).

Evaluation of the Neonate

- After delivery of the neonate, the emergency physician must quickly complete a neonatal assessment based on the three criteria below. If the emergency physician is delivering alone, this must sometimes be done concurrent with the third stage of labor (e.g., delivery of the placenta), and the emergency physician must manage both patients at once.
  - Preterm vs. term
    - Preterm neonates are more likely to require resuscitative interventions due to inadequate ventilation from surfactant deficiency, hypothermia, organ damage upon delivery owing to immature vasculature and higher rates of infection. Thus, it is important to have an estimated gestational age before delivery to prepare for resuscitative efforts.
  - Respiratory status
    - Evaluate for respiratory effort and respiratory distress. If the neonate is in distress, take the following steps:
      - Position airway and clear secretions, as needed.
      - If obvious obstructive respiratory distress is present, suction the mouth and nares.
      - For neonates who fail to respond to initial resuscitative efforts and have signs of persistent respiratory distress, cyanosis, or a heart rate of less than 100 beats/min, further interventions are indicated (Fig. 89.2).
  - Muscle tone
    - Presence of vigorous movements versus flaccid tone may also help guide resuscitative decisions.
- Stable term or near-term neonates with strong respiratory effort and vigorous tone can be managed routinely with recording of Apgar scores and allowing for skin-to-skin contact with the mother as soon as possible.

SUGGESTED READINGS

Jara-Alamonte, G. (2015). Neonatal resuscitation. *emDocs*. Available at: http://www.emdocs.net/neonatal-resuscitation/.

Precipitous birth not occurring on a labor and delivery unit. *UpToDate*. Available at: https://www.uptodate.com/contents/precipitous-birth-not-occurring-on-a-labor-and-delivery-unit?search=obstetric%20emergencies&topicRef=114518&source=see_link#H10.

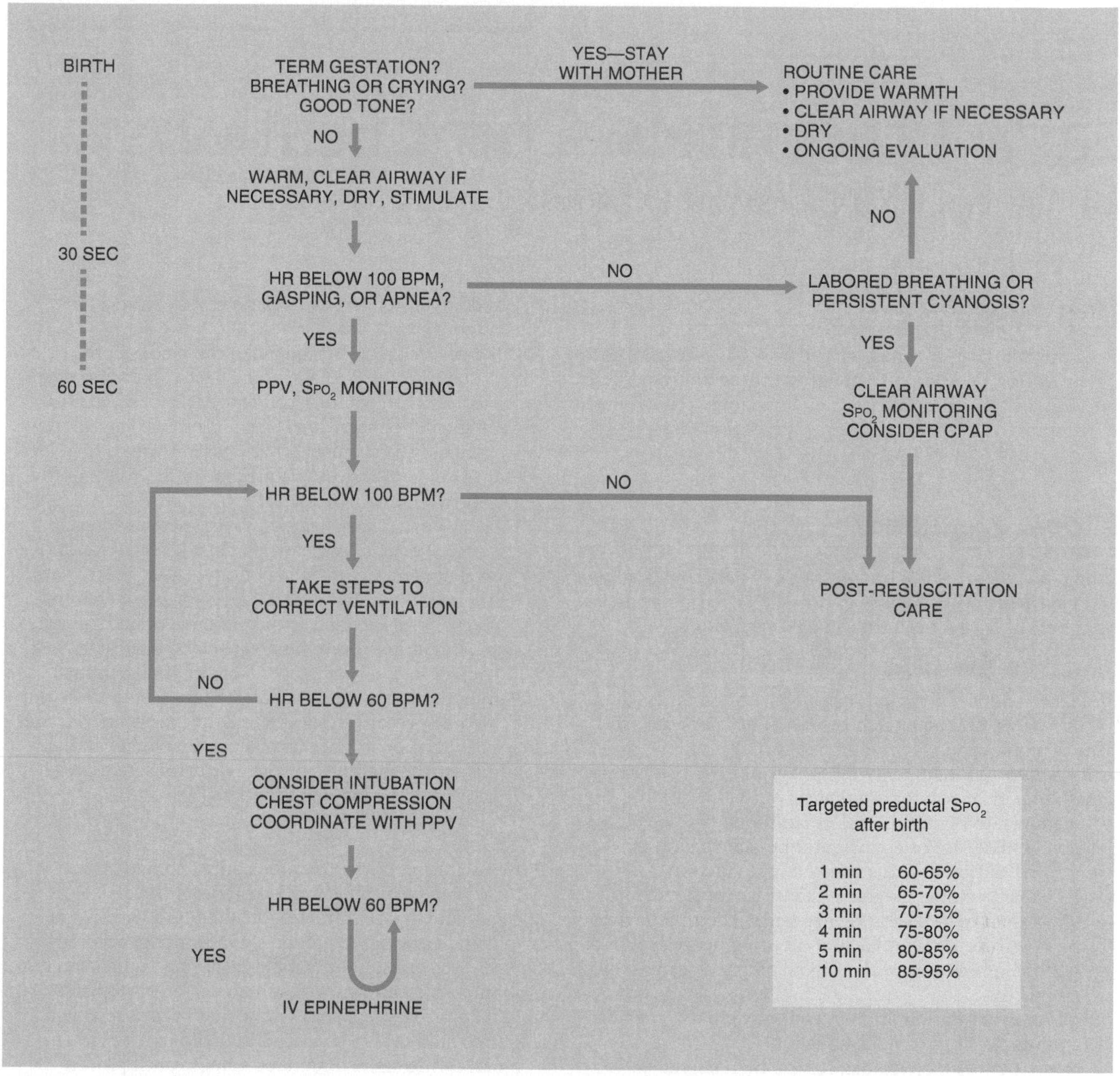

FIG. 89.2 A time-based approach to the resuscitation of a normal and apneic or cyanotic newborn. *BPM*, beats per minute; *CPAP*, continuous positive airway pressure; *HR*, heart rate; *IV*, intravenous; *PPV*, positive pressure ventilation; *SPO_2*, peripheral arterial oxygen saturation. (From American Academy of Pediatrics, American Heart Association. (2011). *Neonatal resuscitation textbook* (6th ed.). American Academy of Pediatrics and American Heart Association; and from Hobel, C. J., & Zakowski, M. (2016). Normal labor, delivery, and postpartum care. In N. F. Hacker, J. C. Gambone, & C. J. Hobel (Eds.), *Hacker and Moore's essentials of obstetrics and gynecology* (6th ed., pp. 96–124, Fig. 8.18). Elsevier.)

CHAPTER 90

BOARD REVIEW

Early Pregnancy Complications

MATTHEW LEVIN, MD, BA, and SAMANTHA PHILLIPS KADERA, MD, MPH, FACEP

Basic Information

Early pregnancy is defined as the first 20 weeks of the partum period. This chapter touches on several important and potentially life-threatening diagnoses that must be recognized by the emergency physician during this period.

Ectopic Pregnancy

Ectopic pregnancy is the leading cause of maternal death in the first trimester. It occurrs in 1%–2% of all pregnancies and more than 90% occur in the Fallopian tubes.

Clinical Presentation

- Classic triad is abdominal pain (90%), vaginal bleeding (50%–80%) and amenorrhea (70%), but patients may be asymptomatic.
- History should include investigation of high-risk factors including prior pelvic inflammatory disease, surgical procedures involving the Fallopian tubes, previous ectopic pregnancy, use of an intrauterine device, and in vitro fertilization or other assisted reproduction.
  - However, ectopic pregnancy must be considered in all women of childbearing age with abdominal/pelvic pain with or without vaginal bleeding because 50% of patients presenting with ectopic pregnancies have no risk factors.
- Physical examination findings can vary greatly, ranging from mild findings to frank shock.
  - If a patient is tachycardic, have a high degree of suspicion for rupture and early hemorrhagic shock.
  - The patient may be bradycardic, however, due to pain and secondary vagal stimulation.
  - Pelvic examination may be normal or show vaginal bleeding.

Diagnosis and Evaluation

- The pregnancy should first be confirmed with a qualitative urine pregnancy test.
- If positive, the patient needs transabdominal and/or transvaginal ultrasonography and a serum quantitative β-human chorionic gonadotropin (β-hCG) test.
  - Ectopic pregnancies are often not seen on ultrasound (US); however, lack of an intrauterine pregnancy (IUP) with an elevated quantitative β-hCG test suggests the diagnosis, especially if secondary signs are seen on US (i.e., increased free fluid in the pelvis), the patient has a concerning physical exam (i,e, significant abdominal tenderness) or known risk factors for ectopic pregnancy.
  - Because ectopic pregnancies can be diagnosed at any quantitative β-hCG level, classic "discriminatory" zone cutoffs for ultrasonography (i.e., when an IUP "should" be seen) are being reconsidered and Ob/Gyn should be consulted for any patient with a high level of concern for ectopic pregnancy regardless of the β-hCG level.
  - Be aware that many ectopic pregnancies, and even ruptured ectopic pregnancies, have low β-hCG, and *no* level of β-hCG can "rule out" an ectopic pregnancy.
  - In patients receiving fertility treatments, heterotopic pregnancies (defined as the presence of both an ectopic and an intra-uterine pregnancy concurrently) happen in approximately 15 out of 1000 patients.
  - In patients who are unstable and for whom there is a high degree of suspicion for ectopic pregnancy, a bedside US showing free intraabdominal fluid can help suggest the diagnosis before a urine or serum pregnancy test is obtained or resulted.

Treatment

- Resuscitation of the unstable patient should be performed by establishing large-bore intravenous (IV) access and rapidly initiating fluid boluses with crystalloid and early blood products. Obstetrics/gynecology (Ob/Gyn) consultants should be notified immediately for unstable patients with a high degree of suspicion (e.g., positive pregnancy test with an acute abdomen or free fluid on US. Hemoperitoneum in a woman of childbearing age is a ruptured ectopic until proven otherwise!).
- In all patients, blood should be drawn for blood typing, quantitative β-hCG, and general chemistry/blood counts. Rh-negative women with an ectopic pregnancy should receive 50 μg of anti-Rho immunoglobulin if at less than 13 weeks' gestation; the full dose of 300 μg should be given if greater than 13 weeks' gestation.
- Methotrexate versus surgery for definitive treatment should be discussed with the Ob/Gyn consultant.
  - The decision will be made based on several factors including the gestational age, size of the embryo, suspicion of tube rupture, and stability of the patient.
- If β-hCG is <1500, US is indeterminate, and clinical suspicion is low based on patient presentation and lack of other secondary US signs (e.g., free fluid, large or complex adnexal mass), patient should be counseled on ectopic precautions and instructed to follow up in 48 hours for a second β-hCG and US.

- Otherwise, if suspicion remains high due to patient presentation and/or US findings, consult with Ob/Gyn *irrespective* of the β-hCG level. There is *no* β-hCG level that rules out an ectopic pregnancy!

First Trimester Vaginal Bleeding

Vaginal bleeding in the first 20 weeks is classified according to degrees of passage of fetal tissue. Bleeding in early pregnancy is extremely common, and although bleeding can be seen in pregnancies that ultimately progress normally, approximately 20% of all pregnancies will spontaneously abort.

Clinical Presentation

- **Threatened abortion:** Closed cervical os, benign examination, no passage of tissue
- **Inevitable abortion:** Dilated cervical os without passage of tissue
- **Incomplete abortion:** Partial passage of products (via history or examination)
- **Complete abortion:** Passage of all fetal tissue
- **Missed abortion:** Fetal demise without passage of any products of conception after 4 weeks' time
- **Septic abortion:** Evidence of infection during any stage; may present with pelvic pain, fever, cervical motion or uterine tenderness, and/or foul-smelling discharge

Diagnosis and Evaluation

- US imaging should be performed to evaluate the location of the pregnancy (IUP vs. ectopic) and to rule out potential mimics such as gestational trophoblastic disease (e.g., molar pregnancies or choriocarcinoma) if the patient has not already had an IUP documented in this pregnancy.
- One can consider an US for fetal viability and risk for miscarriage (e.g., subchorionic hemorrhage, fetal size smaller than dates), depending on local US availability and patient preference, although it is not strictly necessary to perform in the ED if an IUP has previously been documented and the risk of heterotopic is low.
  - Heterotopic pregnancies are almost exclusively seen in patients receiving in vitro fertilization therapy.
- Obtain blood counts, blood typing for Rh factor determination, quantitative β-hCG, and urinalysis.
- Any products of conception found on examination should be sent for pathology.
- Approximately 2% of patients undergoing medical or surgical abortions present with complications. These complications include hemorrhage, uterine perforation, infection/retained products of conception, or hematometra (i.e., uterine distension syndrome secondary to an intrauterine hematoma).
- A patient presenting with significant postprocedural bleeding is concerning for uterine rupture. Evaluate for free fluid in the abdomen with focused assessment with sonography for trauma examination, obtain a pelvic US for uterine rupture (bedside), and immediately consult with Ob/Gyn for likely operative repair.

Treatment

- For the unstable patient, aggressive fluid resuscitation with crystalloids and/or blood products is indicated. Ob/Gyn should be consulted emergently.
  - This is rare in early pregnancy loss (e.g., <12 weeks) unless there is an underlying bleeding disorder.
- For incomplete abortions, the decision for expectant versus medical versus surgical management should be made in conjunction with the patient and the consulting Ob/Gyn.
- Patients with gestational trophoblastic disease should receive especially close follow-up until β-hCG returns to 0.
- Patients with threatened or complete abortions may be discharged with close follow-up and instructions for pelvic rest and return precautions for fever, excessive bleeding, or discharge.
- Septic abortions require broad-spectrum IV antibiotics and an Ob/Gyn consult.
  - Appropriate regimen would include clindamycin IV 900 mg every 8 hours plus gentamycin 1–2 mg/kg three times a day +/− Ampicillin 2 g every 4 hours.
- Significant bleeding after a surgical abortion may require tamponade with a large Foley balloon and/or Bakri balloon as well as other resuscitative measures similar to postpartum hemorrhage (see Chapter 93. Post-Delivery Complications). If uterine rupture is found or highly suspected, the patient will most likely need operative repair by Ob/Gyn.

Hyperemesis Gravidarum

Nausea and vomiting early in pregnancy are expected and, if mild, are often considered to be a normal physiologic response. However, severe degrees of emesis can both be functionally limiting for the patient and cause severe hypovolemia, weight loss, malnutrition, and electrolyte disturbances. Hyperemesis gravidarum is ultimately a diagnosis of exclusion, and one should consider alternative diagnoses unrelated to pregnancy, including intraabdominal or urinary tract infections (particularly if onset is after 10 weeks' gestation).

Clinical Presentation

- Typical onset at 5–6 weeks' gestation with peak symptoms at 9–10 weeks
- Vomiting occurring more than 3 times a day
- Weight loss
- Orthostatic hypotension or associated symptoms (e.g., lightheadedness, syncope)
- Ptyalism (hypersalivation)

Diagnosis and Evaluation

- Ultimately a clinical diagnosis
- An assessment of the patient's volume status and electrolytes is indicated for any pregnant patient presenting to the emergency department with vomiting.
- Consider the diagnosis if patient exhibits:
  - Weight loss more than 3 kg
  - Ketosis (or ketonuria)
  - Hypokalemia

Treatment

- Fluid resuscitation (preferably dextrose 5% in water because the dextrose helps break the ketotic cycle)

- Pyridoxine (vitamin B_6)
- Antihistamines (doxylamine, diphenhydramine, meclizine)
- Antiemetics (e.g., metoclopramide, promethazine, or ondansetron)
  - Note that there are some data on ondansetron use in early pregnancy and birth defects; have a risk/benefit discussion with patient.
- Thiamine to prevent Wernicke's encephalopathy
- Hospital admission if significant electrolyte abnormalities, continued inability to tolerate food by mouth after treatment, persistent ketosis, severe hypokalemia, or weight loss >10% of prepregnancy weight

Urinary Tract Infections

Although the incidence of bacteriuria occurs at similar rates among pregnant and nonpregnant women, rates of progression to pyelonephritis are higher in the pregnant population, likely because of anatomic changes. Some studies have shown correlations between urinary tract infections and adverse pregnancy outcomes, so a screening urinalysis should be checked on all pregnant patients. (Be aware that these guidelines are currently changing based on new data.)

Clinical Presentation

- Asymptomatic or typical urinary tract infection symptoms.
- Be vigilant for subtle signs of pyelonephritis: pregnant women are at high risk of progression!

Diagnosis

- Urinalysis: any bacteriuria and cystitis should be treated.
- As in nonpregnant women, *Escherichia coli* is the predominant pathogen.

Treatment

- Cephalosporins or nitrofurantoin are recommended.
- In patients with pyelonephritis, treat aggressively with IV antibiotics and IV hydration and consider admission owing to the high risk of pregnancy loss, preterm labor, and sepsis.
- Sulfonamides and fluoroquinolones are contraindicated.

Appendicitis

Acute appendicitis is the most common general surgical emergency encountered in pregnant patients (the second most common is biliary disease). Diagnosis can be difficult in the setting of multiple other normal and abnormal potential etiologies of lower abdominal pain in pregnancy as well as changes in the anatomic location of the appendix throughout pregnancy as the uterus expands.

Clinical Presentation

- Right lower or right upper quadrant pain (displacement of appendix upward as gestation progresses), anorexia, and/or fever
- Round ligament pain is a common cause of abdominal pain generally in the second trimester although it can extend to the third trimester and can mimic appendicitis. It is classically unilateral and sharp and occurs during movement or activity. It should not be associated with other systemic symptoms and tends to be intermittent.

Diagnosis and Evaluation

- Ultimately depends on resources available.
- Ultrasonography: high positive predictive value but low negative predictive value.
- Magnetic resonance of the abdomen/pelvis: high sensitivity and specificity.
- Limited protocols with low-dose helical computed tomography can limit fetal radiation exposure to <3 mGy.

Treatment

- Surgical consult; decision can be made for medical vs surgical management

Venous Thromboembolism (Deep Vein Thrombosis and Pulmonary Embolism)

Risk for venous thromboembolism is significantly increased in pregnancy and the early postpartum period. Pulmonary embolism is the seventh leading cause of maternal mortality and accounts for 9% of maternal deaths.

Clinical Presentation

- Patients are at increased risk with increasing gestational age, advanced maternal age, increasing parity, multiple gestations, bedrest, and obesity.
- Risk continues through the early postpartum period.
- Signs and symptoms are similar to those in nonpregnant patients although lower extremity edema in late gestation/early postpartum can complicate the clinical examination for deep vein thrombosis.

Diagnosis

- Utility of D-dimer is controversial and nearly guaranteed to be elevated above the standard 500 ng/mL in all patients by the third trimester.
  - Can consider adjusted reference ranges: >750 ng/mL in first trimester, >1000 ng/mL in second trimester, >1250 in third trimester.
  - A negative D-dimer test has a high negative predictive value in any trimester.
- Imaging options include serial lower extremity compression Doppler US versus computed tomographic angiography of pulmonary arteries.

Treatment

- Treat with subcutaneous low-molecular-weight heparin or intravenous unfractionated heparin.
- Warfarin is contraindicated in pregnancy.

Dysrhythmias

Arrhythmias are the most common cardiac complication in pregnancy and are believed to be due to stretching of the myocardium secondary to increased blood volume. The most common arrhythmia in those with structurally normal hearts is supraventricular tachycardia due to atrioventricular nodal reentrant tachycardia and atrioventricular reentrant tachycardia. Although the diagnostic approach is generally the same as for nonpregnant patients (rule out structural heart disease, especially if atrial fibrillation), antiarrhythmic medications are generally avoided.

Clinical Presentation

- Palpitations, syncope or presyncope, dyspnea, chest pain

Diagnosis

- Electrocardiogram

Treatment

- Supraventricular tachycardia: first-line adenosine
- Atrial fibrillation: rhythm control preferred over rate control and threshold for anticoagulation lowered because of prothrombotic state.
- Also safe to use β-blockers, calcium channel blockers (diltiazem or verapamil), or digoxin.
- Avoid amiodarone unless life-threatening dysrhythmia.
- Electrical cardioversion can be considered; no evidence of harm to the fetus from either cardioversion or most sedation medications, although fetal monitoring is often recommended.

Vaccines and Medications to Avoid

Below is an abbreviated list of commonly used medications that should be avoided in the pregnant patient. For further information on safety of medications in pregnancy, consult a pharmacist or a reputable online resource.

- Antibiotics
  - Tetracyclines
  - Fluoroquinolones
  - Sulfonamides
- Warfarin
- Anticonvulsants
  - Valproic acid
  - Phenytoin
  - Lamotrigine
- Angiotensin-converting enzyme inhibitors
- Live vaccines
  - Measles-mumps-rubella
  - Live attenuated influenza
  - Varicella

SUGGESTED READINGS

American College of Obstetricians and Gynecologists Committee on Practice Bulletins-Gynecology. (2018). ACOG practice bulletin no. 193: Tubal ectopic pregnancy. *Obstetrics and Gynecology, 131*(3), e91–e103. doi:10.1097/AOG.0000000000002560

American College of Obstetricians and Gynecologists Committee on Practice Bulletins-Obstetrics. (2018). ACOG practice bulletin no. 189: Nausea and vomiting of pregnancy. *Obstetrics and Gynecology, 131*(1), e15–e30. doi:10.1097/AOG.0000000000002456

Houry, D. E., & Salhi, B. A. (2014). Acute complications of pregnancy. In J. A. Marx, R. S. Hockberger, & R. M. Walls (Eds.), *Rosen's emergency medicine: Concepts and clinical practice* (8th ed.). Elsevier Saunders.

CHAPTER **91**

BOARD REVIEW

Late Pregnancy Complications

MATTHEW LEVIN, MD, BA, and SAMANTHA PHILLIPS KADERA, MD, MPH, FACEP

Background Information

- Late pregnancy is defined as the partum period after 20 weeks of gestation.
- Although many women will seek care at the labor and delivery (L&D) units for stable or milder symptoms this late in pregnancy, the emergency physician (EP) must be prepared to care for more severe, life-threatening late pregnancy complications, because ambulances will usually bring these women to the emergency department for initial evaluation and treatment.

Vaginal Bleeding in Late Pregnancy

General Principles

- Vaginal bleeding in late pregnancy may have multiple etiologies, including placental abruption, placenta previa, preterm labor, and "bloody show" at the onset of labor.
- Bleeding can range from minimal to life-threatening, depending on the etiology.

Placental Abruption

- Placental abruption (or *abruptio placentae*) is the premature partial or complete separation of the placenta from the uterine wall prior to delivery.

Clinical Presentation

- Painful vaginal bleeding (ranging from mild to life-threatening)
- Abdominal or back pain
- Uterine tenderness and irritability with hypertonic/hyperactive contractions
- Fetal distress as indicated by fetal heart rate (FHR) abnormalities
- Can lead to maternal disseminated intravascular coagulation (DIC) owing to thrombin generation
- Risk factors for placental abruption include prior abruption, increased age/parity, multiple gestations, preeclampsia or hypertension, cigarette smoking, or trauma.

Diagnosis and Evaluation

- Usually a clinical diagnosis based on vaginal bleeding, abdominal pain, and uterine contractions. Physical exam with a tender, contracting uterus (often with frequent or sustained contractions) in contrast to the exam for placenta previa (discussed later), which shows a non-tender, non-contracting uterus.
- Ultrasound: classic finding is retroplacental hematoma, but sensitivity is only 25%–60%.
  - Therefore, a negative ultrasound does **not** rule out abruption.
- FHR abnormality is a sensitive indicator and supports the diagnosis.
- Laboratory findings consistent with DIC are found in 10%–20% of severe abruptions (elevated prothrombin time or partial thromboplastin time, low fibrinogen, elevated D-dimer).

Treatment

- If the mother is unstable, begin volume resuscitation with crystalloids and/or blood products, particularly if DIC is suspected because the patient may need multiple units of blood products (packed red blood cells, platelets, fresh frozen plasma as appropriate) to correct coagulopathies.
- Fetal monitoring of all patients in late pregnancy with bleeding
  - This should be initiated as soon as possible because the degree of maternal bleeding/instability may not correlate with fetal well-being.
- Emergent obstetric (OB) consult
  - If fetal distress, the patient may need an emergent cesarean section.
- Administer Rhogam for patients who are Rh-negative.

Placenta Previa

- Placenta previa is another common cause of vaginal bleeding in late pregnancy; it is caused by implantation of the placenta over the internal cervical os (Fig. 91.1).

Clinical Presentation

- 90% have painless, bright red vaginal bleeding; a small minority have painful bleeding.
- Typically, larger volume than "bloody show" (defined as a small amount of bright red blood with or without passage of a mucus plug at the beginning of labor).
- Soft uterus without tenderness or contractions
- Higher-risk patients include those with prior cesarean sections, multiple gestations, or multiple induced abortions.
- For patients receiving prenatal care, placenta previa is usually found on screening ultrasound. Because 90%

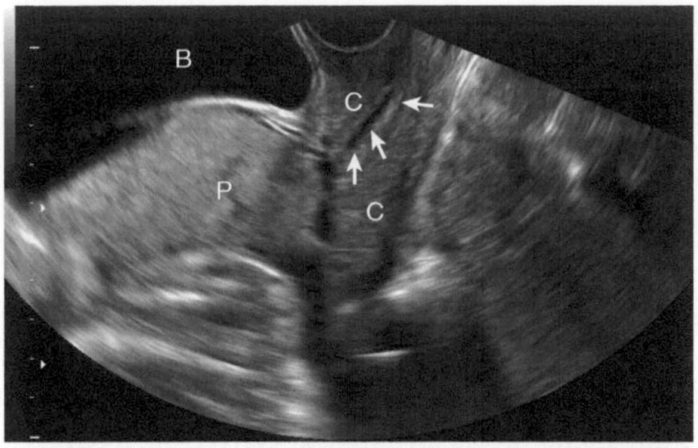

FIG. 91.1 Posterior complete placenta previa.Transvaginal ultrasound showing the placenta completely covering the internal os and extending posteriorly. *Arrows* indicate cervical canal. *B*, maternal bladder; *C*, cervix; *P*, placenta. (From Merriam, A., & D'Alton, M. E. (2018). Placenta previa. In J. Copel (Ed.), *Obstetric imaging: Fetal diagnosis and care* (pp. 455–458.e1, Fig. 106.3.) Elsevier.)

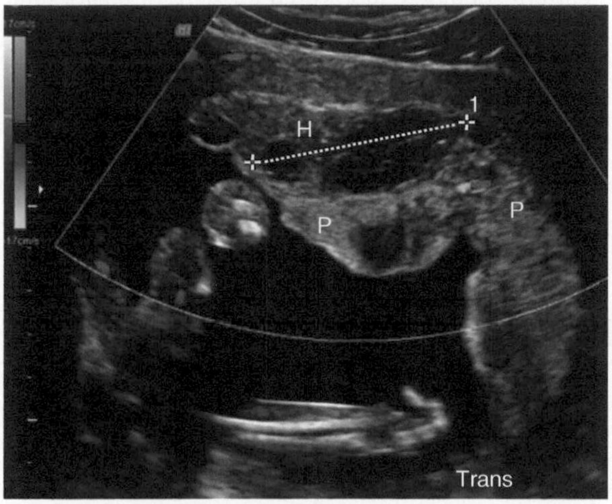

FIG. 91.2 Uterus in transverse view (*Trans*) showing a retroplacental hematoma. Hemorrhage (*H*) with a heterogeneous appearance is located behind the placenta (*P*), with a small subchorionic component. Caliper (*1*) shows measurement of the retroplacental hematoma. (From Merriam, A., & D'Alton, M. E. (2018). Placental abruption. In J. Copel (Ed.), *Obstetric imaging: Fetal diagnosis and care* (pp. 426–429.e1, Fig. 96.3.) Elsevier.)

of placenta previas identified before 20 weeks resolve before delivery, many patients are followed with serial ultrasounds and are aware of their diagnosis.

Diagnosis and Evaluation

- Diagnosis is based on transabdominal ultrasound demonstrating placental tissue over the internal cervical os (Fig. 91.2).
- Pelvic examination (especially bimanual) is contraindicated because it may cause increased bleeding.

Treatment

- Emergent OB consultation for fetal monitoring and consideration of emergent cesarean delivery
- Volume resuscitation with crystalloids and/or blood products, as needed

Premature Rupture of Membranes

- Defined as rupture of membranes prior to the onset of labor.
- Premature rupture of membranes (PROM) can be further specified as preterm PROM (PPROM), which occurs prior to 37 weeks' gestation.

Clinical Presentation

- May present with either a rush of fluid or a continuous leak of fluid from the vagina
- Passage of bloody show with or without a mucous plug
- Risk of uterine infection (presenting as fever, abdominal pain, uterine tenderness, leukocytosis, tachycardia, contractions) is dependent on the duration of rupture.

91

Diagnosis and Evaluation

- The diagnosis of PROM and PPROM is clinical, based on visualizing a pool of amniotic fluid via a sterile speculum examination.
- Confirmed by pH testing using nitrazine paper (dark blue indicates pH greater than 7.0) and/or a ferning pattern on slide smear
- If PROM is suspected, but there is no pooling, then an ultrasound demonstrating oligohydramnios is presumptive evidence of PROM.

Treatment

- Emergent OB consultation
- Obstetric may recommend antibiotic prophylaxis or testing for chlamydia, gonorrhea, and group B streptococcus to guide later antibiotic decisions as well as steroids for fetal lung maturity, depending on gestational age (see below).

Preterm Labor

- Preterm labor is defined as onset of labor before 37 weeks' gestation; it can often be difficult to diagnose accurately in its early stages but has important implications for mother and fetus.

Clinical Presentation

- Regular uterine contractions prior to 37 weeks gestation with effacement and dilation of the cervix

Diagnosis and Evaluation

- Over-diagnosis is common, because diagnosis is based on clinical features. The criteria below are typically used for the enrollment of patients in research studies.
  - Uterine contractions 4 or more every 20 minutes or 8 or more in 60 minutes **plus**
  - Transvaginal ultrasound showing less than 20 mm cervical length **or**
  - 20 to 30 mm cervical length with positive fetal fibronectin **or**
  - Cervical dilation greater than 3 cm

Treatment

- Fetal monitoring and OB consult for admission and potential tocolytic administration

- If EGA (the estimated gestational age) is less than 34 weeks, OB may recommend certain medications, especially if there is a delay to transfer to the labor and delivery unit.
  - Glucocorticoids to reduce neonatal morbidity and mortality related to inadequate lung development (betamethasone is commonly used)
  - Prophylactic antibiotics for group B *Streptococcus*.
  - If fetus is 24 to 32 weeks estimated gestational age, magnesium sulfate for neuroprotection against cerebral palsy

Preeclampsia, Eclampsia, and HELLP

- Hypertension in pregnancy can be related to a number of disorders or simply be a preexisting condition. One should have a high index of suspicion for preeclampsia, eclampsia, or HELLP (Hemolysis, Elevated Liver enzymes, Low Platelets) syndrome in pregnant women presenting to the ED with elevated blood pressures.

Clinical Presentation

Preeclampsia

- Systolic blood pressure greater than 140 mm Hg or diastolic greater than 90 mm Hg, typically sustained over two measurements at least 6 hours apart
- Headache or visual disturbances
- Extremity and/or facial swelling
- Dyspnea
- Decreased urine output
- Abdominal pain, especially right upper quadrant
- Signs of labor or abruption (see above)

Eclampsia

- New seizures in a woman with a hypertensive disorder of pregnancy (preeclampsia, gestational hypertension, or HELLP)
- May have preceding headache or right upper quadrant pain

HELLP Syndrome

- Abdominal pain with or without nausea and vomiting
- Hypertension as above
- Thrombocytopenia-related bleeding (uncommon)

Diagnosis and Evaluation

- All women presenting to the emergency department with hypertension (with or without seizure) near or after 20 weeks' gestation should have urine and laboratory studies obtained to evaluate for preeclampsia (urinalysis for protein or protein to creatinine ratio, complete blood cell count, basic metabolic panel, liver function tests, consider DIC laboratory study for ill-appearing patients or those with HELLP).
- *Pre-eclampsia*: new hypertension in addition to proteinuria OR significant organ dysfunction with or without proteinuria in a patient more than 20 weeks gestation
  - The amount of proteinuria is currently under debate as there have been cases of preeclampsia without proteinuria.
- *Eclampsia*: clinical diagnosis is based on the features of preeclampsia plus seizures.
- *HELLP*: severe variant of preeclampsia meeting particular laboratory criteria (Box 91.1)

BOX 91.1 *Tennessee Criteria for Diagnosis of HELLP Syndrome*

Evidence of hemolysis
Increased lactate dehydrogenase (greater than 600 U/L)
Increased aspartate aminotransferase (less than 70 U/L)
Thrombocytopenia (less than 100,000/μL)

Treatment

- *Chronic or preexisting hypertension* without evidence of preeclampsia can be treated with methyldopa, labetalol, or nifedipine (avoid angiotensin-converting [ACE] inhibitors) in consultation with OB.
- *For severe preeclampsia or eclampsia*, primary initial treatment is magnesium sulfate with a loading dose of 4 to 6 g over 20 minutes followed by an infusion of 1 to 2 g/hr. If this does not correct the blood pressure, labetalol 20 mg intravenous or hydralazine 5 mg intravenous can be added.
  - Patient should be monitored for signs of magnesium toxicity, including hyporeflexia, respiratory depression, and bradydysrhythmias.
- *For HELLP*, correct coagulopathy, as needed, with blood products; treat blood pressures as above.
- Obstetric consult for admission of all patients with preeclampsia, eclampsia, and HELLP. Definitive treatment includes delivery of the fetus. However, note that up to 10% of preeclampsia cases will occur postpartum up to 6 weeks; these cases are medically managed.

Uterine Rupture

- Uterine rupture can be a catastrophic event leading to fetal and/or maternal death. It typically occurs after prior cesarean section or other uterine surgery (e.g., myomectomy) or following significant abdominal trauma.

Clinical Presentation

- Abdominal pain with or without vaginal bleeding
- Loss of station of presenting fetal part
- Change in FHR tracing
- Hematuria
- Maternal hemodynamic instability

Diagnosis and Evaluation

- Diagnosis is typically clinical, based on identification of complete disruption of all uterine layers in the operating room.
- If patient is stable and not in labor, obtain radiologic diagnosis via ultrasound or computed tomography (CT) scan (unlikely in true rupture because most patients are unstable).

Treatment

- May not be clinically distinguishable from severe placental abruption, but urgent delivery of the fetus is the primary management for both diagnoses if signs of fetal or maternal instability.
- Emergent OB consult and preparation for likely surgical delivery and hysterectomy

- Fluid and blood resuscitation of the mother, if hemodynamically unstable

Peripartum Cardiomyopathy

- Peripartum cardiomyopathy is a rare but potentially life-threatening form of heart failure. It typically presents in the last month of pregnancy up to 5 months postpartum.

Clinical Presentation

- Presentations range in severity from mild dyspnea to florid pulmonary edema and cardiogenic shock.
- Presenting symptoms include dyspnea on exertion, fatigue, orthopnea, and paroxysmal nocturnal dyspnea.
- More common in African-American and multiparous women. It also has a high recurrence rate in subsequent pregnancies.

Diagnosis and Evaluation

- Primarily a clinical diagnosis, although as in non-pregnancy-related congestive heart failure (CHF), laboratory studies including brain natriuretic peptide, electrocardiogram, and chest x-ray may be useful to confirm the diagnosis.
- Definitive diagnosis is made with echocardiography (left ventricular ejection fraction is less than 45% in the absence of another cause of CHF).

Treatment

- Treatment is similar to that for nonpregnant CHF, with the additional consideration of drug safety in pregnant or breastfeeding mothers.
  - Diuretics and vasodilators
  - Oxygen and noninvasive positive pressure ventilation
  - ACE inhibitors are contraindicated if during the last month of pregnancy but should be considered postpartum.
- Obstetric and cardiology consult
  - These patients will likely require admission for definitive diagnosis and initiation of treatment.

Neurologic Emergencies in Late Pregnancy (and the Postpartum Period)

Background Information

- Headaches are common in late pregnancy and the postpartum period. They are usually benign secondary to alterations in sleep patterns and hormonal influences. However, late pregnancy and the postpartum period are also high-risk times for several neurologic emergencies.
- Emergency physicians should have a low threshold for imaging in the new onset, severe headache or those headaches associated with neurologic symptoms even if subtle or subjective.

BOX 91.2 *Warning Signs in Postpartum Headache*

- New-onset headaches in pregnancy
- Different than prior headaches
- Worst headache of life or thunderclap headache
- Focal neurologic deficits (including isolated sensory signs)
- Altered mental status
- Fevers or meningismus
- Elevated blood pressure
- Papilledema or evidence of elevated intracranial pressure
- Hyperreflexia

Clinical Presentation

- The warning signs and differential diagnosis for dangerous postpartum headaches are summarized in Box 91.2 and Table 91.1, respectively.
- Presentations can be subtle, so EPs should take new or worsening headaches seriously, especially if they present with neurologic complaints (even those that are subtle).
- Migraines generally get better during late pregnancy but rebound after birth. These will present as typical migraines, and most women will have a history of similar headaches.
- Pregnant, and especially postpartum women up to 6 weeks after delivery, are at higher risk of intracerebral hemorrhage (ICH) (especially subarachnoid hemorrhage) when compared with the general population.
  - ICH will present in a typical fashion with acute-onset severe headache with or without altered mental status and/or neurologic symptoms.
- Additionally, physiologic changes in pregnancy result in a hypercoagulable state, which increases the risk for cerebral infarct and central venous thrombosis.
  - Risk is greatest during the postpartum period.
  - Strokes will present similarly to those in nonpregnant patients.
  - Central venous thrombosis is a difficult diagnosis. It may present with a progressively worsening daily headache (can be of any character) and will only present with neurologic symptoms later in its course. EPs must have a high index of suspicion for this diagnosis.
- Preeclampsia can also present as an isolated headache with elevated blood pressure (see above).

TABLE 91.1 *Differential Diagnosis of Late Pregnancy and Postpartum Headache*

CAUSES OF LATE PREGNANCY AND POSTPARTUM HEADACHES	
Non-Life-Threatening	Life-Threatening
• Headache syndromes (migraine, tension, cluster) • Sinus headaches • Pseudotumor cerebri*	• Intracranial hemorrhage • Ischemic stroke • Central venous thrombosis • Central nervous system tumor • Meningitis/encephalitis • Preeclampsia/eclampsia

*If progresses, may be vision-threatening and debilitating.

Diagnosis and Evaluation

- Initial evaluation of a pregnant (or postpartum) patient with a severe, new onset headache should be a noncontrast CT to rule out ICH (unless the patient is stable and magnetic resonance imaging [MRI] is readily available).
- The EP should consider obtaining a computed tomography (CT) venogram or magnetic resonance (MR) venogram for those patients with presentations concerning for central venous thrombosis; additionally, consider MRI/magnetic resonance angiography to evaluate for stroke in women presenting with headache and acute neurologic findings.
  - Few data exist on the safety of gadolinium in pregnancy, so it is often avoided in the United States. However, it is considered safe in Europe.
  - Contrast (both iodinated and gadolinium) is safe in breastfeeding mothers, and there is no need to counsel patients to "pump and dump" for any length of time (see Chapter 94. The Breastfeeding Mother in the Emergency Department).

Treatment

- Treatment of ICH and subarachnoid hemorrhage is the same in pregnant patients as it is in nonpregnant patients.
- Ischemic stroke should also be treated similarly to nonpregnant patients. Be aware that pregnancy is not an absolute contraindication for tissue plasminogen activator, although risk/benefits should be discussed with the patient in consultation with neurology.
- The treatment for central venous thrombosis is anticoagulation with heparin or low molecular weight heparins.
- Consultation with neurology, neurosurgery, interventional radiology, and obstetrics, as indicated

SUGGESTED READINGS

ACOG Committee Opinion 767: Emergent therapy for acute-onset, severe hypertension during pregnancy and the postpartum period. American College of Obstetricians and Gynecologists. (2019). *Obstetrics and Gynecology, 133*, e174–e180.

American College of Obstetricians and Gynecologists (ACOG). (2016). Practice Bulletin No. 171: Management of preterm labor. *Obstetrics and Gynecology, 128*, e155–e164.

Ananthe, C., & Kinzler, W. (2019). Placental abruption: Pathophysiology, clinical features, diagnosis and consequences. *UpToDate*. Last updated: September 2020. https://www.uptodate.com/contents/placental-abruption-pathophysiology-clinical-featuresdiagnosis-and-consequences

Houry, D. E., & Salhi, B. A. (2014). Acute complications of pregnancy. In Marx, J. A., Hockberger, R. S., & Walls, R. M. (Eds.), *Rosen's emergency medicine: Concepts and clinical practice* (8th ed.). Elsevier.

Complications of Delivery

ANNA NGUYEN, DO, and PAMELA L. DYNE, MD

- Although most prehopital and emergency department deliveries are uncomplicated, emergency physicians must be prepared to manage common delivery complications.
- Common complications include nuchal cords, prolapsed cords, breech deliveries, shoulder dystocias and primary postpartum hemorrhage.
- Cardiac arrest in pregnancy is rare but when it does occur, there are several unique management considerations.

Umbilical Cord Emergencies

NUCHAL CORD

General Principles

- Defined as a loop of umbilical cord around the fetal neck
- Nuchal cord is a relatively common finding.
- Most are easily reduced upon delivery without any significant associated fetal risks or complications.
- Nuchal cords may be single, multiple, tight, or loose. In some cases, tight nonreducible nuchal cords have been associated with impaired fetal growth, ischemic stroke, asphyxia, and even fetal demise.
- Risk factors include long umbilical cords (≥70 cm) and excessive fetal movement in the prenatal period.

Clinical Presentation

- Palpation or visualization of a nuchal cord after delivery of the fetal head

Diagnosis and Evaluation

- Although usually a clinical diagnosis made during delivery, prenatal ultrasound may demonstrate the presence of a nuchal cord.

Treatment

- A loose nuchal cord can be easily reduced by slipping it over the fetal head or back over the shoulders to allow the body to deliver through the loop.
- Tight nuchal cords
  - If unable to reduce, continue to deliver through the cord. Often the cord can be reduced once the fetus is delivered.
  - As a last resort, the nuchal cord can be doubly clamped and cut. However, this is associated with decreased placental blood flow and neonatal anemia.

PROLAPSED UMBILICAL CORD

General Principles

- Umbilical cord slips ahead of the presenting fetal part and protrudes into the vaginal canal becoming vulnerable to compression as labor progresses.
- Risk factors include malpresentation (e.g., breech) or unengaged presenting part of the fetus, prematurity or low birth weight, multiparity, multiple gestation (later born fetuses at risk), low-lying placenta, uterine malformation, prolonged labor, or a long umbilical cord.

Clinical Presentation, Diagnosis, and Evaluation

- Cord prolapse is usually overt and the cord may be visualized and palpated on speculum or digital examination.
- Occult prolapse may present with fetal bradycardia or decelerations.

Treatment

- Definitive treatment is emergent cesarean; however, a few stabilizing measures can be attempted in the interim.
  - Manually elevate the presenting fetal part by placing a hand in vaginal vault and elevate it off the cord.
  - Place mother in Trendelenburg or knee-chest position.
  - Retrofill and distend the bladder with normal saline to elevate the presenting part off the cord.
  - Administer a tocolytic to reduce uterine contraction onto the cord.
  - Keep the prolapsed cord moist with wet gauze and manually replace it in the vagina to avoid exposing it to the cold environment as that may precipitate umbilical artery vasospasms and poor fetal perfusion.

Complications of Fetal Delivery

SHOULDER DYSTOCIA

General Principles

- Shoulder dystocia is a true obstetric emergency because prolonged dystocia can lead to poor fetal outcomes, including anoxic brain injury and even death.
- Most shoulder dystocias will resolve with relatively simple maneuvers if the emergency physician acts quickly.
- Risk factors include maternal diabetes and obesity causing fetal macrosomia, post-term pregnancy, and history of prior shoulder dystocia.

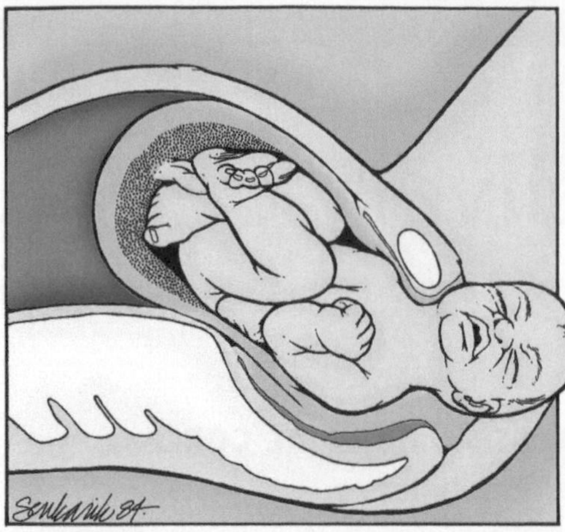

FIG. 92.1 When delivery of the fetal head is not followed by delivery of the shoulders, the anterior shoulder often becomes caught behind the symphysis, as illustrated. The head may retract toward the perineum, and desperate traction on the fetal head is not likely to facilitate delivery and may lead to trauma. (From Lanni, S. M., Gherman, R., & Gonik, B. (2017). Malpresentations. In S. G. Gabbe, J. R. Niebyl, J. L. Simpson, M. B. Landon, H. L. Galan, E. R. M. Jauniaux, D. A. Driscoll, V. Berghella, & W. A. Grobman (Eds.), *Obstetrics: Normal and problem pregnancies* (7th ed., pp. 368–394.e1, Fig. 17.26). Elsevier.)

Clinical Presentation, Diagnosis, and Evaluation

- Entrapment of the fetus' bilateral shoulders within the pelvic inlet, leading to the fetal head retracting back into the perineum ("turtle sign") and inability to deliver the anterior shoulder (Fig. 92.1)

Treatment

- Treatment should be pursued in the following sequential steps:
  - Stop maternal pushing.
  - Assess for and reduce nuchal cord.
  - Drain distended bladder if present.
  - Perform the following maneuvers sequentially until shoulder dystocia is released:
    - ***McRobert's maneuver:*** maternal hip hyperflexion (Fig. 92.2)
    - ***McRobert's maneuver*** with suprapubic pressure
    - Deliver the posterior arm: place hand into vagina, locate the posterior forearm, and pull arm out of the vagina (Fig. 92.3).
    - Rotate the fetus.
      - ***Rubin maneuver:*** manual rotation of fetal posterior shoulder toward the direction the fetal head is facing to displace shoulders from the narrow anteroposterior diameter of pelvic inlet (Fig. 92.4)
      - ***Woods maneuver:*** repeated manual rotation of fetal posterior shoulder toward the fetal back until the anterior shoulder is delivered
    - Fracture of anterior clavicle
- Several last-resort maneuvers can be performed by obstetrics, including the ***Zavanelli maneuver*** (push fetal head back into the uterus and proceed with cesarean section), abdominal rescue (low transverse hysterotomy to allow manual rotation of the anterior shoulder and vaginal delivery), or symphysiotomy (surgical incision

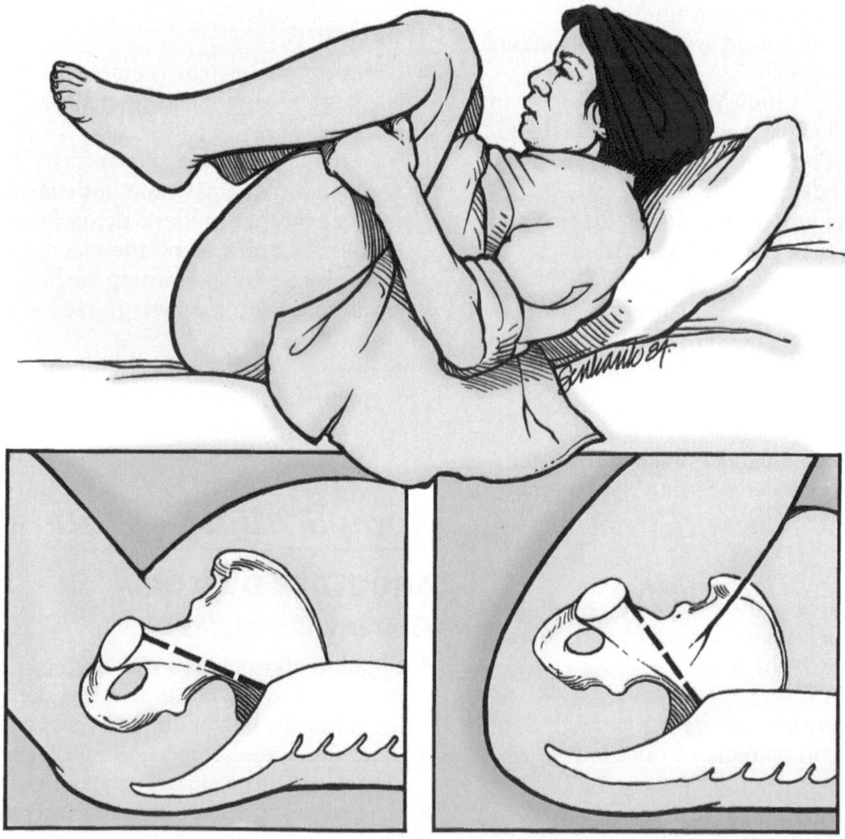

FIG. 92.2 The least invasive maneuver to disimpact the shoulders is the McRobert's maneuver. Sharp ventral flexion of the maternal hips results in ventral rotation of the maternal pelvis and an increase in the useful size of the outlet. (From Lanni, S. M., Gherman, R., & Gonik, B. (2017). Malpresentations. In S. G. Gabbe, J. R. Niebyl, J. L. Simpson, M. B. Landon, H. L. Galan, E. R. M. Jauniaux, D. A. Driscoll, V. Berghella, & W. A. Grobman (Eds.), *Obstetrics: Normal and problem pregnancies* (7th ed., pp. 368–394.e1, Fig. 17.29). Elsevier.)

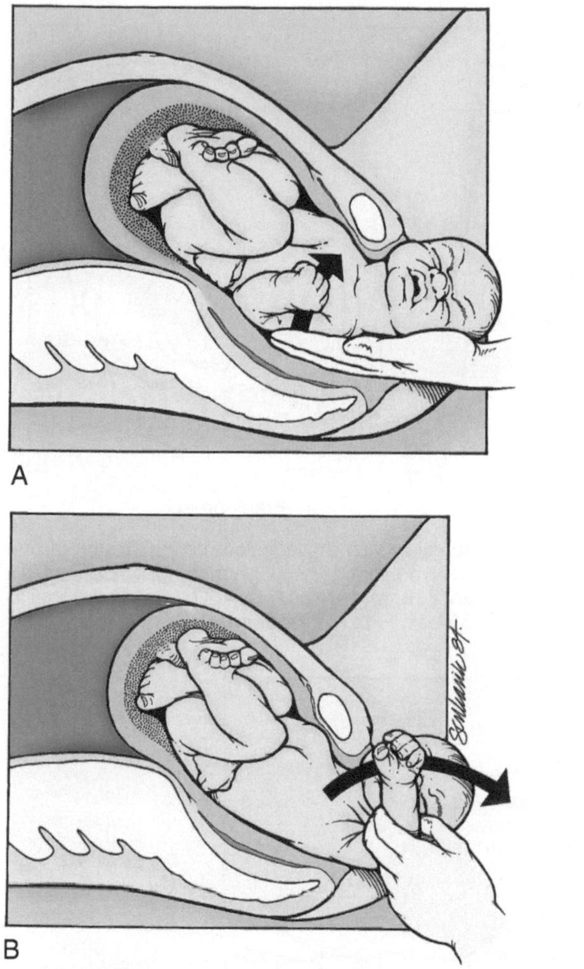

FIG. 92.3 The operator here inserts a hand and sweeps the posterior arm across the chest and over the perineum. Care should be taken to distribute the pressure evenly across the humerus to avoid unnecessary fracture. (From Lanni, S. M., Gherman, R., & Gonik, B. (2017). Malpresentations. In S. G. Gabbe, J. R. Niebyl, J. L. Simpson, M. B. Landon, H. L. Galan, E. R. M. Jauniaux, D. A. Driscoll, V. Berghella, & W. A. Grobman (Eds.), *Obstetrics: Normal and problem pregnancies* (7th ed., pp. 368–394.e1, Fig. 17.31). Elsevier.)

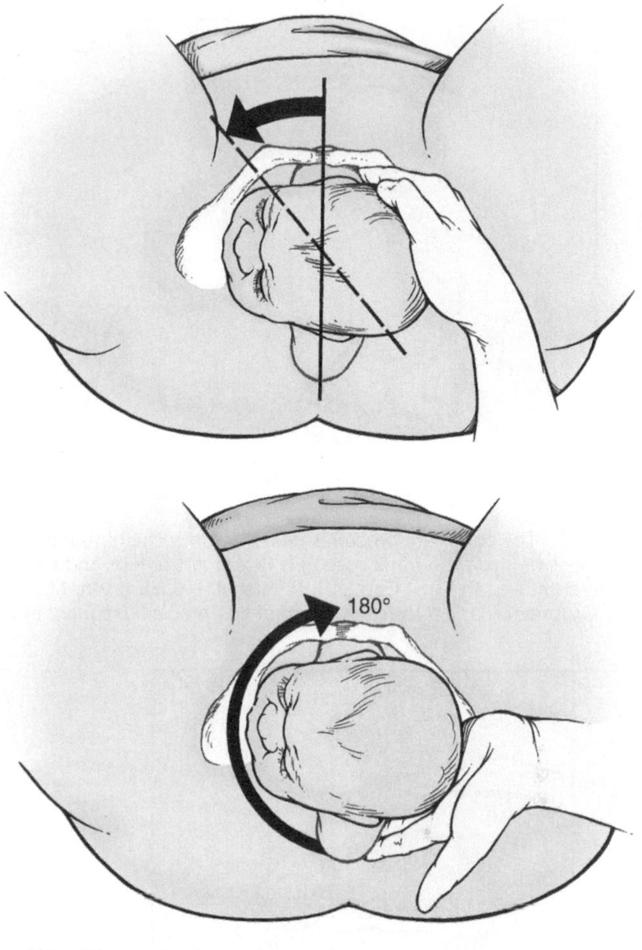

FIG. 92.4 Rotation of the anterior shoulder forward through a small arc or of the posterior shoulder forward through a larger one will often lead to descent and delivery of the shoulders. Forward rotation is preferred, because it tends to compress and diminish the size of the shoulder girdle, whereas backward rotation would open the shoulder girdle and increase its size. (From Lanni, S. M., Gherman, R., & Gonik, B. (2017). Malpresentations. In S. G. Gabbe, J. R. Niebyl, J. L. Simpson, M. B. Landon, H. L. Galan, E. R. M. Jauniaux, D. A. Driscoll, V. Berghella, & W. A. Grobman (Eds.), *Obstetrics: Normal and problem pregnancies* (7th ed., pp. 368–394.e1, Fig. 17.30). Elsevier.)

of the symphysis cartilage, allowing for partial separation of pubic bones to increase pelvic inlet diameter).

BREECH DELIVERY

General Principles

- In the case of a precipitous delivery of a breeched fetus in the emergency department, it is important to involve obstetric specialists immediately. However, given the possibility of a rapidly progressing labor, emergency physicians must be aware of the specific procedural techniques and associated complications, such as prolapsed umbilical cord and dystocia/entrapment of fetal parts, to ensure a safe delivery (see Fig. 92.6A–F).

Clinical Presentation, Diagnosis, and Evaluation

- *Frank or complete breech presentations* (buttocks first) implies that the largest diameter of the fetus will deliver first and subsequent head entrapment is unlikely. Most likely the delivery will progress to at least the torso without physician assistance.
- *Incomplete or footling breech* presentation increases the risk of fetal head entrapment, thus is a contraindication to vaginal delivery and emergent cesarean should be pursued (Fig. 92.5).

Treatment (Fig. 92.6A–F)

- Determine the presenting fetal part (buttocks vs. foot).
- Place mother in the lithotomy position with a wedge under one side of her buttocks.
- Can consider an episiotomy (though it is not always necessary) but only after the fetal anus is visible at the maternal vulva in order to facilitate imminent delivery
- Physician-assisted delivery (Fig. 92.6A)
  - Should only be performed once the fetus is delivered to at least its umbilicus; if done before, this can lead to an ***increased*** risk of head entrapment.
  - Assistance via suprapubic pressure, gentle rotation of trunk, and extraction of limbs as indicated (see below)

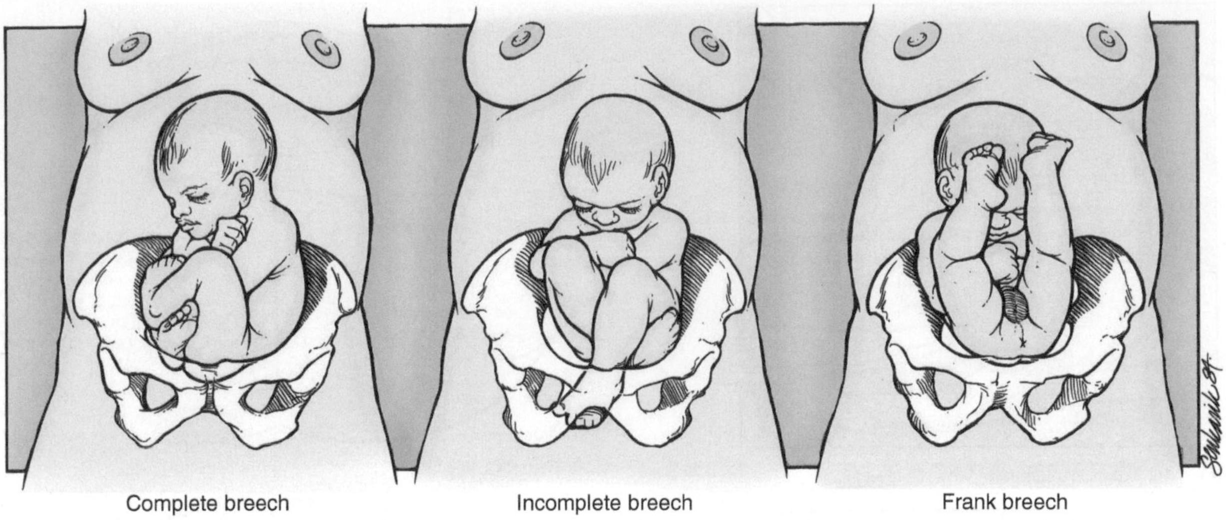

FIG. 92.5 The complete breech is flexed at both the hips and the knees. The incomplete breech shows incomplete deflexion of one or both knees or hips. The frank breech is flexed at the hips and extended at the knees. (From Lanni, S. M., Gherman, R., & Gonik, B. (2017). Malpresentations. In S. G. Gabbe, J. R. Niebyl, J. L. Simpson, M. B. Landon, H. L. Galan, E. R. M. Jauniaux, D. A. Driscoll, V. Berghella, & W. A. Grobman (Eds.), *Obstetrics: Normal and problem pregnancies* (7th ed., pp. 368–394.e1, Fig. 17.14). Elsevier.)

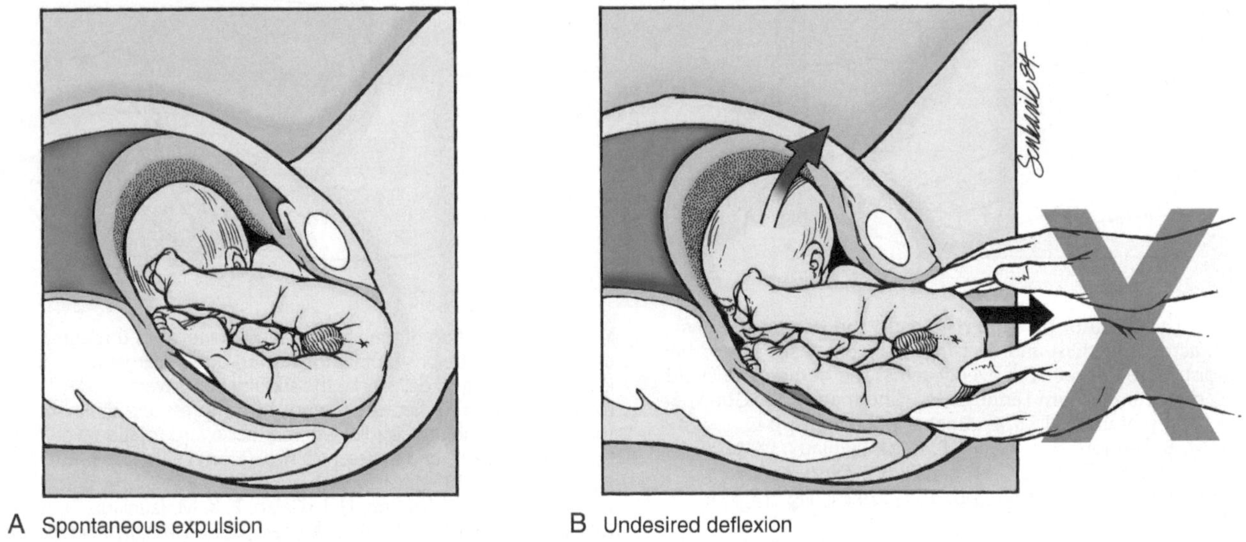

FIG. 92.6A The fetus emerges spontaneously (**A**), whereas uterine contractions maintain cephalic flexion. Premature aggressive traction (**B**) encourages deflexion of the fetal vertex and increases the risk of head entrapment or nuchal arm entrapment. (From Lanni, S. M., Gherman, R., & Gonik, B. (2017). Malpresentations. In S. G. Gabbe, J. R. Niebyl, J. L. Simpson, M. B. Landon, H. L. Galan, E. R. M. Jauniaux, D. A. Driscoll, V. Berghella, & W. A. Grobman (Eds.), *Obstetrics: Normal and problem pregnancies* (7th ed., pp. 368–394.e1, Fig. 17.17). Elsevier.)

- **Note:** to avoid fetal injury and trauma, do *not* apply traction on the trunk. Avoid manually extracting fetus, unless prolonged dystocia is leading to fetal asphyxia.
- Delivery of buttocks and lower limbs (Fig. 92.6B)
  - ***Pinard maneuver:*** if the lower limbs are extended when the breeched fetus is delivered to the level of the umbilicus, apply pressure on the back of the fetal knee to flex and externally rotate at the hips to deliver each lower limb.
- Delivery of upper limbs (Figs. 92.6C and 6D): in breech presentations, fetal arms are usually crossed across the chest and should deliver spontaneously after buttocks/lower limbs. Entrapment of the arms usually occurs when the arms are extended or behind the fetal head, requiring additional interventions to ensure safe delivery.
  - ***Loveset maneuver:*** hold fetus firmly at hips/pelvis, and rotate 180 degrees in opposite directions along the sagittal plane to deliver each arm (Fig. 92.6D).
- Delivery of the head (Figs. 92.6E and 6D)
  - Key procedural point is to deliver the head in a flexed position and avoid overextension of the delivered fetal body to minimize risk of head entrapment.
  - Rotate fetus to face the floor, stabilize the trunk over forearm and parallel to the floor, and apply suprapubic pressure to promote fetal neck flexion. Then, allow maternal contractions to deliver the head. Consider wrapping the fetus in a towel to aid in control of the delivered body.
  - Avoid neck hyperextension because it can occlude the vertebral arteries and will make entrapment more likely.

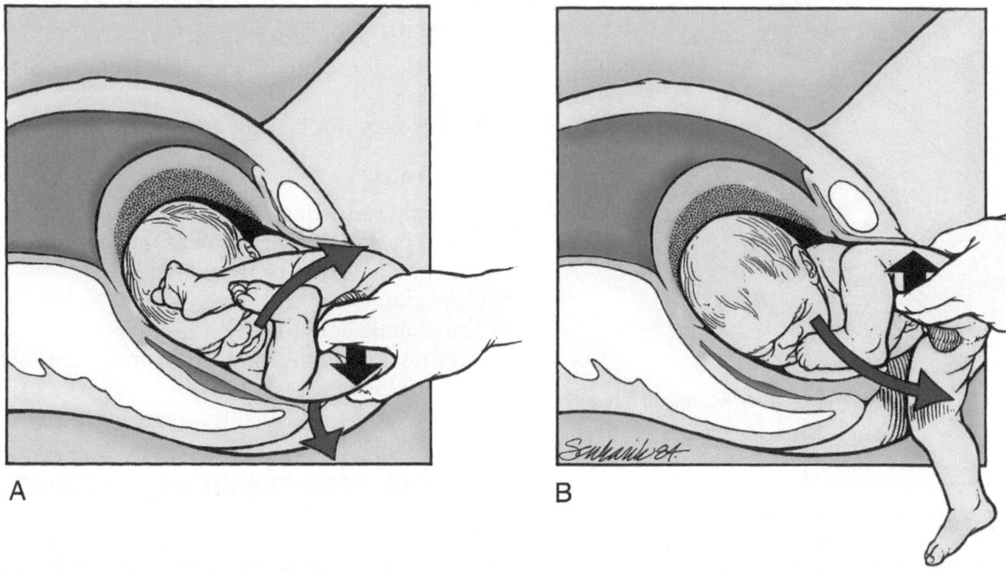

FIG. 92.6B After spontaneous expulsion to the umbilicus, external rotation of each thigh (**A**) combined with opposite rotation of the fetal pelvis results in flexion of the knee and delivery of each leg (**B**). (From Lanni, S. M., Gherman, R., & Gonik, B. (2017). Malpresentations. In S. G. Gabbe, J. R. Niebyl, J. L. Simpson, M. B. Landon, H. L. Galan, E. R. M. Jauniaux, D. A. Driscoll, V. Berghella, & W. A. Grobman (Eds.), *Obstetrics: Normal and problem pregnancies* (7th ed., pp. 368–394.e1, Fig. 17.18). Elsevier.)

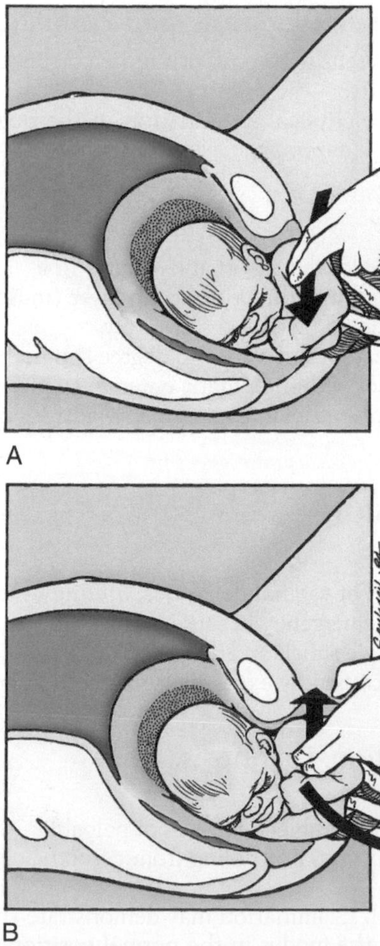

FIG. 92.6C When the scapulae appear under the symphysis, the operator reaches over the left shoulder, sweeps the arm across the chest (**A**), and delivers the arm (**B**). (From Lanni, S. M., Gherman, R., & Gonik, B. (2017). Malpresentations. In S. G. Gabbe, J. R. Niebyl, J. L. Simpson, M. B. Landon, H. L. Galan, E. R. M. Jauniaux, D. A. Driscoll, V. Berghella, & W. A. Grobman (Eds.), *Obstetrics: Normal and Problem Pregnancies* (7th ed., pp. 368–394.e1, Fig. 17.19). Elsevier.)

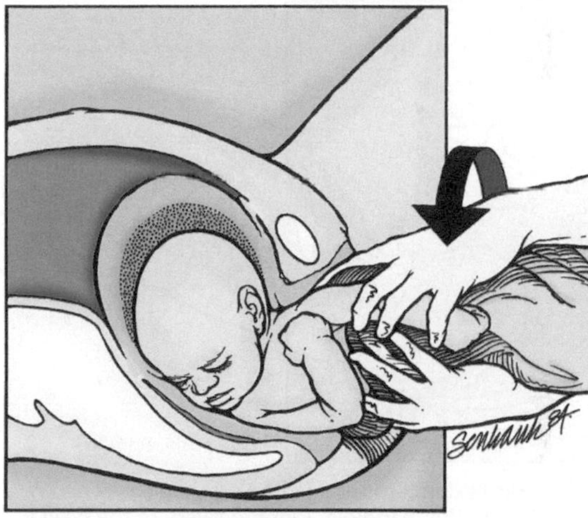

FIG. 92.6D Gentle rotation of the shoulder girdle facilitates delivery of the right arm. (From Lanni, S. M., Gherman, R., & Gonik, B. (2017). Malpresentations. In S. G. Gabbe, J. R. Niebyl, J. L. Simpson, M. B. Landon, H. L. Galan, E. R. M. Jauniaux, D. A. Driscoll, V. Berghella, & W. A. Grobman (Eds.), *Obstetrics: Normal and problem pregnancies* (7th ed., pp. 368–394.e1, Fig. 17.20). Elsevier.)

  - Avoid pulling downward traction because that can result in fetal cervical dislocation.
  - If the head is entrapped, placing the mother in position for the McRobert's maneuver and applying suprapubic pressure may help deliver the head.
- If the breech fetus fails to deliver within 60 minutes of maternal pushing, emergent cesarean is indicated.

Primary Postpartum Hemorrhage

Background Information

- Primary postpartum hemorrhage is defined as more than 500 mL of blood loss immediately after vaginal delivery.

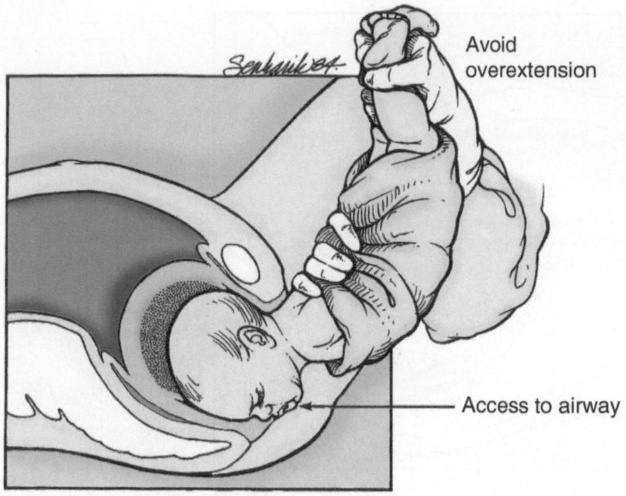

FIG. 92.6E Following delivery of the arms, the fetus is wrapped in a towel for control and is slightly elevated. The fetal face and airway may be visible over the perineum. Excessive elevation of the trunk is avoided. (From Lanni, S. M., Gherman, R., & Gonik, B. (2017). Malpresentations. In S. G. Gabbe, J. R. Niebyl, J. L. Simpson, M. B. Landon, H. L. Galan, E. R. M. Jauniaux, D. A. Driscoll, V. Berghella, & W. A. Grobman (Eds.), *Obstetrics: Normal and problem pregnancies* (7th ed., pp. 368–394.e1, Fig. 17.21). Elsevier.)

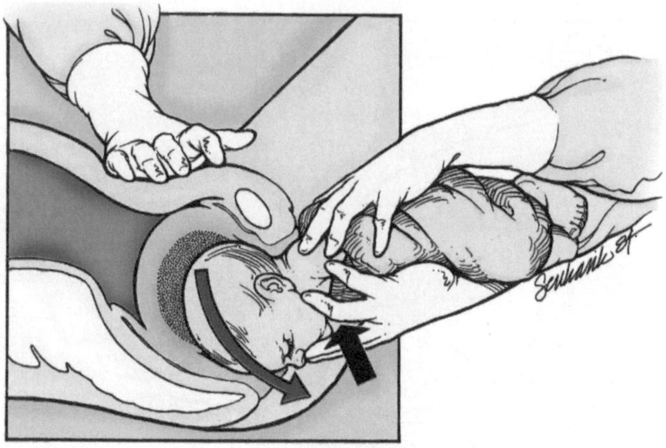

FIG. 92.6F Cephalic flexion is maintained by pressure (*black arrow*) on the fetal maxilla, not the mandible. Often delivery of the head is easily accomplished with continued expulsive forces from above and gentle downward traction.(From Lanni, S. M., Gherman, R., & Gonik, B. (2017). Malpresentations. In S. G. Gabbe, J. R. Niebyl, J. L. Simpson, M. B. Landon, H. L. Galan, E. R. M. Jauniaux, D. A. Driscoll, V. Berghella, & W. A. Grobman (Eds.), *Obstetrics: Normal and problem pregnancies* (7th ed., pp. 368–394.e1, Fig. 17.22). Elsevier.)

Secondary postpartum hemorrhage is defined as "excessive vaginal bleeding" 24 hours or more after delivery (see Chapter 93. Postpartum Emergencies).
- Postpartum hemorrhage has many common causes (see below and Table 92.1), but can also be the first presentation of a bleeding diathesis, most commonly Von-Willebrand disorder.

UTERINE ATONY

General Principles

- Accounts for 80% of primary postpartum hemorrhage cases
- Due to lack of postpartum uterine contractions leading to poor contracture of placental vasculature and persistent bleeding

Clinical Presentation, Diagnosis, and Evaluation

- Dilated, atonic uterus with persistent, excessive vaginal bleeding
- Uterus does not become firm after third stage of labor

Treatment

- Manual uterine massage
- Gauze packing of the fornices, intrauterine balloon tamponade (Bakri or large foley)
- Oxytocin
- Tranexamic acid (TXA)
- Uterine artery embolization by interventional radiology (IR) in severe cases
- Hysterectomy as a final resort by obstetrics/gynecology

VAGINAL AND CERVICAL LACERATIONS

General Principles

- Can be classified as first degree (vaginal mucosa or perineal skin only), second degree (perineal muscles involved), third degree (anal sphincter involved), and fourth degree (anal epithelium involved leading to a communication between vaginal and anal epithelium)

Clinical Presentation, Diagnosis, and Evaluation

- The patient may present with postpartum hemorrhage depending on severity.
- Diagnosis is made by physical examination. A thorough rectal examination is important to ensure there is no anal involvement.

Treatment

- Repair with running locked absorbable sutures in a cephalocaudal (top-down) direction. Each layer (muscular vs. epithelial) should be closed separately.
- Any lacerations greater than a second degree should be repaired by obstetrics, although many emergency physicians will have an obstetrician evaluate any laceration requiring repair.

UTERINE INVERSION

General Principles

- A rare complication of vaginal deliveries, uterine inversion is an obstetric emergency because it can lead to maternal hemorrhagic shock and death.
- It is thought to be caused by excessive cord traction and fundal pressure.

Clinical Presentation, Diagnosis, and Evaluation

- Abdominal pain, vaginal bleeding, loss of palpable fundus with a round mass protruding from cervix/vagina after delivery
- Diagnosis is clinical. Examination may demonstrate the inability to palpate the fundus in the normal position.

Treatment

- Immediately call for assistance from obstetrics/gynecology.
- Do NOT remove the placenta because this can increase bleeding.

TABLE 92.1 Causes, General Principles, Diagnosis and Evaluation, and Treatment of Postpartum Hemorrhage (PPH)

Diagnosis	General Principles	Diagnosis and Evaluation	Treatment
Uterine atony	Most common cause of primary PPH	Examination with a boggy, soft uterus after the third stage of labor	Manual uterine massage Gauze packing of fornices Intrauterine balloon tamponade Oxytocin TXA Uterine artery embolization Hysterectomy
Vaginal and cervical lacerations	Can be classified by degree (1st to 4th) depending on tissue layers involved	Diagnosed by physical examination	1st and 2nd degree: may be repaired by the emergency physician with running locked absorbable sutures Higher than 2nd degree: obstetric consult for repair
Uterine inversion	Rare complication of vaginal delivery	Inability to palpate uterus in normal position May visualize uterus through cervix	Immediate obstetrics consult Do NOT remove placenta If possible, manually replace uterus (may be facilitated with uterine relaxants). If replaced, physically maintain position until obstetrics arrives.
Retained placenta	3 types: trapped placenta, placenta adherens, placenta accreta	Inability to deliver placenta within 30 minutes of fetal delivery	Apply gentle cord traction. Manual extraction may be attempted (except for accrete which is treated with hysterectomy).
DIC	Often secondary to other obstetric complications (e.g., eclampsia/HELLP, amniotic fluid embolism, placental abruption)	Presents as primary PPH with petechiae and/or purpura, bleeding from IV sites Laboratory studies show thrombocytopenia (more than 50% decrease from baseline), schistocytes, increased PT/INR/PTT, decreased fibrinogen, increased d-dimer/LDH/total bilirubin.	Identify and treat underlying cause Transfuse blood products ICU admission

DIC, (disseminated intravascular coagulation); *HELLP*, (hemolysis, elevated liver enzymes, low platelet count); *PT*, (prothrombin time); *INR*, (international normalized ratio); *PTT*, (partial thromboplastin time); *TXA*, (tranexamic acid).

- If possible, manually replace the inverted uterus into the pelvis. However, this often requires general anesthesia.
- Administer uterine relaxants (e.g., terbutaline or magnesium sulfate).
- Once inversion is corrected, administer uterotonics (e.g., oxytocin).
- Do not remove hand until stability is confirmed.
- If above measures fail, surgical correction is indicated.

RETAINED PLACENTA

General Principles

- Defined as the inability to deliver the placenta within 30 minutes after delivery of fetus, a retained placenta can interfere with postpartum uterine contractions (thereby leading to postpartum hemorrhage).
  - Three types of retained placenta:
    - Trapped placenta: placenta has completely separated from the uterus, but is trapped behind a closed cervix.
    - Placenta adherens: placenta adheres to the uterine wall, but is easily separable.
    - Placenta accreta: placenta invades past the decidua into the myometrium.

Clinical Presentation, Diagnosis, and Evaluation

- Diagnosis is made when there is inability to deliver the placenta within 30 minutes after delivery of the fetus.

Treatment

- Apply gentle cord traction.
  - If uterine atony is preventing placental expulsion, administer oxytocin.
  - If cervical contraction is preventing placental expulsion, administer tocolytics to relax cervical smooth muscle.
- If above measures fail, should consult Ob. Can attempt gentle manual extraction with Ob consult if patient continues to have PPH; however, be aware that this can worsen bleeding in placenta accreta so it is not without risk.

DISSEMINATED INTRAVASCULAR COAGULATION (DIC)

General Principles

- In pregnancy, DIC typically occurs in the setting of another obstetric complication, such as placental abruption, severe preeclampsia, eclampsia, the syndrome of Hypertension, Elevated Liver enzymes, Low Platelet count (HELLP syndrome), amniotic fluid embolism, or a septic abortion.
- DIC can present as a primary postpartum hemorrhage if it occurs just before, during, or after delivery.

Clinical Presentation

- Usually presents as petechiae or purpura, bleeding from intravenous or venipuncture sites or excessive bleeding during or after delivery

Diagnosis and Evaluation

- Laboratory findings include the following consistent with hemolysis:
  - Thrombocytopenia (less than 50% from baseline)
  - Schistocytes on peripheral smear
  - Increased prothrombin time or international normalized ratio and partial prothrombin time
  - Decreased fibrinogen
  - Increased D-dimer, lactate dehydrogenase, and total bilirubin

Treatment

- Identify and treat the underlying cause, if possible (e.g., if eclampsia, then delivery of fetus).
- Transfuse blood products, as needed.
- Prompt delivery if fetus has not yet been delivered
- Usually requires intensive care unit-level care

CARDIOPULMONARY ARREST IN PREGNANCY

General Principles

- Causes of cardiopulmonary arrest in pregnant women can be remembered by the mnemonic A–H:
  - A – Anesthesia complications, Accidents/trauma
  - B – Bleeding
  - C – Cardiac
  - D – Drugs
  - E – Embolic disease
  - F – Fever (e.g., sepsis)
  - G – General: hypoxia, electrolyte abnormalities
  - H – Hypertension and sequela (e.g., eclampsia, intracranial hemorrhage)

Diagnosis and Evaluation

- Diagnosis is clinical, although it may not be known or apparent that the mother is pregnant.

Treatment

- The goal of resuscitation should be directed at maternal stabilization because fetal survival is directly related to maternal outcomes.
- Airway
  - Secure airway early, if indicated, because pregnant women are at an increased risk of aspiration owing to decreased lower esophageal tone and increased intraabdominal pressure from a gravid uterus.
  - Prepare for possible difficult intubation because airway edema is common in pregnancy.
- Breathing
  - Optimize ventilation and oxygenation to keep SpO_2 above 95% to ensure adequate fetal oxygenation.
  - Prepare for rapid desaturation given physiologic changes in pregnancy.
  - Avoid hyperventilation and respiratory alkalosis because they can cause uterine vasoconstriction and decrease fetal perfusion.
  - Decrease ventilatory volumes in patients with a large gravid uterus.
- Circulation
  - Manually displace the gravid uterus or tilt the patient to the left to prevent compression of the inferior vena cava and allow for venous return. This can be done by securing a patient to a backboard and tilting it to the left.
  - Assess gestational age.
    - If fundus is at or above the umbilicus, the fetus is likely 20 or more weeks; gestation, and perimortem cesarean delivery is indicated (see below).
  - Perimortem cesarean delivery is indicated if return of spontaneous circulation (ROSC) is not achieved within 4 minutes of initiation of resuscitation. Delivery should be completed within 5 minutes to optimize outcomes (both maternal and/or fetal). The delivery should be done via classic midline (incision made from the xiphoid down to the pubic symphysis) cesarean incision.
    - Perimortem cesarean sections between 20 and 24 weeks' gestation are performed in an attempt to improve maternal hemodynamics (as the fetus is not yet viable).
    - After 24 weeks' gestation, a perimortem cesarean section can be performed in an attempt to salvage the fetus as well as to improve maternal hemodynamics.
  - Chest compressions, defibrillation, and medication dosages follow the same Advanced Cardiac Life Support (ACLS) protocol as in nonpregnant women.

SUGGESTED READINGS

Complicated deliveries (EMDocs: https://emdocs.net/the-complicated-delivery-what-do-you-do/)

Perimortem C-section (EMCrit RACC: https://emcrit.org/emcrit/perimortem-c-section/)

Postpartum hemorrhage (REBELEM: https://rebelem.com/post-partum-hemorrhage/)

CHAPTER **93** BOARD REVIEW

Postpartum Emergencies

TYLER HAERTLEIN, MD, and NATASHA WHEATON, MD

- In the US, at least one-quarter of postpartum women face a potentially high-risk complication.
- There are significant racial disparities in postpartum complication rates and outcomes of those complications.
- Due to sparse postpartum care, variable insurance as well as other factors, women in the US often seek postpartum care in the emergency department (ED).
- Emergency physicians (EPs) must be comfortable with common postpartum emergencies including postpartum hemorrhage (primary and secondary), postpartum depression (PPD), endometritis and amniotic fluid embolism (AFE).
- Mastitis and breast abscess are covered seperately in Chapter 94 (The Breastfeeding Mother in the Emergency Department).

Secondary Postpartum Hemorrhage

General Principles

- Primary postpartum hemorrhage (PPH) occurs within the first 24 hours after delivery and is discussed further in Chapter 92. Complications of Delivery.
- Secondary PPH is defined as "excessive" vaginal bleeding occurring between 24 hours and 12 weeks postpartum (Box 93.1).
- Subinvolution of the placental bed and retained products are the most common causes of secondary PPH.

Clinical Presentation

- Patients with secondary PPH present with vaginal bleeding and may present with abnormal vital signs or in hypovolemic shock, depending on the severity of bleeding.

Diagnosis and Evaluation

- Ultimately, PPH is a clinical diagnosis based on time frame and volume of bleeding as specified above.
- Physical examination, including vaginal examination, is imperative to diagnose the specific etiology of PPH, quantify the amount of bleeding, and tailor an appropriate treatment plan.

BOX 93.1 *Risk Factors for Secondary Postpartum Hemorrhage*

Abnormal placentation (including previa, accreta, increta, percreta)
Placental abruption
Uterine infection (e.g., endometritis)
Complicated pregnancy (e.g., pre-eclampsia, eclampsia, HELLP, diabetes or gestational hypertension)
Retained products of conception
Underlying bleeding disorder (e.g., von Willebrand disease, thrombocytopenia, hemophilia)
Instrumented delivery (e.g., forceps delivery, vacuum delivery) or caesarean delivery
Prolonged labor

- In stable patients with secondary PPH, pelvic ultrasonography can be considered to identify retained products of conception and subinvolution of the placental bed. Other sonographic findings may include a vascular abnormality, such as a pseudoaneurysm or an arteriovascular malformation.
- It is important to consider complications of PPH such as severe anemia, sepsis, and disseminated intravascular coagulation (DIC), although these are more common in primary PPH.

Treatment

- Simultaneous volume resuscitation and hemorrhagic source control are imperative in the initial treatment of PPH.
- Patients with PPH may present with hemorrhagic shock, so the EP must also make an assessment of the patient's airway and breathing.
- All patients with PPH should be placed on continuous cardiac monitoring and those with significant bleeding should have multiple sites of large-bore intravenous access established.
- All patients with PPH also warrant consultation with the obstetrician on call.
- As in all causes of hemorrhagic shock, volume resuscitation should focus on early blood product transfusion.
- Definitive treatment of the most common causes of secondary PPH (retained products of conception) is dilation and curettage, but management is guided by the cause of bleeding. For those with subinvolution, initial treatment may begin with methylergonovine or carbopost, but surgical intervention with laparotomy embolization, vessel ligation, or hysterectomy may be necessary if bleeding is severe.

Postpartum Depression

General Principles

- PPD depression shares the same hallmark characteristics of primary nonperipartum depression but is unique in that it occurs either during pregnancy (usually at the later end) or within 4 weeks of delivery.
- Prevalence numbers vary but best estimates are that between 10% and 15% of pregnancies are complicated by PPD.
- Although PPD is prevalent, the most feared complications—suicide and infanticide—are relatively rare, with rates approximated at 1 per 100,000 live births in the United States.
- There is significant stigma surrounding mental health in pregnancy (especially PPD) so EPs should consider screening all postpartum women in the ED for PPD regardless of presenting complaint because women may present with unrelated complaints (including those for their infants).
- Risk factors for PPD are listed in Box 93.2.

Clinical Presentation

- Although the clinical presentation is similar to that of major unipolar depression, the hallmark of peripartum depression is its temporal association to pregnancy.
- May present primarily with general anxiety or more specifically, anxiety related to the child.
- May also present with mania or psychosis (rare).
- Many PPD symptoms (fatigue, difficulty with sleep, changes in appetite) overlap those experienced in the normal postpartum state, making PPD a difficult diagnosis.
- "Baby blues" presents with less severe symptoms than true PPD beginning on day 2–3 postpartum and self-resolves within 2 weeks.

Diagnosis

- The diagnostic criteria for PPD are the same criteria in *The Diagnostic and Statistical Manual of Mental Disorders*, 5th ed., used to diagnose nonperipartum major depression (see Box 93.3) though th.

Evaluation

- Given the prevalence of PPD and the reluctance of many patients to disclose symptoms, EPs should consider screening all postpartum women.
- Screen adequately for suicidality/homicidality (it may be very difficult to encourage mothers to admit feelings of harm toward their child), psychosis (which may be very subtle), and manic symptoms.
- Be aware that, given the stigma surrounding postpartum mental health issues, it may be difficult for the mother to disclose, so be patient and create a safe space for disclosure.
- Thyroid disease is also common postpartum, and EPs should consider screening for hypothyroidism when making a new postpartum depression diagnosis.

BOX 93.2 *Risk Factors for Postpartum Depression*

Previous episodes of depression or anxiety
Undesired pregnancy
Young age
Drug or alcohol abuse
Intimate partner violence
Poor socio-economic support

BOX 93.3 *Diagnostic Criteria for Major Depressive Disorder*

DEPRESSED MOOD and/or ANHEDONIA with 3 or 4 of the following symptoms:
Sleep disturbances (increase or decrease)
Interest loss
Guilt or feelings of worthlessness
Energy decreased
Concentration decreased
Appetite changes (increased or decreased)
Psychomotor retardation
Suicidal thoughts (or thoughts of harm to infant in case of PPD)

Treatment

- Given the risk of morbidity and even mortality for both mother and infant, EPs should have a very low threshold for involving psychiatry when concern for postpartum depression exists.
- Treatment often involves psychotherapy and antidepressant medications; many are compatible with breastfeeding.
- Inpatient admission should be considered for patients with suicidality, thoughts of harm toward the child, inability to care for self or the child, or evidence of psychosis or mania.

Endometritis

General Principles

- Postpartum endometritis refers to a spectrum of infectious complications involving one or more of the following within 2–10 days after birth: myometrium, parametrium, and the obstetric surgical site (for cesarean deliveries).
- Cesarean delivery is the most important risk factor for developing postpartum endometritis followed by length of labor and/or rupture of membranes.

Clinical Presentation

- History of foul-smelling lochia, pelvic pain and/or incisional pain, redness, or drainage often associated with systemic symptoms such as chills, fevers, and/or malaise
- On examination, patients may have fever and may exhibit uterine tenderness and/or varying levels of cervical discharge.
- If delivered by cesarean section, the wound may or may not look externally infected.

Diagnosis

- Largely a clinical diagnosis based on diagnostic criteria of postpartum fever (not due to another etiology) of oral temperature of ≥38.0°C on any two of the first 10 days postpartum, exclusive of the first 24 hours (fevers are common in the first 24 hours and usually resolve). Additionally, midline uterine and/or abdominal tenderness and leukocytosis support the clinical diagnosis.
- Cultures, both of vaginal discharge and of blood, are often obtained but of questionable value unless the patient appears overtly septic.
- Testing for gonorrhea and chlamydia should be performed if results from pregnancy are not known or available.
- Imaging studies including pelvic ultrasonography and/or computed tomography of the abdomen and pelvis may be considered but are not necessary. They are primarily used to characterize potential complications (e.g., abscess, septic pelvic thrombophlebitis).

Treatment

- The goals of treatment are to prevent the complications of postpartum endometritis, which include peritonitis, pelvic abscess, and septic thrombophlebitis.

- Consult patient's obstetrician or the obstetrician on call.
- Administer broad-spectrum antibiotics, most commonly clindamycin and gentamycin, to cover β-lactam–producing anaerobes. Can consider adding vancomycin if there is significant concern for methicillin-resistant *Staphylococcus aureus* infection (usually post-cesarean section with concurrent wound cellulitis).
- Unstable patients should receive initial ED resuscitation, be evaluated for potential surgical management by the obstetrician on call, and be admitted for intravenous antibiotics.
- Patients post-cesarean section or with significant underlying comorbidities should be treated similarly to unstable patients.
- Stable patients with mild illness may be admitted or discharged home on oral antibiotics with close follow-up. Most commonly, stable patients managed as outpatients receive a 10-day course of clindamycin (300 mg three times per day) or doxycycline (100 mg twice a day).

Amniotic Fluid Embolus

General Principles

- AFE is a rare condition where amniotic fluid and fetal cells enter maternal circulation, usually within 30 minutes of delivery.
- AFE is rare to see in the ED due to its proximity to delivery unless it is a precipitous out-of-hospital or ED delivery.
- Patients are usually critically ill with frank shock and it is important to keep a broad differential including more common conditions as it is a diagnosis of exclusion.
- In addition to AFE, EPs should consider acute respiratory distress syndrome (ARDS), acute myocardial infarction, pulmonary embolism, eclampsia, intracranial hemorrhage, and cerebral vascular events in their critically ill postpartum patients.
- Many of the conditions listed above also occur during late pregnancy and are further discussed in Chapter 91. Late Pregnancy Complications.

Clinical Presentation

- Patients will be critically ill with sudden hypotension, hypoxia, tonic-clonic seizures, altered mental status, or stroke symptoms, depending on which organ system is affected.
- DIC occurs in 80% and may present with bruising, bleeding, or clotting.

Diagnosis and Evaluation

- Ultimately, AFE is a diagnosis of exclusion. It generally presents as acute onset of cardiovascular instability with respiratory involvement during or just after delivery in the absence of another cause. It is often followed by coagulopathy (e.g., DIC).
- Laboratory testing may include a complete blood count, comprehensive metabolic panel, coagulation studies, blood gas, cardiac enzymes, and blood cultures. ECG and chest radiography should also be obtained.
- Further imaging may include bedside ultrasonography, neuroimaging, and, if stable, computed tomographic angiography of the chest, depending on presenting symptoms.

Treatment

- Supportive care is key in the management of AFE as the EP excludes other life-threatening diagnoses.
- Given the rapid progression of the disease, advanced airway management and aggressive circulatory resuscitation are usually needed.
- Circulatory resuscitation is a difficult task in patients with AFE because excessive fluid resuscitation may worsen pulmonary edema, and therefore vasopressors, most commonly norepinephrine, are often included in management algorithms.
- Patients may have bleeding secondary to DIC or may have postpartum hemorrhage from a more common etiology such as uterine atony or lacerations. A focused examination is necessary for distinction.
- Ultimately, in patients who are unresponsive to aggressive supportive care, extracorporeal membrane oxygenation may be considered.
- All patients will need admission to critical care units.

Postdural Headaches

- Headaches are common postpartum and many of the serious etiologies overlap with those in the late postpartum period (see Chapter 91. Late Pregnancy Complications).
- A unique cause of headaches postpartum includes postdural headaches.

General Principles

- Can occur post-epidural in up to 5% of patients and are relatively benign though they can be severely limiting in terms of symptomology.
- Higher risk with inexperienced operator, increased number of attempts, atraumatic pencil point needles, and larger needle size.

Clinical Presentation

- Presenting within 72 hours of delivery, the headaches are generally described as worse with sitting or standing and can be debilitating.
- Patients should be afebrile. Meningitis or osteomyelitis/diskitis may be considered if febrile and/or the patient has accompanying focal back pain or lower neurologic complaints.

Treatment

- Patients who have mild symptoms may benefit from bed rest, oral analgesics, hydration, and antiemetics. Additionally, although the evidence is not high quality, oral or IV caffeine administration may be helpful.
- If symptoms fail to resolve with conservative measures, an epidural blood patch is considered definitive treatment and usually provides immediate relief.

SUGGESTED READINGS

Baldisseri, M. R., & Clark, S. L. Amniotic fluid embolism. *UpToDate*. Available at: www.uptodate.com/contents/amniotic-fluid-embolism

Millsap, G. (2014). Post-dural headaches. *EMDocs*. Available at: www.emdocs.net/post-lp-headache/

Pearlstein, T., Howard, M., Salisbury, A., & Zlotnick, C. (2009). Postpartum depression. *American Journal of Obstetrics and Gynecology*, 200(4), 357–364.

CHAPTER **94**

BOARD REVIEW

The Breastfeeding Mother in the Emergency Department

DIANE D. HSU, MD, and ANDREA W. WU, MD, MMM

- It is important that emergency physicians (EPs) understand the basics of caring for lactating mothers, support lactation while the mother is in the emergency department (ED), and be familiar with how to treat complications of lactation.
- Postpartum women should be asked about lactation status.
- In the early postpartum months, lactating mothers will need to either feed or pump approximately every 2-3 hours (this changes to every 4-6 hours as the baby ages).
- It is important that mothers are allowed to pump or feed on this schedule or they will become engorged (which is painful and also increases the risk of mastitis) and risk losing milk supply which can interrupt the nursing relationship permanently.
- Breast pumpts are readily availably in many hospitals through labor and dlivery or the neonatal intensive care unit.
- Most common ED medications are compatible with continued breastfeeding, including contrast dye, pain medications, conscious sedation medications and many antibiotics.
- "Pumping and dumping" is rarely medically indicated.
- There are multiple resources (including LactMed) that clinicians can use to ensure lactation safety.
- Lack of lactation support and inappropriate advice to "pump and dump" can lead mothers to prematurely wean their infants.
- See Box 94.1 for a summary of these recommendations.

Mastitis

General Principles

- Mastitis is defined as inflammation due to a bacterial infection of the breast that usually occurs in breastfeeding mothers.
- It should be differentiated from blocked or plugged ducts, which almost always resolve spontaneously with hand expression of breast milk and heat application within 24–48 hours.
- If the plugged duct does not resolve after 72 hours, a galactocele or milk retention cyst may have formed, and in this case, aspiration should be performed by a breast surgeon.
- Note that 75% of mastitis occurs within the first 3 months after initiating breastfeeding and may lead a mother to wean her baby before she had intended.

BOX 94.1 *Supporting Breastfeeding Mothers in the Emergency Department*

Encourage frequent nursing or pumping
Try to avoid substituting with formula. Obtain lactation consultation promptly if available
Avoid "pump and dump." Ask about lactation status in all postpartum mothers and remember many women will breastfeed into the toddler years
Check before prescribing
While most medications are safe in lactation, some medications are contraindicated in breastfeeding mothers. Check the LactMed database for safety and therapeutic alternatives for breastfeeding mothers.

Clinical Presentation

- Usually caused by *Staphylococcus aureus* infection predisposed by local skin breakage
- Risk factors include:
  - **Milk stasis resulting from poor drainage and prolonged engorgement**
    - Blocked milk ducts, ineffective latching or not emptying the breast in a timely manner, milk oversupply, not wearing a supportive bra, dehydration, medications that decrease mild production (e.g., antihistamines, pseudoephedrine, etc.).
  - **Local microtrauma**
    - Nipple fissures, infant biting/mouth abnormalities (e.g., short frenulum), fungal infection
  - **Immunocompromised maternal state**
- Presents with fever, chills, malaise, fatigue (flu-like symptoms) and unilateral breast pain, warmth and swelling > 24 hours
  - Before 24 hours, symptoms are likely due to a blocked duct and condition often self-resolves with continued nursing and massage, as mentioned above.

Diagnosis and Evaluation

- The diagnosis of mastitis is made clinically with symptoms listed above in conjunction with breast cellulitis (often wedge-shaped).
- Breast milk cultures are rarely obtained because positive cultures can be from bacterial colonization, and negative cultures do not rule out mastitis.
  - Culture is recommended only when the infection is severe, unusual, refractory to antibiotic treatment, or

when abscess is suspected or is located in high bacterial resistance institution/area.
- May obtain ultrasound (bedside or formal) to evaluate for breast abscess if patient fails to respond to appropriate oral antibiotics or has an examination result concerning for abscess (e.g. area of fluctuance underlying cellulitis, see below)
- Needle aspiration for drainage and culture (rare to need open incision and drainage), may be done by the EP if small and superficial or by a breast surgeon, if large and/or deep (see Treatment).

Treatment

- Continue breastfeeding to prevent engorgement. Alternate feeding positions to make sure breasts are fully emptied. Patient may benefit from lactation consult to evaluate effective latching and troubleshoot other problems.
- Ensure adequate hydration.
- Apply warm compression (warm bottle rolling) and local massage.
- Wear a supportive bra.
- PO antibiotics for 10–14 days to cover for *Staphylococcus aureus*, *Streptococcus*, and *Escherichia coli* although can give a watch-and-wait prescription for those with symptoms less than 24 hours.
  - First line: dicloxacillin 500 mg PO q6hrs, given infant safety profile. Add trimethoprim/sulfamethoxazole two DS tabs by mouth twice a day if MRSA is supected. Consider clindamycin for those with significant PCN allergies.
  - It is important to have close follow-up to monitor response to antibiotic treatment.
- Consider consultation or referral to breast specialist if patient has failed outpatient antibiotics or there is concern for malignancy.
- Inflammatory breast cancer, although rare, carries high morbidity and mortality and cannot always be differentiated from acute mastitis during the initial ED encounter.
- Consider antifungal treatment for both the patient and the infant if there are signs and symptoms consistent with *Candida* infection. The classic symptom presentation is shooting breast pain in a breastfeeding mother whose infant has oral thrush. Physical examination may demonstrate exquisite tenderness with erythema and warmth but also flaky, dry skin changes. Topical antifungal treatment, such as Nystatin cream twice daily, may be applied to the breast (systemic medication may be indicated if the topical agents fail) and oral Nystatin solution may be prescribed to the infant.

Breast Abscess

Clinical Presentation

- Presents as mastitis with a focal area of increased discomfort
- Often re-presents to the ED as a failure of outpatient mastitis treatment

Diagnosis and Evaluation

- Physical examination demonstrates redness, warmth, and an area of fluctuance.
- Bedside ultrasonography can evaluate the depth and size of the abscess as these factors affect treatment.

Treatment

- Percutaneous needle aspiration is recommended over open incision and drainage as initial therapy in lactating women to avoid creating a milk duct fistula.
- The EP may consider needle aspiration of small, superficial abscesses; larger or deeper abscesses require breast surgery consultation and management.
- Breast abscesses may need repeated needle aspiration and/or surgical incision and drainage for definitive treatment. Patients will benefit from follow-up with a breast surgeon or breast diagnostic center radiologist after diagnosis of a breast abscess in the ED.

94

SUGGESTED READINGS

Amir, L. H. (2014). ABM [Academy of Breastfeeding Medicine] clinical protocol #4: Mastitis, revised March 2014. *Breastfeeding Medicine*, 9(5), 239–243.

Amir, L. H., Trupin, S., & Kvist, L. J. (2014). Diagnosis and treatment of mastitis in breastfeeding women. *Journal of Human Lactation*, 30(1), 10–13.

Faust, J., & Westafer, L. (Hosts). (2018, May 1). Emergency care of lactating patients. In *FOAMcast. An emergency medicine podcast*. https://foamcast.org/2018/05/01/emergency-care-of-lactating-patients/

Hendrickson, R. G., & McKeown, N. J. (2012). Is maternal opioid use hazardous to breast-fed infants? *Clinical Toxicology (Philadelphia, Pa)*, 50(1), 1–14.

CHAPTER 95

BOARD REVIEW

Complications of Assisted Reproductive Technology

CLAUDIE BOLDUC, MD, MPH, and NATASHA WHEATON, MD

Background Information

- Assisted reproductive technology (ART) is the use of medical procedures handling both a woman's ova and a man's sperms to treat infertility or to create a viable embryo for future pregnancies.
- In vitro fertilization (IVF) is the most common and effective ART and refers to the process by which an oocyte is harvested, fertilized, and transferred into the uterine cavity. This process commonly lasts 2–3 weeks and is known as one ART cycle.
- IVF has been routinely used since 1981 and is estimated to now account for 1.7% of live births in the United States.
- Women and couples are waiting longer to have children and are opting to freeze their eggs or embryos, thus further increasing demand for IVF.
- The Centers for Disease Control and Prevention estimates that 30% of all ART cycles are completed for egg or embryo banking.
- Nearly 300,000 ART cycles are performed per year in the United States; therefore, emergency physicians must be well versed in the technology and its complications.
- The steps in an ART cycle involve: (1) ovarian hormonal stimulation, (2) ova retrieval, (3) intracytoplasmic sperm injection, (4) embryo culture, and (5) embryo transfer (typically with two embryos).
- The main complications are related to ovarian stimulation, pelvic procedures, and complications related to the pregnancy itself, especially given the risk of multiparity (40% of ART live births are twins). Table 95.1 includes a list of ART complications.
- IVF patients are at least twice as likely to have an ectopic pregnancy, and heterotopic pregnancies (presence of both an ectopic and intra-uterine pregnancies concurrently) are almost always seen in IVF patients.
- In addition to ectopic and heterotopic pregnancies, the main emergent complication that is specific to ART is ovarian hyperstimulation syndrome (OHSS), which is discussed here in more detail. Please see Chapter 90 for further discussion of ectopic pregnancy.

TABLE 95.1 *Complications of Assisted Reproductive Therapy*

	Complications
Ovarian stimulation	Ovarian hyperstimulation syndrome Ovarian torsion Ovarian hemorrhage
Pelvic instrumentation (egg retrieval, embryo transfer)	Damage to surrounding structures Pelvic infection
Pregnancy	Multiparity risks (40% twins) Ectopic pregnancies (IVF doubles the risk) Heterotopic pregnancies

IVF, in vitro fertilization.

Ovarian Hyperstimulation Syndrome

OHSS is an iatrogenic condition caused by the hormonal stimulation during the ART cycle, specifically human chorionic gonadotropin (hCG), and is characterized by bilateral ovarian cysts and fluid shifts.

General Principles

- It is estimated that up to 10% of women undergoing IVF will suffer from OHSS.
- Although most cases are mild, 1%–3% of women will have severe disease, and fatal cases have been reported.
- Risk factors include young age (<35 years), previous exaggerated response/OHSS, polycystic ovarian syndrome, and slender body habitus.
- The pathophysiology involves a fluid shift from the intravascular space to the third compartment ("third spacing"), caused by increased capillary permeability and ovarian neoangiogenesis secondary to vasoactive substances secreted by the ovaries.

Clinical Presentation

- Enlargement of the ovaries causes abdominal pain, nausea, and vomiting, and this is the most common presentation.
- There are two subsets of OHSS: "early-onset" OHSS, which usually begins 4–7 days after administration of hCG, and "late-onset" OHSS, which presents after the pregnancy is established and is typically more severe because of the effect of increasing hCG levels.
- A classification system exists for severity and ranges from mild to severe (see Table 95.2).
- In moderate to severe cases, presentations are characterized by third spacing of fluid or leakage from ruptured

TABLE 95.2 Classification of Ovarian Hyperstimulation Syndrome Severity

Mild	Abdominal distension, discomfort, nausea, vomiting, and/or diarrhea Ovarian enlargement 5–12 cm
Moderate	Mild features + sonographic evidence of ascites Laboratory abnormalities: Hct >41%, elevated WBC >15,000, hypoproteinemia
Severe	Moderate features + clinical evidence of ascites and/or hydrothorax Hypotension and/or hypovolemia (due to third spacing) Dyspnea Laboratory abnormalities: Hct >55%, WBC >25,000, creatinine >1.6, hyponatremia, hyperkalemia, and elevated LFT results)

Hct, hematocrit; *LFT*, liver function test; *WBC*, white blood cell [count].

ovarian follicles and thus includes ascites, edema, hydrothorax, and/or hydropericardium.

- In severe cases, the change in blood volume leads to weight gain of up to 15–20 kg, pleural effusions and hypoxia, leukocytosis, hypercoagulable state, and decreased renal perfusion and function leading to electrolyte abnormalities.
  - Hypercoagulable state
    - Both venous and arterial. Of the venous complications, 83% occur in the veins of the neck, arm, and head (60%). Pulmonary embolism occurs in 4%–12% of cases of OHSS.
  - Electrolyte abnormalities
    - Consistent with prerenal acute kidney injury from third spacing, which can lead to hyperkalemia and acidosis. Can also occur or be worsened by microthrombi from hemoconcentration.
- Enlarged ovaries in OHSS are also at increased risk for torsion and hemorrhagic rupture.

Diagnosis and Evaluation

- Bimanual pelvic examination is contraindicated because of the fragility of ovaries and high risk of rupture/hemorrhage.
- Clinical examination should focus on volume status.
  - Evaluate for distant heart sounds, jugular venous distension, and hypotension (pericardial effusion/tamponade)
  - Decreased breath sounds (pleural effusions)
  - Distended abdomen (ascites)
  - Peripheral edema
- Use bedside ultrasonography to further characterize fluid accumulation.
- Laboratory tests should include serum β-hCG, complete blood count (hemoconcentration), basic metabolic panel (BMP) (evaluate for renal failure and electrolyte abnormalities), liver function tests (abnormalities indicate severe OHSS), prothrombin time, partial thromboplastin time, and international normalized ratio.
- Consider formal ultrasonography of the pelvis to assess for ovarian torsion, ectopic, ascites. or ruptured cysts. Expect to see bilateral enlarged cystic ovaries; size helps determine severity.

Treatment

- Treatment depends largely on the severity of OHSS.
- In mild cases, women can be treated as outpatients with symptomatic control with acetaminophen (avoid nonsteroidal inflammatory drugs). Consult gynecology and ensure patient has close follow-up.
- Mild OHSS can progress to moderate or severe especially if pregnancy occurs. Therefore, patients should be instructed to return to the emergency department for worsening abdominal pain, weight gain (> 1 kg/day) or increasing abdominal girth.
- Moderate OHSS can also occasionally be treated as an outpatient, though often requires admission. If discharged after Ob/Gyn consultation, patients should have complete blood count studies and transvaginal ultrasonography every 48 hours if abdominal pain symptoms are worsening (tracking fluid status and hematocrit). Patients should also be instructed to remain well hydrated (2 liters of fluid intake per day); bed rest may be necessary.
- If patients are unable to maintain their hydration, have hematocrit >45%, white blood cell count >25,000, creatinine >1.6, tense ascites, or hypotension, they should be hospitalized.
- Severe OHSS requires admission to the intensive care unit. The focus of treatment is on reversing such complications as kidney failure, electrolyte abnormalities, and coagulopathies/thrombosis. Patients may require physical removal of fluid (e.g., paracentesis, pleuracentesis, pericardiocentesis). Paracentesis is a high-risk procedure, given enlarged ovaries, and should not routinely be done by the emergency physician.
- Diuresis should be avoided, given the risk of further complicating intravascular depletion and hypotension.

SUGGESTED READING

Cassella, C. (2016, October 23). *In vitro fertilization patient and ED presentations: Pearls and pitfalls*. emDocs. http://www.emdocs.net/vitro-fertilization-patient-ed-presentations-pearls-pitfalls/, 2016.

95

SECTION THIRTEEN BOARD REVIEW

Psychobehavioral

CHAPTER **96**

BOARD REVIEW

Emergency Care of Psychiatric Patients

BRITTANY GUEST, DO, and STEVEN LAI, MD

Clinical Presentation, Diagnosis, and Evaluation

- According to the 2015 National Hospital Ambulatory Medical Care Survey by the Centers for Disease Control and Prevention, mental health disorders accounted for 5.7 million visits to the emergency department (ED).
- As the number of mental health–related visits to EDs continues to increase, it is crucial that physicians know how to safely control the agitated or violent psychiatric patient and quickly evaluate for possible organic causes of the aggressive behavior.
- It is vital to determine whether the change in behavior of your patient is from a primary psychiatric condition or an organic cause. Obtaining collateral information, if available, from friends and family, including medical and psychiatric history, substance use, recent illnesses, and ingestions, may be useful.
- A thorough physical examination, with particular attention to signs of infection, trauma, toxidromes, needle tracks, and focal neurologic deficits, are paramount in determining a confounding or organic etiology. A complete set of vital signs, including pulse oximetry, should be obtained. If available, a point-of-care serum glucose test should be obtained, as well.
- It is prudent to suspect an organic process in the elderly, agitated patient, particularly one without a prior known psychiatric history.

Treatment and Approach

- The approach to the agitated psychiatric patient centers on ensuring the safety of the patient, the treating staff, and the other patients.
- Ensure a safe exit if the patient becomes aggressive.
- All combative patients should be disarmed before physician evaluation and there should be no obstacles between the exit and the provider.
- Verbal deescalation should often be the first technique used when approaching the agitated patient. Use a calm voice, introduce yourself, explain your role, allow the patient to express their concerns, and identify and manage potential causes for aggressive behavior (i.e., pain, hunger, anxiety). This may not be appropriate or effective in an extremely aggressive patient. Physical restraints may be required.
- Physical restraints are a temporary measure and should be used only with frequent monitoring and reassessments. They should be discontinued immediately when the safety of the patient and staff is ensured. When applying physical restraints, one should ideally have a team of at least five people, wear personal protective equipment, and always explain to the patient what you are doing and that everything is being done in the best interest of their safety and the safety of the people around them. Physical restraints may include mittens, spit shields, arm and leg soft restraints, vest and lap belts, and four-point leather restraints, depending on the degree of agitation.
- Chemical restraints may also be indicated. Traditionally, haloperidol (5–10 mg intramuscularly) and/or lorazepam (1–2 mg intramuscularly) is a common regimen. However, the newer atypical antipsychotics (olanzapine, ziprasidone, etc.) generally have a better side effect profile and may be preferred, especially in a patient who has a known psychiatric disorder. For those who are combative or agitated from withdrawal (e.g., alcohol) or intoxication, benzodiazepines alone may be sufficient. By calming the patient, chemical restraints facilitate the performance of a physical examination to assess for any organic cause of behavioral changes. Similar to physical restraints, monitoring and frequent reassessments are necessary when employing chemical restraints.
- Involuntary hospitalization may be warranted if the patient poses a danger to self or others, or if they are unable to provide basic needs of food, clothing, and shelter (i.e., gravely disabled).
- Patients may be *medically detained* if the patient has a psychiatric emergency, but is refusing care and lacks capacity. If psychiatric care is not available at your facility, transfer will need to be arranged. Any licensed physician can *medically detain* a patient to evaluate the patient and provide care.
- *Involuntary detainment* (i.e., civil commitment) is the lawful restraint of a person who is a danger to themselves, is a danger to others, or is gravely disabled.
- Classifications of who can involuntarily detain a patient (separate from medical detainment) vary from state to state, but typically include law enforcement and psychiatrists.

Substance Abuse and Addiction

RANDALL W. LEE, MD, and ADAM R. EVANS, MD

Substance abuse can lead to substance use disorders, depending on the drug of abuse, genetic predisposition, and other demographic variables. The 12-month prevalence of substance use disorders in the United States was 6.2% in 2018, with alcohol comprising approximately 80% of all substances. Substance abuse is linked to higher mortality worldwide and timely recognition of these syndromes is warranted.

Basic Information: Definitions

- *Substance abuse:* substance use leading to adverse consequences (e.g., trouble with work or liver injury from alcohol use)
- *Tolerance:* need for increasing amounts of a substance to produce intoxication or desired effect
- *Substance dependence:* absence of control resulting in compulsive use of a substance and marked by *craving*, *tolerance*, and *withdrawal* symptoms
- *Withdrawal:* physiologic response resulting in symptoms typically opposite of intoxication when the substance is discontinued
- *Substance use disorder:* current unifying term that encompasses all disorders related to substance use and abuse

Clinical Presentation

The clinical picture of a patient who is suffering from a substance use disorder can vary greatly, depending on the substance used. Signs and symptoms of substance use and abuse often result from states of acute intoxication or withdrawal.

Intoxication

- Table 97.1 lists the signs and symptoms of intoxication associated with commonly abused substances.

Withdrawal

Alcohol Withdrawal

- Alcohol withdrawal can occur within as little as 4 hours after last ingestion.
- Symptoms often include nausea, vomiting, tremors, hallucinations, anxiety, altered cognition, ataxia, headache, and seizures.
- Hallucinations and seizures usually present within 24–48 hours from last ingestion.
- *Delirium tremens*, a severe withdrawal syndrome that includes autonomic instability, hallucinations, delirium, and seizures; tends to peak 2–5 days after cessation of alcohol and is relatively rare before 24 hours of cessation.
- *Wernicke encephalopathy* can occur in heavy drinkers and severely malnourished patients secondary to thiamine (vitamin B_1) deficiency. Typically presentation includes altered mental status, nystagmus, ophthalmoplegia, and ataxia. Autonomic and temperature dysregulation can also occur, leading to hypotension and hypothermia. The mainstay of treatment for Wernicke encephalopathy is thiamine administration.
- *Korsakoff syndrome* can follow Wernicke encephalopathy and leads to anterograde and retrograde amnesia and confabulation.

Benzodiazepine Withdrawal

- Rapid reduction in benzodiazepine dose in chronic users can result in withdrawal symptoms and signs, similar in presentation to alcohol withdrawal.
- These may include tremors, anxiety, hallucinations, delusions, and seizures; it is important to realize that benzodiazepine withdrawal can also be life-threatening.
- However, the onset may often be delayed (i.e., days to 1 week after cessation) compared with alcohol withdrawal.

Opioid Withdrawal

- Characterized by mydriasis, rhinorrhea, piloerection, yawning, and increased bowel sounds, opioid withdrawal is usually not life-threatening, except in neonates.
- The onset of withdrawal can occur 6 hours after last ingestion, peaking at 48–72 hours, and symptoms can last several days.
- Adrenergic hyperactivity (i.e., central nervous system excitation, tachypnea, tachycardia, hypertension) and gastrointestinal symptoms (i.e., abdominal cramping, nausea, vomiting, and diarrhea) predominate.

Substance Use Complications

- The use of stimulants (i.e., amphetamines, 3,4-methylenedioxymethamphetamine, cocaine, and phencyclidine) can lead to many complications, including traumatic injuries, rhabdomyolysis, hyperthermia, myocardial injury, acute stroke, electrolyte imbalances, psychosis, delirium, depression, liver injury, and coagulopathies.
- Opiate abuse can lead to such complications as hypothermia, hypoxic brain injury, myocardial injury or infection, electrolyte imbalances, delirium, depression, bacteremia, and other infections, especially with injection drug use.

TABLE 97.1 Substance Intoxication: Clinical Presentation and Treatment

Substance	Cardinal Features	Treatment
Ethanol (sedative/hypnotic)	Respiratory depression Slurred speech Ataxia Unsteady gait Nystagmus Stupor or coma	Supportive IV fluids, dextrose, and electrolyte repletion if indicated Imaging if trauma is suspected
Cannabis/THC/CBD	Conjunctival injection Nausea Nystagmus Tachycardia	Supportive
PCP	Hallucinations Hypertension Hyperthermia Nystagmus Tachycardia Violent behavior	Benzodiazepines Active cooling (hyperthermia) IV fluids (hypovolemia, rhabdomyolysis)
Opioid	Respiratory depression Slurred speech Miosis (pupillary constriction) Impairment in attention or memory Stupor or coma	Naloxone
Cocaine	Tachycardia Hypertension Hyperthermia Mydriasis (pupillary dilation) Psychomotor agitation Confusion, hallucinations, delusions Seizures Stupor or coma Chest pain, myocardial infarction, coronary vasospasm, and cardiomyopathy Cardiac dysrhythmias QRS and QT prolongation Aortic and coronary artery dissection	Benzodiazepines Active cooling IV fluids (hypovolemia, rhabdomyolysis) Phentolamine (HTN emergency) Sodium bicarbonate (wide QRS) **Avoid β-blockers**
Amphetamines, MDMA	Similar to cocaine Hyponatremia	Benzodiazepines Active cooling IV fluids (hypovolemia, rhabdomyolysis)
Benzodiazepines	Ataxia Hypotension Impaired cognition Respiratory depression Slurred speech	Supportive Flumazenil (can precipitate seizures in chronic users)

CBD, cannabidiol; *IV,* intravenous; *MDMA,* 3,4-methylenedioxymethamphetamine; *PCP,* phencyclidine; *THC,* tetrahydrocannabinol.

Diagnosis

History and physical examination remain the best tools available to diagnose a substance use disorder. *The Diagnostic and Statistical Manual of Mental Disorders* (5th ed.) outlines specific diagnostic criteria to diagnose substance use disorder and to determine the severity of a patient's illness.

- There are also many drug and alcohol screening tools that help identify patients who suffer from substance use disorders. Some examples:
  - Alcohol abuse: CAGE questionnaire, Michigan Alcoholism Screening Test (MAST), Alcohol Use Disorders Identification Test (AUDIT)
  - Drug abuse: Drug Abuse Screening Test (DAST)
- These tools, along with brief motivational intervention strategies, result in a short-term reduction of substance abuse, including decreased emergency department visits.

Treatment

Substance Intoxication

- Table 97.1 summarizes basic medical management of selected intoxication syndromes. Medical management can occur in conjunction with referral to inpatient or outpatient rehabilitation centers. These programs focus on symptom control during the acute withdrawal period and provide therapy from trained counselors.
- After the withdrawal period, patients are encouraged to join support groups like Alcoholics Anonymous (AA) and Narcotics Anonymous (NA).
- The success rates of this strategy unfortunately still remain low, especially for alcohol use disorder. One study demonstrated that fewer than 7% of patients were able to refrain from alcohol in the subsequent years after initial sobriety.

Alcohol and Benzodiazepine Withdrawal

- The mainstay of treatment is with aggressive use of benzodiazepines. Diazepam is often recommended as a first-line agent owing to its fast onset and long half-life, but others are often used in the acute setting.
- Phenobarbital can also be used as a primary treatment modality. Some patients have a better response to barbiturates because of the drug's altered mechanism of action on the brain.
- Patients with mild withdrawal who are deemed safe for discharge can be prescribed a benzodiazepine (i.e., chlordiazepoxide) taper. Moderate to life-threatening withdrawal states require admission.
- Ketamine and dexmedetomidine use in alcohol withdrawal may be effective but requires further study at this time.

Opioid Withdrawal

- There is increasing evidence that medication-assisted treatment is effective treatment and improves abstinence rates. Symptom control can be achieved through a variety of classes of agents, including:
  - Opioid agonist therapy: includes methadone and buprenorphine
  - Nonopioid adjunctive medications: includes α_2-adrenergic agonists, such as clonidine
  - Other supportive treatment for symptom control: muscle relaxants (tizanidine, cyclobenzaprine), and antiemetics (ondansetron, metoclopramide)
- Note that there is a risk of QT prolongation when multiple medications that increase the QT interval (methadone and ondansetron) are concomitantly administered, particularly in patients who may have electrolyte abnormalities from vomiting and diarrhea.

SUGGESTED READINGS

American Psychiatric Association. (2013). *Diagnostic and statistical manual of mental disorders* (5th ed.). American Psychiatric Association.

Cutler, J. L. (2014). *Psychiatry* (3rd ed.). Oxford University Press.

Galanter, M., Kleber, H. D., & Brady, K. T. (Eds.). (2014). *The American Psychiatric Publishing textbook of substance abuse treatment* (5th ed.). American Psychiatric Publishing.

Mood and Thought Disorders

BRITTANY GUEST, DO, and STEVEN LAI, MD

General Principles

- Patients who have thought disorders, such as schizophrenia, and mood disorders, such as depression, have a high incidence of emergency department visits.
- In addition to controlling danger to patient and staff from patients' violent and disruptive behavior, the emergency physician must rule out and treat organic etiologies such as endocrine disorders (e.g., thyrotoxicosis), neurologic disorders (e.g., Huntington disease and dementia), infection (e.g., encephalitis), metabolic disturbances (e.g., hypercalcemia and hyponatremia), medication effects, and substance abuse and intoxication or withdrawal—all of which may mimic the presentation of psychiatric illnesses.

Schizophrenia

Clinical Presentation

- Most common type of psychosis
- Symptoms often first manifest in late adolescence and early adulthood; more frequent in males.
- Patients typically present with a deterioration from a normal level of functioning, usually first characterized by social withdrawal, bizarre behavior, and difficulty functioning at school or work.
- Factors associated with schizophrenia include family history, structural abnormalities, and low socioeconomic class.

Diagnosis and Evaluation

- The differential diagnosis is *broad* and can include the following conditions:
  - *Brief psychotic disorder:* defined as psychotic symptoms lasting more than 1 day but less than a month
  - *Schizophreniform disorder:* defined as psychotic symptoms lasting from 1 to 6 months
  - *Schizoaffective disorder:* defined as psychosis occurring exclusively during an episode of mania or depression
  - Schizoid and schizotypal personality disorder
  - Delirium, dementia, or psychosis secondary to substance use and acute intoxication or secondary to a medical condition (i.e., hypoglycemia, metabolic abnormalities, neurologic conditions, endocrine disorders, etc.)
- The *diagnosis of schizophrenia* is based on the presence of two or more of the following symptoms for 6 months:
  - Delusions
  - Hallucinations (auditory more than visual, tactile, olfactory, gustatory)
    - If nonauditory hallucinations occur, suspect organic cause of psychosis (visual hallucinations are more common in children with mood and thought disorders)
  - Disorganized speech
  - Disorganized or catatonic behavior
  - *Negative symptoms*: flat affect, emotional withdrawal, anhedonia, decreased fluency, and social withdrawal

Treatment

- Treatment may include a combination of antipsychotics (typical and atypical, with the latter having more efficacy for negative symptoms, such as blunted affect and social withdrawal) and outpatient/group therapy.
- Psychomotor agitation may warrant chemical and physical restraint, if verbal deescalation is ineffective.
- Consider sedation (i.e., haloperidol and benzodiazepines for severe agitation), and admission/transfer for psychiatric inpatient care if the patient is a danger to self or others, or is gravely disabled.

Major Depression

Clinical Presentation

- Affects about 10%–25% of women and about 5%–10% of men.
- A major depressive episode is characterized by disturbances in mood, cognition, vegetative function, and psychomotor activity.
- Patients may express hopelessness, helplessness, and have decreased capacity to experience pleasure.
- More women suffer from depression, but more men commit suicide. Most completed suicides are by firearms, whereas most attempts are ingestions. The lifetime risk of suicide for a person with major depression is 15%. Box 98.1 delineates some risk factors for suicide (the SAD PERSONS mnemonic).
- Differential diagnosis includes mood disorders secondary to medical conditions, such as hypothyroidism, Huntington disease, Alzheimer disease, multiple sclerosis, substance abuse, bereavement, adjustment disorder, and medication side effects.
- *Bereavement* (grief reaction) after the loss of a loved one is normal. Severe symptoms usually resolve after 2 months, and moderate symptoms can take up to a year to resolve.
- *Persistent depressive disorder* (dysthymia) is a depressive mood disorder characterized by a chronic course and typically an insidious and early onset (in childhood to early adulthood). These patients typically have a depressed mood for most of the day, for more days

BOX 98.1 *Risk Factors for Suicide (SAD PERSONS Mnemonic)*

S = Sex (male)
A = Age (<19 or >45 years)
D = Depression or hopelessness
P = Previous suicide attempt
E = Ethanol/alcohol or drug abuse
R = Rational thinking loss
S = Separated, divorced, or widowed
O = Organized plan
N = No social support
S = Stated future intent (or medical sickness)

than not, for at least 2 years (more than 1 year in children and adolescents). Treatment often involves a combination of drug therapy with individual or group psychotherapy.

Diagnosis and Evaluation

- Diagnosis is clinical; patients suffer from one or more depressive episodes lasting at least 2 weeks and have at least five of the following symptoms (SAD CAGES):
  S = Sleep (too much or too little)
  A = Appetite (change in appetite or weight)
  D = Depressed mood (or anhedonia)
  C = Concentration (poor)
  A = Activity (psychomotor retardation or agitation)
  G = Guilt (thoughts of worthlessness or guilt)
  E = Energy (fatigue)
  S = Suicidal ideation

Treatment

- If the patient is a danger to self (high suicide risk) or others or is gravely disabled, admit or transfer to a facility with inpatient psychiatry.
- If the patient is not suicidal, outpatient follow-up may be considered, as long as there is strong social and family support. Antidepressant medications are generally prescribed by the psychiatrist.

Bipolar Disorder

Clinical Presentation

- Bipolar disorder is characterized by cycles of profound depression that alternate with periods of an excessively elevated or irritable mood, known as mania. Manic symptoms can be characterized by the mnemonic DIG FAST.
  D = Distractible
  I = Impulsive
  G = Grandiose ideas (inflated self-esteem)
  F = Flight of ideas, racing thought
  A = Activity increased
  S = Sleep less
  T = Talkative, pressured speech
- Note that bipolar disorder is associated with comorbidities (anxiety, substance abuse) as well as an increased risk of suicide.

Diagnosis and Evaluation

- The diagnosis is made clinically, after exclusion of other medical conditions.
- Bipolar disorder type I is classically characterized by the pattern of alternating severe depression with episodes of mania.
- Bipolar disorder type II is diagnosed when episodes of severe depression are separated by periods of hypomania, a less severe form of mania that usually does not lead to gross impairment of function or psychosis.
- Differential diagnosis includes thyroid disorders, substance abuse, neurologic tumors and epilepsy (i.e., temporal lobe), metabolic disorders, attention-deficit/hyperactivity disorder, cyclothymic disorders, and psychotic disorders.
- In children, rapid cycling (mood swings) can occur and complicate diagnosis.

Treatment

- Admit or transfer to inpatient psychiatry if there is a concern for danger to self, danger to others, or grave disability.
- In consultation with a psychiatrist, consider administering medications, including mood stabilizers (i.e., lithium), anticonvulsants (i.e., valproate), or antipsychotics (i.e., quetiapine).

General Principles of Anxiety Disorders

- Characterized by an excessive worry or fear that affects a person's daily activities (work, school) and relationships.
- Diagnosis remains clinical; anxiety disorders are frequently associated with various medical illnesses. It is therefore imperative to rule out potential organic precipitants and etiologies.
- See Chapter 103 for details on generalized anxiety disorder, panic disorder, and phobic disorder.

Obsessive-Compulsive Disorder

- Characterized by repetitive **obsessions** (intrusive and repetitive thoughts or images that cannot be eliminated, often causing anxiety or grief) and **compulsions** (behaviors or rituals that temporarily relieve this anxiety).
- Group A hemolytic streptococcal infection may be associated with OCD in children (i.e., pediatric autoimmune neuropsychiatric disorder associated with streptococcal infection [also known as PANDAS]).
- Differential diagnosis includes delusional disorder, schizophrenia, and GAD. Treatment includes CBT (exposure-response therapy) and SSRIs (higher doses than typically used for depression).

Posttraumatic Stress Disorder

- Due to repetitive and intrusive memories of a traumatizing event, most commonly an act of physical or sexual violence, a war, or a death of a loved one
- PTSD results in increased arousal, hypervigilance, avoidance behaviors, and depressed and/or anxious mood for at least 1 month.
- Patients typically have no history of panic attacks.
- Differential diagnosis includes depression, GAD, and adjustment disorder.

- Treatment is multifaceted and can include CBT, psychotherapy (eye movement desensitization and reprocessing), individual or group therapy, SSRIs, and long-acting benzodiazepines.

General Principles of Factitious Disorders

- Patients with factitious disorder deliberately fabricate symptoms to assume a sick role or achieve secondary gain.
- Differential diagnosis includes organic pathologies based on the fabricated symptoms and a balance will have to be achieved between a sufficient and exhaustive workup.
- For more information about factitious disorder imposed on self (formerly Munchausen syndrome) and factitious disorder imposed on another (formerly Munchausen syndrome by proxy) please see Chapter 103

Eating Disorders and Personality Disorders

RACHEL SHING, MD, and JAMES J. MURPHY JR., MD, MPH

Eating Disorders

- Characterized by a persistent disturbance of eating that significantly impairs physical health or psychosocial functioning.
- Includes anorexia nervosa, bulimia nervosa, avoidant/restrictive food intake disorder, pica, binge eating disorder, and rumination disorder. The relevant criteria from *The Diagnostic and Statistical Manual of Mental Disorders*, fifth edition (DSM-5), are outlined in Tables 99.1 and 99.2.

ANOREXIA NERVOSA

Clinical Presentation

- The patient often appears emaciated and can present with significant hypotension, hypothermia, and bradycardia.
- Indicators of physiologic dysfunction include amenorrhea, cold intolerance, lanugo (a fine, downy body hair), or skin yellowing associated with hypercarotenemia.
- The patient typically refuses to maintain a body weight over the minimum normal for age and height (i.e., body mass index [BMI] <17.5); they misperceive body weight,

TABLE 99.1 Diagnostic and Statistical Manual of Mental Disorders, *Fifth Edition, Criteria for Eating Disorders*

Anorexia Nervosa	Bulimia Nervosa	Binge Eating Disorder
Restriction of caloric intake relative to requirements, leading to a lower than expected body weight in the context of age, sex, development, and physical health (<85% predicted)	Recurrent episodes of binge eating characterized by both: • Eating in a discrete time period an amount of food that is larger than most people would eat in the same period under the same circumstance • A feeling of lack of control over eating during an episode	Recurrent episodes of binge eating characterized by both: • Eating in a discrete time period an amount of food that is larger than most people would eat in the same period of time under the same circumstance • A feeling of lack of control over eating during an episode
Fear of weight gain or becoming fat, despite lower than predicted body weight	Recurrent, inappropriate compensatory behaviors to prevent weight gain, including self-induced emesis; abuse of laxatives, diuretics, or other medications; caloric restriction; or excessive exercise	The episodes are associated with three of the following: • Eating much more quickly than normal • Eating until feeling uncomfortably full or overfull • Eating large amounts of food even when not feeling hungry • Eating alone because of embarrassment about how much one is eating • Feeling disgusted, depressed, or guilty afterward
Derangement in the way the patient's body weight or appearance is experienced, undue effects of body weight on self-evaluation, or denial of the dangerousness of the current low body weight.	Bingeing and purging at least one time a week for 3 weeks	The patient exhibits marked distress regarding binge eating
The minimum level of severity is based, for adults, on current BMI (see below) or, for children and adolescents, on BMI percentile. Mild: BMI ≥17 kg/m^2 Moderate: BMI 16–16.99 kg/m^2 Severe: BMI 15–15.99 kg/m^2 Extreme: BMI <15 kg/m^2	Self-evaluation is unduly influenced by body weight and appearance	The binge eating occurs at least one time a week for 3 months
	The disturbance does not occur exclusively during episodes of anorexia	The binge eating is not associated with inappropriate compensatory behavior and does not occur exclusively during the course of anorexia, bulimia, or avoidant/restrictive food intake disorder

BMI, body mass index.
From Bornick, G.L. (2020). Eating disorders. In J. E. Tintinalli, O. J. Ma, D. M. Yealy, G. D. Meckler, J. S. Stapczynski, D. M. Cline, & S. H. Thomas (Eds.), *Tintinalli's emergency medicine: A comprehensive study guide* (9th ed.). McGraw-Hill Education.

TABLE 99.2 Diagnostic and Statistical Manual of Mental Disorders, *Fifth Edition, Criteria for Eating Disorders*

Avoidant/Restrictive Food Intake Disorder	Pica	Rumination Disorder
An eating or feeding disturbance (e.g., apparent lack of interest in eating or food avoidance based on the sensory characteristics of food, concern about aversive consequences of eating) as manifested by persistent failure to meet appropriate nutritional and/or energy needs associated with one (or more) of the following: • Significant weight loss • Significant nutritional deficiency • Dependent on enteral feeding or oral nutritional supplements • Marked interference with psychosocial functioning	Eating of one or more nonnutritive, nonfood substances on a persistent basis over a period of at least 1 month severe enough to warrant clinical attention	Repeated regurgitation of food over a period of at least 1 month Regurgitated food may be rechewed, reswallowed, or spit out
Disturbance is not better explained by lack of available food or by an associated culturally sanctioned practice	Developmentally inappropriate	Regurgitation is not attributable to an associated gastrointestinal or other medical condition (e.g., gastroesophageal reflux, pyloric stenosis)
Does not occur exclusively during the course of anorexia nervosa or bulimia nervosa, and there is no evidence of a disturbance in how one's body weight or shape is experienced	Not part of a culturally supported or socially normative practice	Does not occur exclusively during the course of anorexia nervosa, bulimia nervosa, binge eating disorder, or avoidant/restrictive food intake disorder

shape, and/or size and there is a fear of becoming obese even when severely underweight.

Diagnosis

- According to DSM-5, the diagnosis of anorexia nervosa requires each of the following:
  - Persistent energy intake restriction that leads to a low body weight (BMI <18.5)
  - Intense fear of gaining weight, becoming fat, or persistent behavior that interferes with weight gain
  - Disturbance in self-perceived weight or shape

BULIMIA NERVOSA

Clinical Presentation

- Both anorexia and bulimia are characterized by an obsession with body shape and weight.
- What distinguishes bulimia from anorexia is that bulimic patients are often of normal weight or overweight.
- Common symptoms include syncope, generalized weakness, bloating, edema, persistent nausea, chest pain, hematemesis, palpitations, dysmenorrhea, and stress fractures.
- Clinical signs may include painless swelling of the parotid and submandibular glands, poor dentition, and thickened skin on the back of the knuckles (Russell sign).

Diagnosis

- The DSM-5 criteria for bulimia nervosa include:
  - Recurrent episodes of binge eating
  - Purging behaviors (e.g., vomiting, laxative/diuretic abuse, excessive exercising) to lose weight
  - Excessive concern regarding body shape and weight
  - Binge eating and purging occurring at least once a week for 3 months
  - The binge eating and compensatory behaviors do not occur exclusively during episodes of anorexia nervosa.

Clinical Presentation and Diagnosis in Other Common Eating Disorders

Avoidant/Restrictive Food Intake Disorder

- Characterized by an avoidance or restriction of food intake, leading to failure to meet nutritional and energy needs.
- Restricts food intake because of a lack of interest in food, an aversion to the sensory characteristics of food (i.e., texture, smell), or a conditioned negative response associated with eating (i.e., choking).
- Patients are typically underweight and children may have growth delay or malnutrition.

Pica

- Patients with pica often consume nonnutritive or nonfood substances, or substances that may be inappropriate to the patient's developmental level, not culturally supported, or not socially normal.
- May be a clinical manifestation of iron deficiency anemia.
- Often diagnosed from a medical complication, such as a bezoar causing intestinal obstruction or perforation, or a hazardous ingestion (i.e., lead-based paints, needles, etc.).

Binge Eating Disorder

- Binge eating disorder is typified by recurrent episodes of eating more than what most would consider normal within a discrete period of time (e.g., ≤2 hours), accompanied by at least three of the following: eating more rapidly than normal, eating when not physically hungry and until uncomfortably full, eating alone because of embarrassment by how much one is eating, and/or feeling guilty afterwards.

Rumination Disorder

- Patients with rumination disorder have repeated regurgitation of food (that may be rechewed, reswallowed, or spit up) over the course of 1 month that is not due to an underlying medical condition (i.e., gastroesophageal reflux disease, pyloric stenosis) and that does not occur with another eating disorder. This process can be hazardous to growth and cause malnutrition.

Other Specified or Unspecified Feeding or Eating Disorder

- This category applies to people who have a pattern of disordered eating that causes clinically significant distress or psychosocial impairment, but do not meet full criteria for a specific eating disorder. Some examples include bulimia nervosa or binge eating disorder of low frequency, atypical anorexia nervosa, purging disorder, or night eating syndrome.

General Principles for Diagnosis and Evaluation of Eating Disorders

- Patients should be evaluated for medical complications related to starvation or persistent purging, especially metabolic or cardiac abnormalities.
- Persistent purging can lead to many medical complications, such as dehydration, hypokalemia and other electrolyte derangements, Mallory-Weiss syndrome, ipecac-induced myopathy occurring in both cardiac and skeletal muscle, diabetes, and dental enamel erosion.
- Laboratory evaluation can include a full chemistry panel including: magnesium, calcium, and phosphorus, complete blood count, urinalysis, pregnancy test, hepatic function panel, serum albumin, lipase and amylase, and thyroid-stimulating hormone. Tests should be guided by the symptoms and physical examination findings.
- One meta-analysis reviewing mortality rates for patients with eating disorders found that 1 in 5 people with anorexia who had died had committed suicide.
- It is prudent to screen patients with a suspected eating disorder for coexisting depression, anxiety, substance abuse, self-injurious behavior, or suicidality.

General Principles for Treatment of Eating Disorders

- Focused on stabilization of medical complications, then hospital admission or outpatient referral.
- Characterized by one or more of the features as listed in Box 99.1, medically unstable patients should be hospitalized. There are no evidence-based criteria to indicate which patients with anorexia or bulimia nervosa need initial hospitalization, although the American Psychiatric Association and Society for Adolescent Medicine do have guidelines for hospitalization (Table 99.3).
- Long-term treatment of eating disorders involves a multidisciplinary approach that includes nutritional rehabilitation, psychotherapy, and pharmacotherapy, with involvement of a mental health clinician, dietician, and general medical clinician.
- Refeeding syndrome, a result of electrolyte and fluid shifts, is a potentially fatal complication of nutritional rehabilitation and patients at risk for this syndrome must be closely monitored.
- Cognitive behavior therapy is the psychotherapy of choice for bulimia nervosa and binge eating disorder. Pharmacotherapy alone can be reasonable for both if nutritional rehabilitation and psychotherapy are not available, with selective serotonin reuptake inhibitors (e.g., fluoxetine) used as first-line treatment.
- Pharmacotherapy is not an initial or primary treatment for anorexia nervosa and is used only for patients who do not respond to standard treatment.

BOX 99.1 *Features of Medical Instability in Eating Disorders*

Blood pressure <80/60 mm Hg or symptoms of lightheadedness
Cardiac dysrhythmia (e.g., QTc >0.499 ms), or any rhythm other than normal sinus rhythm or sinus bradycardia
Marked dehydration
Moderate to severe refeeding syndrome characterized by serum phosphorous <2 and marked edema
Serious medical complication of malnutrition (e.g., syncope, seizures, cardiac failure, liver failure, pancreatitis, hypoglycemia, or marked electrolyte disturbance)

Personality Disorders

General Principles

- An enduring, inflexible pattern of inner experience and behavior that markedly deviates from cultural expectations.
- Onset is often during adolescence or young adulthood and is pervasive over time, leading to distress or impairment due to poor interpersonal functioning.
- It is not uncommon for a clinician to feel threatened or angry, or to find it difficult to connect with a patient with a personality disorder, and awareness of this response may be useful in recognizing and managing these patients.
- There are three clusters of personality disorders:
  - Cluster A: "paranoid, odd, eccentric"
  - Cluster B: "dramatic, emotional, and erratic"
  - Cluster C: "anxious, fearful"

Clinical Presentation of Personality Disorders

Cluster A: Paranoid, Schizoid, Schizotypal

Paranoid Personality Disorder

- Often mistrustful and suspicious of others and frequently assume that others will exploit, harm, or deceive them

Schizoid Personality Disorder

- Often appear socially isolated or are "loners"
- Have an extremely restricted emotional range, accompanied by little desire for interpersonal relationships, including with family

Schizotypal Personality Disorder

- Often have discomfort and a reduced capacity for close relationships, which results in inappropriate, stiff, or constricted interpersonal interactions
- May also have unusual mannerisms or speech, magical thinking, and an eccentric or odd appearance

Cluster B: Borderline, Narcissistic, Histrionic, Antisocial

Borderline Personality Disorder

- Marked by unstable interpersonal relationships and self-image, emotional lability, and marked impulsivity, resulting in self-destructive behaviors

Narcissistic Personality Disorder

- Prone to a sense of grandiosity, entitlement, need for admiration, and limited ability to empathize with others

TABLE 99.3 American Psychiatric Association Criteria for Hospital Admission

Medical status	Adults: heart rate <40 beats/min, blood pressure <90/60 mm Hg, serum glucose <60 mg/dL (<3.3 mmol/L), potassium <3 mEq/L, temperature <36.1°C, end-organ compromise requiring acute treatment, poorly controlled diabetes Children: heart rate near 40 beats/min, orthostasis, blood pressure <80/50 mm Hg, hypokalemia, hypophosphatemia, hypomagnesemia
Suicidality	Specific plan with high lethality or intent
Weight	Generally <85% of ideal body weight or acute weight change with food refusal
Motivation to recover	Very poor motivation; patient preoccupied with intrusive repetitive thoughts and/or uncooperative with treatment
Comorbid disorders	Any existing psychiatric disorder requiring hospitalization
Structure required	Needs supervision to ensure caloric intake, prevention of exercise, or prevention of purging behavior
Environmental	Severe family conflict or absence of family, absence of appropriate outpatient resources in patient's geographic region

From Bornick, G.L. (2020). Eating disorders. In J. E. Tintinalli, O. J. Ma, D. M. Yealy, G. D. Meckler, J. S. Stapczynski, D. M. Cline, & S. H. Thomas (Eds.), *Tintinalli's emergency medicine: A comprehensive study guide* (9th ed.). McGraw-Hill Education.

Histrionic Personality Disorder

- Have rapidly shifting, shallow emotions with a proclivity for being the center of attention and overestimation of the intimacy of relationships

Antisocial Personality Disorder

- Demonstrate a disregard for and violate the rights of others. Diagnosis requires individual to be at least 18 years old.
- If under 18 years old, the behavior is considered *conduct disorder*.

Cluster C: Avoidant, Dependent, Obsessive-Compulsive

Avoidant Personality Disorder

- Socially inhibited, these individuals are hypersensitive to criticism and rejection and fear being shamed, ridiculed, or disliked in a relationship

Dependent Personality Disorder

- Characterized by having an overwhelming need to be taken care of, coupled with a fear of being alone, that manifests as submissive, clinging, and indecisive behavior

Obsessive-Compulsive Personality Disorder

- Possess a preoccupation with orderliness, perfectionism, and mental and interpersonal control, at the expense of flexibility, openness, and efficiency

General Principles of Diagnosis and Evaluation of Personality Disorders

- Diagnosis of personality disorders requires an evaluation of the person's long-term patterns of functioning.
- Patients should not be diagnosed with a personality disorder from a single interview; the emergency department environment is inadequate for such diagnoses.

General Principles of Approach and Treatment of Personality Disorders

- Patients can be inherently challenging to evaluate and treat.
- On the basis of the history and physical examination, pursue focused laboratory evaluation and testing for organic pathologic conditions.
- Screen for conditions requiring acute psychiatric stabilization (psychosis, major depression with suicidal ideation) and employ strategies to facilitate patient interaction. A nuanced approach for certain clusters of personality traits is listed below:
  - Cluster A: Approach with genuine curiosity; ask for clarification on any odd terms used.
  - Cluster B: Set firm boundaries early and maintain a direct and professional affect.
  - Cluster C: Maintain direct, empathetic, and relaxed affect toward the patient.

SUGGESTED READINGS

American Psychiatric Association. (2013). Feeding and eating disorders. In *Diagnostic and statistical manual of mental disorders* (5th ed.). American Psychiatric Association.

Bornick, G. L. (2020). Eating disorders. In Tintinalli, J. E., Ma, O. J., Yealy, D. M., Meckler, G. D., Stapczynski, J. S., Cline, D. M., & Thomas, S. H. (Eds.). *Tintinalli's emergency medicine: A comprehensive study guide* (9th ed.). McGraw-Hill Education.

Moukaddam, N., AufderHeide, E., Flores, A., & Tucci, V. (2015). Shift, interrupted: Strategies for managing difficult patients including those with personality disorders and somatic symptoms in the emergency department. *Emergency Medicine Clinics of North America, 33*(4), 787–810. doi:10.1016/j.emc.2015.07.007. Accessed April 2, 2019

Yager, J. (2019). Eating disorders: Overview of prevention and treatment. *UpToDate*. https://www.uptodate.com/contents/eating-disorders-overview-of-prevention-and-treatment. Accessed December 27, 2019

CHAPTER 100

BOARD REVIEW

Violence, Abuse, and Neglect

THERESA H. CHENG, MD, JD, and CAROLYN JOY SACHS, MD, MPH

In the United States, more than 3000 children, women, and elders die yearly from abuse. Additionally, there are 3 million children investigated as potential victims of child abuse, 2–5 million cases of elder abuse, and 2–4 million cases of intimate partner violence (IPV) each year. Emergency physicians are in a unique position to identify abusive situations before they result in permanent physical disability, psychologic disability, or death. Because of the relative isolation of many victims, an emergency department (ED) encounter may be the only opportunity for abuse detection and intervention.

Intimate Partner Violence

General Principles

- Defined as a pattern of assaults on or coercive behavior toward one intimate partner by the other including, but not limited to, physical, sexual, and psychological abuse.
- IPV is repetitive, and victims, most often female, typically suffer six episodes per year.
- One out of three women in the United States will be physically or sexually assaulted by a partner.
- IPV injuries are "criminal acts" in every state and included under many state assault reporting laws.

Clinical Presentation

- Recognition of victimized individuals requires a high degree of suspicion.
- Victims may not disclose the true mechanism of injury.
- The following historical factors may suggest IPV:
  - Frequent physician visits for trauma
  - Delays in seeking medical treatment after an injury
  - Overprotective partner
  - Injuries during pregnancy
  - History of depression or suicide attempts
  - History of prior abuse or abuse in the family

Diagnosis and Evaluation

- ED providers should incorporate IPV screening questions into routine clinical assessment because most cases require investigation on the physician's part, and victims rarely disclose abuse without prompting.
- Patients should be alone when broaching the topic of abuse.
- Clinicians can help patients feel more comfortable disclosing abuse by framing questions in ways that let patients know that they are not alone, that the provider takes this issue seriously, that the provider is comfortable hearing about abuse, and that help is available (Box 100.1).

BOX 100.1 *Suggested Framing Questions/Statements*

"Because violence is common in patients' lives, I now ask every patient I see in the emergency department about violence."

"I don't know if this is a problem for you, but many patients are dealing with abusive relationships. Some are too afraid or uncomfortable to bring it up themselves, so I've started asking about it routinely."

Treatment

- After addressing the trauma or chief complaint that brought the victim to the ED, brief supportive counseling by physicians may result in a dramatic catharsis for a victim who until then has been suffering in silence.

Child Abuse

General Principles

- When a parent or caregiver causes injury, death, emotional harm, or risk of serious harm to a child either through action or failing to act

Clinical Presentation

- Children presenting with injuries that seem incompatible with the given history, a mechanism incompatible with the child's developmental milestones or with injuries that have no logical explanation should raise a red flag for abuse.
- Any child who presents with a change in mental status or seizures must raise concern for intracranial injury from abuse. Other red flag symptoms or physical examination findings are listed in Box 100.2.

Diagnosis and Evaluation

- ED staff must maintain a high index of suspicion to identify children who are abused.
- To encourage disclosure, examiners must obtain the history in a nonaccusatory manner.
- If the child is verbal, a separate history should be obtained from the child and the caretaker when each is alone.
- In cases of suspected child abuse, emergency physicians must evaluate for injuries from prior episodes of abuse, such as a skeletal survey to detect old or healing fractures.

Treatment

- Mandatory reporting of suspected child abuse, and emergency physicians should know the statutes in the jurisdictions in which they practice.

BOX 100.2 Physical Indicators of Abuse

Any unexplained change in mental status should raise concern for occult head injury and "shaken baby syndrome"
Any bruises in infants <6 months of age or more than one bruise in a premobile infant; bruises in unusual locations, like ears
Retinal hemorrhages (the most common manifestation of abusive head trauma in infants)
Symmetric extremity injuries
Multiple injuries at different stages of healing
Scapular, multiple skull, vertebral body, spinous process, metaphyseal (bucket-handle), posterior rib or sternal fractures
Circumferential immersion, patterned, buttock, or cigarette burns
Adult human bite marks
Blunt instrument marks (belts, bats, rods)

- Emergency physicians should know where to locate these protocols and how to utilize them.
- Hospitalization may be indicated for injuries, and to allow time for child protective services to investigate the source of the injury and determine whether or not the child is safe at home. Safety of these children must also be considered.

Elder Abuse/Neglect

General Principles

- Defined as the refusal or failure of a caregiver to fulfill his or her obligations or duties to an elderly person, including, but not limited to, providing food, clothing, medicine, shelter, supervision, medical care, and services deemed essential for the well-being of another.
- Risk factors include female gender, cognitive impairment, social isolation, and increased dependency (disability in self-care).
- Most reported cases of elder abuse involve neglect, which may present with medical problems resulting from poor nutrition, poor hygiene, or lack of needed medications and care.
- 1 in 10 older Americans have experienced some form of elder abuse, but only about 1 in 14 cases of abuse are reported to authorities.
- Currently, all 50 states mandate that providers report child abuse to state authorities, and 47 states require that elder abuse be reported to state or local law enforcement.

Clinical Presentation

- Clinical presentations include injuries, pressure ulcers, falls, malnutrition, dehydration, and functional decline. All of these may be a sign of caregiver abuse or neglect.
- Injuries without a logical explanation should raise suspicion for abuse.

Diagnosis and Evaluation

- It is incumbent upon the emergency provider to gather this information from history and clinical examination to intervene on a potentially dangerous situation.
- To avoid intimidation by possible abusers, the patient should be interviewed by themselves.
- If abuse or neglect is suspected, a comprehensive evaluation as in all medically ill patients, including serum chemistries, urinalysis, and radiographs, should be obtained.
- The physician should carefully document the findings of mistreatment or self-neglect and reasons for declaring the patient incapable of acting in his or her own best interest, if applicable.

Treatment

- If the patient no longer has the capacity to make reasonable decisions for him- or herself, contact law enforcement or adult protective services (APS).
- Documentation of violence or neglect in the medical chart may be the only written evidence of abuse, and thus may play a crucial role in aiding the patient.

Other General Treatment Principles for Violence, Abuse, and Neglect

Evidence Collection and Documentation

- Victims of family violence who are also recent victims of sexual assault must be offered an evidentiary examination and the standard physical evidence collection per state protocol and federal Violence Against Women Act of 1994 funding legislation.
- Documentation of violence or neglect in the medical chart may be the only written evidence of abuse, and thus may play a crucial role in aiding the patient.

Referral

- After identifying abuse, referral is perhaps the physician's most crucial intervention for dealing with victims of family violence.
- Identification, documentation, and treatment of injuries mean little unless a victim or caretaker is given the resources needed to change the situation.
- Emergency physicians typically have neither the time nor the expertise to comprehensively counsel a victim or caretaker.
- Referral services are critical.

Child and elder abuse hotlines are available in all locations but vary by jurisdiction.

There are national hotlines for all three forms of abuse:

- Elder abuse and maltreatment: ElderCare Locator 1-800-677-1116
- Child abuse and maltreatment: Childhelp National Child Abuse Hotline 1-800-4-A-CHILD (1-800-422-4453)
- IPV and abuse: National Domestic Violence Hotline 1-800-799-SAFE (1-800-799-7233)

SUGGESTED READINGS

Anglin, D., & Sachs, C. (2003). Preventive care in the emergency department: Screening for domestic violence in the emergency department. *Academic Emergency Medicine*, *10*, 1118–1127.
Halphen, J. M., Varas, G. M., & Sadowsky, J. M. (2009). Recognizing and reporting elder abuse and neglect. *Geriatrics*, *64*(7), 13–18.
Keshavarz, R., Kawashima, R., & Low, C. (2002). Child abuse and neglect presentations to a pediatric emergency department. *The Journal of Emergency Medicine*, *23*(4), 341–345.

CHAPTER **101**

BOARD REVIEW

Side Effects of Selected Psychiatric Medications

BRITTANY GUEST, DO, and STEVEN LAI, MD

- Many psychiatric patients take multiple medications to control both their psychiatric illness and medical comorbidities.
- These various medications can have many adverse side effects, as well as potentially life-threatening drug interactions, that emergency physicians (EPs) must know how to quickly recognize and treat.

Extrapyramidal Side Effects

Clinical Presentation

- Extrapyramidal side effects (EPSs) due to blockade of dopamine (D_2) receptors in the basal ganglia by the antipsychotic medication occur more frequently with first-generation antipsychotics (i.e., haloperidol) and are less common with use of second-generation (i.e., quetiapine, olanzapine) antipsychotics.
- Risk factors include a family history, history of cocaine or alcohol use, or treatment with a potent dopamine D_2 receptor antagonist (i.e., fluphenazine, haloperidol).
- Clinical manifestations of EPSs are outlined in Table 101.1.
- EPS often occurs shortly after initiation of drug treatment or an increase in drug dose, with 50% occurring within 48 hours of initiation of treatment and 90% within 5 days.
- Patients can have acute dystonic reactions resulting in involuntary spasms of the face, neck, back and extremities, typically within the first several days of treatment with an antipsychotic medication.
- Tardive dyskinesia (TD), a delayed EPS characterized by involuntary hyperkinetic movements, most often in the face, can be irreversible and have a significant negative impact on quality of life.
- The diagnosis of TD can be difficult, because symptoms often first appear after a reduction in dose or after discontinuation of the antipsychotic (unmasking).

Diagnosis

- Rapid resolution of symptoms after treatment often confirms the diagnosis.
- Failure to improve should prompt consideration of alternative diagnoses. As mentioned earlier, TD differs from the other EPSs in that the signs may be irreversible, despite discontinuation of the offending medication.
- The diagnosis of TD can be difficult, because symptoms often first appear after a reduction in dose or after discontinuation of the antipsychotic (unmasking).

Treatment

- For EPS, stop or decrease the dose of the offending agent.
- Acute EPS may be treated with diphenhydramine and anticholinergic agents.
- Benztropine can be used to prevent recurrence.
- Securing the airway is rarely necessary; however, laryngeal and pharyngeal dystonic reactions may place the patient at risk of imminent respiratory arrest and the airway should be controlled.
- If the patient is taking a typical antipsychotic medication, substitution with an atypical antipsychotic medication may prevent recurrence.
- As mentioned above, TD may be irreversible, despite discontinuation of the offending medication.
- Antipsychotic medications can also cause significant QT prolongation and the risk of QT prolongation increases when the drug is given intravenously (IV); therefore, these medications should be given intramuscularly if

TABLE 101.1 *Extrapyramidal Side Effects*

Reaction	Onset	Symptoms
Acute dystonia	Hours to days	Facial grimacing; muscle spasm of tongue, face, and neck; **reversible**
Akathisia	Hours to days	Restless, constant movement; pacing; agitation; **reversible**
Oculogyric crisis	Hours to days	Fixed deviation of the eyes in one direction or continuous rotatory eye movements, **reversible**
Laryngeal dystonia	Hours to days	Potentially life- threatening; rare throat-tightening sensation resulting in difficulty breathing and swallowing; **reversible**
Pseudoparkinsonism	Weeks to months	Shuffling gait, pill-rolling tremor, stooped posture; **reversible**
Tardive dyskinesia	Months to years	Lip smacking, tongue protrusion, involuntary body movements; **potentially irreversible**

possible and the patient should ideally be placed on a cardiac monitor, with IV administration.

Neuroleptic Malignant Syndrome

Clinical Presentation

- Neuroleptic malignant syndrome (NMS) is a rare, life-threatening idiosyncratic reaction to neuroleptic medications and is associated with antipsychotic medications (first generation > second generation) and antiemetics (metoclopramide, promethazine).
- Exact etiology is unknown, but it is likely related to central nervous system (CNS) dopamine receptor blockade by antipsychotic medications.
- Onset of symptoms can be progressive over days to weeks, but can also occur years into therapy. Once the syndrome starts, it usually evolves over 24–72 hours.
- NMS presents with severe muscle rigidity ("lead pipe" rigidity) and hyperthermia, plus at least two other clinical features, such as leukocytosis, rhabdomyolysis, altered mental status, or autonomic instability.
- End-organ effects can include rhabdomyolysis, renal failure, seizures, dysrhythmias, and death.

Diagnosis

- Diagnosis is primarily clinical based on the history and physical examination and requires exclusion of other drug-induced, systemic, or neuropsychiatric illnesses.
- No laboratory test is diagnostic for NMS.
- Laboratory studies can assess severity and complications, e.g., rhabdomyolysis, acute renal injury, increased liver transaminases, leukocytosis, thrombocytosis, and metabolic acidosis.
- The differential diagnoses often include CNS infections, status epilepticus, strokes, cerebral neoplasms, NMS, malignant hypertension, serotonin syndrome, withdrawal syndromes, thyroid storm, sepsis, and heat stroke. Table 101.2 compares the signs and symptoms of NMS versus serotonin syndrome.

TABLE 101.2 *Neuroleptic Malignant Syndrome Versus Serotonin Syndrome*

	Neuroleptic Malignant Syndrome	Serotonin Syndrome
Cause	Dopamine blockade	Increased serotonin activity
Course	Prolonged	Resolves rapidly
Onset	Gradual (days to weeks)	Abrupt (hours)
Vital signs	Fever, ↑ HR, ↑ RR	Fever, ↑ HR, ↑ RR
Muscle tone	"Lead pipe" rigidity	Increased
Reflexes	Decreased	Increased, clonus
Pupils	Normal	Mydriasis

HR, heart rate; *RR*, respiration rate.

- A lumbar puncture may be indicated to rule out meningitis as a cause of fever and altered mental status.

Treatment

- Mainly supportive, with a goal of controlling the rigidity and hyperthermia to prevent complications, such as respiratory and renal failure
- Discontinue all antipsychotics and start cooling measures. Evaporative cooling, ice packs, and cooled IV fluids can be used to reduce hyperthermia.
- Intubation may be indicated because patients can have dysphagia, excessive salivation, depressed mental status, and hypoxemia.
- If patient is profoundly dehydrated from insensible fluid losses, fluid resuscitation can be beneficial.
- Benzodiazepines, amantadine, dantrolene, and bromocriptine may be used, but their value is controversial.

Serotonin Syndrome

Clinical Presentation

- Onset of symptoms tends to be rapid, within 24 hours.
- Myoclonus (most common finding), muscle rigidity (lower extremities > upper extremities), agitation, confusion, hyperthermia, tachycardia, tachypnea, hyperactive bowel sounds, and dilated pupils (Table 101.2 compares NMS to serotonin syndrome)
- Includes autonomic hyperactivity, hemodynamic changes, neuromuscular derangements, and changes in mental status
- Results from increased serotonin activity in the CNS owing to overdose or combination of serotonergic medications (i.e., selective serotonin reuptake inhibitors, tricyclic antidepressants, bupropion, triptans, 3,4-methylenedioxymethamphetamine, tramadol) and the initiation of monoamine oxidase inhibitors ([MAOIs], discussed next)

Diagnosis

- Primarily clinical
- The Hunter serotonin toxicity criteria requires one of the following features: spontaneous clonus, inducible clonus or ocular clonus with agitation or diaphoresis, tremor and hyperreflexia, or a combination of hypertonia, hyperthermia, and ocular or inducible clonus.
- Differential diagnoses are similar to NMS and further workup to rule out alternative causes is prudent.

Treatment

- Mainstay of treatment is the removal of the offending agent, cooling measures, and supportive care.
- Benzodiazepines may be used to control muscle rigidity, agitation, and tremor. IV fluids may be useful to prevent rhabdomyolysis.
- Cyproheptadine, a serotonin 2A antagonist, may also be useful, although it is only available orally.
- Up to 25% of patients require intubation and ventilatory support.

Monoamine Oxidase Inhibitor Toxicity

Clinical Presentation

- Monoamine oxidase (MAO) is an enzyme that inactivates epinephrine, norepinephrine, dopamine, and serotonin. Inhibition of MAO increases the presynaptic concentrations of these neurotransmitters and can be used in the treatment of atypical (increased appetite, sleeping too much) or refractory depression. Examples of MAO inhibitors (MAOIs) are phenelzine and tranylcypromine (antidepressants), selegiline (antiparkinsonian), and procarbazine (antineoplastic). MAOIs are considered second-line agents for depression because of their adverse side effects, which include serotonin syndrome and hypertensive crisis.
- In MAOI overdose, patients can present with agitation, mydriasis, hyperthermia, diaphoresis, hyperreflexia, and tachycardia (hyperadrenergic state).
- Seizures, hypotension, and bradycardia can occur in severe overdoses. These symptoms can be delayed up to 24 hours after the overdose.
- Differential diagnosis can include sympathomimetic intoxication, alcohol or sedative withdrawal, strokes, CNS infections, serotonin syndrome, NMS, malignant hyperthermia, thyroid storm, acute coronary syndrome, and pheochromocytoma.
- Patients taking MAOIs can also present with a tyramine reaction, because MAO typically decreases the availability of absorbed dietary amines (i.e., tyramine) in the body. This occurs in patients on MAOIs who ingest tyramine-containing foods (e.g., aged cheese, beer, wine, pickled fish, cured meats).
  - Onset of symptoms is often rapid, occurring 15–90 minutes after ingestion.
  - Symptoms can include severe occipital or temporal headaches, severe hypertension (hypertensive crisis), diaphoresis, mydriasis, neck stiffness, chest pain, and neuromuscular excitation.
  - May increase risk for myocardial infarctions and intracerebral hemorrhage
  - Differential diagnosis is similar for MAOI overdose.

Diagnosis and Treatment

- Diagnosis of both MAOI overdose and tyramine reaction is clinical, based on the history and physical examination.
- Treatment is largely supportive, with a focus on controlling marked hypertension.
  - In acute overdose, activated charcoal or gastric lavage may be helpful if there are no contraindications.
  - For severe hypertension, phentolamine or nitroprusside can be used; β-blockers can result in unopposed α-receptor stimulation, so they are contraindicated.
  - Benzodiazepines can be used for agitation, IV fluids for rhabdomyolysis, and dantrolene for life-threatening hyperthermia.
  - Ventricular arrhythmias may be treated with lidocaine or procainamide.

101

SUGGESTED READINGS

Boyer, E. W., & Shannon, M. (2005). The serotonin syndrome. *The New England Journal of Medicine*, 352, 1112.

Gottlieb, M., Long, B., & Koyfman, A. (2018). Approach to the agitated emergency department patient. *The Journal of Emergency Medicine*, 54(4), 447–457.

Kim, H. K., Leonard, J. B., Corwell, B. N., & Connors, N. J. (2021). Safety and efficacy of pharmacologic agents used for rapid tranquilization of emergency department patients with acute agitation or excited delirium. *Expert Opinion on Drug Safety*, 20(2), 123–138.

Klein, L. R., Driver, B. E., Miner, J. R., Martel, M. L., Hessel, M., Collins, J. D., Horton, G. B., Fagerstrom, E., Satpathy, R., & Cole, J. B. (2018). Intramuscular midazolam, olanzapine, ziprasidone, or haloperidol for treating acute agitation in the emergency department. *Annals of Emergency Medicine*, 72(4), 374–385.

Yap, C. Y. L., Taylor, D. M., Kong, D. C. M., Knott, J. C., & Taylor, S. E. (2019). Risk factors for sedation-related events during acute agitation management in the emergency department. *Academic Emergency Medicine*, 26(10), 1135–1143.

CHAPTER 102

BOARD REVIEW

Agitated Delirium, Delirium Versus Dementia

CATHERINE WEAVER, MD, and HANNAH WALLACE, MD, MPH

- Altered mental status (AMS) and behavioral changes account for an estimated 10%–20% of emergency department (ED) visits.
  - Significantly higher rates among the elderly and those with known mental health or substance use disorders.
  - Agitated delirium, delirium, and dementia account for a large portion of these visits.
  - Others causes of AMS, such as trauma, frank psychosis, or acute depression, are often, but not always, easier to differentiate than the first three (Table 102.1).
- Differential diagnosis of AMS and behavioral emergencies is incredibly broad (Box 102.1).
  - Patients require a quick but careful assessment of their mental and physical health to determine the best management plan.
- Recognizing signs and symptoms characteristic of each disorder and understanding their pathophysiology and ideal treatment plan are crucial to caring for patients in a busy ED.

Agitated Delirium

General Principles

- Condition that presents with fluctuating level of consciousness in addition to acute psychomotor agitation, aggression, and hyperthermia with significant diaphoresis.

TABLE 102.1 *Comparison of Agitated Delirium, Acute Psychosis, Delirium, and Dementia*

Characteristic	Agitated Delirium	Acute Psychosis	Delirium	Dementia
Onset	Acute	Acute but often history of similar in past	Acute	Progressive; months to years
Vital signs	Abnormal: tachycardia, hyperthermia, tachypnea, may be hypertensive	Typically unaffected	Typically abnormal (fever, tachycardia)	Typically unaffected
Prior psychiatric history	Common + drug abuse history	Common	Uncommon	Uncommon
Course	Rapid, fluctuating	Sometimes stable, sometimes fluctuating	Rapid, fluctuating	Slowly progressive, stable
Psychomotor activity	Highly agitated, aggressive	Variable	Variable: sometimes depressed, sometimes agitated	Typically normal
Cognitive function	Variable, but usually highly disorganized, responding to internal stimuli, with incoherent speech and frequent yelling. Typically will not follow commands or converse with physician.	Sometimes impaired and disorganized, with primarily auditory hallucinations, delusions, paranoia. Speech often, but not always, coherent although disorganized.	Usually impaired; often with visual ± auditory hallucinations, delusions, with sometimes pressured, sometimes slow, sometimes incoherent speech	Memory typically impaired but attention often intact; disturbances in other cognitive functions such as language (aphasia), motor (apraxia), identifying objects (agnosia), and executive functioning
Course	Requires rapid sedation and cooling plus other supportive measures and management of complications, such as acidosis, disseminated intravascular coagulation, rhabdomyolysis. May progress to sudden cardiopulmonary arrest.	Responds to therapy but often recurs	Typically resolves with treatment of underlying pathology	Some secondary dementias respond to therapy; most is slowly progressive despite treatment

BOX 102.1 *Differential Diagnosis of Altered Mental Status and Behavioral Abnormalities in the Emergency Department*

Serotonin syndrome
Neuroleptic malignant syndrome
Malignant hyperthermia
Sympathomimetic syndrome or other acute intoxication
Agitated delirium
Psychotropic drug withdrawal
Alcohol withdrawal, delirium tremens, Wernicke's encephalopathy
Psychiatric illness
Heat stroke
Thyrotoxicosis, myxedema coma
Adrenergic stimulation
Hepatic failure/hepatic encephalopathy
Nutritional deficiencies
Electrolyte and fluid disturbances
Hypoglycemia
Status epilepticus or postictal state
Head injury
Stroke or intracranial bleeding
Infection (especially meningitis, encephalitis, sepsis)
Hypertensive encephalopathy
Medication adverse effects, polypharmacy
Central nervous system mass lesion
Paraneoplastic/autoimmune encephalopathy

- No accepted definition or criteria for this clinical diagnosis.
- Patients are more often male, and the etiology is often multifactorial, related to long-term mental illness, stimulant drug use (most commonly cocaine, although methamphetamine, phencyclidine, and LSD have also been described), withdrawal from alcohol (or benzodiazepines), and sometimes sudden cessation of antipsychotic medications.
- Underlying mechanism is controversial but believed to be related to dysfunction in the brain's dopaminergic system and/or high levels of catecholamines exacerbated by concomitant stimulant use, resulting in hyperactivity and hyperthermia.
- Estimated mortality rate is ~8%–9%, although, given the lack of an accepted definition, the accuracy of the estimate is unclear. Most patients are believed to die of cardiopulmonary arrest related to underlying physiologic changes from chronic drug use, hyperthermia, and high catecholamine stress on the heart.

Clinical Presentation

- Signs include extreme paranoia, disorientation, hallucinations, and dissociation.
- Patients may demonstrate incoherent speech or yelling and are often extremely aggressive and demonstrate seemingly superhuman strength and endurance, frequently while trying to resist restraint. This has been attributed to their failure to recognize painful stimuli.
- Vital signs are often notable for hyperthermia with profuse diaphoresis, tachycardia, and tachypnea.
- Agitated delirium and sympathomimetic toxidromes often present similarly, but patients with agitated delirium are more likely to display bizarre abnormal behavior (i.e., stripping off clothing in front of police) with a lesser amount of recent drug use.

Diagnosis and Evaluation

- Agitated delirium is primarily a clinical diagnosis, and it is crucial to initiate treatment early to ensure the safety of your patient as well as staff.
- Conduct a full trauma survey, check vital signs (including a pulse oximetry and core temperature), and perform electrocardiography.
- Laboratory tests that may support the diagnosis and guide management include point-of-care blood glucose, complete blood count (CBC), comprehensive metabolic panel (CMP), creatine kinase, venous blood gas (VBG), urine drug screen, ethanol level, thyroid studies, ammonia, lactate, troponin, aspirin and acetaminophen levels, a pregnancy test if female, and urinalysis (UA). Obtain chest radiograph (CRX) to assess for infectious etiologies and computed tomography (CT) of the brain to rule out hemorrhage.
- Consider lumbar puncture if there is persistent concern for meningitis, encephalitis, or subarachnoid hemorrhage.

Treatment

- Goals in patient management are to rapidly pharmacologically sedate, use the least amount of physical restraint necessary to subdue the patient, and begin cooling to prevent cardiopulmonary arrest.
- There is limited evidence for the best agent for sedation. Intramuscular administration may be preferred given the rapidity and relative safety of the route. Common agents used in agitated delirium, as well as their potential side effects, are listed in Box 102.2.
- Once the patient is sedated, remove physical restraints as quickly as possible.
- Verbal deescalation should be the first step, although this will likely fail in agitated delirium.

Other Supportive Measures for Agitated Delirium

- Rapid cooling in patients with significant hyperthermia
- Rehydration with intravenous fluids
- Calming measures and reduction of external stimuli
- Management of complications such as disseminated intravascular coagulation (DIC), rhabdomyolysis, acidosis, and hyperkalemia
- If intubating the tachypneic patient who manifests agitated delirium, consider setting a higher initial respiratory rate and tidal volume because the paralytic eliminates the patient's respiratory drive and means of compensating for an underlying metabolic acidosis.

BOX 102.2 *Pharmacologic Sedation in Agitated Delirium*

Midazolam or lorazepam (may need redosing)
Ketamine (potential for laryngospasm, tachycardia, hypertension; optimal dose unknown)
Haloperidol (potential for dopaminergic interaction and QT prolongation)
Ziprasidone (potential for dopaminergic interaction and QT prolongation)
Olanzapine (risk of hypotension, especially with concomitant benzodiazepine use)

Delirium Versus Dementia

General Principles

- Patients presenting with **agitated delirium** as described above differ from those presenting with typical delirium and dementia owing to their high degree of psychomotor agitation.
- Distinguishing **typical delirium** from dementia can be much more difficult, especially if the patient arrives without caretakers or family members who are able to provide a history of baseline mental status.
- 10%–20% of elderly patients who present to the ED have symptoms of delirium and are at high risk for delirium because they are likely to have multiple comorbidities, be on multiple medications, and have preexisting brain disease, such as dementia.
- Several key characteristics distinguish these two often overlapping entities (see Table 102.1).

DELIRIUM

- A symptom rather than etiology of disease, is believed to be the result of significant alteration in cerebral metabolic activity involving both the cerebral cortex and the subcortical structures.
- Characterized by an alteration in consciousness associated with a reduced ability to focus or maintain attention.
- Likely related to derangement of multiple neurotransmitters and electrolytes, sometimes in addition to direct effects of drugs and exotoxins on the central nervous system (CNS).
- Causes of delirium are broad and include infectious etiologies, drug and alcohol intoxication or withdrawal, acute metabolic disturbances, trauma, CNS disease, hypoxia, vitamin deficiencies, thermal and endocrinologic emergencies, acute vascular causes, paraneoplastic or autoimmune processes (such as N-methyl-d-aspartate receptor encephalitis, lupus cerebritis), and heavy-metal intoxications.
- In elderly patients, the most common causes are infection (especially urinary tract infections and pneumonia) and polypharmacy.

Clinical Presentation

- Disturbances in consciousness, memory, cognition, and perception, including inability to focus attention, difficulty with language or speech, disorientation, memory deficits, hallucinations, and delusions
- May manifest sleep-wake reversal, emotional lability, and hypersensitivity to light, may be somnolent (hypoactive, depressed) or agitated (even manic).
- Symptoms develop over a short time (i.e., hours to days) and wax and wane.
- Patients may demonstrate symptoms of the primary disease process, including but not limited to infectious symptoms, evidence of trauma, and clinical toxidrome.

Diagnosis and Evaluation

- History, including careful examination of medications, physical examination (including consideration for a core temperature measurement), laboratory studies, and/or radiographic studies are used to evaluate for the etiology of delirium.
- Tests may include: blood glucose, CBC, CMP, blood cultures, lactate, VBG, ammonia, serum osmolality, ethanol level, drug screen, thyroid studies, UA, CXR, CT or magnetic resonance imaging (MRI) of the brain, and lumbar puncture.

Treatment

- Management of delirium is centered on diagnosing and treating the underlying pathology.
- Screen for and treat easily reversible causes (i.e., hypoglycemia, hypoxia, narcotic overdose, heat stroke).
- Initiate treatment for other identifiable causes (such as fluids and antibiotics for infection; warming for hypothermia or cooling for hyperthermia; blood pressure control for hypertensive encephalopathy or intracranial bleeding; intravenous thiamine for Wernicke's encephalopathy).
- Provide supportive care, including calming measures, reduction of external stimuli, and pharmacologic sedation (preferably with antipsychotics rather than benzodiazepines in the elderly) as needed.
- Avoid benzodiazepines in those at risk for delirium, except in cases of alcohol and benzodiazepine withdrawal.

DEMENTIA

- Gradually progressive deterioration of cognitive function with relatively intact level of consciousness (see Table 102.2 for definition and criteria per the *Diagnostic and Statistical Manual of Mental Disorders*, 5th ed.).
- Causes are multifactorial and can be reversible or irreversible.
- Primary dementias (see Table 102.3) include Alzheimer disease, frontotemporal dementia (Pick disease), Huntington disease, Parkinson disease, and progressive supranuclear palsy.

TABLE 102.2 ***Diagnostic and Statistical Manual of Mental Disorders, 5th ed., Definition and Criteria of Major Neurocognitive Disorder/Dementia***

Diagnostic Criteria	Major Neurocognitive Disorder/ Dementia
A	Significant cognitive decline in one or more cognitive domains (including learning and memory, language, executive function, complex attention, perceptual-motor function, and social cognition) based on: 1. Concern about significant decline, expressed by the individual or knowledgeable informant, or observed by clinician 2. Substantial impairment, documented by objective cognitive assessment
B	Cognitive deficits are sufficient to interfere with independence in everyday activities
C	Not exclusively during episode of delirium
D	Not better explained by another mental disorder such as schizophrenia or major depressive disorder

TABLE 102.3 *Primary Dementias*

Dementia Type	Characteristics
Alzheimer disease (AD)	Early amnesia and impairment in executive functioning with late personality and language disturbances and variable apraxia, agnosia, alexia. Common visuospatial disorientation. Risk increases with age (although familial AD can present early). Neuroimaging often demonstrates widespread atrophy in later stages.
Frontotemporal dementia (Pick disease)	Early personality/behavior changes, including disinhibition, and language disturbances with late amnesia, apraxia, agnosia, and alexia. Develops earlier than AD; mean age of onset is 50 years. Neuroimaging demonstrates frontotemporal atrophy in later stages.
Huntington disease	Uncontrolled movements of arms, legs, head, face, and upper body (chorea), dysarthria, dysphagia, facial twitching, paired with progressive dementia as well as emotional changes such as increasing irritability and depression. Autosomal-dominant with symptoms often presenting between ages 30 and 50.
Parkinson disease	Resting tremors (pill-rolling) and rigidity, as well as bradykinesia, impaired balance, and trouble moving or walking (shuffling gait); later with progressive dementia. May initially present with nonspecific symptoms of tiredness, aching limbs, mental slowness, and depression. Onset typically in late middle age.
Progressive supranuclear palsy	Uncommon. Parkinsonian motor disturbances, dysarthria, dysphagia, pseudobulbar palsy, supranuclear ophthalmoparesis/ophthalmoplegia, mood and behavior changes due to frontal lobe dysfunction, early severe cognitive deficits. Onset typically in late middle age.

102

- Secondary dementias include vascular (most common), endocrinologic, infectious, or nutritional dementias and dementias due to head trauma or mass effect.
- Most patients presenting with dementia do not present emergently.
- ED evaluation is centered around evaluating for potentially reversible causes and identifying any acute disease.

Clinical Presentation

- Patients can present with memory impairment (to both creating new and remembering old memories), difficulty handling complex tasks, and impaired reasoning.
- Cognitive disturbances, such as aphasia, apraxia, agnosia, and altered executive functioning, may be present.
- Patients tend to have a relatively stable level of consciousness, and the deficits do not occur exclusively during the course of acute medical illness.

Diagnosis and Evaluation

- Diagnosis, especially in the ED, is centered around evaluating for reversible causes.
- Consider whether symptoms are actually a presentation of delirium secondary to an underlying disease.
- Screen for depression.
- Review medications, as well as neurologic and mental status examinations.
- Assess cognition by screening with the Mini-Mental State Examination or other brief screening tests for dementia to evaluate orientation, attention and calculation, memory/recall, language, and visual-spatial skills.
- Laboratory tests and imaging may be used for further workup and exclusion of differential diagnoses, including CBC, CMP, thyroid studies, evaluation for syphilis and human immunodeficiency virus (HIV), vitamin B_{12} and folate levels, UA, drug screen, CRX, and CT or MRI of the brain as indicated.

Treatment

- Primarily aimed at the underlying disease
- Initiate treatment for acutely reversible causes in ED. Otherwise, outpatient referral to neurology or admission with placement and subsequent referral as indicated would be appropriate.

SUGGESTED READINGS

Huff, J. S. (2016). Altered mental status and coma. In J. E. Tintinalli, J. S. Stapczynski, O. J. Ma, D. M. Yealy, G. D. Meckler, & D. M. Cline (Eds.), *Tintinalli's emergency medicine: A comprehensive study guide* (8th ed., pp. 1156–1161). McGraw-Hill Education.

Kanich, W., Brady, W. J., Huff, J. S., Perron, A. D., Holstege, C., Lindbeck, G., & Carter, C. T. (2002). Altered mental status: Evaluation and etiology in the ED. *American Journal of Emergency Medicine, 20*(7), 613–617.

Karas, S. (2002). Behavioral emergencies: Differentiating medical from psychiatric disease. *Emergency Medicine Practice, 4*, 1–18.

Marx, J. A., & Rosen, P. (2014). Confusion. In J. A. Marx, R. S. Hockberger, & R. M. Walls (Eds.), *Rosen's emergency medicine: Concepts and clinical practice* (8th ed., pp. 151–155). Elsevier.

Marx, J. A., & Rosen, P. (2014). Delirium and dementia. In J. A. Marx, R. S. Hockberger, & R. M. Walls (Eds.), *Rosen's emergency medicine: Concepts and clinical practice* (8th ed., pp. 1398–1408). Elsevier.

Takeuchi, A., Ahern, T. L., & Henderson, S. O. (2011). Excited delirium. *Western Journal of Emergency Medicine, 12*(1), 77–83.

CHAPTER 103

BOARD REVIEW

Anxiety Disorders, Factitious Disorders, Neurotic Disorders

CATHERINE WEAVER, MD, and JAMES J. MURPHY JR., MD, MPH

- Anxiety disorders are extremely common and can precipitate a visit to an emergency department.
- Panic attacks are a common acute coronary syndrome mimic and an illness anxiety disorder can exacerbate any underlying presentation.
- It is important to be sensitive and, when appropriate, reassuring to these patients and refer them for proper outpatient therapy.
- Neurotic disorders can mimic more serious neurologic or other medical conditions.
- Factitious disorder by proxy can be a serious, reportable form of abuse.

Clinical Presentation, Diagnosis, and Evaluation of Anxiety Disorders

- The general presentation of the following anxiety, factitious, and neurotic disorders can vary widely.
- The criteria determined by the *Diagnostic and Statistical Manual of Mental Disorders*, 5th ed. (DSM-V) for each is summarized.
- These diagnoses can only be made when the behavior is not attributable to the physiologic effects of a substance or another medical condition (unless otherwise specified) and when they are not better explained by another psychiatric disorder.
- Additionally, a psychiatric disorder only exists when the behavioral disturbance causes clinically significant distress or impairment in social, occupational, educational, or other important areas of functioning.
- In general, these disorders are more common in women than in men. Illness anxiety disorder is equally prevalent in both genders.

Separation Anxiety Disorder

Those with separation anxiety disorder exhibit developmentally inappropriate and excessive fear or anxiety concerning separation from those to whom the individual is attached for ≥4 weeks in children or adolescents and ≥6 months in adults as evidenced by three or more of the following:

- recurrent excessive distress when anticipating or experiencing separation from home or other major attachment figures
- persistent and excessive worry about losing major attachment figures or about possible harm to them, such as illness, injury, disasters, or death
- persistent and excessive worry about experiencing an untoward event (getting lost, kidnapped, etc.) that causes separation from a major attachment figure
- persistent reluctance or refusal to go out, away from home, to school, to work, or elsewhere because of fear of separation
- persistent reluctance or refusal to sleep away from home or go to sleep without being near a major attachment figure
- repeated nightmares involving the theme of separation
- repeated complaints of physical symptoms (headaches, abdominal distress, nausea, etc.) when separation from major attachment figures occurs or is anticipated

Selective Mutism

- Selective mutism is a failure to speak for ≥1 month in specific situations in which there is an expectation for speaking (i.e., school or work), despite speaking in other situations, causing a disturbance in educational or occupational achievement or social communication.
- The failure to speak is not attributable to a lack of knowledge or comfort with the spoken language being used, nor a communication disorder, nor does it occur exclusively during the course of autism spectrum disorder, schizophrenia, or another psychotic disorder.

Specific Phobia

- Patients exhibit a fear or anxiety lasting for ≥6 months about a specific object or situation (i.e., flying, heights, seeing blood, or certain animals) that is out of proportion with the actual danger posed by the object or situation.
- The phobic object or situation almost always provokes immediate fear or anxiety and is either actively avoided or endured with intense fear or anxiety.
- In contrast to adults, it is not necessary for children to judge their fear to be unreasonable or excessive.
- Phobias, like separation anxiety, are common in children, and can present with behavioral dysregulation or somatic complaints.
- Differential diagnosis includes panic disorders, PTSD, and GAD.
- Mainstay of treatment is CBT (i.e., desensitization or exposure-response prevention therapy) and can also include short-acting benzodiazepines, SSRIs, beta-blockers (i.e., propranolol), and anxiolytic agents.

Social Anxiety Disorder

- Patients with social anxiety disorder have marked fear or anxiety out of proportion to the threat posed about one or more social situations in which the individual is exposed to possible scrutiny by others, being observed, or performing in front of others (i.e., having conversations, eating, drinking, giving a speech).
- The individual often fears they will act in a way or show anxiety symptoms that will be negatively evaluated.
- This must include peers and not only adults in the case of a child, and these symptoms must last ≥6 months.

Panic Disorder

Those with panic disorder have recurrent unexpected panic attacks with at least one episode followed by 1 month of one or both of the following: a persistent concern or worry about additional panic attacks or their consequences (i.e., fear of "going crazy" or having a heart attack), and/or significant maladaptive change in behavior related to the attacks, such as avoidance of unfamiliar situations, exercise, etc.

Panic attacks are defined as an abrupt surge of intense fear or intense discomfort that reaches a peak within minutes, and during which time four or more of the following symptoms occur:

- palpitations or accelerated heart rate
- sweating
- trembling or shaking
- sensation of shortness of breath or smothering
- sensation of choking
- chest pain or discomfort
- nausea or abdominal distress
- feeling dizzy, unsteady, lightheaded, or faint
- chills or heat sensations
- paresthesias
- derealization or depersonalization
- fear of losing control or "going crazy"
- fear of dying (often absent in children)
- Differential diagnoses include a variety of etiologies, including endocrine (hypoglycemia, thyroid disorders, pheochromocytoma), neurologic (seizures, neoplasms), pharmacologic (acute intoxication or medication side effects), cardiovascular (arrhythmias and myocardial infarctions), and other psychiatric conditions (GAD, obsessive-compulsive disorder [OCD], posttraumatic stress disorder [PTSD]).
- Treatments may include CBT, "flooding therapy," desensitization, or medications including SSRIs, short-acting benzodiazepines, b-blockers, and anxiolytic agents.

Agoraphobia

- Those with agoraphobia have a marked fear or anxiety out of proportion of the actual danger for ≥6 months about two or more of the following situations: using public transportation, being in open spaces, being in enclosed spaces, standing in line or being in a crowd, and/or being outside of the home alone.
- The patient fears these situations because of thoughts that escape may be difficult or that help will not be available in the event of developing panic, embarrassment, or other incapacitating symptoms.

Generalized Anxiety Disorder

Those with generalized anxiety disorder possess an excessive anxiety and worry occurring more days than not for ≥6 months about a wide variety of events, activities, or situations that the individual finds difficult to control. The anxiety and worry are associated with at least three (or more than one in a child) of the following six symptoms that are present for more days than not:

- restlessness or feeling keyed up or on edge
- being easily fatigued
- difficulty concentrating or mind going blank
- irritability
- muscle tension
- sleep disturbances (i.e., difficulty falling or staying asleep or restless, unsatisfying sleep)
- Differential diagnosis includes such organic causes as hyperthyroidism and pheochromocytoma, use of central nervous system stimulants (i.e., caffeine, cocaine, and amphetamines), and other psychiatric conditions, such as depression, schizophrenia, or other anxiety disorders.
- Treatment may include group and cognitive-behavioral therapy (CBT), coupled with medications, such as selective serotonin reuptake inhibitors (SSRIs), longacting benzodiazepines, and anxiolytics.

Substance-Induced or Medication-Induced Anxiety Disorder

- This disorder is predominated by anxiety or panic attacks that occur both during or soon after substance intoxication or withdrawal (including caffeine) or after exposure to a medication (such as pseudoephedrine, diet pills).
- The involved substance or medication is capable of reproducing the symptoms.
- The symptoms must not be better explained by a preexisting anxiety disorder that is not substance- or medication-induced, nor occur exclusively in the course of delirium.

Clinical Presentation, Diagnosis, and Evaluation of Neurotic Disorders

Somatic Symptom Disorder

Of note, this DSM-V diagnosis consolidates the DSM-IV diagnoses of somatization disorder, undifferentiated somatoform disorder, hypochondriasis, and pain disorder. A patient must have at least one somatic symptom(s) that is distressing or that results in a significant disruption of daily life. The specific symptom may change, but the state of being distracted by a somatic symptom must last 6 months. Common somatic symptoms include pain, weakness, tingling, heaviness, or a generalized sense of being unwell.

The patient has excessive thoughts, feelings, or behaviors related to the somatic symptom(s) or health concerns manifested by at least one of the following:
- Disproportionate and persistent thoughts about the seriousness of one's symptoms
- Persistently high level of anxiety about health or symptoms
- Excessive time or energy devoted to these symptoms or health concerns

Patients frequently have a concomitant medical illness. Their symptoms may also be a result of a normal bodily function. However, the illness is diagnosed by the disproportionate level of distress it causes.

Illness Anxiety Disorder

- Illness anxiety disorder is a new disorder that was introduced in DSM-V, derived in part from hypochondriasis, a diagnosis which has been eliminated.
- This disorder includes the preoccupation for ≥6 months with having or acquiring a serious illness.
- The specific illness feared may change, but the fear of something persists.
- Somatic symptoms rarely accompany the disorder and, if present, are only mild.
- If another medical condition is present or if the patient is at high risk for a condition because of family history or other significant risk factor, the preoccupation is clearly excessive or disproportionate.
- There are two recognized subtypes: care-seeking and care-avoidant.
- Those with the care-seeking subtype perform excessive health-related behaviors (i.e., overly vigilant for signs of illness or frequently utilizing health care).
- Patients with the care-avoidant subtype exhibit maladaptive avoidance of situations that are believed to represent health threats (i.e., avoidant of appointments or visiting sick family members).
- These patients are as equally at risk for true medical illness as anyone else and deserve full assessments like any other patient.

Conversion Disorder (Functional Neurological Symptom Disorder)

- Characterized by unintentional loss of function (i.e., blindness, paralysis) with no identifiable organic cause
- Often occurs suddenly after a traumatic or extremely stressful event. *La belle indifférence*, or an inappropriate lack of concern for a neurologic deficit, is no longer believed to help differentiate between a functional and organic neurologic disorder.
- Diagnosis is clinical and the examination is inconsistent with known anatomic or pathophysiologic states.
- Opticokinetic test, which involves placing a mirror in front of the patient and quickly moving it laterally, can be useful to evaluate for blindness. If the patient tracks the image of themselves laterally, they are not truly blind.
- In addition to reassurance and outpatient psychiatric and medical follow-up, avoid telling the patient that their symptoms are not real; doing so can worsen the condition.

Psychological Factors Affecting Other Medical Conditions

For diagnosis, patient must have another underlying medical condition that is not a psychiatric diagnosis for which they have psychological or behavioral factors that adversely affect the medical condition in one or more of the following ways:
- the close temporal association between the psychological factors and the development or exacerbation of or delayed recovery from the medical condition
- the factors interfere with the treatment of the medical condition (e.g., poor adherence)
- the factors constitute additional well-established health risks for the individual
- the factors aggravate the underlying pathophysiology, precipitating or exacerbating symptoms, or necessitate medical attention

Factitious Disorder Imposed on Self (Formerly Munchausen Syndrome)

- Patients feign physical or psychological signs, including symptoms of injury or disease, associated with identified deception.
- The individual presents self as ill, impaired, or injured without obvious external rewards.
- Classically men in their 20s to 40s
- Secondary gain is to subject himself or herself to unnecessary testing to obtain sympathy and attention and to secure the "sick role."
- Treatment is early confrontation and close outpatient follow-up.

Factitious Disorder Imposed on Another (Formerly Munchausen Syndrome by Proxy)

- Patients falsify physical or psychological signs or symptoms and may induce injury or disease in another while presenting the other (victim) as ill, impaired, or injured even in the absence of obvious external reward.
- The diagnosis is applied to the perpetrator, not the victim.
- Examples of behaviors to induce illness or the appearance of illness include simple lies, falsification of medical records, poisoning (i.e., with insulin or excess sodium in children), injection of foreign material (i.e., feces, milk) under the skin or into the bloodstream, or tampering with laboratory specimens (i.e., adding blood to a urine sample to induce a positive result for hematuria).

- Secondary gain is achieved via prolonged contact with health-care providers at the expense of the patient. This is a form of child abuse and the emergency physician must notify child protective services.
- Perpetrators are often quite knowledgeable about the medical history and appear attentive and caring.
- Psychiatric care can also be provided to the perpetrator because there is a high rate of suicide when confronted.

Other Somatic Symptom and Related Disorders

This subset includes presentations of somatic symptom disorders that cause significant distress or impairment in social, occupation, or other important areas of functioning but do not meet full criteria for another disorder within the class. Examples include:

- brief somatic symptom disorder (<6 months)
- brief illness anxiety disorder (<6 months)
- illness anxiety disorder without cession of health-related behaviors
- pseudocyesis, or a false belief of being pregnant associated with objective signs and reported symptoms of pregnancy
- unspecified somatic symptom and related disorder

Treatment

- For most of the anxiety disorders discussed, cognitive-behavioral therapy, with or without selective serotonin reuptake inhibitors, constitutes the mainstay of treatment.
- Benzodiazepines are only appropriate as short-term therapy for panic disorders.
- Long-term, psychiatric follow-up and possibly a selective serotonin reuptake inhibitor are required.
- Treatment modalities can vary for phobic disorders, but sometimes include extinction via exposure therapy, as well as generalized cognitive-behavioral therapy.
- For factitious and neurotic disorders, medication plays a less important role.
- For conversion and somatic disorders, regular follow-up with a primary care physician can be useful to decrease emergency department visits, iatrogenic harm of over-testing, and distress as a therapeutic relationship is established and patients become more open to psychiatric referral.

SUGGESTED READING

American Psychiatric Association. (2013). *Diagnostic and statistical manual of mental disorders* (5th ed.). American Psychiatric Association.

SECTION FOURTEEN

BOARD REVIEW

Renal and Urogenital

CHAPTER **104** BOARD REVIEW

Acute Kidney Injury

AMIR A. ROUHANI, MD, and NASEEM MORIDZADEH, MD

General Principles

- Acute kidney injury (AKI) refers to a rapid decrease in kidney function that leads to retention of nitrogenous waste products (i.e., urea), dysregulation of volume status, and a wide range of metabolic and electrolyte disturbances, leading to increased morbidity and mortality.
- AKI has replaced the term "acute renal failure" because it better reflects the broad spectrum of diseases, beyond failure alone, that can result in clinically relevant kidney damage in the acute setting.

Definition and Staging

- AKI is defined as an abrupt reduction in kidney function within the last 48 hours, defined as an absolute increase in serum creatinine of 0.3 mg/dL, a 50% or greater increase in serum creatinine, or reduction in urine output. Multiple criteria exist for defining and staging of AKI, such as Acute Kidney Injury Network, Risk, Injury, Failure, Loss of Kidney function, and End-stage renal disease, and Kidney Disease Improving Global Outcomes (KDIGO).
- The KDIGO 2012 Clinical Practice Guidelines define AKI as any one of the following:
  - Increase in serum creatinine 0.3 mg/dL or greater within 48 hours *or*
  - Increase in serum creatinine by 1.5 or more times baseline (occurring within last 7 days) *or*
  - Oliguria (urine output less than 0.5 mL/kg/hr for at least 6 hours)
- Beyond providing a formal definition of AKI, KDIGO has also developed criteria to classify the severity of AKI. The KDIGO stages of severity of AKI are as follows:
  - Stage 1
    - Increase in serum creatinine to 1.5 to 1.9 times baseline *or*
    - Increase in serum creatinine by 0.3 mg/dL or more *or*
    - Reduction in urine output to less than 0.5 mL/kg/hr for 6 to 12 hours
  - Stage 2
    - Increase in serum creatinine to 2.0 to 2.9 times baseline *or*
    - Reduction in urine output to less than 0.5 mL/kg/hr for 12 or more hours
  - Stage 3
    - Increase in serum creatinine to 3.0 times baseline *or*
    - Increase in serum creatinine to 4.0 mg/dL or more *or*
    - Reduction in urine output to less than 0.3 mL/kg/hr for 24 or more hours *or*
    - Anuria for 12 or more hours *or*
    - Initiation of renal replacement therapy *or*
    - In patients younger than 18 years: decrease in estimated glomerular filtration rate to less than 35 mL/min/1.73 m^2.
- KDIGO criteria should be applied only after adequate fluid resuscitation has taken place and easily reversible causes of kidney injury, such as obstruction, have been excluded.
- Despite their intended utility in certain situations, the various criteria used for determining the severity of AKI are not without limitations and can pose challenges in the clinical assessment and management of patients with AKI.
- Some of these challenges include the lack of differentiation between the various etiologies of AKI and their reliance on determining a patient's baseline creatinine level when there is no previously documented or available value.
- A simpler approach focuses on determining the changes in urine output and classifies AKI as nonoliguric, oliguric (urine output less than 0.5 mL/kg/hr), or anuric (urine output less than 50 to 100 mL/day).
- The presence of anuria is rare, but may be associated with shock, bilateral renal artery occlusion, rapidly progressive (crescentic) glomerulonephritis, renal cortical necrosis, or complete bilateral urinary tract obstruction.

Pathogenesis

- The etiologies of AKI can be divided into three broad categories: prerenal, intrinsic renal, and postrenal (Fig. 104.1).
- *Prerenal AKI*, which is caused by renal hypoperfusion, may be due to a true loss of intravascular volume, redistribution of volume, decrease in effective cardiac output, and other causes. It is the most common type of AKI in the nonhospital setting. Specific causes include:
  - Intravascular volume depletion: vomiting, diarrhea, blood loss, insensible losses, third spacing, pancreatitis, peritonitis, trauma, burns, diuretic therapy
  - Volume redistribution: sepsis, anaphylaxis, nephrotic syndrome, cirrhosis, other hypoalbuminemic states, hepatorenal syndrome
  - Decreased effective arterial volume: decreased cardiac output (myocardial infarction, valvular disease, cardiomyopathy), decreased renal perfusion (renal artery embolization, stenosis, fibromuscular dysplasia), shock

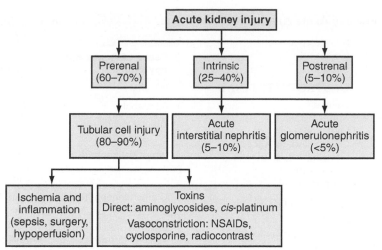

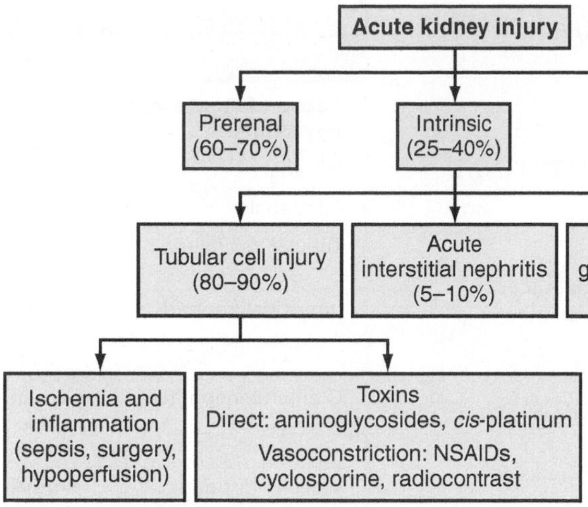

FIG. 104.1 Main categories of acute kidney injury. NSAIDs, nonsteroidal antiinflammatory drugs. (Molitoris, B. A. (2019). Acute kidney injury. In L. S. Goldman & A. I. Schafer (Eds.), *Goldman-Cecil medicine* (26th ed., pp. 748–753, Fig. 112.1). Elsevier Health Sciences.)

  - Medications that limit glomerular perfusion: angiotensin converting enzyme inhibitors, nonsteroidal antiinflammatory drugs (NSAIDs), calcineurin inhibitors (cyclosporin, tacrolimus)
- *Intrinsic AKI* results from pathology involving the glomerulus, interstitium, renal tubule, and/or the blood supply to the kidney. Specific causes are outlined below:
  - Glomerular diseases
    - Systemic diseases
      - Systemic lupus erythematosus
      - Infective endocarditis
      - Systemic vasculitis (e.g., polyarteritis nodosum)
      - Henoch-Schönlein purpura
      - Human immunodeficiency virus (HIV)-associated nephropathy
      - Essential mixed cryoglobulinemia
      - Goodpasture syndrome
    - Primary renal diseases
      - Poststreptococcal glomerulonephritis
      - Other postinfectious glomerulonephritis
      - Rapidly progressive glomerulonephritis
  - Vascular diseases
    - Large-vessel diseases
      - Renal artery thrombosis or stenosis
      - Renal vein thrombosis
      - Atheroembolic disease
    - Small- and medium-vessel diseases
      - Scleroderma
      - Malignant hypertension
      - Hemolytic uremic syndrome
      - Thrombotic thrombocytopenic purpura
      - HIV-associated microangiopathy
  - Tubulointerstitial diseases and conditions
    - Drugs
    - Toxins (e.g., heavy metals, ethylene glycol)
    - Infections
    - Multiple myeloma
  - Acute tubular necrosis
    - Ischemia
      - Shock
      - Sepsis
      - Severe prerenal azotemia
    - Nephrotoxins
      - Antibiotics
      - Radiographic contrast agents (controversial)
      - Myoglobinuria
      - Hemoglobinuria
  - Other diseases and conditions
    - Severe liver disease
    - Allergic reactions
    - NSAIDs
- *Postrenal AKI* results from obstruction at any level of the urinary tract. Specific causes include:
  - Intrarenal and ureteral
    - Kidney stone
    - Papillary necrosis
    - Malignancy (intrinsic or extrinsic)
    - Retroperitoneal fibrosis
    - Crystalline precipitation (uric acid, oxalic acid, or phosphate crystals)
  - Bladder
    - Kidney stone
    - Blood clot
    - Prostatic hypertrophy
    - Bladder carcinoma
    - Neurogenic bladder
  - Urethra
    - Posterior urethral valves
    - Phimosis
    - Stricture

Clinical Presentation

- The clinical manifestations of AKI can vary. Patients may describe symptoms that may be directly related to the underlying cause of AKI or the result of its complications. These include metabolic derangements, disturbances in fluid balance, or effects on specific organ systems (Box 104.1). For example, patients may present with vomiting, volume overload, decreased urine output, or urinary obstruction.
- Symptoms often may be indolent and patients may even be asymptomatic. AKI may not be obvious on initial evaluation and diagnosis may be delayed until laboratory data are obtained.

BOX 104.1 Clinical Features of Acute Kidney Injury

CARDIOVASCULAR
Pulmonary edema
Arrhythmia
Hypertension
Pericarditis
Pericardial effusion
Myocardial infarction
Pulmonary embolism

METABOLIC
Hyponatremia
Hyperkalemia
Acidosis
Hypocalcemia
Hyperphosphatemia
Hypermagnesemia
Hyperuricemia

NEUROLOGIC
Asterixis
Neuromuscular irritability
Mental status changes
Somnolence
Coma
Seizures

GASTROINTESTINAL
Nausea
Vomiting
Gastritis
Gastroduodenal ulcer
Gastrointestinal bleeding
Pancreatitis
Malnutrition

HEMATOLOGIC
Anemia
Hemorrhagic diathesis

INFECTIOUS
Pneumonia
Septicemia
Urinary tract infection
Wound infection

(From Wolfson, A. B. (2018). Renal failure. In R. M. Walls, R. S. Hockberger, & M. Gausche-Hill (Eds.), *Rosen's emergency medicine: Concepts and clinical practice*, (9th ed., pp. 1179–1196, Box 87.1). Elsevier.)

TABLE 104.1 Common Urinalysis Findings in Acute Kidney Injury

Cause of Acute Kidney Injury	Urinalysis
Prerenal	Normal or hyaline casts
Intrarenal	
Tubular cell injury	Muddy-brown, granular, epithelial casts
Interstitial nephritis	Pyuria, hematuria, mild proteinuria, granular and epithelial casts, eosinophils
Glomerulonephritis	Hematuria, marked proteinuria, red blood cell casts, granular proteinuria
Vascular disorders	Normal or hematuria, mild proteinuria
Postrenal	Normal or hematuria, granular casts, pyuria

(From Molitoris, B. A. (2019). Acute kidney injury. In L. S. Goldman & A. I. Schafer (Eds.), *Goldman-Cecil medicine* (26th ed., pp. 748–753, Table 112.6). Elsevier Health Sciences.)

TABLE 104.2 FE_{Na} Values for the Various Causes of Acute Kidney Injury

Cause of Acute Kidney Injury	FE_{Na}	BUN to Serum Creatine Ratio
Prerenal	Less than1%	More than 20
Intrarenal		Less than 10 to -15
Tubular necrosis	1% or greater	
Interstitial nephritis	1% or greater	
Glomerulonephritis (early)	Less than 1%	
Vascular disorders (early)	Less than 1%	
Postrenal	>1% or greater	More than 20

(From Molitoris, B. A. (2019). Acute kidney injury. In L. S. Goldman & A. I. Schafer (Eds.), *Goldman-Cecil medicine* (26th ed., pp. 748–753, Table 112.5). Elsevier Health Sciences.)

Diagnosis and Evaluation

- Diagnosis of AKI and its sequelae can be made through a combination of history and physical examination, laboratory testing, imaging, electrocardiogram, and biopsy.
- All patients with suspected or confirmed AKI should be assessed for volume status and uremic symptoms. Laboratory abnormalities, such as hyperkalemia, hyperphosphatemia, and hypocalcemia should be identified. Acid-base status should also be determined.
- In addition, careful review of medications that may be nephrotoxic is imperative.

Laboratory

Urinalysis

- The various components of the urinalysis can be useful as both a screening and a diagnostic test for AKI. Hematuria without recent instrumentation can be seen in nephrolithiasis, glomerular disease, or vasculitis. The microscopic analysis of urinary sediment can be particularly useful in determining the cause of an AKI.
- The contents of the renal tubule are reflected in the composition of a cast. Hyaline casts are commonly seen in dehydration, after exercise, or in association with glomerular proteinuria. White blood cell casts are suggestive of renal parenchymal inflammation. Red blood cell casts are indicative of glomerular hematuria, typically seen in glomerulonephritis or vasculitis. Fatty casts are associated with heavy proteinuria and nephrotic syndrome (Table 104.1).

Serum and Urine Chemical Analysis

- Metabolic panels may be useful to assess the creatinine and blood urea nitrogen-to-creatinine ratios, electrolyte abnormalities, serum osmolality, and acid–base status of patients with AKI.
- Electrolyte panels should include calcium, magnesium, and phosphorous levels. Creatine kinase levels should also be considered. Urine electrolytes, including Na, K, urine Cr, and urine osmolality, can be utilized in comparison with serum values and to calculate the fractional excretion of sodium or urea. However, these tests often perform poorly in differentiating between the various types of renal failure (Table 104.2).
- Additional laboratory studies that can be considered include creatinine kinase, serum drug levels, and uric acid.

Imaging

- Renal imaging is of limited utility in the initial emergency department evaluation of AKI, particularly if the history and examination demonstrate an obvious etiology. However, it can be particularly helpful in identifying obstructive causes of renal dysfunction.
- Renal ultrasound is a safe, noninvasive, and sensitive imaging modality for the evaluation of obstruction.

- Computed tomography (CT) scanning can be useful to obtain anatomic images of the kidney and urinary tract, although it does not provide information regarding renal function.
- Furthermore, although contrast-enhanced images may provide valuable information in the evaluation of a patient with renal failure, there is a potential risk of additional renal injury from contrast agents (although this is controversial).
- In obstruction, classic contrast CT findings are normal to large-sized kidneys, dense nephrograms, and delayed opacification of dilated collecting systems.
- Noncontrast CT scans, on the other hand, avoid the risk of potentially nephrotoxic agents in obtaining imaging and can also provide valuable information, such as the presence of hydronephrosis, ureteral dilation, renal stones, masses, and fibrosis.
- Gadolinium administration for magnetic resonance imaging has been associated with nephrogenic systemic fibrosis and should be avoided, if possible, in patients with AKI.

Treatment

- The treatment of AKI depends on the underlying etiology. However, the first priority should focus on management of complications related to AKI, namely the potentially life-threatening fluid and electrolyte abnormalities.
- Hypervolemia, hyperkalemia, uremia resulting in pericarditis or altered mental status, and severe metabolic acidosis are the primary life-threatening complications that must be immediately addressed in a patient with AKI. If appropriate medical therapy is ineffective in reversing these complications, hemodialysis is indicated.
- After life-threatening issues have been addressed, attention can then be turned toward the underlying etiology of the AKI. Prerenal and postrenal AKI should be considered and managed first because these tend to be more easily treated and reversible.
- In prerenal AKI, the treatment should focus on correction of the underlying cause of disease. This may involve correcting volume status and augmenting cardiac output and can be accomplished through administration of intravenous fluids, vasopressors or inotropes, blood transfusions, and/or diuresis.
- It is also important to address significant electrolyte abnormalities and discontinue all potentially nephrotoxic agents. Dialysis should be reserved for the life-threatening complications, but is rarely necessary in prerenal AKI.
- Postrenal AKI treatment should focus on resolution of the obstructive cause, including via transurethral or suprapubic catheter placement, ureteral stents, or percutaneous nephrostomy tubes, depending on the site of obstruction.
- Once potential prerenal and postrenal causes of AKI have been considered and addressed, it is important to consider the multitude of intrinsic renal etiologies of AKI. In intrinsic AKI, treatment is initially supportive with optimization of hemodynamics and discontinuation of nephrotoxic agents.
- Treatment with corticosteroids or other immunosuppressants may be indicated in various forms of glomerulonephritis (although not indicated in poststreptococcal glomerulonephritis).
- Corticosteroids may also be used to treat acute interstitial nephritis if no improvement is seen after 3 to 7 days, although this is rarely initiated in the emergency department.
- Renal vascular disease is treated based on the underlying microvascular or macrovascular cause. All nephrotoxic agents should also be discontinued. Drugs that are renally cleared should be dose-adjusted.
- Care should be taken to maintain euvolemia and avoid volume overload while maintaining adequate mean arterial pressure (MAP). MAP goal is generally greater than 65 mm Hg, but MAPs of greater than 80 mm Hg may improve renal outcomes in patients with chronic hypertension.
- Associated electrolyte disturbances and acid–base disorders should also be treated.
- The use of diuretics in the management of AKI is controversial. Studies have demonstrated that even slight fluid overload can lead to increased mortality risk and poor outcomes.
  - Although the administration of diuretics has not been shown to improve renal function or creatinine level, an increase in urine output, either spontaneously or with the use of diuretics, can be suggestive of lower injury severity and increased likelihood for renal recovery.
  - Furthermore, the use of diuretics to increase urine output can help mitigate the negative effects of volume overload or pulmonary edema.
  - Thus, diuretics may be considered, but should be used for only a limited period of time to relieve signs and symptoms of volume overload, not as a prolonged form of therapy or as a replacement for dialysis.
- Dialysis and ultrafiltration remain the most effective method of volume removal in a patient with AKI, regardless of the underlying etiology. Indications for hemodialysis in the management of AKI include:
  - Fluid overload refractory to diuretics (i.e., positive fluid balance)
  - Serum potassium greater than 6.5 mEq/L or rapidly rising potassium refractory to medical therapy
  - pH less than 7.1 owing to metabolic acidosis in a patient who would not tolerate bicarbonate administration (i.e., volume overload) *or* owing to lactic acidosis or ketoacidosis
  - Clinical signs of uremia, including pericarditis, neuropathy, or otherwise unexplained change in mental status
- Beyond potassium derangements, other electrolyte abnormalities to consider are hypocalcemia and hyperphosphatemia.
- Reduced glomerular filtration rate leads to hyperphosphatemia in AKI, which in turn leads to hypocalcemia.
- Because calcium is bound to albumin, it is important to obtain an ionized calcium. Total serum calcium concentrations are an inaccurate reflection of calcium in patients with abnormal albumin levels.
  - In patients with asymptomatic hypocalcemia in the setting of hyperphosphatemia, treatment should be focused on correction of the phosphate.

- In patients with symptomatic hypocalcemia (i.e., paresthesia, tetany, confusion, seizures, Trousseau's sign, Chvostek's sign, or QT prolongation), treatment with intravenous calcium should be initiated.
- If phosphate levels are greater than 8 to 10 mg/dL, the risk of calcium phosphate deposition (typically occurs when the calcium-phosphate product is more than 70) into the vasculature and organs is significantly increased with calcium administration.
- Dialysis to correct both the hyperphosphatemia and the hypocalcemia is indicated.
- Hyperphosphatemia is particularly common in patients with AKI owing to tumor lysis syndrome and rhabdomyolysis. Treatment with dietary phosphate binders is indicated in patients with a phosphate more than 6 mg/dL.
- Calcium-containing phosphate binders, such as calcium acetate or calcium carbonate, may be given in patients who are hypocalcemic.
- If ionized calcium levels are high, non-calcium-containing phosphate binders, such as lanthanum carbonate, sevelamer, or aluminum hydroxide, are preferred to prevent calcium phosphate deposition.

SUGGESTED READINGS

Brady, W. J., & Sudhir, A. (2013). Renal failure. In J. G. Adams, E. D. Barton, J. L. Collings, P. M. C. DeBlieux, M. A. Gisondi, & E. S. Nadel (Eds.), *Emergency medicine: Clinical essentials* (2nd ed.). Elsevier Health Sciences.

Molitoris, B. A. (2019). Acute kidney injury. In L. S. Goldman & A. I. Schafer (Eds.), *Goldman-Cecil medicine* (26th ed.). Elsevier Health Sciences.

Wolfson, A. B. (2018). Renal failure. In R. M. Walls, R. S. Hockberger, & M. Gausche-Hill (Eds.), *Rosen's emergency medicine: Concepts and clinical practice* (9th ed.). Elsevier.

CHAPTER 105

BOARD REVIEW

Chronic Kidney Disease

AMIR A. ROUHANI, MD, and NASEEM MORIDZADEH, MD

General Principles

- Acute kidney injury (AKI) mainfests as a decrease in kidney function occuring over a relatively short time period and can be reversible.
- Chronic kidney disease (CKD) manifests as a slow, progressive decline in renal function owing to nephron loss and scarring over the course of months to years.
- CKD is usually irreversible without renal transplantation.
- End-stage renal disease (ESRD) refers to patients in whom renal function has diminished to a point in which life-threatening manifestations can develop if the patient does not receive renal-replacement therapy, either with dialysis or transplantation.
- Acute complications in CKD are usually seen in the setting of superimposed illness, trauma, or other physiologic stress and are commonly associated with electrolyte and other metabolic derangements, symptomatic volume overload, and complications of uremia.
- Management focuses on identification and treatment of the underlying cause of these acute abnormalities in an attempt to return the patient to a stable, compensated state.

Definitions

- CKD is defined by the presence of *kidney damage* or *decreased kidney function* for **3 months or more**. *Kidney damage* is characterized by pathologic abnormalities defined by the presence of one of the following:
  - Albuminuria: this demonstrates increased glomerular permeability and may be associated with widespread endothelial dysfunction as seen in patients with hypertension, diabetes, dyslipidemia, smoking, and obesity. It can be measured with a "spot" urine albumin-to-creatinine ratio (ACR). ACR 30 mg/g or greater is considered abnormally elevated.
  - Urinary sediment abnormalities (i.e., red or white blood cell casts) suggest glomerular injury or tubular inflammation (Table 105.1).
  - Imaging abnormalities (i.e., polycystic kidneys, hydronephrosis, small or echogenic kidneys)
  - Pathologic abnormalities: based on kidney biopsy, may demonstrate glomerular, vascular, or tubulointerstitial disease
  - Kidney transplantation: any patient with a history of kidney transplantation is considered to have "kidney damage," irrespective of markers of kidney damage or biopsy results.
- *Decreased kidney function* is defined as a decreased glomerular filtration rate (GFR) less than 60 mL/min per 1.73 m^2 for more than 3 months with or without the findings of kidney damage listed above. *Kidney failure* is defined as a GFR less than 15 mL/min per 1.73 m^2 *or* treatment by dialysis. This cutoff of GFR less than 60 mL/min defines a patient as having CKD, signifying an increased risk for all-cause and cardiovascular mortality, ESRD, AKI, and CKD progression as compared with those with GFR 60 mL/min per 1.73 m^2 or greater.
  - Definition of CKD involves a time frame of 3 months or more.

TABLE 105.1 *Complications of Chronic Kidney Disease*

Affected System	Cause for Mechanism	Clinical Syndrome
System symptoms	Anemia, inflammation	Fatigue, lassitude
Skin	Hyperparathyroidism, calcium-phosphate deposition	Rash, pruritis, metastatic calcification
Cardiovascular disease	Hypertension, anemia, hyperchomocysteinemia, vascular calcification	Atherosclerosis, heart failure, stroke
Serositis	Unknown	Pericardial or pleural pain and fluid, peritoneal fluid
Gastrointestinal	Unknown	Anorexia, nausea, vomiting, diarrhea, gastrointestinal tract bleeding
Immune system	Leukocyte dysfunction, depressed cellular immunity	Infections
Endocrine	Hypothalamic-pituitary axis dysfunction	Amenorrhea, menorrhagia, impotence, oligospermia, hyperprolactinemia
Neurologic	Unknown	Neuromuscular excitability, cognitive dysfunction progressing to coma, peripheral neuropathy (restless leg syndrome or sensory deficits)

(From Mitch, W. E. (2020). Chronic kidney disease. In L. S. Goldman & A. I. Schafer (Eds.), *Goldman-Cecil medicine* (26th ed., pp. 799–804, Table 121.4). Elsevier Health Sciences.)

- Time frame may be determined by a review of prior measurements or estimates of GFR, albuminuria, proteinuria, urine dipstick, or sediment examinations, or by imaging findings showing reduced kidney volume, reduction in cortical thickness, or presence of multiple renal cysts.
- Another possible means of determining the chronicity is to obtain repeat measurements within and beyond the 3-month time frame in the course of the evaluation and treatment of a patient with kidney disease.

Staging

- Staging of CKD is important in guiding management and risk stratification for progression and complications. Staging is based on (1) cause of disease, (2) six categories of GFR known as the G stages, and (3) three categories of albuminuria known as the A stages.
  - Cause of disease: by identifying the cause of CKD, treatment may be tailored to prevent further injury as well as to determine the risk of complications and the rate of progression. Causes include, but are not limited to, diabetes, drug toxicity, autoimmune disease, urinary tract obstruction, and kidney transplantation.
  - G stages
    - G1: GFR more than 90 mL/min per 1.73 m^2
    - G2: GFR 60 to 89 mL/min per 1.73 m^2
    - G3a: GFR 45 to 59 mL/min per 1.73 m^2
    - G3b: GFR 30 to 44 mL/min per 1.73 m^2
    - G4: GFR 15 to 29 mL/min per 1.73 m^2
    - G5: GFR less than 15 mL/min per 1.73 m^2 or treatment by dialysis
  - Albuminuria
    - A1: ACR less than 30 mg/g (less than 3.4 mg/mmol)
    - A2: ACR 30 to 299 mg/g (3.4 to 34.0 mg/mmol)
    - A3: ACR 300 mg/g or greater (more than 34.0 mg/mmol)
- There is a graded increase in risk for mortality, progression of CKD, and ESRD at higher levels of albuminuria independent of estimated glomerular filtration rate (eGFR).

Pathogenesis

- Chronic kidney disease is the result of progressive destruction of nephrons manifested by a rising creatinine level.
- For every 50% reduction in GFR, the plasma creatinine level will double.
- Causes of CKD can be divided into prerenal, intrinsic renal, and postrenal causes.
  - Prerenal etiologies are typically vascular in nature, such as renal arterial disease and hypertensive nephrosclerosis.
  - Intrinsic renal etiologies can be either glomerular or tubulointerstitial in nature. Glomerular causes include focal sclerosing glomerulonephritis (GN), membranoproliferative GN, membranous GN, crescentic GN, IgA nephropathy, diabetic nephropathy, collagen vascular disease, amyloidosis, postinfectious, and human immunodeficiency virus (HIV) nephropathy. Tubulointerstitial causes include nephrotoxins, analgesic nephropathy, hypercalcemia or nephrocalcinosis, multiple myeloma, reflux nephropathy, sickle nephropathy, chronic pyelonephritis, and tuberculosis.
  - Postrenal causes are obstructive in nature and include nephrolithiasis, ureteral tuberculosis, retroperitoneal fibrosis, retroperitoneal tumors, prostatic obstruction, and congenital abnormalities (Box 105.1).

Clinical Presentation

- In the early stages, CKD is typically asymptomatic.
- As the disease progresses to later stages, symptoms appear in association with complications.
- Manifestations of advancing renal failure include changes in urine volume, anemia, electrolyte disturbances, metabolic acidosis, hypertension, volume overload, and mineral/bone disorders. There can also be increased risk for systemic drug toxicity, infections, cardiovascular diseases, and other forms of end-organ dysfunction.
- Progressive loss of renal function inevitably results in the recognizable clinical syndrome of uremia.
  - Symptoms of uremia include anorexia, nausea/vomiting, bleeding, mental status changes, peripheral neuropathy, and pericarditis.

BOX 105.1 ***Major Causes of Chronic Kidney Disease***

VASCULAR CAUSES

Renal arterial disease
Hypertensive nephrosclerosis

GLOMERULAR CAUSES

Primary glomerulopathies
Focal sclerosing glomerulonephritis (GN)
Membranoproliferative GN
Membranous GN
Crescentic GN
IgA nephropathy
Secondary glomerulopathies
Diabetic nephropathy
Collagen vascular disease
Amyloidosis
Postinfectious
HIV nephropathy

TUBULOINTERSTITIAL CAUSES

Nephrotoxins
Analgesic nephropathy
Hypercalcemia or nephrocalcinosis
Multiple myeloma
Reflux nephropathy
Sickle nephropathy
Chronic pyelonephritis
Tuberculosis

OBSTRUCTIVE CAUSES

Nephrolithiasis
Ureteral tuberculosis
Retroperitoneal fibrosis
Retroperitoneal tumor
Prostatic obstruction
Congenital abnormalities

HEREDITARY CAUSES

Polycystic kidney disease
Alport's syndrome
Medullary cystic disease

HIV, Human immunodeficiency virus; *IgA*, immunoglobulin A.
(From Wolfson, A. B. (2018). Renal failure. In R. M. Walls, R. S. Hockberger, & M. Gausche-Hill (Eds.), *Rosen's emergency medicine: Concepts and clinical practice* (9th ed., pp. 1179–1196.e1, Box 87.6). Elsevier.)

- Patients may present with hypertension, signs of volume overload, uremic "frost" (white powder on skin owing to deposition of urea), signs of pericarditis, and encephalopathy.
- Although uremia usually correlates with a reduction in GFR to below 15%–20% of normal, the serum blood urea nitrogen (BUN) or creatinine concentrations do not necessarily correlate with the development of this syndrome.
- Once uremic, renal replacement therapy with either hemodialysis, peritoneal dialysis, or renal transplantation is required.

- Uremia can affect multiple organ systems.
  - The cardiovascular system is among the most commonly affected. Cardiovascular complications include chronic volume overload, hyperlipidemia, and myocardial ischemia and infarction. Pericarditis with or without a pericardial effusion is also a common cardiovascular manifestation of CKD, particularly in patients who have not received dialysis.
  - Uremic pleuritis, with or without pleural effusions, can be seen as well, along with pulmonary edema in a "batwing" perihilar appearance on plain radiograph.
  - Neurologic manifestations of uremia include lethargy, altered mental status, asterixis, myoclonic twitching, and seizures.
  - Gastrointestinal effects are commonly seen in the form of anorexia, nausea, and vomiting.
  - Uremia leads to immunosuppression resulting in increased susceptibility to infections, because both humoral and cellular immunity are inhibited.
  - A normocytic, normochromic anemia develops owing to decreased erythropoietin production in the kidneys.
  - Uremia is also associated with decreased platelet function and altered von Willebrand factor resulting in bleeding complications.
  - Metabolic disturbances are prominent and manifest as electrolyte derangements most commonly with potassium, calcium, and phosphorus (see Table 105.1).

Diagnosis and Evaluation

- Many patients who come to the emergency department will already carry the diagnosis of CKD or ESRD.
- Initial laboratory evaluation demonstrating an elevated BUN and creatinine level should be compared with prior values.
- A chronic elevation for 3 months or more helps to establish the diagnosis.
- Other clues may include small, atrophic kidneys on imaging, although the lack of this finding does not exclude the diagnosis.
- ED evaluation of a patient with CKD in the emergency department should first focus on the serious, life-threatening complications associated with this illness.
- Asses for evidence of end-organ complications and laboratory analysis to assess for electrolyte and acid–base abnormalities.
- An electrocardiogram may also be helpful in determining changes associated with specific electrolyte (e.g., potassium) or metabolic disturbances.

BOX 105.2 ***Reversible Factors and Treatable Causes of Chronic Kidney Disease***

REVERSIBLE FACTORS

Hypovolemia
Congestive heart failure
Pericardial tamponade
Severe hypertension
Catabolic state, protein loads
Nephrotoxic agents
Obstructive disease
Reflux disease

TREATABLE CAUSES

Renal artery stenosis
Malignant hypertension
Acute interstitial nephritis
Hypercalcemic nephropathy
Multiple myeloma
Vasculitis (e.g., systemic lupus erythematosus, Wegener's granulomatosis, polyarteritis nodosa)
Obstructive nephropathy
Reflux nephropathy

(From Wolfson, A. B. (2018). Renal failure. In R. M. Walls, R. S. Hockberger, & M. Gausche-Hill (Eds.), *Rosen's emergency medicine: Concepts and clinical practice* (9th ed., pp. 1179–1196.e1, Box 87.7). Elsevier.)

Treatment

- Addressing life-threatening and/or potentially reversible complications, such as volume overload, pericardial tamponade, metabolic derangements, acid-base disorders, electrolyte disturbances, such as hyperkalemia, and severe hypertension.
- Treat reversible causes of AKI, superimposed on CKD, disease attempting to slow progression, and prepare patients for renal replacement therapy. See Box 105.2 for reversible factors and treatable causes of CKD.
- Acute bleeding can be managed with desmopressin (DDAVP) (stimulates release of vWF from endothelial cells), cryoprecipitate, and conjugated estrogens.
- Symptomatic or life-threatening anemia can be treated with transfusion of packed red blood cells.
- Emergent hemodialysis should be initiated for severe metabolic acidosis, severe hyperkalemia or hypercalcemia, refractory volume overload, advanced uremia, and specific toxic ingestions.

105

SUGGESTED READINGS

Brady, W. J., & Sudhir, A. (2013). Renal failure. In J. G. Adams, E. D. Barton, J. L. Collings, P. M. C. DeBlieux, M. A. Gisondi, & E. S. Nadel (Eds.). *Emergency medicine: Clinical essentials* (2nd ed.). Elsevier Health Sciences.

Mitch, W. E. (2019). Chronic kidney disease. In L. S. Goldman & A. I. Schafer (Eds.), *Goldman-Cecil medicine* (26th ed.). Elsevier Health Sciences.

Wolfson, A. B. (2018). Renal failure. In R. M. Walls, R. S. Hockberger, & M. Gausche-Hill (Eds.). *Rosen's emergency medicine: Concepts and clinical practice* (9th ed.). Elsevier.

CHAPTER 106

BOARD REVIEW

Dialysis-Related Emergencies

CAMERON W. HARRISON, MD, and AMIR A. ROUHANI, MD

General Principles

- Dialysis is the process of removing waste products and excess fluid from the body.
- Despite the successes of dialysis as a life-sustaining therapy in the treatment of kidney disease, certain complications can arise that may require evaluation and management in the emergency department (ED).
- Any patient who is on dialysis is at risk, not only from the direct complications of dialysis, but also from complications arising from underlying kidney disease, especially for those that dialysis is unable to correct.
- The two major modalities most commonly used for dialysis are **hemodialysis** and **peritoneal dialysis**.
  - Hemodialysis involves an extracorporeal dialyzer circuit in which the patient's heparinized blood travels through at a high flow rate, allowing the diffusion of solutes and fluid.
  - Peritoneal dialysis
    - Involves infusing sterile dialysis fluid into the peritoneal cavity through a catheter (i.e., Tenckhoff catheter).
    - Dialysis fluid has large amounts of glucose that causes a large osmotic gradient, which forces fluid and solutes from the bloodstream to cross the peritoneal membrane into the peritoneum, where they are then removed by the catheter.
- Each of these processes comes with its own unique complications.

Hemodialysis-Related Emergencies

DIALYSIS DISEQUILIBRIUM SYNDROME

Clinical Presentation

- Dialysis disequilibrium syndrome (DDS) occurs when there are rapid decreases in plasma serum urea nitrogen concentration and other solutes during dialysis.
- Results in cerebral edema and increased intracranial pressure.
- Severity of illness can range from mild disease (i.e., nausea, headache, and muscle cramping) to severe disease (i.e., confusion, seizures, and coma).

Diagnosis, Evaluation, and Treatment

- DDS is a diagnosis of exclusion and all patients who present with mental status or central nervous system changes should be evaluated for other causes such as cerebrovascular accident, intracranial hemorrhage, infection, electrolyte disturbances, and metabolic acidosis.
- Appropriate laboratory and imaging studies should be considered, such as complete blood count (CBC), basic metabolic panel (BMP), blood cultures, chest radiograph, and computed tomography of the brain.
- DDS usually resolves after discontinuation of hemodialysis. In severe cases, hypertonic therapy, such as hypertonic saline or mannitol, can be used to manage central nervous system effects.

HYPOTENSION

Clinical Presentation

- Hypotension is the most common complication associated with hemodialysis.
- Cause may be multifactorial, but often due to hypovolemia from excess ultrafiltration.
- Risk of hypotension is much greater with hemodialysis than peritoneal dialysis.
- The presentation of hemodialysis-associated hypotension may range from asymptomatic to symptoms of dizziness, nausea/vomiting, chest pain, and other nonspecific symptoms.
- On examination, patients may exhibit signs of decreased end-organ perfusion.

Diagnosis, Evaluation, and Treatment

- Evaluation of hypotension should involve consideration of medication side effects, sepsis, blood loss, decreased intake, gastrointestinal losses, cardiac complications, anaphylaxis, thromboembolic disease, and air embolism.
- A broad workup that includes laboratory testing and diagnostic imaging should be considered in patients who do not respond immediately to supportive care.
- Management of dialysis-associated hypotension usually responds to intravenous fluid administration.

AIR EMBOLISM

Clinical Presentation

- Air embolism occurs when air bubbles become trapped at any systemic site in the body, resulting in ischemia and end-organ compromise.
- May result in cerebral ischemia, respiratory failure, and circulatory collapse.
- Given modern safeguards employed during hemodialysis sessions, this complication is exceedingly rare and is generally iatrogenic.
- Symptoms may include chest pain, shortness of breath, and syncope.

- Signs include hypoxia, hypotension, altered mental status, respiratory compromise, and cardiovascular collapse.

Diagnosis and Evaluation

- Diagnostic testing in patients with suspected air embolism involves evaluating for end-organ effects.
- Pertinent laboratory testing may involve blood gas analysis, troponin, and B-type natriuretic peptide (BNP). Imaging studies such as chest radiograph and bedside echocardiography may be obtained.
- Advanced imaging with contrast-enhanced CT can be helpful depending on the organ-system involved.

Treatment

- Administer oxygen.
- Patients may be placed in the left lateral decubitus position (Durant maneuver) and Trendelenburg positions to prevent air from traveling to the right side of the heart and pulmonary arteries.
- All catheters should be clamped.
- Vasopressors and mechanical ventilation may be necessary in severe cases.
- Catheter aspiration may be considered. Direct aspiration from the right ventricle can be attempted if the patient decompensates.
- Hyperbaric treatment can also be considered if available.

HEMOLYSIS

Clinical Presentation

- Hemolysis as a result of hemodialysis can be caused by shear stress from high flow rates through the dialysis apparatus, hyperthermia from warming of blood during dialysis, damage from irregularities in tubing, and osmotic changes.
- In addition to direct effects on red blood cells, complications related to electrolyte disturbances, such as hyperkalemia, can occur.
- Severe hemolysis usually presents with nausea, shortness of breath, abdominal/back pain, and chills. Physical examination may be associated with tachycardia, hypertension, and signs of cardiopulmonary and neurologic compromise.

Diagnosis, Evaluation, and Treatment

- Diagnostic evaluation involves CBC, BMP, haptoglobin, type and screen, peripheral smear, and other hemolysis laboratory tests.
- Electrocardiography (ECG) may be helpful in evaluating for electrolyte and metabolic disturbances.
- Initial management involves immediate discontinuation of hemodialysis until the underlying cause of hemolysis is identified. In severe cases, transfusion of packed red blood cells may be required.

ANAPHYLAXIS

Clinical Presentation

- Patients with end-stage renal disease (ESRD) may be exposed to various allergens, increasing the risk for the development of anaphylaxis.
- Examples of potential allergens are heparin, disinfectants, iron, antibiotics, and dialyzer components.
- Patients with anaphylaxis may present with symptoms of pruritus, urticaria, nausea/vomiting, and dyspnea. On examination, patients may show signs of hemodynamic instability, angioedema, skin changes, and respiratory compromise, such as wheezing and stridor.

Diagnosis, Evaluation, and Treatment

- Diagnosis of anaphylaxis is made clinically, and evaluation should involve the performance of a thorough history and physical examination to determine the presence of skin, mucosal, gastrointestinal, cardiac, pulmonary, and other end-organ involvement.
- Laboratory and radiographic studies are generally not required to make this diagnosis and should not delay management.
- Initial management involves prompt administration of intramuscular epinephrine.
- Adjunctive therapy may involve intravenous corticosteroids and antihistamines. In severe cases, patients may require vasopressors and/or mechanical ventilation.

HYPERKALEMIA

Clinical Presentation

- Hyperkalemia may occur as a result of dietary indiscretion, medication-related complications, and/or inadequate dialysis from patient noncompliance or vascular access dysfunction.
- Patients are often asymptomatic, but may present with muscle weakness or paralysis, dyspnea, or other cardiovascular signs or symptoms.

Diagnosis, Evaluation, and Treatment

- All patients with ESRD on hemodialysis presenting to the ED should have an ECG to evaluate for characteristic changes associated with hyperkalemia.
- In addition, BMP, magnesium, and phosphorus levels should be determined.
- Detailed management of hyperkalemia is discussed elsewhere, but generally involves administration of insulin and glucose, albuterol, bicarbonate, diuretics (if not anuric), and zirconium cyclosilicate. Calcium in the form of calcium gluconate or calcium chloride should be given for serious ECG changes (e.g., widening of the QRS interval).
- Definitive management involves nephrology department consultation for emergent hemodialysis.

CHEST PAIN

Clinical Presentation

- Chest pain is a common complaint in ESRD patients seen in the ED and may be due complications of medical comorbidities, manifestations of ESRD, and/or complications of dialysis.
- The etiology of chest pain in this patient population may be cardiac ischemia, pericarditis, aortic dissection, thromboembolic disease, and rib fractures from renal osteodystrophy.

- Many patients on dialysis for ESRD have either coronary artery disease or comorbidities that place them at high risk for coronary artery disease.
- The clinical presentation varies depending on the underlying etiology of chest pain, but onset of pain may occur during or shortly after dialysis sessions.
- Common symptoms associated with chest pain include shortness of breath, back pain, jaw pain, arm numbness, or other nonspecific symptoms.
- Clinical signs are specific to the underlying etiology. For example, a patient with pericarditis with cardiac tamponade will present with hypotension, a narrow pulse pressure, muffled heart sounds, and jugular venous distension.

Diagnosis, Evaluation, and Treatment

- Evaluation involves appropriate history and physical examination.
- An ECG should be obtained to evaluate for ischemic changes.
- Laboratory analysis may include CBC, BMP, troponin, and BNP. A chest radiograph can aid in evaluating for specific cardiopulmonary disease.
- A bedside echocardiogram is useful to evaluate for changes such as cardiac tamponade and right ventricular dysfunction.
- Treatment involves rapid identification and management of the underlying cause of pain. For example, pericardiocentesis and subsequent pericardiectomy may be required for cardiac tamponade.

HYPERTENSION

Clinical Presentation

- Hypertension is a common problem in patients with ESRD and is typically managed in the outpatient setting.
- Rarely, a rapid rise in blood pressure can lead to acute end-organ dysfunction, resulting in a hypertensive emergency. These patients may present with vision changes, chest pain, dyspnea, nausea/vomiting, headache, and altered mental status.
- Physical examination may be significant for papilledema, changes in level of consciousness and orientation, focal neurologic abnormalities, and pulmonary edema.

Diagnosis and Evaluation

- Evaluation should involve laboratory and radiographic tests to evaluate for acute end-organ damage.
- This may include CBC, BMP, troponin, BNP, urinalysis, and chest radiograph.
- CT and/or magnetic resonance imaging of the brain may be warranted if significant neurologic symptoms are present.

Treatment

- Management of hypertensive emergency involves gradually lowering blood pressure by approximately 15% of mean arterial pressure in the first hour.
- Hypertension in ESRD patients may be extremely difficult to manage medically because this condition may be related to the volume status of the patient. In these cases, urgent dialysis is needed.

Hemodialysis Vascular Access Complications

- Effective hemodialysis requires vascular access that is able to withstand high flow rates.
- Common forms of vascular access include arteriovenous fistulas, vascular grafts, and tunneled catheters. Each of these are prone to specific complications.

THROMBOSIS

Clinical Presentation

- Thrombosis can occur in arteriovenous fistulas and grafts and may result spontaneously or occur iatrogenically. Care should always be taken to avoid obtaining blood pressures from and applying tourniquets to the extremity with the vascular access site.
- Thrombosis should be managed expeditiously to avoid permanent loss of access.
- Thrombosis involving vascular access site usually presents with an inability to complete dialysis. The access site may become firm over time and the vascular thrill may be decreased or absent.

Diagnosis, Evaluation, and Treatment

- Evaluation of thrombosis of the vascular access site involves a detailed examination and confirmatory imaging, generally involving Doppler ultrasonography.
- If there is a high level of concern for thrombosis, confirmatory testing should not delay consultation with a vascular surgeon.
- Emergent vascular surgery consultation should be initiated.
- Definitive therapy involves thrombectomy. Rarely, thrombolytics may be used.

ACCESS SITE INFECTIONS

Clinical Presentation

- Infection is the most common complication of dialysis access catheters.
- Infection generally occurs when bacteria seed the vascular access and gain access to the bloodstream. This is why venous puncture of dialysis access sites is generally avoided.
- Presentations may range from indolent and subtle to rapidly progressive systemic disease, such as sepsis.
- Patients may present with fevers, chills, and pain at the vascular access site.
- Physical examination may reveal signs of local infection as well as clinical signs of sepsis.

Diagnosis, Evaluation, and Treatment

- Initial evaluation involves a detailed history and physical examination to determine the source of infection.
- Diagnostic workup should involve evaluation for sepsis, including CBC, BMP, lactate, and blood cultures (including from access site).
- Initial treatment involves management of sepsis and administration of empiric antibiotic therapy.

BLEEDING INVOLVING VASCULAR ACCESS SITE

Clinical Presentation

- Bleeding involving dialysis access sites can be significant and difficult to control and may be caused by needle dislodgement during dialysis, complications of pseudoaneurysm, and erosion or ulceration.
- Bleeding may be further complicated by anemia and platelet dysfunction commonly associated with ESRD.
- Patients may present with slow oozing or brisk, life-threatening hemorrhage.

Diagnosis and Evaluation

- The diagnosis is typically made clinically, and evaluation focuses on evaluation of anemia and coagulopathy.
- Laboratory analysis may include CBC, BMP, prothrombin time/international normalized ratio, and partial thromboplastin time. Blood should also be sent for type and crossmatch in serious cases that may require transfusion.

Treatment

- Initial management involves attempting to achieve hemostasis by applying firm, manual pressure. A pressure dressing may be applied.
- Emergent vascular surgery consultation should be obtained for serious or life-threatening bleeding.
- Underlying coagulopathy, thrombocytopenia, and/or platelet dysfunction should also be addressed.

Peritoneal Dialysis-Related Emergencies

PERITONITIS

General Principles

- Infection and peritonitis are common complications of peritoneal dialysis.
- The catheter acts as a foreign body connecting the external environment and skin surface to the peritoneal cavity and carries an increased risk of seeding bacteria that may result in an infection.
- Infection is usually caused by gram-positive bacteria, and *Staphylococcus aureus* and *S. epidermidis* are the most common.
- Infection can also result from gram-negative bacteria and fungi.
- A small percentage of infections may be culture-negative.

Clinical Presentation

- Patients may present with fever, abdominal pain, cloudy peritoneal fluid, nausea/vomiting, and sepsis.

Diagnosis, Evaluation, and Treatment

- Evaluation involves sampling peritoneal fluid for cell count and Gram stain and culture. Infection is suggested by the presence of **>100 white blood cells or >50 neutrophil cells/mm^3**.
- Treatment generally involves intraperitoneal antibiotics.
- Empiric treatment with vancomycin AND ceftazidime *or* cefepime *or* gentamicin is recommended until culture results return.

CELLULITIS

Clinical Presentation

- Cellulitis and other skin or soft tissue infections can occur in or around the catheter tunnel and is commonly due to leakage from the catheter itself.
- Patients may present with warmth, erythema, pain, and discharge in or around the catheter site.

Diagnosis, Evaluation, and Treatment

- Evaluation involves Gram stain and culture of any purulent exudate and evaluation for systemic infection.
- Management involves empiric antibiotic treatment with appropriate coverage for skin flora. Cephalexin is considered first-line therapy. If purulence is noted, trimethoprim-sulfamethoxazole may be used.

Other Complications of Peritoneal Dialysis

- Malfunction or obstruction of the peritoneal catheter is another complication associated with peritoneal dialysis. It is important to distinguish these peritoneal dialysis cathter-related issues from decreased flow, which may be secondary to constipation and is easily treatable. True catheter dysfunction may require urgent surgical and nephrology consultation.
- Perforated viscus can also occur and may be due to traumatic puncture of the bowel by the peritoneal catheter. Treatment involves emergent surgical consultation for operative intervention.

106

SUGGESTED READINGS

Chang, Y., & Gilbert, G. H. (2013). Dialysis-related emergencies. In J. G. Adams, E. D. Barton, J. L. Collings, P. M. C. DeBlieux, M. A. Gisondi, & E. S. Nadel (Eds.), *Emergency medicine: Clinical essentials* (2nd ed., pp. 1003–1010). Elsevier.

Wolfson, A. B. (2018). Renal failure. In R. M. Walls, R. S. Hockberger, & M. Gausche-Hill (Eds.), *Rosen's emergency medicine: Concepts and clinical practice* (9th ed., pp. 1179–1196). Elsevier.

CHAPTER **107**

BOARD REVIEW

Renal Transplant Emergencies

JOSHUA J. BAUGH, MD, MPP, MHCM, and ADAM R. EVANS, MD

- Kidneys are the most commonly transplanted organ in the United States: there are more than 20,000 renal transplants per year. Consequently, the number of related visits to the emergency department (ED) has grown substantially in the past few decades.
- Complications of organ transplantation present a unique set of challenges to the emergency physician. One key consideration is time from transplantation, which is often divided into three periods: early (<1 month), intermediate (1–6 months), and late (>6 months).
- Across these time periods, there are a wide variety of complications related to solid organ transplantation, including surgical complications, infections, organ rejection, immunosuppressant regimens (side effects and increased cardiovascular risk), and malignancy.
- Anatomic and physiologic variations that result from transplantation may also change the presentation of common diseases. A primary goal of the emergency physician is to identify and treat transplant-specific complications (Table 107.1).

Infections

General Principles

- Infection is a common complication in renal transplant patients and is most common during the first 6 months after transplant surgery (i.e., when the immunosuppressant doses are the highest).
- Although immunosuppressant drugs dramatically decrease the incidence of graft rejection, they also increase the risk of infection. Immunosuppression alters clinical presentations of many infectious diseases and often makes the signs and symptoms of their presentations atypical or more subtle.
- A wide variety of opportunistic organisms cause infection as a result of immunosuppression and they can escalate and spread rapidly.
- Many patients take prophylactic antimicrobial or antiviral medications, such as trimethoprim-sulfamethoxazole and acyclovir, which lower, but do not eliminate, the risk of infection.
- Definitive diagnosis is often delayed because serologic testing or invasive procedures may be required to identify specific infections. Therefore, rapid initiation of intravenous fluids as tolerated and broad-spectrum antibiotics is an essential step in emergency management if infection is suspected.

Clinical Presentation

- Fever occurs in up to half of transplant patients with an infection, but lack of fever does not exclude an infectious etiology.
- Pain in a specific area without fever should often prompt an infectious workup because immunosuppression can mask the typical presentation of common infections.
- Overall, bacterial infections are the most common. Infections to consider are based on the posttransplant time period.

Early (<1 Month)

- Nosocomial infections: pneumonia, urinary tract infection, vascular access infection, *Clostridium difficile* colitis
- Surgical site infections (i.e., *Staphylococcus*, *Streptococcus*, *Escherichia coli*) and superinfection of graft tissue
- Donor-derived infections
  - Bacteria: methicillin-resistant *S. aureus*, vancomycin-resistant enterococcus, *Mycobacterium tuberculosis*
  - Fungi (*Candida* spp.) or parasites (toxoplasmosis)

Intermediate (1–6 Months)

- During this time, viremia and opportunistic infections predominate, and the latter occurs in up to 25% of all renal transplant patients. Organisms are often hospital-specific and include a wide variety of bacteria, mycobacteria, fungal, and parasitic organisms.
- Cytomegalovirus (CMV) is an infection common to all transplanted organ patients and results in high fever and organ-specific (i.e., pulmonary, gastrointestinal, central nervous system) symptoms with invasive disease.
- There can also be a reactivation of dormant host infections (i.e., cytomegalovirus, varicella-zoster virus, herpes simplex virus, and Epstein-Barr virus) and surgical site infections.

Late (>6 Months)

- In this time period, community-acquired infections and respiratory viruses predominate.

Diagnosis and Evaluation

- Laboratory tests should be obtained for all febrile renal transplant patients. If there is no apparent source, one can start with urinalysis with urine culture, chest radiograph, blood cultures, lactate, complete blood count with differential, and electrolyte panel with serum creatinine.
- Detailed studies should be sent based on suspected source from history and physical examination (e.g., cerebrospinal fluid analysis for suspected meningitis, stool studies for suspected infectious colitis, etc.).
- Serologic tests and tissue biopsy are often required to guide inpatient therapy and provide a definitive diagnosis.

TABLE 107.1 ***Differential Diagnosis of Early Renal Transplant Complications***

Surgical Complications	Vascular Complications	Graft Complications
Perinephric hematoma	Renal artery stenosis	Acute tubular necrosis from prolonged graft ischemic time
Lymphocele	Renal artery thrombosis	Graft rejection
Wound infection	Renal vein thrombosis	Graft infection
Ureteral stenosis		Medication toxicity
Urinary leak		

- Biopsy is not practical to obtain in the ED and many serologic results are unlikely to return within the timeframe of the ED visit (i.e., specific markers of infection), so ED treatment is often empiric.
- Imaging of the suspected site of infection should be performed in most cases, and evaluation may also include Doppler ultrasonography of the transplanted kidney.

Treatment

- For all febrile patients with signs of sepsis, severe sepsis, or septic shock, initiate intravenous (IV) fluid resuscitation and broad-spectrum antibiotics.
- Consider antiviral and antifungal medications when appropriate, particularly if patients are not taking prophylactic agents.
- Corticosteroids (i.e., hydrocortisone 50–100 mg IV) should be given to severely ill renal transplant patients receiving chronic steroid therapy to prevent acute adrenal insufficiency.
- Consultation with a transplant specialist should occur in all cases if feasible. An infectious disease consultation may be considered as well.
- Most patients will be admitted unless the transplant team prefers discharge with close follow-up.

Graft Rejection

General Principles

- Renal graft rejection is a significant cause of transplant dysfunction and loss.
- Although modern immunosuppressive medication regimens have decreased the incidence of this complication, it is prudent to consider renal graft rejection in all transplant patients presenting to the ED.
- In a renal transplant patient with a history of diabetes, the most common cause of graft rejection and death is cardiovascular disease.

Clinical Presentation

- A variety of cellular mechanisms lead to distinctive patterns of graft rejection, which can occur at different times: hyperacute (minutes to hours), acute (first 6 months), or chronic (months to years).
- Patients may also present with a spectrum of symptoms. Patients can be asymptomatic, with rejection found only on routine biopsy. Patients can also present with nonspecific symptoms (i.e., fever, malaise) or with graft pain and tenderness over the graft site.
- Be aware that fever can be a symptom of both infection and graft rejection. It is important to investigate and treat for both possibilities simultaneously.
- It is also important to pay particular attention to hypertension and decreased urine output (oliguria) because these can be signs of renal graft rejection.

Diagnosis and Evaluation

- Laboratory testing may demonstrate a rise in serum creatinine, and electrolyte abnormalities (i.e., uremia, hyperkalemia) may be present.
- Ultrasound imaging may demonstrate increased graft size, loss of the corticomedullary junction, prominent hypoechoic pyramids, and elevated vascular resistance indices in graft rejection.
- Graft biopsy is usually not indicated in the ED, but is required for definitive diagnosis.

Treatment

- Treatment of graft rejection is typically made in conjunction with renal transplant service consultation in the inpatient setting, with the mainstay of treatment being high-dose corticosteroids (i.e., methylprednisolone 500–1000 mg IV).

Drug Toxicity

General Principles

- Renal transplant patients require lifelong immunosuppression to prevent graft rejection.
- Medication regimens are divided into two phases: induction (period of highest incidence of rejection) and maintenance.
- Maintenance therapy consists of an initial three-drug regimen that is then tapered down to two drugs to limit medication side effects. Often the agent removed is a steroid.
- All immunosuppressants increase the risk for opportunistic infections and certain cancers, such as lymphoma, cervical cancer, and skin cancer.
- Each medication class also has its own unique set of side effects (Table 107.2).
- Newer biologic agents, such as monoclonal and polyclonal antibodies, are better tolerated overall, but introduce the risk of serum sickness and anaphylaxis.

Clinical Presentation

- Immunosuppressant medications contribute to the development of infections and malignancies that lead to ED presentations. Medication side effects can also become the primary reason for an ED visit.
- The presence of any new coagulopathy, liver or renal dysfunction, central nervous system disturbance, or electrolyte imbalance should prompt the provider to consider the role of medication side effects and toxicity.
- Common medication side effects are listed in Table 107.2. There are myriad medication interactions that may affect immunosuppressant drug levels.

Diagnosis and Evaluation

- A thorough history, medication review, and physical examination all remain paramount.

TABLE 107.2 Common Immunosuppressant Medications and Side Effects

Drug	Side Effects
Azathioprine	Bone marrow suppression, hepatotoxicity, pancreatitis
Cyclosporine[a]	Nephrotoxicity (acute or chronic), electrolyte derangements (e.g., hyperkalemia), neurotoxicity, hepatotoxicity
Mycophenolate	GI symptoms (abdominal pain, nausea, vomiting, diarrhea), bone marrow suppression
Tacrolimus	Similar to cyclosporine BUT prominent *neurotoxicity* (headache, tremor, seizures)
Sirolimus	Pancytopenia, interstitial pneumonitis
Biologics (mono- and polyclonal antibodies)	Fever, serum sickness, anaphylaxis, anemia, thrombocytopenia
Corticosteroids	Weight gain, Cushingoid appearance, GI bleeding, avascular necrosis, psychologic effects

[a]Calcineurin inhibitors such as cyclosporine have multiple drug-drug interactions.
GI, gastrointestinal.

- Drug levels can be obtained for tacrolimus and sirolimus.
- Laboratory testing, such as complete blood count, serum creatinine, liver function tests, and coagulation assays, may provide clues about drug toxicity, but the diagnosis is largely clinical.

Treatment

- Acute management of drug toxicity is largely supportive because commonly used agents do not have specific antidotes.
- Long-term management may involve dose reduction, switching immunosuppressant classes, or modifying other medications to reduce drug-drug interactions.
- Changes in the immunosuppressant regimen should only be made in conjunction with specialist consultation.

Surgical Complications

General Principles

- There are unique surgical complications of the renal graft itself that occur in addition to general transplant complications, such as infection, rejection, and drug toxicity.
- Most of these complications occur within the immediate postoperative period, although they can occur up to 3 months post transplantation.
- Surgical anastomotic sites, including the renal vessels and the ureter, are at particular risk for stenosis and obstruction.
- Mass effect from hematomas and lymphoceles can compromise graft function as well.

Clinical Presentation

- The clinical presentation varies, owing to the underlying surgical complications.
  - Renal artery or vein occlusion: oliguria or acute anuria, pain and erythema over graft site, abdominal pain, nausea and vomiting
  - Renal artery stenosis: oliguria, hypertension, and peripheral edema
  - Peritransplant hematoma: pain over graft site, decrease in hemoglobin/hematocrit, rise in serum creatinine
  - Urinary leak: disruption of the graft ureter at urinary bladder leads to urine extravasation; can cause acute renal failure
  - Lymphocele: leaking lymphatics leading to a peritransplant fluid collection, causing pain over graft site, acute renal failure, ipsilateral lower extremity edema
  - Obstructive uropathy: obstruction of ureter by ureteral stenosis or mass effect from lymphocele or hematoma, causing acute renal failure ± pain and swelling at graft site
  - Bleeding after biopsy: obstructive uropathy due to blockage of bladder outlet or ureter by a blood clot; may cause hematuria

Diagnosis and Evalaution

- Evaluation and testing may also vary based on the suspected surgical complication.
  - Chemistry panel assessing renal function and electrolytes (signs of renal failure)
  - Complete blood count to assess for hemoglobin and hematocrit (hematoma, postbiopsy bleed)
  - Urinalysis to assess for hematuria, proteinuria (signs of renal failure)
  - Renal ultrasonography (urinary leak, lymphocele, hematoma, obstructive uropathy)
  - Doppler ultrasonography (renal artery or vein occlusion)
  - Computerized tomography (peritransplant hematoma, lymphocele, urinary leak)

Treatment

- Treatment is directed toward the specific etiology found on diagnostic workup and should be chosen in consultation with the patient's urologist and transplant nephrologist.
  - Surgical exploration (renal artery/vein thrombosis, hematoma, urinary leak, lymphocele)
  - Percutaneous transluminal angioplasty (renal artery stenosis)
  - Percutaneous drainage (lymphocele, hematoma)
  - Percutaneous nephrostomy tube + ureteral stent (obstructive uropathy)
  - Transfusion + angiographic occlusion of bleeding vessel (biopsy-related bleeding)

SUGGESTED READINGS

Aktas, S., Boyvat, F., Sevmis, S., Moray, G., Karakayali, H., & Haberal, M. (2011). Analysis of vascular complications after renal transplantation. *Transplantation Proceedings*, *43*(2), 557–561.

Fishman, J. A. (2007, December 20). Infection in solid-organ transplant recipients. *The New England Journal of Medicine*, *357*(25), 2601–2614.

Hamandi, B., Husain, S., Humar, A., & Papadimitropoulos, E. A. (2014, October 15). Impact of infectious disease consultation on the clinical and economic outcomes of solid organ transplant recipients admitted for infectious complications. *Clinical Infectious Diseases*, *59*(8), 1074–1082.

Long, B., & Koyfman, A. (2016, November). The emergency medicine approach to transplant complications. *American Journal of Emergency Medicine*, *34*(11), 2200–2208.

Sugi, M. D., Albadawi, H., Knuttinen, G., Naidu, S. G., Mathur, A. K., Moss, A. A., & Oklu, R. (2017). Transplant artery thrombosis and outcomes. *Cardiovascular Diagnosis and Therapy*, *7*(Suppl. 3), S219.

Turtay, M. G., Oğuztürk, H., Aydın, C., Colak, C., Işık, B., & Yılmaz, S. (2012, March). A descriptive analysis of 188 liver transplant patient visits to an emergency department. *European Review for Medical and Pharmacological Sciences*, *16*(Suppl. 1), 3–7.

United States Renal Data System. (2015). 2015 USRDS annual data report: Epidemiology of kidney disease in the United States. National Institutes of Health, National Institute of Diabetes and Digestive and Kidney Diseases.

Venkat, K. K., & Venkat, A. (2004, October). Care of the renal transplant recipient in the emergency department. *Annals of Emergency Medicine*, *44*(4), 330–341.

CHAPTER **108**

BOARD REVIEW

Nephrolithiasis

VANESSA CAMILLE KREGER, MD, MPH, and ANDREW GROCK, MD

- Kidney stones are a common cause of emergency department visits for abdominal pain with a prevalence of 6%–12%.
- Kidney stones occur more often in Caucasians than in African Americans, and more commonly in men.
- Various conditions, such as diabetes, obesity, hyperparathyroidism, and gout, increase the risk of developing renal stones, as does the use of certain medications (i.e., indinavir and carbonic anhydrase inhibitors).
- Additionally, a history of nephrolithiasis increases the risk of recurrence with 10-year rates up to 50%.
- Kidney stones typically develop as a result of supersaturation of salts in the kidneys. Stones are predominately composed of calcium (oxalate or phosphate) salts, as well as struvite, uric acid, and cystine. Small variations in urine saturation, pH, and crystal concentration can contribute to kidney stone formation.

Clinical Presentation

- Clinical symptoms relate to stone location. Stones forming in the kidney are typically asymptomatic (patients may be diagnosed with nephrolithiasis when an imaging examination is performed for other reasons), whereas stones that enter the ureter result in severe waxing and waning pain from ureteral inflammation, prostaglandin release, and ureteral dilatation.
- Therefore patients typically present with significant distress from acute onset, colicky abdominal pain, often involving the flank, lower abdomen, or groin. Patients are classically unable to find a position of comfort, in contrast to patients with acute appendicitis or peritonitis, who classically maintain a rigid posture to minimize movement and thus pain.
- Hematuria is sometimes not a reliable indicator of the presence of stones, because in up to 15% of cases there are no microscopic red blood cells on urinalysis.
- Concomitant urinary tract infection (UTI) can also occur and patients can present with symptoms of pyelonephritis or sepsis.

Diagnosis and Evaluation

- The differential diagnosis for abdominal or flank pain should be broad and include numerous potentially life-threatening diseases (Table 108.1).
- Nephrolithiasis is diagnosed by both clinical gestalt and imaging.
- A low-radiation-dose noncontrast computed tomography (CT) scan of the abdomen and pelvis is the most specific and sensitive imaging modality. However, even low-radiation CT exposes patients to ionizing radiation and it may be prudent to avoid CT imaging in young (age ≤50 years), otherwise healthy patients with a history of ureterolithiasis, presenting with symptoms consistent with uncomplicated renal colic.
- Alternatively, ultrasonography can evaluate for hydronephrosis (nephrolithiasis-induced obstruction) and for other such pathologies as cholecystitis and abdominal aortic aneurysms. Ultrasonography rarely, however, identifies exact location and/or stone size, both of which are important prognostic factors in predicting likelihood of and time to stone passage.
- Therefore the choice of imaging should be tailored to the clinical presentation and risk factors.
- A urinalysis to evaluate for a concurrent UTI and pregnancy testing in women of childbearing age is recommended.
- Although often obtained, a serum creatinine test is not strongly recommended unless the patient has unilateral or horseshoe kidneys, a renal allograft, clinical dehydration from emesis, baseline kidney disease, or stones not passed for more than 1 month.

Treatment

- The mainstay of treatment is symptom control.
- Pain control can be achieved by nonsteroidal antiinflammatory drugs such as ketorolac because these inhibit prostaglandin synthesis and reduce ureteral spasm.
  - Nonsteroidal antiinflammatory drugs may be contraindicated in those with an allergy, underlying kidney disease, or history of a gastrointestinal bleed, or in the elderly.
- Second-line treatment may include other such modalities as acetaminophen, intravenous lidocaine, opiates, or low-dose ketamine.
- Nausea is routinely treated with antiemetics, such as ondansetron or metoclopramide.
- If the patient is clinically volume depleted, intravenous fluids may be indicated.
- UTIs should be treated with antibiotics.
- Patients may be discharged if their pain is adequately controlled and there is no evidence of a UTI with an obstructing stone.
- Kidney stones ≤5 mm are likely to pass spontaneously (Table 108.2), whereas larger stones are less likely to pass spontaneously. Proximal ureteral stones are also less likely to pass than distal ureteral stones.
- Consider consultation with urology department and inpatient management for patients with signs of high-grade obstruction, concomitant infection, urinary extravasation, hypercalcemic crisis, solitary or transplanted kidneys, intractable pain, or large obstructing stones that are unlikely to pass spontaneously (i.e., ≥7 mm).

TABLE 108.1 Nephrolithiasis Mimics

Urologic Disease	GI	Vascular	Gynecologic	Other
Pyelonephritis	Appendicitis	AAA	Ovarian cyst	Tumor
Tumors	Diverticulitis		Ovarian or testicular torsion	Lymphadenopathy
Papillary necrosis	Biliary colic		Endometriosis	Musculoskeletal pain
Renal infarct	Cholecystitis		Ectopic pregnancy	Herpes zoster
Hematoma	Bowel obstruction			
Ureteral stricture	Mesenteric ischemia			
Urinary retention				

AAA, abdominal aortic aneurysm; *GI*, gastrointestinal.

TABLE 108.2 Rates of Spontaneous Ureteral Stone Passage by Size

Stone Size (mm)	Percentage of Spontaneous Passage
1	87
3	83
5	60
7	47
10	27

- If there is evidence of an infection with an obstructing stone, emergent urology department consult is indicated for possible ureteral stent or percutaneous nephrostomy tube placement. Without urinary diversion, these patients can rapidly decompensate due to overwhelming sepsis.
- Medical expulsion therapy with α-blockers, such as tamsulosin (i.e., Flomax) remains controversial; however, current urology guidelines continue to advise tamsulosin to aid in stone passage.

SUGGESTED READINGS

Alelign, T., & Petros, B. (2018). Kidney stone disease: An update on current concepts. *Advances in Urology*, 3068365.

Golzari, S. E., Soleimanpour, H., Rahmani, F., Zamani Mehr, N., Safari, S., Heshmat, Y., & Ebrahimi Bakhtavar, H. (2014). Therapeutic approaches for renal colic in the emergency department: A review article. *Anesthesiology and Pain Medicine*, 4(1), e16222.

Gottlieb, M., Long, B., & Koyfman, A. (2018). The evaluation and management of urolithiasis in the ED: A review of the literature. *The American Journal of Emergency Medicine*, 36(4), 699–706.

108

CHAPTER 109

BOARD REVIEW

Urogenital Infections

KELLIE KITAMURA, MD, and STEVEN LAI, MD

Urinary Tract Infections

PEDIATRICS

General Principles

- In children who are not toilet-trained, catheterization or suprapubic aspiration should be used for urine collection.
- Urinary tract infections (UTIs) are the most common serious bacterial infections in immunized infants and young children.
- Most frequently occur within the first year of life for both boys and girls, although girls have a three times higher risk than boys.
- Risk factors include uncircumcised status, vesicoureteral reflux, urolithiasis, poor hygiene, and urinary retention.
  - Risk of UTIs is 4 to 20 times higher in boys who are not circumcised.
  - In neonates, the presence of congenital anomalies of the kidney and urinary tract increases the risk of UTI, and UTIs typically are the result of hematogenous spread.
  - In children, UTIs are the result of retrograde contamination from perineal or periurethral organisms, with *Escherichia coli* being the most common causative organism. *Klebsiella*, *Proteus*, and *Enterobacter* species are also common. In children who are not toilet-trained, catheterization or suprapubic aspiration should be used for urine collection.

Clinical Presentation

- Presentation varies with age.
  - Neonates may be septic and present with only symptoms of fever, poor feeding, irritability, and/or lethargy.
  - Older children may complain of dysuria along with abdominal pain and vomiting. High or prolonged fevers are suggestive of UTI. Although identifying another source of fever lowers the likelihood of UTI, it does not rule out concomitant UTI.
  - Physical examination may demonstrate abdominal tenderness or costovertebral angle tenderness (in pyelonephritis). Genitalia should be inspected for anatomic abnormalities that may predispose to UTI.

Diagnosis

- In infants less than 2 months of age, a positive urine culture is the gold standard.
- For children between 2 to 24 months of age, the American Academy of Pediatrics (AAP) guidelines state that both pyuria and bacteriuria on urinalysis are highly suggestive of a UTI, whereas a positive culture is necessary for definitive diagnoses (Table 109.1).
- In febrile infants 2 to 24 months of age, the prevalence of a UTI is approximately 5%–7%.
- AAP recommends identification of specific risk factors to help providers determine whether they should screen for a UTI (Table 109.2).
- In older children, the presence of symptoms with a consistent physical examination combined with a urine dip positive for pyuria and/or nitrites is diagnostic, although the urine culture is definitive.
- Pelvic examinations should be done on sexually active adolescent females to rule out pelvic inflammatory disease (especially if the urinalysis is negative).
- Imaging from the emergency department is rarely necessary, although patients should follow up with their primary pediatrician to evaluate for structural abnormalities, as indicated.

Treatment

- Neonates should be admitted to the hospital for intravenous antibiotics with further workup, including possible lumbar puncture and blood cultures.

TABLE 109.1 American Academy of Pediatrics: Diagnosis of UTI

Urinalysis suggestive of infection	Pyuria as defined by: Positive leukocyte esterase (≥1+) on dipstick analysis, or ≥5 WBC/hpf with standardized or automated microscopy, or ≥10 WBC/mm^3 on a hemocytometer with an enhanced urinalysis
	OR Bacteriuria (note: Pyuria is absent in approximately 10%–20% of children with UTI)
AND Positive urine culture	At least 50,000 colony-forming units (CFUs) per mL of a uropathogen cultured from a urine specimen obtained through catheterization or SPA

WBC, White blood cell; *UTI*, urinary tract infection; *SPA*, suprapubic aspiration.

(Adapted from Subcommittee on Urinary Tract Infection, Steering Committee on Quality Improvement and Management. Roberts, K. B. (2011). Urinary tract infection: Clinical practice guideline for the diagnosis and management of the initial UTI in febrile infants and children 2 to 24 months. *Pediatrics, 128*, 595–610.)

TABLE 109.2 *Probability of UTI in Febrile Infants 2 to 24 Months of Age Based on Gender and Risk Factors*

		UTI PROBABILITY	
Gender	**Risk Factors**	**Less than 1%**	**Less than 2%**
Female	• White race • Less than 12 months of age • Temperature 39°C or higher • Fever 48 or more hours • No other infectious source	1 or more risk factor	2 or more risk factors
Circumcised male	• Nonblack race • Temperature 39°C or higher • Fever 24 or more hours • No other infectious source	2 or fewer risk factors	3 or fewer risk factors
Uncircumcised male	Uncircumcised febrile males' probability of UTI is greater than 1% just from being uncircumcised, even without taking into account other risk factors.		

(Adapted from Subcommittee on Urinary Tract Infection, Steering Committee on Quality Improvement and Management. Roberts, K. B. (2011). Urinary tract infection: Clinical practice guideline for the diagnosis and management of the initial UTI in febrile infants and children 2 to 24 months. *Pediatrics, 128*, 595–610.)

- Most children can be treated as outpatients with oral antibiotics so long as they are able to tolerate orals, are euvolemic, and not immunocompromised.
  - Oral antibiotic regimens include 7 to 14 days of either amoxicillin, trimethoprim-sulfamethoxazole, cefpodoxime, or cephalexin.
  - Intravenous antibiotics include ceftriaxone and other third-generation cephalosporins, cefazolin, ampicillin in cases of *Enterococcus faecalis*, gentamicin, and tobramycin.

ADULTS

General Principles

- UTIs are common emergency department diagnoses in both men and women and can be classified based on anatomic sites involved.
  - Urethritis and cystitis are infections of the lower urinary tract.
  - Pyelonephritis is an infection of the upper tract involving the renal parenchyma and pelvicalyceal system.
- UTIs are also classified as uncomplicated and complicated.
  - Uncomplicated infection is a diagnosis limited to healthy, young, nonpregnant patients with normal anatomy.
  - Complicated urinary tract infections include patients who are male, or have anatomic abnormalities, ureteral stents, or indwelling catheters; or suffer from recurrent infections, are immunosuppressed, have advanced neurologic disease, significant comorbid conditions, or have a known history of antibiotic-resistant pathogens.
- Recurrent UTIs are defined by two uncomplicated UTIs within 6 months or three or more UTIs in the past year.
- Similar to pediatrics, *E. coli* is the most common pathogen, followed by *Klebsiella*, *Proteus*, *Enterobacter*, and *Pseudomonas* species.

Clinical Presentation

- In males, dysuria without presence of urethral discharge suggests a UTI.
- Lower urinary tract symptoms include dysuria, frequency, urgency, hesitancy, and suprapubic pain or tenderness on examination.
- Patients may also complain of hematuria.
- Vaginal discharge or irritation is more suggestive of vaginitis, cervicitis, or pelvic inflammatory disease (PID) rather than UTI.
- Unlike in pyelonephritis, fever is uncommon in simple cystitis.
- Flank pain and costovertebral angle tenderness may be seen in both simple cystitis as referred pain or in pyelonephritis.
- Presence of systemic symptoms, including fever, chills, nausea, or vomiting, is diagnostic of pyelonephritis; and there may not be any lower urinary tract symptoms.

Diagnosis

- Based on clinical findings as well as urinalysis and culture
- Positive nitrites on the urinalysis has a high specificity for UTI caused by bacteria that convert nitrates to nitrite, including *E. coli*. Nitrites have a low sensitivity for detection of *Enterococcus*, *Pseudomonas*, and *Acinetobacter* species, because these pathogens do not convert nitrates to nitrites and thus result in negative nitrites.
- Positive leukocyte esterase has poor sensitivity and specificity. Thus, a positive result supports the diagnosis of UTI, but a negative result does not rule it out. The presence of bacteria is highly associated with positive urine culture results.
- Imaging is not helpful for simple UTIs and may only aid diagnosis when there is concern for complicated UTIs, such as infected ureteral stones, renal abscesses, or emphysematous cystitis or pyelonephritis.

Treatment

- Uncomplicated cystitis can be treated with a 3 day course of ciprofloxacin, a 3 to 5 day course of trimethoprim-sulfamethoxazole, or a 5 day course of cephalexin or nitrofurantoin.
- Complicated UTIs and pyelonephritis can be treated as an outpatient in patients who are otherwise healthy and can tolerate oral medication with a 10- to 14-day course of ciprofloxacin, trimethoprim-sulfamethoxazole, cefdinir, or cefpodoxime.

- Patients requiring inpatient hospitalization may be treated with ceftriaxone, ciprofloxacin, cefotaxime, gentamicin, cefepime, or carbapenems.
- Pregnant patients should be treated for asymptomatic bacteriuria (with a positive urine culture) or simple cystitis with cephalexin or fosfomycin. Pregnant patients with pyelonephritis should be admitted and started on a second- or third-generation cephalosporin.

Male-Specific Infections

BALANITIS/BALANOPOSTHITIS

General Principles

- Balanitis refers to inflammation of the glans of the penis, whereas posthitis refers to inflammation of the foreskin. Balanoposthitis refers to the presence of both.
- Most often these conditions are caused by infection with *Candida* (most commonly), *Staphylococcus*, *Streptococcus* species, and less commonly *Mycoplasma genitalium*. It is rarely caused by *Neisseria gonorrhoeae* or *Chlamydia*.
- Contributing risk factors include poor hygiene (particularly in uncircumcised males), external irritation or trauma, contact dermatitis, obesity, or diabetes.
- Balanoposthitis may be the presenting sign of new-onset diabetes, particularly if recurrent.

Clinical Presentation

- Erythema, excoriation, and edema may be present at the glans and foreskin (Fig. 109.1). Patients may complain of pain and itching and occasionally malodorous discharge. Curd-like discharge suggests a candidal etiology, whereas foul smelling and purulent discharge suggests a bacterial cause. The foreskin may be difficult to retract, although concurrent phimosis is rare (Fig. 109.2).
- Systemic symptoms are rare, unless balanitis is a manifestation of reactive arthritis, in which case, there may be associated joint inflammation, eye symptoms, and mouth sores.

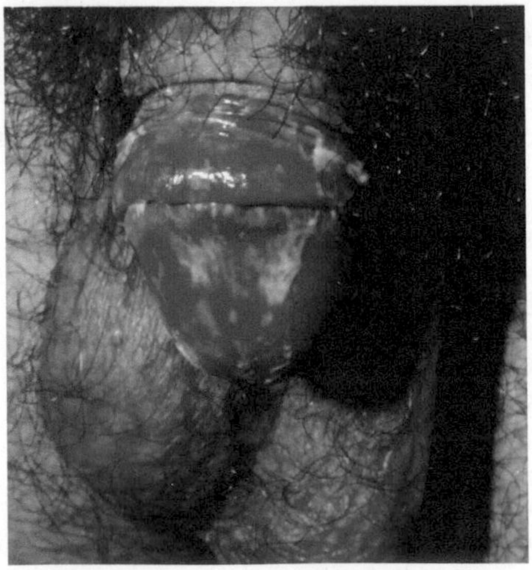

FIG. 109.1 Balanoposthitis. (From Dinulos, J. G. H. (2018). Fungal infections. In T. Habif, J. G. H. Dinulos, M. S. Chapman, & K. Zug (Eds.), *Skin disease: Diagnosis and treatment* (4th ed., pp. 241–281, Fig. 9.13). Elsevier.)

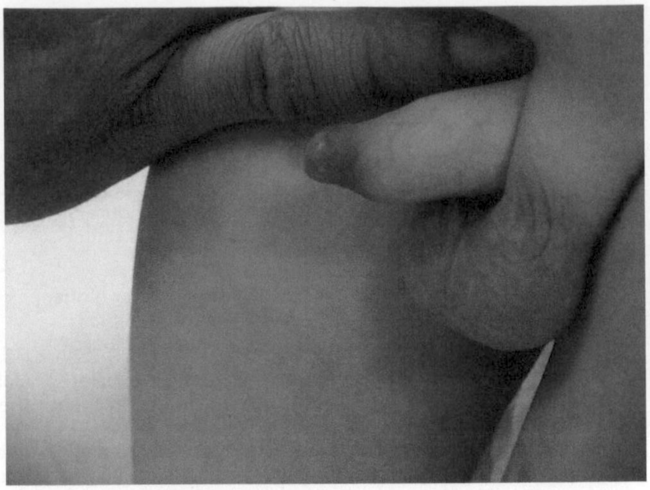

FIG. 109.2 Pediatric phimosis with balanoposthitis. (From Huang, C. J. (2009). Problems of the foreskin and glans penis. *Clinical Pediatric Emergency Medicine, 10*(1), 56–59, Fig. 1.)

Diagnosis

- Balanitis and balanoposthitis are clinical diagnoses based on the physical examination.
- Severe or persistent cases may warrant a culture or biopsy with urology.
- Consider point-of-care glucose check to screen for undiagnosed diabetes.

Treatment

- Genital hygiene is paramount, with emphasis on retraction of the foreskin and twice-daily bathing of the involved area with saline solution.
- Sitz baths may also reduce inflammation.
- Consider empiric treatment for candidal infection with clotrimazole or miconazole for 7 days.
- Treat severe inflammation with topical 0.5% hydrocortisone cream applied sparingly twice daily for 7 days. If a bacterial etiology is suspected, oral amoxicillin-clavulanic acid or cephalexin for 7 days, combined with topical mupirocin or metronidazole, is appropriate.
- Oral metronidazole or clindamycin may be necessary for severe cases. Circumcision should be considered as an outpatient.

EPIDIDYMITIS

General Principles

- Acute epididymitis is a one of the most common causes of scrotal pain.
- Although it is caused by infection from retrograde transit of organisms from the vas deferens, epididymitis may also be secondary to trauma or autoimmune disease.
- In younger boys, it may be the result of congenital anatomic anomalies of the lower urinary tract and caused by reflux of urine or coliform bacteria.
- *N. gonorrhoeae* and *C. trachomatis* are common in sexually active males younger than 35, whereas *E. coli* and *Pseudomonas* species are more common in older males.

Clinical Presentation

- Patients will complain of the gradual onset of pain.

- On examination, there is localized testicular pain and tenderness to palpation of the epididymis that is relieved with scrotal elevation (Prehn sign).
- Patients may also complain of abdominal, inguinal, or scrotal pain, and urinary symptoms may be present.
- Involvement of the testicle (epididymo-orchitis) occurs quickly and may result in diffuse testicular pain and swelling and may result in scrotal erythema or a reactive hydrocele. Older patients may have urinary obstruction.
- Systemic symptoms are rare, although they may be present with concomitant acute bacterial prostatitis.

Diagnosis

- Epididymitis is a clinical diagnosis.
- Urinalysis and culture should be performed in those with lower urinary tract symptoms and consider testing for *N. gonorrhoeae* and *C. trachomatis* in high-risk patients.
- Testicular ultrasound may demonstrate enlarged and hypoechoic epididymis and may help rule out testicular torsion.

Treatment

- Sexually active males under the age of 35 or those who participate in high-risk sexual behavior should be treated for presumed *N. gonorrhoeae* and *C. trachomatis*. Please refer to the Sexually Transmitted Infection section for treatment recommendations.
- Older patients without any risk factors for sexually transmitted infections should be treated with ciprofloxacin or levofloxacin for 10 days.
- Patients who practice insertive anal intercourse should receive both a one-time dose of ceftriaxone IM and levofloxacin for 10 days.
- Conservative treatments, such as ice, nonsteroidal antiinflammatory drugs, and scrotal elevation may be done for symptomatic relief.

ORCHITIS

Clinical Presentation

- Isolated orchitis is a rare infection of the testis; usually seen in conjunction with systemic viral infections, such as mumps, or Epstein-Barr virus.
- Bacterial orchitis is typically associated with epididymitis (epididymo-orchitis) and thus caused by similar pathogens, including *N. gonorrhoeae, C. trachomatis*, and *E. coli*.
- Pain is gradual in onset over a few days and the testicle is swollen and tender on examination.
- Patients may also have fever, nausea, vomiting, and malaise.

Diagnosis and Treatment

- It is a clinical diagnosis.
- Testicular ultrasound may be warranted to rule out testicular torsion or abscess.
- Treatment: antibiotics with similar coverage as epididymitis listed above

BACTERIAL PROSTATITIS

General Principles

- Bacterial prostatitis is an infection of the prostate most commonly caused by gram-negative organisms, primarily *E. coli*. Other causative organisms include *Klebsiella*, *Enterobacter*, *Proteus*, and *Pseudomonas* species. Gonorrhea and chlamydia should be considered in younger men who are sexually active.
- Risk factors include being immunocompromised, urinary tract obstruction (physiologic or neurologic), concurrent acute epididymitis or urethritis, presence of an indwelling catheter, recent instrumentation, and receptive anal intercourse.

Clinical Presentation

- Often ill-appearing, patients complain of fever, chills, and myalgias, often associated with penile, perineal, suprapubic, pelvic, or lower back pain. Other lower urinary tract symptoms include frequency, urgency, and obstructive symptoms.
- If patients are experiencing urinary retention, urethral catheterization may risk rupture of a potential abscess or may induce septic shock, thus suprapubic catheter catheterization with urology consultation is preferred.

Diagnosis

- Physical examination will reveal perineal tenderness and a painful and boggy prostate that is warm to touch. Examination should be gentle to prevent precipitating bacteremia.
- Urine culture is recommended, but the diagnosis is clinical, because urinalysis and culture may be negative. Bacteriuria and pyuria are common. Gram stain of the urine may help guide antibiotic choice.
- Consider testing for *N. gonorrhoeae* and *C. trachomatis* in sexually active males younger than 35 or those who engage in high-risk sexual behaviors.

Treatment

- If patients are experiencing urinary retention, urethral catheterization may risk rupture of potential abscess or may induce septic shock, thus suprapubic catheter catheterization with urology consultation is preferred.
- Mainstay for outpatient treatment is antibiotics. First-line empiric treatment is either trimethoprim-sulfamethoxazole or a fluoroquinolone (i.e., ciprofloxacin or levofloxacin) for 4 to 6 weeks.
- Younger patients (less than 35 years) who are sexually active, patients who engage in high-risk sexual activities, or those with concomitant epididymitis or urethritis should also be treated empirically for *N. gonorrhoeae* and *C. trachomatis* with a one-time ceftriaxone IM dose and a 2-week course of doxycycline.
- Admit patients who are toxic appearing, have signs of severe sepsis, or cannot tolerate oral antibiotics. Intravenous levofloxacin or ciprofloxacin, possibly with an aminoglycoside (i.e., gentamicin or tobramycin) is preferred.
- If there is a high suspicion for enterococcus (i.e., gram-positive cocci on gram stain), ampicillin would be first-line treatment and, if the patient has risk factors or history of methicillin-resistant *Staphylococcus aureus*, vancomycin may be used.
- If toxic appearing, the occurrence of a complication of prostatitis should be considered, such as prostatic abscess or metastatic infection of the sacroiliac or vertebral bones.

CHRONIC PROSTATITIS

General Principles

- Characterized by prolonged or recurrent prostatitis, although a history of previous acute prostatitis may be absent
- May be secondary to inadequate treatment of acute bacterial prostatitis
- Most common cause of recurrent UTIs in males; *E. coli* is the most common bacterial pathogen.

Clinical Presentation

- Patient may be entirely asymptomatic but more commonly have irritative voiding symptoms and may have pelvic or genital pain.
- No physical examination findings are pathognomonic, as prostate may be normal or may be tender and boggy.
- Overall, these patients do not appear to be ill, in contrast to those with acute bacterial prostatitis.

Diagnosis and Treatment

- A clinical diagnois
- Urine culture is helpful in guiding antibiotic choice because recurrence of bacterial strains as previous episode(s) is common.
- Fluoroquinolones are first-line antibiotics, with trimethoprim-sulfamethoxazole, doxycycline, or azithromycin as second line. Refer to previous urine culture sensitivities, if available. Duration of antibiotics should be for at least 6 weeks, although occasionally a 6- to 12-week course is necessary.

URETHRITIS

General Principles

- Infectious urethritis results in urethral inflammation most often caused by sexually transmitted pathogens, which are covered in detail later in the chapter.
- Most commonly owing to *C. trachomatis* or *N. gonorrhoeae*, although species of *Ureaplasma*, *Mycoplasma*, *Trichomonas*, and *Candida* are also common pathogens

Clinical Presentation

- Dysuria or painful urination is the most common presenting symptom.
- Penile itching or burning and urethral discharge may also be present. Patients can be asymptomatic (5%–10% of men with gonococcal urethritis are asymptomatic) with laboratory evidence of disease.
- On examination the meatus may be edematous or inflamed and mucopurulent discharge may be present.

Diagnosis

- Generally a clinical diagnosis based on symptoms and examination.
- Gram stain of urethral discharge may demonstrate the presence of white blood cells (WBCs) (fewer than two, indicating low suspicion for sexually transmitted infection [STI]) and any organisms.
- First-void urine that is positive for leukocyte esterase or has fewer than 10 WBC per high power field (hpf) is suggestive of urethritis.
- Gonorrhea and chlamydia testing should also be performed.

Treatment

- Refer to the STI section for treatment of gonococcal urethritis.
- If concerned for non-gonococcal urethritis, patients may receive either a single dose of azithromycin or a 1-week course of doxycycline.

Female-Specific Infections

VULVOVAGINITIS

Bacterial Vaginosis (BV)

General Principles

- Most common cause of malodorous vaginal discharge.
- BV is the result of a change in vaginal flora resulting in a reduction of normal *Lactobacillus* to an increase of organisms, such as *Gardnerella vaginalis*, *Mycoplasma hominis*, and *Prevotella* and *Bacteroides* species. This reduction of *Lactobacillus* also results in an increase of vaginal pH.
- Not associated with chronic medical conditions or immunosuppression.
- Risk factors include: sexual activity (presence of other sexually transmitted infections increases risk), women who have sex with women are at higher risk (although it is not yet classified as a sexually transmitted infection), douching, and cigarette smoking.
- Pregnant women with untreated bacterial vaginosis are at risk for preterm delivery.
- May increase the risk of transmission of human immunodeficiency virus (HIV), gonorrhea, chlamydia, and herpes

Clinical Presentation

- 50%–75% of patients can be asymptomatic; symptomatic women may complain of malodorous "fishy smelling" vaginal discharge that is off-white and thin.
- Patients typically do not have urinary symptoms, pruritus, pain, vaginal irritation, or dyspareunia.

Diagnosis

- Amsel criteria can help with the diagnosis. Three of the four following criteria must be present:
  - Thin and white homogenous discharge that coats the vaginal walls
  - Presence of clue cells on wet mount
  - Vaginal fluid pH greater than 4.5
  - Positive whiff test (defined as fishy odor to the vaginal discharge with addition of 10% KOH)
- Gram stain of the vaginal discharge can also be done.

Treatment

- Symptomatic women should be treated with metronidazole or clindamycin. Both oral metronidazole for 7 days and intravaginal metronidazole gel for 5 days are appropriate first-line treatments. Oral clindamycin or intravaginal clindamycin cream for 7 days is another treatment option.
- Asymptomatic women and sexual partners do not need to be treated. Topical or intravaginal treatments should be avoided in pregnant patients.

Candida Vaginitis

General Principles

- Second most common cause of vaginitis symptoms, most often caused by *Candida albicans*
- Most often occurs after menarche, although it is also common in younger females less than 2 years of age.
- Risk factors include diabetes, immunosuppression, states of increased estrogen levels (including pregnancy), and recent antibiotic use.
- Uncomplicated candidiasis, which is most common, is characterized by a sporadic or infrequent episode with only mild symptoms in otherwise healthy and nonpregnant patients.
- Complicated infections are characterized by severe signs or symptoms, pregnancy, immunosuppression, multiple comorbid conditions, or recurrent infection (more than three per year).
- It is not considered a sexually transmitted infection.

Clinical Presentation

- Vulvar pruritus and irritation are the most common symptoms, and patients may also complain of dysuria or dyspareunia.
- Physical examination, there may be vulvar erythema and edema.
- Vaginal discharge is classically white and curd-like, although it is not always present (Fig. 109.3). Usually no odor is present.

Diagnosis

- Clinical diagnosis, based on history and physical examination

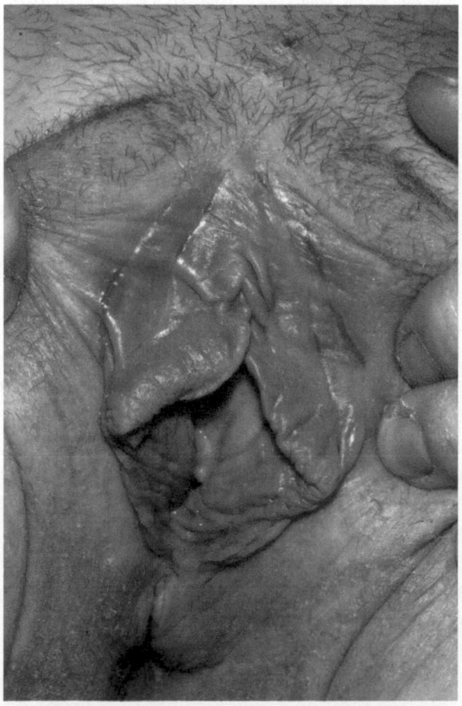

FIG. 109.3 Candida vulvovaginitis. (From Dinulos, J. G. H. (2018). Fungal infections. In T. Habif, J. G. H. Dinulos, M. S. Chapman, & K. Zug (Eds.), *Skin disease: Diagnosis and treatment* (4th ed., pp. 241–281, Fig. 9.11). Elsevier.)

- Wet mount or Gram stain may demonstrate yeast or pseudohyphae and help rule out alternative diagnoses (e.g., trichomonas, bacterial vaginosis) or coinfection.

Treatment

- One-time dose of oral fluconazole is adequate as treatment for uncomplicated infections.
- A 1- to 3-day course of topical azoles (e.g., clotrimazole, miconazole) have similar cure rates to oral medications for uncomplicated infections.
- Complicated infections require longer treatment.
  - If the symptoms are severe, oral fluconazole is preferred, once every 72 hours, repeated for two or three doses. Topical therapy should be extended for 7 to 14 days.
  - Recurrent candidiasis treatment requires three doses of oral fluconazole every 72 hours and maintenance fluconazole weekly for 6 months.
  - Patients who are immunocompromised should receive oral therapy for 7 to 14 days.
  - Pregnancy is considered complicated candida vaginitis; however, these patients should avoid oral medication and instead use topical azoles for 7 days.

Trichomonas Vaginitis

General Principles

- Most common non-viral sexually transmitted infection; parasite infects both men and women
- Associated with pelvic inflammatory disease and preterm birth; and appears to facilitate HIV transmission

Clinical Presentation

- Women may have vaginal irritation and pruritus; vaginal discharge is classically frothy, green-yellow, thin, and malodorous. Punctate hemorrhages ("strawberry cervix") are characteristic.
- Males are typically asymptomatic, although they may have pruritus or irritation of the penis, dysuria, pain with ejaculation, or urethral discharge.

Diagnosis

- Can be diagnosed via wet mount; an elevated vaginal pH greater than 4.5 is not diagnostic, but is more common.

Treatment

- A one-time dose of metronidazole or tinidazole are the only effective treatments.
- Gel and topical ointments are less effective than oral medications and are not recommended.
- Pregnant patients should be treated with oral metronidazole despite risks of drug adverse effects given the associated risk of preterm birth and low-birth-weight infants may result if left untreated.
- Patients with HIV should be treated for 7 days.
- Sexual partners must be treated.

CERVICITIS

General Principles

- Cervicitis is the inflammation of the cervix, most often secondary to infection, although may also be owing to a noninfectious etiology.

- *C. trachomatis* and *N. gonorrhoeae* are most common causes, chlamydia being more common. *Herpes*, *Trichomonas*, and *Mycoplasma* are less-common causative organisms.
- Identification and treatment of cervicitis is important because it may result in endometritis or pelvic inflammatory disease if left untreated.
- Cervicitis in pregnancy may cause low birth weight or preterm birth.

Clinical Presentation

- Symptoms include purulent or mucopurulent vaginal discharge, postcoital bleeding, and intermenstrual bleeding (Fig. 109.4).
- Dysuria, dyspareunia, or vaginal irritation may be present, although typically cervicitis is painless unless there is coexistent endometritis or pelvic inflammatory disease.

Diagnosis

- Cervicitis diagnosis found on examination
- Pelvic examination reveals mucopurulent or purulent discharge and a friable cervix.
- Test for chlamydia and gonorrhea and obtain a wet mount for *Trichomonas*.

Treatment

- Treat empirically for chlamydia and gonorrhea. Please refer to STI segment.

PELVIC INFLAMMATORY DISEASE (PID)

General Principles

- A spectrum of inflammation of the female reproductive tract
- Includes endometritis, myometritis, parametritis, oophoritis, and may extend into the pelvic peritoneum
- Can also spread to result in periappendicitis, pelvic peritonitis, and perihepatitis in Fitz-Hugh-Curtis syndrome
- *N. gonorrhoeae* and *C. trachomatis* account for many cases; other pathogens include *Herpes*, *Trichomonas*, *Mycoplasma*, and *Ureaplasma*.
- PID may be a polymicrobial infection and anaerobic (e.g., *Bacteroides*, *Peptostreptococcus*, *Prevotella*) and aerobic (e.g., *Gardnerella*, *Haemophilis*, *Streptococcus*, *E. coli*) bacteria may contribute.

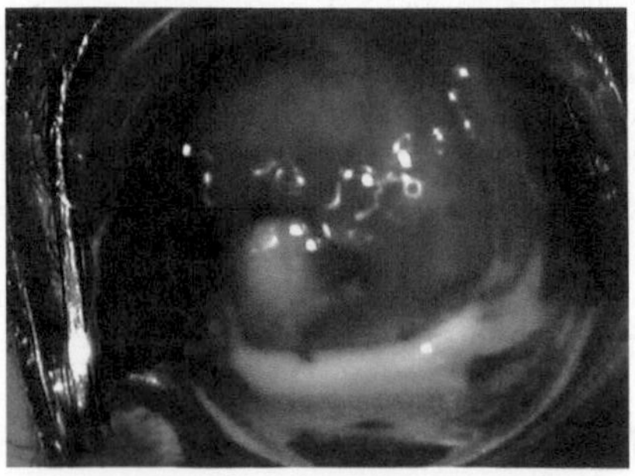

FIG. 109.4 Mucopurulent discharge from cervical os concerning for pelvic inflammatory disease. (From Clutterbuck, D. (2019). Pelvic infection and STIs. In B. A. Magowan, P. Owen, & A. Thomson (Eds.), *Clinical obstetrics and gynaecology* (4th ed., pp. 155–168, Fig. 18.5). Elsevier.)

- Most cases are thought to originate as sexually transmitted infections that ascend the reproductive tract.
- Risk factors include multiple sexual partners, history of STI, frequent vaginal douching, and the recent placement of an intrauterine device less than 3 weeks prior.
- Nearly 50% of patients diagnosed with PID do not have risk factors, and 15% of cases may be owing to nonsexually transmitted organisms.
- Appropriate diagnosis and management of PID is necessary to prevent sequelae including tuboovarian abscesses, ectopic pregnancy, infertility, and chronic pelvic pain and dyspareunia.

Clinical Presentation

- Symptoms range from patients being asymptomatic to having lower abdominal or pelvic pain, abnormal vaginal discharge, intermenstrual or postcoital bleeding, dyspareunia, dysuria, and systemic symptoms (although less common) may also be present, including fever, malaise, nausea, and vomiting.
- In Fitz-Hugh-Curtis syndrome (perihepatitis), right upper quadrant pain is present and is more often associated with gonococcal and chlamydial salpingitis.
- On examination, patients may have cervical motion tenderness and uterine or ovarian tenderness (unilateral or bilateral). Mucopurulent discharge is often present on examination. Rebound tenderness may be present if infection has spread to the peritoneum.

Diagnosis

- A clinical diagnosis and a spectrum of disease
- No single test, or historical or physical finding on examination can offer a definitive diagnosis of PID. Providers must maintain a high index of suspicion.
- Absence of WBCs on wet mount or lack of mucopurulent discharge on examination makes PID less likely, and other causes of abdominal pain should be considered.
- Ultrasonography may be useful in suspected cases of tuboovarian abscess.
- All patients should be screened for *N. gonorrhoeae* and *C. trachomatis*.

Treatment

- Antibiotic regimens are targeted to treat gonorrhea, chlamydia, anaerobes, gram-negative organisms, and *Streptococcus*.
- Inpatient treatment should be considered for pregnant patients, in those with tuboovarian abscesses, or with severe illness or inability to tolerate oral antibiotics.
  - Inpatient regimens include combination of cefoxitin or cefotetan, plus doxycycline. Clindamycin and gentamicin comprise an alternative combination regimen.
  - Outpatient regimens include a one-time dose of ceftriaxone intramuscularly with a 2-week course of doxycycline, with or without metronidazole.
  - Patients should be reevaluated within 2 days to assess for clinical response, because admission for parenteral antibiotics may be necessary for persistent or worsening of symptoms.
  - Sexual partners should be treated and patients should avoid sexual activity until treatment is completed.

- In patients with IUDs, removal does not expedite treatment, and these are usually left in place with close outpatient follow-up.

POSTPARTUM ENDOMETRITIS

General Principles

- Endometritis is the inflammation of the uterine lining.
- Acute nonpostpartum infectious endometritis is secondary to PID or an invasive gynecologic procedure (see PID section regarding treatment for endometritis unrelated to pregnancy).
- Postpartum endometritis may also extend into the myometrium or parametrium and is a common cause of fever greater than 24 hours after delivery.
  - *N. gonorrhoeae* and *C. trachomatis* are less-common causative organisms in endometritis related to pregnancy. Most often, postpartum endometritis is a polymicrobial infection of aerobic and anaerobic organisms. Rarely it may be caused by *C. sordellii* or *perfringens*, Streptococcal or Staphylococcal species.
  - Delivery by cesarean section is the biggest risk factor, along with concomitant bacterial vaginosis.
  - Other risk factors include prolonged labor or rupture of membranes, use of vacuum or forceps extraction, presence of chorioamnionitis, internal fetal monitoring, HIV infection, or in group B *Streptococcus* carriers.
  - Postpartum endometritis is classified as early (24 to 48 hours) or late (more than 48 hours).

Clinical Presentation

- Postpartum fever and midline lower abdominal pain are present in most women with endometritis, along with chills, headache, and malaise.
- Physical examination may reveal uterine tenderness and foul smelling and purulent lochia.
- Clostridia, Streptococci, and Staphylococci can cause toxic shock syndrome with patients presenting with high fever, hypotension, and evidence of end-organ damage.

Diagnosis

- Clinical diagnosis
- Signs and symptoms are nonspecific.
- Blood, cervical, and endometrial cultures are not routinely performed.
- Ultrasonography may identify retained products.

Treatment

- Mild cases can be treated with an oral 14-day antibiotic regimen of clindamycin or augmentin (with or without metronidazole).
- Most cases require hospitalization with parenteral treatment of clindamycin plus gentamicin. Ampicillin-sulbactam is a second-line option.

BARTHOLIN'S ABSCESS

General Principles

- Bartholin's glands are located in the vulva at the 4 and 8 o'clock positions on each side of the vaginal introitus.
- No known risk factors other than a history of prior abscesses.
- Obstruction of the ducts may result in cyst or abscess formation.
- Abscesses are usually polymicrobial; incidence of methicillin-resistant *Staphylococcus aureus* is increasing and *N. gonorrhoeae* and *C. trachomatis* have also been implicated.

Clinical Presentation

- Cysts are generally painless, although they may be symptomatic because of the size.
- Abscesses are associated with severe pain and swelling to the lower medial labia majora (Fig. 109.5).
- Systemic symptoms are rare.

Diagnosis

- Bartholin's abscess is a clinical diagnosis.
- Biopsy is rarely needed, except in cases of postmenopausal women (to rule out a malignancy) because Bartholin's glands typically shrink with age.
- Some sources recommend biopsy after age 40.

Treatment

- Mainstay of treatment is incision and drainage under local anesthesia using local anesthesia and a #11 scalpel.
- An incision, no larger than a few millimeters to prevent displacement of the Word Catheter, is made on the mucosal surface within the introitus, but external and lateral to the hymenal ring.
- The Word Catheter is a 1-inch catheter with the diameter of a 10 French Foley catheter and an inflatable balloon at the tip. The catheter is inserted into the abscess cavity after the incision and drainage, and the balloon is

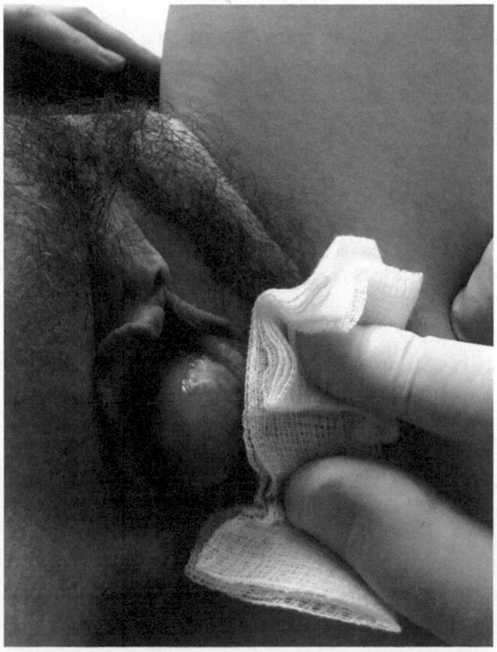

FIG. 109.5 Bartholin abscess. (From Di Donato, V., Bellati, F., Casorelli, A., Giorgini, M., Perniola, G., Marchetti, C., Palaia, I., & Benedetti Panici, P. (2013). CO_2 laser treatment for Bartholin gland abscess: Ultrasound evaluation of risk recurrence. *Journal of Minimally Invasive Gynecology, 20*(3), 346–352, Fig. 1.)

109

filled with 2 to 3 mL of saline. It is meant to stay in place for 4 to 6 weeks to prevent recurrence.

- Sitz baths several times a day are also recommended.
- Antibiotics are usually unnecessary unless there is concomitant cellulitis or systemic symptoms, for recurrence, or if the patient is at high risk for developing complicated infection. Trimethoprim-sulfamethoxazole or amoxicillin-clavulanate plus clindamycin for 7 days are appropriate treatment options.
- Follow-up with gynecology is recommended.
- If there are multiple recurrences, operative marsupialization by the gynecologist may be warranted.

Sexually Transmitted Infections

CHLAMYDIA

Clinical Presentation

- Most commonly reported sexually transmitted infection in the United States, caused by C. *trachomatis*
- Can clinically present as urethritis, cervicitis, epididymitis, orchitis, proctitis, prostatitis, and PID. Gonorrhea is a common coinfectant.
- Commonly, males complain of symptoms of urethritis or epididymitis, and women complain of pelvic pain and vaginal discharge. Patients may also be asymptomatic.

Diagnosis

- Nucleic acid amplification tests are the diagnostic test of choice performed on endocervical or urethral swab specimens or on urine specimens (for males, urine specimens demonstrate equal sensitivity and specificity as urethral swab specimens).

Treatment

- A one-time dose of azithromycin or a 1-week course of doxycycline is usually sufficient, except in cases of epididymitis and PID where a prolonged treatment course is necessary.

GONORRHEA

Clinical Presentation

- Second most common sexually transmitted infection in the United States, is caused by N. *gonorrhoeae*, a gram-negative dipolococcus.
- Can clinically present as urethritis, cervicitis, epididymitis, orchitis, proctitis, prostatitis, and PID.
- Males with gonorrhea most often present with urethritis with profuse purulent penile discharge.
- Women most often complain of pelvic pain and vaginal discharge, although most women are asymptomatic. Oropharyngeal and conjunctival involvement is also possible.
- Disseminated gonococcal infection may present with fever, chills, monoarticular arthritis or arthralgias, rash, and tenosynovitis. The rash is usually composed of tender necrotic pustules with an erythematous base. Disseminated gonococcal infection may also result in hepatitis, myocarditis, endocarditis, and meningitis. Patients may also be asymptomatic.

Diagnosis

- Nucleic acid amplification is the diagnostic test of choice performed on endocervical or urethral swab specimens or on urine specimens.
- Cultures are necessary for diagnosis of cerebrospinal fluid, rectal, oropharyngeal, conjunctival, or synovial fluid infections.

Treatment

- Updated CDC guidelines as of December 2020 now recommend an increased dose from 250 mg to 500 mg of intramuscular ceftriaxone. The CDC no longer recommends adding azithromycin for dual coverage and recommends a 1-week course of doxycycline only if concomitant chlamydia cannot be ruled out. Patients who weigh greater than 150 kg should receive 1 g of intramuscular ceftriaxone.
- Disseminated gonorrhea should be treated on an inpatient basis with daily ceftriaxone intravenously or intramuscularly.

Syphilis

Clinical Presentation

- Caused by *Treponema pallidum*, a spirochete
- Primarily transmitted through exposure of moist skin to an infected area and usually involves the genitalia
- Primary stage: presents as a single painless ulcer, known as a chancre, at the site of inoculation.
  - Ulcer usually begins as a papule and develops into a clean-based ulcer with sharp borders (Fig. 109.6). Although classically taught to be a solitary ulcer, it can present as multiple ulcers.
  - If left untreated, the ulcer resolves after 2 to 6 weeks.
  - Lymphadenopathy may or may not be present, and there are no associated systemic symptoms.
- Secondary syphilis: rash is the most common manifestation associated with lymphadenopathy.
  - Typically occurs 1 to 2 months after resolution of the primary stage

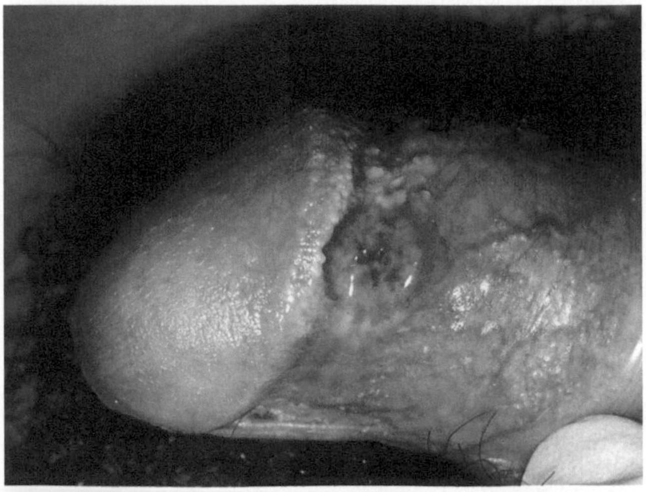

FIG. 109.6 Painless syphilis chancre. (From Sukthankar, A. (2014). Syphilis. *Medicine, 42*(7), 394–398, Fig. 3.)

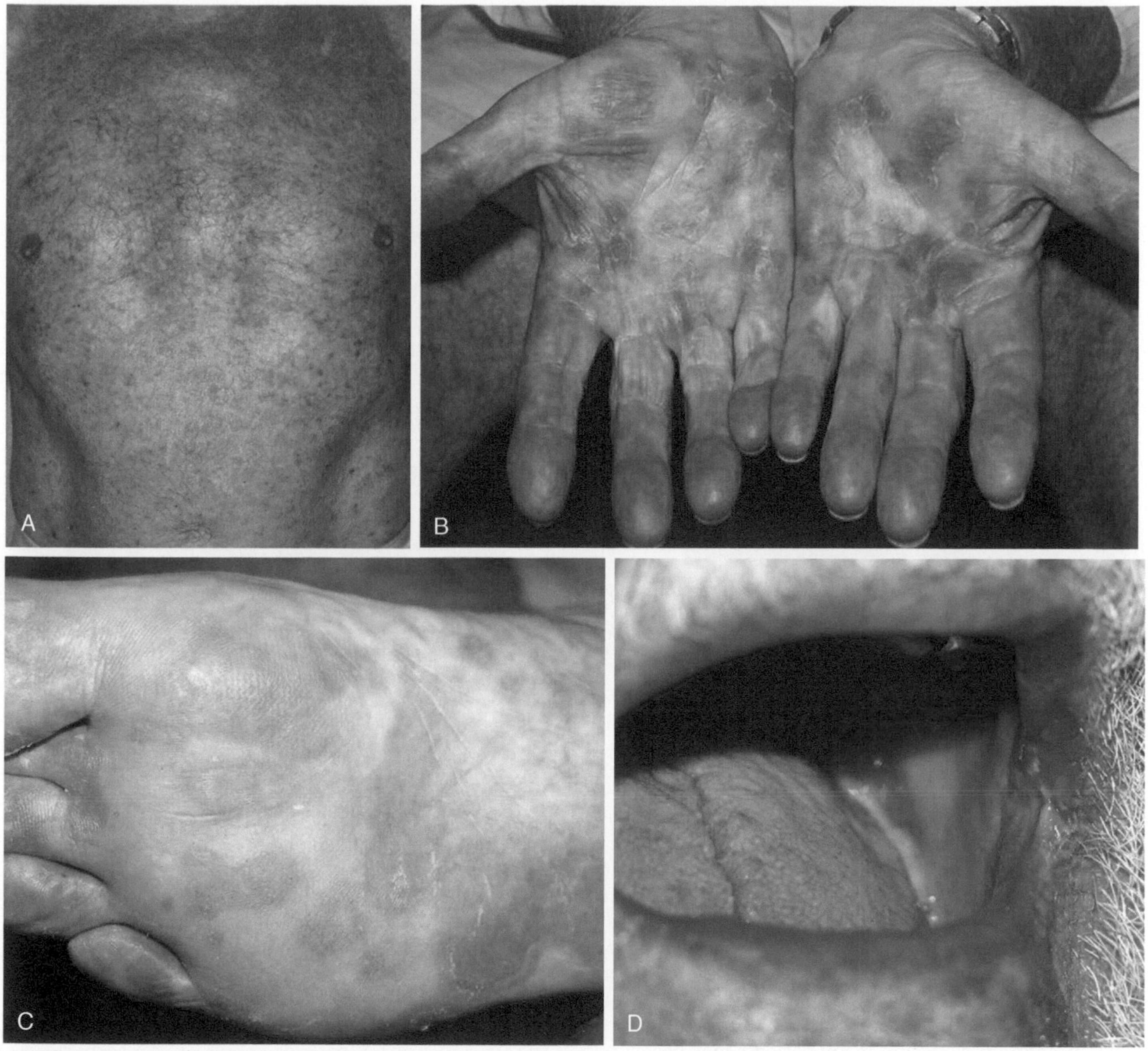

FIG. 109.7 Secondary syphilis maculopapular rash. (From Wickremasinghe, S., Ling, C., Stawell, R., Yeoh, J., Hall, A., & Zamir, E. (2009). Syphilitic punctate inner retinitis in immunocompetent gay men. *Ophthalmology, 116*(6), 1195–1200, Fig. 2.)

  - Rash classically begins on the torso and spreads to the extremities involving the palms and soles. Lesions are usually macular; however, they may become papulosquamous and dull red in color (Fig. 109.7).
  - Condylomata lata are flat papules that may develop in the labia, perineum, or around the anus (Fig. 109.8).
  - Systemic symptoms may occur during the secondary stage, including fever, malaise, fatigue, headache, and generalized lymphadenopathy.
  - Symptoms of secondary syphilis can also self-resolve if left untreated.
- Tertiary syphilis may occur after latent periods of at least 3 to 4 years.
  - Nervous system and cardiovascular systems are classically affected and the disease may manifest as peripheral neuropathy (tabes dorsalis), meningitis, thoracic aortic aneurysm, or as gummatous lesions in the mucous membranes.

Diagnosis

- Two tests are necessary for the diagnosis: nontreponemal Venereal Disease Research Laboratory (VDRL) becomes positive 2 to 4 weeks after the primary chancre appears. VDRL test is nonspecific (resulting in false–positive screening).
- Rapid plasma reagin (RPR) is necessary for confirmation.

Treatment

- Primary and secondary syphilis can be treated with a one-time dose of IM long-acting penicillin G benzathine. Sexual partners need to be evaluated and treated. Tertiary syphilis is treated with three doses (1 week apart) of the same IM form of penicillin.

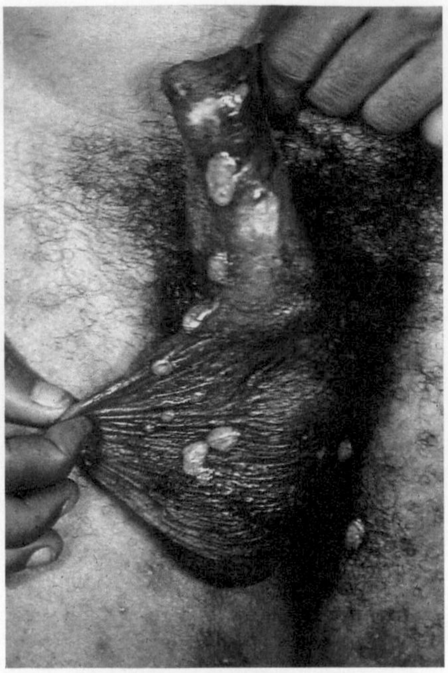

FIG. 109.8 Condylomata lata. (From James, W. D., Elston, D. M., McMahon, P. J. (2018). Syphilis, yaws, bejel, and pinta. In: W. D. James, D. M. Elston, & P. J. McMahon. *Andrews' diseases of the skin clinical atlas* (pp. 251–261, Fig. 18.34). Elsevier.)

Herpes Simplex Virus (HSV)

CLINICAL PRESENTATION

- Classically more commonly caused by HSV-2, which tends to have a tropism for genital mucosa; however, it may also be caused by HSV-1.
- Clinical course of both HSV-1 and HSV-2 are indistinguishable; however, HSV-2 may lead to more recurrence.
- Estimated that one in five sexually active adults is infected with the virus.
- Viral shedding occurs during both symptomatic and asymptomatic periods and many patients may become infected without symptoms.
- Symptoms may be caused by either primary infection or recurrence.
  - Primary genital herpes (first infection without preexisting antibodies to HSV-1 or HSV-2) is characterized by severe and prolonged systemic and local symptoms. Preexisting antibodies to HSV-1 (i.e., nonprimary first infection) can decrease the severity of the clinical presentation caused by HSV-2. In primary infection, patients have genital lesions that initially begin as vesicles and develop into painful shallow ulcers usually in groups (Fig. 109.9). Bilateral painful lymphadenopathy may also be present. Symptoms typically peak around 7 days and lesions usually heal between 2 and 4 weeks. Patients may also have systemic infections, including fever, malaise, myalgias, and headache.
  - In recurrence, patients usually only develop the genital vesicles and ulcers and do not have systemic symptoms. Recurrence occurs in 60%–90% of patients.

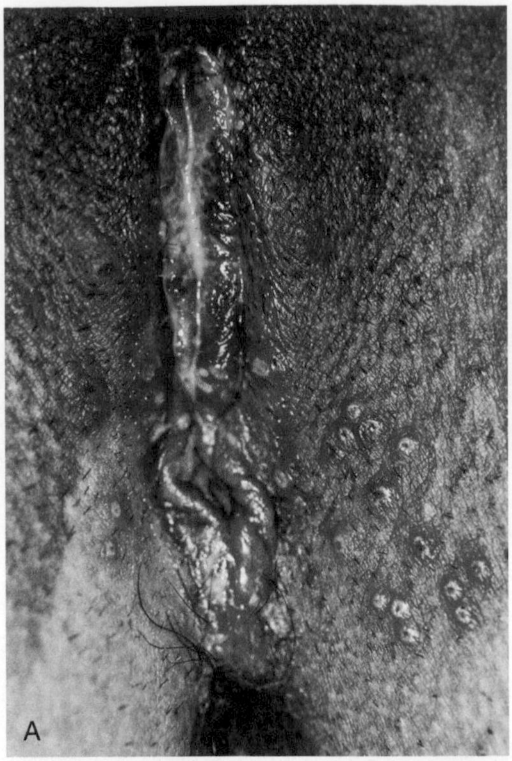

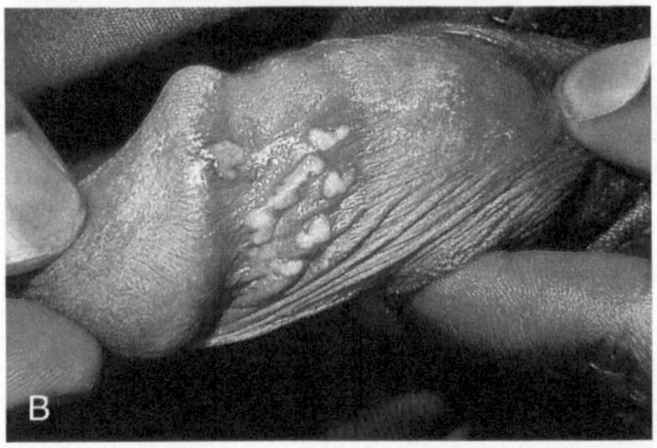

FIG. 109.9 Painful ulcers characteristic of herpes simplex virus infection. (**A**, From Downing, C., Mendoaz, N., Sra, K., & Tyring, S. K. (2019). Human herpesviruses. In J. L. Bolognia, J. V. Schaffer, & L. Cerroni, L. (Eds.), *Dermatology* (4th ed., Fig. 80.3). Elsevier. **B**, Adapted from White, G. M., & Cox, N. H. (2006). *Diseases of the skin* (2nd ed.). Mosby.)

Diagnosis

- Usually a clinical diagnosis; confirmatory testing should be done.
- Viral culture remains the gold standard, it takes several days with a relatively high frequency of false-negatives.
- PCR testing is preferred.

Treatment

- Antiviral medication is not curative, although may decrease the duration of symptoms in primary HSV and may shorten or prevent recurrence.
- Acyclovir, valacyclovir, and famciclovir are options for both a primary episode and for recurrence or as suppressive medication.
- Antivirals are typically prescribed for 7 to 10 days for primary episodes and 2 to 5 days for recurrence.

Chancroid

Clinical Presentation

- Caused by *Haemophilus ducreyi*
- Rare in the United States and more commonly seen in developing countries
- Patients have multiple painful ulcers that begin as painful papules, accompanied by fluctuant and tender lymphadenitis.
- May be yellow necrotic-appearing exudate from the ulcers
- Classically, there is one unilateral lymph node and it may rupture (Fig. 109.10).
- Overall clinical presentation is similar to herpes; however, the large and fluctuant lymph node involvement suggests chancroid.

Diagnosis

- A clinical diagnosis (especially because neither PCR nor culture testing of *H. ducreyi* is routinely available) after exclusion of herpes and syphilis
- The CDC has developed a case definition for definite and probable chancroid for reporting purposes (Table 109.3).

Treatment

- A one-time dose of azithromycin, a one-time IM injection of ceftriaxone, or ciprofloxacin for 3 days are all acceptable treatment options.
- Lymph nodes should be drained.
- Sexual partners should be evaluated and treated.

Lymphogranuloma Venereum (LGV)

Clinical Presentation

- Caused by specific serotypes of *C. trachomatis*
- Rare in the United States and more prevalent in tropical countries
- Risk factors include patients who have traveled to endemic areas and in men who have sex with men (MSM).

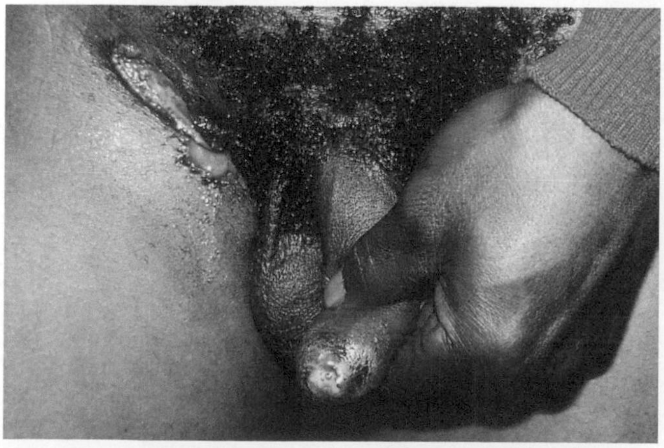

FIG. 109.10 Chancroid ulcer of glans of penis with weeping lymphadenopathy. (From Spinola, S. (2010). Chancroid. In S. A. Morse, K. K. Holmes, & R. C. Ballard (Eds.), *Atlas of sexually transmitted infections and AIDS* (4th ed., pp. 141–156, Fig. 8.11B). Elsevier.)

TABLE 109.3 *Chancroid (Haemophilus ducreyi) CDC Definitions*

Clinical description	A sexually transmitted infection, caused by infection with *Haemophilus ducreyi,* characterized by painful genital ulceration and inflammatory inguinal adenopathy
Laboratory criteria for diagnosis	Isolation of *H. ducreyi* from a clinical specimen
Case classification	
Probable	A clinically compatible case with both (a) no evidence of *Treponema pallidum* infection either by dark field microscopic examination or serologic test AND (b) no clinical evidence or culture negative for herpes simplex virus (HSV)
Confirmed	A clinically compatible case that is laboratory confirmed

- Initial infection is usually a transient lesion that is small and painless and self-resolves; thus, it is commonly missed by patients.
- The secondary stage begins anywhere from 1 week to a month after the primary lesion resolves. Patients complain of painful lymphadenopathy, classically unilateral (Fig. 109.11). The lymph nodes can form sinus tracts or firm inguinal masses.
- Can also cause proctitis (especially in MSM), leaving patients with abnormal rectal discharge, pain, tenesmus, and constipation

Diagnosis

- Usually diagnosed clinically based on presentation and risk factors, although serologic testing is available

Treatment

- Patients can be cured with a 3-week course of doxycycline.

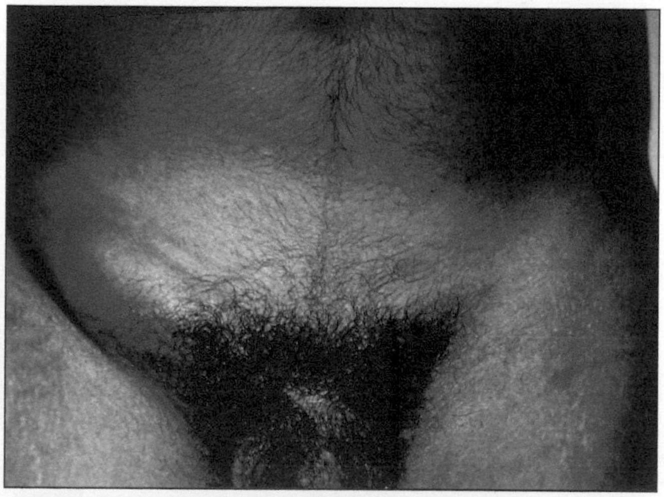

FIG. 109.11 Painful unilateral lymphadenopathy of lymphogranuloma venereum. (From Lupi, O., Hozannah, A, Romero, M., Leal Passos, M. R., De Queiroz Varella, R., Pellegrini Nahn, E., Jr., de Souza Salles, R., Eleutério, J., Jr., Mariano, P. C., Bitencourt, P. T., de Barros, L. K. C., de Sousa Padilha, C. B., Jardim, M. L., Talhari, S., & Talhari, C. (2017). Bacterial sexually transmitted infection. In S. K. Tyring, O. Lupi, & U. R. Hengge (Eds.). *Tropical dermatology* (2nd ed., pp. 313–345, Fig. 26.3). Elsevier.)

- Erythromycin is an alternative for patients who cannot tolerate doxycycline.
- Sexual partners should be tested.

Granuloma Inguinale

Clinical Presentation

- Caused by *Klebsiella granulomatis*
- Rare in developed countries and the United States and more often seen in tropical and semitropical regions
- Not highly contagious; thus repeated exposure is necessary to contract it.
- Patients will have multiple firm, painless ulcers on the genitalia and perineum.
- Ulcers are highly vascular and bleed easily (Fig. 109.12). There is no lymphadenopathy. If left untreated, the ulcers may result in urethral stenosis and lymphatic obstruction, resulting in leg elephantiasis.

Diagnosis

- *Klebsiella granulomatis* can be identified via bipolar staining of biopsy specimens.

Treatment

- Three-week regimens of doxycycline (first-line), azithromycin, ciprofloxacin, or bactrim may be used as treatment, although relapse can occur.

Condylomata Acuminata

Clinical Presentation

- Also known as anogenital warts, condylomata acuminata is caused by human papillomavirus (most commonly types 6 and 11).
- Vary in presentation—may be either soft or firm, pedunculated or broad based, painful or painless, and some lesions may be friable (Fig. 109.13).

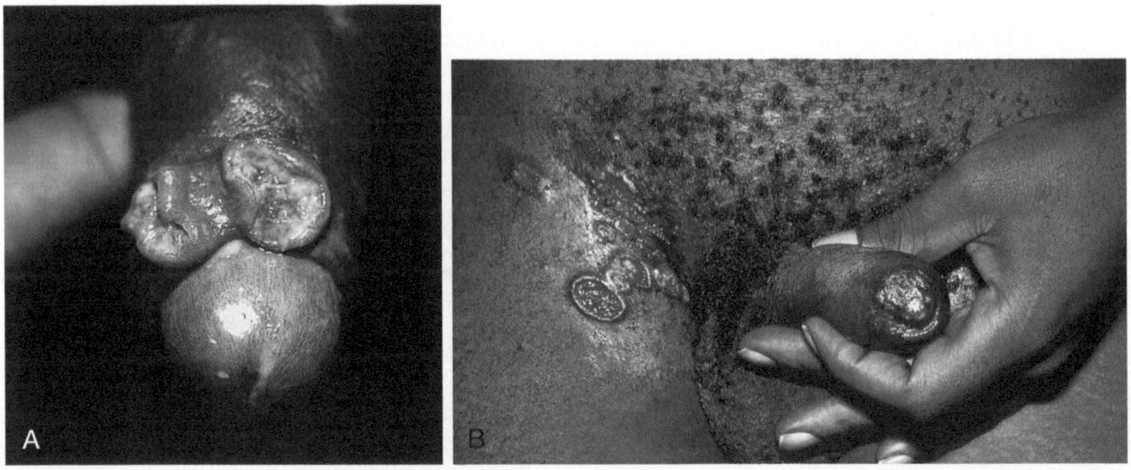

FIG. 109.12 Multiple painful ulcers of granuloma inguinale. (From James, W. D., Berger, T. G., & Elston, D. M. (2016). *Andrews' diseases of the skin: Clinical dermatology* (12th ed., pp. 266–267). Elsevier.)

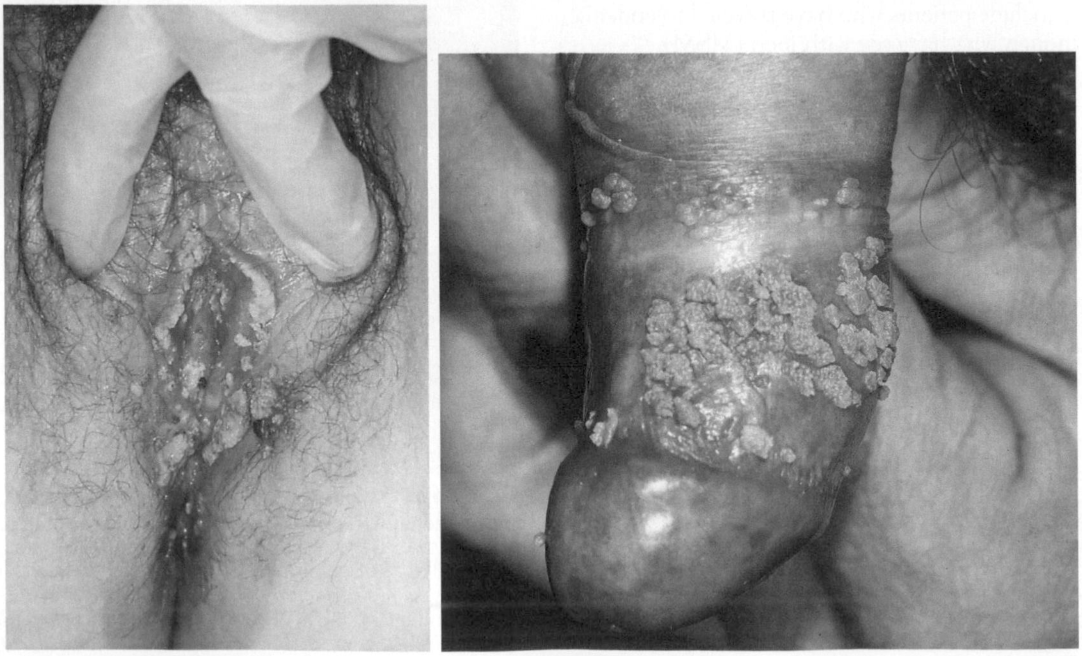

FIG. 109.13 Genital warts. (From Dinulos, J. G. H. (2018). Sexually transmitted viral infections. In J. G. H. Dinulos (Ed.), *Habif's clinical dermatology: A color guide to diagnosis and therapy* (7th ed., Figs 11.6 and 11.14). Elsevier.)

Diagnosis

- Primarily a clinical diagnosis
- Syphilis may need to be ruled out, given there is often confusion with condylomata lata.
- A speculum examination is necessary to evaluate for intravaginal or cervical lesions.

Treatment

- Mainstay of treatment is the removal of symptomatic warts, although all options have high failure rates.
- Patients can apply podofilox solution for 3 days, imiquimod cream 3 times a week, or sinecatechins ointment 3 times a day.
- In-office treatments include cryotherapy, surgical removal, trichloroacetic acid, or bichloroacetic acid.
- Biopsy to exclude cancerous lesions is indicated in those who are immunocompromised, postmenopausal women, or those who do not respond to standard treatment.

SUGGESTED READINGS

Brunham, R. C., Gottlieb, S. L., & Paavonen, J. (2015). Pelvic inflammatory disease. *The New England Journal of Medicine, 372*, 2039–2048.

Davis, J. E., & Schneider, R. E. (2009). An evidence-based approach to male urogenital emergencies. *Emergency Medicine Practice, 11*(2).

Pfennig, C. (2019). Sexually transmitted infections in the emergency department. *Emergency Medicine Clinics of North America, 38*(2), 165–192.

CHAPTER 110

BOARD REVIEW

Structural Urogenital Findings and Emergencies

ANNA YAP, MD, BA, and RACHEL SHING, MD

General Principles

Penile Anatomy. The penis (Fig. 110.1) consists of paired corpora cavernosa (erectile bodies) that lie dorsal to the corpus spongiosum, which surrounds the urethra. These three structures are wrapped by the tunica albuginea, a thin connective tissue layer.

- Glans: distal head of the penis
- Prepuce: the distal foreskin, which in uncircumcised males, lies over the glans and can be retracted to expose the glans
- The coronal sulcus distinguishes the glans penis from the penile shaft

Scrotal Anatomy (see Fig. 110.2)

- Made of two halves that each contain a separate testicle, spermatic cord, and epididymis.
- Each testicle is encapsulated by a fibrous tunica albuginea, which is then surrounded by the tunica vaginalis.

Priapism

Clinical Presentation

- An erection of the penis for longer than 4 hours in the absence of sexual desire or stimulation.

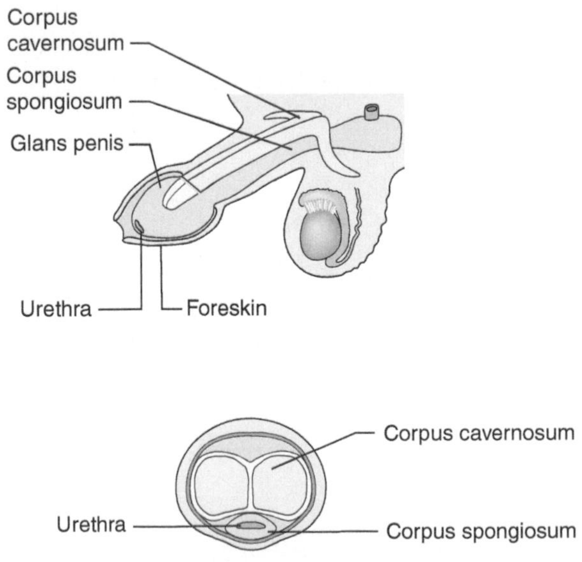

FIG. 110.1 Anatomy of the penis. (Modified from Stewart, G. D. (2018). Urological surgery. In O. J. Garden & R. W. Parks (Eds.), *Principles and practice of surgery* (7th ed., pp. 429–460, Fig. 23.21). Elsevier.)

- More than one-third of patients with severe priapism may have permanent erectile dysfunction despite treatment.
- There are two types of priapism: ischemic (low flow) and nonischemic (high flow).
- Ischemic (low flow), the most common form of priapism, is also known as anoxic or venoocclusive priapism.
  - Smooth muscle of the corpora cavernosa is unable to relax, resulting in a penile compartment syndrome leading to hypoxia and acidosis of the tissue.
  - Has many causes, including medications, illicit drugs, hematologic disorders, central nervous system disorders, infections, toxins, carbon monoxide, hypertriglyceridemia, cancer, or idiopathic.
  - Patients typically present shortly after onset. Examination reveals a painful, rigid shaft with a soft glans.
- In children, this is seen most commonly in patients with Sickle Cell Anemia and is managed in the standard fashion for priapism.
- Nonischemic (high flow) priapism, which is rare, results from arterial inflow from an arterial-cavernosal fistula.
  - Fistula formation can be secondary to perineal or penile trauma, or a result of congenital arterial malformations.
  - Gradual in onset and may present up to 72 hours after a traumatic event
  - Can be painless and nonischemic priapism is less painful than the ischemic form
  - Examination reveals a partial or fully rigid shaft with a firm glans. Patients may demonstrate a "Piesis sign," where perineal compression decreases erection.

Diagnosis and Evaluation

- The history will differentiate between ischemic and nonischemic priapism.
- Blood gas analysis can be run on blood aspirated from the corpora cavernosa. A pH less than 7.25, PaO_2 less than 30 mm Hg, and PCO_2 greater than 60 mm Hg suggest ischemic priapism.
- Color Doppler ultrasound of the cavernosal arteries can also be used to identify normal, increased, or absent flow.

Treatment

- Acute ischemic priapism requires emergent urology consult.
- Management should progress in a stepwise fashion to achieve prompt detumescence.
  - First-line therapy is aspiration of blood, with or without irrigation of the corpora cavernosa. Anesthesia is

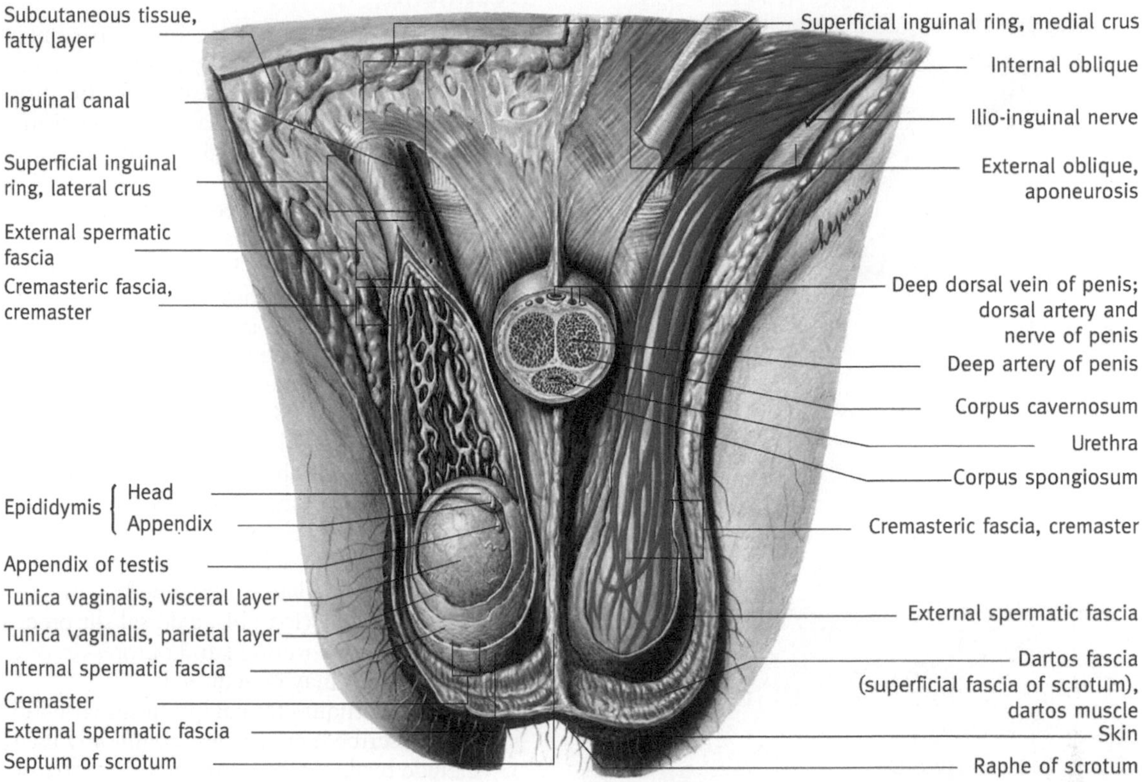

FIG. 110.2 Anatomy of the scrotum. (With permission from Waschke, J., & Paulsen, F. (2013). *Sobotta atlas of human anatomy* (15th ed.). Elsevier/Urban & Fischer.)

achieved by a dorsal penile block with 1% lidocaine at the 10:30 and 1:30 position (Fig. 110.3). For aspiration, a 19- or 21-gauge needle with a 50 mL syringe is inserted directly into the corpus cavernosum at the penoscrotal junction laterally at the 3 or 9 o'clock position to avoid the neurovascular bundle. Aspirate 20 to 30 mL of blood at a time until blood appears red and freshly oxygenated. Irrigation can be done with sterile saline.

- Intracavernous injection of sympathomimetic drugs should be performed if priapism persists following aspiration/irrigation, or if the priapism is greater than 4 hours duration. Phenylephrine is the recommended agent owing to its minimal risk of cardiovascular side effects when compared with other sympathomimetic medications. Dilute phenylephrine with normal saline to a concentration of 100 to 500 µg/mL and give 1-mL injections every 5 minutes for up to 1 hour or detumescence. Lower concentrations in smaller volumes should be used in children and patients with severe cardiovascular disease. During and following intracavernous injection, observe patients for adverse side effects of sympathomimetic drugs, such as acute hypertension, headache, reflex bradycardia, tachycardia, palpitations, and cardiac arrhythmia. Blood pressure and cardiac monitoring are recommended for patients with high cardiovascular risk.
- If not improving, the patient may require urgent surgical shunt procedures by a urologist.
- In addition to direct treatments for relieving the painful tumescence, provide treatment for other underlying causes, such as intravenous fluids for individuals with sickle cell disease. Discontinue any offending medications.

- In contrast, the initial management of nonischemic priapism is typically observation.
  - Up to two-thirds of patients will have spontaneous resolution of symptoms.
  - Aspiration has only a diagnostic role and injectable medications are not recommended or effective as treatment.
  - If resolved, patients can follow up with a urologist within 1 week.

Phimosis and Paraphimosis

Clinical Presentation, Diagnosis, and Evaluation

- Phimosis and paraphimosis only occur in uncircumcised males because these conditions involve the foreskin.
- The diagnosis is made primarily by history and physical examination.
- Phimosis is the inability to retract the prepuce (distal foreskin).
  - May be normal (physiologic phimosis owing to circumferential adhesions between the foreskin and the glans) as a newborn and many resolve with age

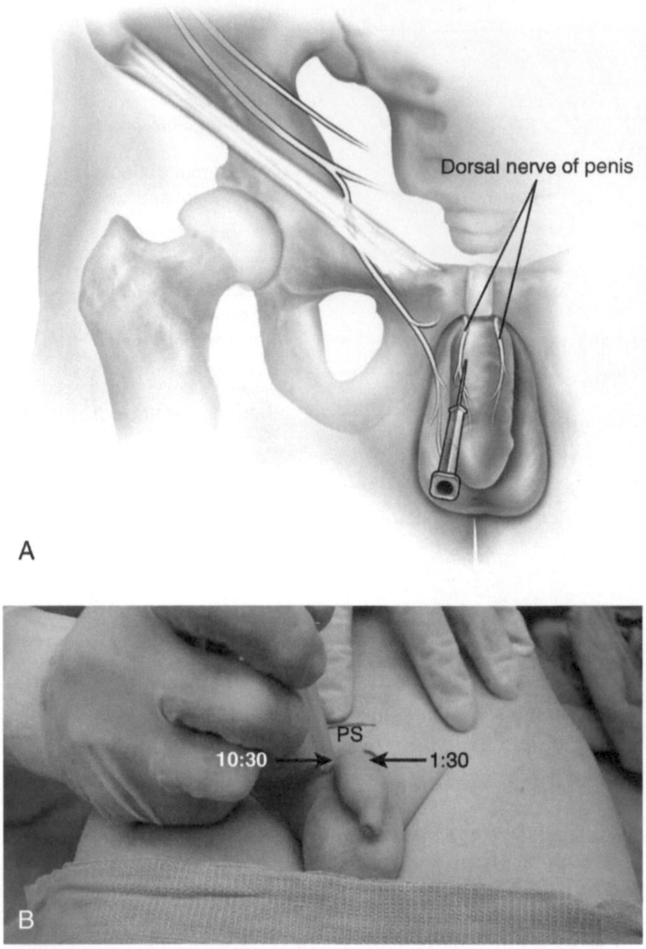

FIG. 110.3 Anatomy for dorsal penile block at the 10:30 and 1:30 position. (From Flack, S., & Lang, R. S. (2017). Regional anesthesia. In P. J. Davis & F. P. Cladis (Eds.), *Smith's anesthesia for infants and children* (9th ed., pp. 461–511.e6). Elsevier.)

- Less than 10% of uncircumcised males have phimosis by age 3 and almost none by late adolescence.
- On examination, the foreskin is unretractable.
- Preputial stone formation and urinary obstruction may occur if there is pathologic phimosis, often secondary to infection and inflammation.

- Paraphimosis, a urologic emergency, is the inability to reduce the foreskin distally to its natural position overlying the glans penis.
  - The foreskin creates a constricting band on the penile shaft, inhibiting venous and lymphatic drainage, causing progressive edema that obstructs arterial inflow, leading to necrosis and gangrene.
  - Appears as a red, painful, swollen glans penis with an edematous, proximally retracted foreskin
  - The penile shaft proximal to the constricting band is usually soft (Fig. 110.4A).
  - Often occurs in the elderly, very young, or developmentally delayed, when the foreskin is not noticed to have returned to its natural position; it can be associated with urinary catheterization, poor hygiene, infection, or following sexual activity.

Treatment

- Phimosis seldom requires emergency treatment.
  - If there is resultant urinary obstruction, a dorsal slit procedure is performed to allow for free urine flow.
- Paraphimosis requires manual reduction of the constricting foreskin back over the glans penis to prevent glans necrosis (see Fig. 110.4).
  - Multiple methods for reduction exist, all centering around decreasing glans edema. The most commonly used initial maneuver involves manual compression of the distal glans penis.
  - Pain control, which is paramount to the procedure's success, may include topical or parenteral medication, as well as local or regional anesthesia. Young children may require procedural sedation.
  - If time permits, other strategies to decrease glans swelling include the application of ice packs, osmotic agents (20% mannitol, 50% dextrose, granulated sugar), or compressive band.
  - Omit these approaches if urgent reduction is necessary or procedural sedation is planned.
  - If manual reduction fails, a dorsal slit procedure to incise the constricting band of foreskin or formal circumcision may be required.
  - Other techniques for paraphimosis reduction have been described, but are less commonly used. They include hyaluronidase injection into the swollen retracted foreskin, traction with forceps, puncture of foreskin with a needle, and glans penis aspiration.
- Discharge patients once the foreskin remains reduced for at least 30 minutes, with absolutely no foreskin retraction for at least 1 week.
- Refer all patients to urology for follow-up, because many develop recurrence.
- Consult urology or a surgeon with similar expertise for patients who present with penile necrosis, complete urinary obstruction, or unsuccessful reduction by the manual technique.

Entrapment (Tourniquet, Foreskin/Penile Zipper)

Clinical Presentation, Diagnosis, and Evaluation

- May visually mimic paraphimosis.
- If not treated quickly, the penis or scrotum is at risk for ischemia, gangrene, or amputation.
- Diagnosis is made primarily by history and physical examination.
- Zipper injury results in localized edema, superficial abrasions, bruising, and pain.
  - Skin loss or necrosis is rare.
  - Most common in uncircumcised children when the foreskin becomes caught and can occur even when wearing underwear
- Hair tourniquet may be nearly invisible because it often hides within the coronal sulcus of the penis.
  - In severe cases the hair tourniquet may cause complete transection of the urethra. The most common

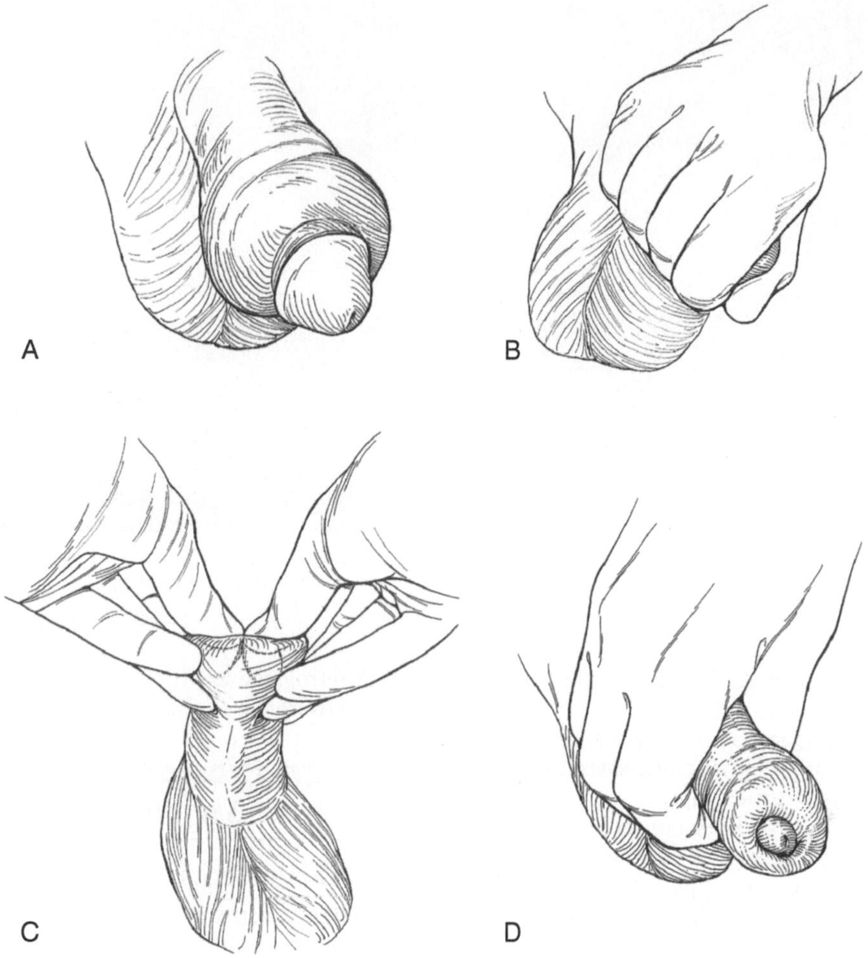

FIG. 110.4 Reduction of paraphimosis. Reduce edema of distal penile skin with manual compression to allow for replacement of distal penile preputial tissue over the glans penis. **A**, Typical appearance of edematous penis with paraphimosis. **B**, Firm manual pressure is applied to reduce edema. **C**, Gentle counter-traction is applied to reduce foreskin. **D**. Fully reduced paraphimosis with normal appearance of the penis. (Reprinted from Vilke, G. M., Ufberg, J. W., Harrigan, R. A., & Chan, T. C. (2008). Evaluation and treatment of acute urinary retention. *Journal of Emergency Medicine, 35*(2), 193–198.)

presentation is an inconsolable crying male infant with an edematous penis.

- A penile tourniquet refers to any ring-like object used for self-stimulation or to maintain an erection.
  - Patients may present with an edematous penis with a constricting ring present at the base or along the shaft.

Treatment

- Pain control is essential to relieving entrapment.
- Use topical anesthetics such as EMLA cream or provide regional anesthesia with a dorsal penile nerve block (see Fig. 110.3).
- After relieving the entrapment, the urethra should be closely inspected.
- Painful urination is normal 1 to 2 days after injury.
- Patients should return if they are unable to void or have hematuria.

ZIPPER INJURY

- Lubricants, such as mineral oil, or application of gentle traction on the zipper may work to free the skin.
- If the penile skin is entrapped without the fastener involved, cut the cloth of the zipper on each side between each tooth to separate them.
- If the fastener is involved, a bone or wire cutter can be used to cut the median bar of the zipper, allowing the two sides to fall apart.
- If none of these techniques are successful, consult urology for emergent circumcision.

HAIR TOURNIQUET

- If the hair tourniquet appears to be superficially embedded, mechanical removal under magnification may be attempted.
- If there is no mucosal involvement, a chemical depilatory agent may be tried. However, deeply embedded tourniquets that are associated with ischemia or necrosis will require emergent surgical consultation.

PENILE TOURNIQUET

- If only mild penile edema is present, the string method may be used to remove the object.
  - String is passed under the ring, wrapped distally, and then the proximal end of the string is pulled up to move the object distally (Fig. 110.5).

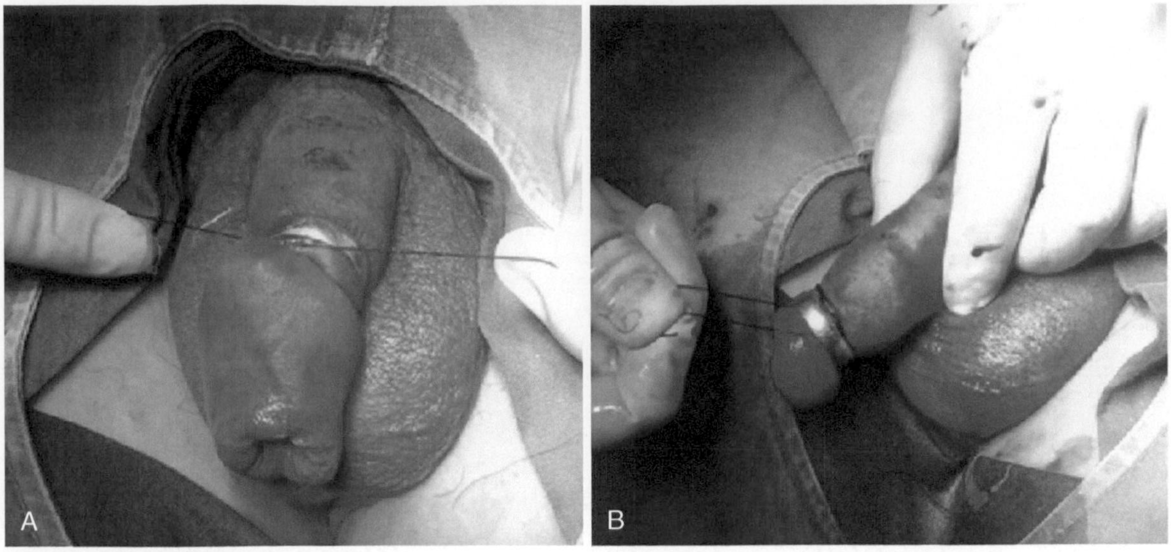

FIG. 110.5 String technique for penile ring removal. (From Dong, C., Dong, Z., Xiong, F., Xie, Z., & Wen, Q. (2013). Successful removal of metal objects causing penile strangulation by a silk winding method. *Case Reports in Urology*, 2013 (1, article 137) 434397.)

- If there is a large amount of penile edema, the object will need to be cut with a tool.
  - Use glass saws to cut glass, oscillating cast saws for plastic, ring cutters or parapneumatic saws for metal (be careful regarding overheating).
  - Always ensure a protective layer between the tool and penis, such as a tongue depressor or a metal sheet.
  - Aspiration of blood from entrapped corpora cavernosa may be required to relieve edema prior to cutting.

Penile/Urethral Foreign Bodies

Clinical Presentation

- Urethral sounding is the act of purposefully placing foreign objects, such as rods, usually for sexual gratification.
- Men also may inject substances, such as petroleum jelly, oil, silicone, or paraffin, directly into the penile shaft to attempt to enlarge the penis or enhance sexual stimulation.
- Patients may present early with pain and bleeding, or later, with infection.
- If substances have been injected directly into the penis, there may be abscesses, fistulas, pain with erection, swelling, or phimosis.

Diagnosis and Evaluation

- Diagnosis is usually made clinically via history and examination.
- If the object is not smooth and readily visualized at the meatus, a radiograph or retrograde urethrogram may be necessary.
- A radiograph is often useful to help characterize the object's shape, if it is radiopaque.

Treatment

- If readily visible, the object may be grasped with a needle driver or clamp and removed with gentle traction.
- Urology should be consulted if the object is not easily removed, if there are signs of infection, or a granuloma has formed.
- A retrograde urethrogram should be done after removal to ensure no urethral damage.

Benign Prostate Hypertrophy and Urethral Stricture

Clinical Presentation

- Benign prostate hypertrophy (BPH) and urethral stricture should be considered when men present with a urinary tract infection (UTI).
- Severe BPH and urethral strictures can result in bladder outlet obstruction, hydronephrosis, renal insufficiency, or recurrent infection.
- BPH is seen in approximately 50% of men at age 50 and 80% of men at age 80.
- Urethral strictures are relatively common in men.
  - Most common causes are idiopathic in developed countries, and trauma in undeveloped countries.
  - Other causes include infection, hypospadias, skin conditions, prior instrumentation, and radiation therapy.
- Symptoms of both include increased urinary frequency, hesitancy, nocturia, urinary incontinence, urgency, straining to void, terminal dribbling, and weak urinary stream. When severe, patients may have acute urinary retention and present with abdominal distention, suprapubic tenderness, and an inability to urinate.

Diagnosis and Evaluation

- Obtain a urinalysis and microscopy to rule out UTI, a creatinine to measure kidney function, and a postvoid residual to evaluate for urinary retention.
- Perform a digital rectal examination if suspecting infection (e.g., prostatitis) or malignancy.

Treatment

- Consider placing a Foley catheter for patients with a postvoid residual greater than 100 to 200 mL or for patients presenting with acute urinary retention.

- Initiate medications, such as alpha-1-adrenergic antagonists (i.e., tamsulosin) or 5-alpha-reductase inhibitors (i.e., finasteride).
- Treat concurrent UTI if present.
- Urology should be consulted if there is difficulty with placing a necessary Foley catheter.
- Consult urology prior to catheter insertion if there is a recent history of urologic surgery (radical prostatectomy or complex urethral reconstruction).
- If urology is not immediately available and there is need for emergency decompression of the bladder, a percutaneous suprapubic catheter may be placed.
- Patients with longstanding obstruction require at least 4 hours of monitoring for post-obstructive diuresis.
- If a patient does have post-osbtructive diuresis, ensure that they can increase oral fluid intake to compensate for the increase in urine output. Patients who are unable to do so, or have urine output of more than 200 mL/hour, should be admitted and one-half the urine output should be replaced with one-half isotonic saline and electrolyte repletion if necessary.
- Other patients with urinary retention in whom hospitalization would be indicated include those with urosepsis or acute renal failure.

Testicular Torsion

Clinical Presentation, Evaluation, and Diagnosis

- Testicular torsion results from inadequate fixation of the lower pole of the testes to the tunica vaginalis.
- Testis can torse on the spermatic cord, causing ischemia from reduced arterial inflow and venous outflow obstruction.
- Irreversible damage and infertility can occur after 6–12 hours of torsion.
- Most common in the neonatal and adolescent groups (secondary to undescended testicles, rapid increase in testicular size), but may occur at any age
- Patients present with sudden and severe onset of pain, often with nausea and vomiting.
- Patients may have a history of prior similar episodes of pain that resolved on their own.
- Fever and dysuria are less likely.
- Examination is notable for an asymmetrically high-riding testis with transverse lie, exquisite tenderness, and absent cremasteric reflex. However, the presence of the cremasteric reflex is not sufficiently reliable to exclude torsion.
- Patient with a compelling history and examination does not require any diagnostic tests and urology should be immediately consulted.
- Color flow Doppler ultrasonography may help to evaluate testicular blood flow, but should not delay definitive management.

Treatment

- Urgent urologic consult is indicated for surgical detorsion and fixation of the testicle.
- If surgery is not available within 2 hours, manual detorsion is warranted.
- With torsion, the testis typically rotates medially, and is detorsed by rotating outward ("opening the book").
- Degree of twisting of the testis may range from 180 to 720 degrees, requiring multiple rounds of detorsion.
- If pain increases or there is no relief, consider reversing direction because one-third of cases can be torsed laterally.
- Successful detorsion is suggested by pain relief, longitudinal orientation, lower position of testis in scrotum, and return of normal arterial pulsations on color Doppler ultrasound.
- Patients require surgical evaluation, regardless of the outcome of manual detorsion, for stabilization by orchiopexy.

Scrotal and Testicular Masses

Clinical Presentation

- Inguinal hernias, acute hydroceles, and varicoceles should be considered in the differential of an acute scrotal mass. A painless testicular mass should raise concern for testicular carcinoma.
- Indirect hernias protrude at the internal inguinal ring, where the spermatic cord exits the abdomen. An inguinal hernia may have an intermittent bulge in the groin that appears with straining (e.g., anything that increases intra-abdominal pressure, valsalva, etc.), or a palpable inguinal mass that extends to the scrotum. Suspect incarcerated hernia if the overlying skin is edematous or erythematous.
- Hydroceles are caused by an accumulation of fluid between the two layers of the tunica vaginalis. Hydroceles may present with gradual progression of swelling, ranging from small, soft collections to containing several liters of fluid. Scrotal transillumination will be bright, which differentiates it from a hematocele, hernia, or solid mass. Neonates can have non-communicating hydroceles where the processus vaginalis has closed and fluid will resorb over time without treatment.
- Varicoceles are enlarged spermatic cord (i.e., pampiniform plexus, see Fig. 110.2) veins and may cause impaired fertility owing to an increase in testicular temperature. Varicoceles usually present gradually, with unilateral painless swelling. Patients may also be symptomatic with dull aching pain that is worse with standing.
  - Varicoceles are usually left-sided, given the venous anatomy.
  - Unilateral right varicocele is uncommon and concerning for underlying pathology causing inferior vena cava obstruction or right renal vein compression/obstruction.
  - On physical examination varicoceles may feel like a "bag of worms" superior to the testicle that decreases in size when in the recumbent position. Varicoceles that do not decompress with the recumbent position are concerning for venous obstruction.
- Testicular carcinoma usually presents as a symptomatic testicular mass with firmness or induration. Of tumors, 10% will present with pain caused by hemorrhage within the tumor. Metastatic tumors can be insidious and should be suspected in males with unexplained supraclavicular lymphadenopathy.

Diagnosis and Evaluation

- Testicular ultrasound is diagnostic of these conditions.
- Computed tomography scan of the abdomen with contrast is indicated when venous obstruction is suspected.

Treatment

- Hydroceles and varicoceles can be managed in the outpatient setting with referral to urology. Emergency department urology consult is indicated if the swelling caused by the hydrocele is large enough to compromise scrotal skin integrity.
- Incarcerated hernias require prompt reduction to prevent strangulation and bowel infarction.
- Testicular carcinomas require urgent urologic referral.

SUGGESTED READINGS

Davis, J., & Silverman, M. (2011). Scrotal emergencies. *Emergency Medicine Clinics of North America*, 29(3), 469–484. https://www.sciencedirect.com/science/article/pii/S0733862711000459.

Dubin, J., & Davis, J. (2011). Penile emergencies. *Emergency Medicine Clinics of North America*, 29(3), 485–499. https://www.sciencedirect.com/science/article/pii/S073386271100040X.

Levey, H., Segal, R., & Bivalacqua, T. (2014). Management of priapism: An update for clinicians. *Therapeutic Advances in Urology*, 6(6), 230–244.

Proteinuria and Hematuria

CASEY KREBS, MD, and ANDREW GROCK, MD

Proteinuria

General Principles

- Proteinuria generally originates from the kidneys and can be divided into glomerular disease, tubular disease, and overflow proteinuria.
- Each can result from an array of diverse etiologies, ranging from benign to pathologic. Miscellaneous (i.e., nonrenal) causes include urinary tract infections, fevers or systemic inflammatory responses, and pregnancy, among others.
- Emergency evaluation centers on evaluation of renal function and evaluation of systemic disease.

Clinical Presentation

- **Nephrotic syndrome** is defined by hypoalbuminemia (< 3 g/dL), peripheral edema, and proteinuria, as measured by greater than 3.5 g in 24 hours, 3+ to 4+ protein on urine dipstick, or a urine protein:creatinine ratio greater than 2. Patients often present with generalized edema due to low oncotic pressure and "foamy" urine from proteinuria. Marked proteinuria can result in:
  - **Hyperlipidemia** as the liver enters an anabolic state to replace lost albumin, which also leads to accelerated atherosclerosis.
  - **Hypercoagulable state** due to the loss of anticoagulants in the urine; can thereby present with venous and/or arterial thromboembolism.
  - **Hypogammaglobulinemia** secondary to the loss of antibodies in the urine resulting in an increased susceptibility to infection.
- Nephrotic syndrome can result from different etiologies:
  - **Minimal change disease** is common in pediatrics and is typically preceded by upper respiratory tract symptoms or immunization.
  - **Focal segmental glomerulonephritis** is more common in African Americans and is usually idiopathic. It is often associated with HIV, heroin, and sickle cell disease, and generally progresses to chronic renal failure.
  - **Membranous nephropathy** is the most common nephrotic syndrome in Caucasians age 30–60 years. It is associated with hepatitis B and C, syphilis, malaria, systemic lupus erythematosus, penicillamine use, and, frequently, neoplasms. There is spontaneous remission in 25% of patients.
  - **Membranoproliferative glomerulonephritis** is associated with various infections, hepatitis C, and cryoglobulin deposition, and results in complement activation, renal damage, and low circulating C3 levels. It carries a poor prognosis with a 50% mortality or end-stage renal disease within 5 years of diagnosis.
  - **Diabetes** can cause arteriosclerosis of the glomerulus' efferent arteriole, which induces chronically high filtration pressures and microalbuminuria. This can then progress to nephrotic syndrome and chronic renal failure.
  - **Systemic amyloidosis** results in amyloid deposits around glomerular capillaries.
- **Nephritic syndrome** is defined by gross hematuria, often dysmorphic erythrocytes and red blood cell (RBC) casts in the urine, and may include proteinuria less than 3.5 g over 24 hours. Stemming from glomerular inflammation and bleeding, nephritic syndrome can also cause acute kidney injury, oliguria, and azotemia. Patients often present with sodium retention, often resulting in elevated blood pressure and edema, especially periorbital edema.
- Nephritic syndrome can result from different etiologies:
  - **Poststreptococcal glomerulonephritis** can appear 2–3 weeks after Group A β-hemolytic streptococcal infection. Patients often present with hypertension, cola-colored urine, oliguria, and periorbital edema. Children rarely progress to chronic kidney disease, whereas ~25% of adults develop rapidly progressive glomerulonephritis (RPGN) (see next paragraph).
  - **RPGN** results from antibody deposition activating the complement system. Patients often progress to renal failure in weeks to months. Goodpasture syndrome results from deposition of an anti–basement membrane antibody and patients present with both hematuria and hemoptysis. Vasculitides, such as microscopic polyangiitis, Churg-Strauss syndrome (often presenting with eosinophilia and asthma), and granulomatosis with polyangiitis (formerly Wegener granulomatosis), can also result in RPGN.
  - **IgA nephropathy** is the most common nephropathy worldwide and usually occurs after acute gastroenteritis, resulting in IgA deposition in the kidneys.
  - **Alport syndrome** is a collagen IV defect, most commonly X-linked–inherited. This condition results in the classic triad of hematuria, sensory hearing loss, and ocular disturbances.
- **Tubular sources** of proteinuria result from a defect in proximal tubule reabsorption and produce less than 2 g per 24 hours. Patients often present with asymptomatic acute renal failure or with nonspecific symptoms or signs. This type of proteinuria can result from hypertensive nephrosclerosis or various tubulointerstitial diseases such as uric acid nephropathy, Fanconi syndrome, acute hypersensitivity interstitial nephritis, heavy metals,

sickle cell disease, nonsteroidal antiiflammatory drugs, antibiotics (classic triad of rash, fever, and eosinophilia).

- **Overflow proteinuria** occurs when serum protein exceeds the capacity to reabsorb it. Proteinuria varies based on etiology. Renal injury results from decreased renal perfusion, direct cytotoxicity, and/or obstruction with intratubular casts from hemoglobinuria, myoglobinuria, multiple myeloma, or amyloidosis.
- **Functional proteinuria** is not associated with renal disease or renal injury and produces less than 2 g per 24 hours. Etiologies include urinary tract infections, fever, heavy exertion or stress, orthostatic proteinuria, congestive heart failure, and pregnancy (i.e., preeclampsia or hemolysis, elevated liver enzymes, and low platelet count occurring in association with preeclampsia).

Diagnosis and Evaluation

- The diagnosis and treatment of proteinuria varies depending on the etiology. A thorough history can help identify the underlying etiology (i.e., recent viral or systemic illnesses, change in medications, or a history of comorbidities [i.e., hypertension, diabetes, cardiac, or renal disease]). Obtain serum urea nitrogen and creatinine levels, particularly in patients with evidence of underlying renal disease. Urinalysis may demonstrate casts, which can help with the diagnosis:
  - Muddy brown: acute tubular necrosis
  - Fatty: nephrotic syndrome
  - RBCs: glomerular disease
  - White blood cells: interstitial nephritis
  - Waxy/granular: chronic kidney disease
  - Hyaline: dehydration
- Serum electrophoresis may demonstrate a monoclonal spike in multiple myeloma. A positive urine pregnancy test may suggest preeclampsia. Additionally, serologic studies such as antinuclear antibody, C3, C4, total complement, hepatitis B and C, and cryoglobulin tests can indicate a rheumatologic or infectious etiology. Lastly, a renal biopsy is the gold standard for adult patients. However, in pediatrics, an empiric trial of steroids is often used and, if the nephrotic syndrome resolves, a biopsy is precluded.

Treatment

Transient, resolved proteinuria requires no follow-up or further testing. The remainder of clinical decisions centers around symptoms (i.e., fevers, edema, thrombosis, hypertension, etc.), degree of proteinuria, and creatinine clearance.

- In asymptomatic patients with non–nephrotic range proteinuria and a normal creatine clearance, discharge with primary care doctor or nephrology follow-up is appropriate.
- In patients with non–nephrotic range proteinuria and an elevated creatinine level, consider emergency department nephrology consultation and further workup.
- Patients with nephrotic range proteinuria do not require routine anticoagulation, but anticoagulation may be indicated if there are additional hypercoagulable risk factors or if thrombosis occurs. Treatment of hypertension may be indicated, particularly in the setting of end-organ damage. In particular, diabetic nephropathy may benefit from treatment with tight glucose control and angiotensin-converting enzyme inhibitors, which may slow progression of disease by reducing filtration rate. Lastly, hyperlipidemia may improve with disease resolution. If not, a statin or other lipid-lowering agent should be given by the primary care provider.

Hematuria

General Principles

Gross hematuria refers to visible blood in the urine and can be as little as 1 mL/L. *Microscopic* hematuria refers to the laboratory diagnosis with more than three erythrocytes per high-power field on urinalysis. Generally, gross hematuria originates in the lower urinary tract. If gross hematuria occurs at the beginning of micturition with subsequent clearing, suspect a urethral source. Alternatively, if there are clots and hematuria throughout the urine stream, suspect a ureteral or bladder source. Lastly, hematospermia indicates a source in the male ejaculatory system. Casts, concurrent protein, or dysmorphic RBCs indicate renal, especially glomerular, pathologies. If the patient is over 50 years old, the patient should, at minimum, receive an outpatient urology referral for a malignancy evaluation.

Clinical Presentation

- Hematuria can present with a variety of clinical syndromes:
  - Acute-onset flank pain and hematuria: nephrolithiasis and renal infarction.
  - Fever, flank pain, hematuria: pyelonephritis (i.e., emphysematous, septic emboli), acute glomerulonephritis, or acute interstitial nephritis.
  - Painless hematuria: urologic malignancy (primary risk factors being over 50 years old, male, smoking history, family history of bladder cancer, occupational exposures [e.g., chemicals, rubber, leather industry], and excessive analgesic use), vascular lesions, vasculitis, and schistosomiasis.
  - Hematospermia is often self-limited. In patients younger than 40 years, most cases are often due to an infection or a benign cause.
  - Abdominal aortic aneurysm classically results in microscopic hematuria with abdominal, flank, or back pain in those older than 50 years and who have a history of smoking. Hematuria results from bladder inflammation secondary to direct pressure from the aneurysm.
- Special populations to consider:
  - HIV-positive patients: have a higher incidence of hematuria from urinary tract or sexually transmitted infections, glomerulonephritis, neurogenic bladder, thrombocytopenia, Kaposi sarcoma, or urethral trauma.
  - Pediatric patients: hematuria most commonly occurs from urinary tract infections, perineal or urethral irritation, congenital anomalies, trauma, acute nephritis (especially postinfectious glomerulonephritis), coagulopathy, nephrolithiasis, and hypercalciuria. Poststreptococcal glomerulonephritis can occur and is associated with low C3 and elevated antistreptolysin titers. Henoch-Schönlein purpura is a vasculitis with a clinical triad of nonthrombocytopenic palpable purpura, arthritis, and abdominal pain. Renal involvement is an important prognostic factor.

BOX 111.1 ***Differential Diagnosis for Hematuria***

- Glomerular
  - Nephritic syndrome
  - Preeclampsia/eclampsia
  - Serum sickness
  - Erythema multiforme
- Nonglomerular renal
  - Interstitial nephritis
  - Pyelonephritis
  - Papillary necrosis (sickle cell anemia, diabetes, NSAID use)
  - Arteriovenous malformations
  - Emboli
  - Polycystic kidney disease
  - Medullary sponge disease
  - Tuberculosis
  - Trauma
- Extrarenal
  - Trauma
  - Iatrogenic/postprocedure
  - Foreign body
  - Urinary epithelial diverticulum
  - Strictures
  - **Nephrolithiasis**
  - **Urinary tract infection**
  - Chemical or radiation cystitis (cyclophosphamide, salicylates, sulfonamides)
  - Endometriosis
  - Benign prostatic hyperplasia
  - **Prostatitis**
  - **Malignancy: transitional cell carcinoma**
  - Erosion or obstruction by other tumor
  - Erosion or obstruction by expanding aortic aneurysm
  - Vascular lesions/malformations
  - Loin pain hematuria syndrome
- Systemic disease
  - Hemophilia or other coagulopathy
  - Pharmacologic anticoagulation
  - Hypertensive emergency
  - Renal vein thrombosis
  - Exercise-induced hematuria
  - Cantharidin (Spanish fly) poisoning
  - Vasculitis/autoimmune/systemic inflammatory
    - Lupus
    - Rheumatic fever
    - Henoch-Schönlein purpura
    - Granulomatosis with polyangiitis
    - Hemolytic-uremic syndrome
    - Goodpasture syndrome
    - Polyarteritis nodosum

NSAID, nonsteroidal antiinflammatory drug.
Bold is for the most common etiologies.

Diagnosis and Evaluation

The diagnosis and treatment of hematuria varies depending on the etiology (Box 111.1). Thorough history and examination can help identify the underlying etiology. Laboratory and radiographic studies may also be helpful.

- Urinalysis
  - Microscopic hematuria: urine micro >3 erythrocytes per high-power field.
  - Urine dipstick false-positive results can be caused by myoglobin (rhabdomyolysis), hemoglobin, and porphyrins.
  - Suspect glomerular disease if there are dysmorphic erythrocytes, RBC casts, and concurrent proteinuria.
- Renal ultrasonography
  - Hydronephrosis and smaller kidney size may indicate obstruction and chronic kidney disease, respectively.
- Bladder ultrasonography
  - Acute urinary obstruction, defined as a postvoid residual greater than 100–150 mL.
  - Clotted blood can lead to urinary outlet obstruction.
- Computed tomography scan
  - A noncontrast scan can identify nephrolithiasis, renal masses, and obstruction.
  - Intravenous contrast (i.e., urogram) may be helpful in identifying structural lesions within the urogenital tract.
- Renal biopsy: standard for adults to identify the true etiology of the nephritic syndrome.

Treatment

The emergency department workup of hematuria should focus on appropriate screening for abdominal aortic aneurysm, systemic disease, acute intrinsic renal disease, and urinary obstruction. Treatment itself depends on the source or cause of hematuria but, generally speaking, *gross* hematuria requires follow-up with the urology department within 2 weeks, and within 1 month for *microscopic* hematuria with no identified cause. Patients with findings consistent with a urinary tract infection (e.g., fever, dysuria, nitrite-positive on urine dipstick with pyuria) should be treated with antibiotics and urine culture may be indicated. If the patient is over age 50 years, even with an identifiable cause of hematuria, they require follow-up for further malignancy evaluation.

SECTION FIFTEEN

BOARD REVIEW

Thoracic/ Respiratory

CHAPTER **112** BOARD REVIEW

Pleura, Mediastinum, and Chest Wall

PATRICIA FERMIN, MD, and GREGORY SAMPSON POWELL, MD, BS

The pleura is a thin serous membrane divided into two parts, visceral and parietal. The visceral pleura lines the lung surface and is poorly innervated. The parietal pleura lines the inner surface of the chest wall and is highly innervated. This lining also separates the pleural cavity from the mediastinum. The mediastinum lies between the lungs and contains the heart, aorta, great vessels, esophagus, thymus, trachea, bronchi, and lymph nodes. The chest wall consists of the rib cage, articulations between the ribs and vertebra, the diaphragm, and intercostal muscles. These parts are crucial for generating the negative intrathoracic pressures necessary for normal alveolar ventilation.

Pleura

PLEURAL EFFUSION

General Principles

- An abnormal accumulation of fluid in the pleural space
- Commonly owing to congestive heart failure, malignancy, bacterial pneumonia, and pulmonary embolism (PE). Tuberculosis (TB) is the leading cause worldwide.
- Classified as either transudative or exudative, based on testing of the fluid (Box 112.1)

Clinical Presentation

- The most common presenting symptom is dyspnea. Pleurisy or cough may also be present depending on the underlying etiology.
- It is asymptomatic in 25% of patients.
- Examination will often reveal dullness to percussion and decreased breath sounds.

Diagnosis and Evaluation

- Chest x-ray (CXR) is first line. Computed tomography (CT) imaging can visualize smaller effusions or assess for loculation.
- Thoracentesis can be performed to help determine the etiology.

Treatment

- Effusions owing to heart failure usually respond well to diuresis alone.
- Therapeutic thoracentesis is indicated if the effusion is large and symptomatic.
  - Risk of reexpansion pulmonary edema with removal of large volumes—more than 1.2 L
- Indwelling pleural catheter or talc pleurodesis for recurrent symptomatic effusions

EMPYEMA

General Principles

- Infection of the pleural space. Most commonly results from bacterial pneumonia.
- Other causes include chest surgery, trauma, esophageal perforation, complications of chest tubes/thoracenteses, or extensions from a subdiaphragmatic injury.
- *Pneumococcus* and *Staphylococcus aureus* are the most common pathogens.

Clinical Presentation

- Often patients will present with symptoms of pneumonia, including pleurisy.
- Onset may be insidious and may be associated with hemoptysis.

Diagnosis and Evaluation

- Made by pleural fluid sampling with return of pus or a positive Gram stain or culture.
- Suspect esophageal perforation in patients who develop effusion after retching.

Treatment

- Drainage with tube thoracostomy and antibiotics are definitive treatments.
- After 48 hours, organization of contents may occur and may require multiple chest tubes, fibrinolytics, or video-assisted thoracoscopic surgery (VATS). Rarely, thoracotomy is necessary.

PNEUMOTHORAX (PTX)

General Principles

- Occurs with accumulation of air in the pleural space with several defining categories:
  - Can be spontaneous, traumatic, or iatrogenic.
  - Can be primary or secondary to underlying lung disease (chronic obstructive pulmonary disease, lung cancer, etc.).

BOX 112.1 Causes of Pleural Effusion

Transudates
- Congestive heart failure
- Cirrhosis with ascites
- Nephrotic syndrome
- Hypoalbuminemia
- Myxedema
- Peritoneal dialysis
- Glomerulonephritis
- Superior vena cava obstruction
- Pulmonary embolism

Exudates

Infections
- Bacterial pneumonia
- Bronchiectasis
- Lung abscess
- Tuberculosis
- Viral illness

Neoplasms
- Primary lung cancer
- Mesothelioma
- Pulmonary or pleural metastases
- Lymphoma

Connective Tissue Disease
- Rheumatoid arthritis
- Systemic lupus erythematosus

Abdominal or Gastrointestinal Disorders
- Pancreatitis
- Subphrenic abscess
- Esophageal rupture
- Abdominal surgery

Miscellaneous Conditions
- Pulmonary infarction
- Uremia
- Drug reactions
- Postpartum
- Chylothorax

(From Kosowsky, J. M, & Kimberly, H. H. (1988). Pleural disease. In P. Rosen & F. J. Baker II (Eds.), *Rosen's emergency medicine: Concepts and clinical practice* (2nd ed., pp. 881–889, Box 67.2). Mosby.)

- Can be simple, open (Fig. 112.1), or tension (Fig. 112.2):
  - Simple means that there is no communication with the atmosphere or a mediastinal shift.
  - Open/communicating means that there is a large defect in the chest wall.
  - Tension PTX occurs when the mediastinum is shifted toward the opposite hemithorax and compresses the contralateral lung and great vessels, causing obstructive shock.
    - In tension PTX, the injury acts as a one-way valve where air enters on inspiration, but cannot leave on expiration.

112

Clinical Presentation

- Dyspnea and chest pain are the most common complaints.
- Decreased or absent breath sounds on the affected side with hyperresonance to percussion
- May display tachycardia, hypotension, hypoxia, jugular vein distention (JVD), and tracheal deviation with tension.

Diagnosis and Evaluation

- Tension PTX should be diagnosed by clinical findings alone.
- Upright CXR for all other pneumothoraces.
  - Supine films may reveal a deep sulcus sign.
  - Do not confuse with pulmonary blebs (seen in chronic lung disease).
- Ultrasound has been shown to have greater sensitivity than x-ray and may be quicker.
  - Absence of lung sliding
  - In M-mode this is represented by a "barcode" sign rather than a "seashore sign."
- CT imaging may reveal extremely small pneumothoraces of unclear significance.

Treatment

- Most occult pneumothoraces (seen only on CT) can be observed.
- For small pneumothoraces (pleural line less than 2 cm), supplemental oxygen alone

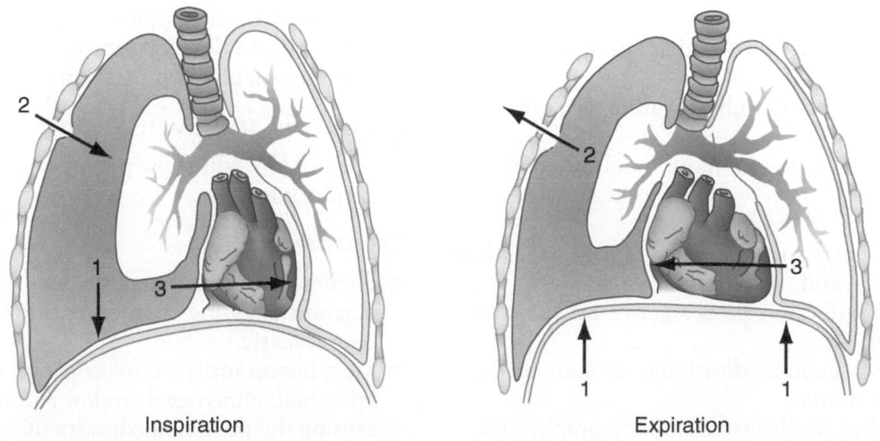

FIG. 112.1 A communicating pneumothorax. (From Raja, A, S. (1988). Thoracic trauma. In P. Rosen & F. J. Baker II (Eds.), *Rosen's emergency medicine: Concepts and clinical practice* (2nd ed., pp. 382–403, Fig. 45.7). Mosby.)

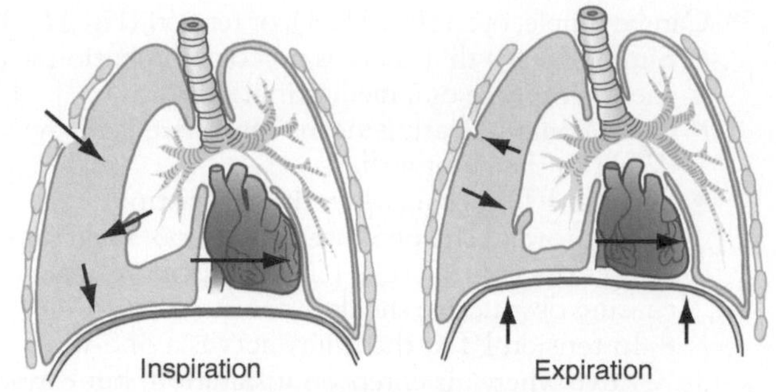

FIG. 112.2 A tension pneumothorax. (From Raja, A. S. (1988). Thoracic trauma. In P. Rosen & F. J. Baker II (Eds.), *Rosen's emergency medicine: Concepts and clinical practice* (2nd ed., pp. 382–403, Fig. 67.1). Mosby.)

- For primary spontaneous pneumothoraces (pleural line more than 2 cm), either needle aspiration or pigtail catheter placement is recommended.
- If secondary, will need either a small-bore tube thoracostomy or a pigtail catheter.
- Associated hemothorax will require tube thoracostomy.
- Consider single-dose prophylactic intravenous (IV) antibiotics (such as cefazolin) during placement of a chest tube in trauma patients.
- For tension pneumothorax, a long large-bore angiocatheter may be inserted prior to thoracostomy. Insert at second intercostal space in the midclavicular line or (preferred) fourth to fifth intercostal space in the midaxillary line.

Mediastinum

MEDIASTINITIS

General Principles

- Most commonly caused by bacterial infection from esophageal rupture.
  - Either iatrogenic during surgery/endoscopy or secondary to retching (Boerhaave syndrome).
- Infection may also come from the neck, retroperitoneum, lung, pleura, chest wall or hematogenous spread.

Clinical Presentation

- Presents with acute fever, tachycardia, chest pain, dysphagia, or respiratory distress.
- Crepitance and edema of the chest wall or neck may be present as well.
- Chronic mediastinitis follows a more indolent course.

Diagnosis and Evaluation

- Causes for chronic mediastinitis include fungal infection, tuberculosis, tumors, and sarcoidosis.
- Laboratory testing will often show signs of infection in acute mediastinitis.
- CXR can show a widened mediastinum, pneumomediastinum, or pneumothorax.
- Chest CT has higher sensitivity than radiography and can guide drainage.
- See Fig. 112.3.

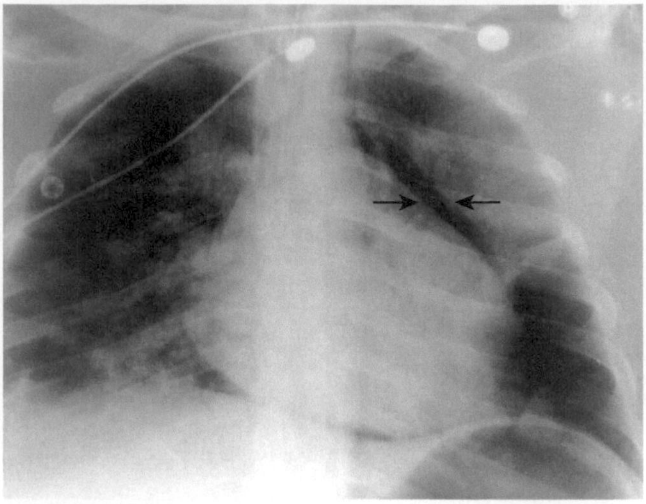

FIG. 112.3 Mediastinitis on chest x-ray. (From Durack, D. T. (2015). Prophylaxis of infective endocarditis. In J. E. Bennett, R. Dolin, & M. J. Blaser (Eds.), *Mandell, Douglas, and Bennett's principles and practice of infectious diseases* (8th ed., Fig. 85.2). Elsevier Saunders.)

Treatment

- Requires broad-spectrum IV antibiotics and surgical evacuation of necrotic tissue.
- May also require pleural drainage, endoscopy, bronchoscopy, or neck exploration.
- Chronic mediastinitis may also need long-term antifungal or antitubercular medications.

PNEUMOMEDIASTINUM

General Principles

- Usually results from a rupture of the esophagus, trachea, or lung.
- It can occur spontaneously, but most often is secondary to trauma.
- Other etiologies include asthma exacerbation, violent coughing, or violent emesis.

Clinical Presentation

- May present as sore throat, dyspnea, or neck pain.
- May dissect into the soft tissues, resulting in subcutaneous emphysema and crepitus.
- Rarely, it can develop tension physiology and cause right ventricular compression.

Diagnosis and Evaluation

- CXR or CT will show pneumomediastinum or pneumopericardium.

Treatment

- Pneumomediastinum alone does not require further diagnostic testing or intervention unless the patient is symptomatic.
- Most important is an investigation for laryngeal, tracheal, bronchial, pharyngeal, and/or esophageal injuries that are causing the pneumomediastinum.
- Tension pneumomediastinum is very rare, but requires emergent surgical decompression.

Chest Wall

COSTOCHONDRITIS

General Principles

- Pain/tenderness of the anterior chest wall, in the costochondral and costosternal regions.
- It is estimated that up to 10% of presentations for chest pain are caused by costochondritis.
- Tietze syndrome involves the costosternal articulations and can cause visible swelling.

Clinical Presentation

- Pain can be sharp, pressure-like, or pleuritic and may radiate down the arms.
- The pain should be highly localized, positional, and completely reproducible.
- There may be a history of overuse, trauma, or autoimmune disorder.

Diagnosis and Evaluation

- Costochondritis is a clinical diagnosis. Studies are only for excluding other diagnoses.

Treatment

- Once more serious pathology has been excluded, the focus of the clinician should be on reducing pain with nonsteroidal antiinflammatory drugs or acetaminophen and reassuring the patient.

SUGGESTED READINGS

Fort, G. G. (2018). Mediastinitis. In Ferri, F. (Ed.), *Ferri's clinical advisor* (p. 802–803.e1). Elsevier.

Inaba, K., Lustenberger, T., & Recinos, G. (2012). Does size matter? A prospective analysis of 28-32 versus 36-40 French chest tube size in trauma. *Journal of Trauma and Acute Care Surgery, 72*(2), 422–427.

Kosowsky, J. M., & Kimberly, H. H. (2018). Pleural disease. In R. M. Walls, R. S. Hockberger, & M. Gausche-Hill (Eds.), *Rosen's emergency medicine: Concepts and clinical practice* (9th ed., p. 881–889.e2). Elsevier.

Acute Respiratory Distress Syndrome and Pulmonary Hypertension

MANUEL AMANDO CELEDON, MD, and CAROLYN SHOVER, MD

Acute Respiratory Distress Syndrome

Acute respiratory distress syndrome (ARDS) is a constellation of symptoms in which a patient develops noncardiogenic pulmonary edema, hypoxia, and diffuse lung findings. The pathophysiology is multifactorial and often related to an identifiable inciting event, such as infection (most commonly pneumonia, sepsis, or aspiration) or trauma. Management is largely supportive and involves a multisystem approach.

General Principles

- Definition: the Berlin definition of ARDS is the most commonly accepted.
  1. Acute respiratory symptoms
  2. Bilateral pulmonary opacities on imaging (*not explained by another cause*)
  3. Respiratory failure not fully explained by heart failure or volume overload
  4. Impairment of oxygenation must be present.
- Pathophysiology: lung injury leads to fluid buildup within alveoli and pulmonary interstitial space. Fluid buildup interferes with normal gas exchange and lung compliance and leads to elevated pulmonary arterial pressures.
- Mechanisms: multifactorial causes lead to lung injury.

Clinical Presentation

- Patients usually present with shortness of breath, typically after an inciting event.
- Patients have respiratory distress, such as tachypnea, tachycardia, or hypoxemia.
- On general examination the patients may have an altered sensorium. The pulmonary examination may reveal crackles or ronchi.
- An inciting event or underlying cause, such as trauma or infection, may be apparent on presentation.

Diagnosis and Evaluation

- On imaging, chest radiograph reveals bilateral alveolar infiltrates.
- Computed tomography shows similar disease as chest radiograph, with worse disease apparent in the dependent area of the lungs.
- Laboratory tests are not specific for ARDS. There may be evidence of an underlying process, such as infection. Arterial blood gas shows hypoxemia.
- Most of the diagnostic workup (e.g., B-type natriuretic peptide test, electrocardiogram, and/or an infectious workup) helps exclude other etiologies of respiratory distress.

Treatment

- Supportive care (such as sedation, neuromuscular blockade, nutrition, prevention of iatrogenic complications)
- Managing inciting event or underlying condition
- When the patient is intubated, use lung-protective ventilation, which includes low tidal volumes (4–8 mL/kg of ideal body weight), high positive end-expiratory pressures, and permissive hypercapnia.
- Conservative fluid resuscitation and prone positioning are other emerging aspects of ARDS management. Steroid use is controversial, but is recommended in severe cases.
- In some specialty centers, extracorporeal membrane oxygenation may be used as a rescue option.
- May present similar to congestive heart failure, but does not respond to same treatments

Pulmonary Hypertension

Pulmonary hypertension is a group of various disease processes in which there are elevated pressures within the pulmonary arterial system. Patients with pulmonary hypertension are divided into five groups:

- Group 1: pulmonary arterial hypertension (drugs, connective tissue disorder)
  - The term pulmonary arterial hypertension (PAH) refers to those patients who fall in Group 1 and is the focus of this discussion.
- Group 2: pulmonary hypertension due to left-sided heart disease
- Group 3: pulmonary hypertension due to chronic lung disorders, hypoxemia (usually chronic obstructive pulmonary disease or interstitial lung disease)

- Group 4: pulmonary hypertension due to pulmonary artery obstructions, such as in a pulmonary embolism
- Group 5: pulmonary hypertension due to unclear or multifactorial mechanisms

General Principles

- Definition: a group of conditions in which the mean arterial pressure of the pulmonary artery is >20 mm Hg at rest (as measured using catheterization of the right side of the heart)
- Pathophysiology: etiologies for patients with PAH fall into several main classes: inherited, toxin exposure, disease-associated (such as HIV), or idiopathic. Thus a wide array of pathophysiology may ultimately lead to PAH. The pathophysiology is multifactorial and involves ultimate remodeling of the pulmonary artery vessel walls, thereby increasing vascular resistance and pressure.

Clinical Presentation

- Patients report shortness of breath, dyspnea on exertion, fatigue.
- On examination, the pulmonic component of the cardiac examination is increased.
- If patients have right-sided heart failure, they may have hepatomegaly, peripheral edema, and elevated jugular venous pressure.
- Patients are very sensitive to fluid status.
  - Hypervolemia rapidly leads to right-sided heart failure.
  - Hypovolemia rapidly leads to hypotension because of preload dependence.

Diagnosis and Evaluation

- Assess mean arterial pressure of pulmonary artery with catheterization of the right side of the heart.
- Assess for other causes of pulmonary hypertension, such as left-sided heart failure or pulmonary embolism.
- Workup may include electrocardiogram, chest radiograph, B-type natriuretic peptide test, troponin test, possibly computed tomography angiography, cardiac catheterization, echocardiogram.

Treatment

The management of patients in respiratory distress related to PAH is challenging because they are sensitive to rapid changes in hemodynamics. Early specialty consultation can be useful.

- Avoid hypoxemia because it causes pulmonary arterial vasoconstriction.
- Optimize right ventricular (RV) preload and reduce RV afterload. This strategy may involve cautious diuresis in RV failure, noting that blood pressure is highly preload-dependent.
- Improve cardiac output (inotropes may be needed).
- Manage arrhythmias (cautious rate control).
- Medications include pulmonary arterial vasodilators such as sildenafil, bosentan, or epoprostenol. These are started in consultation with a specialist.
  - Patients may present in heart failure, but avoid nitrates in patients on phosphodiesterase type 5 inhibitors (sildenafil) because of the risk of hypotension.
- Patients are difficult to manage if intubated, so it is important to use low positive end-expiratory pressures so as not to further decrease preload.

113

SUGGESTED READINGS

NHLBI [National Heart Lung and Blood Institute] ARDS Network. (n.d.) Available at: www.ardsnet.org/

Fan, E., Brodie, D., & Slutsky, A. S. (2018). Acute respiratory distress syndrome: Advances in diagnosis and treatment. *Journal of the American Medical Association, 319*(7), 698–710. doi:10.1001/jama.2017.21907

Wilcox, S. R., Kabrhel, C., & Channick, R. N. (2015). Pulmonary hypertension and right ventricular failure in emergency medicine. *Annals of Emergency Medicine*, 66(6), 619–631.

CHAPTER 114

BOARD REVIEW

Obstructive and Restrictive Lung Disease

THOMAS E. BLAIR, MD

Obstructive lung disease is characterized by resistance to airflow owing to airway obstruction. Restrictive lung disease is characterized by decreased lung volumes. The restrictive process and subsequent decreased lung capacity may be extrinsic or intrinsic to the lungs. In spirometry, obstructive lung disease reveals a decreased forced expiratory volume at one second (FEV_1) with near normal forced vital capacity (FVC) and therefore a decreased FEV_1/FVC ratio. Restrictive diseases are defined by a decreased forced vital capacity and normal or elevated FEV_1/FVC. In emergency medicine, however, it is most important simply to recognize the different pathophysiologic changes between restrictive lung disease in comparison with obstructive lung diseases. In reality there is substantial overlap between the two categories.

Restrictive Lung Disease

- Decreased lung volumes/lung capacity with a multitude of causes:
  - Intrinsic: acute respiratory distress syndrome, pulmonary fibrosis, sarcoidosis, pneumonitis, etc.
  - Extrinsic: obesity hypoventilation syndrome, pleural effusion, pneumothorax, ascites, kyphoscoliosis, neuromuscular disorders (Guillain-Barre syndrome, muscular dystrophy, etc.).
- Evaluation and treatment of restrictive lung disease should focus on assessing and reversing the underlying etiology (such as identifying and draining a pleural effusion). Because there is rarely an immediately reversible cause, emergency management is often focused on support of oxygenation and ventilation, as needed. Important causes of restrictive lung disease are discussed in detail throughout this section.

Obstructive Lung Disease

ASTHMA

General Principles

- Asthma is a chronic recurrent respiratory disorder characterized by repeated bouts of dyspnea/wheezing secondary to bronchospasm and airway inflammation.
- Asthma is caused by a complex interaction between the immune system, the environment, and genetic factors.

Clinical Presentation

- Patients present with a constellation of dyspnea, wheezing, cough, and chest tightness. Episodes may be spontaneous or triggered by an allergy, the environment, or an infection. Episodes with a rapid onset (fewer than 6 hours) tend to have a more bronchospastic component. These episodes may be more severe, but respond better to therapy. Episodes that peak over days tend to have a more inflammatory component and are slower to respond. Patients with a prior need for mechanical ventilation or intensive care admissions are at higher risks for mortality.

Diagnosis and Evaluation

- Asthma is formally diagnosed using spirometry, which reveals reversible airflow obstruction. Spirometry is not feasible in the emergency setting, so clinical diagnosis is usually established using history and physical examination along with a response to therapy.
- Peak expiratory flow rate can be used to determine quantitatively the severity of the airway obstruction.
  - Its use does not reliably predict admission nor does it decrease morbidity or mortality.
- Chest radiography is not routinely indicated, but should be considered in patients with fever, hypoxia, atypical features, significant comorbid conditions, or possible complications, or in patients requiring hospital admission.
- Blood gas analysis is not routinely indicated, but can help detect worsening status when clinical assessment and peak flow alone are not sufficient. Venous blood gas along with pulse oximetry is usually sufficient and arterial blood gas is rarely warranted.
  - Hyperventilation is typical during asthma exacerbations; therefore hypocapnia is often present. The presence of a normal $PaCO_2$ may actually indicate impending respiratory failure. Hypercapnia is a late finding.
- Other laboratory testing is not routinely indicated.
  - Lactate, if measured, is commonly elevated during albuterol therapy, but is not associated with hypoperfusion or worse outcomes (type B lactic acidosis).
  - Leukocytosis may be seen with corticosteroid therapy.

Treatment

- Inhaled short-acting beta-2 adrenergic agonists (albuterol) are the mainstay of treatment to reverse bron-

chospasm. Albuterol can be administered as intermittent nebulization, metered dose inhaler, or continuous nebulization.
- Inhaled anticholinergics (ipratropium) are added for moderate to severe disease, up to three doses.
- Systemic glucocorticoids (e.g., prednisone or methylprednisolone) are indicated whenever symptoms persist despite inhaled therapies. Oral and intravenous therapies are equivalent, except in critically ill patients when intravenous (IV) therapy is preferred.
- Magnesium sulfate (2 g IV over 20 minutes) causes smooth muscle relaxation and bronchodilation. Indicated in severe exacerbations, it decreases the need for admission.
- Epinephrine (nonselective beta-agonist) or terbutaline (selective beta-2 agonist) is indicated only when air movement is so poor that inhaled beta-agonists are ineffective.
- A trial of noninvasive mechanical ventilation (BiPAP) may be appropriate in patients while medications are taking effect and may prevent the need for intubation.
- Mechanical ventilation is indicated for impending respiratory failure, but does not address the underlying pathophysiology of asthma.
  - Continued aggressive postintubation medical treatment is necessary.
  - Ventilator settings should be set to avoid barotrauma and breath stacking (Fig. 114.1).
  - Management may require permissive hypercapnia with relatively low respiratory rates to optimize inspiratory-to-expiratory (I:E) ratios.
  - If an intubated asthmatic patient becomes hemodynamically unstable, immediately disconnect from the ventilator and manually compress the chest until all air has escaped. Then slowly mechanically ventilate with 100% O_2.
    - If the patient remains unstable, assess for the DOPE mnemonic: *D*islodgement of tube, *O*bstruction of tube, *P*neumothorax, and *E*quipment failure.
- Intravenous ketamine, general anesthesia with inhaled anesthetics, and extracorporeal membrane oxygenation (ECMO) can be considered in the most severe or refractory cases.
- The following medication classes are not currently recommended as standard care for acute asthma exacerbations: long-acting beta-2 agonists (salmeterol), long-acting anticholinergics (tiotropium), inhaled corticosteroids, methylxanthines (theophylline), leukotriene modifiers (montelukast), and heliox.

CHRONIC OBSTRUCTIVE PULMONARY DISEASE (COPD)

General Principles

- As with asthma, COPD is caused by chronic airway inflammation leading to airway obstruction. Unlike asthma, parenchymal damage in the form of emphysema is a hallmark of COPD.
- The chronic inflammation and parenchymal damage are caused by chronic exposure to environmental irritants, especially tobacco smoke.

Clinical Presentation

- As with asthma, patients will present with a combination of dyspnea, wheezing, cough, and chest tightness. Patients usually have a history of chronic exposure to irritants such as tobacco smoke. Patients may also meet criteria for chronic bronchitis: a productive cough lasting at least 3 months and recurring over at least 2 consecutive years. As disease progresses, chronic hypoxemia, pulmonary hypertension (group 3 PH), and cor pulmonale (right-sided heart failure) may develop.

Diagnosis and Evaluation

- COPD is formally diagnosed with spirometry revealing persistent airflow limitation that is incompletely reversed using bronchodilators. Formal diagnosis is not feasible in the emergency department. Clinical diagnosis is suggested in patients with a typical history and physical examination findings, especially when there is a known chronic exposure to environmental irritants (e.g., tobacco).
- Unlike in asthma, chest radiography should be routinely performed in patients with COPD exacerbations because it may reveal complications and alternative diagnoses, such as infiltrates, pneumothoraces, and masses.

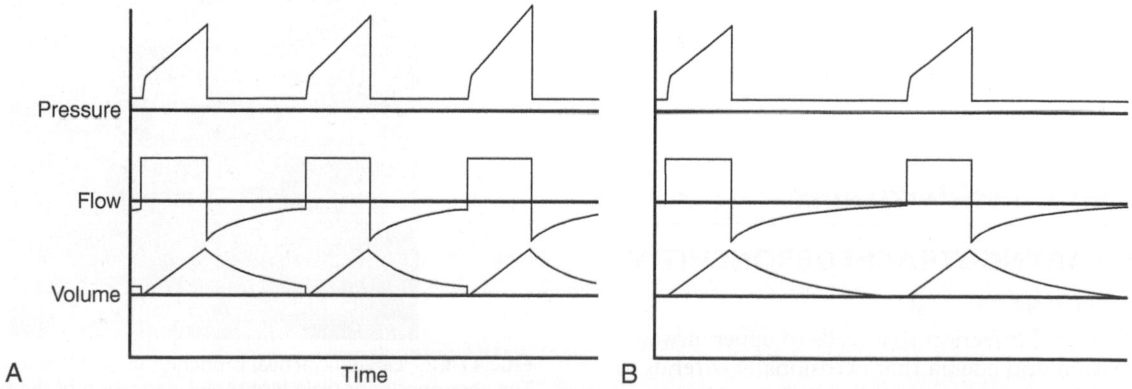

FIG. 114.1 **A**, Air trapping is evident by progressively increasing inspiratory pressures, failure of expiratory flow to return to zero before the next breath, and an inspiratory volume greater than expiratory volume in a flow-volume targeted mode of ventilation. **B**, Decreasing the respiratory rate allows for complete exhalation before the next breath, thus alleviating air trapping. (From Bergin, S. P., & Rackley, C. R. (2016). Managing respiratory failure in obstructive lung disease. *Clinics in Chest Medicine, 37*(4), 659–667, Fig. 3.)

- As in asthma, blood gas analysis is not routinely indicated.
- Although both bacterial and viral infections play a frequent role in COPD exacerbations, neither viral testing nor sputum cultures should play a routine role in the emergency department. The one possible exception is influenza testing during influenza season because a positive result may prompt use of antivirals.

Treatment

- A substantial overlap exists in the treatment of COPD and asthma, with major differences highlighted below.
  - Titrate oxygen to approximately 92%: overuse of supplemental oxygen may decrease respiratory drive.
  - Inhaled short-acting beta-2 adrenergic agonists (albuterol)
  - Inhaled anticholinergics (ipratropium)
  - Systemic glucocorticoids (e.g., prednisone or methylprednisolone)
  - Antibiotics should be considered in patients with two of the three findings: (1) increased dyspnea, (2) increased cough, and (3) increased sputum purulence. Antibiotics are also used for patients requiring invasive or noninvasive ventilation. Typical regimens are 5 to 7 days of therapy with macrolides (azithromycin), tetracyclines (doxycycline), or aminopenicillins (amoxicillin-clavulanic acid).
  - Magnesium sulfate, unlike in asthma, has not been shown to be beneficial.
  - Noninvasive mechanical ventilation (BiPAP) is strongly supported by the literature to decrease the need for mechanical ventilation.
- Intubation has similar indications and cautions as it does in asthma.

ACUTE BRONCHITIS

General Principles

- Acute bronchitis is a common mimic of pneumonia and may present with cough (with or without sputum).
- Diagnosis is clinical, but in patients with abnormal vital signs or abnormal breath sounds on auscultation, a chest x-ray can usually differentiate bronchitis from pneumonia.
- Of cases, 90% are viral and antibiotics should not be prescribed. Treatment is with supportive care alone, with or without albuterol for bronchospasm.
- Notably, bronchitis is the most common cause of hemoptysis.

Pediatric Considerations

CROUP (LARYNGOTRACHEOBRONCHITIS)

General Principles

- Croup is a viral infection that leads to upper airway inflammation and edema that occasionally extends to the bronchi.
- Parainfluenza virus is responsible for the majority of cases. Respiratory syncytial virus and influenza are less-common causes.

Clinical Presentation

- The defining features of croup are a barking cough, inspiratory stridor, and hoarseness.
- Occurs in children 6 months to 3 years of age.
- Usually preceded by 1 to 3 days of a viral prodrome and upper respiratory symptoms.
- The presence of drooling, dysphagia, high fevers, torticollis, or toxic appearance should prompt consideration of alternative diagnoses, such as epiglottitis, bacterial tracheitis, retropharyngeal abscess, or foreign body.

Diagnosis and Evaluation

- Diagnosis is clinical.
- Radiographs should not be routinely used because they are not sensitive or specific enough to change management. If obtained, however, they may reveal a "steeple sign," named for the appearance of the subglottic tracheal narrowing (Fig. 114.2).
- Laboratory testing is rarely indicated.

Treatment

- Glucocorticoids, such as oral dexamethasone (0.15 to 0.6 mg/kg; max 16 mg), decrease symptoms, emergency department length of stay, and need for admission.
- Nebulized epinephrine reduces airway edema through local vasoconstriction. It is indicated for patients with stridor at rest. Onset is within 10 minutes and duration is 2 to 3 hours. Treatments can be repeated if needed.

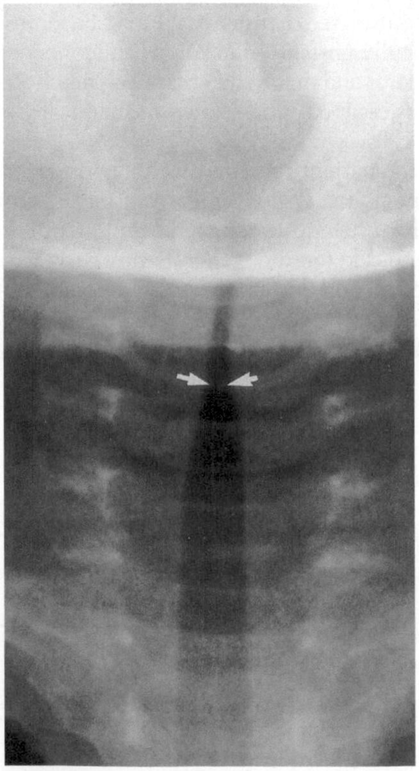

FIG. 114.2 Laryngotracheal bronchitis in an 11-month-old boy. The anteroposterior plain film shows narrowing of the subglottic region, also called the steeple sign (*arrows*). (From Hudgins, P. A., Robson, C. D., & Friedman, E. R. Pediatric airway disease. In P. M. Som & H. D. Curtin. *Head and neck imaging* (5th ed., Fig. 30.82). Elsevier.)

Patients should be observed 2 to 3 hours after the last dose to monitor for return of symptoms.

- Cool mist does not improve clinical outcomes, but may provide modest symptom relief.
- In the rare case that intubation is necessary, an endotracheal tube one-half size smaller than calculated may be needed to account for the inflamed airway.
- Admit patients with persistent stridor at rest, persistent respiratory distress, or hypoxia.

BRONCHOPULMONARY DYSPLASIA (BPD)

General Principles

- Bronchopulmonary dysplasia is a pulmonary disease of prematurity, usually defined as the need for supplemental oxygen at 28 days postnatally.
- It is caused by the underdeveloped premature lung and may be worsened by the detrimental effects of subsequent oxygen toxicity and mechanical ventilation.
- Incidence increases with decreasing gestational age and decreasing birth weight.

Clinical Presentation

- Patients usually present to the emergency department for acute exacerbations of previously diagnosed BPD.
- Exacerbations may be characterized by increasing oxygen requirements, pulmonary edema, airway reactivity, infection, or pneumothorax.

Diagnosis and Evaluation

- Physical examination may reveal tachypnea, wheezing, crackles, or respiratory distress.
- At baseline, chest radiography is variable and may reveal hyperinflation, atelectasis, or an interstitial pattern. During exacerbations, it can reveal the cause of decompensation, such as infiltrates, pulmonary edema, or pneumothorax.
- During acute exacerbations of BPD, there should be a low threshold for obtaining blood gas analysis, complete cell count, and blood cultures (if infection is suspected).

Treatment

- The treatment of acute exacerbations of BPD should be targeted at the acute trigger.
- Bronchospasm may respond to inhaled beta-agonists (albuterol), pulmonary edema to loop diuretics (furosemide), and infection to antibiotics.

CYSTIC FIBROSIS (CF)

General Principles

- Cystic fibrosis is an autosomal-recessive condition caused by a mutation in the CF transmembrane conductance regulator, a chloride channel.
- This defect causes thickened secretions primarily resulting in progressive respiratory disease, including chronic bronchitis, bronchiectasis, obstructive lung disease, and progressive respiratory failure.
- Patients are particularly at risk for infection with *Pseudomonos aeruginosa*, *Staphylococcus aureus* (including methicillin-resistant *S. aureus*), and *Haemophilus influenzae*.
- Thickened secretions also cause extrapulmonary manifestations, including chronic sinusitis, pancreatitis, meconium ileus, bowel obstruction, cholelithiasis, and male infertility.

Clinical Presentation

- Patients with known CF will often present to the emergency department with acute pulmonary exacerbations. Signs and symptoms of exacerbation may include productive cough, dyspnea, fever, fatigue, and chest congestion.

114

Diagnosis and Evaluation

- Emergency department evaluation of CF exacerbations should include blood cultures, sputum cultures, and chest radiographs.

Treatment

- Antibiotics are almost always indicated in CF exacerbations. Antibiotic selection can be based on prior culture results, but severe exacerbations almost always include double coverage for *Pseudomonas*. A common empiric inpatient regimen is piperacillin-tazobactam plus tobramycin.
- There should be a low threshold for treatment with antiinfluenza drugs, such as oseltamivir during the flu season.
- Systemic glucocorticoids are often used if there appears to be a component of bronchospasm.
- Chronic treatments should be continued, such as inhaled hypertonic saline, chest physiotherapy, and chronic oral azithromycin.

SUGGESTED READINGS

Tintinalli, J. E., Stapczynski, J. S., Ma, O. J., Yealy, D. M., Meckler, G. D., & Cline, D. M. (2016). *Tintinalli's emergency medicine: A comprehensive study guide* (8th ed.). McGraw-Hill Education.

Walls, R. M., Hockberger, R. S., & Gausche-Hill, M. (2018). *Rosen's emergency medicine: Concepts and clinical practice* (9th ed.). Elsevier.

CHAPTER 115 BOARD REVIEW

Pulmonary Embolism/Infarct—Septic Embolic, VTE, and Fat Emboli

MANUEL AMANDO CELEDON, MD, and CAROLYN SHOVER, MD

Venous Thromboembolism

General Principles

- Venous thromboembolisms (VTE) occur when factors disrupt the homeostasis between thrombosis and anticoagulation, leading to increased fibrin deposition and decreased elimination. These factors can be categorized as either provoked (acquired) or unprovoked (idiopathic, hereditary). The underlying mechanism of thrombosis results from the triad of hypercoagulability, vascular endothelial injury, and stasis (referred to as the Virchow triad). Patients diagnosed with a thrombotic event often have at least one identifiable risk factor for thrombosis (many patients have multiple factors). About half of VTEs in patients with a hereditary thrombophilia are associated with the additional existence of an acquired risk factor.

1. Hereditary factors include factor V Leiden mutation, protein C/S deficiency, antithrombin III deficiency, and prothrombin gene mutation (prothrombin G20210A).
2. Acquired factors include immobility (long distance travel, bed rest, casts), advanced age, malignancy, recent surgery or trauma, pregnancy or postpartum period, obesity, oral contraceptives (estrogens), noninfectious inflammatory conditions (lupus, antiphospholipid syndrome, nephrotic syndrome), and intravenous catheters. The main presentations of VTEs include:

- Deep vein thrombosis (DVT)
- Pulmonary embolism (PE)
- Superficial thrombophlebitis

Deep Venous Thrombosis

General Principles

- The deep venous system of the lower extremity is divided into above the knee (proximal) and below the knee (distal) veins. Immobilization, especially of the knee or hip, confers the biggest risk of DVT to the patient.
- The proximal deep venous system includes:
  - Femoral vein (previously named the superficial femoral vein)
  - Deep femoral vein
  - Common femoral vein
  - External iliac vein
- The distal deep venous system includes:
  - Calf veins: anterior tibial, posterior tibial, and peroneal veins
  - Popliteal vein
- Untreated DVTs have the potential for embolization and may cause PEs.
- Distal greater saphenous vein clots are considered a superficial thrombosis, whereas a clot in the greater saphenous vein near its connection with the femoral vein is considered a proximal DVT.
- Upper extremity DVT (UEDVT) is associated with intravenous catheters. Limited data exist regarding the efficacy of treatment of UEDVT for preventing embolization of clot from an upper extremity source.
- Guidelines from the American College of Chest Physicians recommend anticoagulation therapy for UEDVTs, with or without catheter removal, depending on the situation.

Clinical Presentation

- Primary symptoms of a DVT include unilateral extremity swelling, pain, fullness, or cramping.
- Some patients will present with erythema that may mimic cellulitis; however, concurrent DVT in patients with clinical evidence of cellulitis is rare.
- A positive Homan sign, discomfort behind the knee on forced foot dorsiflexion, has limited predictive value because it is neither sensitive nor specific.
- *Phlegmasia alba dolens* is a painful white leg that represents significant iliofemoral vein occlusion with associated arterial insufficiency that may be limb-threatening.
- *Phlegmasia cerulea dolens* is a painful blue leg representing significant iliofemoral vein occlusion that may be limb-threatening (at risk for compartment syndrome).

Diagnosis and Evaluation

- Centers around developing pretest probability (PTP) using the clinical gestalt of an experienced practitioner or by using a clinical decision tool (i.e., Wells score).
  - Patients are divided into three risk groups based on probability of disease: low (5%), intermediate (17%), and high (17%–53%).

- The D-dimer is a fibrin breakdown product that acts as a surrogate marker for detecting the presence of a thrombotic event within the past 72 hours.
- The compression ultrasound is the gold standard imaging study to confirm the diagnosis of a DVT.
- Diagnostic scenarios:
  - A negative D-dimer alone essentially rules out a DVT in patients with low pretest probability (PTP).
  - A negative high-sensitivity D-dimer is sufficient to rule out DVT in a patient with moderate PTP (posttest probability of less than 1%).
  - A negative D-dimer, when used in conjunction with a negative three-point ultrasound, is sufficient to exclude DVT in patients with any PTP.
  - Patients with a high PTP, positive D-dimer, and a negative ultrasound at the index visit should receive a follow-up ultrasound in 7 days to rule out definitively a DVT.
- If you suspect a pelvic vein or inferior vena cava (IVC) thrombus, obtain a computed tomography (CT) venogram with contrast or magnetic resonance venography.
- Venography was previously the gold standard for diagnosis, but it is rarely used because it is invasive and costly.

Treatment

- Immediate systemic anticoagulation is the cornerstone for treatment of VTE, with most patients qualifying for outpatient management. Anticoagulation should be initiated empirically, unless contraindicated, in patients with a high PTP for DVT if ultrasound is not available emergently.
- The selection of anticoagulant is based on a variety of factors, including risks of bleeding, patient comorbid conditions, convenience, and physician experience and preferences.
- Initial anticoagulation depends on patient characteristics.
  - Warfarin requires bridging with low-molecular-weight heparin (LMWH).
  - Oral factor Xa inhibitors should be avoided with a very low glomerular filtration rate.
  - Malignancy-associated VTE likely has lower recurrence with LMWH than warfarin; data on oral factor Xa inhibitors are not yet sufficiently strong.
  - Pregnancy-associated VTE should be treated with LMWH.
- Indications for thrombectomy or catheter-directed thrombolysis:
  - Massive DVTs such as seen in phlegmasia cerulea dolens and phlegmasia alba dolens. These conditions represent vascular emergencies that require immediate treatment with thrombectomy or thrombolysis (if thrombectomy unavailable).
- Indications for an IVC filter:
  - Patients with absolute contraindications or complications of anticoagulation (i.e., active bleeding, recent surgery, etc.)
  - Propagation or recurrence of a DVT despite adequate anticoagulation
  - Patients with massive clot burden and limited cardiopulmonary reserve
- Patients with uncomplicated DVTs, low risk for bleeding, and no significant comorbid conditions can be considered for discharge from the emergency department.

Pulmonary Embolism

General Principles

- A PE is the second leading cause of sudden, unexpected, nontraumatic death in outpatients.
- PEs result primarily from dislodgment of a clot that formed in the deep veins of the body. Most emboli develop from the lower extremity proximal veins (iliac, femoral, and popliteal), but they may also originate from the pelvic veins, inferior vena cava, upper extremity veins, and right side of the heart.
  - Other possible types of emboli include septic, fat, amniotic fluid, and tumors.
- The clot travels through the right ventricle (RV) into the low-resistance pulmonary vasculature leading to obstruction, acute pulmonary hypertension, pulmonary ischemia, and infarction.
- There is poor correlation between the size of pulmonary vascular obstruction and severity of symptoms. However, patients with evidence of right-sided heart strain (seen on electrocardiogram [ECG]), right-sided heart dilation (seen via echocardiography, CT, or an elevated B-type natriuretic peptide [BNP]), or myocardial injury (elevated troponin) are at increased risk of circulatory shock and death.
- The mechanism of death from PE is believed to be from near-total pulmonary artery occlusion (obstructive shock) leading to pulseless electrical activity. Asystole is thought to arise from the ischemic effect on the atrioventricular node and infranodal conduction system.
- Hypotension is an ominous finding that represents a fourfold increase in risk of death relative to normotensive patients.

Clinical Presentation

- The presentation is variable, ranging from asymptomatic to shock or sudden death.
- The most common symptom is dyspnea unexplained by physical examination, ECG, or chest x-ray (CXR).
  - The second most common symptom is chest pain with pleurisy.
- Clinical signs of a DVT occur in about half of patients with a PE.
- Tachycardia and tachypnea are seen in about half of patients coming to the emergency department with a PE.
- The presence of unexplained hypoxemia increases the probability of PE; however, a normal oxygen saturation, although reassuring, is not sufficient to rule out a PE.
- Other signs and symptoms include hemoptysis, low-grade fever, syncope.

Diagnosis and Evaluation

- Centers around developing PTP using the clinical gestalt of an experienced practitioner or by using validated

BOX 115.1 *Pulmonary Embolism Rule-out Criteria (PERC)*

Inclusion criteria: must meet all criteria and have a clinical gestalt pretest probability of under 15%; if PERC negative, no further workup for PE indicated

- Age <50 years
- Heart rate <100 beats per minute
- SaO_2 <95% on room air
- Unilateral leg swelling
- Hemoptysis
- Recent surgery or trauma
- Prior pulmonary embolism or deep venous thrombosis
- No estrogen use

clinical tools (i.e., Modified Wells, Geneva score, Pulmonary Embolism Rule-out Criteria [PERC], [Box 115.1]).
  - Clinical tools categorize patients using either a two-tier model (low-risk and non-low-risk) or a three-tier model (low, moderate, or high-risk).
    - Recent guidelines favor the more conservative two-tier model.
- Suggested algorithm to evaluate PE in the emergency department using a two-tier model:
  - Low-risk group
    - The PERC may be used to exclude PE at bedside in patients considered to have a low PTP. All elements of the rule must be satisfied in order to identify this very low-risk population.
    - In patients where the PERC criteria are not applicable (such as when all elements of the rule are not satisfied), but are considered low risk based on PTP a negative D-dimer is used to exclude PE.
    - Patients at low risk with a positive D-dimer must proceed to CT pulmonary angiography (CTPA) in order to exclude PE.
  - Non-low-risk group
    - A negative D-dimer alone is not sensitive enough to rule out PE in these patients; therefore CTPA is the recommended initial test and physicians should consider empiric anticoagulation in the absence of contraindications.
- ECG is abnormal in most patients with a PE, but findings are nonspecific. The ECG is most helpful to evaluate for alternative causes of the patient's symptoms. When PEs cause ECG changes, it is usually owing to acute or subacute pulmonary hypertension. The most common finding is tachycardia, but T-wave inversions in the anterior leads (right-sided heart strain) and incomplete or complete right bundle branch block may also be seen. The S1Q3T3 pattern is uncommon, occurring in less than 10% of patients.
- CXR is most helpful to evaluate for alternative causes of the patient's symptoms and to determine eligibility for ventilation perfusion (V/Q) scanning. The CXR findings in PE are nonspecific.
  - Hampton hump is a rare sign that should raise suspicion for PE. It describes a wedge-shaped density in the periphery of the lung where the narrow end of the wedge is facing the hilum.
  - Westermark sign is a rare sign that should raise suspicion for PE. It describes the abrupt disappearance of pulmonary vessels distal to the PE (oligemia) and is the CXR version of a filling defect.
- Echocardiogram is mostly helpful for risk stratifying the severity of PE, because it may provide visual evidence of right-sided heart strain or dysfunction.
- Laboratory studies:
  - D-dimer is used in conjunction with clinical scoring tools to help exclude PE in low-risk patients.
    - Age-adjusted D-dimer is increasingly used in patients with low to intermediate PTP to exclude PE (to account for the fact that D-dimer levels rise with age).
      - Age (if over 50 years) × 10 = cutoff value in ng/mL
  - The D-dimer has a half-life of 8 hours and can be elevated for at least 3 days after symptomatic VTE.
  - B-type natriuretic peptide has limited diagnostic value. It is useful to risk stratify the severity of a PE.
  - Troponin has limited diagnostic value. It is useful to risk stratify the severity of a PE.
  - Arterial blood gas may reveal respiratory alkalosis, hypoxemia, or a widened alveolar-arterial gradient. If normal, it does not rule out PE.
- Diagnostic imaging:
  - CTPA is the study of choice, if available, and if the patient has adequate kidney function.
  - Ventilation-perfusion (V/Q) scan is used in patients with borderline kidney function. However, the patient must have a normal baseline CXR (will be nondiagnostic in pleural effusion, pneumonia, or other pulmonary disease).
  - Lower extremity ultrasound may be used in patients with suspected PE in whom definitive imaging is contraindicated or indeterminate. If lower extremity ultrasound is positive, patients can be treated with anticoagulation. If ultrasound is negative, proceed to other methods of excluding PE.
- Pregnant patients with a suspected PE require a nuanced approach that focuses on minimizing fetal radiation (Fig. 115.1).
  - More than half of pregnant patients with VTE present in the third trimester.
  - The pulmonary vascular imaging modality of choice to exclude PE in pregnancy is controversial. The decision should be discussed with your local radiologist because radiation exposure is highly dependent on local techniques and protocols. CTPA is probably the most reasonable test.
- Massive PE (high-risk PE):
  - Sustained hypotension (below 90 mm Hg) for at least 15 minutes or requiring inotropic support
  - A 40-mm Hg reduction in baseline systolic blood pressure
  - Symptomatic bradycardia
  - Cardiac arrest
- Submassive PE (intermediate risk PE):
  - Acute PE, without hypotension, but with signs of cardiopulmonary stress as evidenced by any of the following:
    - Right ventricular strain or dysfunction on imaging:
    - RV dilation seen on CT or "D sign" on echocardiogram RV dysfunction on echocardiogram

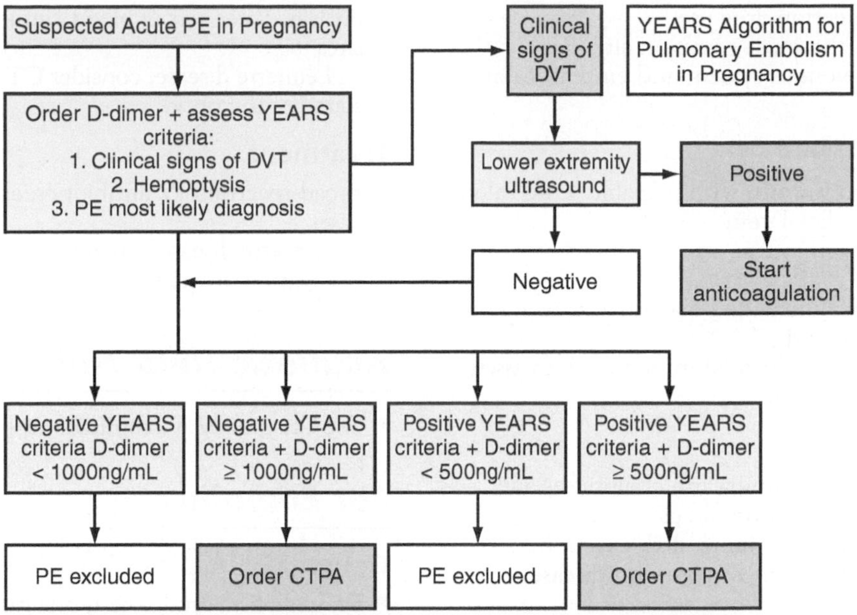

FIG. 115.1 Pregnancy-Adapted YEARS Algorithm for Diagnosis of Suspected Pulmonary Embolism. *PE*, pulmonary embolism; *DVT*, deep venous thrombosis; *CTPA*, CT pulmonary angiography. (Modified from van der Pol, L. M., Tromeur, C., Bistervels, I. M., et al; Artemis Study Investigators. (2019). Pregnancy-adapted YEARS algorithm for diagnosis of suspected pulmonary embolism. *New England Journal of Medicine, 380*(12), 1139–1149. doi: 10.1056/NEJMoa1813865. PubMed PMID: 30893534.)

- Surrogate markers for RV strain or dysfunction:
  - BNP elevation
  - ECG showing new complete or incomplete right bundle branch block, anteroseptal ST-depressions, or T-wave inversions
  - Troponin elevation
- Less severe PE
  - Normotensive and no signs of RV strain

Treatment

- Anticoagulation is the cornerstone of treatment with the same considerations as for DVT (Table 115.1).
- Thrombolysis is indicated in patients without contraindications to fibrinolysis and clinical evidence of massive PE.
  - Standard dose:
    - Systemic fibrinolysis is achieved with 100 mg of alteplase over 2 hours.
  - Cardiac arrest dose:
    - 50 mg of alteplase by IV push.
  - The use of fibrinolytics is controversial in submassive PE, but is generally not recommended.
  - Catheter-directed thrombolysis is an emerging treatment, but it has limited evidence to support its use (may decrease risk of significant hemorrhage).
  - Thrombolytics are not indicated in patients with less severe PEs.
- Thrombectomy is indicated in critically ill patients when thrombolysis is contraindicated.
- An IVC filter is indicated in patients with recurrent PE while on adequate anticoagulation or to prevent PE in those with contraindications to anticoagulation.
- Some patients diagnosed with a PE may be stable and can be treated as outpatients. If the patient meets low-risk criteria and has appropriate access to expedited follow-up, discharging from the emergency department is an option. All other patients should be admitted.

Superficial Thrombophlebitis

General Principles

- Similar risk factors as DVT or PE

TABLE 115.1 *Emergency Department Anticoagulation for Deep Vein Thrombosis or Pulmonary Embolism*

Anticoagulant	Initial Dose	Restriction	Time to Peak (Hrs)
Unfractionated heparin	80 U/kg, then 18 U/kg/h, IV	Heparin-induced thrombocytopenia	1
Enoxaparin	1 mg/kg subcutaneously*	Creatinine clearance less than 30 mL/min	3
Dalteparin	200 U/kg subcutaneously*	Creatinine clearance less than 30 mL/min	4
Fondaparinux	5–10 mg subcutaneously*	Creatinine clearance less than 30 mL/min	3
Rivaroxaban	15 mg orally with food	Creatinine clearance less than 30 mL/min	2–4
Apixaban	10 mg orally, with or without food	Creatinine clearance less than 30 mL/min	3–4

*Although low-molecular-weight heparin compounds are usually injected subcutaneously, no trials have been conducted to justify this route over intravenous injection. Intravenous injection achieves more rapid anticoagulation and does not produce more bleeding.

(From Kline, J.A. (2017). Pulmonary embolism and deep vein thrombosis. In R. M. Walls, R. S. Hockberger, & M. Gausche-Hill (Eds.) *Rosen's emergency medicine: Concepts and clinical practice* (9th ed., Table 78.3). Elsevier.)

- Associated with injection drug use.
- Saphenous vein is the most common site. Rarely extends into deep venous system and embolization is rare.

Clinical Presentation

- Pain, erythema, and warmth with palpable "cord" along the course of a superficial vein

Diagnosis and Evaluation

- Diagnosis is usually clinical and may require exclusion of DVT using ultrasound.
- Examination should be repeated in one week to assess for progression of thrombosis.

Treatment

- Largely supportive, including warm compresses and nonsteroidal antiinflammatory drugs
- Anticoagulation is not recommended, except in extensive (more than 5 cm) or recurrent disease.

Other Embolic Diseases

- Venous thromboembolism is the most common form of embolism encountered in the emergency department. However, there are other rare but clinically significant types of embolism.

SEPTIC EMBOLISM

General Principles

- Septic emboli are primarily associated with endocarditis and infective thrombophlebitis.
- Injection drug users are at an increased risk of septic emboli from peripheral veins or from infected heart valves.
- Lemierre syndrome is a rare form of thrombophlebitis (usually caused by *Fusobacterium necrophorum*) of the internal jugular vein, usually in setting of oropharyngeal infection.

Clinical Presentation

- May present with a variety of nonspecific symptoms that may mimic other primary processes, such as multilobar pneumonia, acute stroke, and so forth.
- Fever, generalized weakness, cough, dyspnea, neurologic deficits
- New cardiac murmur, arterial emboli, pulmonary infarct, conjunctival hemorrhage, petechial rash, Osler nodes, Roth spots, Janeway lesions
- Should consider Lemierre syndrome in ill-appearing patients with severe oropharyngeal infection and neck pain.

Diagnosis and Evaluation

- Similar diagnosis and evaluation as endocarditis
- Transesophageal echocardiogram is most sensitive and specific to evaluate for valvular vegetations.
- Advanced imaging to evaluate for pulmonary, cerebral, renal, or other emboli
- At least three sets of blood cultures from three separate sites
- In Lemierre disease, consider CT venography or ultrasound of the neck.

Treatment

- Broad-spectrum IV antibiotics; embolectomy in select cases
  - Lemierre disease may require surgical intervention (ligation or excision of the jugular vein).

Amniotic Fluid Embolism

- See Chapter 92: Complications of Delivery

Fat Embolism

General Principles

- Fat embolism syndrome is a clinical diagnosis that is defined by the presence of fat globules within the pulmonary circulation. It is a rare event that usually occurs after trauma (almost all cases are associated with long bone or pelvic fractures).

Clinical Presentation

- Usually presents 24 to 72 hours after the inciting event.
- The classic triad includes hypoxemia, neurologic abnormalities, and petechial rash.

Diagnosis and Evaluation

- A diagnostic challenge because many findings are nonspecific and no biomarker has been validated for the diagnosis of the syndrome.
- Laboratory results may reveal anemia, thrombocytopenia, and lipiduria. CXR is usually normal, with some patients having interstitial edema.
- CTPA or V/Q scanning is helpful to rule out alternative causes of hypoxemia.
- Diagnosis of exclusion in patients who present with unexplained hypoxemia and neurologic impairment (petechial rash occurs in less than half of patients) in the right clinical setting with an otherwise negative workup.

Treatment

- Supportive care. There are no definitive treatments for fat embolism syndrome.

SUGGESTED READINGS

Kline, J. A. (2018). Pulmonary embolism and deep vein thrombosis. In R. M. Walls, R. S. Hockberger, & M. Gauche-Hill (Eds.). *Rosen's emergency medicine: Concepts and clinical practice* (9th ed., pp. 1051–1066). Elsevier.

Stein, P. D., Yaekoub, A. Y., Matta, F., & Kleerekoper, M. (2008). Fat embolism syndrome. *American Journal of the Medical Sciences, 336*(6), 472–477. doi:10.1097/MAJ.0b013e318172f5d2.

Tritschler, T., Kraaijpoel, N., Le Gal, G., & Wells, P. S. (2018, October 16). Venous thromboembolism: Advances in diagnosis and treatment. *Journal of the American Medical Association, 320*(15), 1583–1594. doi:10.1001/jama.2018.14346. Review. Erratum in: (2018, December 18). *Journal of the American Medical Association, 320*(23), 2486. PubMed PMID: 30326130.

CHAPTER 116

BOARD REVIEW

Pulmonary Infections

THOMAS E. BLAIR, MD, and SUSANNAH EMPSON, MD

The lungs consist of the bronchioles, alveolar ducts, alveolar sacs, and alveoli. Pulmonary infections can lead to impairments in oxygenation, ventilation, and significant insensible losses. Pulmonary infections are common in the emergency department. They can range from mild and self-limiting necessitating only supportive care to life-threatening with high morbidity and mortality.

Pneumonia

General Principles

- Pneumonia is an acute infection of the pulmonary parenchyma and a leading cause of death worldwide.
- Respiratory pathogens are transmitted via droplets or aerosol inhalation and subsequently colonize the nasopharynx. Microaspiration of these pathogens into the sterile lower respiratory tract can result in clinically significant disease.
- Less commonly, pneumonia can result from direct penetration/instrumentation or hematogenous seeding. Pneumonia is often characterized based on the location of acquisition (community vs. nosocomial) or causative organism.
  - **Community-acquired pneumonia (CAP):** acquired outside of the healthcare setting
    - Typical pneumonia
      - Most commonly *Streptococcus pneumoniae*, but occasionally *Haemophilus influenzae* (HiB) or *Moraxella catarrhalis*
    - Atypical pneumonia
      - Most commonly *Mycoplasma pneumoniae*, but occasionally *Legionella, Chlamydophila pneumoniae*, or *Chlamydia psittaci*
  - **Nosocomial pneumonia:** acquired in the hospital setting. Additional consideration should be given to organisms such as methicillin-resistant *Staphylococcus aureus* (MRSA) and *Pseudomonas*.
    - **Hospital-acquired pneumonia (HAP):** acquired more than 48 hours after hospital admission.
    - **Ventilator-associated pneumonia:** acquired more than 48 hours after endotracheal intubation.
    - **Healthcare-associated pneumonia (HCAP):** The Infectious Diseases Society of America no longer recognizes this type of pneumonia as a separate entity. Previously this distinction served to identify those at risk for multidrug-resistant pathogens; however, the categorization was non-specific and led to excessively broad antibiotic coverage. Coverage for *Pseudomonas*, MRSA, and other multidrug-resistant organisms now requires a more nuanced approach, including assessment of prior cultures, recent antibiotic exposure, structural lung disease, and severity of illness.
  - **Aspiration pneumonia:** oral or gastric contents are aspirated into the lungs in patients with poor glottic closure, cough reflex, or clearing mechanisms. Risk factors include periodontal disease, alcohol/drug use, sedation, and neurologic disorders.
    - Aspiration pneumonitis from gastric acid may precede aspiration pneumonia.
      - Antibiotics are not usually indicated during this early stage.
      - Anaerobes and other constituents of the normal oral flora are common pathogens.
      - *Klebsiella* is classically the causative organism in alcoholics.
  - **Viral pneumonia:** accounts for approximately 20% of cases in which a pathogen is identified.
    - Most commonly influenza and parainfluenza. Occasionally rhinoviruses, adenoviruses, respiratory syncytial virus (RSV), metapneumovirus, and varicella. Coronaviruses such as SARS-CoV-1 and SARS-CoV-2 may cause severe acute respiratory syndrome (SARS).
  - **Fungal pneumonia:** organisms include *Histoplasma capsulatum, Coccidioides immitis, Blastomyces dermatitidis, Pneumocystis jirovecii*, and *Aspergillus fumigatus*. (See Chapter 61. Fungal Infections.)

Clinical Presentation

- History may reveal:
  - Fever/chills, fatigue, cough, sputum production, dyspnea, pleuritic chest pain.
  - Prior viral upper respiratory infection can progress to viral pneumonia or predispose to bacterial pneumonia.
  - Atypical pneumonia generally presents more indolently than typical pneumonia.
- Physical examination findings may include:
  - Fever, tachycardia, tachypnea, hypoxia, and/or hypotension. Tachypnea is the most sensitive finding for pneumonia.
  - Increased work of breathing, rales/crackles, rhonchi.
  - Tactile fremitus, egophony, and dullness to percussion signify consolidation.
  - Decreased breath sounds may signify a parapneumonic effusion.

Diagnosis and Evaluation

Imaging

- Chest x-ray (CXR) alone is usually sufficient to confirm a clinical suspicion of pneumonia.
  - Typical pneumonia: CXR may show segmental or subsegmental infiltration, air bronchograms, and lobar consolidation (Fig. 116.1).
  - Atypical pneumonia: interstitial pattern or patchy infiltrates corresponding to the spread of the infection along the intralobular airway (Fig. 116.2).
  - Aspiration pneumonia: findings occur in dependent areas of the lungs (lower lobes or posterior segments of upper lobes in supine patient). Abscesses may occur.
  - MRSA pneumonia: CXR may reveal cavitary or necrotizing pneumonia.
  - Coronavirus disease 2019 (COVID-19) pnuemonia: CXR may reveal bilateral and peripheral ground-glass opacities.
  - Additional findings: hilar/mediastinal adenopathy, pneumatoceles, pneumothorax, pleural effusions, empyema.
- Chest computed tomography is more sensitive than plain films, and can be considered in those with highly abnormal CXR findings, or for those with high clinical suspicion of pneumonia and negative CXR.

Laboratory Studies

- Laboratory testing may support the diagnosis of pneumonia, point to a causative organism, or identify complications.
  - White blood cell count above 15,000/mm^3 increases the probability of a bacterial cause.
  - Basic metabolic panel (BMP): may identify end-organ dysfunction. Clinical decision rules for risk stratification often require measurement of serum urea nitrogen (e.g., PSI/PORT score or CURB-65).
  - Lactate dehydrogenase: can be elevated in *Pneumocystis jirovecii* pneumonia (PCP) (sensitive, but not specific).

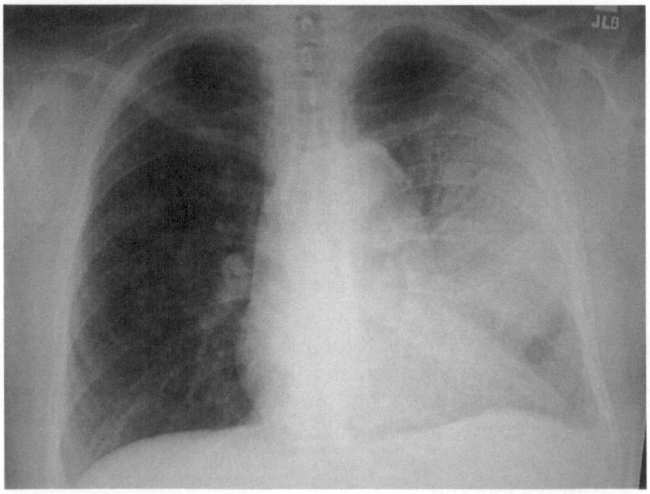

FIG. 116.1 Posteroanterior chest radiograph showing left upper lobe opacification and air bronchograms in typical pneumonia. (From Moran, G., & Waxman, M. (2018). Pneumonia. In R. M. Walls, R. S. Hockberger, & M. Gausche-Hill M (Eds.), *Rosen's emergency medicine: Concepts and clinical practice* (9th ed., p. 874, Fig. 66.1). Elsevier.)

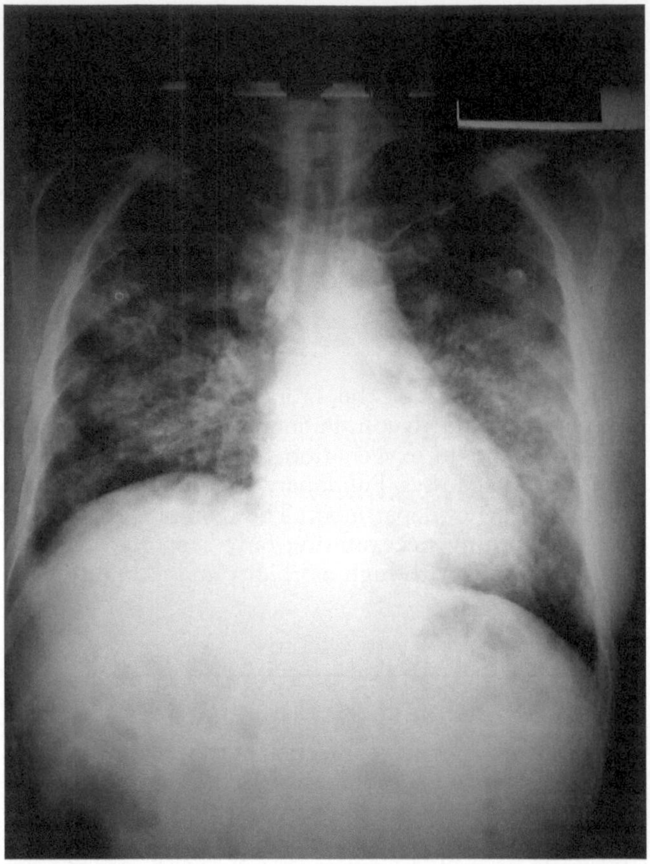

FIG. 116.2 Posteroanterior chest radiograph with patchy infiltrates in atypical pneumonia. (From Moran, G., & Waxman, M. (2018). Pneumonia. In R. M. Walls, R. S. Hockberger, & M. Gausche-Hill M (Eds.), *Rosen's emergency medicine: Concepts and clinical practice* (9th ed., p. 875, Fig 66.2). Elsevier.)

  - ABG: not routinely necessary, but helpful in critically ill patients or for those in whom PCP is suspected (A-a gradient can predict the need for steroids).
  - Blood cultures should be drawn for severe cases and all inpatients empirically treated for MRSA or *Pseudomonas aeruginosa*.
  - Sputum gram stain/culture: American Thoracic Society/Infectious Diseases Society of America guidelines for the management of CAP support limiting sputum gram stain/culture to patients with severe disease or high likelihood of unusual pathogens.
  - Other considerations: influenza testing, *Legionella/S. pneumoniae* urine antigen, viral antigen testing, or viral polymerase chain reaction (PCR)
  - Despite microbiologic testing, causative pathogens are only identified in 50% of cases.

Treatment

- Resuscitation with oxygen/ventilation support, intravenous (IV) fluids, and vasopressors as indicated
- Empiric antibiotics based on overall clinical presentation and local antibiograms (Table 116.1 and Table 116.2)
- In addition to antibiotic recommendations in Tables 116.1 and 116.2, consider:
  - Aspiration pneumonia: add anaerobic coverage, such as clindamycin OR metronidazole if severe disease or

TABLE 116.1 Community-Acquired Pneumonia in Adolescents and Adults: Outpatient Treatment

Clinical Setting	Antibiotic Regimen	Comments
Previously healthy, no antimicrobials in last 3 months	Doxycycline 100 mg orally twice a day	Preferred for adolescent or young adult when likelihood of *Mycoplasma* is high; variable activity vs. *Streptococcus pneumoniae*
	Azithromycin. 500 mg once, followed by 250 mg daily for 4 days	Treats common typical bacterial and atypical pathogens; clarithromycin can be substituted.
Comorbid conditions or antimicrobials in last 3 months	Levofloxacin, 750 mg orally daily for 5 days	Can substitute moxifloxacin, 400 mg daily for 7 to 14 days; treat common typical and atypical bacterial pathogens; active against DRSP; use fluoroquinolone if recently received β-lactam or macrolide
	Cefpodoxime, 200 mg orally twice a day, plus azithromycin, 500 mg orally daily	Use if fluoroquinolones recently received; can substitute cefdinir, cefprozil, or amoxicillin-clavulanate for cefpodoxime; variable activity against DRSP

DRSP, Drug-resistant *S. pneumoniae.*

(From Moran, G., & Waxman, M. (2018). Pneumonia. In R. M. Walls, R. S. Hockberger, & M. Gausche-Hill M (Eds.), *Rosen's emergency medicine: Concepts and clinical practice* (9th ed., p. 8747, Table 66.1). Elsevier.)

TABLE 116.2 Community-Acquired Pneumonia in Older Children and Adults: Inpatient Antimicrobial Treatment

Clinical Setting	Antibiotic Regimen*	Comments
Community-acquired, non-immunocompromised	Ceftriaxone 1 g every 24 hours ± azithromycin, 500 mg every 24 hours IV or orally	Can substitute cefotaxime, ceftaroline, ampicillin-sulbactam, or ertapenem for ceftriaxone
	Respiratory fluoroquinolone (levofloxacin, 750 mg IV every 24 hours, or moxifloxacin, 400 mg IV every 24 hours)	Treats most common bacterial and atypical pathogens; active against DRSP
Severe pneumonia (ICU)	Ceftriaxone, 1 g IV every 24 hours + levofloxacin, 750 mg IV every 24 hours + vancomycin, 1 g IV every 12 hours	Can substitute cefotaxime, cefepime, ceftaroline, ertapenem, or ß-lactam or ß-lactamase inhibitor for ceftriaxone; can substitute moxifloxacin for levofloxacin; can substitute linezolid for vancomycin
Patients at risk for *Pseudomonas* and MRSA	Cefepime, 2 g IV very 12 hours + ciprofloxacin, 500 mg IV every 12 hours + vancomycin, 1 g IV every 12 hours	Can substitute other antipseudomonal ß-lactams, such as piperacillin-tazobactam, imipenem, meropenem, or doripenem, for cefepime; can substitute aminoglycoside plus macrolide for ciprofloxacin
Presumed PCP	TMP-SMX, 240/1200 mg IV every 6 hours	Add ceftriaxone to TMP-SMX, if severe, until PCP confirmed; alternatives for sulfa allergy include clindamycin + primaquine

DRSP, drug-resistant *S. pneumoniae; ICU,* intensive care unit; *IV,* intravenously; *PCP, Pneumocystis* pneumonia; *TMP-SMX,* trimethoprim-sulfamethoxazole.

(From Moran, G., & Waxman, M. (2018). Pneumonia. In R. M. Walls, R. S. Hockberger, & M. Gausche-Hill M (Eds.), *Rosen's emergency medicine: Concepts and clinical practice* (9th ed., p. 878, Table 66.2). Elsevier.)

concerned for lung abscess or empyema (2019 guidelines do not recommend routinely adding anaerobic coverage for suspected aspiration pneumonia).
  - Postviral, severe, cavitary, or necrotizing pneumonia: add MRSA coverage, such as vancomycin.
  - For suspected influenza, add oseltamivir.
  - For COVID-19 pneumonia, add dexamethasone if patient is hypoxic.
- Most adult patients with CAP do not require respiratory isolation.
  - Droplet precautions for *Mycoplasma*, pertussis, plague, influenza
  - Airborne precautions for tuberculosis and varicella
- Disposition should be dictated by the severity of the illness, likelihood of deterioration, underlying medical conditions, and reliability of home care/follow-up.
- The pneumonia severity index and CURB-65 clinical decision tools help risk stratify patients with regard to 30-day mortality.

High-Yield Associations

- *Legionella* pneumonia is an atypical pneumonia associated with diarrhea and hyponatremia. It may occur in outbreaks, especially from contaminated water sources. Diagnosis is with urine antigen testing. Treatment is similar to other atypical pneumonias with macrolides (azithromycin) or fluoroquinolones (levofloxacin).
- *Chlamydia psittaci* pneumonia (psittacosis) is an atypical pneumonia acquired from inhalation of bird feces. Serologic testing is confirmatory, but expect psittacosis in any examination question that mentions birds. Treat with doxycycline. Azithromycin is second-line treatment.

116

Lung Abscess

General Principles

- A lung abscess is a localized area of necrosis of lung parenchyma; it is usually caused by suppurative microbial infection. Lung abscesses are typically a result of aspiration of oral contents (a complication of aspiration pneumonia), but may also be caused by atypical fungal/parasitic infections, hematogenous spread (endocarditis), lung infarct, penetrating trauma, and neoplasms.
  - Anaerobic bacteria are the most common cause of lung abscesses in immunocompetent individuals and are typically community acquired.
    - *Peptostreptococcus*, *Fusobacterium*, and *Bacteroides*
  - Aerobic bacteria include
    - *S. aureus* and *Klebsiella*
    - *Pseudomonas* and *Nocardia* may occur in immunocompromised hosts.

Clinical Presentation

- Lung abscesses take 7 to 14 days to evolve after an aspiration event; therefore, presentation is indolent.
- Symptoms include cough (often productive of putrid tasting sputum), hemoptysis, fever, pleuritic chest pain, weight loss, and night sweats.
- Physical examination may reveal fever, tachycardia, tachypnea, or hypoxia. Lung examination may be unremarkable or patients may have focal rackles/rhonchi/wheezing or decreased breath sounds.

Diagnosis and Evaluation

- Evaluation and diagnostic workup are similar to that of pneumonia (described above).

Imaging

- Chest x-ray is usually diagnostic. Findings include:
  - Dense cavitary lesion that may have air fluid levels if the abscess communicates with a bronchiole (Fig. 116.3).
  - Multiple abscesses can be seen in septic emboli.
- Chest CT is more sensitive, but not necessarily warranted for diagnosis.

Laboratory Studies

- Laboratory studies are not required to confirm the diagnosis and are largely nonspecific.
  - Complete blood cell count: leukocytosis
  - Elevated inflammatory markers: erythrocyte sedimentation rate, C-reactive protein
  - Expectorated sputum Gram stain and cultures may reveal causative organism.

Treatment

- Most lung abscesses resolve with medical management. Antibiotic coverage should include coverage of anaerobes as well as consideration of MRSA coverage (vancomycin) in the appropriate clinical scenario (postviral, endocarditis, postsurgical, and so forth). Some initial treatment options include:
  - Ampicillin-sulbactam
  - Piperacillin-tazobactam
  - Meropenem
  - Clindamycin
  - Add vancomycin if concern for MRSA.
- Drainage usually occurs spontaneously into the tracheobronchial tree and can be confirmed with the development of air-fluid levels on a chest radiograph.
  - For nondraining abscesses, surgical options include image-guided percutaneous drainage or thoracotomy with pulmonary resection.

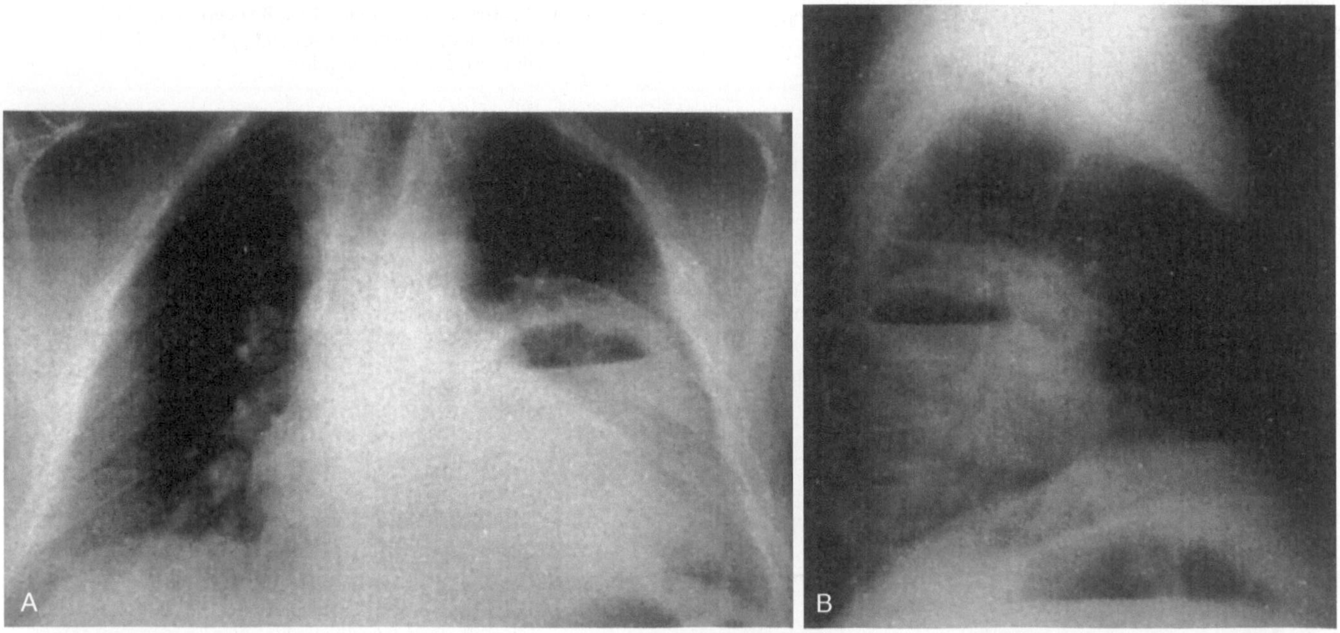

FIG. 116.3 Posteroanterior (**A**) and lateral (**B**) chest radiographs with abscess showing cavitary lesion with air fluid levels. (From Moran, G., & Waxman, M. (2018). Pneumonia. In R. M. Walls, R. S. Hockberger, & M. Gausche-Hill M (Eds.), *Rosen's emergency medicine: Concepts and clinical practice* (9th ed., p. 875, Fig. 66.4). Elsevier.)

- Most abscesses require inpatient hospitalization until symptoms resolve followed by oral antibiotics for 4 to 8 weeks.
- CXR findings typically lag behind clinical improvement and can take more than 2 months to resolve.

Pediatric Considerations

PERTUSSIS

General Principles

- Pertussis is an infection of the upper and lower respiratory tracts caused by the aerobic gram-negative coccobacillus *Bordetella pertussis*.
- Transmission is via aerosolized respiratory droplets with an incubation phase of 7 to 10 days. Bacteria adhere to the ciliated respiratory cells and produce a toxin that damages the respiratory epithelium.
- Immunization is approximately 80% effective after three doses of the diptheria, tetanus, and pertussis (DTaP) vaccine, which is administered at 2, 4, 6, and 18 months followed by a booster at 4 to 6 years and tetanus, diphtheria, and pertussis (Tdap) vaccine administration at 11 to 12 years.
- The disease is most common and severe in infants (less than 1 year of age), but can also affect adolescents and adults owing to waning immunity.

Clinical Presentation

- Clinical case definition is a cough lasting more than 2 weeks that includes one of the four following characteristics: (1) paroxysms of cough, (2) inspiratory whoop, (3) posttussive emesis, or (4) apnea (infants).
- Pertussis is characterized by three clinical stages, and symptoms depend on the stage at presentation.
  - Catarrhal stage (1 to 2 weeks): nonspecific upper respiratory infection symptoms and mild cough; greatest infectivity.
  - Paroxysmal stage (2 to 4 weeks): paroxysms of staccato cough sometimes associated with cyanosis. Coughing fits can be followed by "inspiratory whoop" or posttussive emesis.
  - Convalescent stage (2 or more months): cough decreasing in severity.
- Physical examination may reveal conjunctival hemorrhage or facial/palatal petechiae from prolonged Valsalva maneuver during coughing fits.
- Classic clinical manifestations are present in only a small minority of patients, and infants (particularly those younger than 6 months) can present with isolated apneic/cyanotic episodes.
- Serious complications can include superimposed bacterial infection/pneumonia, rib fractures, pneumothorax, and apnea in infants.
- Infectivity wanes after 3 weeks of disease or 5 days of antibiotics.

Diagnosis and Evaluation

- Diagnosis and the decision for treatment are initially made based on clinical criteria.
- Laboratory/microbiologic testing is often required to confirm the diagnosis and identify sick contacts. Choice of testing is based on duration of symptoms.
  - 0 to 4 weeks of symptoms
    - Send sputum culture and PCR assay. PCR has an increased sensitivity and more rapid turnaround when compared with culture and is not affected by antibiotic use.
  - More than 4 weeks of symptoms
    - Serologic testing
- CXR: not routinely recommended, except to exclude other etiologies. Findings are nonspecific and may include peribronchial thickening, atelectasis, and consolidation.
- Pertussis is a nationally notifiable disease and all confirmed cases or cases that meet the clinical case definition must be reported to local health departments.

Treatment

- Antibiotics reduce infectivity, but are not helpful in reducing disease severity or the duration (unless given in the first week).
  - Azithromycin is usually the drug of choice.
- Postexposure prophylaxis (PEP) should be considered for the following:
  - Household contacts
  - High-risk individuals: infants, women in the third trimester of pregnancy, immunocompromised persons, severe asthmatics, and those with close contacts to infants.

Disposition

- Most patients do not require hospitalization unless there is respiratory distress, inability to tolerate oral feeds, or hypoxia.
- Infants younger than 6 months of age typically are admitted to the hospital owing to high apnea risk.
- Neonates with apnea should be admitted to the intensive care unit (ICU).

BRONCHIOLITIS

General Principles

- Bronchiolitis is an infectious respiratory syndrome in children younger than 2 years of age affecting the upper and lower airways, particularly bronchioles. It is almost always caused by viral infection, particularly by RSV.
- Bronchiolitis is seasonal, with most infections occurring in the winter months. It is usually benign and self-limiting, but rarely may have severe complications.

Clinical Presentation

- Characterized by a prodromal upper respiratory infection (cough/rhinorrhea) followed by lower respiratory/bronchiole inflammation (wheezing or crackles).
- One-third of patients will have an associated fever.
- May clinically resemble reactive airway disease.
  - Personal or family history of wheezing and atopic conditions makes diagnosis of reactive airway disease/asthma more common, especially in older infants.

- Most disease is mild and self-limited. Severe disease may present with:
  - Tachypnea, respiratory distress, and hypoxia.
  - Difficulty feeding, insensible losses, dehydration, and lethargy.
  - Apnea in neonates and young infants.
- Prematurity, low birth weight (less than 2500 g), and comorbid conditions can increase severity.
- Disease severity peaks around days 3 to 5, but symptoms can last up to 2 weeks with a nagging cough and noisy breathing for 1 month.

Diagnosis and Evaluation

- Diagnosis is clinical. Respiratory viral panels (point-of-care, antigen-based, polymerase chain reaction [PCR]) are not usually indicated, except for purposes of cohorting admitted patients or to obviate the need for additional testing.
- Testing positive for RSV does not necessarily eliminate the need for fever workup.
  - Consider urinalysis/culture in infants younger than 8 weeks of age with concomitant fever, because the incidence of serious bacterial infection has been reported at approximately 7% in RSV-positive patients. The vast majority (82%) of these serious bacterial infections are attributed to urinary tract infections.
  - Full fever workup should be obtained in febrile infants younger than 4 weeks of age, regardless of viral testing.
- Chest radiographs are not routinely indicated, but may reveal peribronchial thickening or hyperinflation.

Treatment

- Many patients/families only require reassurance. Moderate to severe cases are generally treated with supportive measures alone.
  - Supplemental oxygen, as needed, for SaO_2 less than 90%
    - In severe cases, noninvasive or invasive positive pressure ventilation may be warranted.
  - Hydration
    - Children well enough to tolerate oral hydration can be hydrated orally.
    - In those who are ill appearing or have significantly increased work of breathing, IV fluids may be necessary at increments of 10 to 20 mg/kg of crystalloid solution.
  - Suction: bulb suctioning or deep suctioning can clear respiratory secretions, but there is no evidence that this changes the clinical outcomes.
  - Generally, avoid using bronchodilators, steroids, nebulized epinephrine, hypertonic saline (in the emergency department), antibiotics, and chest physiotherapy.
    - A trial of nebulized albuterol or epinephrine can be considered in severe disease, although this is controversial and therefore unlikely to be on an exam.
  - Nebulized hypertonic saline has been shown to reduce hospital length of stay, but not admission rates and therefore is not recommended in the emergency department.
  - Palivizumab, a monoclonal antibody against RSV, is recommended as prophylaxis for children less than 1 year of age with chronic lung disease of prematurity or significant congenital heart disease.
    - It is not indicated for emergency department management or acute infections.

Disposition

- Most patients will meet discharge criteria if they are well appearing, tolerate oral intake, have oxygen saturations greater than 90% on room air, and do not require frequent deep suctioning.
- Special consideration should be given to children younger than 3 months, infants with a history of prematurity, congenital cardiac disease, chronic lung disease, or immunodeficiency.

SUGGESTED READINGS

Anderson, E., & Mace, S. E. (2016). Lung empyema and abscess. In J. E. Tintinalli, J. S. Stapczynski, O. J. Ma, D. M. Yealy, G. D. Meckler, & D. M. Cline (Eds.), *Tintinalli's emergency medicine: A comprehensive study guide* (8th ed.). McGraw-Hill.

Moran, G., & Waxman, M. (2018). Pneumonia. In R. M. Walls, R. S. Hockberger, & M. Gausche-Hill (Eds.), *Rosen's emergency medicine: Concepts and clinical practice* (9th ed.). Elsevier.

Roosevelt, G. E. (2018). Pediatric respiratory emergencies: diseases of the lungs. In R. M. Walls, R. S. Hockberger, & M. Gausche-Hill (Eds.), *Rosen's emergency medicine: Concepts and clinical practice* (9th ed.). Elsevier.

Scarfone, R. J., & Seiden, J. A. (2018). Pediatric respiratory emergencies: lower airway obstruction. In R. M. Walls, R. S. Hockberger, & M. Gausche-Hill (Eds.), *Rosen's emergency medicine: Concepts and clinical practice* (9th ed.). Elsevier.

Breast and Lung Tumors

THOMAS E. BLAIR, MD, and SUSANNAH EMPSON, MD

Globally, lung and breast cancers are the most commonly diagnosed malignancies, and lung cancer is the leading cause of cancer deaths worldwide among both men and women. Patients may present to the emergency department with symptoms and complications of local, metastatic, or paraneoplastic disease.

Breast Tumors

General Principles

Neoplasms of the breast are most commonly ductal and lobular, but inflammatory disease carries the highest mortality. Neoplasms may be either in situ or invasive, and staging is based on the TNM system. Estrogen/progesterone receptor expression and HER2 overexpression are important for therapeutic considerations.

Clinical Presentation

- Local symptoms: palpable mass or skin/nipple changes.
- Metastatic disease
  - Bone: bone pain, bony swelling
  - Lungs: dyspnea, cough, chest pain
  - Brain: headache, vision changes, nausea/vomiting, focal neurologic deficit, seizure
  - Liver: jaundice, anorexia, abdominal pain

Diagnosis and Evaluation

- Historical features: age, obesity, family/personal history of breast cancer, age at menarche/menopause, parity, hormone therapy.
- Physical examination: hard, immobile single lesion with irregular borders, skin changes (erythema, thickening, dimpling), nipple retraction/discharge, axillary adenopathy.
- Diagnostic workup includes both imaging (ultrasonography or mammography) and tissue sampling (fine-needle aspiration or biopsy) and can be done as an outpatient.
- Conditions requiring emergent workup include spinal metastasis with cord compression, brain metastasis with cerebral edema, and hypercalcemia of malignancy.

Treatment

Treatment is based upon staging and involves a multimodal approach including surgery, radiation, and drug therapy (hormonal agents, chemotherapy, biologic modifiers) and typically does not involve acute hospitalization.

Lung Tumors

General Principles

Bronchogenic carcinoma refers to any malignancy arising in the airways and pulmonary parenchyma. Eighty-five percent of bronchogenic carcinoma is non–small cell lung cancer (NSCLC), including both adenocarcinoma and squamous cell carcinoma. Small cell lung cancer (SCLC) accounts for roughly 10% of bronchogenic carcinoma and is a more aggressive neuroendocrine tumor. Both NSCLC and SCLC can be associated with paraneoplastic syndromes.

Clinical Presentation

- Intrathoracic manifestations: cough, dyspnea, hoarseness (recurrent laryngeal nerve involvement), dysphagia (esophageal compression)
  - Superior vena cava (SVC) syndrome (SVC compression/invasion): facial plethora and edema, dilated neck veins
  - Pancoast syndrome (apical tumors): Horner syndrome (sympathetic ganglion compression causing ptosis, miosis, anhidrosis), brachial plexus compression
  - Hemoptysis: usually scant, but may become massive if tumor erodes into blood vessels. Massive hemoptysis has variable definitions, but usually includes patients with airway/respiratory compromise or >100 mL/h.
- Metastatic manifestations
  - Liver and adrenal: largely asymptomatic and diagnosed via laboratory tests and imaging
  - Bone: bone and back pain
  - Brain: headache, vision changes, nausea/vomiting, focal neurologic deficit, seizure
- Paraneoplastic syndromes
  - Symptomatic hypercalcemia due to tumor parathyroid hormone-related protein or calcitriol secretion (squamous cell)
  - Symptomatic hyponatremia due to syndrome of inappropriate antidiuretic hormone secretion (small cell)
  - Cushing syndrome due to ectopic adrenocorticotropic hormone production
  - Neurologic: cerebellar ataxia, neuropathy, encephalitis, retinopathy, opsomyoclonus (dancing eyes-dancing feet syndrome), Lambert-Eaton syndrome (autoantibodies attack calcium channels at the neuromuscular junction leading to muscle weakness).
  - Hematologic: anemia, leukocytosis, thrombocytosis, eosinophilia, hypercoagulability
  - Dermatomyositis and polymyositis

Diagnosis and Evaluation

- High-risk historical features: age, cigarette smoking (accounts for 90% of lung cancer), radiation therapy, environmental toxins, pulmonary fibrosis, HIV
- Physical examination: guided by chief complaint, but should include complete cardiac, pulmonary, musculoskeletal, and neurologic examinations
- Diagnostic workup
  - Laboratory studies: complete blood count, basic metabolic panel, liver function tests, calcium level, lactate dehydrogenase
  - Chest radiograph can show pulmonary mass/nodule, widened mediastinum (adenopathy or primary tumor burden), postobstructive atelectasis or consolidation, pleural effusions, etc.
  - Significantly abnormal chest radiograph findings may warrant contrast-enhanced computed tomography scan with addition of computed tomography scan of the abdomen/pelvis to visualize spine, adrenal glands, and liver. There is no evidence to suggest that brain imaging is emergently warranted in patients without neurologic complaints.
  - Tissue biopsy for histopathology, immunohistochemistry, and genetic mutations
- Conditions that require urgent/emergent attention include postobstructive pneumonia, massive hemoptysis, SVC syndrome, spinal metastasis with cord compression, brain metastasis with cerebral edema, hypercalcemia of malignancy, and symptomatic or severe hyponatremia.

Treatment

In stable patients who do not warrant hospitalization for complications of primary/metastatic malignancy or paraneoplastic syndrome, treatment can be arranged on an outpatient basis. SCLC is aggressive, so consideration of hospitalization for further staging and initiation of treatment may be warranted. Treatment is based on the type of malignancy (NSCLC or SCLC), staging, genetic mutations, and immunohistochemistry. It involves a multimodal approach including surgery, radiation, and drug therapy (chemotherapy, molecularly targeted therapy, immunotherapy).

- SVC syndrome: patients with airway compromise may require emergent endovascular evaluation for stenting or thrombectomy. Emergent radiation therapy may also be needed in severe/refractory cases.
- Massive hemoptysis
  - Place patient in the lateral decubitus position with bleeding side down.
  - Intubate with a large endotracheal tube.
    - If left-sided source, consider right main-stem intubation. If right-sided source, can attempt left main-stem intubation with bougie or fiberoptic assistance.
    - Reverse anticoagulation and consider nebulized tranexamic acid (randomized data support nebulized tranexamic acid for non-massive hemoptysis).
  - May require multimodal definitive treatment including interventional bronchoscopy, interventional radiology, and/or cardiothoracic surgery

SUGGESTED READINGS

Joe, B. N. (2019). Clinical features, diagnosis, and staging of newly diagnosed breast cancer. *UpToDate*. Retrieved May 30, 2019, from https://www.uptodate.com/contents/clinical-features-diagnosis-and-staging-of-newly-diagnosed-breast-cancer

Midthun, D. E. (2019). Overview of the initial treatment and prognosis of lung cancer. *UpToDate*. Retrieved May 31, 2019, from https://www.uptodate.com/contents/overview-of-the-initial-treatment-and-prognosis-of-lung-cancer

Midthun, D. E. (2019). Overview of the risk factors, pathology, and clinical manifestations of lung cancer. *UpToDate*. Retrieved May 31, 2019, from https://www.uptodate.com/contents/overview-of-the-risk-factors-pathology-and-clinical-manifestations-of-lung-cancer

Thomas, K. W., & Gould, M. K. (2019). Overview of the initial evaluation, diagnosis, and staging of patients with suspected lung cancer. *UpToDate*. Retrieved May 31, 2019, from https://www.uptodate.com/contents/overview-of-the-initial-evaluation-diagnosis-and-staging-of-patients-with-suspected-lung-cancer

SECTION SIXTEEN

BOARD REVIEW

Toxicology

CHAPTER 118

BOARD REVIEW

General Toxicologic Principles

THOMAS E. BLAIR, MD

Given the overwhelming number of medications, illicit drugs, and toxins in the environment, it can be daunting to approach the poisoned patient. Toxicology can be greatly simplified by focusing on the commonalities in treating all poisoned patients and a few specifics about commonly encountered/tested toxins. This chapter discusses the general approach to toxicology; subsequent chapters in this section detail a focused approach to specific toxins/poisonings.

Clinical Presentation

Each substance has its own unique clinical presentation; however, many have telltale toxidromes that provide significant clues to the offending agent.

- Anticholinergic
  - Flushing, anhidrosis, hyperthermia, mydriasis, and delirium
  - "Red as a beet, dry as a bone, hot as a hare, blind as a bat, mad as a hatter"
- Cholinergic
  - SLUDGE (salivation, lacrimation, urination, defecation, gastrointestinal cramping, emesis)
  - "Killer Bs": bronchorrhea, bronchoconstriction, and bradycardia
- Sympathomimetic:
  - Agitation, mydriasis, diaphoresis, hypertension, tachycardia
    - Similar to anticholinergic, but with diaphoresis not anhidrosis
- Serotonergic: Similar to sympathomimetic but with hyperreflexia/clonus
- Opiate: Miosis, respiratory depression, and mental status depression
- Other high-yield associations may give critical clues clinically and during the examination.
  - Phosgene gas: smells of freshly mown hay
  - Cyanide: smells of bitter almonds
  - Methyl salicylate (oil of wintergreen): smells of wintergreen mint
  - Isopropyl alcohol: smell of acetone
  - Arsenic and organophosphates: smell of garlic
  - Hydrogen sulfide: smells of rotten eggs. Occurs in oil refinery or sewage workers
  - Hydrofluoric acid: used in glass etching
  - Carbon monoxide: entire household with flu-like symptoms
  - Methemoglobinemia: pulse oximeter continuously reads 85%
- "One Pill Can Kill": A few medications are notoriously toxic in pediatrics:
  - Ca^{2+} channel blockers, clonidine, tricyclic antidepressants, opiates, sulfonylureas, chloroquine/quinine

Diagnosis and Evaluation

- For significant toxicities, consider assessing the following factors:
  - Point-of-care glucose
  - Chemistry panel for renal function, anion gap, and electrolyte abnormalities
  - Blood gas and lactate if acid–base disturbance is present
  - Complete blood count
  - Hepatic panel/coagulation panel for hepatotoxic medications
  - Electrocardiogram for dysrhythmia or conduction abnormalities
  - Acetaminophen/salicylate levels to assess coingestions
  - Other specific drug levels as indicated (lithium, valproic acid, phenytoin, digoxin, etc.)
  - Serum osmoles, basic metabolic panel and ethanol to calculate osmolar gap for toxic alcohol ingestions
  - Urine drug screens are notoriously insensitive and nonspecific. Use with caution
  - Computed tomography of the brain to assess for other causes of altered mental status

Treatment

Supportive Care

- The cornerstone of toxicologic treatment is "aggressive supportive care." Although there may be different focuses for different toxidromes, the following is a general guideline:
  - Address airway, breathing, circulation, and decontamination (the "ABCDs").
  - Neurologic
    - Benzodiazepines for seizure. Generally, avoid phenytoin for toxin-mediated seizures.
    - Cooling measures for hyperthermia. Acetaminophen/nonsteroidal antiinflammatory drugs are less useful.
    - Sedation for severe motor agitation
  - Cardiovascular
    - Intravenous fluids or vasopressors (usually norepinephrine) for hypotension
    - Treat hypertensive emergency with titratable agents (nicardipine, etc.).
    - In general, bicarbonate bolus for wide QRS or ventricular tachycardia (e.g., tricyclic antidepressants, propranolol toxicity). Generally, avoid procainamide.
    - In general, magnesium bolus if QT is prolonged
  - Pulmonary
    - Intubate if coma or respiratory depression.
      - Acidemic patients may require increased minute ventilation to provide respiratory compensation.

- Renal/electrolytes
  - Monitor and manage electrolytes.
  - Hemodialysis for renal failure
- Fluids, electrolytes, nutrition/gastrointestinal
  - Proton pump inhibitors for gastritis
  - Gastroenterology department consult for consideration of endoscopy if gastrointestinal bleed
- Endocrine: manage hyperglycemia/hypoglycemia.
- Hematology: transfuse for significant anemia.
- Psychiatric
  - Verbal deescalation, benzodiazepines, and/or antipsychotics for agitation
  - Legal hold for intentional overdose

Decontamination

- In toxicology, decontamination should be an early part of the primary survey. Standard decontamination procedure includes the following:
  - Brush away any dry or powdered agents.
    - Especially lime, which creates an alkali solution when exposed to water
  - Remove contaminated clothing.
  - Irrigate affected areas thoroughly with water or saline irrigation.
    - Exception: metal compounds (lithium, sodium, etc.) should be decontaminated using mineral oil because harmful chemical reactions may occur with water.

Gastrointestinal Decontamination

- Administer activated charcoal (AC) if the airway is intact or secured and the ingestion happened <1–2 hours before presentation. Do not intubate just to give AC.
  - Avoid AC in substances that are not well adsorbed such as alcohols, acids, alkalis, heavy metals, hydrocarbons, and inorganic ions (including lithium).
  - Consider multiple-dose AC in medications that may be adsorbed during enterohepatic circulation. Notable drugs include theophylline, phenobarbital, dapsone, carbamazepine, and quinine (mneumonic: These People Drink Charcoal Quickly).
  - Consider whole bowel irrigation with polyethylene glycol for medications that are enteric-coated, delayed-release, or not adsorbed with AC. Also consider in "body packers" of illicit drugs. Notable examples are remembered by the mnemonic *LIMPS*.
    - *LIMPS*: Lithium, Iron, Metals (lead), Packers, Sustained-release medications
  - Avoid inducing emesis with agents such as ipecac.

Hemodialysis

- Drugs are generally dialyzable if they have smaller molecular weight, smaller volume of distribution, and are not highly protein-bound.
  - Most commonly dialyzed toxins are remembered by the mnemonic *MEAL*.
    - *MEAL*: Methanol, Ethylene glycol, Aspirin, Lithium
  - Other rarely dialyzed toxins include theophylline, carbamazepine, dabigatran, isoniazid, and massive ingestions of acetaminophen, barbiturates, or valproic acid.

Antidotes

- Several antidotes are important clinically and are highly testable (Table 118.1).

TABLE 118.1 *Toxins and Their Associated Antidotes*

Toxin	Antidote
β-Blockers	Glucagon, calcium, high-dose insulin, lipid emulsion therapy
Ca^{2+} channel blockers	Calcium, high-dose insulin, glucagon, lipid emulsion therapy
Digoxin	Digoxin-specific antibodies
Acetaminophen	*N*-Acetylcysteine
Salicylates	Bicarbonate and HD
Opiates	Naloxone
Local anesthetics	Lipid emulsion therapy
Heparin	Protamine
Warfarin	Vitamin K, four-factor PCCs
Dabigatran	Idarucizumab
Factor Xa inhibitors	Andexanet alfa; if unavailable, four-factor PCCs
Valproic acid	L-carnitine
SSRIs	Cyproheptadine
TCAs	Bicarbonate
Isoniazid	Pyridoxine
Anticholinergics	Physostigmine (rarely indicated)
Cholinergics	Atropine and pralidoxime (2-PAM)
Lead	BAL, EDTA, succimer
Methanol	Fomepizole, ethanol (if fomepizole unavailable), HD
Ethylene glycol	Fomepizole, ethanol (if fomepizole unavailable), HD
Carbon monoxide	O_2/hyperbaric O_2
Cyanide	Hydroxocobalamin
Methemoglobin	Methylene blue
Hydrofluoric acid	Calcium gluconate topical, consider intraarterial calcium

BAL, British anti-lewisite; *EDTA*, ethylenediaminetetraacetic acid; *HD*, hemodialysis; *PCCs*, prothrombin complex concentrates; *SSRIs*, selective serotonin reuptake inhibitors; *TCAs*, tricyclic antidepressants.

118

SUGGESTED READINGS

American Academy of Clinical Toxicology, European Association of Poisons Centres and Clinical Toxicologists. (1999). Position statement and practice guidelines on the use of multi-dose activated charcoal in the treatment of acute poisoning. *Journal of Toxicology: Clinical Toxicology*, 37(6), 731–751. https://doi:10.1081/CLT-100102451.

Hoffman, R. S., Howland, M. A., Lewin, N. A., Nelson, L. S., Goldfrank, L. R., & Flomenbaum, N. E. (Eds.). (2015). *Goldfrank's toxicologic emergencies* (10th ed.). McGraw-Hill Education.

Walls, R. M., Hockberger, R. S., & Gausche-Hill, M. (Eds.). (2018). *Rosen's emergency medicine: Concepts and clinical practice* (9th ed.). Elsevier.

CHAPTER **119** BOARD REVIEW

Cardiovascular Drugs

MICHAEL T. JORDAN, MD, and CYNTHIA KOH, MD

β-Blockers

General Principles

- β-Blockers inhibit the endogenous effects of catecholamines, such as epinephrine and norepinephrine, at the β_1 and β_2 receptors.
- β_1 receptors, when bound to an agonist, increase inotropy (heart contractility), chronotropy (heart rate), and dromotropy (cardiac conduction velocity).
- β_2 receptors, when bound to an agonist, can cause a multitude of effects: vascular smooth muscle relaxation, bronchodilation, glycogenolysis, gluconeogenesis, uterine relaxation, neutrophil demargination, and release of free fatty acids.
- β-Blockers have many uses today, including in the treatment of myocardial infarction, congestive heart failure, coronary artery disease, tachydysrhythmias, migraines, benign essential tremors, hyperthyroidism, and glaucoma.
- β-Blockers have unique properties that help to differentiate them.
  - β_1-Specific antagonists are considered cardioselective, thus decreasing inotropy, chronotropy, and dromotropy.
  - β_1/β_2 antagonists are considered noncardioselective and have similar cardiac effects as β_1 antagonists but include β_2-blocking effects such as peripheral vasoconstriction and bronchoconstriction.
  - Several β-blockers also have α-receptor blockade activity leading to peripheral vasodilation.
- Propranolol is the most common β-blocker to cause severe overdoses due to its lipophilic properties and cardiac sodium channel-blocking properties.
- At toxic levels, even selective β-blockers inhibit both β_1 and β_2 receptors regardless of their affinity for specific receptors at therapeutic levels.

Clinical Presentation

- The most prominent effects in overdose are seen from toxicity at the β_1 receptors.
  - Bradycardia and hypotension are the most common presenting signs.
- Effects of toxicity are typically seen within 6 hours of ingestion, except for sotalol, which can have a delayed and prolonged toxicity.
- Propranolol's sodium channel-blocking effect makes it notably dangerous within the class.
  - A Brugada-like pattern may be seen on electrocardiogram (ECG) with propranolol overdose.
- Sotalol has type III antiarrhythmic activity (potassium channel blockade) and thus prolongs the QT interval, leading to torsades de pointes and ventricular fibrillation.

Diagnosis and Evaluation

- Diagnosis is based on history of exposure and clinical symptomatology.
- There are no readily available tests for β-blocker levels in the blood.
- Serum glucose should be measured in all patients because β-blocker toxicity can lead to hypoglycemia through interference with glycolysis and gluconeogenesis (more commonly seen in children and diabetic patients).
- Respiratory rate should be monitored, especially if there is concern for propranolol or other lipophilic β-blocker toxicities because these may induce central apnea.

Treatment

Initial Management

- Standard supportive care and activated charcoal if recent ingestion.
- Whole-bowel irrigation if sustained-release formulation.
- Atropine 0.5–1 mg every 2–3 minutes up to a maximum dose of 3 mg if the patient is bradycardic, typically for heart rate less than 50 beats/min.
- Vasopressors have no antidotal action, but are often needed to maintain satisfactory perfusion.
- Often, the therapies just stated are only temporizing and should be used only if it will not delay the following therapies.

Glucagon

- Glucagon acts independently of β-adrenergic receptors in cardiac tissue.
- Glucagon increases inotropy and chronotropy by increasing intracellular cyclic adenosine monophosphate levels which leads to increased heart rate and stroke volume which leads to increased cardiac output addressing both bradycardia and hypotension.
- Bolus 3–10 mg over 1–2 minutes; if there is a response, start an infusion at the response dose over 1 hour.
- Half-life of glucagon is about 20 minutes; if boluses are effective, a continuous infusion should be started shortly thereafter.
- A common complication after the glucagon bolus is vomiting. Coadminister antiemetics or consider intubation if mental status is questionable.
- Other side effects include hypocalcemia, hypokalemia, and allergic reactions.
- Tachyphylaxis occurs quickly with glucagon so the infusion may need to be uptitrated.

Calcium

- β-Antagonism decreases intracellular calcium, leading to smooth muscle relaxation; supplementation may reverse hypotension by increasing intracellular calcium levels.

- Start at 1–2 g of calcium chloride (through central access only because of the risk of vascular injury) or 3–6 g of calcium gluconate (up to 9 g) over 10 minutes but may be pushed quicker if necessary.
- Repeat doses can be given every 20 minutes, and a calcium drip can be started.
- Aim for calcium level of 14 mg/dL, and measure at least 30 minutes after administration.

High-Dose Insulin

- Unclear mechanism, but increases cardiac output by increasing heart rate and stroke volume, addressing both bradycardia and hypotension
- Typically start at 1 U/kg bolus followed by 1 U/kg per hour infusion.
- Check glucose and administer dextrose if the patient becomes hypoglycemic; continue close monitoring and consider continuous dextrose infusion if persistently hypoglycemic.

Other

- Consider lipid emulsion therapy or extracorporeal membrane oxygenation in extreme cases.

Calcium Channel Blockers

General Principles

- The primary action of calcium channel blockers (CCBs) is to inhibit the slow L-type (long-acting) voltage-gated calcium channels in myocardium and smooth muscle leading to decreased calcium-induced calcium release. They are used therapeutically for atrial fibrillation, angina, hypertension, migraines, Raynaud phenomenon, Prinzmetal angina, and subarachnoid hemorrhage, among others.
  - CCBs are associated with the most fatalities in overdose, and verapamil is the most toxic.
  - CCB blockade leads to decreased inotropy, decreased chronotropy, slowed atrioventricular (AV) nodal conduction, depressed sinoatrial nodal activity, and arterial vasodilation.
  - The nondihydropyridine CCBs, verapamil and diltiazem, exert most of their effects on the myocardium and AV node, causing bradycardia and decreased contractility.
  - The dihydropyridine CCBs, amlodipine and nifedipine, among others, exert most of their effects on the peripheral vasculature. Note that dihydropyridine drugs have the suffix *-dipine*.
  - In overdose, however, the specificity of the two classes decreases, leading to compromise of both the myocardial function and peripheral vasculature.
  - Onset of toxicity after overdose is usually seen within the first 1–6 hours for most CCBs; however, proceed with caution because these drugs are widely available in sustained- or delayed-release preparations.

Clinical Presentation

- Nondihydropyridine CCB toxicity presents as hypotension and bradycardia.
- Dihydropyridine CCB toxicity presents as hypotension, often with a reflex tachycardia as a response to the peripheral vasodilation.
- Hyperglycemia occurs because of inhibition of insulin release as a result of L-type calcium channel blockade in the pancreas. It has been found to correlate with severity of poisoning and poor outcomes.
  - CCB toxicity causes the heart to use carbohydrates for energy rather than the typical fatty acids.
  - Hypoinsulinemia and decreased glucose uptake into the myocardium lead to decreased myocardial contractility in this state.
  - *Note that hyperglycemia is a testable distinction from β-blocker toxicity, which can cause hypoglycemia.*

Diagnosis and Evaluation

- Like β-blockers, no useful diagnostic test exists for CCBs.
- The presentation of hypotension and bradycardia with AV block in a patient with altered mental status with hyperglycemia should suggest CCB overdose.
- Toxicity from nondihydropyridine receptors leads to bradycardia and hypotension, thus the differential diagnosis should include β-blocker toxicity, cardiogenic shock, and myocardial infarction.

Treatment

- Standard supportive care and activated charcoal if recent ingestion
- Whole-bowel irrigation if sustained-release formulation
- Intravenous fluids, atropine, and vasopressors should be used only if it will not delay the specific therapies.
- Management is similar to β-blocker toxicity, although glucagon is used less.
- Calcium and high-dose insulin therapy are specific treatment modalities and dosing is like β-blocker toxicity.
- Consider glucagon, lipid emulsion therapy, or extracorporeal membrane oxygenation in extreme cases.

Digoxin

General Principles

- Digoxin is a cardioactive glycoside, a subset of cardioactive steroids, that comes from the foxglove plant *Digitalis lanata* and has a variety of effects on the cardiovascular system. It may be prescribed to patients with congestive heart failure or atrial fibrillation with rapid ventricular response.
  - The mechanism of action is inhibition of the sodium–potassium adenosine triphosphatase, leading to increased intracellular sodium and increased extracellular potassium.
  - With elevated intracellular sodium, the transmembrane gradient of the sodium–calcium ion exchange channel is decreased, leading to less calcium efflux which results in increased calcium-induced calcium release, and increased inotropy.
  - Digoxin increases vagal activity, and at toxic levels can block the sinoatrial node's intrinsic impulses and AV nodal conduction.
  - Digoxin also acts on the Purkinje fibers by decreasing the resting potential, shortening the action potential duration, and causing enhanced automaticity, leading to ventricular dysrhythmias.

TABLE 119.1 Acute versus Chronic Digoxin Toxicity

Acute Toxicity	Chronic Toxicity
Lower mortality	Higher mortality
Hyperkalemia (best predictor of mortality in acute toxicity)	Hyperkalemia or hypokalemia
AV blocks and bradycardia are the most common ECG changes	Ventricular dysrhythmias are the most common ECG changes
GI symptoms CNS depression	GI symptoms CNS depression Visual changes including xanthopsia (yellow halos around lights) and chromatopsia (aberrations in color vision)
Responsive to atropine	Not responsive to atropine

AV, atrioventricular; *CNS*, central nervous system; *ECG*, electrocardiogram; *GI*, gastrointestinal.

Clinical Presentation

- Significant differences can be seen in acute versus chronic toxicity, outlined in Table 119.1.
- Acute toxicity is overall rare; most cases arise because of chronically supratherapeutic levels secondary to worsening renal function or a recent uptitration in dose.
- In chronic toxicity, visual changes may occur, including xanthopsia (yellow halos around lights) and chromatopsia (aberrations in color vision).
- Symptoms are often initially nonspecific, such as fatigue and gastrointestinal symptoms.
- The most common ECG finding in a patient taking digoxin is premature ventricular contractions. Therapeutic levels may also cause the digoxin effect (downsloping ST depressions with a "Salvador Dali mustache" appearance). At toxic levels, digoxin can cause almost any dysrhythmia, including AV block, atrial tachycardia, and ventricular dysrhythmia.

Diagnosis and Evaluation

- Obtain a digoxin level, electrolytes, and serial ECGs in all suspected overdoses.
- Steady-state level (6–8 hours after ingestion) and not peak level is used to guide therapy.
- Often it is not practical to wait 6–8 hours to treat for digoxin overdose, so the clinical picture should guide decision-making and treatment.

Treatment

- Standard supportive care and activated charcoal if recent ingestion
- The mainstay treatment for digoxin poisoning is digoxin-specific fragment antigen-binding antibodies (digoxin-specific antibodies) and is used in both acute and chronic poisonings; guidelines for its use are outlined in Box 119.1.
- Dosing for digoxin-specific antibodies can be calculated based on known dose or serum drug concentration. If these are unknown, empiric dosing in life-threatening presentations is 10 vials for acute poisoning and 6 vials for chronic.
  - Adverse effects include allergic reactions and hypokalemia.
- The goal is to replete potassium in a hypokalemic patient to a normal range.
- Standard hyperkalemia management is warranted if clinically appropriate.
- Historically, intravenous calcium pushes for cardiac arrest or as a treatment for hyperkalemia were once believed to cause "stone heart" by increasing the already elevated intracellular calcium; however, data shows that it is safe to give intravenous calcium in digoxin toxicity (and has been done even before digoxin toxicity was identified without adverse effect).
- Hypomagnesemia enhances digoxin's effects, so a level should be measured and repleted if low.
- In pulseless electrical activity arrest with hyperkalemia from suspected digoxin toxicity, sodium bicarbonate should be administered immediately for hemodynamic stabilization.

BOX 119.1 Indications for Digoxin-Specific Antibodies

Hyperkalemia >5.0 mEq/mL in acute toxicity
Life-threatening dysrhythmias
Chronic elevation of SDC associated with severe GI disturbances, altered mental status, or dysrhythmias
SDC >15 ng/mL or >10 ng/mL 6 h post ingestion
Acute ingestion of 10 mg in an adult or 4 mg in a child
Associated poisoning with other cardioactive steroids, β-blockers, CCBs, TCAs

CCBs, calcium channel blockers; *GI*, gastrointestinal; *SDC*, serum digoxin concentration; *TCAs*, tricyclic antidepressants.

Clonidine

General Principles

Clonidine is a centrally acting antihypertensive medication that acts by stimulating the α_2 and imidazoline receptors in the brain.

- α_2 agonism leads to activation of inhibitory neurons in the nucleus tractus solitarius causing decreased norepinephrine release, precipitating decreased sympathetic outflow.
- Agonism of imidazoline receptors in the brain can cause unconsciousness, hypotension, and bradycardia.
- Clonidine is used therapeutically for hypertension, opioid abuse, posttraumatic stress disorder, and tobacco withdrawal; criminally, it has been used for drug-facilitated sexual assault.

Clinical Presentation

- Clonidine overdose typically presents with usual signs of decreased sympathetic outflow: central nervous system depression (most common), hypotension, bradycardia, and sometimes hypothermia or bradypnea.
- Can mimic an opioid overdose with obtundation, miosis, respiratory depression, and hypothermia

TABLE 119.2 Cardiovascular Drug Toxicities

Medication	Basic Information	Clinical Presentation	Treatment
ACE ARBs	Inhibit effects of renin-angiotensin system	Angioedema	Airway management Drugs have weak evidence to support use.
Diuretics	Thiazides and loop diuretics	Electrolyte abnormalities Thiazides: hyperglycemia, gout, pancreatitis	Standard therapies
Nitrates and nitrites	Vasodilation	Hypotension Reflex tachycardia Methemoglobinemia	IV fluids Vasopressors O_2 and methylene blue
Nitroprusside	Vasodilation	Cyanide poisoning	Thiosulfate Hydroxocobalamin

ACE, angiotensin-converting enzyme inhibitor; *ARBs,* angiotensin receptor blockers; *IV,* intravenous.

- Can mimic digoxin, β-blocker, or CCB toxicity, with hypotension and bradycardia
- A patient taking clonidine who stops suddenly can undergo withdrawal and present with tachycardia, hypertension, tremors, and agitation.

Diagnosis and Evaluation

- Diagnosis is largely based on history and clinical picture.
- Naloxone can be given to differentiate from opioid overdose.

Treatment

- Standard supportive care and activated charcoal if recent ingestion.
- Case reports of naloxone therapy for treatment exist, although evidence is weak.

Miscellaneous Cardiovascular Drug Toxicities

See Table 119.2 for a list of miscellaneous cardiovascular drug toxicities.

SUGGESTED READINGS

Hoffman, R. S., Howland, M. A., Lewin, N. A., Nelson, L. S., Goldfrank, L. R., & Flomenbaum, N. E. (2015). *Goldfrank's toxicologic emergencies* (10th ed.). McGraw-Hill Education.

Wolfson, A. B. (2018). Cardiovascular drugs. In R. M. Walls, R. S. Hockberger, & M. Gausche-Hill (Eds.), *Rosen's emergency medicine: Concepts and clinical practice* (9th ed., pp. 1886). Elsevier.

CHAPTER 120

BOARD REVIEW

Analgesic Toxicity

LISA ZHAO, MD, and MICHAEL TETWILER, MD, MPH

Pain is the most common presenting symptom for patients coming to the emergency department. Analgesia refers to the relief of pain. Many analgesics are prescribed but a vast amount are available over the counter. Easy access makes analgesics culprits of overdose and toxicity, especially if patients are not aware of their dangerous potential.

Acetaminophen

General Principles

- Acetaminophen (*N*-acetyl-*p*-aminophenol [APAP]) is an effective agent for moderate pain with few side effects when used in appropriate dosages. Although its mechanism is unknown, APAP has known analgesic and antipyretic activity and few antiinflammatory properties.
- Recommended daily maximum of 3000 mg/day. Hepatic toxicity is rare with ingestions less than 10 g in a 24-hour period unless patients have underlying liver disease or concomitant alcohol abuse.
- APAP is metabolized primarily in the liver, into toxic and nontoxic products through glucuronidation, sulfation, and a minor pathway in which the hepatic cytochrome P450 enzyme system metabolizes APAP (mainly CYP2E1), forming a minor yet significant alkylating metabolite known as *N*-acetyl-*p*-benzoquinone imine (NAPQI), which normally is eliminated by glutathione (Fig. 120.1). When glutathione pathways are overwhelmed, an increase in NAPQI can lead to hepatic cell necrosis, resulting in hepatic failure, and acute tubular necrosis, resulting in renal failure.

Clinical Presentation

- Stage 1 (day 1): Often asymptomatic or nonspecific symptoms of nausea, vomiting, anorexia, and malaise. No hepatic injury has occurred at this stage.
- Stage 2 (days 2–3): Right upper quadrant abdominal pain. Elevated liver enzymes correlate with hepatic injury, usually with aspartate aminotransferase rising before alanine aminotransferase. Patients with mild to moderate toxicity may still recover from this.
- Stage 3 (days 3–4): Fulminant hepatic failure and compromised synthetic function leading to coagulopathy, jaundice, encephalopathy, metabolic acidosis. Laboratory results vary, but liver enzymes may be elevated to the thousands. Prothrombin time and international normalized ratio may also be elevated. Metabolic acidosis, elevated lactate, and renal failure may be present. Death occurs from multiorgan failure usually between days 3 and 5. Overall mortality is less than 0.5%; most ingestions do not cause toxicity or injury.
- Stage 4 (day 7): Patients who survive to this point will recover completely without any residual hepatic sequelae.

Diagnosis and Evaluation

- Historical information of time of ingestion and dosage is important. Toxic ingestion occurs with dosage >150 mg/kg within a 24-hour period.
- Serum APAP levels should be checked at 4 hours.
  - Plot serum level on the Rumack-Matthew nomogram (Fig. 120.2) to determine likelihood of toxicity and need for treatment with *N*-acetylcysteine (NAC). The nomogram is only helpful in a single acute ingestion. For multiple doses, use the most conservative time of ingestion and the cumulative dose.
  - A serum acetaminophen level measured at 4 hours can exclude acetaminophen ingestion if negative.
- Check hepatic panel for hepatotoxicity, coagulation panel for synthetic function, chemistry panel for metabolic acidosis. Screen for co-ingestants.
- For chronic ingestions or uncertain time of ingestion, check liver function tests (LFTs) and an APAP level.
  - If LFTs and acetaminophen levels are both within normal limits, hepatic injury is unlikely. Otherwise, initiate treatment.

Treatment

- GI decontamination via activated charcoal is beneficial within 4 hours of ingestion. Whole-bowel irrigation is less useful because acetaminophen is rapidly absorbed.
- NAC is given to increase the availability of glutathione for the elimination of NAPQI.
  - Indications for NAC
    - Ingestion of ≥150 mg/kg or serum level >150 μg/mL at 4 hours
    - Clinical suspicion of acetaminophen ingestion with no available serum test results within 8 hours of the ingestion.
    - Treatment recommended by the Rumack-Matthew nomogram
    - In intravenous (IV) acetaminophen overdose, treat if >60 mg/kg exposure until acetaminophen levels are undetectable.
  - Dosing
    - Oral: 140 mg/kg by mouth loading, maintenance of 70 mg/kg every 4 hours for a total of 17 doses
    - IV: 150 mg/kg IV loading, maintenance dose of 50 mg/kg over 4 hours, then 100 mg/kg over 16 hours

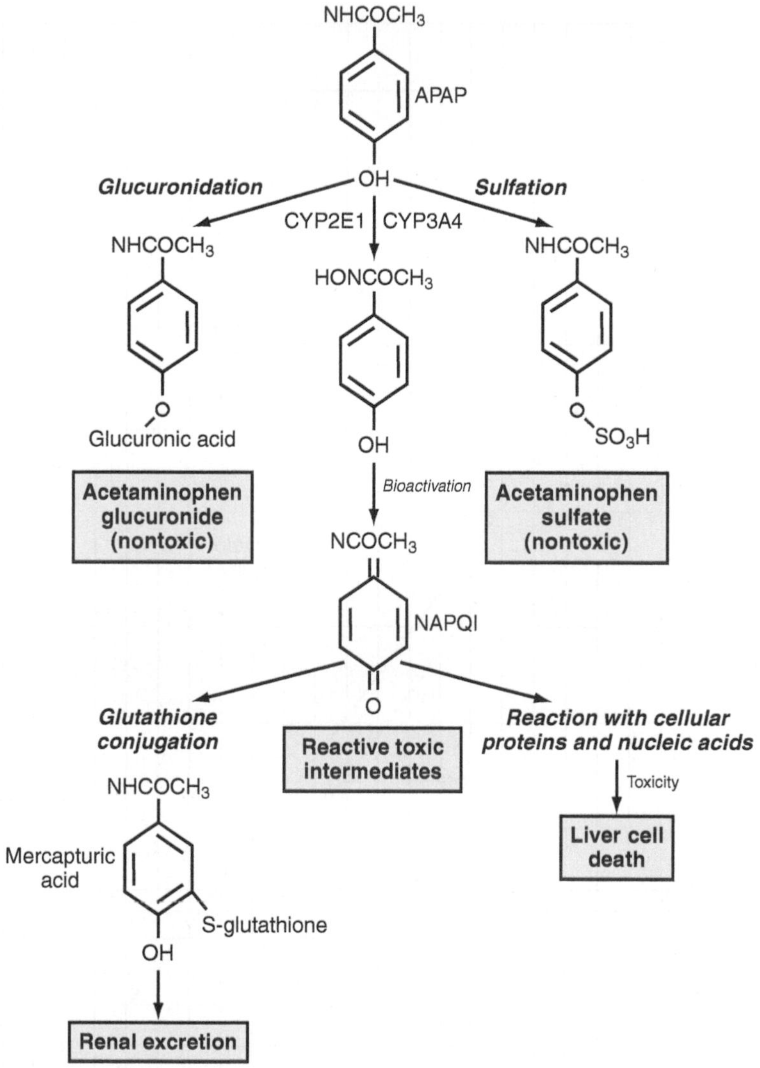

FIG. 120.1 Acetaminophen metabolism. (From Ogilvie, J. D., Rieder, M. J., & Lim, R. (2012). Acetaminophen overdose in children. *Canadian Medical Association Journal, 184*(13), 1492–1496. https://doi:10.1503/cmaj.111338.)

  - IV versus treatment by mouth: IV is easier to use, has a shorter duration of treatment, and patients prefer it. It is preferred over the oral course in patients already in fulminant hepatic failure. IV NAC has a risk of anaphylactoid reactions and is costlier.
  - NAC is almost 100% effective if given within 8 hours and may prevent hepatotoxicity up to 24 hours after ingestion. For patients presenting >24 hours after ingestion or with an unknown ingestion time, NAC should be given at any detectable acetaminophen level or elevation of serum transaminases while in consultation with a toxicologist. In patients already in fulminant hepatic failure, NAC may decrease the incidence of complications.
- Hemodialysis reduces serum acetaminophen levels in massive overdoses.
- Disposition
  - Patients require admission if receiving NAC. Treatment is considered complete once APAP is undetectable and LFTs have normalized.
  - Those who do not require NAC or are low risk for hepatotoxicity based on the nomogram can be discharged after a 4–6-hour period of observation.

Pediatric Considerations

- Maximum daily dose of acetaminophen is 75 mg/kg in children <12 years old.
- Children have an increased ability to metabolize acetaminophen and therefore may be at lower risk of developing hepatotoxicity.

Nonsteroidal Antiiflammatory Drugs

General Principles

- Nonsteroidal antiinflammatory drugs (NSAIDs) reversibly inhibit cyclooxygenase (COX), which synthesizes prostaglandin. The decrease in prostaglandin raises the

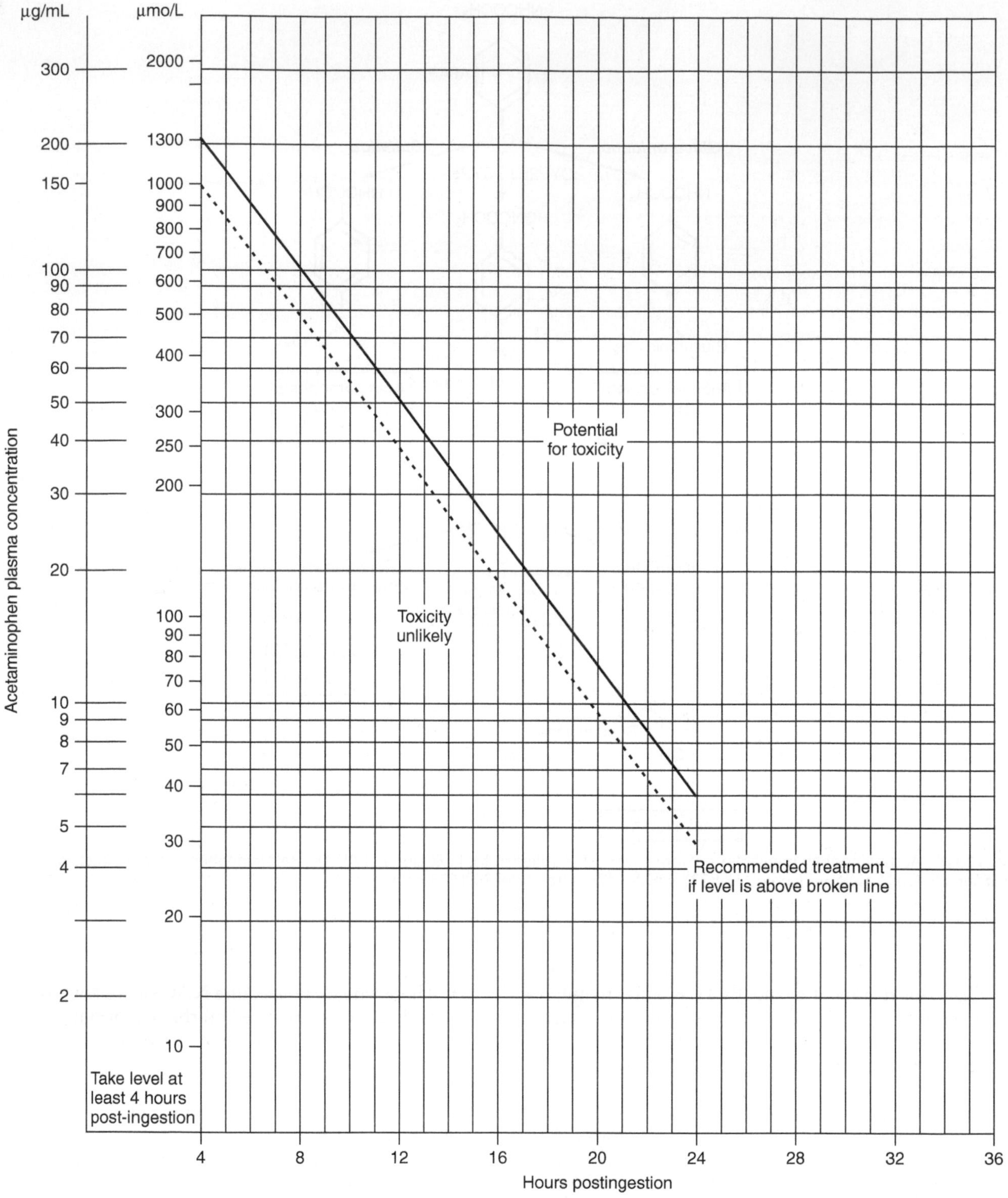

FIG. 120.2 Nomogram. (From Mofeson, H. C., Carraccio, T.R., McGuigan, M., & Greensher, J. (2019). Medical toxicology. In R. D. Kellerman & D. P. Rakel (Eds.), *Conn's current therapy 2019* (pp. 1273–1324). Elsevier.)

threshold of activation of nociceptors leading to analgesia. NSAIDs inhibit two different COX enzymes.

- COX-1 is found in all cells and plays an important role in homeostatic functions. COX-2 is activated by injury or inflammation, and generates prostaglandins as part of the inflammatory process.

- There are two types of NSAIDs:
  - Nonselective COX inhibitors are responsible for more adverse events, particularly GI bleeding, than other analgesics because of their wide use.
  - COX-2 selective inhibitors were developed in the hopes of decreasing ulceration and GI bleeding. However,

COX-2 inhibitors may increase adverse cardiovascular events.

Clinical Presentation

- Acute overdose: usually morbidity is minimal and fatalities are rare. Ibuprofen is by far the most common culprit.
  - Patients are usually asymptomatic upon presentation unless massive overdose.
  - Nausea, vomiting, abdominal pain within 4 hours of ingestion of >100 mg/kg
  - GI bleeds may occur and are dose-dependent.
  - Acute renal injury may occur in susceptible individuals.
  - Severe symptoms include metabolic acidosis, hypotension, arrhythmias, apnea, and coma in cases of ingestion of >400 mg/kg.
- Chronic use may cause kidney injury, gastritis, myocardial infarction, or stroke.

Diagnosis and Evaluation

- Diagnosis is historical; minimal workup is usually required.
- Consider complete blood cell count, basic metabolic panel, electrocardiogram, and screening for coingestants.

Treatment

- Standard supportive care and activated charcoal if recent ingestion
- Hemodialysis not usually effective for removal because NSAIDs are highly protein bound
- Discharge if stable after 4 hours of observation and discussion with poison control center.

Salicylates

General Principles

- Active ingredient is salicylic acid. Used to treat pain, fever, and inflammation, and for its cardioprotective and antiplatelet effects.
- Aspirin is an NSAID and works by inhibiting COX in an irreversible manner.
- Also comes in topical forms for dermatologic purposes such as salicylic acid or methyl salicylate (oil of wintergreen). Toxicity does not usually occur with topical use except in children.
- Bismuth subsalicylate (Pepto-Bismol) may become toxic with long-term chronic use.
- Fatal aspirin intoxication can occur after the ingestion of 10–30 g by adults and as little as 3 g by children. The acute toxic dose of acetylsalicylic acid is 300 mg/kg, and 500 mg/kg is potentially lethal.
- Typically, salicylates are metabolized by the liver but during cases of overdose, the kidney becomes a major route of clearance.

Clinical Presentation

- Early signs of toxicity
  - Ototoxicity leading to tinnitus, muffled hearing, or deafness
  - Abdominal pain, nausea, and vomiting. In severe cases, GI bleeding can occur owing to disruption of protective mucosal barrier.
  - Subtle tachypnea due to activation of the medullary respiratory center
- Later and severe signs of toxicity
  - Seizures, coma, and cerebral edema may occur and are more commonly found in chronic ingestions by elderly patients.
  - Hyperthermia from uncoupling of oxidative phosphorylation
  - Acute lung injury in the form of noncardiogenic pulmonary edema can occur owing to increased capillary permeability.

Diagnosis and Evaluation

- History of time of ingestion and dosage
- Laboratory evaluation including serum chemistries, blood gases, salicylate levels
  - Salicylates cause a mixed acid-base picture.
    - Respiratory alkalosis due to hyperventilation
    - Anion gap metabolic acidosis due to the acid itself and from interference with oxidative phosphorylation leading to lactate and pyruvate formation
    - Respiratory acidosis may be a late finding in the case of altered mental status from salicylates or coingestants.
  - Salicylate levels >30 mg/dL are usually associated with symptoms; however, the level rarely correlates with the degree of toxicity. Salicylate levels are more useful if tests are repeated every 1–2 hours.

Treatment

- Activated charcoal if ingestion within 2 hours. Consider even beyond 2 hours especially if enteric-coated.
- Consider whole-bowel irrigation in enteric-coated or delayed-release formulations.
- Standard supportive measures including hyperventilation of the intubated patient to correct acidosis and maintain compensatory mechanisms. Avoid oversedation so that the patient may overbreathe the ventilator.
- Correct fluid deficits and acid-base abnormalities.
- Alkalinization of serum and urine with sodium bicarbonate is the treatment of choice for symptomatic moderate toxicity. Alkalinization shifts the salicylate out of the brain and other tissues into the serum, where it can be cleared by the kidneys. Goal for serum pH is 7.5. Goal for urine pH is 7.5–8.
- Replete electrolytes, especially potassium, given shifts from alkalinization.
- Hemodialysis is the treatment of choice for severe toxicity. Indications include:
  - Renal failure, altered mental status, acute lung injury, worsening clinical condition despite alkalinization, refractory or severe acid-base disturbances
  - Serum levels >100 mg/dL in acute ingestion or >60 mg/dL in chronic ingestion
- Disposition
  - In minor ingestions, patients can be discharged after observation. In longer-release formulations, patients may need to be observed for >24 hours.
  - In major ingestions that require alkalinization or hemodialysis, patients will need to be admitted.

Pediatric Considerations

- Whereas transdermal toxicity is uncommon in adults, just 5 mL of oil of wintergreen can be fatal in a toddler.
- Salicylates can lead to Reye syndrome in children, leading to fatty acid infiltration in liver cells, ultimately causing hepatic encephalopathy.

Opioids

General Principles

- Opiates are agents structurally related to natural alkaloids found in opium such as morphine and codeine. Opioid refers to anything with pharmacologic activity similar to opiates.
- Opioids act by binding to endorphin receptors (μ, κ, and δ) throughout the nervous system to suppress pain detection peripherally, modify pain transmission in the spinal cord and thalamus, and alter perception of pain at the level of the cortex. The μ receptor is agonized by all current known opioids.
- Opioid-related addiction has increased dramatically and is responsible for the growing epidemic of opioid abuse and accidental death.

Clinical Presentation

- Classic symptoms are miosis, respiratory depression, and mental status depression.
- Decreased smooth muscle activity in the GI tract and bladder can lead to constipation and urinary retention.
- Specific effects
  - Heroin can cause acute lung injury up to 24 hours after use that is characterized by noncardiogenic pulmonary edema.
  - Morphine and meperidine can cause mast cell release of histamine, which can lead to urticaria, bronchospasm, and orthostatic hypotension.
  - Morphine can cause nausea and vomiting by activating the chemoreceptor trigger zone of the medulla.
  - Meperidine, tramadol, or dextromethorphan used in conjunction with other serotonergic agents can lead to serotonin syndrome.
  - Meperidine and tramadol lower the seizure threshold.
  - Meperidine may cause mydriasis (not miosis).
  - Fentanyl can cause muscle rigidity, especially in the trunk and chest wall, making ventilation difficult during anesthesia induction.
  - Methadone and propoxyphene prolong the QT interval and can lead to cardiac arrhythmias.
  - Consider acetaminophen toxicity based on suspected drug formulation.
  - Black tar heroin, a crude and impure variety, has been linked to outbreaks of wound botulism.

Diagnosis and Evaluation

- Diagnosis is primarily clinical and is based on history and the presence of miosis along with altered mental status and respiratory depression.
- Chest radiograph may be beneficial if pulmonary examination findings are abnormal to assess for acute lung injury.
- Urine drug screens are not generally useful in the acute setting.
  - False-positive results can be seen from poppy seeds, rifampin, diphenhydramine, dextromethorphan, and fluoroquinolones.
  - False-negative results can be seen with certain semisynthetic and synthetic drugs like methadone, fentanyl, and oxycodone.
  - The screen can be positive for up to 2–3 days after use.

Treatment

- Standard supportive care
- Activated charcoal can be considered if given early once mental status has improved for oral overdoses. Whole-bowel irrigation is necessary in the case of body packers who transport illicit drugs.
- Naloxone: competitive opioid antagonist
  - Dosing: 2 mg IV if apneic or near apneic; 0.4 mg IV in those who are opioid naïve or in whom respiratory depression is not severe. In opioid-dependent patients, an even smaller dose in increments is indicated to avoid withdrawal. May repeat every 3 minutes up to 15 mg. After initial reversal, may require continuous infusion.
  - IV is the preferred route, but inhaled and intranasal forms (for bystander and emergency medical services) are also available.
- Buprenorphine, a partial μ-receptor agonist, can be considered for maintenance therapy to treat chronic opiate dependence. It is not used in acute toxicity.
- Disposition
  - Because the half-life of naloxone is shorter than that of most opioids, patients generally require observation with possible repeat doses or infusion.
  - Methadone is very long-acting and usually requires admission.
  - If no repeat doses are used, an observation period of 4–6 hours is usually adequate.

SUGGESTED READINGS

Bella, J. G., & Carter, W. A. (2016). Nonsteroidal anti-inflammatory drugs. In J. E. Tintinalli, J. S. Stapczynski, O. J. Ma, D. M. Yealy, G. D. Meckler, & D. M. Cline (Eds.), *Tintinalli's emergency medicine: A comprehensive study guide* (8th ed., pp. 1276–1279). McGraw-Hill Education.

Burillo-Putze, G., & Miro, O. (2016). Opioids. In J. E. Tintinalli, J. S. Stapczynski, O. J. Ma, D. M. Yealy, G. D. Meckler, & D. M. Cline (Eds.), *Tintinalli's emergency medicine: A comprehensive study guide* (8th ed., pp. 1251–1255). McGraw-Hill Education.

Hendrickson, R. G., & McKeown, N. J. (2019). Acetaminophen. In L. S. Nelson, M. A. Howland, N. A. Lewin, S. W. Smith, L. R. Goldfrank, & R. S. Hoffman (Eds.), *Goldfrank's toxicologic emergencies* (11th ed., pp. 472–491). McGraw-Hill Education.

Holubek, W. J. (2019). Nonsteroidal antiinflammatory drugs. In L. S. Nelson, M. A. Howland, N. A. Lewin, S. W. Smith, L. R. Goldfrank, & R. S. Hoffman (Eds.), *Goldfrank's toxicologic emergencies* (11th ed., pp. 511–518). McGraw-Hill Education.

Hung, O. L., & Nelson, L. S. (2016). Acetaminophen. In J. E. Tintinalli, J. S. Stapczynski, O. J. Ma, D. M. Yealy, G. D. Meckler, & D. M. Cline (Eds.), *Tintinalli's emergency medicine: A comprehensive study guide* (8th ed., pp. 1269–1275). McGraw-Hill Education.

Levitan, R., & LoVecchio, F. (2016). Salicylates. In J. E. Tintinalli, J. S. Stapczynski, O. J. Ma, D. M. Yealy, G. D. Meckler, & D. M. Cline (Eds.), *Tintinalli's emergency medicine: A comprehensive study guide* (8th ed., pp. 1265–1268). McGraw-Hill Education.

Lugassy, D. M. (2019). Salicylates. In L. S. Nelson, M. A. Howland, N. A. Lewin, S. W. Smith, L. R. Goldfrank, & R. S. Hoffman (Eds.), *Goldfrank's toxicologic emergencies* (11th ed., pp. 555–566). McGraw-Hill Education.

Marx, J. A., Hockberger, R. S., & Walls, R. M. (Eds.). (2014). *Rosen's emergency medicine: Concepts and clinical practice* (8th ed.). Elsevier.

Nelson, L. S., & Howland, M. A. (2019). Opioids. In L. S. Nelson, M. A. Howland, N. A. Lewin, S. W. Smith, L. R. Goldfrank, & R. S. Hoffman (Eds.), *Goldfrank's toxicologic emergencies* (11th ed., pp. 519–537). McGraw-Hill Education.

CHAPTER **121** BOARD REVIEW

Local Anesthetics

JONIE HSIAO, MD

General Principles

Local anesthetics (LAs) reversibly block sodium channels, thereby disrupting depolarization and transmission of pain signals. Pain fibers are preferentially inhibited over touch, temperature, and motor nerves. LAs include two classes of drugs: amino amides and amino esters (Table 121.1).

- Role of pH
  - LAs are weak organic bases, prepared in an acidic solution to extend shelf-life.
  - Less effective in acidic environments such as infected tissue.
  - Sodium bicarbonate buffering enhances effectiveness and decreases pain with injection.
- Epinephrine preparations
  - Vasoconstriction
    - Decreases the systemic absorption of LAs and increases maximum safe dose.
    - Increases local concentration and prolongs duration of effect.
    - Promotes hemostasis.
    - Traditionally not recommended at distal sites (e.g., tip of the nose, finger, penis, and ear) because of theoretical risk of iatrogenic ischemic necrosis, although not supported in large studies.

TABLE 121.1 *Types of Local Anesthetics*

Class	Drugs	Differences
Am**i**no am**i**des (generic names contain two "*i*"s)	L**i**doca**i**ne Bup**i**vaca**i**ne Pr**i**loca**i**ne Mep**i**vaca**i**ne	Metabolized by the liver More stable Fewer hypersensitivity reactions
Amino esters	Cocaine Procaine (Novocaine) Tetracaine Benzocaine	Metabolized through hydrolysis

Clinical Use

- Choice of LA depends on type of procedure, duration needed, site, need for hemostasis and patient's allergies (Table 121.2).
- Dosing expressed as a percentage of 1000 mg/mL
  - 1% = 0.01 × 1000 mg/mL = 10 mg/mL
  - Can therefore multiply the percentage of the local anesthetic by 10 to get milligrams per milliliter
- Modalities
  - Direct subcutaneous infiltration such as in wound repair, limited by volume required and risk of systemic toxicity
  - Regional nerve blockade, preferred if anatomically feasible
  - Topical such as lidocaine, epinephrine, and tetracaine (LET) for wounds or eutectic mixture of local anesthetics (EMLA) for intact skin

Toxicity

- Referred to as local anesthetic systemic toxicity (LAST) and is due to sodium channel blockade of cardiac or central nervous system sodium channels and impaired function.
  - Classically presents as perioral paresthesias followed by altered mental status, seizures, and eventually refractory dysrhythmias (Table 121.3)
- Uncommon unless exceeding maximum dosing or iatrogenic intravascular injection.
- Central nervous system symptoms usually precede cardiac.
  - Lipophilicity increases susceptibility.
  - Bupivacaine is the most cardiotoxic.
    - Longer-acting
    - May not have preceding central nervous system symptoms

TABLE 121.2 *Comparison of Common Local Anesthetic Agents*

Agent	Approximate Duration (min)	Onset	Maximum Dosing	Maximum Dosing with Epinephrine
Lidocaine	60–120	Rapid	4.5 mg/kg	7 mg/kg
Mepivacaine	120–240	Very rapid	4.5 mg/kg	7 mg/kg
Bupivacaine	240–480	Intermediate	2 mg/kg	3 mg/kg
Procaine	15–45	Slow	7 mg/kg	9 mg/kg

Adapted from McGee, D. L. (2019). Local and topical anesthesia. In J. R. Roberts, C. B. Custalow, & T. W. Thomsen (Eds.), *Roberts and Hedges' clinical procedures in emergency medicine and acute care* (7th ed., Table 29.6). Elsevier. Adapted from Milner, J. R., & Burton, J. H. (2018). Pain management. In R. M. Walls, R. S. Hockberger, & M. Gausche-Hill (Eds.), *Rosen's emergency medicine: Concepts and clinical practice* (9th ed., Tables 3.6, 3.7). Elsevier.

TABLE 121.3 Local Anesthetic Systemic Toxicity

System	Signs and Symptoms	Treatment
Central nervous	Paresthesia, often circumoral Lightheadedness Visual or auditory hallucinations, tinnitus Anxiety, restlessness Muscle spasms Decreased level of consciousness Seizures Coma	Supportive Benzodiazepines for seizures
Cardiac	Initial hypertension and tachycardia Peripheral vasodilation and hypotension Bradycardia and atrioventricular block Ventricular dysrhythmias Cardiovascular collapse	Supportive Advanced Cardiovascular Life Support (ACLS) Lipid emulsion therapy

- Lipid emulsion therapy is used for patients with signs of cardiotoxicity and can be considered in patients with seizures.
  - Works by creating an intravascular "lipid sink" for these lipophilic medications
  - Side effects of lipid rescue include pancreatitis and deep vein thrombosis. It also interferes with many laboratory tests.
- Hematologic considerations
  - Benzocaine spray may cause methemoglobinemia (treated with methylene blue).

SUGGESTED READINGS

McGee, D. L. (2019). Local and topical anesthesia. In J. R. Roberts, C. B. Custalow, & T. W. Thomsen (Eds.), *Roberts and Hedges' clinical procedures in emergency medicine and acute care* (7th ed.). Elsevier.

Milner, J. R., & Burton, J. H. (2018). Pain management. In R. M. Walls, R. S. Hockberger, & M. Gausche-Hill (Eds.), *Rosen's emergency medicine: Concepts and clinical practice* (9th ed.). Elsevier.

Schwartz, D. R., & Kaufman, B. (2015). Local anesthetics. In R. S. Hoffman, M. A. Howland, N. A. Lewin, L. S. Nelson, L. R. Goldfrank, & N. E. Flomenbaum (Eds.), *Goldfrank's toxicologic emergencies* (10th ed.). McGraw-Hill Education.

Hypoglycemics and Insulin

PATRICIA FERMIN, MD, and GREGORY SAMPSON POWELL, MD, BS

Hypoglycemia is defined as symptoms such as anxiety, nervousness, palpitations, alteration in consciousness, lethargy, and/or confusion associated with a low glucose level (usually <50 mg/dL) that resolve with glucose administration. Insulin is the most common cause of hypoglycemia, but several oral hypoglycemic agents can cause it as well.

General Principles

- Insulin, incretin analogs, and amylin are parenteral, whereas the other agents are oral.
- There are many types of oral hypoglycemic agents, including sulfonylureas (e.g., glyburide, glipizide), meglitinides (e.g., nateglinide, repaglinide), biguanides (e.g., metformin), thiazolidinediones (e.g., rosiglitazone, pioglitazone), α-glucosidase inhibitors (e.g., acarbose), sodium glucose cotransporter 2 inhibitors (e.g., empagliflozin, canagliflozin).
- The only oral agents associated with hypoglycemia are sulfonylureas and meglitinides because they stimulate the pancreas to release insulin.
- Biguanides such as metformin can cause lactic acidosis, especially in renal impairment.
- Sodium-glucose cotransporter-2 inhibitors can cause euglycemic diabetic ketoacidosis because these medications increase renal excretion of glucose, but do not address insulin insufficiency.
- Rosiglitazone has been linked to an increased risk of acute coronary syndrome.
- Insulin overdose may have delayed and/or prolonged onset of hypoglycemia, depending on the type of insulin utilized.

Clinical Presentation

- Clinical manifestations are divided into two categories: neuroglycopenic and autonomic.
- Neuroglycopenic symptoms include altered mental status, lethargy, confusion, combativeness, seizures, focal neurologic deficits, and unresponsiveness.
- Autonomic symptoms include anxiety, diaphoresis, nausea/vomiting, palpitations, hypothermia, paresthesias, and tremor.
- The most common dysrhythmias are sinus tachycardia, atrial fibrillation, and premature ventricular contractions.
- Hypokalemia may occur with insulin overdose.
- The rate of drop in blood glucose levels may dictate which category of symptoms manifests primarily (sudden drops produce autonomic symptoms and gradual drops produce neuroglycopenic symptoms); however, this is not always reliable.

Diagnosis and Evaluation

- Early suspicion is critical because confirmatory testing is readily available with a glucometer.
- Hypoglycemia should always be considered as a potential cause of altered mental status.
- Consider the underlying cause of hypoglycemia
  - Drug interactions (ethanol, quinidine, β-blockers, monoamine oxidase inhibitors, angiotensin-converting enzyme inhibitors, salicylates, haloperidol).
  - Decreased metabolism or renal clearance (obtain liver and renal function testing).
  - Sepsis/infection
  - Decreased oral intake
- If concern for surreptitious exposure, obtain insulin and C peptide levels (C peptide indicates endogenous insulin production because C peptide is not present on injectable insulin).
- In those suspected of self-harm, consider testing for coingestants.

Treatment

- Address hypoglycemia and anticipate recurrence.
- Adults: if alert and able to tolerate, provide rapidly metabolized carbohydrates orally. If not, give 50 mL (1 ampule) of dextrose 50% intravenously (IV)/intraosseously, which contains 25 g of dextrose
  - Expect a temporary glucose rise of 100 mg/dL after 1 ampule.
- Pediatric rule of 50
  - Dextrose 50%, 1 mL/kg for 8+ years old ($50 \times 1 = 50$), maximum 1 ampule (50 mL, adult dose)
  - Dextrose 25%, 2 mL/kg for children 2 months to 8 years ($25 \times 2 = 50$)
  - Dextrose 10%, 5 mL/kg for neonates 0–2 months ($10 \times 5 = 50$)
- If unable to obtain IV/intraosseous access, consider glucagon 1 mg as an intramuscular injection, which usually takes 7–10 minutes to take effect; anticipate vomiting as a side effect.
- Once patient improves, treatment can continue with oral administration of long-acting carbohydrates or IV infusion of dextrose (usually dextrose 10% in water at a maintenance rate).
- Continue to check blood glucose level every 30 minutes for the first 2 hours.
- If patient fails to improve despite adequate carbohydrates, consider other causes.
- Octreotide is the drug of choice for those with sulfonylurea-induced hypoglycemia that is recurrent. It does not correct hypoglycemia. Rather, it reduces the risk

of recurrent episodes once the hypoglycemia has already been treated by decreasing endogenous insulin production.

- Diazoxide is another option in the treatment of refractory sulfonylurea-induced hypoglycemia. It inhibits insulin secretion from the pancreas but may cause hypotension.
- Admission is indicated in the following conditions
  - In the setting of starvation, alcohol, liver or kidney failure, sulfonylurea use.
  - Long-acting insulin use.
  - Continued episodes of hypoglycemia after observation for 4–6 hours.
  - Intentional overdose.

SUGGESTED READING

Su, M. K. (2013). Hypoglycemic agent overdose. In J. G. Adams, E. D. Barton, J. L. Collings, P. M. C. DeBlieux, M. A. Gisondi, & E. S. Nadel (Eds.), *Emergency medicine: Clinical essentials* (2nd ed., pp. 156, 1329–1333.e1). Elsevier.

Anticoagulants

MANUEL AMANDO CELEDON, MD, and JASKARAN SINGH, MD

Anticoagulants are used to prevent clot formation and are the cornerstone of treatment in venous thromboembolism. Although the mechanism of action is slightly different for each class of anticoagulant, they all work by interrupting a step in the coagulation cascade. The main side effect of anticoagulants, by definition, is increased risk of bleeding.

Heparin (Unfractionated and Low-Molecular-Weight Heparin)

General Principles

- Binds antithrombin III (ATIII), which creates a heparin-antithrombin III complex that inhibits multiple steps in the intrinsic and extrinsic coagulation pathway; inhibits thrombin and factors IXa, Xa, XIa, and XIIa.
- Low-molecular-weight heparin (LMWH) is derived from heparin but has a longer half-life and greater activity against factor Xa.
- Heparin-induced thrombocytopenia is a known complication of heparins that results in antibody-mediated thrombocytopenia. It is more commonly associated with heparin than LMWH.

Clinical Presentation

- Patient may present with spontaneous or traumatic bleeding.

Diagnosis and Evaluation

- Diagnosis is based on history. May see elevation of prothrombin, international normalized ratio (INR), and partial thromboplastin time.

Treatment

- Standard supportive care
- The antidote is protamine sulfate. It is indicated in clinically significant bleeding and its dosage is calculated based on the dose of heparin that the patient is taking
  - It reverses the effect of heparin but only partially inactivates LMWH.
  - Protamine sulfate is associated with anaphylactic and anaphylactoid reactions and therefore must be used with caution.
  - The onset of action is within 1 minute with a duration of action up to 2 hours.

Vitamin K Antagonist (Warfarin)

General Principles

- Warfarin is an oral anticoagulant that inhibits the production of vitamin K–dependent clotting factors (II, VII, IX, and X).
- Inhibits vitamin K epoxide reductase, effectively blocking conversion of vitamin K to its active form.
- The effects of warfarin are delayed until body stores of preformed clotting factors are depleted. Peak effect not seen until 2–3 days.
- Warfarin also blocks the production of proteins C and S, which promote thrombolysis, thereby initially creating a prothrombotic period as preformed vitamin K–dependent clotting factors are depleted.

Clinical Presentation

- Patient may present with spontaneous or traumatic bleeding.

Diagnosis and Evaluation

- Diagnosis is based on history. May see elevation of prothrombin time and INR.
- In a single acute ingestion, a normal INR at 48 hours rules out significant ingestion.

Treatment

- Standard supportive care and activated charcoal if recent ingestion.
- Vitamin K will reverse warfarin's effect over several hours to a day.
- Fresh frozen plasma (FFP), which contains active vitamin K–dependent clotting factors, allows for partial reversal of anticoagulation.
- Prothrombin complex concentrate ([PCC]; concentrated II, VII, IX, and X) allows for immediate and complete reversal of anticoagulation and is the agent of choice in life-threatening bleeding.
- The approach to anticoagulation reversal is guided by the INR level and the presence of active bleeding
  - Life-threatening bleeding: hold warfarin, give vitamin K 10 mg intravenously, and give PCC.
  - No bleeding and INR >10: hold warfarin and give vitamin K 2.5 mg by mouth.
  - No bleeding and INR 4.5–10: hold warfarin.
- Vitamin K administration in life-threatening bleeding is important because it helps regenerate clotting factors for sustained warfarin reversal.

- PCC leads to a more rapid and complete INR reversal, has less risk of transfusion-related circulatory overload, and has equivalent risks of thromboembolic events when compared with FFP, so FFP should be used only if PCC is unavailable.

Direct Thrombin Inhibitors

General Principles

- Inhibit the enzyme thrombin (factor IIa), which is responsible for converting fibrinogen to fibrin.
- They include the direct oral anticoagulant dabigatran (Pradaxa) and the hirudin derivatives.

Clinical Presentation

- Patient may present with spontaneous or traumatic bleeding.

Diagnosis and Evaluation

- Diagnosis is based on history. There is no clinical test available for monitoring drug activity.

Treatment

- Standard supportive care and activated charcoal if recent ingestion.
- Idarucizumab 5 g IV (Praxbind), a monoclonal antibody fragment that binds dabigatran, should be administered if there is life-threatening bleeding while taking dabigatran.
- If it is not available and for all other direct thrombin inhibitor ingestions, four-factor PCC should be administered.
- Consider an antifibrinolytic agent (tranexamic acid).
- Hemodialysis can be considered for dabigatran ingestion as well.

Direct Factor Xa Inhibitors

General Principles

- Inhibit the enzyme factor Xa, which is responsible for converting prothrombin to thrombin.
- They include the direct oral anticoagulants known as the "-xabans" (rivaroxaban [Xarelto], apixaban [Eliquis], edoxaban, etc.).
- Note that generic name of "**Xa**bans" has the mechanism of action in the name **Xa**.
  - Unfortunately, dabigatran's brand name (Pradaxa) also contains those letters.

Clinical Presentation

- Patient may present with spontaneous or traumatic bleeding.

Diagnosis and Evaluation

- Diagnosis is based on history. There is no clinical test available for monitoring drug activity.

Treatment

- Gastrointestinal decontamination with activated charcoal is recommended if the dose was taken within the past 2 hours in addition to an antifibrinolytic agent (tranexamic acid).
- Andexanet alfa, recombinant factor Xa, administration is recommended for reversal of these agents if it is needed. If unavailable, treatment with four-factor PCC is recommended.
- Hemodialysis is not effective for direct factor Xa inhibitors.

SUGGESTED READINGS

Ageno, W., Gallus, A. S., Wittkowsky, A., Crowther, M., Hylek, E. M., & Palareti, G. (2012). Oral anticoagulant therapy: Antithrombotic therapy and prevention of thrombosis, 9th ed: American College of Chest Physicians evidence-based clinical practice guidelines. *Chest, 141*(Suppl. 2), e44S–e88S. https://doi:10.1378/chest.11-2292.

Holbrook, A., Schulman, S., Witt, D. M., Vandvik, P. O., Fish, J., Kovacs, M. J., Svensson, P. J., Veenstra, D. L., Crowther, M., & Guyatt, G. H. (2012). Evidence-based management of anticoagulant therapy: Antithrombotic therapy and prevention of thrombosis, 9th ed: American College of Chest Physicians evidence-based clinical practice guidelines. *Chest, 141*(Suppl. 2), e152S–e184S. https://doi:10.1378/chest.11-2295.

Lee, C. J., & Ansell, J. E. (2011). Direct thrombin inhibitors. *British Journal of Clinical Pharmacology, 72*(4), 581–592. https://doi:10.1111/j.1365-2125.2011.03916.x. Review. Erratum in: (2011). *British Journal of Clinical Pharmacology*, 72(4), 718. Dosage error in article text. PubMed PMID:21241354; PubMed Central PMCID: PMC3195735. https://doi:10.1111/j.1365-2125.2011.03916.x.

Anticonvulsants and Antidepressants

PATRICIA FERMIN, MD, and GREGORY SAMPSON POWELL, MD, BS

Anticonvulsants or antiepileptics are used to treat acute seizures and prevent recurrent seizures. First-generation antiepileptics have a therapeutic serum range that is monitored for long-term treatment and are used to determine acute toxicity with an overdose. The "second- and third-generation" antiepileptics have fewer serious side effects and drug interactions. Therapeutic levels are not monitored for these medications.

Benzodiazepines

General Principles

- Therapeutic uses include treatment of anxiety, seizures, insomnia and alcohol/sedative-hypnotic withdrawal.
- γ-Aminobutyric acid (GABA) agonist
- Rarely fatal with isolated overdose; increased morbidity with mixed overdoses

Clinical Features

- Predominant neurologic symptoms: dizziness, slurred speech, somnolence, ataxia, confusion, incoordination, general impairment of intellectual function
- Respiratory depression and hypotension with intravenous (IV) administration or coingestions
- Enhanced/prolonged symptoms in elderly, children, patients with hepatic disease
- Paradoxical reactions such as excitation, anxiety, aggression, hostile behavior, and delirium may occur especially in children and the elderly.
  - Paradoxical reactions are believed to be due to loss of cortical inhibition.
  - Treat with observation or alternative agents such as antipsychotics.

Diagnosis

- Limited value for testing; serum levels do not correspond to clinical presentation.

Treatment

- Consider activated charcoal (AC) within 1 hour of ingestion.
- Gastric lavage, forced diuresis, and hemodialysis are ineffective.
- Flumazenil is a selective antagonist to central effects of benzodiazepines.
  - Beneficial for iatrogenic benzodiazepine oversedation during procedures
  - Contraindicated in chronic use because it may precipitate seizures
  - Treat flumazenil-induced seizures with phenobarbital or propofol, avoiding benzodiazepines because they are likely to be ineffective.
- Indication for admission: significant altered mental status, hypotension, respiratory depression

Phenytoin and Fosphenytoin

General Principles

- Serious complications after intentional overdose are rare if supportive care is provided.
- Fosphenytoin: soluble in aqueous solutions, nonirritating to tissues, and can be given intramuscularly
- Mechanism of action is neuronal sodium channel blockade.
  - At higher concentrations, delays activation of neuronal potassium currents

Clinical Presentation

- Toxicity typically presents as nystagmus, ataxia, dysarthria, and depressed mental status.
- Hypotension and cardiovascular complications are most seen in IV administration owing to the propylene glycol diluent, which is a potent myocardial depressant and vasodilator. Hypotension is less common with fosphenytoin.

Diagnosis and Evaluation

- Phenytoin level: therapeutic range is 10–20 μg/mL.
- Monitor serum levels every few hours because of long and erratic absorption orally.
- Isolated oral ingestions do not need cardiac monitoring.

Treatment

- Standard supportive care and AC if recent ingestion
- Gastric lavage and whole-bowel irrigation not indicated
- Hemodialysis/hemoperfusion may improve severe and persistent toxicity.

- Mild symptoms can be observed and the patient discharged if phenytoin levels are trending downward.
- Symptomatic chronic intoxication in general should be admitted for observation.

Carbamazepine

General Principles

- Inhibits sodium and acetylcholine receptors
- Central antidiuretic effects, which may lead to syndrome of inappropriate antidiuretic hormone
- Therapeutic concentration is 4–12 μg/mL.
- Metabolized in the liver, with active metabolite responsible for neurotoxicity

Clinical Presentation

- Mental status depression, ataxia, nystagmus, ileus, hypertonicity with increased deep tendon reflexes, dystonic reactions, and anticholinergic toxidrome
- Clinical deterioration can be delayed or have a crescendo-decrescendo course.
- Can cause wide QRS interval and seizures
- Laboratory test abnormalities: hyponatremia, hyperglycemia, transient elevation of liver enzymes
- Increased incidence of aplastic anemia with long-term use

Diagnosis

- Serum concentrations of higher than 40 μg/mL are associated with more serious complications such as seizures, respiratory failure, coma, cardiac conduction defects.
- Serum concentrations higher than 60–80 μg/mL may be fatal.

Treatment

- Standard supportive care and AC if recent ingestion
- Hemodialysis/hemoperfusion for severe toxicity with multiorgan dysfunction
- Sodium bicarbonate for cardiac conduction delay (wide QRS on electrocardiogram)

Valproate, Valproic Acid, and Divalproex Sodium

Clinical Presentation

- The most frequent sign of toxicity is central nervous system depression.
- Respiratory depression, hypotension, hypoglycemia, hypocalcemia, hyponatremia, hypophosphatemia, anion gap metabolic acidosis, elevation of liver function tests, **hyperammonemia**, elevated lactate, pancreatitis, and thrombocytopenia can occur.

Diagnosis and Evaluation

- Valproic acid level: therapeutic concentrations are 50–100 μg/mL.

Treatment

- Standard supportive care
- Single-dose AC or multidose charcoal and whole-bowel irrigation for ingestion of enteric-coated and delayed-release preparations
- High-dose naloxone may reverse neurologic depression.
- **L-Carnitine** is given to increase valproate metabolism, especially in large overdoses, hepatotoxicity, or valproate-related hyperammonemic encephalopathy.
- Hemoperfusion and hemodiafiltration for severe overdose

Second- and Third-Generation Anticonvulsants

General Principles

- Less toxic than first-generation agents; most serious complications with mixed ingestion
- Management is with AC and supportive care.
- Table 124.1 shows atypical anticonvulsants and their toxicity.
- **Lamotrigine** overdose treatment includes AC, sodium bicarbonate for QRS widening, magnesium sulfate for QT prolongation, and IV lipid emulsion.

Antidepressants

- Antidepressants are used to treat major depression, obsessive-compulsive disorder, panic disorders, and eating disorders. They are primarily metabolized by the liver; therefore, hepatic dysfunction can lead to increased drug levels and consequently drug toxicity.

Bupropion

General Principles

- Inhibition of neuronal reuptake of norepinephrine and dopamine

TABLE 124.1 *Atypical Anticonvulsants and Toxicity*

Anticonvulsant Drug	Clinical Features of Poisoning
Gabapentin and pregabalin	Lethargy, ataxia, slurred speech, gastrointestinal symptoms
Lamotrigine	Lethargy, coma, ataxia, nystagmus, seizures, cardiac conduction abnormalities
Levetiracetam	Lethargy, coma, respiratory depression
Tiagabine	Lethargy, facial grimacing, nystagmus, posturing, agitation, coma, hallucinations, seizures
Topiramate	Lethargy, ataxia, nystagmus, myoclonus, coma, seizures, metabolic acidosis (secondary to carbonic anhydrase inhibition)

From Vale, J. A., & Bradberry, S. M. (2016). Poisoning. In P. Kumar & M. Clark (Eds.), *Kumar and Clark's clinical medicine* (9th ed., pp. 63–85). Elsevier.

Clinical Presentation

- Significant toxicity is not expected in adult ingestions less than 450 mg.
- Agitation, dizziness, tremor, nausea, vomiting, drowsiness, and tachycardia
- Seizures are more common with toxicity compared with other antidepressants.

Treatment

- Standard supportive care and AC if recent ingestion
- More than 450 mg of extended-release preparations require at least 24 hours of monitoring.

Mirtazapine

General Principles

- Increases central norepinephrine and serotonin neurotransmission; histamine blocker

Clinical Features

- Most common features: sedation, confusion, sinus tachycardia, and mild hypertension

Treatment

- Standard supportive care and AC if recent ingestion

Trazodone

General Principles

- Selective serotonin reuptake inhibitor, α-adrenergic, and histamine receptor blockers
- Used more commonly for its side effect of sleep than its antidepressant effect
- One of the most common causes of drug-induced priapism

Clinical Features

- Central nervous system depression, orthostatic hypotension
- Prolonged QT interval

Treatment

- Standard supportive care and AC if recent ingestion
- IV magnesium for a prolonged QT

Selective Serotonin Reuptake Inhibitors

General Principles

- Most frequent class for overdoses given their more frequent prescription as therapy for depression
- Fatalities are uncommon.

Clinical Features

- Hyponatremia believed to be due to syndrome of inappropriate antidiuretic hormone
- Sexual dysfunction, headache, sedation, insomnia, dizziness, weakness, tremor, anxiety

TABLE 124.2 *Symptoms of Serotonin Syndrome*

Cognitive	Altered level of consciousness, agitation, restlessness, anxiety, insomnia, stupor
Autonomic	Hyperthermia, diaphoresis, hypertension/hypotension, tachycardia, tachypnea, mydriasis, incontinence, nausea, vomiting, diarrhea
Neuromuscular	Myoclonus (distinguishing feature), muscle rigidity, hyperreflexia, tremor, akathisia, incoordination

124

TABLE 124.3 *Serotonergic Agents*

Antidepressants	Monoamine oxidase inhibitors, selective serotonin reuptake inhibitors, serotonin/norepinephrine reuptake inhibitors, cyclic antidepressants
Atypical antipsychotics	Quetiapine, olanzapine, clozapine
Drugs of abuse	Cocaine, amphetamines, mescaline
Opioids/opiate-like medications	Meperidine, tramadol, fentanyl
Antibiotics	Linezolid
Others	Lithium, dextromethorphan, triptans, bromocriptine, levodopa, trazodone, bupropion
Supplements	L-Tryptophan, St. John's wort

Modified from Fricchione, G. L., Beach, S. R., Gross, A. F., Huffman, J. C., Bush, G., & Stern, T. A. (2017). Catatonia, neuroleptic malignant syndrome, and serotonin syndrome. In T. A. Stern, O. Freudenreich, F. A. Smith, G. L. Fricchione, & J. F. Rosenbaum (Eds.), *Massachusetts General Hospital handbook of general hospital psychiatry* (7th ed., pp. 253–265). Elsevier.

- Gastrointestinal: nausea, diarrhea, constipation, vomiting, anorexia
- Citalopram and escitalopram more associated with cardiotoxicity and dysrhythmias
- **Serotonin syndrome**
  - Classically presents as agitation, tachycardia, hyperthermia, hyperreflexia, and **myoclonus** (most distinguishing feature). See Table 124.2.
  - Majority occur within 2–24 hours after increasing or adding a serotonin agonist.
  - See Table 124.3 for a list of serotonergic agents.

Treatment

- Standard supportive care and AC if recent ingestion
- Cyproheptadine, a serotonin receptor antagonist, for severe cases
- Observe for at least 6 hours.
- Admit if the patient is having persistent cardiac abnormalities, altered mental status, or serotonin syndrome.

Serotonin Norepinephrine Reuptake Inhibitors

Clinical Features

- Tachycardia, hypertension, tremors, diaphoresis, mydriasis

- Venlafaxine has higher incidence of seizures, rhabdomyolysis, and cardiotoxicity.
- Electrocardiogram (ECG) abnormalities: sinus tachycardia most commonly, widened QRS, prolonged QT

Treatment

- Standard supportive care and AC if recent ingestion
- Whole-bowel irrigation for large venlafaxine ingestion
- Observe for at least 6 hours for asymptomatic patients.
- Admit patients with symptoms or ingestion of extended-release formulas.

Tricyclic Antidepressants

General Principles

- Also used to treat obsessive-compulsive disorder, attention-deficit disorder, anxiety disorder, and panic and phobia disorders
- Highly lipophilic; poor response to hemodialysis/hemoperfusion, diuresis
- Toxicity: life-threatening symptoms: 10 mg/kg in adults; commonly fatal if more than 1 g
- Sodium channel and potassium blockade, α-receptor blockade, serotonin and norepinephrine inhibition, anticholinergic activity

Clinical Presentation

- Mild to moderate symptoms: drowsiness, confusion, slurred speech, ataxia, dry mucous membranes and axillae, sinus tachycardia, urinary retention, myoclonus, and hyperreflexia
- Cardiotoxicity is the most concerning feature and may be detected on ECG.
  - Terminal R wave in aVR
  - Brugada pattern on ECG (note cardiac sodium channels role in tricyclic antidepressant overdose and Brugada syndrome)
  - Prolonged PR interval and QRS duration, right axis deviation, bradycardia, heart blocks, ventricular dysrhythmias
- Serious toxicity almost always occurs within the first 6 hours of ingestion.

Diagnosis and Evaluation

- Diagnosis is based on history of exposure and clinical symptomatology.
- Serial ECGs and continuous cardiac monitoring should be obtained to monitor for cardiotoxicity.

Treatment

- Standard supportive care and AC if recent ingestion
- No role for multidose charcoal or whole-bowel irrigation
- Sodium bicarbonate indicated for widened QRS, arrhythmia, hypotension, and acidosis
  - Start with 1 ampoule (50 mEq) and repeat until QRS narrows, then convert to drip.
  - Close monitoring for 6 hours
  - Consider lipid emulsion for refractory dysrhythmias.
  - Admission for all symptomatic patients
  - Patients asymptomatic for 6 hours do not require admission.

Monoamine Oxidase Inhibitors

General Principles

- Used to treat atypical and refractory cases of depression and Parkinson disease
- Associated with tyramine reactions and serotonin syndrome
- Caution prescribing medications to anyone who is taking monoamine oxidase inhibitors because of numerous drug interactions

Clinical Features

- Significant drug toxicity with ingestions slightly greater than therapeutic doses
- Produces hyperadrenergic state with stimulation of β- and α-adrenergic receptors
- **Tyramine reaction**
  - Tyramine is an amine commonly found in higher concentrations in aged, cured, smoked, pickled, or fermented dietary products.
  - Tyramine is metabolized by monoamine oxidase and accumulates when taking monoamine oxidase inhibitors.
  - Produces severe occipital or temporal headache and sympathomimetic effects
  - May lead to hypertensive emergency
  - Phentolamine (peripheral α-blocker) is the drug of choice, although alternative titratable antihypertensives are also acceptable (e.g., nitroprusside).

Diagnosis and Evaluation

- Diagnosis is based on history of exposure and clinical symptomatology.
- Leukocytosis and thrombocytopenia are commonly seen.
- Hypotension may occur in severe cases and is a poor prognostic sign.

Treatment

- Standard supportive care and AC if recent ingestion
- Phentolamine is the drug of choice for hypertensive emergency.

SUGGESTED READINGS

Guttman, J. (2018). Nausea and vomiting. In R. M. Walls, R. S. Hockberger, & M. Gausche-Hill (Eds.), *Rosen's emergency medicine: Concepts and clinical practice* (9th ed., p. 230–241.e1). Elsevier.

Olson, K. R., Anderson, I. B., Benowitz, N. L., Blank, P. D., Clark, R. F., Kearney, T. E., Kim-Katz, S. Y., & Wu, A. H. B. (Eds.). (2018). *Poisoning & drug overdose* (7th ed., Section II: Specific poisons and drugs: Diagnosis and treatment). McGraw-Hill Medical.

Tintinalli, J. E., Stapczynski, J. S., Ma, O. J., Yealy, D. M., Meckler, G. D., & Cline, D. M. (Eds.) (2016). *Tintinalli's emergency medicine: A comprehensive study guide* (8th ed.). McGraw-Hill Education.

CHAPTER **125**

BOARD REVIEW

Antipsychotics, Antiemetics, and Lithium

CAROL LEE, MD, and KATHLEEN YIP, MD

Antipsychotics

General Principles

- Classification
  - Typical or first-generation (e.g., haloperidol, chlorpromazine)
  - Atypical or second-generation (e.g., olanzapine, aripiprazole, clozapine, quetiapine, risperidone, ziprasidone)
- Mechanism
  - Dopamine D_2 receptor antagonist

Clinical Presentation

- Due to potent antihistamine and antimuscarinic activity, symptoms such as sedation, blurry vision, tachycardia, dry mouth, and urinary retention can occur, especially with second-generation agents.
- Extrapyramidal symptoms
  - Dystonic reactions including torticollis (neck) and oculogyric crisis (eye deviation)
  - Akathisia: psychomotor restlessness
  - Higher incidence in typical compared with atypical antipsychotics (Table 125.1)
- Neuroleptic malignant syndrome (NMS)
  - Abrupt reductions in central dopaminergic neurotransmission, leading to the tetrad of (1) altered mental status, (2) hyperthermia, (3) rigidity, and (4) dysautonomia (tachycardia and labile blood pressures)
  - Rigidity is usually severe and classically described as "lead-pipe" rigidity.
  - Most cases of NMS are in the context of therapeutic use, not overdose.
  - Usually occurs shortly after initiation of therapy, but may occur at any time.

Diagnosis and Evaluation

- Diagnosis is based on history of exposure and clinical symptomatology.
- Nonspecific laboratory findings include elevated levels in creatine kinase, white blood cells, and liver function tests.
- A lumbar puncture is often indicated to rule out meningitis and may reveal elevated protein.

Treatment

- Standard supportive care. Gastrointestinal decontamination is not likely to be helpful.
- Other treatments are more controversial because the magnitude of benefit is unclear.
  - Dantrolene: a direct skeletal muscle relaxant
  - Bromocriptine and amantadine: dopaminergic agonists

Antiemetics

- The antiemetics metoclopramide (Reglan) and prochlorperazine (Compazine) are both dopamine receptor antagonists and have toxicities similar to those of antipsychotics including akathisia, dystonic reactions, and

TABLE 125.1 *Extrapyramidal Symptoms*

Reaction	Onset	Features	Treatment
Acute dystonia	Within the first week	Sustained muscle spasms (e.g., torticollis, oculogyric crisis)	Anticholinergics (e.g., benztropine, diphenhydramine)
Parkinsonism	1 week to 1 month	Bradykinesia, shuffling gait, resting tremor, masklike facies, rigidity	Dose reduction, anticholinergics (e.g., benztropine, diphenhydramine)
Akathisia	1 week to 2 months	Motor restlessness	Dose reduction, switching to alternative drug, benzodiazepines
Tardive dyskinesia	Months to years	Choreoathetosis (e.g., lip smacking)	Stop offending antipsychotic, often irreversible
Neuroleptic malignant syndrome	Any time, but commonly in first 2 weeks of initiation	Muscle rigidity, hyperthermia, autonomic instability, altered mental status	Stop offending antipsychotic, provide supportive care

rarely NMS. Ondansetron (Zofran), on the other hand, is a serotonin antagonist. It is not associated with extrapyramidal symptoms or NMS, but may prolong the QTc.

Lithium

General Principles

- Eliminated almost entirely by the kidneys unchanged. Medications that alter renal function (e.g., angiotensin-converting enzyme inhibitors, nonsteroidal antiinflammatory drugs, thiazide diuretics) can lead to toxicity.

Clinical Presentation

- Acute: predominant early gastrointestinal symptoms similar to those of ingestions of other metal salts
- Chronic: neurologic symptoms
  - Confusion, ataxia, tremors, fasciculations, clonus, hyperreflexia
  - Nephrogenic diabetes insipidus (inability of kidney to concentrate urine)
  - Hypothyroidism due to competition and concentration in the thyroid gland
- Acute on chronic: features of both types

Diagnosis and Evaluation

- Lithium level, serum electrolytes, renal function, and thyroid levels

Treatment

- Standard supportive care and serial monitoring of sodium and lithium levels
- Gastrointestinal decontamination is not helpful because activated charcoal does not bind to lithium.
- Hemodialysis is indicated with severe signs and symptoms of neurotoxicity (e.g., altered mental status, seizures), renal dysfunction, and lithium level > 4 mEq/L in acute toxicity (>2.5 mEq/L in chronic toxicity).

SUGGESTED READINGS

Greller, H. A. (2015). Lithium. In R. S. Hoffman, M. A. Howland, N. A. Lewin, L. S. Nelson, L. R. Goldfrank, & N. E. Flomenbaum (Eds.), *Goldfrank's toxicologic emergencies* (10th ed.). McGraw-Hill Education.

Juurlink, D. (2015). Antipsychotics. In R. S. Hoffman, M. A. Howland, N. A. Lewin, L. S. Nelson, L. R. Goldfrank, & N. E. Flomenbaum (Eds.), *Goldfrank's toxicologic emergencies* (10th ed.). McGraw-Hill Education.

CHAPTER 126

BOARD REVIEW

Antimicrobials

THOMAS E. BLAIR, MD, and SUSANNAH EMPSON, MD

- Antimicrobial toxicity can occur secondary to side effects of therapeutic dosing, acute overdose, or subacute/chronic effects from sustained use. Side effects are either immunologic or nonimmunologic. Table 126.1 lists some common antibacterial toxicities. What follows is a more detailed discussion of selected antimalarial, antituberculous, and antiretroviral toxicities.

Isoniazid

General Principles

- Isoniazid (INH) is a first-line treatment of latent and active tuberculosis. It works by inhibiting the synthesis of mycolic acids, a component of bacterial cell walls. INH is metabolized in the liver and excreted by the kidneys. Toxicity occurs in one of several ways:
- Direct hepatotoxicity
- Functional deficiency of pyridoxine (vitamin B_6)
  - Reduction in γ-aminobutyric acid (GABA) production
  - Peripheral neuropathy

TABLE 126.1 *Selected Antimicrobial Toxicities and Their Specific Treatments*

Drug	Acute Toxicity
Penicillin	Seizures (50 million units or more IV)
Amoxicillin	Crystalluria, hematuria, rash if given in mononucleosis
Nitrofurantoin	Methemoglobinemia, contraindicated in G6PD deficiency
Chloramphenicol	Gray baby syndrome and cardiovascular collapse in newborns
Fluoroquinolones (e.g., ciprofloxacin)	Tendinopathy, QT prolongation, seizure, neurologic symptoms
Macrolides (e.g., azithromycin)	Prolonged QT
Sulfonamides	Methemoglobinemia, Stevens-Johnson syndrome
Vancomycin	Red man syndrome (nonimmunologic anaphylactic response, previously termed anaphylactoid reaction), nephrotoxicity
Tetracyclines (e.g., doxycycline)	Photosensitivity
Rifampin	Cytochrome P450 inducer, decreasing other drugs' efficacy, including contraceptives
Metronidazole	Disulfiram-like reaction: flushing, nausea and vomiting with ethanol

G6PD, glucose-6-phosphate dehydrogenase; *IV*, intravenously.
Adapted from Rella, J. G., & Carter, W. A. (2016). Antimicrobials. In: J. E. Tintinalli, J. S. Stapczynski, O. J. Ma, D. M. Yealy, G. D. Meckler, & D. M. Cline (Eds.), *Tintinalli's emergency medicine: A comprehensive study guide* (8th ed., p. 1346). McGraw-Hill Education.

Clinical Presentation

- Acute overdose typically occurs between 30 minutes and 2 hours after ingestion of >20 mg/kg. Symptoms begin with nausea, altered mental status, and ataxia. Symptoms can progress to seizure, metabolic acidosis, and coma. Seizures are generalized tonic-clonic in nature and refractory to typical anticonvulsive therapy.

Diagnosis and Evaluation

- Diagnosis is based on history and presentation of refractory status epilepticus. INH level tests are not clinically relevant given that they take days to weeks to return a result. INH can cause both a direct anion-gap metabolic acidosis and an indirect anion-gap acidosis through the production of lactate.

Treatment

- Standard supportive care and activated charcoal if recent ingestion.
- Seizure management
  - **Pyridoxine (vitamin B_6):** 1 g intravenously for every gram of INH ingested OR 5 g intravenously if ingested amount is unknown. Pediatric dosing is 70 mg/kg with a maximum of 5 g.
  - **Benzodiazepines:** phenytoin and fosphenytoin have no role in the treatment of INH-induced seizures.

Antimalarials

General Principles

- Malaria is a protozoal infection transmitted via the female *Anopheles* mosquito with *Plasmodium* species including *falciparum*, *ovale*, *vivax*, *malariae*, and *knowlesi*. Antimalarial medications typically target the parasite's digestive vacuole and affect either the hepatic or erythrocytic stage of infection. Life-threatening toxicities in acute overdose typically manifest with cardiac and neurologic symptoms. The medications discussed below are those with the most severe and/or common toxicities.

Clinical Presentation

- Chloroquine
  - Neurologic: headache, altered level of consciousness, visual disturbances, seizures
  - Cardiac: tricyclic antidepressant–like toxicity: hypotension, QRS and QT prolongation, atrioventricular block
  - Pulmonary: respiratory depression
  - Gastrointestinal: nausea, vomiting, diarrhea
  - Metabolic/endocrine: hypokalemia
- Quinine/quinidine
  - Toxicity attributed to Na/K channel blockade, α-adrenergic antagonism, and hyperinsulinemia
  - Neurologic: coma, neuromuscular paralysis
  - Head, eyes, ears, nose, and throat: ocular toxicity (acute blindness), ototoxicity (tinnitus/deafness)
  - Cardiac: wide QRS, prolonged QT, torsades de pointes, hypotension
  - Endocrine: hypoglycemia
  - Hematologic: Coombs-positive hemolysis
- Mefloquine
  - Neurologic: hallucinations, psychosis, insomnia, vivid dreams, headache, seizures
    - Contraindicated in patients with seizures or psychiatric disorders
- Primaquine
  - Hemolytic anemia and methemoglobinemia (contraindicated in glucose-6-phosphate dehydrogenase deficiency)

Diagnosis and Evaluation

- Diagnosis is based on history of exposure and clinical symptomatology.

Treatment

- All agents: standard supportive care and activated charcoal if recent ingestion.
- Quinine
  - Sodium bicarbonate (to maintain pH >7.55) to prevent cardiac toxicity
  - Octreotide for hypoglycemia to reduce endogenous insulin production
- **Chloroquine:** treat wide QRS-like tricyclic antidepressant toxicity with sodium bicarbonate.
- **Primaquine:** methylene blue for methemoglobinemia

Antiretrovirals

General Principles

- Antiretroviral therapies used to treat HIV infection target the major viral enzymes (reverse transcriptase, protease, integrase) and their attachment and fusion sites. Categories include nucleoside reverse transcriptase inhibitors, nonnucleoside reverse transcriptase inhibitors, protease inhibitors, entry and fusion inhibitors, and integrase inhibitors. Initial regimens typically include two nucleoside reverse transcriptase inhibitors and another agent. Side effects from antiretroviral medications are common.

Clinical Presentation

- Table 126.2 lists the major adverse effects of selected antimicrobial medications.

TABLE 126.2 *Antiretroviral Medications, Major Adverse Effects*

Antiretroviral Medications	Adverse Effects
Nucleoside reverse transcriptase inhibitors	
Abacavir	Stevens-Johnson syndrome, hypersensitivity reaction (fever, rash, myalgia)
Didanosine	Peripheral neuropathy, lactic acidosis, hepatic steatosis (rare)
Lamivudine	Lactic acidosis, hepatic steatosis (rare)
Stavudine	Pancreatitis, lactic acidosis, peripheral neuropathy, ascending muscle weakness, dyslipidemia
Tenofovir	Pancreatitis, headache, renal failure, diarrhea, nausea, vomiting
Zidovudine	Bone marrow suppression
Nonnucleoside reverse transcriptase inhibitors	
Delavirdine	Transaminitis rash (blisters), headache
Efavirenz	Depression, psychosis, suicidal ideation
Nevirapine	Stevens-Johnson syndrome, hepatic failure
Protease inhibitors	
Amprenavir	Toxicity from propylene glycol diluent
Atazanavir	Increased indirect bilirubin, prolonged PR interval
Darunavir	Headache, nausea, diarrhea, rash
Fosamprenavir	Hyperlipidemia, rash
Indinavir	Urolithiasis, nephrotoxicity, indirect hyperbilirubinemia
Nelfinavir	Secretory diarrhea
Ritonavir	Hyperlipidemia, nausea, vomiting, hyperglycemia
Saquinavir	Hyperglycemia, lipodystrophy
Tipranavir	Intracerebral hemorrhage, hepatotoxicity
Entry and fusion inhibitors	
Enfuvirtide	Pneumonia, injection site reaction
Maraviroc	Abdominal pain, postural hypotension
Integrase inhibitors	
Raltegravir	Increased creatine phosphokinase, nausea, headache

From Rothman, R., Marco, C.A., & Yang, S. (2016). Human immunodeficiency virus infection. In J. E. Tintinalli, J. S. Stapczynski, O. J. Ma, D. M. Yealy, G. D. Meckler, & D. M. Cline (Eds.), *Tintinalli's emergency medicine: A comprehensive study guide* (8th ed., p. 1056). McGraw-Hill Education.

Treatment

- Treatment typically consists of supportive care and ceasing the offending agent. This is usually done in consultation with an infectious disease specialist.

SUGGESTED READINGS

Bella, J. G., & Carter, W. A. (2016). Antimicrobials. In J. E. Tintinalli, J. S. Stapczynski, O. J. Ma, D. M. Yealy, G. D. Meckler, & D. M. Cline (Eds.), *Tintinalli's emergency medicine: A comprehensive study guide* (8th ed., pp. 1345–1347). McGraw-Hill Education.

Molyneaux, M. (2016). Malaria. In J. E. Tintinalli, J. S. Stapczynski, O. J. Ma, D. M. Yealy, G. D. Meckler, & D. M. Cline (Eds.), *Tintinalli's emergency medicine: A comprehensive study guide* (8th ed., pp. 1070–1076). McGraw-Hill Education.

Rao, R. B. (2019). Isoniazid (INH) poisoning. *UpToDate*. Retrieved May 28, 2019, from https://www.uptodate.com/contents/isoniazid-inh-poisoning

Rothman, R., Marco, C. A., & Yang, S. (2016). Human immunodeficiency virus infection. In J. E. Tintinalli, J. S. Stapczynski, O. J. Ma, D. M. Yealy, G. D. Meckler, & D. M. Cline (Eds.), *Tintinalli's emergency medicine: A comprehensive study guide* (8th ed., pp. 1047–1056). McGraw-Hill Education.

Takhar, S. S., & Chin, R. L. (2018). HIV infection and AIDS. In R. M. Walls, R. S. Hockberger, & M. Gausche-Hill (Eds.), *Rosen's emergency medicine: Concepts and clinical practice* (9th ed., pp. 1626–1638). Elsevier.

Travassos, M., & Laufer, M. K. (2019). Antimalarial drugs: An overview. *UpToDate*.

Anticholinergic Toxicity

LISA ZHAO, MD, and EUGENIE COMO, MD

Anticholinergic toxicity is a commonly seen toxidrome owing to the ubiquity of anticholinergic agents. Presenting symptoms can be vague and may resemble other toxidromes or delirium from organic illnesses. Fatality is rare.

General Principles

- Anticholinergics competitively inhibit acetylcholine at muscarinic receptors in the central nervous system, smooth muscle, ciliary body of the eye, and salivary and sweat glands. In contrast, nicotinic receptors occur at neuromuscular junctions and are not antagonized by anticholinergics.
- A list of common anticholinergic agents is shown in Box 127.1. Over-the-counter antihistamines such as diphenhydramine are the most common agents. *Datura* (jimsonweed) is readily found in the environment and is used recreationally for its hallucinogenic properties.
- Toxicity occurs most commonly by ingestion, although it may rarely occur transdermally (scopolamine), or topically (atropine ophthalmic drops).

Clinical Presentation

- "Red as a beet": flushing from cutaneous vasodilation
- "Dry as a bone": anhidrosis due to peripheral inhibition of sweat glands
- "Hot as a hare": anhidrotic hyperthermia as a result of impaired cooling
- "Blind as a bat": nonreactive mydriasis from inhibition of pupillary constriction
- "Mad as a hatter": delirium and hallucinations from central nervous system effects. In higher doses, central nervous system depression may occur, leading to lethargy and coma.
- "Full as a flask": urinary retention from detrusor and urethral sphincter dysfunction

BOX 127.1 ***Agents That Produce Anticholinergic (Antimuscarinic) Poisoning Syndrome***

Anticholinergic syndrome can be caused by many agents, including atropine, diphenhydramine, and scopolamine.

Plants
- *Atropa belladonna* (deadly nightshade)
- *Datura stramonium* (jimsonweed)
- *Mandragora officinarum* (mandrake)
- *Hyoscyamus niger* (henbane)

Belladonna alkaloids (natural) and related synthetic compounds
- Atropine
- Homatropine
- Scopolamine
- Glycopyrrolate (peripheral effects only)

Antispasmodics
- Clidinium bromide (Librax)
- Cyclobenzaprine (Flexeril)
- Dicyclomine (Bentyl)
- Propantheline bromide (Pro-Banthine)
- Methantheline bromide (Banthine)
- Orphenadrine (Norflex)
- Flavoxate (Urispas)
- Oxybutynin (Ditropan)

Antiparkinsonian medications
- Benztropine mesylate (Cogentin)
- Biperiden (Akineton)
- Trihexyphenidyl (Artane)

Topical mydriatics (Ocular)
- Cyclopentolate (Cyclogyl)
- Homatropine (Isopto Homatropine)
- Tropicamide (Mydriacyl)

Antihistamines
- Brompheniramine (Dimetane)
- Chlorpheniramine (Ornade, Chlor-Trimeton)
- Cyclizine (Marezine)
- Dimenhydrinate (Dramamine)
- Diphenhydramine (Benadryl, Caladryl)
- Hydroxyzine (Atarax, Vistaril)
- Meclizine (Antivert)
- Doxylamine (Unisom)
- Promethazine (Phenergan)

Antipsychotics
- Clozapine (Clozaril)
- Chlorpromazine (Thorazine)
- Prochlorperazine (Compazine)
- Thiothixene (Navane)
- Thioridazine (Mellaril)
- Trifluoperazine (Stelazine)
- Perphenazine (Trilafon)

Others
- Amantadine (Symmetrel)
- Disopyramide (Norpace)
- Glutethimide (Doriden)
- Procainamide (Pronestyl)
- Quinidine (Quinidex)

From Fulton, J.A., & Nelson, L. S. (2012). Anticholinergics. In J. G. Adams, E. D. Barton, J. Collings, P. M. C. DeBlieux, M. A. Gisondi, & E. S. Nadel (Eds.), *Emergency medicine: Clinical essentials* (2nd ed., pp. 1239–1245.e1). Saunders.

- Cardiac effects: tachycardia (often the first sign seen), QRS and QT prolongation.
- Gastrointestinal effects: reduced or absent bowel sounds, ileus due to decreased gastrointestinal motility.
- Many drugs have multiple pharmacologic effects and are not "pure anticholinergics."
  - Tricyclic antidepressants can cause cardiac arrhythmias due to sodium channel blockade.
  - Atypical antipsychotics cause mental status fluctuations rather than agitation.
- To distinguish from sympathomimetic toxidrome, look for reduced bowel sounds and anhidrosis (as opposed to diaphoresis).
- Serotonin syndrome may look similar but has clonus, increased muscle tone, and diarrhea.
- Diagnosis is based on history of exposure and clinical symptomatology.
- Specific tests to consider
  - Serum drug levels of anticholinergics are rarely helpful or easily available.
  - Glucose, acetaminophen, and salicylate levels, pregnancy testing, creatine kinase (to assess for rhabdomyolysis), serum chemistry tests
  - Electrocardiogram is essential to rule out arrhythmias, such as prolonged QRS or QTc.

Treatment

- Standard supportive care and activated charcoal if recent ingestion.
- Sodium bicarbonate for QRS prolongation or arrhythmias.
- Physostigmine is a reversible acetylcholinesterase inhibitor used in cases with refractory agitation or hemodynamic instability. It should be used in consultation with a poison control center and/or toxicologist
  - Physostigmine should be used only in pure anticholinergic overdose. Cases of asystole have been described in patients with tricyclic antidepressant overdoses with prolonged QRS interval who were given physostigmine.
  - Relative contraindications include patients with cardiac conduction abnormalities, reactive airway disease, intestinal obstruction, and epilepsy.
  - Dosing is 0.5–1 mg intravenously slowly over 5 minutes. Reversal of anticholinergic effects occurs fairly quickly and may prevent the need for intubation. Repeat dose after 20–30 minutes if severe symptoms recur.
  - Cholinergic toxicity, as well as seizures and bradyarrhythmias, may occur. Atropine should be readily available at the bedside as an antidote.
- Disposition: observe patients with mild to moderate toxicity for 6 hours. Patients with more persistent symptoms should be admitted for cardiac monitoring and further observation.

SUGGESTED READINGS

Hoffman, R. S., Howland, M. A., Lewin, N. A., Nelson, L. S., Goldfrank, L. R., & Flomenbaum, N. E. (Eds.). (2015). *Goldfrank's toxicologic emergencies* (10th ed.). McGraw-Hill Education.

Tintinalli, J. E., Stapczynski, J. S., Ma, O. J., Yealy, D. M., Meckler, G. D., & Cline, D. M. (Eds.). (2016). *Tintinalli's emergency medicine: A comprehensive study guide* (8th ed.). McGraw-Hill Education.

Walls, R. M., Hockberger, R. S., & Gausche-Hill, M. (Eds.). (2018). *Rosen's emergency medicine: Concepts and clinical practice* (9th ed.). Elsevier.

CHAPTER **128**

BOARD REVIEW

Cholinergics: Nerve Agents and Organophosphates

ZAHIR BASRAI, MD, and JASKARAN SINGH, MD

General Principles

- Cholinergic agents are acetylcholinesterase inhibitors that result in an accumulation of acetylcholine at muscarinic and nicotinic receptors. They have been used in chemical warfare (G agents, V agents) and as insecticides (organophosphate and carbamate insecticides). They are readily absorbed via dermal, gastrointestinal, and respiratory routes and can accumulate in body fat, even causing toxicity after gradual exposure.

Clinical Presentation

- Patients present with a cholinergic syndrome. The muscarinic effects result in SLUDGE (*s*alivation, *l*acrimation, *u*rination, *d*efecation, *g*astrointestinal cramping, and *e*mesis). The "killer B's" are the fatal complications of cholinergic syndrome and include: *b*ronchorrhea, *b*ronchoconstriction, and *b*radycardia. Ocular effects of the toxicity (miosis) are the most consistent finding.

Diagnosis and Evaluation

- Diagnosis is made clinically usually after exposure to insecticides or nerve agents.
- A 1-mg atropine challenge can be performed. Mild syndromes may resolve with this small dose; however, very large doses may be necessary in some exposures.
- Confirmation testing involves sampling plasma and erythrocyte cholinesterase levels, which typically do not give results immediately.

Treatment

- Decontamination and standard supportive care.
- Activated charcoal is rarely useful.
- If necessary, intubate using a nondepolarizing paralytic (rocuronium).
- Atropine is the definitive treatment because it competitively antagonizes acetylcholine at muscarinic receptors. Suggested dosing is 1–3 mg of intravenous atropine, followed by a doubling of each subsequent dose every 5 minutes until "atropinization" has been achieved, as evidenced by control of hypersecretions.
- Oximes, such as pralidoxime (2-PAM), are the other part of the definitive treatment to enhance acetylcholinesterase regeneration but are time-sensitive and should therefore be given early.
- Significant exposures require hospitalization for monitoring, given the potential for delayed syndromes that require repeated atropine dosing.

SUGGESTED READINGS

Tintinalli, J. E., Stapczynski, J. S., Ma, O. J., Yealy, D. M., Meckler, G. D., & Cline, D. M. (Eds.). (2016). *Tintinalli's emergency medicine: A comprehensive study guide* (8th ed.). Chapter 195 – Pesticides. McGraw-Hill Education.

Welker, K., & Thompson, T. M. (2018). Pesticides. In Walls, R. M., Hockberger, R. S., & Gausche-Hill, M. (Eds.), *Rosen's emergency medicine: Concepts and clinical practice* (9th ed., pp. 1947–1956). Elsevier.

CHAPTER **129** BOARD REVIEW

Mushrooms, Poisonous Plants, and Nutritional Supplements

JONIE HSIAO, MD, and EUGENIE COMO, MD

Mushroom Poisoning

Mushroom poisonings are common and usually have a self-limited course. However, lethal ingestions can occur, in particular when amatoxin-containing species are mistakenly foraged and ingested.

General Principles

Most toxic mushrooms only cause self-limited gastroenteritis. Some contain the chemical psilocybin and are consumed recreationally for their hallucinogenic properties. Cyclopeptide-containing mushrooms such as *Amanita phalloides* are highly lethal.

- Amatoxins
  - Toxic cyclopeptides that are heat stable and insoluble in water
  - Bind to DNA-dependent RNA polymerase II and inhibit protein transcription, resulting in cell death.
  - Act on organs with rapid cell turnover such as the gastrointestinal tract, hepatocytes, and renal tubules.
  - Minimum lethal dose is 0.1 mg/kg; for *Amanita phalloides*, approximately one to two medium-sized mushroom caps.

Clinical Presentation

- Ingestion of nonfatal mushrooms usually results in a self-limited gastrointestinal illness with a rapid onset of symptoms, *within 6 hours* of ingestion.
- Amatoxin poisoning has a *delayed* onset after ingestion, beginning with the following:
  1. Severe gastrointestinal symptoms including nausea, vomiting, diarrhea, and diffuse abdominal pain, resulting in massive fluid loss and often renal failure at 6–24 hours
  2. A period of transient improvement between 12 and 36 hours
  3. Progression to fulminant liver injury, encephalopathy, and multiorgan failure over the next 2–6 days
- Gyromitrin-containing mushrooms, also known as false morels, cause amatoxin-like hepatotoxicity, but are notable in that they can additionally cause refractory seizures and methemoglobinemia.

Diagnosis and Evaluation

- Mushroom identification may not be possible if there is no sample left or if the culprit is unclear when multiple mushrooms are foraged and eaten.
- Delayed onset of symptoms should raise suspicion for amatoxin ingestion.
- For amatoxins
  - Amatoxin levels are not routinely available.
  - Comprehensive laboratory testing should include liver function tests, coagulation panel, and renal function tests.
  - Aspartate transaminase/alanine transaminase levels peak at 60–72 hours after ingestion.

Treatment

- General mushroom poisoning
  - Standard supportive care and consider activated charcoal if recent ingestion
- For amatoxins
  - No proven effective treatment is available.
  - Proposed therapies include silibinin dihemisuccinate and high-dose penicillin (both potentially inhibit amatoxin uptake), *N*-acetylcysteine, and early hemodialysis.
  - Consultation with poison control and early referral to a tertiary care center with liver transplant capabilities should be initiated.
  - Mortality rate is approximately 10%–25%.
- For gyromitrin-containing mushrooms, seizure mechanism is similar to isoniazid toxicity.
  - Administer pyridoxine for seizures along with benzodiazepines.
  - Methylene blue for methemoglobinemia

Plant Poisoning

Ingestion of potentially toxic plants is a commonly reported cause of accidental poisoning, especially among children. For most, the clinical course is self-limited. Severe illness occurs when specific plants are intentionally consumed recreationally or in a suicide attempt.

General Principles

There are many varieties of toxic plants (Table 129.1) and therefore many mechanisms by which they can cause poisoning. Toxicity is related to the amount of toxin, which is determined by several factors.

- The amount and part of the plant ingested (e.g., flower, stem, seed, or roots)
- The method of preparation or consumption (e.g., if concentrated and brewed as a tea)

TABLE 129.1 Notable Toxic Plants

Name	Toxin	Toxic Effects
Peace lily (*Philodendron*)	Raphides (insoluble calcium oxalate)	Localized mucosal swelling
Jimsonweed (*Datura*), nightshade (*Belladonna*)	Alkaloids	Anticholinergic, hallucinogenic
Oleander, foxglove, lily of the valley	Cardiac glycosides	Digitalis toxicity
Water hemlock, *Cicuta* spp.	Cicutoxin (GABA antagonist)	Seizure
Ackee fruit (unripe)	Hypoglycin A	Hypoglycemia
Castor beans (chewed or crushed)	Ricin	GI, hypovolemic shock, multiorgan failure
Wild saffron (*Colchicum autumnale*)	Colchicine (antimitotic)	GI, multiorgan failure
Poison hemlock, tobacco	Alkaloids	Nicotinic cholinergic
Fruit pits (cherries, peaches, plums, chewed or crushed)	Cyanogenic glycosides (amygdalins)	Cyanide poisoning (in large ingestions)

GABA, γ-aminobutyric acid; *GI,* gastrointestinal.

- Typically, an ingestion of a substantial amount of the plant is required to cause serious toxicity.

Clinical Presentation

- Most cause mild to moderate self-limited gastroenteritis.
- Some cause localized dermatologic reactions.
- Systemic toxicity is uncommon but can occur with specific plants.

Diagnosis and Evaluation

- Misidentification of the plant reported by the patient and family is common.
- For unclear and potentially toxic exposures, a full panel of laboratory studies should be considered: electrolytes, renal function, complete blood cell count, creatine kinase, liver function tests, partial thromboplastin time/international normalized ratio, urinalysis, and an electrocardiogram.
- Digoxin level may be elevated for plants containing cardiac glycosides, but *does not correlate with toxicity. In the context of plant ingestion, the digoxin level should be considered a qualitative and not quantitative test.*

Treatment

- Symptom-based and generally only requires supportive care.
- Digoxin-specific antibodies for plants containing cardiac glycosides; may require high doses.
- If exposure is unclear, hemodynamically stable patients with minimal or no symptoms should be observed for at least 6 hours.

Vitamins, Herbal Supplements, and Performance-Enhancing and Weight Loss Drugs

With passage of the Dietary Supplement Health and Education Act in 1994, US Food and Drug Administration oversight of dietary supplements was significantly reduced. There are few restrictions in terms of the safety, quality, and purported benefits of these products. As a result, toxicity from intended or unintentional compounds in these products can occur.

TABLE 129.2 Vitamin Toxicity

Name	Adverse Effects
Vitamin A	CNS: psychosis, headache, visual symptoms Gastroenteritis Liver injury
Vitamin D	Hypercalcemia Hyperphosphatemia
Vitamin E	Gastroenteritis Coagulopathy

CNS, central nervous system.

General Principles

- Vitamins
  - Generally, toxicity occurs only with fat-soluble vitamins (A, D, E) because water-soluble vitamins are excreted in the urine (Table 129.2).
- Herbal supplements, performance-enhancing drugs, and weight loss drugs
  - Toxicity may be caused by the intended components, misidentified or impure product, intentional adulterants, or drug-drug interactions (Table 129.3).

SUGGESTED READINGS

Nelson, L. S., Howland, M. A., Lewin, N. A., Smith, S. W., Goldfrank, L. R., & Hoffman, R. S. (Eds.). (2019). *Goldfrank's toxicologic emergencies* (11th ed.). McGraw-Hill.

Olson, K. R., Anderson, I. B., Benowitz, N. L., Blanc, P. D., Clark, R. F., Kearney, T. E., Kim-Katz, S. Y., & Wu, A. H. B. (Eds.). (2018). *Poisoning and drug overdose* (7th ed., Section II: Specific poisons and drugs: Diagnosis and treatment, pp. 73–497). McGraw-Hill.

Walls, R. M., Hockberger, R. S., Gausche-Hill, M., Bakes, K., Baren, J. M., Erickson, T. B., Jagoda, A. S., Kaji, A. H., VanRooyen, M., & Zane, R. D. (Eds.). (2018). *Rosen's emergency medicine: Concepts and clinical practice* (9th ed.). Elsevier.

TABLE 129.3 *Notable Toxic Supplements*

Name	Intended Use	General Mechanism	Adverse Effects
Anabolic steroids	Physical performance	↑Testosterone	Virilization Acne Aggression, mania, psychosis Hypertension Hyperlipidemia Cholestatic hepatitis Immunosuppression
Ephedra (ma huang)	Physical performance Weight loss	Sympathomimetic	Cardiovascular (e.g., AMI, stroke) Psychosis Seizures Liver toxicity
Kava	Anxiolysis Insomnia	GABA	Liver toxicity
Kratom	Mood enhancement Opioid withdrawal	Opioid (mostly) Stimulant (low dose)	Psychosis Addiction Seizures Coma Respiratory depression
St. John's wort	Depression	Unclear Induces CYP450	Drug-drug interactions Serotonin syndrome

AMI, acute myocardial infarction; *CYP450,* cytochrome P450; *GABA,* γ-aminobutyric acid.

Toxic Alcohols

LISA ZHAO, MD, and JAMES JIANG, MD

Toxic alcohols are compounds found in household and industrial products and are often ingested accidentally or in suicide attempts. Alcohols are rapidly absorbed from the gastrointestinal (GI) tract and then metabolized by alcohol dehydrogenase and aldehyde dehydrogenase. In some instances, toxicity is caused by the parent compound (isopropyl alcohol) and in others, by their metabolites (methanol and ethylene glycol; Fig. 130.1).

Methanol and Ethylene Glycol

General Principles

- Methanol
  - Colorless, volatile liquid found in windshield wiper fluid, solid cooking fuel, solvents, and some perfumes.
  - Most poisoning occurs by ingestion. Exposure can occur through inhalation or skin, but this rarely causes toxicity.
  - Worldwide, poisoning occurs because of contaminated alcoholic beverages or when it is used as an alternative to ethanol, intentionally or unintentionally.
  - Metabolized into formaldehyde, then formic acid, which is toxic to the retinal epithelial cells, optic nerve cells, and basal ganglia cells.
  - At lower pH, the nondissociated form of formic acid is favored, which crosses the blood-brain barrier more readily, worsening central nervous system (CNS) effects.
- Ethylene glycol
  - Colorless, odorless, and sweet-tasting; found in car radiator antifreeze and some metal cleaners
  - Poisoning occurs exclusively by ingestion because it does not penetrate skin well.
  - Metabolized into glycolic acid, then to oxalic acid
    - Glycolic acid causes most of the metabolic acidosis.
    - Oxalic acid binds serum calcium, forming calcium oxalate crystals.
  - Can also be metabolized to nontoxic metabolites. Thiamine and pyridoxine are cofactors in this pathway.
  - Crystals precipitate in renal tubules, leading to acute renal failure, or in other tissues, leading to multiorgan dysfunction.

Clinical Presentation

- Methanol
  - Neurologic effects
    - Inebriation in a dose-dependent manner, less inebriating than ethanol.
    - Can lead to CNS depression to the point of coma
    - Seizures, delayed parkinsonism (from effects on basal ganglia), and polyneuropathies can occur.

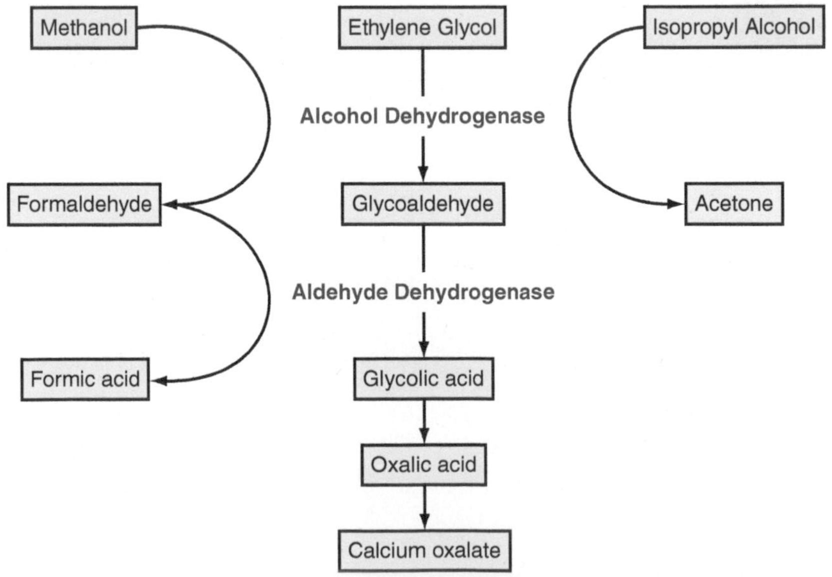

FIG.130.1 Metabolic pathways of methanol, ethylene glycol, and isopropyl alcohol.

- Computed tomography scan may demonstrate basal ganglia hemorrhages.
- Visual changes
  - Impairment of color vision, "snowstorm" vision (spots with blurred vision), total blindness in severe cases. Permanent visual impairment can occur with just one mouthful.
  - On physical examination: papilledema, nystagmus, central scotoma, optic disc pallor, afferent pupillary defect.
- Cardiovascular effects: tachycardia and hypotension; hemodynamic collapse in severe cases.
- Usually effects can be reversible if treated, but blindness and parkinsonism may be permanent.

- Ethylene glycol
  - Neurologic effects
    - Intoxication is due to parent compound, more inebriating than alcohol.
    - Seizure and coma in severe cases. Seizures can be due to hypoglycemia.
    - Late findings include parkinsonism and isolated cranial nerve abnormalities.
  - Cardiopulmonary effects
    - Tachycardia and hypertension
    - Tachypnea for metabolic acidosis compensation
    - Heart failure, acute lung injury from glycolic acid and calcium oxalate crystal formation
    - Arrhythmias from QT prolongation secondary to hypocalcemia due to calcium oxalate crystal formation
  - Renal effects
    - Calcium oxalate crystal deposition leading to renal impairment
    - Temporary dialysis is often needed. Resolution takes weeks to months.

Diagnosis and Evaluation

- Serum chemistries (including calcium), osmolality, blood gas, and electrocardiogram. Lactate and ketone levels are also useful. Ethanol level is required to calculate osmolar gap.
- Immediately after ingestion, anion gap is normal and osmolar gap will be elevated because most of the ingested alcohol is parent alcohol and has not yet been metabolized into acid (Fig. 130.2).
  - Serum osmolarity is calculated by 2 × [sodium mmol/L] + ([glucose mg/dL]/18) + ([serum urea nitrogen mg/dL]/2.8) + ([ethanol mg/dL]/3.7); be sure to use correct units.
  - Osmolar gap (serum osmoles – calculated serum osmolarity) is significant if >10 mOsm/L, suggesting acute toxic alcohol poisoning.
  - Moderate elevations of osmolar gap (10–20) can occur in alcoholic ketoacidosis and lactic acidosis and may complicate the picture.
- Once metabolized, anion gap rises and osmolar gap normalizes. Metabolic acidosis may take up to 16–24 hours to develop.
- Serum levels are not widely available but may be helpful, specifically methanol, formate, ethylene glycol, oxalate concentrations. Once obtained, levels are not necessarily indicative of toxicity and are controversial.

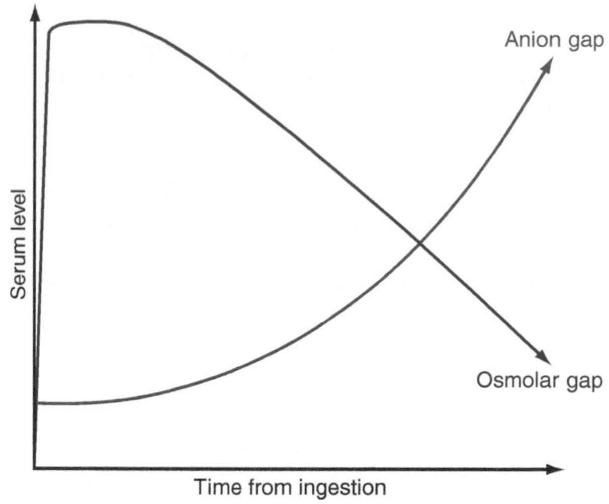

FIG. 130.2 Progression of anion gap and osmolar gap over time after methanol or ethylene glycol ingestion.

- Imaging studies such as computed tomography or magnetic resonance imaging of the head are not necessary unless there are neurologic deficits.
- In ethylene glycol toxicity, urine may fluoresce with a Wood lamp (because of the fluorescein in antifreeze) and may reveal calcium oxalate crystals. These findings are neither sensitive nor specific.

Treatment

- Standard supportive care
- No role for GI decontamination because alcohols are very rapidly absorbed.
- Block conversion of parent compounds to toxic metabolites.
  - Fomepizole: competitive inhibitor of alcohol dehydrogenase. Dosage is 15 mg/kg intravenously, then 10 mg/kg every 12 hours for 4 doses, then 15 mg/kg every 12 hours until ethylene glycol and methanol levels are undetectable. Indications:
    - Methanol or ethylene glycol level >20 mg/dL if laboratory results are available
    - Coma or decreased mental status in patient with osmolar gap >10 mOsm/L
  - Ethanol may be used if fomepizole is not available to a target of 100–150 mg/dL serum alcohol level.
  - Goal of therapy is to resolve metabolic acidosis or decrease levels of methanol and ethylene glycol to <20 mg/dL (if available).
  - Eventually parent compound will be cleared by kidneys or will need to be dialyzed if patient is in renal failure.
- Correct acidosis, and eliminate toxic metabolites.
  - Sodium bicarbonate is used to reverse acidosis to target pH of 7.35–7.45. Evidence is not robust to support urine alkalinization, but if no contraindications, there could be a theoretical benefit.
  - Hemodialysis indications
    - Refractory metabolic acidosis with pH <7.25, or anion gap >30
    - Visual changes in methanol poisoning

  - Acute renal failure
  - Hemodynamic instability despite supportive care
  - Ethylene glycol or methanol level >50 mg/dL (if available)
  - Electrolyte abnormalities not responsive to conventional treatment
- Repletion of cofactors and adjunctive therapy
  - Limited evidence to indicate efficacy but unlikely to cause harm
  - Folate and folinic acid may help metabolize formic acid from methanol toxicity to CO_2 and water.
  - Pyridoxine, thiamine, magnesium may prevent formation of oxalic acid.

Isopropyl Alcohol

General Principles

- Found in rubbing alcohol and hand sanitizer, and is used as a common solvent for cosmetic and household use.
- Most commonly poisoning occurs by ingestion but can also occur by inhalation if poor ventilation, or transdermally during alcohol sponge bath.
- Metabolized into acetone by alcohol dehydrogenase, which does not cause toxic effects. The toxic effects of isopropyl alcohol are due to the parent compound itself. It is not metabolized by aldehyde dehydrogenase.

Clinical Presentation

- Roughly twice as intoxicating as ethanol because of its large molecular weight, which may cause respiratory depression
  - Rapid onset within 30–60 minutes due to rapid absorption
  - Delayed effects due to lingering acetone
- Ketones may cause fruity-smelling breath.
- Hypoglycemia may occur due to decreased NADH/NAD^+ ratio.
- Nausea, vomiting, and abdominal pain; may cause hemorrhagic gastritis.
- If aspirated, can lead to hemorrhagic tracheobronchitis.
- In massive ingestion, hypotension occurs owing to systemic vasodilation.

Diagnosis and Evaluation

- Laboratory studies, including point-of-care glucose, chemistry for osmolar gap, and serum osmoles
  - Does NOT cause a metabolic acidosis or elevated anion gap.
  - Osmolar gap will be elevated.
- Serum isopropyl not available in all hospitals.
- Ketosis will occur owing to acetone formation (ketosis without acidosis).

Treatment

- Supportive care. Manage airway if obtunded, and give intravenous fluids if patient is hypotensive. Give proton pump inhibitors for gastritis and arrange consult with gastroenterology department for consideration of endoscopy if GI bleed.
- No role for fomepizole or ethanol—they may actually prolong effects by preventing metabolism.
- If patient is refractory to fluids, consider vasopressors and hemodialysis.
- Discharge if asymptomatic after 4–6 hours of observation. If CNS effects, consider admission.

Pediatric Considerations

- Children can develop symptoms with as little as three sips of 70% isopropyl alcohol.
- Dermal absorption is more common in infants because of greater body surface area. Methanol and isopropanol are easier to absorb than ethylene glycol.

SUGGESTED READINGS

Cohen, J. P., & Quan, D. (2016). Alcohols. In J. E. Tintinalli, J. S. Stapczynski, O. J. Ma, D. M. Yealy, G. D. Meckler, & D. M. Cline (Eds.), *Tintinalli's emergency medicine: A comprehensive study guide* (8th ed.). McGraw-Hill. https://accessemergencymedicine.mhmedical.com/content.aspx?bookid=1658&sectionid=109437660

Helman, A. (Host), Thompson, M., & Austin, E. (2018, January). Toxic alcohols—Minding the gaps (Episode 106) [Audio podcast episode]. In *Emergency medicine cases*. https://emergencymedicinecases.com/toxic-alcohols/

Wiener, S. W. (2011). Toxic alcohols. In L. S. Nelson, N. A. Lewin, M. A. Howland, R. S. Hoffman, L. R. Goldfrank, & N. E. Flomenbaum (Eds.), *Goldfrank's toxicologic emergencies* (9th ed.). McGraw-Hill. https://accesspharmacy.mhmedical.com/content.aspx?bookid=454&sectionid=40199520

Recreational Drugs

JONIE HSIAO, MD, and ROBERT CAREY, MD

Recreational drugs are psychoactive legal and illegal drugs that induce an altered mental state for a nonmedical purpose. They are often categorized as depressants, stimulants, and/or hallucinogens. Based on 2018 data, in the United States, about 53.2 million persons, nearly 1 in 5 people, aged 12 years and older have used illicit drugs, including prescription drugs, in the past year.[1] In 2017, there were 70,237 drug overdose deaths in the United States. Marijuana is the most widely used drug, at a prevalence of 15.9%. Opioids, including prescription painkillers, heroin, and synthetic drugs, have a combined prevalence of less than 5%, but are involved in more than half of fatal overdoses.[2]

Marijuana

General Principles

- Marijuana is derived from the cannabis plant. It is typically smoked or ingested. Δ^9–Tetrahydrocannabinol is the main active agent, acting primarily on cannabinoid receptors (cannabinoid type 1 receptors) in the central nervous system (CNS). Marijuana is a schedule 1 drug in the United States, but has been legalized for recreational or medicinal use in many states.

Clinical Presentation

- Inhaled onset 5–10 minutes, duration 2–4 hours.
- Ingested onset 1–3 hours, duration 2–12 hours. Because effects are delayed, patients are more likely to redose, causing higher likelihood of undesirable effects, especially in children.
- Most common findings
  - Tachycardia and conjunctival injection.
  - Euphoria, mild alterations in sensory perception, cognitive slowing.
- Less common and more likely in children
  - Ataxia, vomiting, agitation, CNS depression.
- Cannabinoid hyperemesis syndrome (Box 131.1)

BOX 131.1 *Cannabinoid Hyperemesis Syndrome*

Patient: heavy marijuana user, multiple times daily for months to years
Presentation: severe abdominal pain and cyclic nausea + vomiting that improves with very hot showers
Treatment: fluids, electrolyte repletion, antiemetics, haloperidol, and/or topical capsaicin
Definitive therapy: cessation of marijuana use

Diagnosis and Evaluation

- Tachycardia typically the only vital sign abnormality.
- Urine drug testing for marijuana is not typically helpful in the acute setting; it remains positive days after use (up to weeks in chronic users).

Treatment

- Acute intoxication rarely requires medical intervention.
- Benzodiazepines as needed for agitation or anxiety.

Synthetic Cannabinoids

General Principles

- Synthetic cannabinoids include an expanding number of products, typically smoked. Like marijuana, synthetic cannabinoids target cannabinoid type 1 receptors. However, because of a lack of oversight, they contain a wide variety of cannabinoid and noncannabinoid psychoactive ingredients in unpredictable concentrations. This leads to potentially more serious toxicity than marijuana. Common street names include Spice and K2.

Clinical Presentation

- Euphoria, sensory perception alterations, and tachycardia.
- Severe agitation, tremulousness, nausea, and vomiting.
- Hallucinations, psychosis, and altered mental status.
- Rarely: seizures, cardiac toxicity, and ischemic stroke.
- Rarely: severe coagulopathy due to adulterant ingredient brodifacoum (vitamin K antagonist).

Diagnosis and Evaluation

- Not detectable in routine urine drug screens.

[1] Substance Abuse and Mental Health Services Administration. (2019). Key substance use and mental health indicators in the United States: Results from the 2018 National Survey on Drug Use and Health (HHS Publication No. PEP19-5068, NSDUH Series H-54). Center for Behavioral Health Statistics and Quality, Substance Abuse and Mental Health Services Administration. Retrieved from https://www.samhsa.gov/data/ Accessed 11/5/2020.
[2] Wilson, N., Kariisa, M., Seth, P., Smith, H. IV, & Davis, N. L. (2020). Drug and opioid-involved overdose deaths—United States, 2017–2018. *MMWR Morbidity and Mortality Weekly Report*, 69, 290–297. DOI:http://dx.doi.org/10.15585/mmwr.mm6911a4 Accessed 11/5/2020.

Treatment

- Similar to marijuana acute intoxication, rarely requires medical intervention.
- Benzodiazepines or antipsychotics as needed for agitation or anxiety.

Opioids

See Chapter 120. Analgesic Toxicity.

Cocaine

General Principles

Cocaine, a sympathomimetic drug, is a commonly abused stimulant derived from the coca plant. It can be ingested, snorted, smoked, or injected. Cocaine causes CNS stimulation and inhibits the reuptake of catecholamines and to some extent serotonin. It is also a local anesthetic agent and blocks Na^+ channels, which can cause conduction abnormalities leading to dysrhythmias. Sold illicitly, it may be combined with other drugs (e.g., with heroin, termed "speedballing") and/or adulterated with other compounds.

Clinical Presentation

- Onset when inhaled, snorted, or by intravenous route is seconds to minutes, lasting 10–90 minutes.
- Onset with ingestion can take 30–60 minutes and has a less predictable duration (Box 131.2).
- May provoke hypertensive emergencies.
- Cardiac dysrhythmias including ventricular fibrillation or tachycardia, other tachyarrhythmias, and QRS widening or QT prolongation (class 1A antidysrhythmic).
- Rhabdomyolysis from increased muscle tone and psychomotor agitation.
- Seizure from CNS stimulation.
- Pneumothorax or pneumomediastinum from inhalation.
- Acute lung injury from inhalation "crack lung" (hemorrhagic alveolitis).
- Nasal septal perforation from intranasal use.

Diagnosis and Evaluation

- Urine drug screening positive up to 72 hours but may only indicate prior use and unrelated to active intoxication.
  - Consider electrocardiogram and comprehensive laboratory testing including electrolytes, glucose, serum urea nitrogen, creatinine, creatine kinase, urinalysis, and troponin.
  - Chest radiography, abdominal imaging (body stuffers), and/or computed tomography of the head as indicated.
  - Levamisole (antiparasitic medication) is a common adulterant; it can cause agranulocytosis and vasculitis.

BOX 131.2 *Sympathomimetic Toxidrome*

CNS stimulation: agitation, psychosis or combativeness
Hypertension
Hyperthermia
Increased motor tone
Mydriasis
Tachycardia
Diaphoresis[a]

[a]Key feature not found in anticholinergic toxidromes.

Treatment

- Benzodiazepines are the mainstay of treatment.
- If the above are not effective for hypertension, phentolamine, a direct α-adrenergic antagonist, can be considered.
- Nitrates for cardiac chest pain.
- β-Blockers generally avoided due to theoretical risk of unopposed α-adrenergic stimulation.
- Sodium bicarbonate for widened QRS and dysrhythmias.
- Seizures are usually self-limited.
- Standard rapid cooling measures for severe hyperthermia.
- Decontamination with activated charcoal and whole-bowel irrigation may be considered for body stuffers.
- Disposition and period of observation required are highly variable depending on clinical manifestations.
- After acute intoxication, patients may become conversely extremely lethargic because of catecholamine depletion.

Methamphetamines, Methylenedioxymethamphetamine (Ecstasy), and Synthetic Cathinones ("Bath Salts")

General Principles

- Methamphetamines are another class of commonly abused stimulants that can be smoked, ingested, or injected. Methylenedioxymethamphetamine (MDMA, also known as Ecstasy) is a designer drug notably used at rave parties. Synthetic cathinones (called "bath salts") are a noteworthy newer class of designer drug. All are sympathomimetics chemically related to amphetamines. They work by increasing the release of catecholamines to varying degrees, especially dopamine, and serotonin.

Clinical Presentation

- Sympathomimetic toxidrome similar to cocaine.
- Hypertensive crisis, seizure, rhabdomyolysis.
- Methamphetamines have a longer duration of action and may result in a prolonged drug-induced psychosis (>12 hours).
- MDMA can cause severe acute hyponatremia due to antidiuretic hormone secretion as well as increasing intake of hypotonic fluids and therefore may present with profound altered mental status and seizures.
- Bath salts can cause severe psychomotor agitation and prolonged psychotic behavior. Some reported cases of psychosis have lasted days to weeks.

Diagnosis and Evaluation

- Urine drug screening can detect amphetamines but is of limited use in the acute setting given potential false-positive and false-negative results; it is not available for designer drugs.
- Hemodynamic monitoring including continuous cardiac monitoring.

- Consider cardiac monitoring, comprehensive laboratory testing including electrolytes, glucose, serum urea nitrogen, creatinine, creatine kinase, and/or urinalysis.

Treatment

- Benzodiazepines are the mainstay treatment for sympathomimetic manifestations.
- Antipsychotics such as haloperidol as needed for severe psychosis.

Lysergic Acid Diethylamide

General Principles

- Lysergic acid diethylamide (LSD) is a psychedelic drug. Commonly called acid, it is formulated as a liquid, tablet, powder, or blotter, and ingested or absorbed sublingually. Doses as small as 20 μg have a significant effect. The primary mechanism is agonism of 5-HT_{2A} serotonin receptors.

Clinical Presentation

- Intense and prolonged (8–12 hours) alterations in sensory and time perception, hallucinations, euphoria.
- Powerful dysphoric hallucinations and delusions ("bad trips") may prompt medical care.
- Tachycardia, hypertension, mild hyperthermia.
- Mydriasis, piloerection, mild gastric distress, and hyperreflexia.
- Large ingestions can cause serotonin syndrome and result in vomiting, diaphoresis, hyperthermia, seizures, rhabdomyolysis, and hematologic dysfunction.

Diagnosis and Evaluation

- Not routinely tested in urine drug screens.

Treatment

- Medical intervention is not typically needed.
- Verbal deescalation, reality testing, and placement in an environment with minimal stimuli.
- Benzodiazepines or antipsychotics as needed for agitation or anxiety.

Phencyclidine

General Principles

- Phencyclidine (PCP) was originally developed as a dissociative agent used in anesthesia, but was recalled because it caused severe agitation during emergence. It is primarily an *N*-methyl-D-aspartate receptor antagonist, but has multiple secondary sites of action: nicotinic anticholinergic, indirect opioid agonist, and dopamine agonist and reuptake inhibitor. PCP can be injected, ingested, snorted, or smoked, often in combination with other drugs.

Clinical Presentation

- Onset depends on method of consumption (<5 minutes with smoking); duration is typically 4–8 hours but can be significantly prolonged.
- Toxidrome is mixed (cholinergic, anticholinergic, sympathomimetic), resulting in variable presentation.
- Tachycardia, hypertension, hyperthermia.
- Extreme agitation, often with aggressive and violent behavior.
- Altered mental status, bizarre delusions, and psychosis.
- Nystagmus: all types, but vertical and rotary are more specific to PCP intoxication.
- Ataxia, muscle rigidity, increased secretions, rhabdomyolysis.
- Other severe side effects include seizures, bronchospasm, life-threatening hyperthermia, apnea, coma, and cardiac arrest.

Diagnosis and Evaluation

- Urine toxicology remains positive 2–4 days after use, but frequent false-positive results occur due to cross-reactivity with many drugs, including diphenhydramine, ketamine, and dextromethorphan.
- Dissociative and analgesic effects make it difficult to control these patients, increasing the likelihood of self-harm and harm to staff; early physical (involving at least four staff) and chemical restraint is often necessary.
- Evaluate for coingestions and potential mimics.
- Consider laboratory testing for renal function and creatine kinase level.
- Perform a thorough trauma survey because patients frequently injure themselves or are injured during restraint by law enforcement or health-care personnel.

Treatment

- Antipsychotics and benzodiazepines for chemical restraint; ketamine should be avoided given its similar mechanism of action to PCP.
- Sedation, intubation, and cooling measures for severe hyperthermia.
- Benzodiazepines for seizures.
- Intravenous fluid therapy and urine output monitoring for rhabdomyolysis.
- Monitoring for 4–6 hours is typically needed before medical clearance.

γ-Hydroxybutyrate

General Principles

- γ-Hydroxybutyrate or GHB is used off-label as a bodybuilding supplement and illicitly in sexual assault (date rape). It acts on endogenous GHB receptors; with ingestion, these receptors are overwhelmed and GABA receptors are stimulated. GHB is formulated as a liquid, pill, tablet, or powder. It has a narrow therapeutic window and can be easily overdosed. It is rapidly absorbed and then cleared within 12 hours.

Clinical Presentation

- Bradycardia and hypothermia.
- Amnesia, drowsiness, cardiac/respiratory depression, and coma.
- *Rapid emergence and return to baseline;* alcohol coingestion can amplify and prolong effects.
  - Patients classically present obtunded, requiring intubation, then rapidly return to baseline and attempt to self-extubate.

- Agitation and emergence delirium.
- GHB withdrawal can occur with chronic use and is similar to alcohol withdrawal.

Diagnosis and Evaluation

- GHB is not detected on routine urine drug screens; if suspected and confirmation is needed for legal purposes, blood and urine samples can be collected as soon as possible given its rapid metabolism.

Treatment

- Airway support and vasopressors for severe intoxication, apnea, and hypotension.
- Once a patient has returned to baseline mental status, he or she can usually be safely discharged.

Inhalants

General Principles

- Inhalants are a broad category of commonly abused drugs, typically hydrocarbons, among children and adolescents. They are found in many household products such as glue, lighter fluid, and spray paint. They are sniffed, bagged, or huffed (saturated on a cloth). Nitrous oxide (N_2O) is another commonly abused inhalant that is used by inhaling whippets, small compressed-gas containers used in whipped-cream makers.

Clinical Presentation

- Table 131.1 presents the negative effects of select hydrocarbon inhalants.
- Nitrous oxide notably can cause peripheral neuropathy and loss of proprioception due its inactivation of vitamin B_{12} (subacute combined degeneration of the spinal cord).
- Chronic huffing, bagging, or sniffing of hydrocarbons may cause cerebellar degeneration.

Diagnosis and Evaluation

- Perioral dermatitis ("sniffer's rash") may be seen on examination.
- Not detectable in routine urine drug screens.

TABLE 131.1 *Acute Inhalant Toxicity (Hydrocarbons)*

System	Effects
CNS	Euphoria, confusion, agitation, hallucinations, seizures, ataxia CNS depression
Cardiac	Myocardial sensitization leading to Ventricular dysrhythmias (sudden sniffing death)
Pulmonary	Hypoxia Aspiration and chemical pneumonitis Bronchospasm
Dermatologic	Perioral dermatitis ("sniffer's rash") Chemical burns

CNS, central nervous system.

- Chest radiograph findings may be delayed for hours.
- 12-Lead electrocardiogram and continuous cardiac monitoring.

Treatment

- Supportive, especially respiratory care.
- Caution with use of β agonists, given myocardial sensitization.
- Caution with albuterol in setting of bronchospasm.
- For ventricular fibrillation or tachycardia, amiodarone and lidocaine are favored over epinephrine.
- For refractory ventricular fibrillation or tachycardia, consider intravenous propranolol or esmolol to counteract sensitization.

SUGGESTED READINGS

Olson, K. R., Anderson, I. B., Benowitz, N. L., Blanc, P. D., Clark, R. F., Kearney, T. E., Kim-Katz, S. Y., & Wu, A. H. B. (Eds.). (2018). *Poisoning and drug overdose* (7th ed., Section II: Specific poisons and drugs: Diagnosis and treatment, pp. 73–497). McGraw-Hill.

Tintinalli, J. E., Stapczynski, J. S., Ma, O. J., Yealy, D. M., Meckler, G. D., & Cline, D. M. (Eds.). (2016). *Tintinalli's emergency medicine: A comprehensive study guide* (8th ed.). McGraw-Hill Education.

Walls, R. M., Hockberger, R. S., & Gausche-Hill, M. (Eds.). (2018). *Rosen's emergency medicine: Concepts and clinical practice* (9th ed.). Elsevier.

Cellular Asphyxiants

ZAHIR BASRAI, MD, and JASKARAN SINGH, MD

In general, the high oxygen-utilizing tissues, such as the heart and brain, are the most sensitive to cellular asphyxiants. Although methemoglobinemia is better categorized as a congenital or acquired hemoglobinopathy, it is included in this chapter.

Carbon Monoxide

General Principles

Carbon monoxide (CO) poisoning is the most common cause of acute poisoning morbidity and mortality in developed nations. It is an odorless and colorless gas that results from the incomplete combustion of nearly all carbon-containing products. It has a much higher affinity for binding hemoglobin than oxygen does. It manifests its toxicity by binding deoxyhemoglobin to form carboxyhemoglobin (COHb), which cannot carry oxygen, and by preventing cellular metabolism through binding a mitochondrial cytochrome complex.

Clinical Presentation

- Mild/early symptoms mimic a viral syndrome, with headache, nausea, dizziness, and myalgias.
- Severe poisoning presents similarly, with altered mental status, coma, hypotension, seizure, and cardiac arrest.
- Patients with prolonged "soaking periods" (exposure durations) and coma are at highest risk of developing delayed neurologic sequelae after days to weeks of an asymptomatic period.
  - Cognitive decline, psychiatric complaints, and movement disorders.
- Of note, methylene chloride (used in paint stripper) is metabolized by the liver to CO and can cause CO toxicity with a delayed onset and prolonged recovery course.

Diagnosis and Evaluation

- Assess for potential exposures (wood fires, indoor gasoline-powered generators).
- Pulse oximetry is unable to detect CO poisoning because it cannot differentiate COHb from O_2Hb.
- Arterial blood gas (ABG) or venous blood gas shows a normal PAO_2 but may reveal metabolic acidosis from lactate production.
- Cooximetry is the test of choice as it directly measures COHb.
  - A normal COHb level in nonsmokers is < 2%, whereas it can be as high as 5%–10% in smokers.
- Additional evaluation includes electrocardiogram, basic metabolic panel, and troponin and creatine kinase levels to evaluate for ischemia and end-organ damage.

Treatment

- Normobaric oxygen delivered by a nonrebreather mask. The duration of therapy is unclear and an end point of symptom resolution in addition to a COHb level < 5% is reasonable.
- The half-life of COHb on room air is about 4–5 hours; this can be decreased to 45–60 minutes with administration of 100% FiO_2 via endotracheal tube, and 20–30 minutes through hyperbaric oxygen therapy.
- Candidates for hyperbaric oxygen therapy to decrease the incidence of delayed neurologic sequelae include:
  - Signs of neurologic abnormalities: altered mental status, syncope
  - Signs of cardiovascular abnormalities: dysrhythmias, myocardial ischemia
  - Institutions have COHb level cutoffs that range from 25% to 40%
  - Special consideration is given for pregnancy, often with a lower COHb threshold, such as 15%
- The decision to initiate hyperbaric oxygen therapy should occur quickly, because a delay of > 6 hours has been shown to decrease its efficacy.

Cyanide

General Principles

Cyanide exposure can occur with smoke inhalation, *Prunus* species pit ingestion (e.g., apricots, peaches, cherries), prolonged nitroprusside drip administration, and during laboratory and industrial accidents. Hydrogen cyanide is noted to have an *odor of bitter almonds*. It prevents cellular metabolism through inhibition of the electron transport chain and as a result inhibits the tissues' extraction of oxygen from blood.

Clinical Presentation

Patients often present with seizures, dysrhythmias, coma, and cardiovascular collapse. Venous blood will appear bright red given its higher than normal oxygen concentration.

Diagnosis and Evaluation

An anion gap metabolic acidosis, high lactate, and arterialization of venous blood as measured by a high central venous oxygen saturation are suggestive. A serum lactate level >8 mmol/L in the appropriate clinical context has good test characteristics for the diagnosis. Serum cyanide levels have a limited role in the emergency department.

Treatment

The goal of treatment is to provide an alternative binding site for the cyanide ion, so that the cytochrome oxidase system can be reactivated.

- The cyanide antidote kit contains sodium nitrite, amyl nitrite, and sodium thiosulfate. The nitrites are used to induce methemoglobin, which has a high affinity for the cyanide ion, and then sodium thiosulfate scavenges the cyanide ion by donating sulfur. The process can cause hypotension and tachycardia and has been replaced by the safer hydroxocobalamin.
- Hydroxocobalamin is a metalloprotein with a central cobalt atom that complexes with the cyanide ion to form cyanocobalamin (vitamin B_{12}), which is excreted in the urine.
- All symptomatic patients should be admitted to an intensive care unit.

Hydrogen Sulfide

General Principles

- Hydrogen sulfide exposures typically occur in petroleum refinery and sewage storage tank workers or during environmental disasters. The gas has a noxious *odor similar to rotten eggs*. It acts as a pulmonary irritant and a cellular asphyxiant, having a mechanism of action that is similar to cyanide. It has a rapid disassociation from the mitochondria, allowing many patients to survive after brief exposure.

Clinical Presentation

- The presentation is similar to that of cyanide toxicity except that most transported patients will have recovered by the time of their arrival to the emergency department. In the field, rescuers often become victims of hydrogen sulfide poisoning.

Diagnosis and Evaluation

- Rapid testing is not available. An ABG test generally reveals a metabolic acidosis and elevated serum lactate levels.

Treatment

- Removal from the exposure and standard resuscitative efforts are generally sufficient.
- All symptomatic patients should be admitted to the intensive care unit.

Methemoglobinemia

General Principles

Methemoglobinemia (MetHb) is a hemoglobinopathy that can be caused by congenital or acquired causes (Box 132.1). It occurs when hemoglobin goes from its reduced, ferrous (Fe^{2+}) state to an oxidized, ferric (Fe^{3+}) state. This change impairs its ability to carry oxygen and also shifts the oxygen-dissociation curve to the left, resulting in tissue hypoxia and lactic acidosis.

BOX 132.1 *Common Causes of Methemoglobinemia*

Hereditary

Hemoglobin M
NADH methemoglobin reductase deficiency (homozygote and heterozygote)
G6PD deficiency

Acquired

Medications

Amyl nitrite
Antineoplastics (e.g., cyclophosphamide, ifosfamide, flutamide)
Dapsone
Local anesthetics (e.g., benzocaine, lidocaine, prilocaine)
Nitroglycerin
Nitroprusside
Phenacetin
Phenazopyridine (Pyridium)
Quinones (e.g., chloroquine, primaquine)
Sulfonamides (e.g., sulfanilamide, sulfapyridine, sulfamethoxazole)

Chemical Agents

Aniline dye derivatives (e.g., shoe dyes, marking inks)
Butyl nitrite
Chlorobenzene
Fire (heat-induced denaturation)
Food adulterated with nitrites
Food high in nitrates
Isobutyl nitrite
Naphthalene (mothballs)
Nitrophenol
Nitrous gases (seen in arc welders)
Paraquat
Silver nitrate
Trinitrotoluene
Well water (nitrates)

Pediatric Cases

Reduced NADH methemoglobin reductase activity in infants (<4 mo)
Seen in association with low birth weight, prematurity, dehydration, acidosis, diarrhea, and hyperchloremia

G6PD, glucose-6-phosphate dehydrogenase; *NADH*, reduced nicotinamide adenine dinucleotide.

Modified from Nelson, L. S., Lewin, N. A., Howland, M. A., Hoffman, R. S., Goldfrank, L. R., & Flomenbaum, N. E. (Eds.). (2011). *Goldfrank's toxicologic emergencies* (9th ed.). McGraw-Hill.

Clinical Presentation

- Patients present with signs and symptoms consistent with hypoxia such as shortness of breath, cyanosis, altered mental status, and cardiac arrhythmias.
- Cyanosis that does not respond to supplemental O_2.

Diagnosis and Evaluation

- Cooximetry measuring for MetHb is the diagnostic test of choice.
- Pulse oximetry is inaccurate because it is unable to differentiate species of hemoglobin other than oxyhemoglobin and deoxyhemoglobin.
  - The pulse oximetry saturation (SpO_2) will read between 75% and 85% regardless of the MetHb level and actual oxygen saturation on ABG (SaO_2).

- The difference between the SaO_2 and SpO_2 is known as a saturation gap and can help with diagnosis.

Treatment

- Discontinue offending agent and start supplemental oxygen.
- Methylene blue (1–2 mg/kg intravenously over 5 minutes) is indicated for patients with symptomatic hypoxia or MetHb >25%.
  - Converts ferric (Fe^{3+}) iron back to ferrous (Fe^{2+}) state.
  - Improvement should be noted within minutes and the dose can be repeated if cyanosis has not disappeared after 1 hour.
  - In patients with glucose-6-phosphate dehydrogenase (G6PD) deficiency, it may cause hemolysis and is not recommended. Exchange transfusion can be used to treat symptomatic patients with G6PD deficiency. Vitamin C is also a direct reducing agent that can be used in patients with G6PD deficiency with methemoglobinemia.
- Asymptomatic patients with methemoglobinemia less than 15% can be discharged home. All other patients should be admitted.

CHAPTER 133

BOARD REVIEW

Heavy Metals

JENNIFER FANG, MD, and CYNTHIA KOH, MD

- There are many elements that comprise the label of "heavy metals," but only a few that an emergency medicine physician is likely to come across. This chapter reviews these most testable presentations. Decontamination with removal of the source of intoxication, if known, is paramount; then, gastrointestinal (GI) decontamination with whole-bowel irrigation should be pursued if any retained material is suspected. In general, activated charcoal does not adsorb heavy metals well but should be considered in inorganic mercury poisoning.

Iron

General Principles

- Iron is available in multiple forms, particularly as supplements for anemia and in prenatal vitamins. Iron salts readily undergo redox reactions with various proteins and enzymes, primarily in hemoglobin for oxygen transfer; in overdose, its primary mechanism of toxicity is through diffuse oxidative damage, resulting in cell death. Iron overdose occurs at doses of 10–20 mg/kg elemental iron.

Clinical Presentation

There are five clinical stages of acute iron toxicity.

1. Marked GI symptoms due to corrosive damage to the GI tract. Patients present with nausea, vomiting, diarrhea, and abdominal pain, sometimes accompanied by GI bleeding and resultant shock. If no GI symptoms occur within the first 6 hours of iron ingestion, serious toxicity is unlikely.
2. Often called the "latent" phase due to apparent resolution of GI symptoms. Although patients may clinically appear improved, toxicity is often still ongoing and may manifest as metabolic acidosis, lethargy, and tachycardia. Patients should be monitored to determine whether they are progressing to systemic disease or have resolution of mild iron toxicity.
3. Progression of systemic toxicity. Widespread tissue damage results in worsening metabolic acidosis, coagulopathy, acute respiratory distress syndrome, shock, seizures, and/or coma.
4. Fulminant hepatic failure. Occurs 2–3 days after ingestion.
5. Delayed sequelae after rare survival of stage four. Bowel obstruction (commonly gastric outlet obstruction) due to scarring from damaged tissue occurs 2–8 weeks after ingestion.

Patients with chronic iron toxicity (e.g., patients receiving chronic transfusions) are at higher risk for *Yersinia enterocolitica* sepsis.

Diagnosis and Evaluation

- Complete blood cell count, blood chemistries, liver function tests, partial prothrombin time, international normalized ratio, and lactate level tests should be ordered to evaluate for leukocytosis, anemia, anion gap acidosis, liver failure, and coagulopathy.
- Total serum iron level >300 μg/dL results in significant GI and systemic toxicity. Peak concentrations occur 4–6 hours after ingestion and should be monitored until downtrending.
- Radiography is not sensitive for iron ingestion because radiopacity is variable. Tablets tend to be radiopaque, whereas liquid and chewable iron preparations are radiolucent.

Treatment

- Standard supportive care. Charcoal is not recommended because iron does not adsorb well.
- Deferoxamine chelates free iron, forming a complex that is renally excreted and creates orange or reddish urine. Should be administered intravenously to patients with signs of significant toxicity or serum iron concentration greater than 500 μg/dL, but infusion rate may be limited by the development of hypotension. Oral deferoxamine is not recommended and can enhance iron absorption.
- In patients with significant toxicity, those with evidence of ongoing absorption should be treated with bowel decontamination using whole-bowel irrigation. Retained iron tablets after whole-bowel irrigation may require endoscopic or surgical removal.

Lead

General Principles

- Lead exposures come from three main sources. Environmental exposures are more common in children, primarily from lead paint in pre-1978 homes. Occupational exposures occur in many industries, such as pottery glazers, construction workers, or people who work with lead bullets. Imported sources include spices, jewelry, toys, and cosmetics. In the United States, lead toxicity, or plumbism, has higher prevalence among minorities and immigrants. Once absorbed, lead binds to erythrocytes and deposits in bones. Over time, redistribution of bone lead contributes to chronically elevated blood lead levels and toxicity. Lead is chemically similar to iron, calcium, and zinc, so it produces widespread effects by affecting calcium-gated channels and enzymes.

Clinical Presentation

- Acute toxicity: encephalopathy (often with cerebral edema on imaging), seizures, hepatitis, vomiting, and hemolytic anemia.
- Subclinical toxicity: growth and neurocognitive development may be affected.
- Chronic toxicity: most common presentation. Should be suspected in those with multisystem complaints (Table 133.1) in the context of exposure risk factors.
- Symptoms of mild toxicity overlap with other common childhood presentations such as viral syndrome, constipation, abdominal colic, seizures, and developmental delay.

Diagnosis and Evaluation

- Physical examination for foreign bodies or retained bullets.
- Complete blood cell count, blood chemistries, liver function tests, urinalysis, peripheral smear showing basophilic stippling (Fig. 133.1).
- Whole-blood lead level.
- Computed tomography or magnetic resonance imaging of the brain, if patient has altered mental status, to evaluate for cerebral edema.
- Radiographs may reveal radiopaque lead foreign bodies or "lead lines" in radiographs (Fig. 133.2) from increased calcium deposition in metaphyses.

TABLE 133.1 *Clinical Manifestations of Chronic Lead Toxicity*

Organ/System	Presentation
Blood	Affects heme synthesis and decreases erythrocyte lifespan which results in anemia
Bone	Growth is stunted and exposed children may have short stature
Cardiac	Hypertension, decreased contractility, dysrhythmias, QT prolongation, wide QRS
Endocrine	Hypothyroid, decreased pituitary hormone secretion
Gastrointestinal	Abdominal pain, constipation, hepatitis, pancreatitis
Neurologic	Gray matter in the brain with certain areas such as the hippocampus affected more than others, headache, peripheral neuropathy (preferentially affecting motor nerves, especially upper extremities and extensor muscles, causing wrist or foot drop), tremor, mood changes
Renal	Interstitial fibrosis; Fanconi-like syndrome with amino acid, glucose, and phosphate losses; decreased uric acid excretion (leads to saturnine gout)
Reproductive	Decreased hormone secretion, chromosome abnormalities, infertility, crosses placenta (abnormal fetal development, miscarriage, preterm delivery)

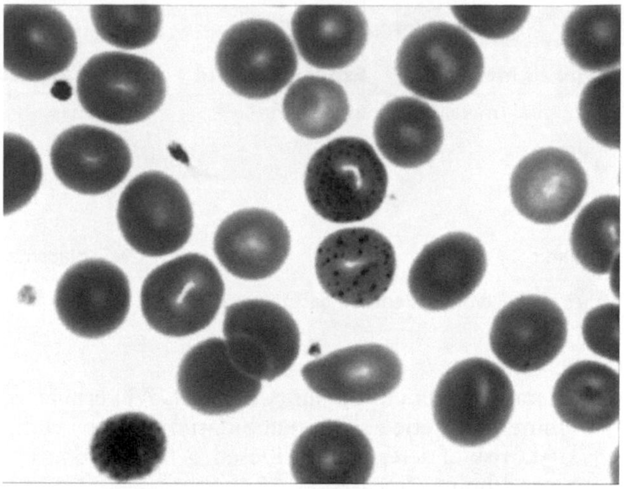

FIG. 133.1 Basophilic stippling on peripheral blood smear. (From Bachmeyer, C., Bagur, E., Lenglet, T., Maier-Redelsperger, M., & Lecomte, I. (2012). Lead poisoning mimicking amyotrophic lateral sclerosis: An adverse effect of rituals. *The American Journal of Medicine, 125*(6), e5–6, Fig. 1.)

- Blood lead level (BLL) at which follow-up is recommended is 5 μg/dL.

Treatment

- Remove from exposure (can be challenging if exposure is from housing).
- Improve nutrition and decrease GI absorption by supplementing with iron, calcium, and vitamin C. Avoid fasting.
- Decontamination with whole-bowel irrigation. Consider endoscopic or surgical removal.
- Chelation—binds lead and increases urinary and fecal excretion.
  - Dimercaprol (British anti-Lewisite [BAL]) for encephalopathy or BLL >100 μg/dL in adults or >70 μg/dL in children.

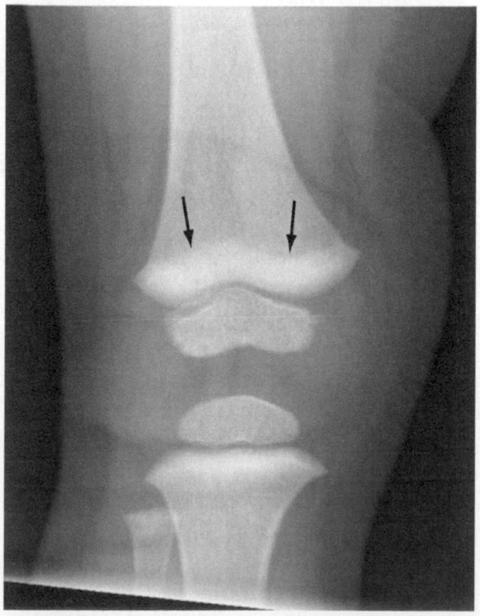

FIG. 133.2 Lead lines. (From Towbin, A. J. (2017). Musculoskeletal. In L. F. Donnelly (Ed.), *Fundamentals of pediatric imaging* (2nd ed., Fig. 7.85). Elsevier.)

TABLE 133.2 *Mercury Toxicity*

Type of Mercury	Exposure Route	Main Distribution	Presentation
Elemental (metallic)	Inhalation	Pulmonary	Respiratory symptoms
Inorganic	Oral	Blood, renal, CNS (late)	Acute: GI symptoms, notably hemorrhagic gastroenteritis Chronic: renal failure, neuropsychiatric symptoms, acrodynia
Organic	Oral	CNS, placenta, renal, skin, liver, blood	Delayed neurologic symptoms

CNS, central nervous system; *GI*, gastrointestinal.

- Edetate calcium disodium (CaNa2EDTA) ethylenediaminetetraacetic acid in combination therapy with BAL, risk of deterioration if used as monotherapy. Start 4 hours after BAL.
- Succimer for mild symptoms or BLL 70–100 μg/dL in adults or 45–70 μg/dL in children.
- BLLs of 5–45 μg/dL do not require chelation. Manage exposure source.
- Chelation recommended for pregnant women and newborns with elevated BLLs.

Mercury

General Principles

- Mercury exposures occur in seafood or such industries as photography, painting, and agriculture. Household items with mercury include older thermometers or fluorescent light bulbs. Mercury is also used in alternative medicine and as a component of imported skin lighteners. The forms of mercury and their toxicities are found in Table 133.2. Organic mercury has the largest volume of distribution because it is the most lipophilic. In the body, the different forms convert between one another. Mercury binds to sulfhydryl groups and disrupts cell membranes and enzymes.

Clinical Presentation

Elemental Mercury

- Liquid but extremely volatile at room temperature. Poor GI absorption.
- If liquid form is aerosolized and inhaled, patients can develop cough, dyspnea, and fever, which may progress to severe injury (pneumonitis, acute respiratory distress syndrome, or bronchial hemorrhage).
  - Aerosolization classically occurs during *vacuuming* in an attempt to clean the spill.

Inorganic Mercury

- Acute ingestion typically intentional, classically in laboratory workers. Patients experience metallic taste, oropharyngeal and abdominal pain, nausea, and hemorrhagic gastroenteritis, which leads to shock and renal failure.
- Chronic toxicity presents with metallic taste, gingivostomatitis, intention tremor that can progress to choreiform movements, hypersalivation, blushing, shyness, renal failure, narrowed visual fields, neuropathy, ataxia, and other neuropsychiatric complaints.
- Acrodynia, or "pink disease," is erythema and edema of hands, feet, and face that can progress to desquamation and is accompanied by sweating, tachycardia, tremors, paresthesias, and irritability.

Organic Mercury

- Methylmercury is present in such large carnivorous fish as swordfish, shark, mackerel.
- The US Food and Drug Administration advises pregnant women, women who may become pregnant, nursing mothers, and young children to avoid fish with high mercury levels.
- Predominantly permanent neurologic symptoms with delayed presentation of weeks to months after exposure. Also causes contact dermatitis and GI symptoms.

Diagnosis and Evaluation

- Complete blood cell count, blood chemistries, liver function tests, urinalysis, and arterial blood gas.
- Whole-blood mercury level and 24-hour urine mercury level, although specific values do not correlate with degree of toxicity.
- Chest radiograph, electrocardiogram, formal visual field testing.

Treatment

- Decontamination
  - If mercury is solid, open windows, adsorb with decontamination kit or sand, and sweep into sealed container. *Do not vacuum because mercury could volatilize further.*
  - Wash skin exposures with water; consider surgical excision if localized area.
  - Standard supportive care and activated charcoal (inorganic mercury may adsorb well).
  - Whole-bowel irrigation.
- Chelation—increases urinary elimination.
  - Elemental and inorganic mercury: use dimercaprol (BAL) intramuscularly or succimer by mouth.
  - Organic mercury toxicity is more difficult to treat because of lipophilicity.
    - BAL should not be used because it can increase mercury in the brain.
    - Succimer may decrease central nervous system mercury levels.

SUGGESTED READINGS

Hoffman, R. S., Howland, M. A., Lewin, N. A., Nelson, L. S., Goldfrank, L. R., & Flomenbaum, N. E. (Eds.). (2015). *Goldfrank's toxicologic emergencies* (10th ed.). McGraw-Hill Education.

Olson, K. R., Anderson, I. B., Benowitz, N. L., Blanc, P. D., Clark, R. F., Kearney, T. E., Kim-Katz, S. Y., & Wu, A. H. B. (Eds.). (2012). *Poisoning & drug overdose* (6th ed.). McGraw-Hill Education.

CHAPTER 134

BOARD REVIEW

Physical and Chemical Irritants

ANDREW GROCK, MD, and JAMES JIANG, MD

Irritants are physical or chemical agents that cause cellular damage after sufficient direct contact with skin or mucosal surfaces. A direct cytotoxic effect or localized trauma can create inflammation and cellular damage. Unlike immune-mediated allergic reactions, irritant reactions lack an immunologic or antibody response. Presentations vary based on the properties of the irritant, host factors, and environmental factors. Common irritants are noted in Tables 134.1 and 134.2.

General Principles

Pathogenesis of Skin Irritants

- Chemical irritants provoke local inflammation by disrupting the epidermal barrier and epidermal cell membrane, direct cytotoxicity, and inciting cytokine release.
- Acids cause coagulation necrosis. Alkalis cause the more severe liquefactive necrosis.
  - Hydrofluoric acid (used in glass etching) causes coagulation necrosis like other acids, but also binds calcium and magnesium.
- Physical irritants induce injury by performing chronic repetitive microtraumas to the stratum corneum.

Pathogenesis of Pulmonary Irritants

- Pulmonary irritants generate inflammation by:
  - Damage to type I and type II pneumocytes → cytokine release → influx of neutrophils → capillary endothelial cell disruption → accumulation of cellular debris and exudate in alveolar sacs → acute respiratory distress syndrome.
- Patients often present after industrial exposure although they may also be victims of terrorism or chemical warfare.
- Notably, phosgene gas is converted to hydrochloric acid and carbon monoxide in the lung and thus has a delayed onset with severe effects.

Clinical Presentation

Skin Irritants

- Presentation varies based on potency:
  - Weaker irritants (chronic dermatitis): scaly skin changes, mild erythema, skin fissuring.
  - Stronger irritants: immediate burning → erythema/bullae formation → ulceration of the skin surface with localized skin necrosis.
  - Hydrofluoric acid: severe coagulation necrosis, pain out of proportion, hypomagnesemia, and hypocalcemia.
- Risk for dysrhythmia from electrolyte abnormalities.

Pulmonary Irritants

- Presentation depends on the speed of resulting mucosal injury.
- With rapid irritants, symptoms develop quickly. Thus, patients usually remove themselves from the exposure before lower respiratory tract involvement.
  - Rapidly acting agents
    - Nasal and oropharyngeal pain and edema.
    - Drooling, cough, and stridor.
    - Concomitant eye and skin irritation.

TABLE 134.1 *Common Chemical and Physical Irritants*

Common Chemical Irritants	Common Physical Irritants
Acids and alkalis	Metals, including tools
Fertilizers and pesticides	Wood
Cleaning agents (detergents, alcohols, etc.)	Fiberglass
Oils	Plant parts (thorns, spines, leaves)
Construction agents (cement, wood treatments, fiberglass, paints, sawdust, plastics)	Paper
Wet work	Dust, soil, dirt
Solvents and glues	

TABLE 134.2 *Common Pulmonary Irritants*

Common Pulmonary Irritants	Source
Ammonia	Fertilizer, refrigerants, industrial use
Copper dioxide, cadmium oxide, zinc oxide	Welding fumes
Chloramine	Bleach with ammonia
Formaldehyde	Chemical disinfectant
Methane, propane	Heating gases
Methyl bromide	Fumigation
Phosgene	Chemical/industrial synthesis or chemical warfare (smells of freshly mowed hay)
Ozone	Disinfectant, electrical equipment
Sulfur dioxide	Exhaust

- Slower acting pulmonary irritants often reach the lower respiratory tract, which causes tracheobronchitis or bronchiolitis and can lead to acute lung injury or ARDS.
- Clinical signs and symptoms include
  - Dyspnea, cough, chest tightness, and adventitious lung sounds.
- Some agents have classic/testable features
  - Phosgene: smells of freshly mowed hay. Chemical terrorism agent. Delayed onset of symptoms.
  - Chlorine gas: greenish gas, chlorine odor.
  - Chloramine is formed from mixing bleach and ammonia, classically while mixing cleaning supplies in an enclosed space.

Diagnosis and Evaluation

- Diagnosing irritant contact dermatitis and irritant pulmonary disease is purely clinical for both.
- Skin irritants
  - Localized inflammatory skin rash develops with a history of irritant exposure.
  - Important components of the history include:
    - Occupational exposures/use of protective equipment
    - Wet work exposure (dishwashers, hairdressers, etc.).
  - For hydrofluoric acid exposure, place patient on cardiac monitor and measure electrolytes.
- Pulmonary irritants
  - Acute or delayed respiratory symptoms after exposure to inhalant gases.
  - Chest radiograph may show alveolar consolidation from pulmonary edema.
  - Blood gas can clarify oxygenation and ventilation status.

Treatment

Skin Irritants

- Prevention by avoidance of offending agents and use of protective equipment.
- Decontamination/irrigation (see Chapter 118. General Toxicologic Principles).
- For irritant contact dermatitis, use topical occlusive emollients and consider topical steroids.
- Hydrofluoric acid
  - Liberally apply topical calcium gluconate gel to exposed skin, to bind fluoride ions.
  - If symptoms persist, locally infiltrate intradermal calcium gluconate.
  - For severe burns, consider intravenous, intraarterial, or Bier block infusion of calcium gluconate.
- Bier block involves “exsanguinating” the extremity using a venous compression bandage, applying a proximal tourniquet, and injecting intravenous medications (in this case calcium gluconate).

Pulmonary Irritants

- Decontamination.
- Mainly supportive: maintain airway patency and adequate oxygenation.
- If indicated: bronchodilators and suctioning.
- Lung-protective ventilation strategies ARDSnet protocols for mechanical ventilation.
- Diuretics and venodilators are unhelpful because the pulmonary edema is noncardiogenic.
- Systemic corticosteroids lack convincing evidence of treatment success. Given some evidence of benefit and relatively little risk, they continue to be commonly used.
- If chlorine or chloramine gas, treat with nebulized 2% sodium bicarbonate for neutralization.
- If phosgene, ozone, fluorine, and oxides of nitrogen, the patient should be observed for 8–12 hours because these irritants reach the lower respiratory tract and can result in delayed symptoms.

SUGGESTED READINGS

Gorguner, M., & Akgun, M. (2010). Acute inhalation injury. *Eurasian Journal of Medicine, 42*(1), 28–35. Retrieved May 23, 2019, from https://www.ncbi.nlm.nih.gov/pmc/articles/PMC4261306/pdf/eajm-42-1-28.pdf

Gresham, C., & LoVecchio, F. (2016). Industrial toxins. In J. E. Tintinalli, J. S. Stapczynski, O. J. Ma, D. M. Yealy, G. D. Meckler, & D. M. Cline (Eds.), *Tintinalli's emergency medicine: A comprehensive study guide* (8th ed.). McGraw-Hill. Retrieved April 23, 2019, from http://accessmedicine.mhmedical.com.libproxy2.usc.edu/content.aspx?bookid=1658&sectionid=109438290

Nelson, L., & Odujebe, O. (2011). Simple asphyxiants and pulmonary irritants. In L. S. Nelson, N. A. Lewin, M. A. Howland, R. S. Hoffman, L. R. Goldfrank, & N. E. Flomenbaum (Eds.), *Goldfrank's toxicologic emergencies* (9th ed.). McGraw-Hill.

SECTION SEVENTEEN

BOARD REVIEW

Trauma

CHAPTER **135**

BOARD REVIEW

Multiple Trauma

MICHAEL T. JORDAN, MD, and JACKIE SHIBATA, MD, MS

The emergency clinician plays a critical role in coordinating a multidisciplinary team to stabilize, resuscitate, and manage the patient with multiple trauma. A structured assessment, namely the ABCDE method, can be used to systematically assess the trauma patient to quickly identify and prioritize injuries, simplifying the thought process in a chaotic environment.

Basic Principles

Definition

Multiple trauma is defined as any trauma associated with two or more injuries, of which one injury is classified as life-threatening. The ABCDE method is used to assess trauma patients: *a*irway and cervical stabilization, *b*reathing, *c*irculation, *d*isability, and *e*xposure and environmental control.

General Approach to Multiple-Trauma Patients

1. Prehospital and triage
2. Primary survey
3. Secondary survey
4. Laboratory and radiographic evaluation
5. Disposition

Mechanisms of Multiple Trauma

Table 135.1 lists mechanisms and common associated injuries of multiple trauma.

- The two most common classifications of multiple trauma are blunt vs. penetrating.
- Thermal injuries and hazardous exposures are less common.
- Mechanisms of injury may be known before arrival during the prehospital and triage stage.

Prehospital and Triage

Prearrival information provides the clinician with insights regarding expected injuries and associated pathology. The following steps can help hospital providers before the patient's arrival.

1. Receive report. Communication between providers in the field and the receiving hospital should include mechanism of injury, vital signs, Glasgow Coma Scale score, suspected injuries based on physical exam and symptoms, treatments provided, intravenous (IV) access, airway interventions, and an estimated time of arrival.
2. Prepare the necessary equipment for stabilization and resuscitation for the incoming trauma.
3. Determine and prioritize the ancillary and specialty services needed upon arrival such as respiratory therapy, trauma surgery, neurosurgery, orthopedic surgery, etc.
4. Assign roles and identify the leader of the trauma resuscitation during a team huddle.

Primary Survey

Basic Principles

- The goal of the primary survey is to immediately identify and manage life-threatening injuries.
- There are five components of the ABCDE evaluation: airway and cervical stabilization, breathing, circulation, disability, exposure and environmental control.
- As critical conditions are encountered, initiate treatment without delay before continuing to the next step of the assessment.
- After the primary survey, evaluate whether the patient needs to be transferred to a facility that can provide definitive treatment not available at the initial hospital.
- Continually reassess components of the primary survey.

AIRWAY AND CERVICAL STABILIZATION

Box 135.1 lists indications for intubation.

Clinical Presentation

- Patients can present with poor respiratory effort, altered mental status, inability to phonate, hypoxia, tachypnea, bradypnea, etc.
- Look for signs of airway obstruction: blood, hematoma, edema, vomitus, facial or neck trauma, and foreign bodies.

Diagnosis and Evaluation

- Assess airway patency, phonation, and ability to protect airway.
  - If a patient can clearly phonate and protect their airway, move to "B" (breathing), but continually reassess the airway.
  - If airway is not patent or patient cannot phonate or protect airway, intubation is likely warranted.
- If there is any concern for a cervical spine (c-spine) injury based on history or examination, take care to limit c-spine movement and place a cervical collar on the patient.
  - If intubation is warranted, have a second provider maintain c-spine immobilization during procedure.
- If time permits, perform a neurologic examination before intubation and sedation; however, the need for

TABLE 135.1 *Mechanisms and Common Associated Injuries of Multiple Trauma*

Mechanism of Injury	Common Associated Injuries
BLUNT TRAUMA	
Motor vehicle collision	
Frontal MVC	Facial fractures Hemothorax/pneumothorax Myocardial/pulmonary contusion Anterior flail chest Aortic injury Splenic or liver laceration Cervical spine fractures Posterior dislocation/fracture of hip or knee
Rear MVC	Hyperextension and fracture of cervical spine Central cord syndrome
Side MVC	Facial fractures Thoracic injuries Splenic, kidney or liver laceration depending on side of impact Hip fracture/dislocation Pelvic fracture
Rollover MVC	High chance of significant injury Crush injuries and compression injuries to spine
Ejection MVC	Likely unrestrained; thus, high chance of significant morbidity and mortality
Motor vehicle vs. pedestrian	Waddell triad: tibia and fibula or femur fractures, craniofacial injuries, truncal injuries Pedestrian at high risk for multiple trauma
Special considerations for MVC	
Windshield damage Steering wheel damage 3-point seat belt restraint	Skull fractures, coup and contrecoup injuries Sternal/rib fractures, flail chest, cardiac contusion, aortic injuries Seat belt sign: bruising corresponding to position of seat belt with increased risk for vascular or visceral injury
Fall from height	Aortic injuries; renal injuries; calcaneal, vertebral, hand/wrist, and pelvic fractures, depending on horizontal or vertical fall
PENETRATING TRAUMA	
Stab wounds	
Anterior chest Lateral thoraco-abdominal area Abdomen Extremities	Cardiac tamponade, hemothorax, pneumothorax Hemothorax, pneumothorax, diaphragmatic injury, liver laceration, splenic laceration Visceral injury if object penetrates peritoneum Neurovascular injuries, fractures, compartment syndrome
Gunshot wounds	
Trunk Extremities	Follow trajectory of bullet to determine possible injuries, evaluate for entrance and exit wounds Neurovascular injuries, compartment syndrome
BURNS AND HAZARDOUS TRAUMA	
Burns	
Electrical Inhalational Thermal	Arrhythmias, compartment syndrome, rhabdomyolysis CO poisoning, cyanide poisoning, airway edema Circumferential eschars, loss of skin leading to hypovolemia
Hazardous	Toxins, chemicals, and radiation can lead to multisystem organ morbidity; call Poison Control: 1-800-222-1222

CO, carbon monoxide; *MVC*, motor vehicle collision.

BOX 135.1 *Indications for Intubation*

A Glasgow Coma Scale score ≤8 in trauma patients (inability to protect airway)
Failure to oxygenate
Failure to ventilate
Expected clinical course (such as impending airway compromise from an expanding hematoma)

an emergent airway always takes priority and need not be delayed.

Treatment

- Although not a definitive airway, a supraglottic airway may be used when a patient has significant facial trauma or is difficult to intubate or ventilate; these devices are contraindicated in awake patients and

those in whom the mouth cannot be opened to insert the device.
- Avoid nasal airway if maxillofacial fracture or basilar skull fracture are suspected.
- Suction the airway of blood and vomitus, and remove foreign bodies and dentures before laryngoscopy.
- Video laryngoscopy with rapid sequence intubation is the recommended first-line approach to minimize c-spine motion and provide superior laryngeal views.
- Provide in-line stabilization by a second provider during endotracheal intubation.
- A cricothyrotomy or other surgical airway may be necessary if endotracheal intubation fails or there is significant facial trauma or airway obstruction.
- Use capnography, auscultation, and postintubation chest radiograph to confirm tube placement.

BREATHING

Clinical Presentation

- Awake patients may complain of difficulty breathing.
- The mechanisms of injury, such as penetrating chest trauma or blunt force trauma to the chest, may signal impending respiratory failure.
- Presentation may include deviated trachea, flail chest, sucking chest wounds, asymmetric breath sounds, chest wall crepitus, etc.
- If patient is adequately ventilating and oxygenating, then proceed to "C" (circulation).

Diagnosis and Evaluation

- Ventilation
  - Assess mental status, chest wall rise, and respiratory rate, and check end-tidal CO_2 or blood gas.
  - If poor ventilation identified, consider naloxone and check glucose.
  - If persistent altered mental status, consider computed tomography (CT) of the head, send toxicology workup, and have a second provider obtain collateral history for exposure to toxins and identify comorbidities.
  - Intubate if unable to identify or reverse the cause of hypoventilation and the patient is retaining significant CO_2 and is obtunded.
- Oxygenation
  - If there is respiratory distress or hypoxia, consider flail chest, pulmonary contusion, pneumothorax, or massive hemothorax.
  - If there are unequal breath sounds, and you identify pneumothorax, hemothorax, or hemopneumothorax, perform a tube thoracostomy.

Use the Extended Focused Assessment with Sonography for Trauma (eFAST) to assess for pneumothorax and hemothorax; presence of B lines may be a sign of lung contusion.

Treatment

- For suspected tension pneumothorax, perform needle decompression with 14-gauge needle at the fourth or fifth intercostal space along the mid- or anterior axillary line, and follow this with the placement of a chest tube at the fourth or fifth intercostal space along the mid- or anterior axillary line.
- If you detect asymmetric breath sounds or unilateral lung sliding (generally on the right) immediately after intubation, the endotracheal tube may be positioned in the mainstem bronchus; measure depth on chest radiograph and reposition tube above the carina.
- Treat toxidromes appropriately when present.

CIRCULATION

Clinical Presentation

- Assess the patient's level of consciousness, skin perfusion, blood pressure, heart rate, pulse pressure, and quality of pulse.
- If the patient has good peripheral pulses, normal mental status, and adequate peripheral perfusion without obvious signs of shock, then proceed to "D" (disability).
- Signs of shock include pallor, tachycardia, hypotension, altered mental status, and rapid and thready pulse.
- Do not transport unstable patients to the CT scanner.

Diagnosis and Evaluation

- In penetrating trauma, use eFAST to assess for pneumothorax, free fluid in the abdomen, and cardiac tamponade.
- The FAST examination has a high specificity, but poor sensitivity for identifying clinically important hemorrhage.
- Serial FAST examinations should be performed if initial FAST is negative in an unstable patient.
- Look for hemorrhage before considering other causes of shock (e.g., neurogenic).
- For hemorrhagic shock, locate the source of hemorrhage using physical examination, radiographs, eFAST, and CT imaging.
- For nonhemorrhagic shock, consider tension pneumothorax, cardiac tamponade, cardiogenic shock, neurogenic shock, septic shock, or hypovolemic shock not due to blood loss.

Treatment

- Identify the culprit source of hemorrhage (Table 135.2) and if possible, obtain control (direct pressure, tourniquet, ligation, interventional radiology for embolization, etc.).
- Establish a minimum of two large-bore IVs (16 gauge or larger); consider central venous or intraosseous access if peripheral IVs cannot be obtained quickly.
- If hemorrhagic or unclear source of shock, transfuse blood products as soon as possible.

While awaiting blood products, permissive hypotension can be considered. No more than 1 liter of balanced crystalloid solution is recommended. More fluid may contribute to dilutional coagulopathy and hypothermia. Balanced crystalloid over normal saline is recommended to avoid non-anion gap metabolic acidosis and renal insufficiency.

- There is no advantage of giving colloids over crystalloid.
- If further resuscitation is required, consider 2:1:1 or 1:1:1 infusion of packed red blood cells (pRBCs) to plasma to platelets.
- Massive transfusion protocol can be initiated when a patient is suspected to require more than 10 U of pRBCs in the first 24 hours of admission OR more than 4 U of pRBCs in 1 hour. Massive transfusion protocol should follow the 2:1:1 or 1:1:1 ratio discussed above.

TABLE 135.2 *Identifying and Controlling Hemorrhage in the Multiple-Trauma Patient*

Hemorrhage Location	Assessment and Management
Superficial hemorrhage	Physical examination, auscultate for bruits or thrills Apply direct pressure Tourniquet if direct pressure not adequate or there is massive exsanguination
Thoracoabdominal hemorrhage Pericardial tamponade Pneumothorax Free fluid in abdomen	Utilize physical examination, eFAST, XR, CT scan If stable, take to operating room for pericardial window. If pulseless, perform thoracotomy for pericardiotomy. Pericardiocentesis can be considered but is generally ineffective in traumatic tamponade. Needle decompression followed by tube thoracostomy Emergent surgical consultation
Retroperitoneal hemorrhage	Uncommon to identify on eFAST, will likely need CT scan Suspect kidney or aortic injury Will likely need operative or IR intervention for embolization
Pelvic hemorrhage	Pelvic XR and CT scan Assess for hematuria and pelvic instability Pelvic binder IR intervention for embolization
Long-bone fractures	Reduce and splint and check neurovascular exam post-reduction Mindful of femur fractures as compartment can tolerate up to 1.5 L of blood Continue to monitor for compartment syndrome, especially in forearm and lower leg injuries

CT, computed tomography; *eFAST*, Extended Focused Assessment with Sonography for Trauma; *IR*, interventional radiology; *XR*, radiograph.

- If the patient is male or a female not of childbearing age, and requires emergent blood transfusion before type and screen, O-positive blood should be administered.
- For women who might be of childbearing age, administer O-negative blood to prevent formation of anti-RhD antibodies.
- Consider tranexamic acid as a 1-g bolus over 10 minutes, ideally administer within 1 hour of injury (although beneficial within 3 hours); then infuse 1 g over 8 hours if hemorrhage is not controlled.
- Consider permissive hypotension, with a mean arterial pressure (MAP) goal of 50 mm Hg, unless there is concern for traumatic brain or spinal cord injury, for which the MAP goal is 80–85 mm Hg.
- Ensure adequate tissue perfusion, identified by mental status, vital signs, physical examination, urine output, lactate level, and base excess.
- Avoid hypothermia; use fluid warmers for infusions and external warming measures.
- Reverse known coagulopathies; for example, if there is a history of warfarin use, administer 4-factor prothrombin complex concentrate and vitamin K.
- Give platelets if thrombocytopenic.
- If indicated, consider administration of the reversal agents for direct thrombin (for dabigatran, give idarucizumab) and factor Xa inhibitors (andexanet alfa).
- Four-factor prothrombin complex concentrate can be used for factor Xa inhibitors if the reversal agent is unavailable.
- Dialysis should be considered in patients taking direct thrombin inhibitors with severe hemorrhage if a reversal agent is unavailable.
- Consider emergency department thoracotomy in patients with penetrating trauma if any signs of life are present in the field or in the emergency department, such as presence of carotid pulse, measurable or palpable blood pressure, spontaneous respiration, extremity movement, pupillary reflex, or cardiac electrical activity who have cardiac arrest during transport or in the emergency department.
- Consider resuscitative endovascular occlusion of the aorta if readily available and indicated (i.e., pelvic hemorrhage).

DISABILITY

Clinical Presentation

- Assess the patient's level of consciousness and evaluate for neurologic deficits.
- The Glasgow Coma Scale (GCS) is a 15-point scale that determines the patient's level of consciousness (see Box 135.2).
- GCS score of 15 does not exclude the possibility of a traumatic brain injury.
- The GCS motor component best correlates with patient outcomes.

BOX 135.2 *Glasgow Coma Scale*

Eye opening

Spontaneous: 4 points
To voice: 3 points
To pain: 2 points
None: 1 point

Verbal response

Oriented: 5 points
Confused/disoriented: 4 points
Inappropriate words: 3 points
Incomprehensible sounds: 2 points
None: 1 point

Motor response

Follows commands: 6 points
Localizes pain: 5 points
Withdraws from pain: 4 points
Flexion posturing: 3 points
Extension posturing: 2 points
None: 1 point

BOX 135.3 *Traumatic and Nontraumatic Causes of Altered Mental Status*

Traumatic

Epidural hematoma, subdural hematoma, subarachnoid hemorrhage, cerebral contusion
Diffuse axonal injury
Poor cerebral perfusion secondary to shock

Nontraumatic

Intoxication
Hypoglycemia
Electrolyte disturbances
Mental health conditions
Previous stroke or intracranial injury

Diagnosis and Evaluation

- Altered mental status can occur from traumatic or nontraumatic causes (see Box 135.3).
- If there is a decrease in GCS score, always assume there is a central nervous system injury until proven otherwise.
- Perform pupillary examination and brief motor examination of extremities as part of disability assessment.
- Perform appropriate CTs, generally noncontrast head and c-spine.

Treatment

- If GCS score is <8, consider intubation to protect airway.
- Reverse any obvious cause of altered mental status, e.g., dextrose for hypoglycemia, volume resuscitation for hypoperfusion, and oxygen for hypoxia.
- Consult a neurosurgeon when a brain or spinal cord injury is identified.
- If elevated intracranial pressure suspected, elevate the head of the bed, infuse mannitol or hypertonic saline, and hyperventilate (PCO_2 goal 35 mm Hg).

EXPOSURE AND ENVIRONMENTAL CONTROL

Clinical Presentation

- Completely disrobe patient to assess all anatomic areas for injury.
- Hypothermia can be present on arrival or quickly develop in the emergency department and is a preventable, potentially lethal complication.

Diagnosis and Evaluation

- Look for signs of penetrating trauma, burns, ecchymosis (Grey Turner sign, Cullen sign), foreign bodies (do not remove until sure it is not penetrating a vessel), open fractures, etc.
- To assess for spinal injury, logroll patients with c-spine stabilization and check the back. Also check axilla, groin, and buttocks because injuries in these areas can be easily missed.
- All patients should be removed from long backboards to prevent decubitus ulcers and aspiration pneumonia.
- Continually monitor patient's temperature.

Treatment

- Place blankets or external warming devices to prevent hypothermia.
- Use warmed crystalloid fluids and blood products if warming transfuser available (can microwave crystalloid fluids but not blood products).
- Decontaminate patient if exposed to toxic chemicals.
- Order diagnostic tests as appropriate for identified injuries.

Secondary Survey

- After the primary survey, the clinician can obtain pertinent medical history and perform a more detailed and complete physical examination to find injuries not observed on the primary survey (Table 135.3).

TABLE 135.3 *Secondary Survey of Trauma Patients*

Region or System	Assessment or Examination	Critical Diagnoses	Emergent Diagnoses
General	Level of consciousness	GCS ≤8	
	GCS score	Focal motor deficit	
	Specific complaints		
Head	Pupils (size, shape, reactivity, visual fields)	Herniation syndrome	Globe rupture
	Contusions		
	Lacerations		
	Evidence of skull fracture (hemotympanum, Battle sign, raccoon eyes, palpable defects)		Open skull fracture Cerebrospinal fluid leak
Face	Contusions		
	Lacerations		
	Midface instability	Airway obstruction due to bleeding	Facial fractures
	Malocclusion		Mandible fracture

TABLE 135.3 *Secondary Survey of Trauma Patients—cont'd*

Region or System	Assessment or Examination	Critical Diagnoses	Emergent Diagnoses
Neck (maintain cervical immobilization)	Penetrating injury, lacerations		
	Tracheal deviation	Carotid injury	
	Jugular venous distention	Pericardial tamponade	
	Subcutaneous emphysema	Tracheal, laryngeal fracture	
	Hematoma	Vascular injury	
	Midline cervical tenderness	Cervical fracture, dislocation	
Chest	Respiratory effort, excursion	Impending respiratory failure	
	Contusions		Cardiopulmonary injury
	Lacerations		Intrathoracic injury
	Focal tenderness, crepitus		Rib fractures
	Subcutaneous emphysema	Flail chest	Pneumothorax
	Heart tones (muffled)	Cardiac tamponade	
	Breath sounds (symmetric)	Tension pneumothorax	Pneumothorax Hemothorax
Abdomen, flank	Contusions		Solid, hollow viscous injury
	Penetrating injury, lacerations	Intraabdominal hemorrhage	Solid, hollow viscous injury
	Tenderness	Intraabdominal hemorrhage	Solid, hollow viscous injury
	Peritoneal signs	Abdominal catastrophe	
Pelvis, genitourinary	Contusions	Pelvic hemorrhage	
	Lacerations		Urogenital injury
	Stability, symphyseal tenderness	Unstable pelvic fracture Pelvic hemorrhage	
	Blood (urethral meatus, vaginal bleeding, hematuria)	Unstable pelvic fracture	Urethral injury
	Rectal examination	Colorectal injury (bleeding)	Urethral injury (high-riding prostate)
Neurologic, spinal cord	Midline bony spinal tenderness	Spinal fracture, dislocation	
	Mental status	Epidural hematoma Subdural hematoma	Cerebral contusions Shear injury
	Paresthesias		Spinal cord injury, contusion Nerve root injury
	Sensory level	Spinal fracture, dislocation	
	Motor function, including sphincter tone	Spinal fracture, dislocation	
Extremities	Contusions	Compartment syndrome	Rhabdomyolysis
	Lacerations	Vascular injury	
	Deformity	Neurovascular injury	Fracture
	Focal tenderness		Fracture
	Pulses	Arterial injury	
	Capillary refill	Hemorrhagic shock Arterial injury	
	Evaluation of compartments	Compartment syndrome	

GCS, Glasgow Coma Scale.
From Wolfson, A. B. (2018). Multiple trauma. In R. M. Walls, R. S. Hockberger, & M. Gausche-Hill (Eds.), *Rosen's emergency medicine: Concepts and clinical practice* (9th ed., p. 294, Table 33.2). Elsevier.

- Roll the patient to assess for spinal tenderness, injuries, step-offs, and rectal tone if indicated.
- Providers can refer to the AMPLE mnemonic, as depicted in Box 135.4, to obtain history.
- Continually reassess the components of the primary survey.

Laboratory and Radiographic Evaluation

Laboratory Evaluation

- Clinical assessment and presentation should guide which diagnostic tests to order (Table 135.4).

BOX 135.4 AMPLE in the Secondary Survey

Allergies
Medications
Past medical history and pregnancy
Last meal
Events and environment surrounding the trauma

TABLE 135.4 Laboratory Testing in the Multiple-Trauma Patient

Laboratory Test	Clinical Importance
Complete blood cell count	Hemoglobin and hematocrit (but note that value may be falsely reassuring, due to time necessary to equilibrate following acute blood loss) Thrombocytopenia
Electrolyte panel	Potassium in CKD, often elevated in crush injuries Sodium in head injury or altered mental status
Liver function tests and lipase	Determine blunt injury to these organs, underlying liver disease, or shock liver in setting of hypoperfusion
PT/INR and PTT	Determine developing or underlying coagulopathies Provide clues to anticoagulation use and need for reversal such as INR and warfarin
Pregnancy test in women	May change medication management May need to consult OB/GYN
Blood type and screen or type and cross depending on injury severity	Prevent transfusion reactions Prevent anti-RhD antibody formation in women of childbearing age
Urine studies	Gross hematuria or microscopic hematuria > 20–50 RBC in urine suggests urinary tract injury Toxicology screen may identify cause of AMS
Lactate, arterial blood gas, base excess, anion gap	Assess tissue perfusion and help guide fluid resuscitation Assess pH
Troponin	Myocardial damage if concern for cardiac contusion

AMS, altered mental status; *CKD*, chronic kidney disease; *INR*, international normalized ratio; *OB/GYN*, obstetrics/gynecology; *PT*, prothrombin time; *PTT*, partial thromboplastin time.

- Laboratory testing can provide a baseline assessment of metabolic derangements to guide resuscitation (e.g., base deficit and lactate).

Radiographic Evaluation

- Radiographic evaluation of the multiple-trauma patient is crucial in identifying acute injuries that may not be elucidated on physical examination.
- eFAST should be performed as part of the primary survey (Box 135.5) to help identify source of blood loss and etiology of hypotension in the trauma patient.
- eFAST is not appropriate (sensitivity is low) to assess for retroperitoneal fluid.
- During the secondary survey, inferior vena cava ultrasonography can help assessment of volume status.

BOX 135.5 Extended Focused Assessment with Sonography for Trauma

Right upper quadrant view
Free fluid in hepatorenal fossa (Morrison pouch) or between diaphragm and liver

Suprapubic view
Free fluid in pelvis

Left upper quadrant view
Free fluid between the splenorenal fossa or between the spleen and diaphragm

Subxiphoid view
Pericardial effusion and/or tamponade
General function/squeeze of left ventricle

Lung views
Pneumothorax
Pleural effusion/hemothorax (Check each lung base when performing right and left upper quadrant views)

BOX 135.6 National Emergency X-Radiography Utilization Study (NEXUS) Criteria

Focal neurologic deficit
Posterior midline cervical spine tenderness
Altered mental status
Intoxication
Distracting injury

- Chest and pelvic radiographs are standard examinations for multiple-trauma patients.
- Although operator-dependent, ultrasonography is superior to chest radiograph to screen for hemothorax, pneumothorax, and cardiac tamponade.
- Perform CT scans based on clinical judgment after completion of the primary survey.
- If c-spine injury is suspected, apply decision rules such as National Emergency X-Radiography Utilization Study (NEXUS) criteria (Box 135.6) or Canadian C-spine Rule to help determine whether CT of the c-spine is indicated.

Disposition

- Decide whether to observe in the emergency department, admit to inpatient, transfer to a tertiary care facility with resources that the current facility does not have, or redline to the operating room.
- Continually reassess all multiple-trauma patients because their disposition and clinical status can change rapidly.

SUGGESTED READINGS

Cameron, P., & Knapp, B. (2016). Trauma in adults. In J. E. Tintinalli, J. S. Stapczynski, O. J. Ma, D. M. Yealy, G. D. Meckler, & D. M. Cline (Eds.), *Tintinalli's emergency medicine: A comprehensive study guide* (8th ed., Kindle locations 80405–80406). McGraw-Hill Education.
Gross Eric, A., & Martel, M. L. (2018). Multiple trauma. In R. M. Walls, R. S. Hockberger, & M. Gausche-Hill (Eds.), *Rosen's emergency medicine: Concepts and clinical practice* (9th ed., pp. 287–300). Elsevier.
Henry, S. (2018). *ATLS advanced trauma life support student course manual* (10th ed.). American College of Surgeons.

CHAPTER 136

BOARD REVIEW

Abdominal Trauma

PUNEET GUPTA, MD, and DENISE WHITFIELD, MD, MBA

Abdominal trauma is a leading cause of mortality and morbidity, accounting for 15%–20% of all trauma-related deaths. Identification of serious intraabdominal injury may be difficult, because clinical signs and symptoms may not be present on initial assessment. The peritoneal cavity can accommodate a trauma patient's entire circulating blood volume. Therefore, recognition of life-threatening hemorrhage with prompt resuscitation and surgical management is paramount.

General Principles

- Abdominal trauma is classified as blunt or penetrating.

Blunt Abdominal Trauma

- Greater risk of mortality compared with penetrating abdominal trauma.
- All abdominal structures are at risk (abdominal wall, solid organs, hollow viscus).
- Motor vehicle collisions are the most common mechanism of injury.
- Spleen is the most commonly injured solid organ in blunt trauma, followed by the liver.

Penetrating Abdominal Trauma

- Gunshot and stab wounds are most common, but any foreign body violating the abdominal wall can result in penetrating trauma.
- Liver is the most commonly injured organ in stab wounds.
- The extent of injury can be difficult to determine based on physical examination.
- Any penetrating injury from the lower chest to the pelvis should be assumed to have penetrated the abdominal cavity until proven otherwise.

Clinical Presentation

- Clinical presentations in abdominal trauma are often clouded by factors that can affect initial examination.
- Distracting injuries or altered mental status owing to head injury, hypoperfusion, or intoxication can confound the clinical presentation.
- Patients may have normal initial examination findings that degrade over time.
- The mechanism of injury and associated factors related to the injury must be considered.

Clinical Features

- May include:
  - Visible trauma (abrasions, lacerations, ecchymoses, hematomas, penetrating wounds, and evisceration)
  - Abdominal tenderness, rigidity, or distension
  - Gastrointestinal hemorrhage
  - Hemodynamic instability: an elevated shock index (heart rate ÷ systolic blood pressure, normal range 0.5 to 0.7) suggests hypovolemic shock before overt vital sign abnormalities manifest.

Diagnosis and Evaluation

General Approach to Abdominal Trauma

- Clinical assessment
  - A complete trauma survey should be performed with abdominal examination as part of the secondary survey.
  - Clinical assessment integrating physical examination, local wound exploration, ultrasonography, and computed tomography (CT) imaging, as appropriate, will determine the need for surgical intervention.
- Physical examination
  - Inspection should be followed by palpation of the abdomen.
  - Abrasions, contusions, ecchymosis, or penetrating wounds may be visible.
  - Patients with equivocal trauma workups, but high clinical suspicion for intraperitoneal injury, warrant serial examinations.
- Diagnostic tests
  - Diagnostic peritoneal lavage (DPL)
    - Not commonly used, given advances in ultrasound technology.
    - Historically, aspiration was undertaken, followed by 1 L normal saline instilled into the peritoneum via catheter.
    - More than 10 mL gross blood or enteric contents on initial aspiration, or more than 100,000 red blood cells (RBC)/mm^3 (blunt trauma) or more than 15,000 to 25,000 RBC/mm^3 (penetrating trauma) in aspirate suggests intraperitoneal hemorrhage.
    - Clinical decision-making based on DPL results alone is no longer indicated.
  - Focused Assessment with Sonography for Trauma (FAST) examination (Fig. 136.1)
    - FAST examination is frequently done in traumatically injured patients. The main indication for use is in hypotensive patients with blunt abdominal injury to elucidate if the etiology of the hypotension is caused by intraperitoneal hemorrhage. It is also used in penetrating injury to the chest to rule out pericardial tamponade.
    - Allows rapid identification of intraperitoneal fluid by examination of dependent portions of the intraperitoneal cavity (Morrison pouch, the splenorenal recess, and the pelvis).

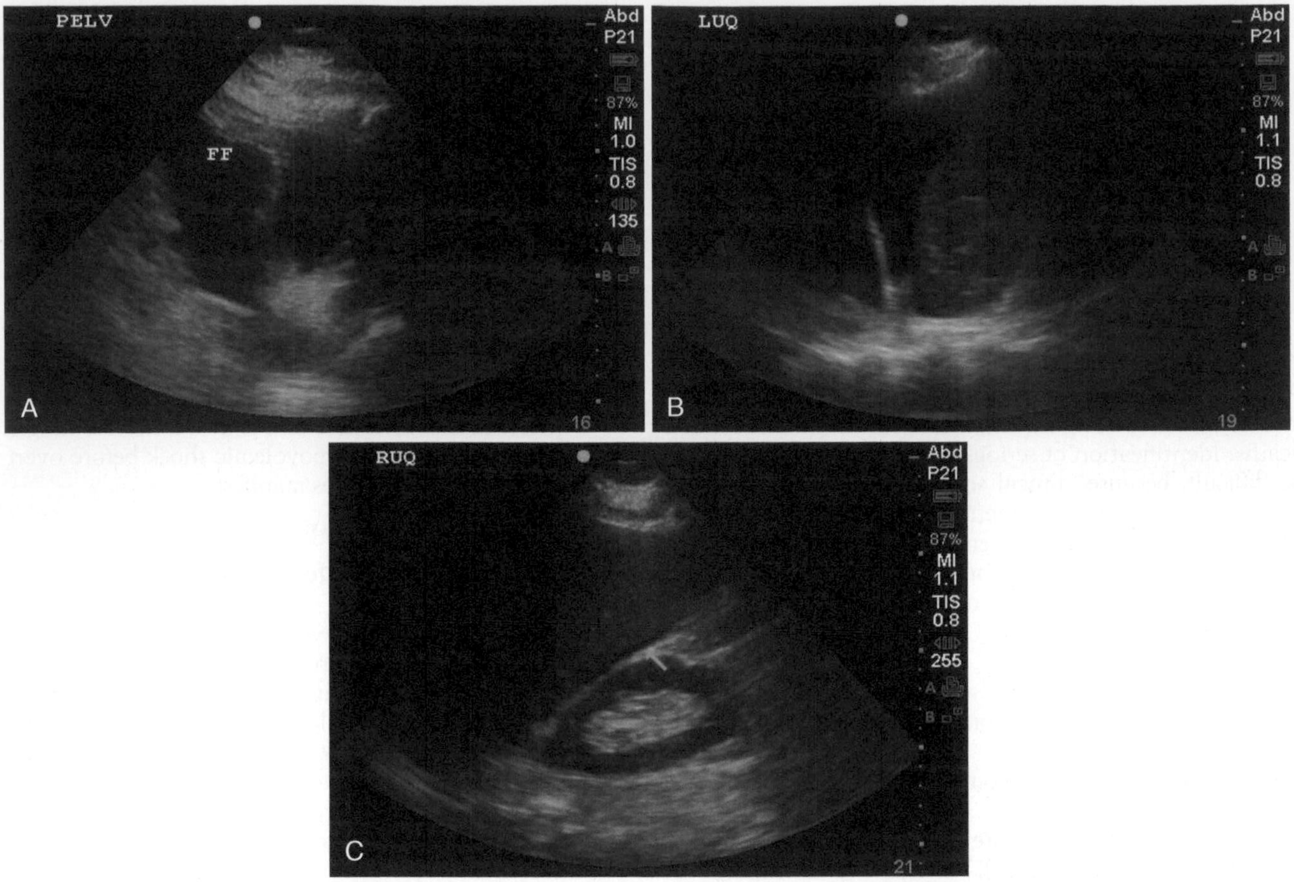

FIG. 136.1 Positive FAST examination. **A**, Free fluid in the pelvis. **B**, Free fluid in the perisplenic space. **C**, Free fluid in Morison pouch. (From Yiju Teresa Liu, MD, RDMS.)

    - Can detect 200 mL or more of intraperitoneal fluid.
    - Extended FAST (eFAST) includes an evaluation for lung sliding to rule out a pneumothorax.
- CT scan
    - CT of the abdomen/pelvis with intravenous contrast is the primary diagnostic imaging test to evaluate abdominal traumatic injury.
    - Hemodynamically stable patients with clinical assessments concerning for abdominal injury should undergo CT imaging.

Treatment

- Treatment and management of abdominal trauma is determined by clinical assessment, including clinical presentation, physical examination, and radiologic imaging (Figs. 136.2–136.4).
- Immediate resuscitation with blood products is indicated for hemodynamically unstable patients.
- Laparotomy is indicated for ongoing hemodynamic instability, peritoneal signs, and specific injuries requiring surgical evaluation and management (Box 136.1). Angioembolization can be considered for splenic injuries and pelvic fracture-related hemorrhage.
- Temporary aortic occlusion by resuscitative endovascular balloon occlusion of the aorta is utilized at select trauma centers for patients with blunt or penetrating injuries below the diaphragm who respond poorly to initial resuscitation.

Specific Abdominal Injuries

ABDOMINAL WALL INJURIES

- Contusions to the abdominal wall usually result from direct force.
- Abdominal wall hematomas may mimic intraabdominal injury, presenting as pain or a palpable mass.
- CT scans are reasonable for patients with abdominal wall injury to evaluate for concomitant intraperitoneal injury.
- Expectant management is appropriate if workup is otherwise negative.

DIAPHRAGMATIC INJURIES

- Diaphragmatic rupture may result from penetrating or blunt injury.
- Diaphragmatic rupture is uncommon and usually left-sided.
- Failure to diagnose and treat may result in herniation and strangulation of the abdominal contents.
- Identification can be made on CT scan, but may not be evident on initial imaging.
- Surgical management is indicated.

SOLID ORGAN INJURIES

- The liver and spleen are the most commonly injured solid intraperitoneal structures in abdominal trauma.

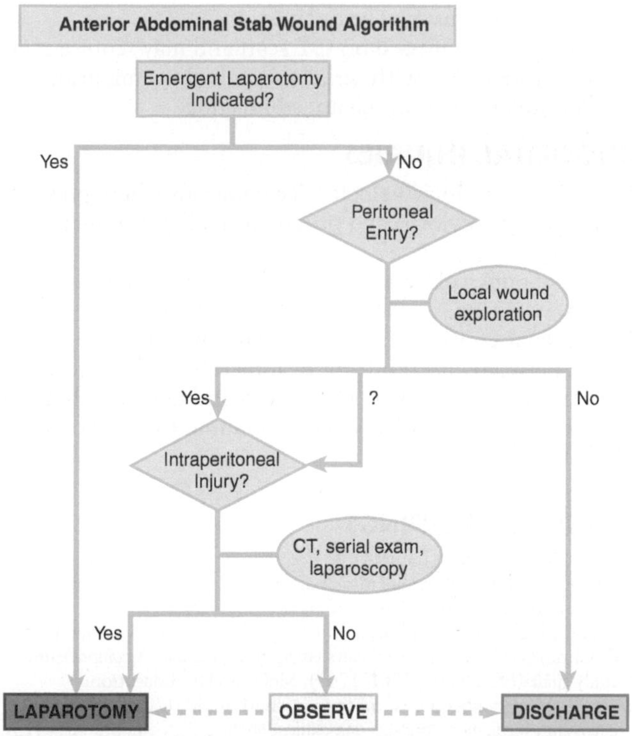

FIG. 136.2 Algorithm for evaluation of anterior abdominal stab wounds. (Adapted from Nichols, J. R., & Puskarich, M. A. (2018). Abdominal trauma. In R. M. Walls, R. S. Hockberger, & M. Gausche-Hill (Eds.), *Rosen's emergency medicine: Concepts and clinical practice* (9th ed., pp. 404–418, Fig. 39.6). Elsevier.)

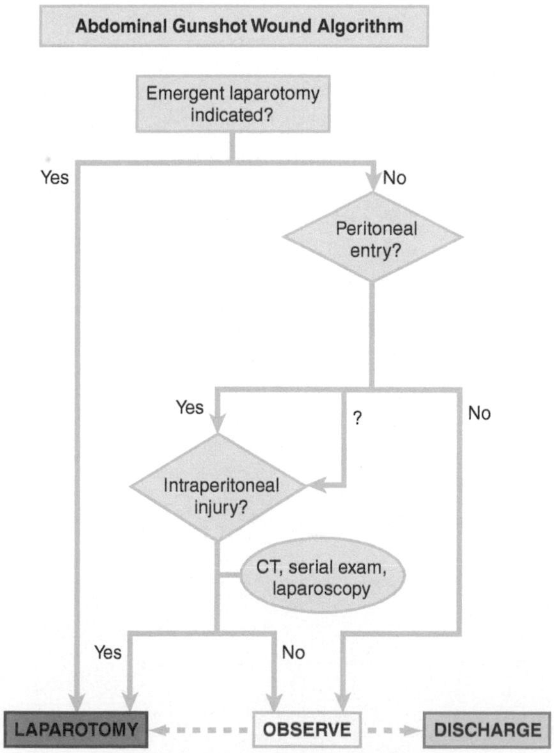

FIG. 136.3 Algorithm for evaluation of abdominal gunshot wounds. (Adapted from Nichols, J. R., & Puskarich, M. A. (2018). Abdominal trauma. In R. M. Walls, R. S. Hockberger, & M. Gausche-Hill (Eds.), *Rosen's emergency medicine: Concepts and clinical practice* (9th ed., pp. 404–418, Fig. 39.7). Elsevier.)

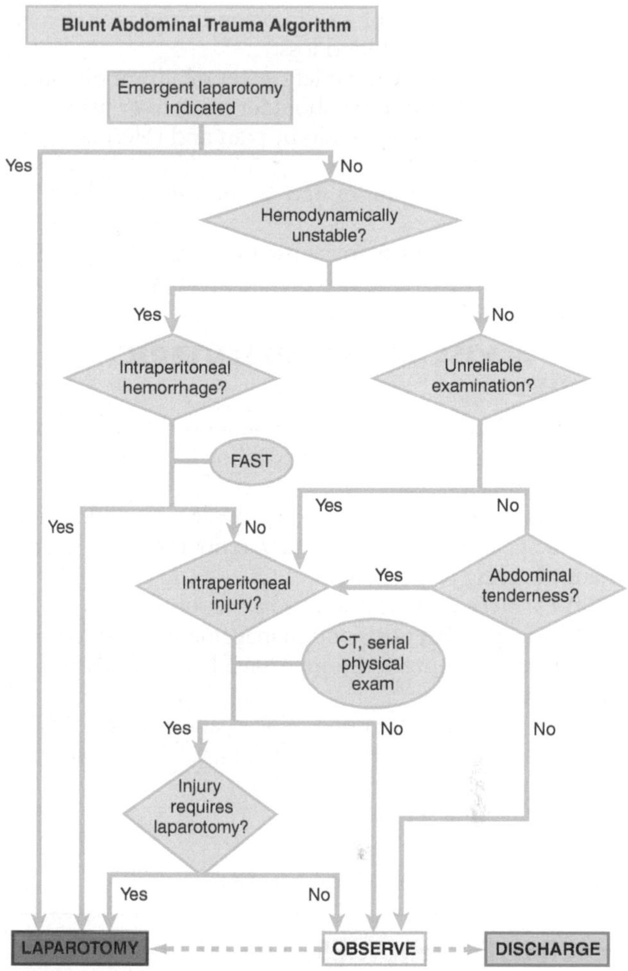

FIG. 136.4 Algorithm for evaluation of blunt abdominal trauma. (Adapted from Nichols, J. R., & Puskarich, M. A. (2018). Abdominal trauma. In R. M. Walls, R. S. Hockberger, & M. Gausche-Hill (Eds.), *Rosen's emergency medicine: Concepts and clinical practice* (9th ed., pp. 404–418, Fig. 39.8). Elsevier.)

BOX 136.1 *Indications for Laparotomy After Trauma*

Penetrating Trauma

Emergent Laparotomy Indicated

Hemodynamic instability
Peritoneal signs
Evisceration
Diaphragmatic injury

Laparotomy Requires Additional Clinical Evidence

Gastrointestinal hemorrhage
Intraperitoneal air

Blunt Trauma

Laparotomy Indicated

Hemodynamic instability with strongly suspected abdominal injury
Unequivocal peritoneal irritation
Intraperitoneal air
Diaphragmatic injury
Significant gastrointestinal bleeding

(From Nichols, J. R., & Puskarich, M. A. (2018). Abdominal trauma. In R. M. Walls, R. S. Hockberger, & M. Gausche-Hill (Eds.), *Rosen's emergency medicine: Concepts and clinical practice* (9th ed., pp. 404–418, Tables 39.2 and 39.3). Elsevier.)

- Signs and symptoms of a solid organ injury include pain and clinical signs of blood loss.
- Splenic injuries may have left upper quadrant abdominal pain and referred left shoulder pain; liver injuries may have right upper quadrant pain and referred right shoulder pain.
- Liver and splenic injuries may be identified on FAST or CT scan.
- Whether expectant management or surgical management is indicated, depends on the severity of injury and the patient's clinical status.

HOLLOW VISCUS AND MESENTERIC INJURIES

- Hollow viscus injury in blunt trauma is the third most common intraperitoneal injury following liver and splenic injuries.
- Symptoms usually present from ongoing blood loss and/or leakage of gastrointestinal contents into the peritoneum leading to peritonitis.
- Clinical signs and symptoms may be subtle.
- Delays in the diagnosis and management of hollow viscus and mesenteric injuries have been shown to increase mortality.
- Injuries may be missed on CT scan and require high clinical suspicion with serial abdominal examination or advanced imaging.
- Management is surgical.

Retroperitoneal Injuries

PANCREATIC INJURIES

- Most common mechanism is rapid deceleration with blunt force to the epigastrium (bicycle handlebars, steering wheel injuries).
- Initial symptoms may be delayed.
- Injuries can be missed on CT scan and may require high clinical suspicion with serial abdominal examination, laboratory studies, or advanced imaging.

DUODENAL INJURIES

- Occur during high-velocity decelerations where pressure between the pylorus and proximal small bowel increases rapidly.
- Gastric outlet obstruction may develop, presenting as pain, vomiting, and abdominal distension.
- Duodenal contents can extravasate into the retroperitoneum, resulting in infection and peritonitis.
- Injuries can be missed on CT scan and may require high clinical suspicion with serial abdominal examination or advanced imaging.

SUGGESTED READINGS

Brenner, M., & Hicks, C. (2018). Major abdominal trauma: Critical decisions and new frontiers in management. *Emergency Medicine Clinics of North America, 36*(1), 149–160.

Tintinalli, J. E., Stapczynski, J. S., Ma, O. J., Yealy, D. M., Meckler, G. D., & Cline, D. M. (2016). *Tintinalli's emergency medicine: A comprehensive study guide* (8th ed., pp. 1761–1765). McGraw-Hill Education.

Walls, R. M., Hockberger, R. S., & Gausche-Hill, M. (2018). *Rosen's emergency medicine: Concepts and clinical practice* (9th ed., pp. 404–418). Elsevier.

Chest Trauma

LAUREN FRYLING, MD, and KATIE REBILLOT, DO

General Principles

- Chest trauma accounts for 10%–15% of all trauma patients coming to the emergency department, and 20% of trauma deaths. Rapid interventions, such as tube thoracostomy, can be life-saving in thoracic trauma and the majority of these critical interventions are done in the emergency department.
- In recent years, there has been a surge in use of computed tomography (CT) scans and ultrasound to diagnose chest trauma. To minimize unnecessary CT use, the National Emergency X-Radiology Utilization Study (NEXUS) group derived a decision instrument to guide the use of CT imaging in blunt chest trauma (Box 137.1).

Chest Wall Trauma

RIB FRACTURES

General Principles

- Rib fractures predispose patients to pneumonia. Musculoskeletal pain from fractures leads to chest wall splinting, which results in lower tidal volumes, stagnant air, and atelectasis. Those at highest risk include older individuals, patients with chronic obstructive pulmonary disease, and those with multiple rib fractures.
  - Flail chest is a fracture of three or more adjacent ribs in at least two places.
  - First rib fracture, without signs of hemodynamic instability, neurologic deficit, examination findings concerning for fracture displacement, or initial chest x-ray abnormalities, are not associated with an increased risk for major neurovascular injury and do not necessitate immediate angiography.

BOX 137.1 *NEXUS Chest Decision Instrument: (Chest CT-All)*

If criteria 1 to 7 are not present, the patient is unlikely to have any major or minor chest trauma.

1. Abnormal chest x-ray (any thoracic injury or wide mediastinum)
2. Distracting injury (using the same criteria as Nexus C-spine)
3. Chest wall tenderness (excluding isolated clavicle tenderness)
4. Sternal tenderness
5. Thoracic spine tenderness
6. Scapular tenderness
7. Mechanism of blunt trauma that exerts rapid deceleration force on the patient:
   A. Fall from a height more than 20 feet, or
   B. Motor vehicle accident at speeds greater than 40 mph with sudden deceleration

(From Rodriguez, R. M., Langdorf, M. I., Nishijima, D., Baumann, B. M., Hendey, G. W., Medak, A. J., Raja, A. S., Allen, I. E., & Mower, W. R. (2015). Derivation and validation of two decision instruments for selective chest CT in blunt trauma: A multicenter prospective observational study (NEXUS chest CT). *PLoS Medicine, 12*(10), e1001883.)

Clinical Presentation

- Rib fracture: chest wall tenderness, bony crepitus, ecchymosis.
- Flail chest: paradoxical motion of the chest wall during respiration with complaints of severe pain, crepitus, and hypoxia, often associated with an underlying pulmonary contusion.

Diagnosis and Evaluation

- Chest x-ray: initial screening tool for rib fractures, but can miss up to 50% of fractures.
- CT scan: more sensitive than plain films for identifying rib fractures, but is not routinely indicated for an isolated rib fracture. CT scan is indicated when there is suspicion of multiple rib fractures or to identify associated injuries, such as pulmonary contusions, pneumothorax, and hemothorax.

Treatment

- Treatment should be aimed at adequate analgesia and preservation of pulmonary function. Most rib fractures heal spontaneously within 3 to 6 weeks. Patients with multiple rib fractures, underlying pulmonary disease such as chronic obstructive pulmonary disease and congestive heart failure, and elderly patients have increased mortality rates and there should be a low threshold for admission and monitoring. Treatment should include the following:
  - Pain control with opioids, nonsteroidal antiinflammatory drugs, and acetaminophen, as well as intercostal nerve blocks, patient-controlled analgesia, and thoracic epidurals
  - Incentive spirometry and breathing exercises
  - Flail chest typically requires more aggressive treatment. Most patients with this diagnosis require intubation owing to chest wall instability and associated pulmonary contusions. A trial of noninvasive, positive-pressure ventilation and aggressive pain management may

be attempted prior to intubation. Surgical fixation is occasionally done for patients with significant chest wall instability, but not in the acute period.

STERNAL FRACTURE

General Principles

- Sternal fractures are frequently a result of motor vehicle collisions when the steering wheel impacts the sternum at high speeds. It can also be seen in restrained passengers owing to the force of the upper seatbelt. This risk is increased if airbags do not deploy.

Clinical Presentation

- Pain over the sternum, ecchymosis, point tenderness, crepitus.

Diagnosis and Evaluation

- Chest x-ray: misses between 50% and 94% of sternal fractures.
- CT scan: more sensitive than x-ray for diagnosing sternal fractures and associated injuries, such as retrosternal hematomas.

Treatment

- Stable patients with isolated sternal fractures can be treated with pain control and outpatient follow-up. Operative fixation is typically reserved for more severe sternal fractures.

Pulmonary Injuries

PNEUMOTHORAX

General Principles

- Simple pneumothorax: air in the pleural space.
- Occult pneumothorax: pneumothorax seen on CT scan, but not on chest x-ray.
- Tension pneumothorax: when air continues to fill the pleural cavity without an exit pathway, the pressure in the cavity builds, which puts pressure on the vena cava and contralateral lung leading to obstructive shock.
- Open pneumothorax: also called a sucking chest wound, this injury is a large defect in the chest wall causing sucking of air into the pleural cavity. Without intervention, it can quickly decompensate into a tension pneumothorax if there is a flap that allows air in but not out.

Clinical Presentation

- Simple pneumothorax: chest pain, hypoxia, tachycardia, dyspnea, subcutaneous emphysema, absent breath sounds.
- Tension pneumothorax: simple pneumothorax findings plus elevated jugular venous pressure, respiratory failure, tracheal deviation, hypoxia, and eventually cardiac arrest.

Diagnosis and Evaluation

- Tension pneumothorax should always be a clinical diagnosis.
- X-ray: supine chest x-ray is the least sensitive modality for diagnosing pneumothorax and may be visualized as a deep sulcus sign. Sensitivity is increased in the upright position when gas accumulates in the apices.
- Ultrasound: provides immediate diagnostic information for prompt intervention. The linear probe is used to look for lung sliding, which indicates a normal interface between the lung and pleura. Lack of lung sliding indicates pneumothorax or hemopneumothorax.
- CT scan: most accurate modality for diagnosing pneumothorax. In major trauma, one of the above modalities is done prior to CT scan so that large pneumothoraces can be treated immediately.

Treatment

- Observation: asymptomatic patients with small apical pneumothoraces can be observed and placed on oxygen to facilitate the resolution of the pneumothorax.
- Simple aspiration: stable, symptomatic patients with small pneumothorax less than 15% of hemithorax or less than 3 cm from apex to cupola.
- Pigtail catheter placement: treatment for spontaneous or traumatic pneumothorax greater than 15% of hemithorax or more than 3 cm from apex to cupola, with no evidence of hemothorax.
- Tube thoracostomy: definitive treatment for hemothorax with or without pneumothorax.
- Heimlich valve: one-way flutter valve that attaches to the chest tube catheter and allows air to exit the chest cavity with exhalation, and closes with inhalation, preventing air entry back into space and thus reexpansion of the pneumothorax. May leave valve open to air or attached to wall suction. Treatment for smaller, spontaneous pneumothorax with no evidence of hemothorax.
- Three-sided dressing: initial management for an open pneumothorax. It allows air to leave the pleural space during expiration. Eventually a chest tube must be placed on the ipsilateral side, but it should not be placed through the open pneumothorax, because such intervention can precipitate empyema or other infection by introducing contaminated contents into the chest cavity. Once the chest tube is placed, the open wound can be repaired.
- Needle thoracostomy: treatment of choice for tension pneumothorax, because it can be performed quickly to relieve pressure and decrease complications. It is typically performed with a long 14- or 16-gauge angiocatheter. It should always be followed with a tube thoracostomy.

HEMOTHORAX

General Principles

- Hemothorax is an accumulation of blood in the pleural space, which can accommodate more than 4 liters of blood. The most common source of bleeding is laceration of lung parenchyma. When the source of bleeding is a low-pressure system, such as the pulmonary vasculature, the bleeding typically will cease on its own. However, when the source is a systemic vessel, such as the bronchial or intercostal artery, surgical intervention is usually required to stop the bleeding.
  - Massive hemothorax: immediate chest tube drainage more than 1500 mL or continuous bleeding at 200 mL/hr for 3 to 4 hours.

Clinical Presentation

- Tachycardia, hypoxia, decreased breath sounds, dullness to percussion, hypovolemic shock.

Diagnosis and Evaluation

- Chest x-ray: blunting of costophrenic angles is seen with 200 to 300 mL of blood on an anteroposterior (AP) view. Supine view is less sensitive and shows blood layering causing a diffuse haziness.
- Ultrasound: hypoechoic or anechoic fluid is seen above the diaphragm. Called the "spine sign" (Fig 137.1), the vertebral bodies can be seen above the diaphragm.
- CT scan: can better quantify the size and identify the cause of hemothorax, such as a lung parenchymal laceration (Fig 137.2) and rib fractures.

Treatment

- Tube thoracostomy: for a traumatic hemothorax, a chest tube (usually 36F to 40F, although smaller sizes have been shown to also be effective) should be inserted between the third and fifth rib space.
- Thoracotomy: surgical intervention is indicated for a massive hemothorax.
- Resuscitation: blood products should be considered early in the setting of severe trauma. Autotransfusion can also be considered in hemothorax owing to blunt trauma, using the chest tube collection system and autotransfusion canister. Autotransfusion is contraindicated in penetrating trauma where the blood may be contaminated.

PULMONARY CONTUSION

General Principles

- Pulmonary contusions occur owing to blunt force injury to the chest wall or from blast injuries. This impact to the lung parenchyma results in alveolar edema and hemorrhage. Edema results from increased alveolar capillary

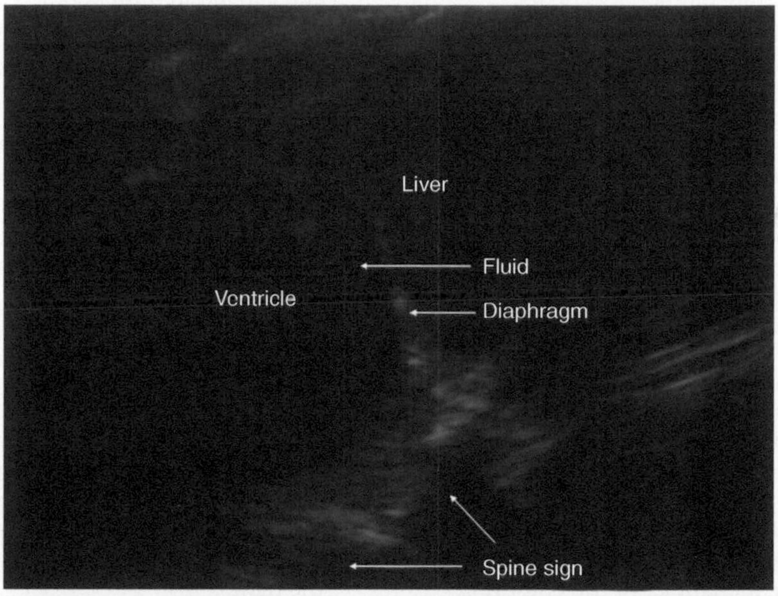

FIG. 137.1 Spine sign. (From Berkowitz, R. (2015). Shortness of breath and unexpected imaging findings. *American Journal of Emergency Medicine, 34*(5), 938.e5–938.e6, Fig 1.)

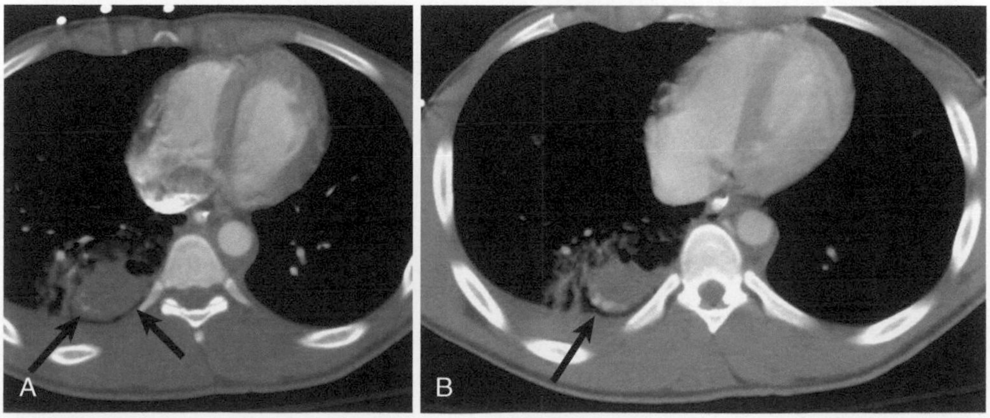

FIG. 137.2 Pulmonary laceration, arterial phase of chest computed tomography. (From Miller, L. A. (2015). Blunt chest trauma. In S. E. Mirvis (Ed.), *Problem solving in emergency radiology* (p.175, Fig. 8.9). Elsevier.)

permeability and activation of systemic inflammatory cascades that can cause acute respiratory distress syndrome.

Clinical Presentation

- Tachypnea, dyspnea, tachycardia, chest wall bruising, respiratory distress, and acute respiratory distress syndrome. Patients may have rales or absent breath sounds and occasionally hemoptysis.

Diagnosis and Evaluation

- Chest x-ray: pulmonary contusions are not always present on the initial x-ray, but usually develop within 6 hours of injury. Findings include patchy opacities and lobar consolidation localized to one part of the lung.
- CT scan: can detect pulmonary contusions (Fig. 137.3) that are not visualized on initial x-ray.

Treatment

- Supportive measures: pain control, suctioning, oxygen, incentive spirometry, and restriction of intravenous fluids to prevent worsening pulmonary edema.
- Noninvasive positive pressure ventilation: continuous positive airway pressure and bilevel positive airway pressure can both be used to support respirations in patients with pulmonary contusions.
- Intubation: in patients with severe pulmonary contusion, intubation should be considered. Lung protective strategy should be employed with low tidal volumes and high positive end-expiratory pressure.

TRACHEOBRONCHIAL INJURY

General Principles

- Tracheobronchial injuries are uncommon. They occur from blunt or penetrating trauma of the chest or neck. Cervical tracheal injuries typically occur owing to penetrating trauma, whereas intrathoracic injuries occur from blunt trauma.
  - Air leak: the flow of air into the pleural space, usually from alveolar-pleural fistula, often detected as bubbling in the water seal chamber of the chest tube drain. Persistent pneumothorax despite chest tube placement should raise suspicion of tracheobronchial injury.
  - Massive air leak: air leak that is present during all phases of respiration that prevents full expansion of the affected lung. These findings suggest major tracheobronchial injury.

Clinical Presentation

- Cervical tracheal injury: dyspnea, hoarseness, subcutaneous emphysema.
- Thoracic tracheal injury: subcutaneous emphysema, and hemoptysis. The most specific finding is a massive air leak and pneumothorax that reaccumulates despite chest tube placement.

Diagnosis and Evaluation

- Chest x-ray: may show subcutaneous emphysema, pneumothorax, air surrounding the bronchus, and pneumomediastinum (Fig 137.4).
- CT scan: can diagnose tracheobronchial injury as well as associated findings, such as esophageal injury or mediastinitis, although sensitivity is not well known.
- Flexible bronchoscopy is the gold standard for diagnosis and can aid in intubation.
- Endoscopy: should be performed to evaluate for concomitant esophageal injury

Treatment

- Intubation: use video laryngoscope or bronchoscope to ensure that the tube has passed the site of injury and avoid creating a blind tract or further tearing of the tracheal injury.
- Surgical repair: for large tracheal tears, mediastinitis, or massive air leaks.

DIAPHRAGM INJURY

General Principles

- Diaphragm injuries can occur after blunt or penetrating injuries. Any stab wound that passes through the chest or abdominal wall from T4 through T12 has the potential to injure the diaphragm. Injury typically occurs on the left side, thought to be because of the liver's presence on the right.
- Diaphragm injuries can be missed initially and not present until months or years later when abdominal organs herniate through the defect. Delayed diagnosis

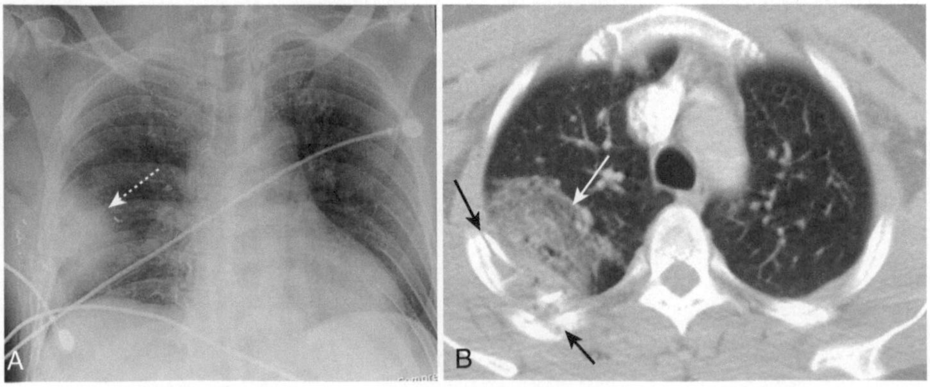

FIG. 137.3 Pulmonary contusions, chest radiography and computed tomography. (From Herring, W. (2020). Recognizing the imaging findings of trauma to the chest. In W. Herring (Ed.), *Learning radiology: Recognizing the basics* (4th ed., pp. 341, Fig. 25.15). Elsevier.)

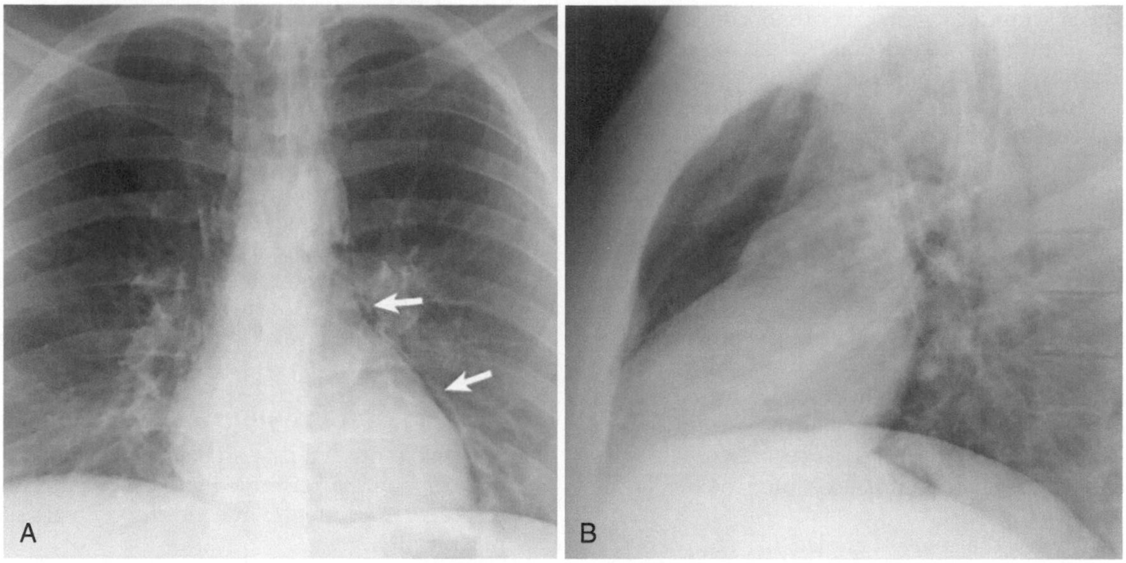

FIG. 137.4 Pneumomediastinum present between left cardiac border and left mediastinal pleura. (Franquet, T. (2019). Pneumomediastinum. In C. M. Walker & J. H. Chung (Eds.), *Muller's imaging of the chest* (pp. 1030–1038.e2). Elsevier.)

is associated with an increased risk for herniation and strangulation of abdominal organs.

Clinical Presentation

- Diaphragm injuries must be considered both in asymptomatic patients with acute thoracoabdominal trauma as well as in symptomatic patients with a remote history of trauma.
  - Abdominal pain, referred shoulder pain, shortness of breath, vomiting, dysphagia, or shock.

Diagnosis and Evaluation

- Chest x-ray: has poor sensitivity, but in severe diaphragm rupture, abdominal contents can be seen in the chest cavity.
- CT: misses about 20% of cases, but may detect diaphragm discontinuity and "collar sign" (Fig. 137.5), which is a waist-like constriction of abdominal viscera through the diaphragm.
- Thoracoscopy or laparoscopy: the gold standard for diagnosing diaphragm rupture.

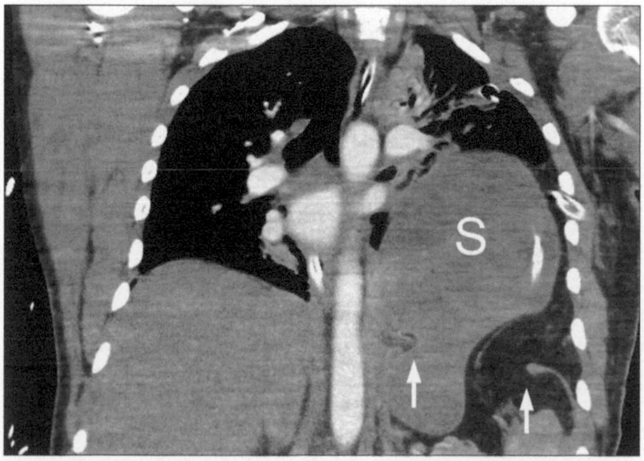

FIG. 137.5 Collar sign. (From Leung, V. A., Patlas, M. N., Reid, S., Coates, A., & Nicolaou, S. (2015). Imaging of traumatic diaphragmatic rupture: Evaluation of diagnostic accuracy at a level 1 trauma centre. *Canadian Association of Radiologists Journal, 66*(4), 310–317, Fig. 1).

Treatment

- Laparoscopy: both diagnostic and therapeutic.

ESOPHAGEAL INJURY

General Principles

- There are multiple etiologies of esophageal laceration and perforation, including the following:
  - Iatrogenic injury, such as upper endoscopy, which is the most common iatrogenic etiology
    - Location: cervical esophagus
  - Boerhaave syndrome, also known as spontaneous esophageal rupture and postemetic rupture, results in esophageal perforation caused by forceful vomiting.
    - Location: distal esophagus
  - Ingested foreign bodies in the esophagus can cause rupture owing to direct laceration, pressure necrosis, or caustic burns.
    - Location: cervical esophagus
  - Traumatic injuries of the esophagus are usually caused by penetrating trauma, such as gunshot or stab wounds, and are commonly associated with tracheal injuries.
    - Location: cervical esophagus

Clinical Presentation

- The presentation of esophageal injury depends on both the location and the etiology of the injury. Although small lacerations from ingested foreign bodies can be relatively benign, perforations from Boerhaave syndrome and trauma are typically life-threatening.
  - Cervical esophageal perforation
    - Initial symptoms: neck pain and stiffness, dysphagia, dysphonia.
    - Delayed symptoms: fluid and air enter into the retropharyngeal space, leading to sepsis and subcutaneous emphysema of the neck and face.
  - Intrathoracic esophageal perforation
    - Initial symptoms: severe chest pain after vomiting.

- Delayed symptoms: gastric contents contaminate the mediastinum and pleura, leading to subcutaneous emphysema of the chest wall and neck, fever, tachypnea, tachycardia, cyanosis, and hypotension.
- Hamman crunch: mediastinal emphysema leads to crunching sound on cardiac auscultation.

Diagnosis and Evaluation

- X-ray: subcutaneous emphysema, pleural effusions, mediastinal or peritoneal free air, pneumothorax, and a widened mediastinum can be seen. With cervical esophageal perforations, there can be air in the prevertebral space.
- Contrast esophagram: the study of choice for esophageal rupture. Water-soluble contrast, such as gastrografin, is used initially to detect perforations because it causes less inflammation than barium if it leaks into the mediastinal space.
- CT: although not the study of choice, CT scan can identify some esophageal perforations and help identify fluid collections in the mediastinum and pleura.
- Flexible endoscopy: extremely sensitive for detecting perforation, but has some associated risks. Insufflation of the esophagus and direct trauma from the endoscope can extend the perforation or cause more air to infiltrate into the mediastinum.

Treatment

- Small esophageal perforations in patients with minimal symptoms can sometimes be managed medically with nothing by mouth status, total parenteral nutrition, and antibiotics. More commonly, perforations are treated with open surgical repair, although it is occasionally repaired endoscopically. In the emergency department, treatment should focus on the following interventions:
  - Nothing by mouth
  - Broad-spectrum antibiotics
  - Volume resuscitation
  - Airway management
  - Surgical consultation
  - Avoid blind placement of nasogastric tubes

Cardiovascular Trauma

BLUNT CARDIAC INJURY

General Principles

- Blunt cardiac injury (BCI) is a term used to describe a range of cardiac injuries, from myocardial concussion to myocardial rupture.
  - Myocardial concussion, also called *commotio cordis*, occurs when blunt injury to the chest stuns the myocardium, which can lead to ventricular tachycardia and fibrillation.
  - Myocardial contusion is the most common type of BCI. It is caused by compression of the heart between the vertebrae and the sternum, resulting in myocardial necrosis. The right ventricle is most commonly affected owing its proximity to the anterior chest wall.

Clinical Presentation

- Myocardial concussion: occurs most frequently in adolescents who are hit in the chest with a small object at high speeds, such as a hockey puck or baseball. It usually results in a brief dysrhythmia, such as ventricular fibrillation/tachycardia, but may lead to cardiac arrest and death.
- Myocardial contusion: the most frequent mechanism involves motor vehicle crashes in which the patient's chest strikes the steering wheel. Patients can present with a range of symptoms, including arrhythmias, wall motion abnormalities, and coronary artery dissection, resulting in myocardial infarction and cardiogenic shock.

Diagnosis and Evaluation

- It is recommended that an electrocardiogram (ECG) and troponin be performed for patients in whom BCI is suspected. A normal ECG and troponin are sufficient to rule out BCI.
  - ECG: the most common, but least specific, finding is sinus tachycardia. Other arrhythmias include supraventricular and junctional tachycardia, atrial flutter or fibrillation, ventricular tachycardia/fibrillation, bundle branch blocks (most common owing to anterior location of the right ventricle), and acute ischemic changes.
  - Cardiac biomarkers: elevated troponin indicates a higher risk of dysrhythmias and left ventricular dysfunction. An elevated troponin should prompt serial testing and an echocardiogram.
  - Bedside echocardiography can be helpful in initial evaluation of hypotensive patients with chest trauma to look for pericardial tamponade.

Treatment

- Aspirin and other antiplatelet agents should be avoided in blunt cardiac injury-related chest pain.
  - Observation/telemetry: patients with cardiac contusion with abnormal ECG or positive biomarkers should be admitted for telemetry and consideration for echocardiography.
  - Arrhythmia: any arrhythmias should be treated by standard Advanced Cardiovascular Life Support (ACLS) protocol. There is no evidence for prophylactic antiarrhythmics.
  - Emergency department thoracotomy for traumatic cardiac arrest is less effective in blunt trauma than in penetrating trauma. The Eastern Association for the Surgery of Trauma recommends against resuscitative thoracotomy for patients with blunt trauma who have no signs of life in the field, although they report that it can be attempted if the patient still has signs of life in the emergency department.

PENETRATING CARDIAC TRAUMA/ACUTE CARDIAC TAMPONADE

General Principles

- Penetrating wounds of the heart can cause cardiac tamponade or hemorrhagic shock. As little as 50 mL of blood trapped in the pericardial space can increase pressure on the right atrium and ventricle, resulting in decreased filling of the heart and tamponade physiology. Pericardial tamponade is more common in the setting of stab wounds to the chest, because gunshot wounds typically create too large a pericardial defect to produce cardiac tamponade.

Clinical Presentation

- Chest pain, tachycardia, dyspnea, hypotension, narrow pulse pressure, pulseless electrical activity arrest.
- Beck triad: distended neck veins, muffled heart sounds, and hypotension. This triad is relatively uncommon because many trauma patients also experience hemorrhage resulting in flat neck veins.
- Pulsus paradoxus: an abnormally large (more than 10 mm Hg) drop in systolic blood pressure during inspiration.

Diagnosis and Evaluation

- Ultrasound: as part of the FAST examination, it is the preferred method to detect cardiac tamponade. Any size effusion in the setting of trauma is highly suggestive of pericardial tamponade. Direct signs include diastolic collapse of the right ventricle.

Treatment

- Immediate tracheal intubation of patients with pericardial tamponade can exacerbate hypotension and cause cardiovascular collapse. Therefore, evacuation of the pericardial effusion and fluid resuscitation should be performed prior to intubation.
  - Pericardiocentesis: in situations where thoracotomy is not possible, pericardiocentesis under ultrasound can be attempted as a temporizing measure. Because blood in the pericardial space is frequently clotted, aspiration is not always possible.
  - Emergency department thoracotomy: the Eastern Association for the Surgery of Trauma strongly recommends a resuscitative thoracotomy for patients who arrive to the emergency department with signs of life who become pulseless after a penetrating thoracic injury, and a conditional recommendation for patients with a pulseless penetrating trauma without signs of life.
  - Operative repair: preferred in stable patients.

BLUNT AORTIC INJURY

General Principles

- Blunt aortic injury results from trauma involving rapid deceleration, such as motor vehicle accidents, falls, and pedestrians struck by automobiles.
- The descending aorta is a fixed structure, whereas the aortic arch is more mobile. When the body decelerates, the aortic arch jerks forward and pulls on the descending aorta causing a tear or rupture. This happens most commonly at the aortic isthmus, just distal to the takeoff of the left subclavian artery.

Clinical Presentation

- The majority of blunt aortic injuries are immediately fatal, resulting in aortic transection and rupture. When patients do survive to the emergency department, it is typically because a pseudoaneurysm is contained by the outer walls of the aorta, but they are at high risk of rupture within 24 hours. These patients typically have vague and nonspecific symptoms.
  - Retrosternal chest pain, upper extremity hypertension, new murmur, pulse deficit.

Diagnosis and Evaluation

- Chest x-ray: a widened mediastinum is present in the majority of blunt aortic injuries. Less-common findings include tracheal deviation, indistinct aortic knob, and left apical pleural cap.
- CT scan: the gold standard for diagnosing aortic injury.

137

Treatment

- Blood pressure control: should be maintained at a systolic of 100 to 120 mm Hg and a heart rate of 60 to 80 beats/min. Esmolol is the first-choice agent, with nitroprusside added as a second agent, if needed.
- Endovascular repair: initial treatment of choice.
- Open repair: has a higher complication than endovascular repair.

SUGGESTED READINGS

Ali, R. S. (2018). Thoracic trauma. In R. M. Walls, R. S. Hockberger, & M. Gausche-Hill (Eds.), *Rosen's emergency medicine: Concepts and clinical practice* (9th ed., Vol. 1). Elsevier.

Morley, E. J., English, B., Cohen, D. B., & Paolo, W. F. (2019). Blunt cardiac injury: Emergency department diagnosis and management. *Emergency Medicine Practice*, *21*(3), 1–20.

Morley, E. J., Johnson, S., Leibner, E., & Shahid, J. (2016). Emergency department evaluation and management of blunt chest and lung trauma. *Emergency Medicine Practice*, *18*(6), 1–20.

CHAPTER 138

BOARD REVIEW

Head Trauma

CHINWE ONU, MD, and BRADLEY CHAPPELL, DO, MHA, FACOEP

This chapter briefly reviews both blunt and penetrating traumatic brain injury (TBI). TBI is a major cause of morbidity and mortality in the United States, causing roughly 2.5 million emergency department visits and over 50,000 deaths annually.

General Principles

- Traumatic brain injury can be caused by primary and secondary insults.
- Primary causes include direct injury by striking the head or indirect injury via acceleration/deceleration movements, whereas secondary injuries consist of factors that worsen clinical outcomes, such as hypoxia, hypoglycemia, hypotension, and cerebral edema.

Clinical Presentation

- A rapid focused neurologic examination is paramount. The Glasgow Coma Scale (GCS) is often used to estimate TBI severity (Table 138.1).
- Complications of TBI include midline shift, increased intracranial pressure (ICP), herniation, seizures, and delayed cerebral ischemia (Fig. 138.1, Table 138.2).
- High-risk groups include the elderly, children, and alcoholics. Manifestations of TBI include:
  - Subdural hematoma (SDH) mostly occurs from blunt trauma that leads to tearing of bridging cortical veins. Alcoholics and elderly patients are predisposed to SDH owing to brain atrophy; infants are also at high risk. A SDH appears concave or crescent-shaped on a

TABLE 138.1 *Glasgow Coma Scale (GCS)*

Response	Score	Significance
Eye Opening		
Spontaneously	4	Reticular activating system in intact; patient may not be aware
To verbal command	3	Opens eyes when told to do so
To pain	2	Opens eyes in response to pain
None	1	Does not open eyes to any stimuli
Verbal Stimuli		
Oriented, converses	5	Relatively intact CNS, aware of self and environment
Disoriented, converses	4	Well articulated, organized, but disoriented
Inappropriate word	3	Random exclamatory words
Incomprehensible	2	Moaning, no recognizable words
No response	1	No response or intubated
Motor Response		
Obeys verbal commands	6	Readily moves limbs when told to
Localizes to painful stimuli	5	Moves limb in an effort to remove painful stimuli
Flexion withdrawal	4	Pulls away from pain in flexion
Abnormal flexion	3	Decorticate rigidity
Extension	2	Decerebrate rigidity
No response	1	Hypotonia, flaccid; suggests loss of medullary function or concomitant spinal cord injury
Severity Scale		
Mild TBI	13 or greater	
Moderate TBI	9–13	
Severe TBI	8 or greater	

(From Papa, L., & Goldberg, S. A. (2018). Head trauma. In R. M. Walls, R. S. Hockberger, & M. Gausche-Hill (Eds.), *Rosen's emergency medicine: Concepts and clinical practice* (9th ed., p. 311, Table. 34.2). Elsevier.)

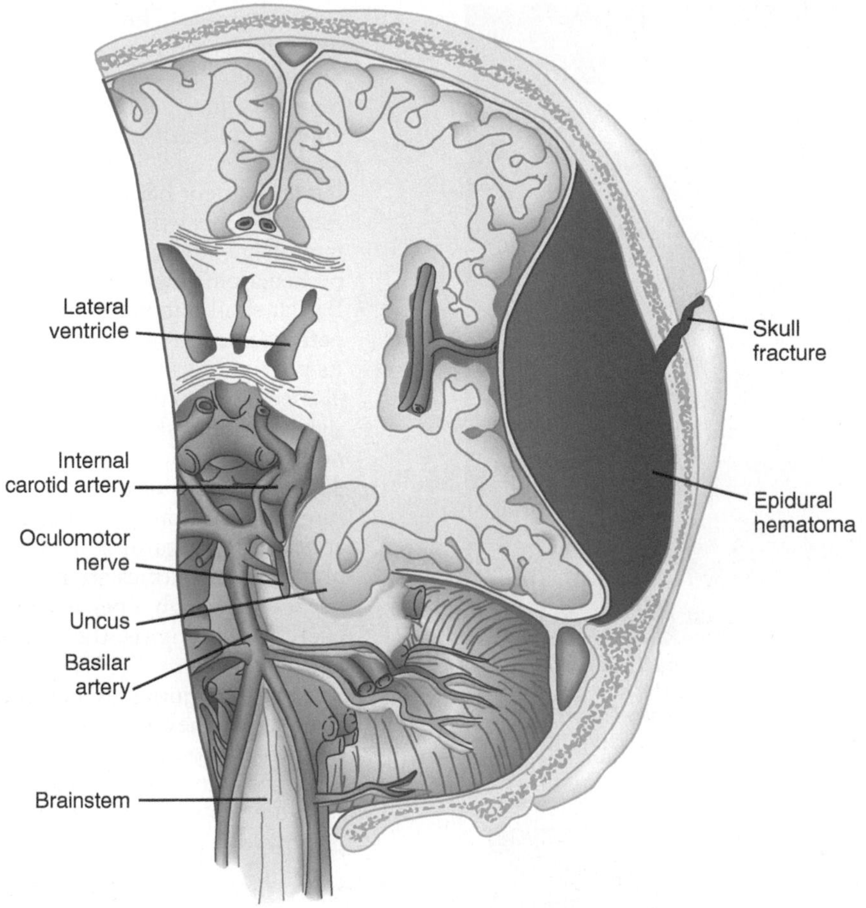

FIG. 138.1 Transtentorial herniation caused by a hematoma. (From Papa, L., & Goldberg, S. A. (2018). Head trauma. In R. M. Walls, R. S. Hockberger, & M. Gausche-Hill (Eds.), *Rosen's emergency medicine: Concepts and clinical practice* (9th ed., p. 308, Fig. 34.4). Elsevier.)

TABLE 138.2 *Herniation Syndromes*

Syndrome	Mechanism	Clinical Manifestations
Transtentorial: Uncal	Ipsilateral uncus pushes downward toward the tentorium compressing the midbrain	• Ipsilateral pupil dilatation and nonreactivity • Contralateral Babinski response • Contralateral hemiparesis • Decerebrate posturing
Transtentorial: Central	Cerebral hemisphere and basal nuclei downward displacement through the tentorium	• Bilateral dilated fixed pupil • Bilateral increased motor tone • Decorticate posturing • Cheyne-Stokes respiration
Subfalcine: Cingulate	Brain displacement of the cingulate gyrus under adjacent flax cerebri	• Headache • Contralateral leg paralysis
Tonsillar	Cerebellar tonsils push downward through the foramen magnum	• Cardiopulmonary collapse from medulla compression • Flaccid quadriplegia from corticospinal tract compression

noncontrast head computed tomography (CT). Any patient with an acute subdural more than 10 mm in thickness, associated with more than 5-mm midline shift, or with a GCS less than 9 warrants a neurosurgical consultation, because surgical evacuation and ICP monitoring may be indicated (Fig. 138.2).

- Epidural hematoma (EDH) classically presents with loss of consciousness after a lateral skull impact, followed by a short period of alertness (the lucent period) before rapid neurologic decompensation. It occurs when the middle meningeal artery is lacerated, leading to blood accumulation between the dura and the skull. On noncontrast head CT, EDH appears convex or lenticular shaped.
- Cerebral contusions and intraparenchymal hemorrhages (IPH) are secondary to direct injury to the brain parenchyma. Hyperdense in appearance on noncontrast head CT, cerebral contusions and IPHs are most commonly located at the base of the frontal and temporal lobes.

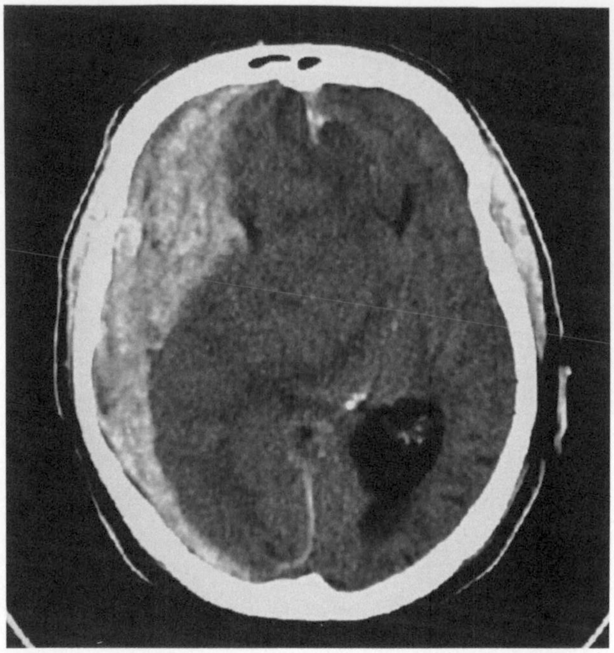

FIG. 138.2 Subdural hematoma. (From Papa, L., & Goldberg, S. A. (2018). Head trauma. In R. M. Walls, R. S. Hockberger, & M. Gausche-Hill (Eds.), *Rosen's emergency medicine: Concepts and clinical practice* (9th ed., p. 314, Fig. 34.9). Elsevier.)

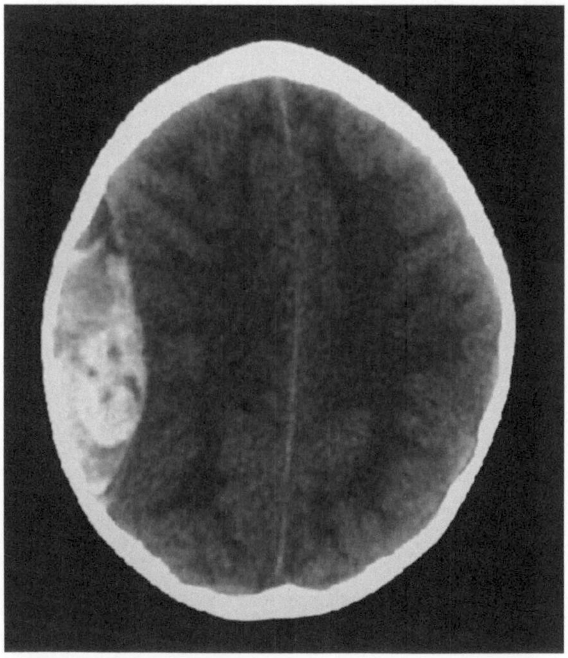

FIG. 138.3 Epidural hematoma. (From Papa, L., & Goldberg, S. A. (2018). Head trauma. In R. M. Walls, R. S. Hockberger, & M. Gausche-Hill (Eds.), *Rosen's emergency medicine: Concepts and clinical practice* (9th ed., p. 313, Fig. 34.7). Elsevier.)

- Traumatic subarachnoid hemorrhages (SAH) occur from injuries to vessels below the arachnoid mater and present similarly to aneurysmal bleeds. On a noncontrast head CT, they appear hyperdense.
- Diffuse axonal injury (DAI) occurs when acceleration-deceleration and rotational forces cause irreversible axonal damage. The head CT commonly appears normal, but can have small hyperdense areas representing multiple punctate hemorrhages. Magnetic resonance imaging (MRI) is the imaging study of choice, and DAI should be considered in all patients where the head CT appears relatively unremarkable, but the patient has a significant neurologic deficit. Also, patients who do not have marked neurologic improvement after evacuation of a subdural or epidural hematoma may have DAI.
- Basilar skull fractures commonly occur at the petrous portion of the temporal bone. Owing to its proximity to the meningeal vessels, there may also be a concomitant epidural hematoma. Clinical signs of basilar skull fracture include hemotympanum, raccoon eyes, battle sign, and cerebrospinal fluid rhinorrhea or otorrhea. In addition to neurosurgical consultation, consider infectious disease consultation regarding initiation of antibiotics. Prophylactic antibiotics are not always recommended because although a persistent CSF leak is a risk for bacterial meningitis, the role of antibiotic prophylaxis is unclear.
- Penetrating injuries are not as common as blunt head trauma, but they are usually from gunshot wounds, stab wounds, and blast injuries (shrapnel). Infection is the most common secondary injury, so antibiotics should be considered when retained shrapnel is present.

Diagnosis and Evaluation

- Imaging is the most important tool in the diagnosis of TBI because it directs subsequent management of the injury. Not all traumatic head injuries require CT imaging, but use of clinical decision rules, such as those outlined by the American College of Emergency Physicians (ACEP) Clinical Policy statement (Box 138.1) or the Canadian Head CT Rules, are helpful in guiding this decision. A noncontrast head CT can be quickly obtained in the emergency department. When there is a significant mechanism of injury, consider obtaining CT imaging of the cervical spine as well, because there is a high likelihood of cervical injury with severe TBI (refer to Chapter 141. Spine and Neck Trauma). The Eastern Association for the Surgery of Trauma (EAST) Blunt Cerebrovascular Injury Guidelines and Denver Criteria support obtaining a CT angiogram of the brain and neck for patients with unexplained neurologic deficit as well as those with a GCS of 8 or less, a petrous bone fracture, diffuse axonal injury, cervical spine fracture, or Lefort II or III facial fractures.
- Laboratory tests are not necessary for the initial diagnosis; however, they can aid in management.
  - Point-of-care glucose is used to rule out hypoglycemia as a cause of altered mentation and further manage blood sugar levels.
  - Prothrombin time, international normalized ratio, or thromboelastography (if available) are especially helpful in patients with unknown medications or those on anticoagulants who need reversal to prevent further intracranial bleeding (refer to Chapter 123. Anticoagulants).

BOX 138.1 ***American College of Emergency Physicians Clinical Policy Regarding Neuroimaging in Adults with Mild Traumatic Brain Injury***

A noncontrast head CT is indicated (Level one recommendation) in adults with LOC or posttraumatic amnesia, only if one or more of the following is present:

- Headache
- Vomiting
- Age older than 60 years
- Deficits in short-term memory
- Physical evidence of trauma above the clavicle
- Posttraumatic seizure
- GCS score below 15
- Focal neurologic deficit
- Coagulopathy

A nonconstract head CT should be considered (Level two recommendation) in patients with head trauma with no LOC or posttraumatic amnesia if there is:

- Focal neuroloci deficit
- Vomiting
- Severe headache
- Age 65 years or older
- Physical sign of a basilar skull fracture
- GCS score below 15
- Coagulopathy
- A dangerous mechanism (e.g., ejection from motor vehicle, pedestrian struck, fall of more than 3 feet or 5 stairs)

(Adapted from J. A. Marx, R. S. Hockberger, & R. M. Walls (Eds.). (2014). *Rosen's emergency medicine: Concepts and clinical practice* (8th ed.). Elsevier.)

Treatment

- Initial management for TBI should focus on airway, breathing, circulation, and establishing a baseline neurologic examination. Upon arrival, place the patient on a monitor, establish large-bore intravenous (IV) lines, immobilize the cervical spine (if appropriate), and elevate the head of the bed (if there is concern for increased intracranial pressure) to 30 degrees to facilitate cerebral venous outflow. For most cases of TBI, neurosurgery consultation and admission are usually indicated (Fig. 138.4).
  - Airway: Intubation is indicated if the patient is hypoxic, hypercarbic (failure to ventilate), unable to protect the airway, or for an anticipated clinical course. It is imperative to maintain cervical spine immobilization during intubation; video-assisted laryngoscopy or fiberoptic intubation can reduce c-spine movement. Patients with a GCS of 8 or less should generally be intubated. Little evidence indicates that pretreatment or choice of rapid sequence induction agents affects outcomes.
  - Breathing/ventilation: The goal is to prevent both hypoxia (PaO_2 less than 60 mm Hg or SpO_2 less than 90%) and hyperoxia because cerebral oxygen toxicity/free radical damage occurs with a PaO_2 greater than 200 mm Hg. Provide supplemental oxygenation if intubation is not indicated, but the SpO_2 is less than 93%. Hypercarbia increases intracranial pressure by causing cerebral vasodilatation and increased cerebral perfusion. Continuous end-tidal carbon dioxide is helpful for titrating the ventilator to prevent hypercarbia and maintain normal $PaCO_2$ (35 to 40 mm Hg). With signs of impending herniation, consider a short trial of hyperventilation with the goal end-tidal carbon dioxide of 30 to 35 mm Hg. Prolonged hyperventilation can be detrimental because it causes cerebral ischemia from cerebral vasoconstriction and reduced cerebral blood flow.
  - Circulation: Hypotension and hypovolemia should be avoided because they are associated with cerebral ischemia and increase mortality and morbidity. Isotonic crystalloid or balanced electrolyte solutions

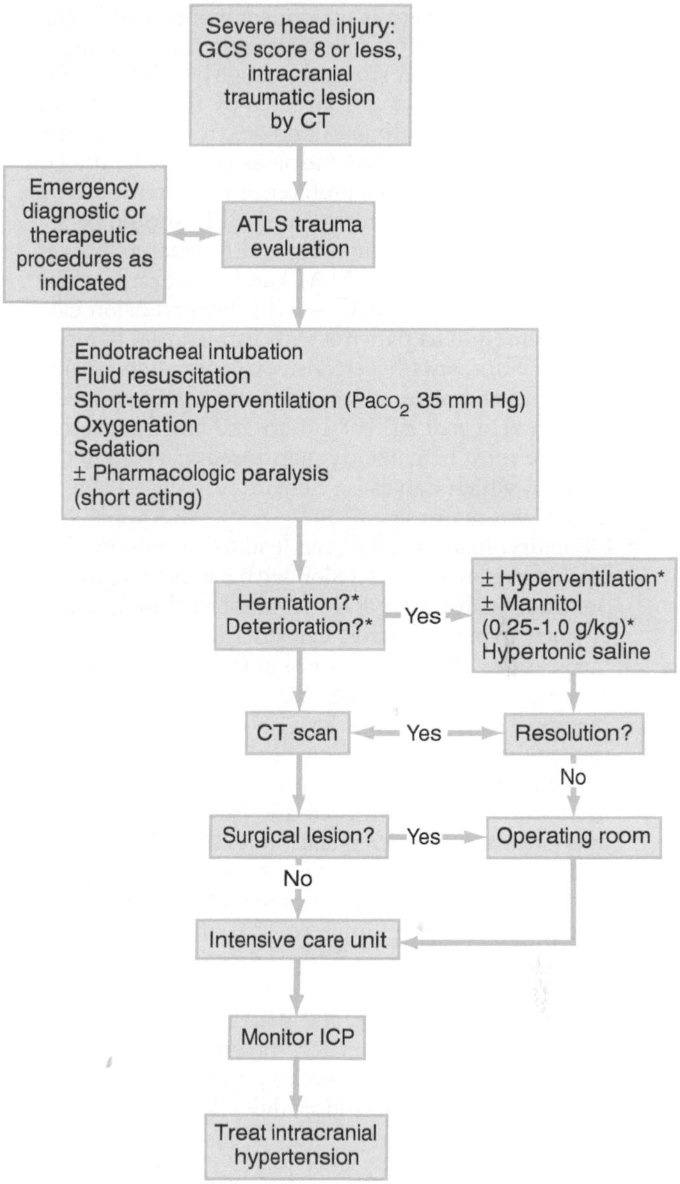

*Only in the presence of signs of herniation or progressive neurologic deterioration not attributable to extracranial factors.

FIG. 138.4 Severe head injury resuscitation. (From Papa, L., & Goldberg, S. A. (2018). Head trauma. In R. M. Walls, R. S. Hockberger, & M. Gausche-Hill (Eds.), *Rosen's emergency medicine: Concepts and clinical practice* (9th ed., p. 317, Fig. 34.14). Elsevier.)

are preferred if there is no evidence of hemorrhagic shock. For those with a hemorrhagic source of hypotension, transfusion should be roughly 1pRBC:1FFP:1 platelet unless otherwise directed by thromboelastography. In general, albumin and dextrose-containing fluids should be avoided; vasopressors may be used, as needed, with an initial preference for norepinephrine. The cerebral perfusion pressure (CPP) should be maintained above 70 mm Hg and is affected by both mean arterial pressure (MAP) and intracranial pressure (ICP) [CPP = MAP – ICP]. Hypertension can be detrimental to patients with intracranial hemorrhages. Thus, anti-hypertensive agents, such as nicardipine, clevidipine, or labetolol, are recommended to achieve a goal SBP of 140 to 160 mm Hg. Blood pressure must be carefully monitored to avoid hypotension, which can cause ischemic damage if the CPP is not maintained.

- Disability: Increased ICP can lead to herniation, the Cushing reflex (hypertension with a widened pulse pressure, bradycardia, and irregular breathing), and changes in mental status. Consider ICP-lowering medications, such as mannitol at 0.5 to 1.0 g/kg and/or 3% saline at 1 to 3 mL/kg. A common side effect of mannitol is hypotension, so it should be avoided in patients with borderline or low blood pressures. Likewise, to reduce progression of intracranial bleeding, reversal agents should be administered to patients taking anticoagulants. Anticoagulation reversal should be undertaken (See Chapter 123. Anticoagulants).
- Seizure prophylaxis: Development of early posttraumatic seizures occurs in up to 12% of patients with blunt head trauma and 50% of those with penetrating head trauma. Seizures cause cerebral hypoxia, hypercarbia, cytokine release, and increased ICP. Phenytoin and levetiracetam have been shown to reduce early posttraumatic seizures; however, they do not prevent late seizures or decrease mortality (Box 138.2).

BOX 138.2 ***Indications for Acute Seizure Prophylaxis in Severe Head Trauma***

Depressed skull fracture
Paralyzed and intubated patients
Seizure at the time of injury
Seizure at emergency department presentation
Penetrating brain injury
Severe head injury (Glasgow Coma Scale score 8 or lower)
Acute subdural hematoma
Acute epidural hematoma
Acute intracranial hemorrhage
Prior history of seizure

(Adapted from J. A. Marx, R. S. Hockberger, & R. M. Walls (Eds.). (2014). *Rosen's emergency medicine: Concepts and clinical practice* (8th ed.). Elsevier.)

BOX 138.3 ***AVPU System***

A—Alert
V—Responds to *v*erbal stimuli
P—Responds to *p*ainful Stimuli
U—*U*nresponsive

(Adapted from Murray, B. L., & Cordle, R. J. (2018). Pediatric trauma. In R. M. Walls, R. S. Hockberger, & M. Gausche-Hill (Eds.), *Rosen's emergency medicine: Concepts and clinical practice* (9th ed., p. 2044), Box 165.5). Elsevier.)

Pediatric Head Trauma

- Annually, in the United States, about 500,000 children 14 years of age or older with a TBI visit the emergency department. Falls are the most common mechanism; however, non-accidental trauma must be considered with all pediatric injuries. Shaken baby syndrome occurs when children are violently shaken when held by the torso or extremity. Injuries can include SDH, SAH, and diffuse retinal hemorrhages. Compared with adults, infants' skulls are more distensible because cranial sutures are still open (less risk of herniation or increased ICP). When evaluating younger pediatric patients, the AVPU (*a*lert, *v*erbal, *p*ain, and *u*nresponsive) acronym is used rather than GCS (Box 138.3).
- Additionally, specific criteria have been defined by the Pediatric Emergency Care Applied Research Network to provide guidance for when neuroimaging is necessary following blunt head injury in children (Fig. 138.5). (Refer to Chapter 143. Pediatric Trauma and Pediatric Fractures.)

SUGGESTED READINGS

Cryer, H. et al. (2015). American College of Surgeons Trauma Quality Improvement Program Guidelines, Traumatic Brain Injury.
Rajajee, Venkatakrishna et al. *Management of Acute Severe Traumatic Brain Injury*. Available at: https://www.uptodate.com/contents/management-of-acute-severe-traumatic-brain-injury?search=traumatic%20brain%20injury&source=search_result&selectedTitle=2~150&usage_type=default&display_rank=2#H26.
Zammit, C., & Knight, W. A., IV. (2013). Severe traumatic brain injury in adults. *Emergency Medicine Practice*, *15*(3), 1–28. Available at: https://www.ebmedicine.net/topics.php?paction=showTopic&topic_id=522.

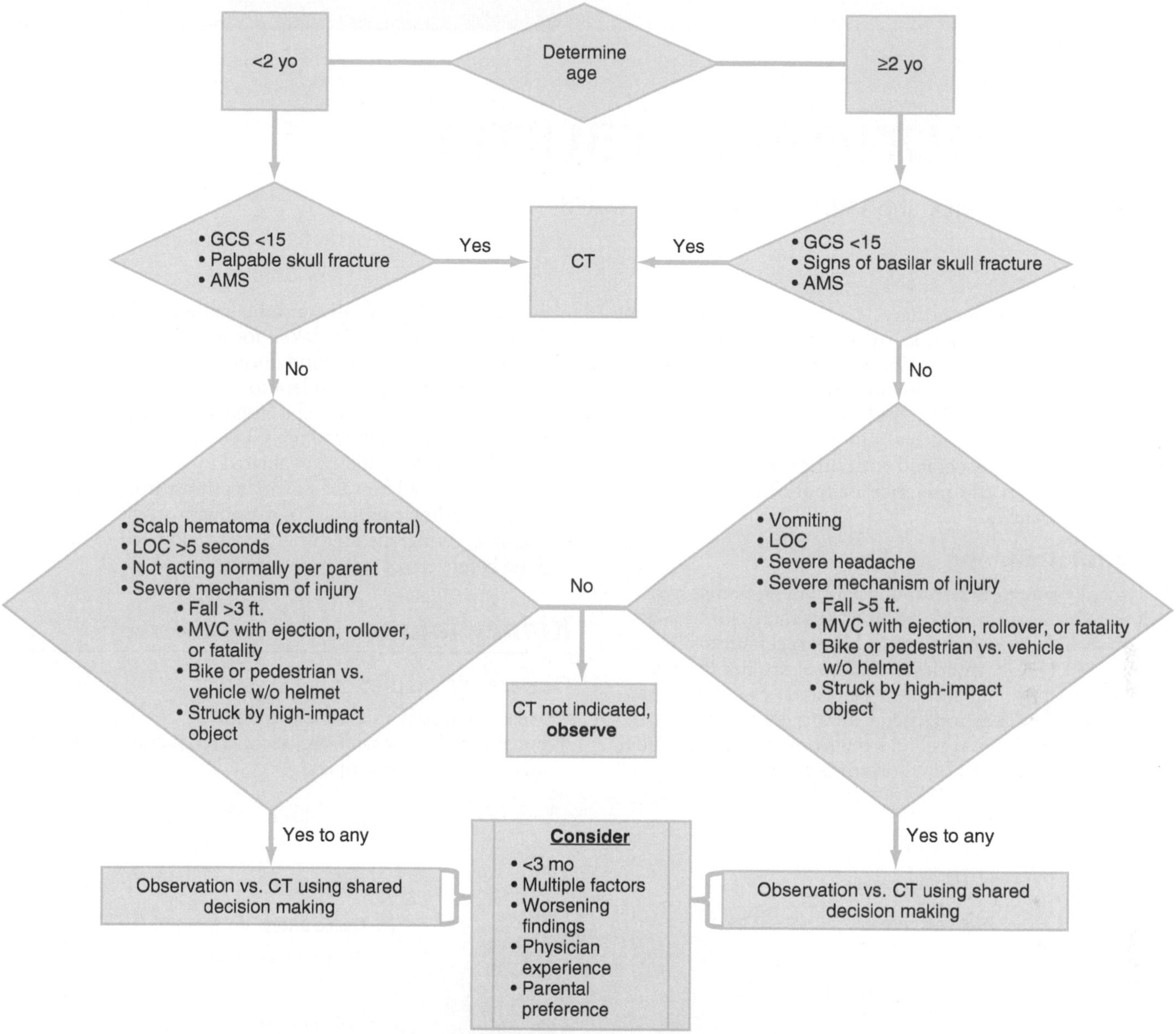

FIG. 138.5 Computed tomography decision rule for pediatric blunt head injury. (From Murray, B. L., & Cordle, R. J. (2018). Pediatric trauma. In R. M. Walls, R. S. Hockberger, & M. Gausche-Hill (Eds.), *Rosen's emergency medicine: Concepts and clinical practice* (9th ed., p. 2047, Fig. 165.1). Elsevier.)

CHAPTER 139

BOARD REVIEW

Genitourinary Trauma

JENNIFER FANG, MD, and JAIME JORDAN, MD, MAEd

Identification of genitourinary (GU) injuries is important to reduce morbidity, such as hypertension, kidney disease, recurrent infections, incontinence, fistulas (i.e., arteriovenous, urethrocutaneous, vesiculocutaneous, vesicovaginal, rectovaginal, colovesical), and sexual dysfunction. The mortality associated with these injuries is generally low, but GU trauma can be associated with other severe injuries and may be missed in the presence of more immediately life-threatening injuries.

Basic Information

- Typically categorized into upper (kidneys, ureters) vs. lower (bladder, urethra, external genitalia), GU trauma can occur from penetrating or blunt mechanisms (Fig. 139.1). GU injuries include, but are not limited to, contusions, hematomas, lacerations, vascular injury (resulting in dissection, pseudoaneurysm, thrombosis, or extravasation), renal pedicle avulsions, collecting system injuries (such as urinomas or urinary extravasation), and burns. Hemodynamically unstable patients with intraabdominal trauma who are taken for immediate laparotomy may have GU injuries found during exploration. Hematuria should prompt consideration of GU injury; further studies should be performed if suspicion for injury is high. For stable patients in whom a GU injury is suspected, the GU system should be evaluated in a retrograde manner to avoid forward-flowing contrast from obscuring or confounding the results of subsequent studies. For example, retrograde urethrography would need to be done before retrograde cystography.

Kidney Injury

General Principles

- Most commonly injured GU organ.
- Preexisting structural issues, such as renal cysts or tumors, increase the risk for injury.

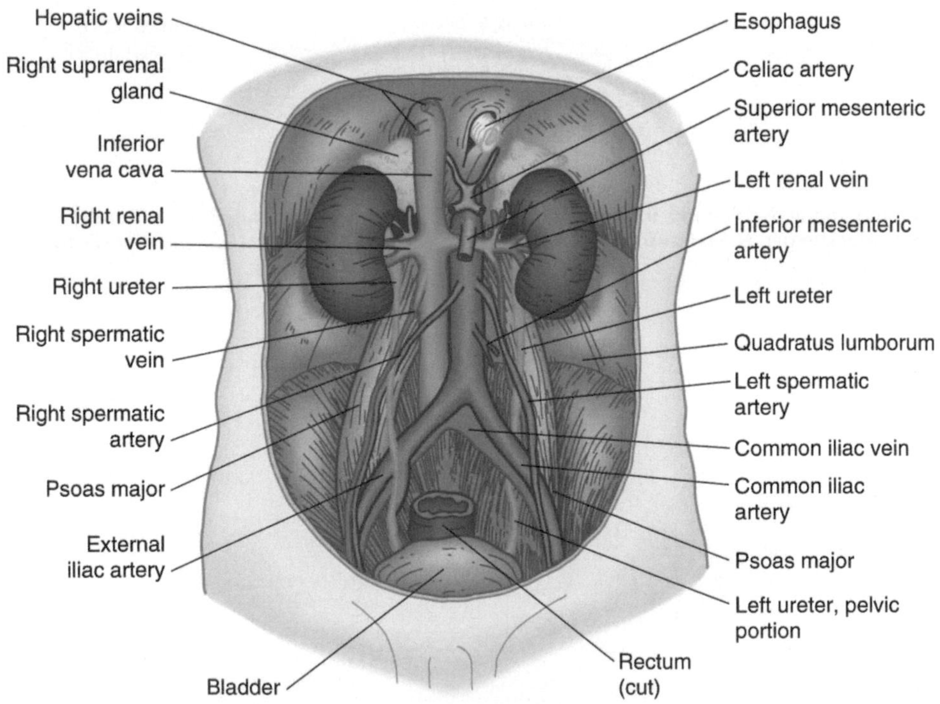

FIG. 139.1 Genitourinary anatomy and surrounding retroperitoneal structures. (From Shewakramani, S. (2018). Genitourinary system. In R. M. Walls, R. S. Hockberger, & M. Gausche-Hill (Eds.), *Rosen's emergency medicine: Concepts and clinical practice* (9th ed., p. 420, Fig. 40.1). Elsevier.)

- Causes include:
  - Penetrating injury in proximity to kidney
  - Blunt force to back or flank
  - Rapid deceleration injury

Clinical Presentation

- Flank pain or tenderness
- Flank ecchymosis
- Hematuria
- Can be associated with posterior or lower rib fractures.

Diagnosis and Evaluation

- Computed tomography (CT) of the abdomen/pelvis with IV contrast.
- CT urography
- American Association for the Surgery of Trauma (AAST) details five grades of renal trauma (Table 139.1 and Fig. 139.2).

Treatment

- Generally should be admitted for observation and serial evaluations.
- Penetrating trauma: low-grade injury may be managed conservatively; surgery for active bleeding or expanding hematoma.
- Blunt trauma: hemodynamically stable patients initially can be treated conservatively. Embolization or surgery should be considered for active bleeding.
- Clinical deterioration within 48 to 72 hours should prompt repeat CT.

TABLE 139.1 ***Renal Trauma Grading Scale by the American Association for the Surgery of Trauma (AAST)***

Grade	Type of Injury	Description
I	Contusion	Microscopic or gross hematuria; urologic studies normal
	Hematoma	Subcapsular, nonexpanding without parenchymal laceration
II	Hematoma	Nonexpanding perirenal hematoma confined to renal retroperitoneum
	Laceration	Less than 1.0 cm parenchymal depth of renal cortex without urinary extravasation
III	Laceration	More than 1.0 cm parenchymal depth of renal cortex without collecting system rupture or urinary extravasation
IV	Laceration	Parenchymal laceration extending through renal cortex, medulla, and collecting system
	Vascular	Main renal artery or vein injury with contained hemorrhage
V	Laceration	Completely shattered kidney
	Vascular	Avulsion of renal hilum which devascularizes kidney

(From Lee, Y. J., Oh, S. N., Rha, S. E., & Byun, J. Y. (2007). Renal trauma. *Radiologic Clinics of North America, 45*(3), 581–592, Table 1.)

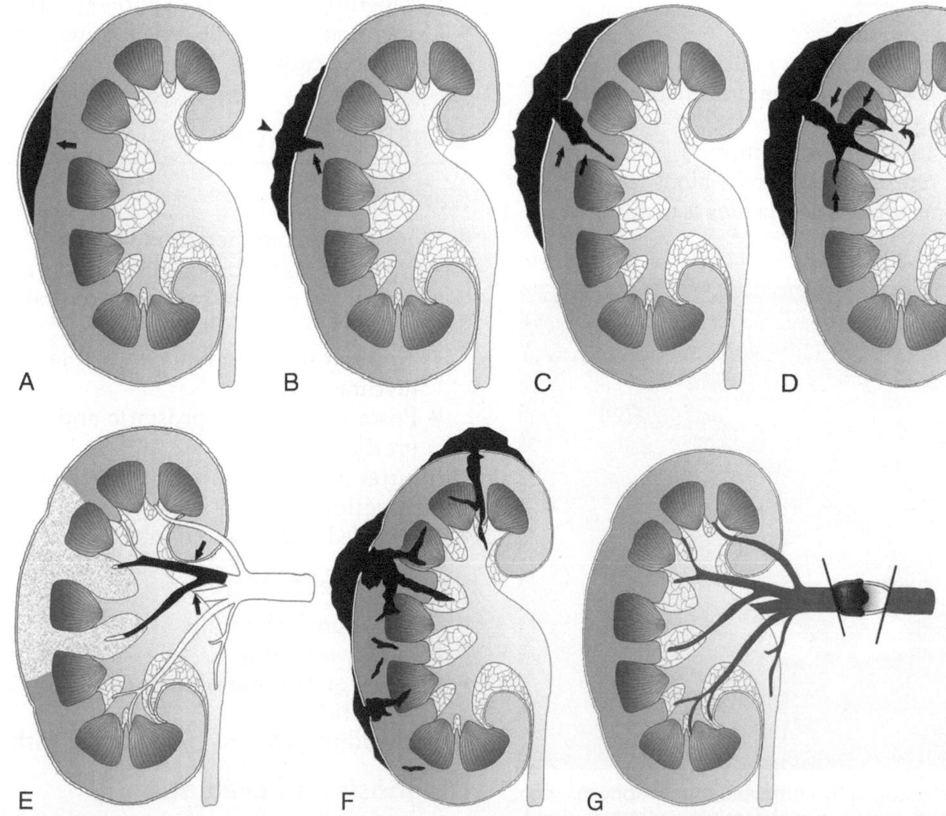

FIG. 139.2 Depiction of renal trauma grading scale by the American Association for the Surgery of Trauma (AAST). A: Grade I. B: Grade II. C: Grade III. D and E: Grade IV. F and G: Grade V. (From Lee, Y. J., Oh, S. N., Rha, S. E., & Byun, J. Y. (2007). Renal trauma. *Radiologic Clinics of North America, 45*(3), 581–592, Fig. 1.)

Ureteral Injury

General Principles

- The ureters are well insulated by surrounding structures, so isolated injury is rare.

Clinical Presentation

- Flank pain or tenderness
- Flank ecchymosis
- Hematuria
- Can be associated with lower rib or spinal fractures.
- No reliable or specific markers of ureteral injury, so these may have delayed presentations (e.g., acute renal insufficiency, fever, increasing flank pain or palpable mass suggestive of urinoma, hydronephrosis, abdominal distension, hemodynamic instability, sepsis without another source).

Diagnosis and Evaluation

- CT of the abdomen/pelvis with IV contrast
- CT urography
- Injuries described based on location and partial or complete transection.

Treatment

- Depending on the type of injury, ureteral stents, percutaneous nephrostomy tubes, or open reconstruction may be indicated.

Bladder Injury

General Principles

- Typically blunt mechanism.
- Associated with pelvic fractures: multirami pelvic fractures and anterior-posterior disruptions are higher risk for genitourinary injury.
- Extraperitoneal or intraperitoneal rupture
  - Intraperitoneal ruptures occur from blunt lower abdominal trauma when the bladder is distended because the bladder dome is the weakest part of the bladder.
  - Extraperitoneal ruptures typically occur from shearing forces in pelvic fractures.

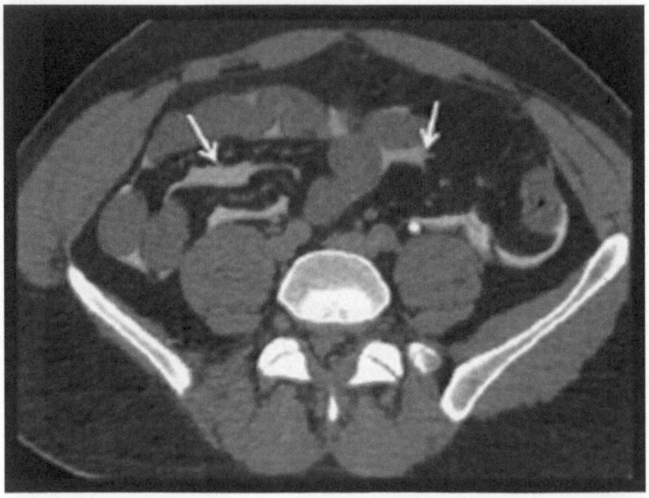

FIG. 139.3 Retrograde cystography computed tomography showing intraperitoneal bladder rupture with intraabdominal contrast visualized. (From Shewakramani, S. (2018). Genitourinary system. In R. M. Walls, R. S. Hockberger, & M. Gausche-Hill (Eds.), *Rosen's emergency medicine: Concepts and clinical practice* (9th ed., p. 428, Fig. 40.15C). Elsevier.)

Clinical Presentation

- Abdominal pain and tenderness
- Hematuria
- Difficulty urinating

Diagnosis and Evaluation

- Retrograde cystography: evaluates for bladder rupture (Fig. 139.3).
  - Can be performed with x-ray or CT (CT more sensitive).
  - Indications
    - Penetrating lower abdominal or pelvic trauma
    - Gross hematuria
    - Pelvic fracture with microscopic hematuria
  - Should instill bladder with contrast rather than passive bladder filling with excreted IV contrast. Instilling contrast distends the bladder and demonstrates extravasation if injury is present; passive filling may miss injuries.
  - With concern for pelvic vascular injury, delay cystography until after angiography, because contrast from cystography can obscure pelvic vessels.

Treatment

- Extraperitoneal injuries are typically nonoperative unless there are also bladder neck or concomitant intraabdominal injuries that require surgical exploration or repair.
- Intraperitoneal injuries require operative repair.
- Urine should be drained via a urinary catheter or a suprapubic catheter.

Urethral Injury

General Principles

- More common in men than women.
- Anterior or posterior segments of the male urethra anatomically divided by the urogenital diaphragm (Fig. 139.4).
  - Anterior segment: bulbous, penile, and glandular urethra
  - Posterior segment: prostatic and membranous urethra
- Injuries may be classified as partial or complete transections.
- Associated with straddle injuries and pelvic fractures.

Clinical Presentation

- Blood at urethral meatus
- Difficulty urinating
- Perineal or external genitalia hematomas, ecchymoses, or lacerations
- High-riding prostate (rare finding with low sensitivity)

Diagnosis and Evaluation

- Retrograde urethrography (RUG)
  - A partial transection (Fig. 139.5) will show both bladder contrast and extravasation, whereas a complete

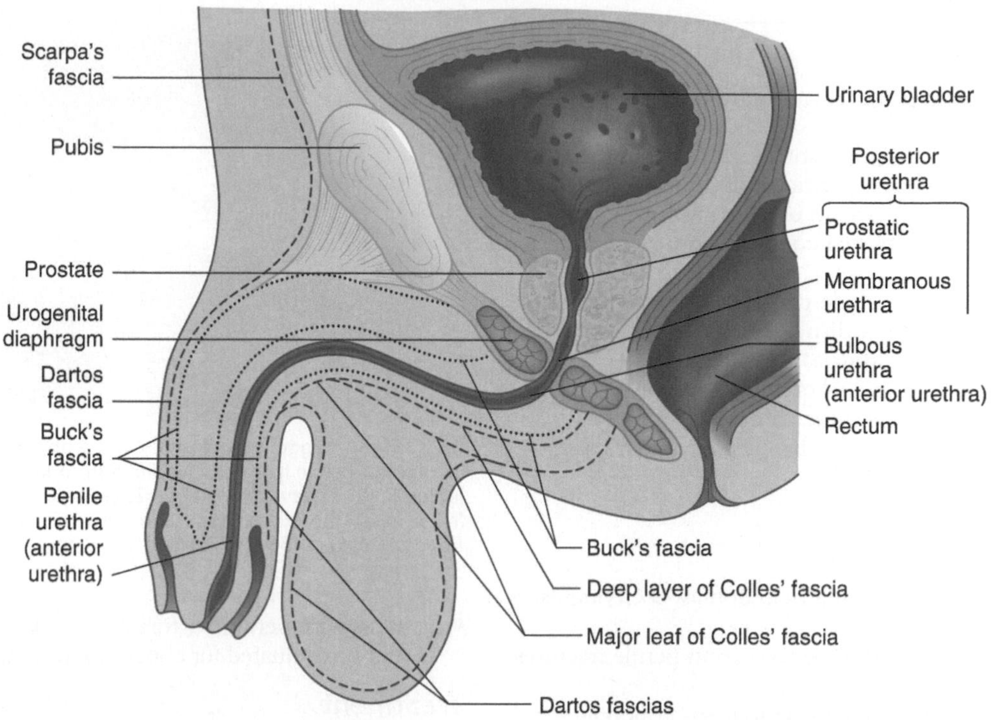

FIG. 139.4 Male lower genitourinary anatomy. (From Shewakramani S. (2018). Genitourinary system. In R. M. Walls, R. S. Hockberger, & M. Gausche-Hill (Eds.), *Rosen's emergency medicine: Concepts and clinical practice* (9th ed., p. 421, Fig. 40.3). Elsevier.)

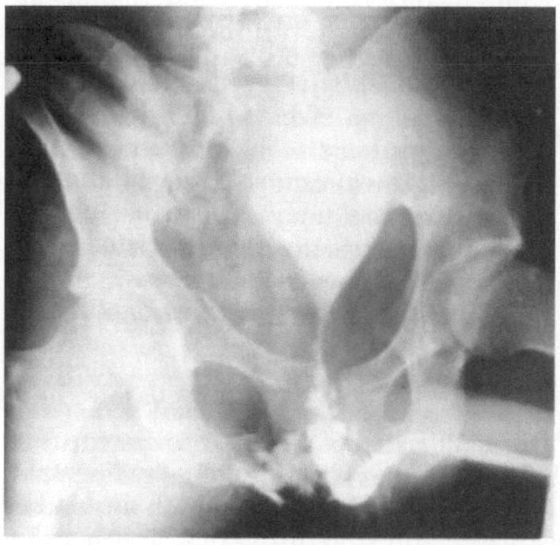

FIG. 139.5 Retrograde urethrogram showing a partial urethral disruption. (From Spirnak, J. P. (1988). Pelvic fracture and injury to the lower urinary tract. *Surgical Clinics of North America, 68*, 1057.)

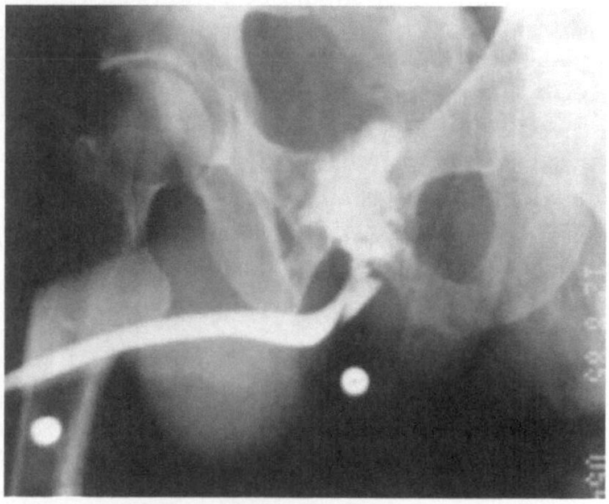

FIG. 139.6 Retrograde urethrogram showing a complete urethral disruption. (From Spirnak, J. P. (1988). Pelvic fracture and injury to the lower urinary tract. *Surgical Clinics of North America, 68*, 1057.)

transection (Fig. 139.6) will not show any bladder contrast.

- Female urethras are short, so rather than performing a RUG, perform a vaginal examination and consider diagnostic urethroscopy by urology.
- With concern for pelvic vascular injury, consider delaying RUG until after vascular imaging, because contrast from the RUG can obscure pelvic vessels.

Treatment

- Typically managed conservatively unless there is a penetrating injury or concomitant bladder or rectal injury. Delayed repair is associated with better outcomes in men.
- Urine should be drained via urinary catheter or suprapubic catheter; in general, if a urethral injury is diagnosed, consult urology regarding urinary catheter placement, because the act of placing the catheter can potentially exacerbate the urethral injury.
- Patients with partial anterior urethral injuries with a urinary or suprapubic catheter in place may be discharged home with outpatient follow-up
- In female patients, if a urinary catheter does not pass, diagnostic urethroscopy and possible surgical repair if a urethral injury is found.

139

External Genitalia

General Principles

- Includes injuries to penis, scrotum, testes, labia, and vagina.
- Female patients with significant external genital trauma are highly likely to have additional injuries. Missed vaginal injuries can be a source of significant hemorrhage in addition to delayed complications, such as fistulas.
- Male genital injuries include penile fracture or amputation, testicular rupture or displacement, hematoceles or hydroceles, and zipper injuries. Penile fractures, typically caused by sexual intercourse, and testicular ruptures occur when the tunica albuginea ruptures. The tunica albuginea covers the corpora cavernosa and the testicles (Fig. 139.7).

Clinical Presentation

- Pain and tenderness
- Perineal or external genitalia hematomas, ecchymoses, or lacerations
- "Eggplant deformity" of the penis seen in penile fractures (Fig. 139.8)
- Difficulty urinating or hematuria suggests concomitant urethral injury.

Diagnosis and Evaluation

- Vaginal examinations should be performed with pelvic injuries to assess for vaginal bleeding, lacerations, or bone fragments. Female patients who do not tolerate bedside examination may require an examination under anesthesia.
- Scrotal or penile ultrasound to evaluate blunt male GU trauma, looking for fascial defects and changes in blood flow. Loss of testicular contour or heterogeneous appearance is consistent with testicular rupture.

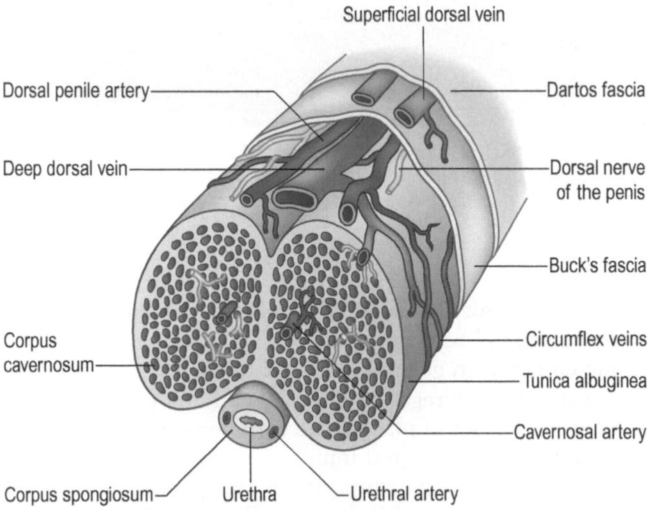

FIG. 139.7 Penile anatomy. (From Edey, A. J., Wilkins, C. J., & Sidhu, P. S. (2011). Ultrasound of the penis. In P. L. Allan, G. M. Baxter, & M. J. Weston (Eds.), *Clinical ultrasound* (3rd ed., p. 622, Fig. 32.1). Elsevier.)

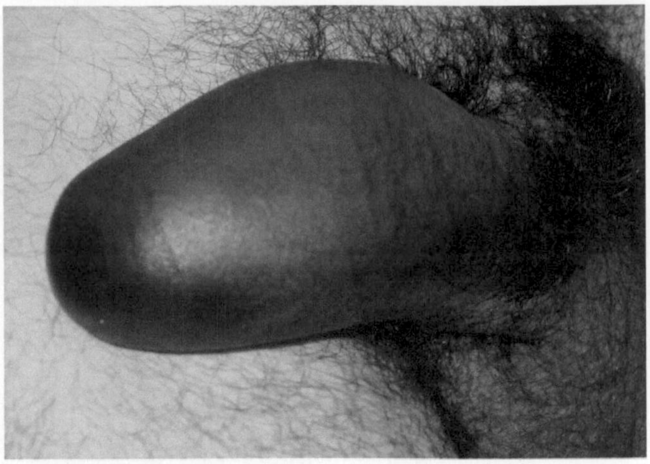

FIG. 139.8 "Eggplant deformity" on a physical examination concerning for penile fracture. (Modified from Koifman, L., Barros, R., Júnior, R. A. S., Cavalcanti, A. G., & Favorito, L. A. (2010). Penile fracture: Diagnosis, treatment and outcomes of 150 patients. *Urology, 76*(6), 1488–1492, Fig. 1.)

- Patients with penile fracture or penetrating penile trauma should be evaluated for concomitant urethral injury.

Treatment

Female GU Injury

- Unless rapidly expanding, vulvar and vaginal hematomas typically can be managed conservatively.
- Superficial lacerations to vulva and vagina can be repaired with absorbable sutures. Deep vaginal lacerations and injuries may require operative repair and washout.

Male GU Injury

- Superficial penile hematomas may be managed conservatively.
- Superficial lacerations can be repaired with absorbable suture.
- Testicular torsion, testicular rupture, testicular displacement, penile fractures, or penetrating injuries with violation of the corpora cavernosa require immediate operative repair.
- An amputated penis requires expedient evaluation for reimplantation. The amputated part should be wrapped in moist gauze and stored in a plastic bag and placed in an ice water bath (tissue should not have direct contact with ice). Reimplantation should occur within 6 hours of warm ischemia and 16 hours of cold ischemia.
- Zipper injuries require zipper removal, pain control (consider dorsal penile nerve block), and local wound care.

SUGGESTED READINGS

Bryant, W. K., & Shewakramani, S. (2017). Emergency management of renal and genitourinary trauma: Best practices update. *Emergency Medicine Practice, 19*(8), 1–20.

Morey, A. F., Brandes, S., Dugi, D. D., et al. (2017). *Urotrauma Guideline*. American Urologic Association. Available at: https://www.auanet.org. Accessed May 31, 2019.

Shewakramani, S. (2018). Genitourinary system. In R. M. Walls, R. S. Hockberger, & M. Gausche-Hill (Eds.), *Rosen's emergency medicine: Concepts and clinical practice* (9th ed., pp. 419–434). Elsevier.

CHAPTER **140**

BOARD REVIEW

Facial Trauma

MICHAEL TETWILER, MD, MPH, and DENNIS HSIEH, MD, JD

Special consideration is warranted when facial trauma occurs, because cosmesis and function are of heightened importance. Trauma to the face is highly associated with assaults, motor vehicle crashes, falls, sports, and gunshot wounds. The injuries can range from simple abrasions requiring no treatment to sight- or life-threatening polytrauma involving globe rupture, traumatic brain injury, cervical (c-spine) injury, and airway compromise. Note that the mechanism predicts severity of injury. Nonaccidental trauma should always be considered as an etiology of the injury.

General Principles

- History is important but can be limited. Pay special attention to motor, sensory, visual, hearing, taste, or smell changes. Consider associated intracranial and neck injury. For any fluid seen, consider cerebral spinal fluid (CSF) leak.
- Airway should be assessed first. After airway, assess for lacerations, contusions, symmetry, function, abnormal motion, crepitus, tenderness, step-offs. The face has many bones (Fig. 140.1). Concern for fracture necessitates imaging: noncontrast head computed tomography (CT) is 90% sensitive for fractures and only goes down to near the orbits. If high suspicion for injury and head CT is negative or fracture location is below where head CT would image, dedicated maxillo facial imaging is recommended. Children are more likely to have associated brain and c-spine injuries.
- Outside of airway compromise and life-threatening exsanguination, treatment of facial injuries can be deferred until after life-threatening injuries are addressed. Nondisplaced or minimally displaced closed fractures can be addressed on an outpatient basis within 7 days for adults and within 3 days for children. Open fractures or those that violate sinuses should get antibiotics (first generation cephalosporin or amoxicillin clavulanate for 7 to 10 days). Ensure tetanus vaccination is up to date.

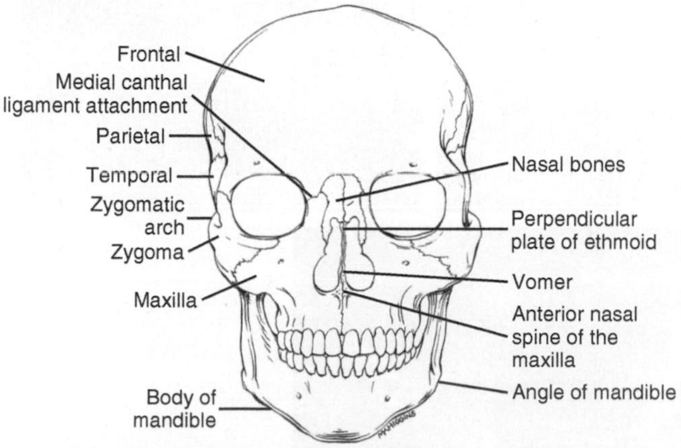

FIG. 140.1 Anterior view of the skull and facial bones. (From Eiff, M. P. (2020). Facial and skull fractures. In M. P. Eiff & R. L. Hatch (Eds.), *Fracture management: For primary care and emergency medicine* (4th ed., Fig. 17.1). Elsevier.)

Skin/Soft-Tissue, Nerve, and Vascular Trauma

Clinical Presentation

- Skin/soft tissue
  - Abrasions, lacerations, contusions: evident on physical examination; may have debris that will have to be cleaned.
- Nerves
  - Numbness: consider fractures causing neuropraxia, compression by hematoma, or nerve laceration.
  - Paralysis: consider peripheral neuropraxia or nerve laceration if acute, but also central causes, including strokes, intracranial hemorrhage, and mechanical obstruction of function.
- Vasculature
  - Rapid bleeding/massive bleeding: consider arterial injury.

Diagnosis and Evaluation

- Skin/soft tissue
  - Assess for depth, location, injury to underlying structures, including arteries and cartilage, and foreign bodies.
- Nerves
  - Assess motor and sensory function.
- Vascular
  - Assess amount and rapidity of bleeding.

Treatment

- Skin/soft tissue: cosmesis is key. Address contamination/potential for tattooing; definitive treatment can be undertaken as long as 24 hours after injury.
  - Abrasions: topical lidocaine for anesthesia, clean, then antibiotic ointment
  - Contusions: ice/elevation
  - Open wound: explore for foreign body, fractures.
    - Deeper than dermis: close with sutures.
    - Shallow: apply skin adhesive.
  - Simple facial lacerations: no antibiotics, except for bites or lacerations through the buccal mucosa, cartilage, or in presence of extensive contamination

- Nerves: if deficits, address underlying injuries; otherwise, outpatient follow-up.
- Vascular: most are self-limited and do not require specialized treatment.
  - Significant bleeding: ligate vessel, but be careful not to injure nerves or ducts.
  - Massive, uncontrollable bleeding: arterial embolization, external carotid ligation (last resort)

Eye/Orbital/Lacrimal Duct Trauma

Clinical Presentation

- Emphysema of orbit and eyelids: consider fracture into sinus.
- Telecanthus (increased distance between medial canthi): consider medial canthal tendon laceration/avulsion and naso-orbitoethmoid fracture.
- Infraorbital anesthesia: consider fracture of orbital floor with resulting damage to infraorbital nerve.
- Enophthalmos: consider orbital wall fracture, which may be masked by edema.
- Exophthalmos: consider retrobulbar hematoma, which may be associated with decreased visual acuity and increased intraocular pressure owing to ischemic neuropathy.
- Diplopia, limited extraocular movement, or pain with extraocular movement: consider global orbital edema, nerve paresis, entrapment of inferior rectus (cannot look upward; see Fig. 140.2), or other extraocular muscles.
- Decreased/loss of visual acuity: consider globe rupture (also teardrop-shaped pupil, severe subconjunctival hemorrhage, extrusion of intraocular contents), retinal detachment, lens dislocation, corneal abrasion/edema, traumatic iritis, intraocular bleed/vitreous hemorrhage, retrobulbar hematoma, and optic nerve injury.
- Bilateral orbital ecchymosis (raccoon eyes): consider basilar skull fracture.
- Epiphora (excessive tearing): consider lacrimal duct obstruction owing to trauma, ocular surface irritation/injury, and nerve (CN VII) dysfunction.

Diagnosis and Evaluation

- Evaluate from above for symmetry of the globes.
- Complete ocular examination: visual acuity, extraocular movements, visual fields, fluorescein, anterior chamber, pressure, fundoscopy, swinging flashlight test to evaluate for afferent pupillary defect.
- If concern for chemical exposure, test pH.
- If concern for retinal detachment or vitreous hemorrhage, bedside ultrasound.
- Assess for lacerations in the medial aspect of eyelids, especially if medial to the lacrimal punctum for duct injury. If high suspicion, consult ophthalmology.
- If high concern for orbital fracture, CT of the face or orbits.

Treatment

- Eyebrow laceration: realign the brow (without shaving), and close the deep muscle layer.
- Simple eyelid laceration: single-layer repair
- Globe rupture: shield; obtain emergent ophthalmology consultation.
- Retrobulbar hematoma: lateral canthotomy with cantholysis if intraocular pressure is greater than 40 or compromised vision (decreased visual acuity or afferent pupillary defect), After canthotomy with cantholysis, emergent ophthalmology consult.
- Isolated orbital fracture: follow up within 1 week.
  - Antibiotics, nasal decongestants, precautions regarding nose blowing.
  - Entrapment or facial asymmetry: follow up within 24 hours.
  - Nasoorbitoethmoid fractures: specialty consultation.
  - Lacrimal duct injury (Fig. 140.3): consult ophthalmology.

Forehead/Nose/Midface Trauma (Fig. 140.4)

Clinical Presentation

- Lacerations may overlie frontal sinus fractures or skull fractures. Fluid leak: concern for CSF leak.

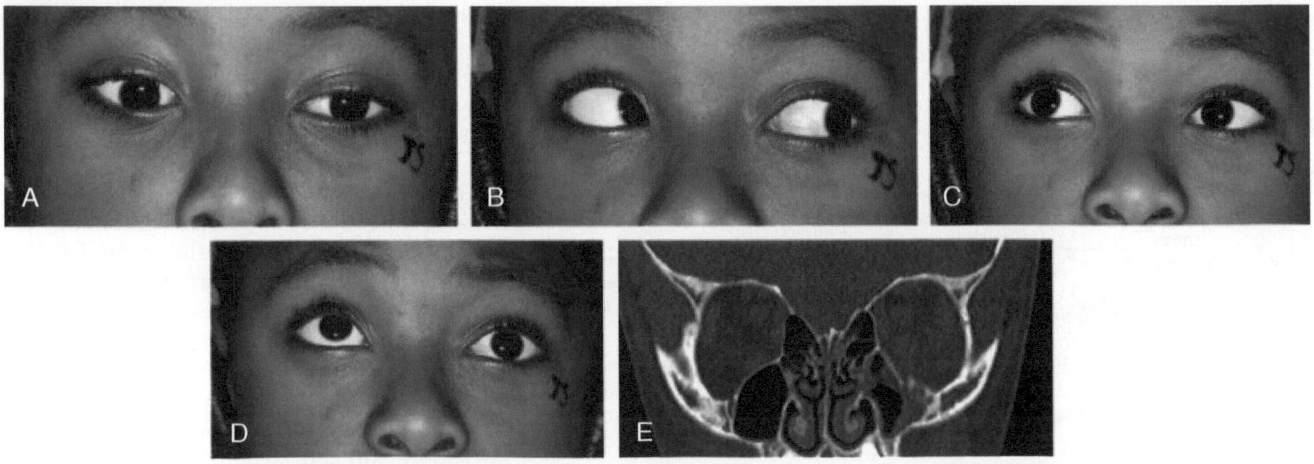

FIG. 140.2 Patient with entrapment of inferior rectus muscle caused by left orbital floor fracture. Note classic description of white eye blowout fracture. **A**, No restriction in downward gaze. **B**, No restriction on lateral gaze. **C**, No restriction on medial gaze. **D**, Restriction of upward gaze owing to physical entrapment of inferior rectus muscle. **E**, Coronal CT demonstrating left orbital floor "trap-door" fracture with entrapment of inferior rectus muscle. (From Kholaki, O., Hammer, D. A., & Schlieve, T. (2019). Management of orbital fractures. *Atlas of the Oral and Maxillofacial Surgery Clinics*, 27(2), 157–165, Fig. 2.)

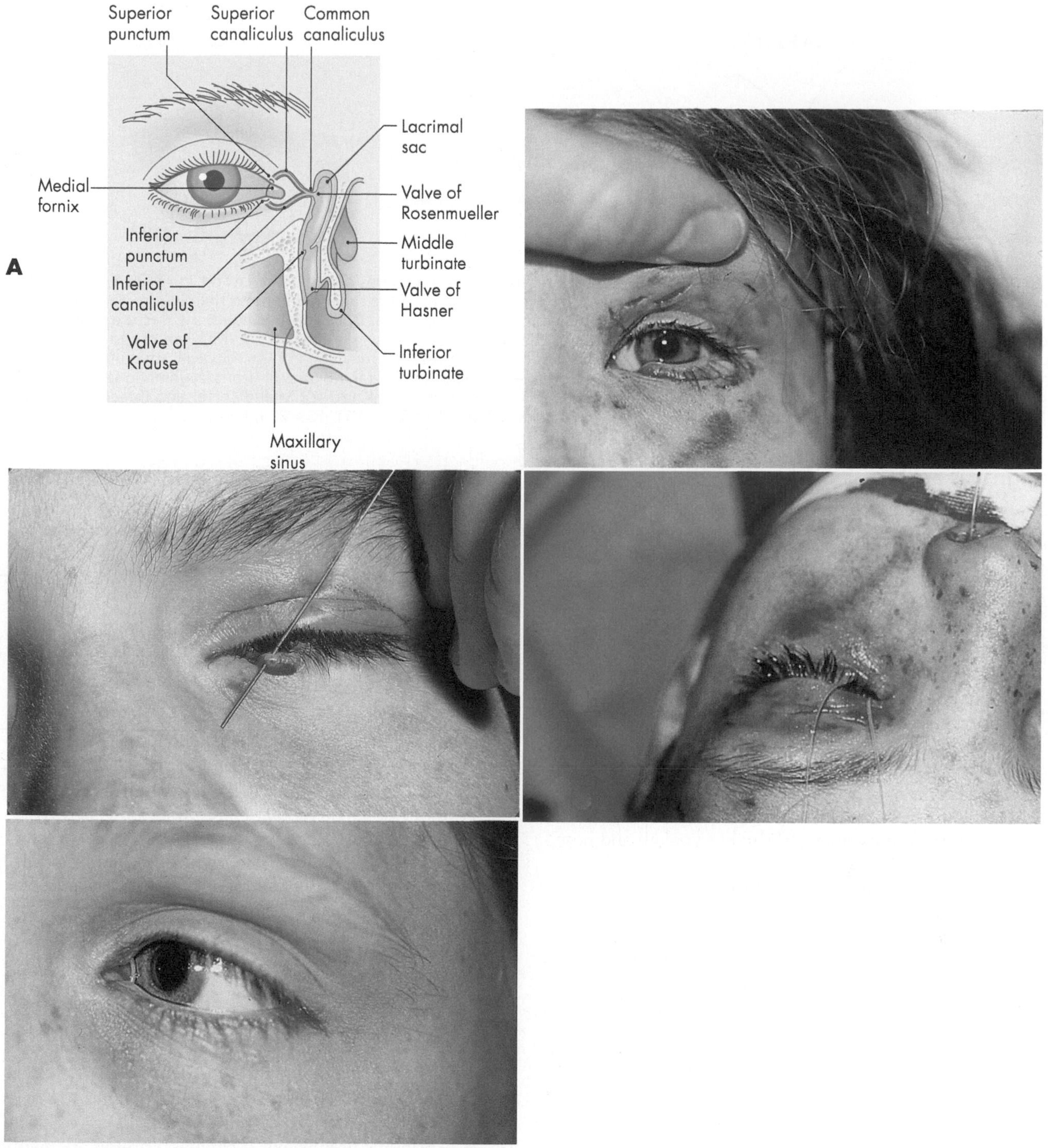

FIG. 140.3 Repair of lacrimal duct injuries. A, Anatomy of the nasolacrimal system. **B**, Medial laceration of the lower eyelid in a 9-year-old girl caused by a dog bite. **C**, Cannulation with a probe confirms the lacrimal transection in a different patient. **D**, Anterograde cannulation of nasolacrimal system through the upper and lower eyelid puncta with Crawford tubes. **E**, The tubes are kept in place for 3 months after repair of the laceration. The Silastic loop can be seen in the medial aspect of the eye between the puncta. (From Eppley, B. L. (2012). Primary repair of facial soft tissue injuries. In P. W. Booth, B. L. Eppley, & R. Schmelzeisen (Eds.), *Maxillofacial trauma and esthetic facial reconstruction* (2nd ed., pp. 342–367, Fig. 19.14). Elsevier Saunders.)

- Contusions over cheekbones, enophthalmos, malocclusion of upper teeth, and/or movement of hard palate while forehead is stabilized: consider midface fractures.
  - Le Fort I: transverse fracture separating the body of the maxilla from the pterygoid plate and nasal septum
  - Le Fort II: pyramidal fracture through the central maxilla and hard palate
  - Le Fort III: craniofacial dysfunction when the entire face is separated from the skull owing to fractures of the frontozygomatic suture line, the orbits, and through the base of the nose and ethmoids
- Epistaxis, nasal tenderness, crepitus, abnormal movement, trouble breathing through nares: consider nasal bone fracture; examine for nasal septal hematoma.
- Rhinorrhea: consider CSF leak.

140

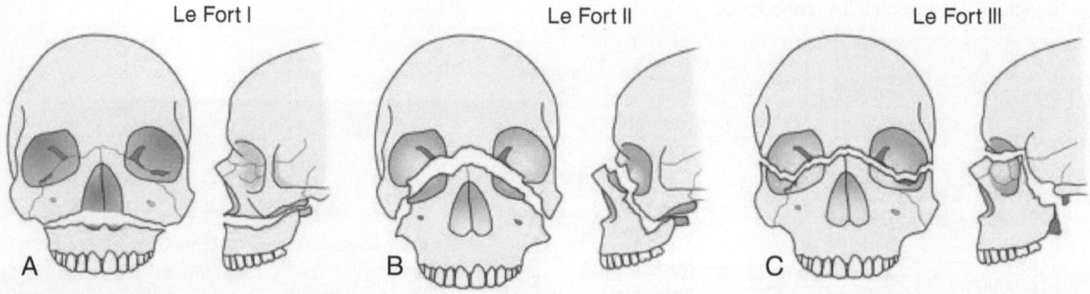

FIG. 140.4 Le Fort fractures, levels I–III. This figure depicts the classic fracture patterns described by Le Fort in 1901. **A,** Le Fort I level fracture: the horizontal plane of the fracture extends between the pterygoid plates of the sphenoid bone to the piriform aperture and lateral nasal wall. The Le Fort I fracture involves the maxilla, including the maxillary sinus. **B**, Le Fort II fracture: the fracture propagates from the pterygoid plates posteriorly, through the orbital floor, to the nasofrontal suture. In bilateral cases, this gives rise to the classic "pyramidal" pattern. **C**, Craniofacial disjunction, or the Le Fort III fracture: involves total separation of the midfacial structures from the cranial base. This level of fracture propagates from the pterygoid plates, through the lateral orbital wall (frontozygomatic suture), by the orbital floor, to the nasofrontal suture. (From Avery, L. L., Susarla, S. M., & Novelline, R. A. (2011). Multidetector and three-dimensional CT evaluation of the patient with maxillofacial injury. *Radiologic Clinics of North America, 49*(1), 183–203, Fig. 13.)

Diagnosis and Evaluation

- Frontal bone
  - If concern for fracture, CT is needed to distinguish.
    - Skull fracture
    - Frontal sinus with anterior table fracture
    - Frontal sinus with anterior and posterior table fracture
  - Supraorbital ridge involvement: maxillofacial CT
- Midface: if suspecting fracture, can go straight to CT without pulling on face
  - For standardized test purposes: if you wish to examine (instead of going straight to imaging), hold the hard palate by the upper incisors and pull anteriorly/rock with one hand while stabilizing the forehead with the other.
    - Le Fort I: only the hard palate/teeth (upper alveolar ridge) move
    - Le Fort II: movement of the hard palate and nose, but not the eyes
    - Le Fort III: entire face will shift with globes held in place only by the optic nerve
    - Note that the clear distinctions of the Le Fort classifications above are somewhat theoretic, because most patients present with mixed fracture types (e.g., Le Fort II on the left and Le Fort III on the right).
- Nose
  - Hold each nare closed and check for air flow through the contralateral nare.
  - Check for nasal cartilage involvement.
  - Visualize the septum to check for septal hematoma.
  - If suspecting a nasal fracture, x-rays or CT of the face can be done to document injury, but will unlikely change management.

Treatment

- Frontal bone
  - Isolated anterior table fractures: nasal/oral decongestants, oral antibiotics, and close follow-up with facial surgeon
  - Posterior table fractures require neurosurgery consultation.
  - Patient with depressed fractures should be admitted for intravenous (IV) antibiotics and operative repair.
- Midface
  - Isolated Le Fort I or stable Le Fort II fractures without concerning features
    - Consult and consider discharge.
  - Le Fort III: admission and IV antibiotics
  - CSF leak: elevate head of bed 40 to 60 degrees, antibiotics, neurosurgery consultation.
- Nose
  - Epistaxis: compression for at least 10 minutes, packing if needed
  - Nasal septal hematoma: incision, drainage, and packing
  - Isolated nasal bone fracture: outpatient follow-up

Zygoma Trauma

Clinical Presentation

- Loss of cheek projection/flattening of malar eminence: consider isolated zygomatic arch fracture versus zygomaticomaxillary fracture (quadripod fracture, formally tripod fracture) that involves the lateral orbital wall, separation of maxilla and zygoma, zygomatic arch, orbital floor.

Diagnosis and Evaluation

- Evaluate by looking from above.
- CT of the face to define extent of injury if asymmetry is appreciated

Treatment

- Isolated zygomatic arch fractures: discharge with follow-up.
  - Antibiotic prophylaxis if paranasal sinuses are involved
- Quadripod fracture with presence of loss or change of vision requires surgical consultation, admission for IV antibiotics, and operative repair.

Oropharynx/Airway/Mandible Trauma

Clinical Presentation

- Intraoral trauma (bleeding, dysphonia, excessive drooling, swelling of tongue, avulsed teeth): consider airway compromise.
- Dysarthria: consider tongue trauma, mandibular fracture/dislocation, and neurologic deficit.

- Expanding facial/extraoral hematoma: consider predicted course and airway compromise.
- Teeth malocclusion/jaw asymmetry (deviation): consider maxilla and mandibular fractures (including alveolar ridge), mandible dislocation, and dental trauma in addition to Le Fort fracture and zygoma fracture.
- Trismus: consider soft-tissue hematoma interfering with jaw opening and fractures of the coronoid process, neck, rami, or zygoma.
- Mucosal ecchymosis and lacerations: consider underlying fracture and open fracture, respectively.
- Contusion or injury to cheek, bloody discharge from duct: consider injury to gland or duct (may not be obvious).

Diagnosis and Evaluation

- Assess ability to maintain airway and listen to the patient's voice (dysphonia, dysarthria).
- Inspect/palpate surface anatomy and ensure no expanding hematoma.
- Inspect vermillion border.
- Intraoral examination, including inspection of teeth, mouth opening
- Tongue blade test: check for malocclusion/fracture: instruct patient to bite down on tongue blade and sustain the hold as examiner pulls on and breaks the tongue blade away (95.7% sensitivity for mandibular fracture).
- Place finger into external auditory canal while opening/closing mouth to check for condyle fracture.
- Externally assess for injury in the area of the parotid and explore any laceration.
- Internally assess for the opening of the Stenson (parotid) duct opposite to the second molar. Compress the gland and look for bloody discharge (abnormal).
- Imaging (Fig. 140.5)
  - Mandible: panorex superior to plain films for fracture detection
  - Facial/mandible CT if complex fracture suspected
  - Chest x-ray for associated dental trauma to check for tooth aspiration

Treatment

- Airway
  - Jaw thrust, head tilt, and chin lift may mitigate partial obstruction.

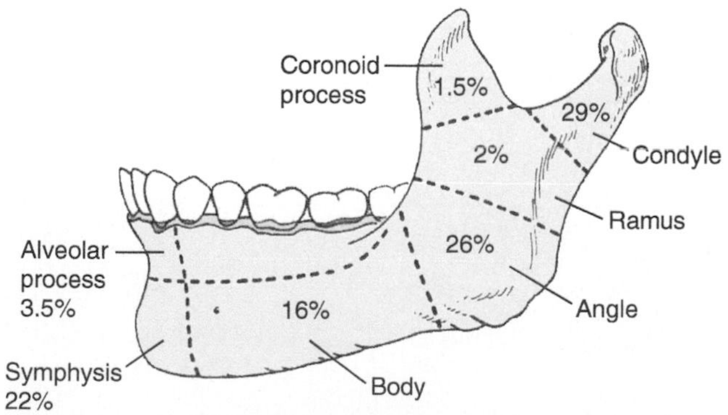

FIG. 140.5 Anatomic classification and percent distribution of mandibular fractures in dentate adult patient. (From Chung. W., & Shah, G. A. (2018). Fractures of the mandible. In E. N. Myers & C. H. Snyderman (Eds.), *Operative otolaryngology: Head and neck surgery* (3rd ed., Fig. 185.1). Elsevier.)

  - Clear out debris.
  - Have double suction available.
  - If unable to maintain airway, perform orotracheal intubation or surgical airway.
    - Gunshot wound/trauma to lower third of face often requires surgical airway.
  - Rapidly expanding hematoma that affects neck/supraclavicular area: awake orotracheal intubation
  - Blind nasotracheal intubation is not recommended in the setting of facial trauma and contraindicated in those with skull base or cribiform plate fractures.
- Lips
  - Mark vermillion border with pen before injecting local anesthesia or, ideally, use a nerve block to prevent distortion of the anatomy (mental nerve block for lower lip, infraorbital nerve block for upper lip).
  - Use nonabsorbable suture for superficial layer.
  - If deep, perform multilayer closure.
- Perioral electrical burns
  - Evaluate for other injuries; delayed labial artery hemorrhage (in 5 to 21 days) may occur; rapid follow-up indicated (within 24 to 48 hours).
- Through and through laceration involving oral mucosa
  - Close in layers: start intraorally and work outward.
  - Irrigate between each layer.
- Intra-oral lacerations/tongue lacerations
  - If small (less than 2 cm), no repair is required: instruct the patient to swish and spit with antiseptic at home.
  - Larger lacerations (more than 2 cm) or those deep enough to trap food require repair with absorbable sutures.
  - Deep tongue lacerations require two- to three-layer repair (deep muscle, submucosa, mucosa).
- Mandible
  - Dislocation: relocate using intraoral or extraoral technique.
  - Closed fractures: apply a Barton bandage (ace wrap around top of head and under mandible or splinting (wiring jaw shut and outpatient follow-up). Children should have follow-up within 24 to 48 hours, given rapid remodeling.
  - Open fractures: IV antibiotics (covering gram-negative rods and anaerobes) and admission for operative repair
- Salivary gland injury
  - Consult ear, nose, and throat or plastic surgery: Stenson (parotid) or Wharton (submandibular) duct may need repair over a stent to prevent formation of cutaneous fistula.

Auricular Trauma

Clinical Presentation

- External: laceration, abrasion, subcutaneous hematomas
- Internal: external canal trauma, hemotympanum; if otorrhea, consider CSF leak.
- Mastoid ecchymosis: consider basilar skull fracture.

Diagnosis and Evaluation

- External: assess for hematoma and lacerations/cartilage involvement.

- Internal: otoscopy to examine for fluid leak, hemotympanum, ruptured tympanic membrane, canal trauma
- NOTE: Fluid on filter paper does not distinguish CSF from saline, saliva, or other clear fluids, but classic teaching has the "halo" effect where CSF makes an additional ring outside of the blood on the filter paper.

Treatment

- Auricular hematoma: drain and place pressure dressing.
- Cartilage: repair with 4-0 absorbable suture and give oral antibiotics, with consideration for *Pseudomonas*.
- Degloving/significant injury: consult specialist to save the cartilage.

SUGGESTED READINGS

Mayersak, R. J. (2018). Facial trauma. In R. M. Walls, R. S. Hockberger, & M. Gausche-Hill (Eds.), *Rosen's emergency medicine: Concepts and clinical practice* (9th ed., pp. 330–344). Elsevier.

Roth, F. S., Koshy, J. C., Goldberg, J. S., & Soparker, C. N. S. (2010). Pearls of orbital trauma management. *Seminars in Plastic Surgery, 24*(4), 398–410. doi:10.1055/s-0030-1269769.

Stewart, C. (2008). Maxillofacial trauma: Challenges in ED diagnosis and management. *Emergency Medicine Practice, 10*(2), 1–20.

Spine and Neck Trauma

ROBERT CAREY, MD, and KIAN PRESTON-SUNI, MD, MPH

Traumatic injuries of the spine and neck are commonly seen in the emergency department, most often from motor vehicle accidents, gunshot wounds, stab wounds, and falls. Although much of the eventual management of significant neck and spine trauma is surgical, the role of the emergency physician in stabilization, resuscitation, targeted physical examination, and appropriate diagnostic workup is essential.

On initial presentation, spine and neck trauma are typically divided by mechanism into blunt or penetrating trauma; neck trauma can also be classified as a hanging/strangulation injury.

Spine Injuries

General Principles

- Cervical spine and thoracolumbar junction are the most commonly injured areas.

Clinical Presentation

- Denis 3-column model: injuries to two or more columns are unstable (Fig. 141.1).
  - **Anterior column:** ant. vertebral body + disk, ant. longitudinal ligament. **Middle column:** post. vertebral body + disk, post. longitudinal ligament. **Posterior column:** laminae, pedicles, facets, transverse processes, ligaments, spinous processes, and so forth.
- Unstable cervical spine (C-spine) fractures mnemonic: **J**efferson **B**it **O**ff **A** **H**angman's **T**humb
  - **J**efferson (C1 burst), **B**ilateral facet dislocation, **O**dontoid (types II and III), **A**tlanto-occipital dissociation, **H**angman fracture (C2 pedicle fracture), **F**lexion teardrop (Table 141.1)

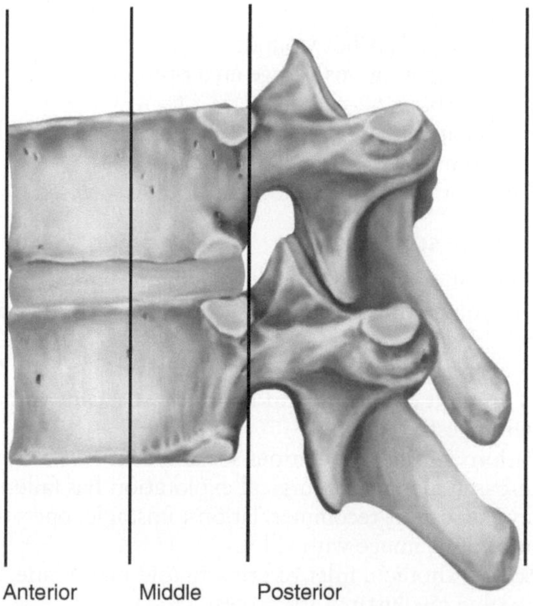

FIG. 141.1 Denis three column model of the spine. (From Dahdaleh, N., Viljoen S., et al. (2013). Surgical stabilization techniques for thoracolumbar fractures. In D. H. Kim, A. R. Vaccaro, C. A. Dickman, D. Cho, S. Lee, & I. Kim (Eds.), *Surgical anatomy and techniques to the spine* (2nd ed., pp. 365–374). Elsevier.)

TABLE 141.1 Classification of Cervical Spine Injuries

Mechanism of Spinal Injury	Stability
Flexion	
Wedge fracture	Stable
Flexion teardrop fracture	Extremely unstable
Clay shoveler fracture	Stable
Subluxation	Potentially unstable
Atlantooccipital dislocation	Unstable
Anterior atlantoaxial dislocation with or without fracture	Unstable
Odontoid fracture with lateral displacement	Unstable
Fracture of transverse process	Stable
Flexion Rotation	
Unilateral facet dislocation	Stable
Rotary atlantoaxial dislocation	Unstable
Extension	
Posterior neural arch fracture (C1)	Unstable
Hangman fracture (C2)	Unstable
Extension teardrop fracture	Usually stable in flexion; unstable in extension
Posterior atlantoaxial dislocation, with or without fracture	Usually stable in flexion; unstable in extension
Vertical Compression	
Bursting fracture of vertebral body	Stable
Jefferson fracture (C1 burst fracture)	Extremely unstable
Isolated fractures of articular pillar and vertebral body	Stable

(From Kaji, A. H., & Hockberger, R. S. (2018). Spinal injuries. In R. M. Walls, R. S. Hockberger, & M. Gausche-Hill (Eds.), *Rosen's emergency medicine: Concepts and clinical practice* (9th ed., pp. 345–371). Elsevier.)

BOX 141.1 Clinical Features Associated With Blunt Cerebrovascular Injury

Clinical Features and Risk Factors

Unexplained neurologic deficit
Arterial bleeding from head and neck
Large or expanding neck hematoma
Cervical bruit in patient younger than 50 years of age
Glasgow Coma Score less than 9
Hanging or strangulation
Diffuse axonal injury seen on computed tomography
Fracture near a vessel:

- Basilar skull near carotid canal (petrous bone)
- Transverse foramen of cervical vertebrae

High-risk cervical spine injuries:

- Fractures of C1-C3
- Subluxation

- Blunt cerebrovascular injury (BCVI): diagnosis frequently delayed until after admission when neurologic deficit develops (Box 141.1).
- Thoracolumbar spine fractures
  - Thoracic: often pathologic, but generally stable; held in place by rib cage
  - Wedge compression fractures: anterior vertebral body compression, intact posteriorly
    - Unstable: more than 50% vertebral body height loss
  - Chance fracture: flexion and distraction causing transverse fracture through vertebra
    - Can be unstable: associated with intraabdominal injuries, lap belts
  - Burst fracture: compressive force pushes fragments outward
    - Posterior fragments displaced into spinal canal
    - Often missed on plain film
  - Flexion-distraction: like the chance fracture, but axis of rotation behind anterior longitudinal ligament, causing anterior compression
    - Failure of middle and posterior columns: unstable
  - Translational injuries: "slice" fracture, associated with tuck and roll from moving vehicle
    - Involves all three columns: unstable

Diagnosis and Evaluation

- Canadian C-spine Rule (CCR) 99.4% sensitive, 45.1% specific (Box 141.2)
  - No high-risk feature, *any* one low-risk feature, and able to rotate neck 45 degrees left and right: negative predictive value 100% for C-spine fracture
  - If CCR criteria met, clinically clear C-spine without imaging
- Thoracolumbar spine
  - Low risk for fracture if absence of back pain, spine tenderness, neurologic deficit, age more than 60, high-risk mechanism
- Plain films: largely replaced by computed tomography (CT) owing to superior sensitivity.
- CT
  - C-spine: highly sensitive for bony injury
  - Chest/abdomen/pelvis with reconstructions: adequate for thoracolumbar spine evaluation
  - CT angiography (CTA) neck: if concerned for BCVI

BOX 141.2 Canadian C-Spine Rule

No High-risk Features

- Age over 65 years
- Dangerous mechanism (fall more than 1 m, axial loading, high-speed motor vehicle collision, rollover, or ejection, recreational vehicle or bicycle accident)
- Presence of paresthesias

Any Low-risk Features

- Minor rear-end crash
- Sitting in the emergency department
- Ambulatory on scene or in emergency department
- Delayed-onset neck pain
- No midline tenderness

Treatment

- Maintain C-spine immobilization for C-spine fractures.
- Remove from backboard (risk for pressure sores and aspiration).
- Spinal motion restriction for thoracolumbar fracture (firm mattress okay).
- Surgical stabilization for unstable fractures
- BCVI: anticoagulation if minor (mild intimal injury, dissection with minimal luminal narrowing), surgery if major (occlusion, pseudoaneurysm, or transection).

Penetrating Neck Injuries

General Principles

- Penetrating neck trauma, defined as violation of the platysma, most commonly involves injury to vascular structures, followed by aerodigestive and spinal cord injuries. The injury mechanism determines which structures are likely affected, and the extent of involvement.
- High-velocity gunshot wounds (e.g., hunting rifles, military-style weapons): large area of injury with a straight path.
- Low-velocity gunshot wounds (e.g., handguns): smaller area of injury with unpredictable path.
- Stabbing or impalement: local structures affected.

Clinical Presentation

- Significant vascular or aerodigestive injury indicated by hemodynamic instability or by one or more "hard" or "soft" signs (Box 141.3).
- 80% of patients presenting with any hard sign and 20% with any soft sign are found to have significant vascular or aerodigestive injury.
- Location of injury determines structures at risk, although zone-based mandatory surgical exploration has fallen out of favor. Current recommendations: unstable, operating room; stable, image with CTA.
  - Zone I: thoracic inlet to cricothyroid membrane. May involve mediastinal structures.
  - Zone II: cricothyroid membrane to angle of mandible. Most penetrating injuries. Affects vascular, aerodigestive structures, spine, and spinal cord.
  - Zone III: above angle of mandible. May involve cranial structures.

BOX 141.3 *"Soft" and "Hard" Signs of Penetrating Neck Trauma*

Soft Signs

- Minor hemoptysis
- Hematemesis
- Dysphonia, dysphagia
- Subcutaneous or mediastinal air
- Nonexpanding hematoma
- Oropharyngeal bleeding
- Neurological findings
- Proximity wound

Hard Signs

- Rapidly expanding/pulsatile hematoma
- Massive hemoptysis
- Air bubbling from wound
- Severe hemorrhage
- Shock not responding to fluids
- Decreased or absent radial pulse
- Vascular bruit or thrill
- Stridor/hoarseness or airway compromise
- Cerebral ischemia
- +/– Massive subcutaneous emphysema

(From Claudius, I., & Newton, K. (2018). Neck. In R. M. Walls, R. S. Hockberger, & M. Gausche-Hill (Eds.), *Rosen's emergency medicine: Concepts and clinical practice* (9th ed., pp. 372–381). Elsevier.)

Diagnosis and Evaluation

- Obtain imaging in patients with significant trauma but with no hemodynamic instability or hard signs.
  - High-resolution CTA of neck is the test of choice for penetrating neck injuries.
  - Zone I: add CTA of chest. Zone III: add CTA of head
  - Esophagram and/or esophagoscopy: indicated within 24 hours if significant injury found or if high suspicion for aerodigestive injury
  - X-rays: poor sensitivity, but can demonstrate pneumomediastinum, pleural effusion, retropharyngeal air, foreign body, or bony/cartilaginous injury

Treatment

- Early intubation for suspected airway or vascular injury, any hard signs. Anticipate difficult airway: edema, tissue distortion common. Prepare for surgical airway. Awake fiberoptic oral intubation, if time allows.
- Direct pressure or Foley balloon in wound for active bleeding.
- Emergent surgical exploration for hemodynamic instability, hard signs, injury identified on CTA.
- Aerodigestive injury: admit, parenteral antibiotic prophylaxis, nothing by mouth, possible surgical debridement and repair versus esophageal diversion and exclusion.
- Cervical collar: associated with increased mortality, no impact on neurologic outcomes.

Hanging and Strangulation Injuries

General Principles

- Judicial hanging (larger drop height) associated with C2 pedicular (Hangman) fracture, cord transection.
- Nonjudicial hanging associated with venous occlusion.

Clinical Presentation

- Venous occlusion leading to cerebral edema, arterial occlusion causing stroke or ischemic injury, arrhythmia from carotid body compression, noncardiogenic pulmonary edema. Hanging associated with thyroid cartilage and hyoid bone fractures. Cricoid cartilage fracture is seen in strangulation.

Diagnosis and Evaluation

- CTA of head and neck to evaluate for vascular injury.

Treatment

- Early airway management.
- Lung-protective ventilation strategy with higher positive end-expiratory pressure and low tidal volumes.

Spinal Cord Injuries

General Principles

- Primary injury: occurs at time of trauma
  - Transection of neural elements: irreversible
  - Compression of cord between vertebrae and ligamentum flavum
    - Increased risk in cervical osteoarthritis and spondylosis in the elderly
  - Primary vascular damage: arterial injury or extradural hematoma
- Secondary injury: delayed progression of neurologic injury. Worsened by 4 H's: *h*ypoxia, *h*ypotension, *h*yperthermia, and *h*ypoglycemia

Clinical Presentation (Fig. 141.2, Table 141.2)

- Complete cord injury: associated with complete motor and sensory levels
  - Often transection or ischemia of the entire cord diameter
  - Difficult to differentiate acutely from spinal shock
    - Concussive injury to cord
    - Absence of reflexes (especially bulbocavernosus) may indicate spinal shock as opposed to complete lesion.
- Incomplete: certain mechanisms of injury to a single region of the spinal cord can result in specific neurologic syndromes (Fig. 141.3).
  - Central cord syndrome: hyperextension in a patient with cervical spine stenosis
    - Upper extremity weakness; sensory effects and lower extremity weakness are variable; fibers innervating more distal structures are more peripheral.
  - Anterior cord syndrome: seen in hyperflexion injuries
    - Caused by disruption of the unpaired anterior spinal artery, resulting in ischemia to the anterior part of the cord
    - Can be seen in aortic injury, damage to anterior column as in teardrop fracture, or anterior displacement of a disk or vertebra
    - Bilateral loss of motor function, pain and temperature sensation; autonomic dysfunction is also common.
  - Brown-Sequard syndrome: commonly from direct penetrating injury
    - Hemisection of the spinal cord
    - Ipsilateral loss of motor function and proprioception, contralateral loss of pain and temperature sensation

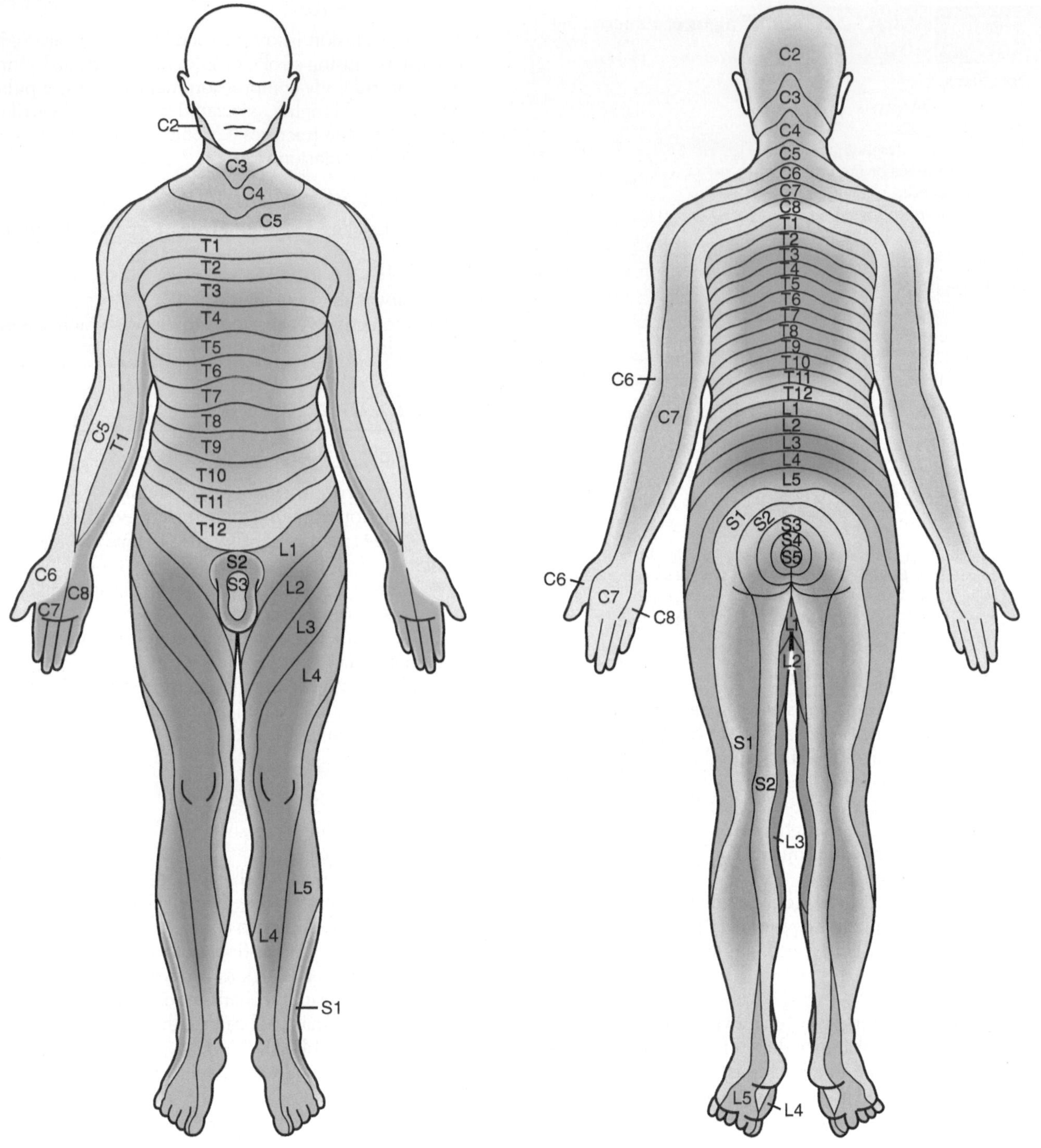

FIG. 141.2 Sensory dermatomes. (From Kaji, A. H., & Hockberger, R. S. (2018). Spinal injuries. In R. M. Walls, R. S. Hockberger, & M. Gausche-Hill (Eds.), *Rosen's emergency medicine: Concepts and clinical practice* (9th ed., pp. 345–371). Elsevier.)

- Additional incomplete cord syndromes are characterized by the location of injury and clinical presentation (Table 141.3).
- Neurogenic shock: high C-spine injuries affecting sympathetic fibers
  - Loss of vasomotor tone and fluid-resistant hypotension, with or without bradycardia
  - Extremities are typically warm and flushed.
- Ascending hypoesthesia may precede respiratory failure.

Diagnosis and Evaluation

- Physical examination documenting motor and sensory levels. Paralysis with
  - Intact reflexes: suggest upper motor neuron
  - Diminished reflexes: associated with lower motor neuron (nerve root or cauda equina)
- Magnetic resonance imaging is the study of choice to evaluate for spinal cord injury.

TABLE 141.2 Spinal Motor Examination

Level of Lesion	Resulting Loss of Function
C4	Spontaneous breathing
C5	Shrugging of shoulders
C6	Flexion at elbow
C7	Extension at elbow
C8-T1	Flexion of fingers
T1-T12	Intercostal and abdominal muscles
L1-L2	Flexion at hip
L3	Adduction at hip
L4	Abduction at hip
L5	Dorsiflexion of foot
S1-S2	Plantar flexion of foot
S2-S4	Rectal sphincter tone

(From Kaji, A. H., & Hockberger, R. S. (2018). Spinal injuries. In R. M. Walls, R. S. Hockberger, & M. Gausche-Hill (Eds.), *Rosen's emergency medicine: Concepts and clinical practice* (9th ed., pp. 345–371). Elsevier.)

TABLE 141.3 Other Incomplete Spinal Injury Syndromes

Syndrome	Location of injury	Presentation
Cauda equina Syndrome	Cauda equina (bundle of nerve fibers distal to conus medullaris)	Saddle anesthesia, urinary retention, asymmetric lower extremity weakness, back pain
Conus Medullaris Syndrome	Conus medullaris (typically at L1-2)	Symmetric lower extremity numbness and mild weakness, urinary and fecal incontinence, impotence, back pain
Posteroinferior Cerebellar Artery (PICA) Syndrome	PICA	Ataxia, vertigo, dysphagia, dysphonia
Horner Syndrome	Cervical sympathetic chain (or upstream fibers)	Ipsilateral ptosis, miosis, anhidrosis
Spinal Cord Injury Without Radiographic Abnormality (SCIWORA)	Anywhere in spinal cord	Delayed onset of neurologic deficits, typically in pediatric patients, without imaging abnormalities

Treatment

- Maintain C-collar.
- Avoid hyperthermia, hypoxia, hypotension, hypoglycemia.
- Foley catheter for bladder distension or atonia.
- Neurogenic shock (diagnosis of exclusion): low-dose pressors with mean arterial pressure goal of approximately 85
- Steroids are not recommended for spinal injury.
- Hypothermia is not recommended for spinal injury or hanging/strangulation.

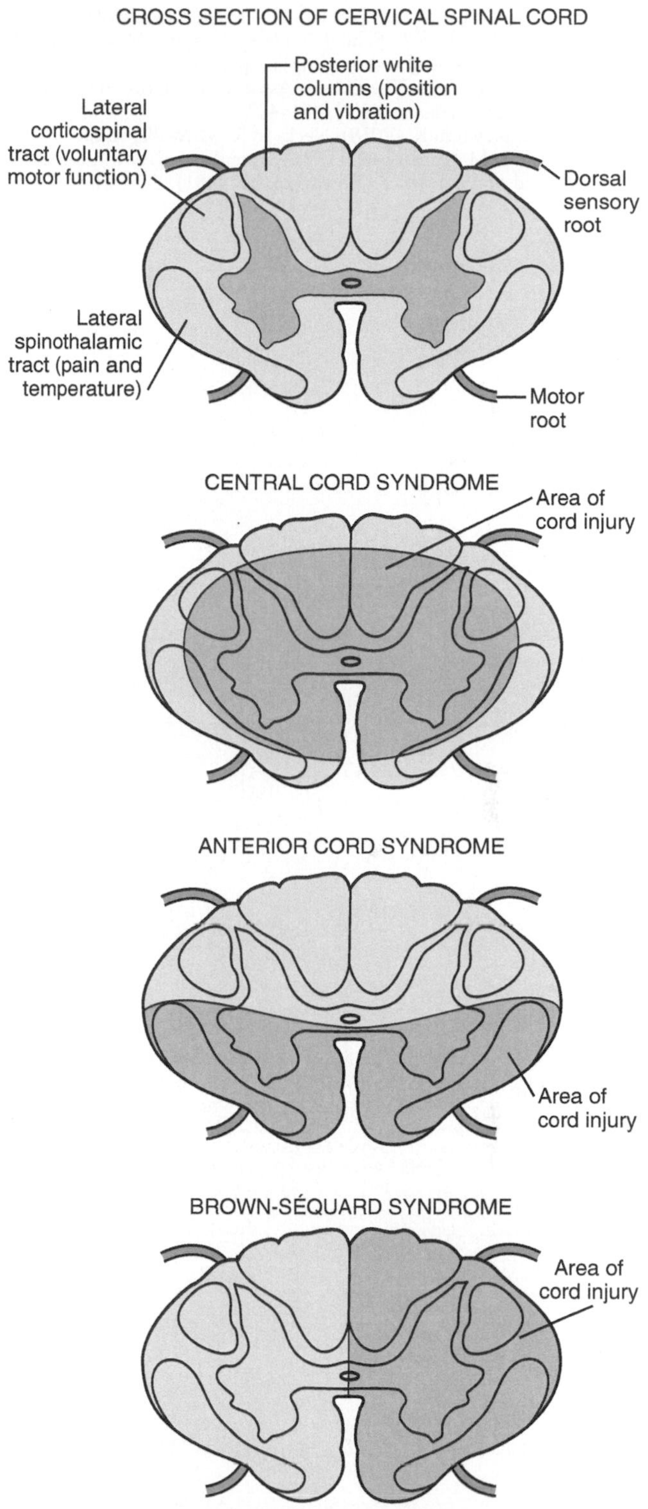

FIG. 141.3 Incomplete cord lesions. (From Kaji, A. H., & Hockberger, R. S. (2018). Spinal injuries. In R. M. Walls, R. S. Hockberger, & M. Gausche-Hill (Eds.), *Rosen's emergency medicine: Concepts and clinical practice* (9th ed., pp. 345–371). Elsevier.)

SUGGESTED READINGS

American College of Surgeons Committee on Trauma. (2018). Spine and spinal cord trauma. *Advanced trauma life support for doctors: Student course manual* (10th ed., pp. 128–146). American College of Surgeons.

141

Bromberg, W. J., Collier, B. C., Diebel, L. N., Dwyer, K. M., Holevar, M. R., Jacobs, D. G., Kurek, S. J., Schreiber, M. A., Shapiro, M. L., & Vogel, T. R. (2010). Blunt cerebrovascular injury practice management guidelines: The Eastern Association for the Surgery of Trauma. *Journal of Trauma*, 68(2), 471–477.

Claudius, I., & Newton, K. (2018). Neck. In R. M. Walls, R. S. Hockberger, & M. Gausche-Hill (Eds.), *Rosen's emergency medicine: Concepts and clinical practice* (9th ed., pp. 372–381). Elsevier.

Kaji, A., & Hockberger, R. S. (2018). Spinal injuries. In R. M. Walls, R. S. Hockberger, & M. Gausche-Hill (Eds.), *Rosen's emergency medicine: Concepts and clinical practice* (9th ed., pp. 345–371). Elsevier.

Sperry, J. L., Moore, E. E., Coimbra, R., Croce, M., Davis, J. W., Karmy-Jones, R., McIntyre, R. C., Jr., Moore, F. A., Malhotra, A., Shatz, D. V., & Biffl, W. L. (2013). Western trauma association critical decisions in trauma: Penetrating neck trauma. *Journal of Trauma and Acute Care Surgery*, 75(6), 936–940.

CHAPTER **142** BOARD REVIEW

Ophthalmologic Trauma

RYAN DEVIVO, DO, MS, and ANDREA W. WU, MD, MMM

Ophthalmologic Trauma

- Patients who have sustained eye trauma should undergo an assessment of visual acuity, the anterior chamber, integrity of the globe, pupil shape and reactivity, lids and lacrimal duct, extraocular movements, presence of a foreign body, and intraocular pressures (IOP), when safe to do so. Bent paperclips or an eyelid speculum may be used to open a swollen eye. An examination under procedural sedation or anesthesia may be warranted for pediatric or agitated patients.

EYELID AND LACRIMAL DUCT INJURIES

General Principles

- The lacrimal apparatus consists of the puncta on the medial aspect of the upper and lower lid, the canaliculi and common canaliculus, the lacrimal sac, and the nasolacrimal duct.
- The upper and lower eyelids have tarsal plates located directly adjacent to the lid margins, which are thick connective tissue that contribute to form and support (Fig. 142.1).

Clinical Presentation

- Lacerations or injury to the eyelid and lacrimal duct may present with pain, excessive tearing, or bleeding. Isolated injuries to the eyelid and lacrimal duct should not affect visual acuity.

Diagnosis and Evaluation

- Assess whether the injury is marginal (e.g., involving the lid margin) or extramarginal, and if there is associated tissue loss. Marginal lacerations typically involve the tarsal plate.
- Exposure of periorbital fat suggests an orbital septal injury.
- Laterally displaced puncta or excessive tearing suggests a canalicular laceration or other lacrimal apparatus injury.
- Ptosis or impaired lid dynamics may be caused by lid edema from a contusion, but be aware of levator or canthal tendon lacerations, which may present similarly.

Treatment

- Small, extramarginal wounds, approximately < 1 mm, heal well without repair.
- Extramarginal, simple lacerations along tension lines may be repaired with simple sutures, preferably 6-0 nylon, with removal in 3 to 5 days.
- Complex lacerations involving the lid margins, canalicular system, levator or canthal tendons, or lacerations with septal exposure or tissue loss require immediate plastics or ophthalmologic consultation in the emergency department.

CHEMICAL BURNS

General Principles

- The degree of injury is determined by the chemical's pH, concentration, volume, and duration of contact. Alkaline injuries typically have greater potential for long-term damage and vision loss.
  - Alkaline: severe and associated with liquefactive necrosis; used in bleach, oven cleaners, drain openers, toilet cleaners, and certain hair products.
  - Acidic: less severe, associated with coagulation necrosis, which limits depth of injury; found in metal cleaners, drain openers, swimming pool cleaners, rust removers, and nail primers.

Clinical Presentation

- Patients may complain of eye pain, burning, tearing, and blurred vision with or without visual acuity loss. Conjunctival injection and chemosis most commonly occur with possible subconjunctival hemorrhage, conjunctival edema, corneal defects, and corneal tissue loss. Corneal cloudiness and perilimbal ischemia (white ring around iris) suggest more severe injury (Fig. 142.2).

Diagnosis and Evaluation

- Use topical anesthetics and pain medications to optimize evaluation.
- A normal ocular pH is 7.0 to 7.2; check ocular pH using pH strips.
- Use fluorescein to evaluate for corneal abrasions, ulcerations, and perforations.
- Check IOP: an elevated IOP occurs more commonly with alkali injuries.

Treatment

- Irrigate the eyes with Normal Saline (NS) or Lactated Ringer (LR); a Morgan lens may be used to facilitate

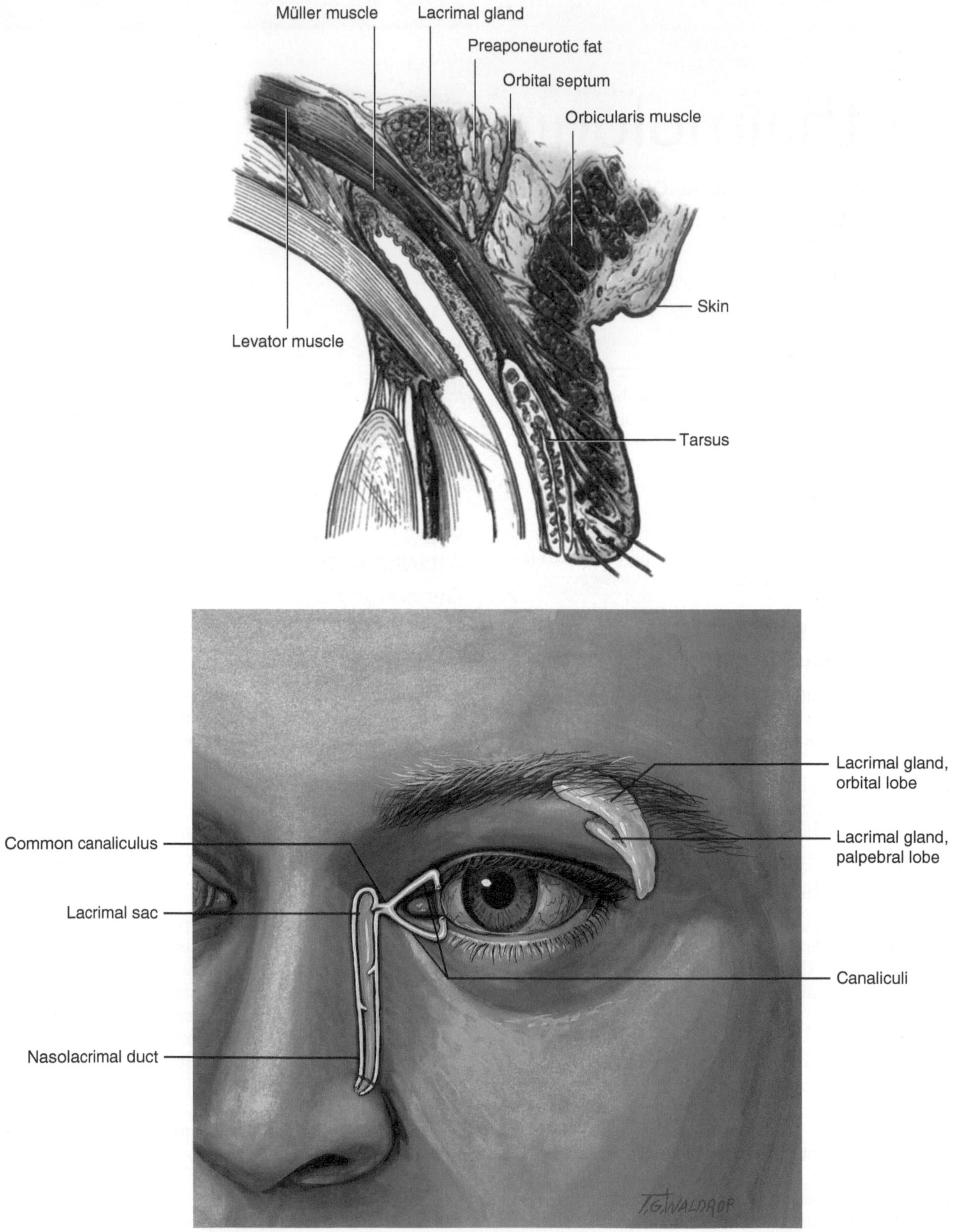

FIG. 142.1 Anatomy of lacrimal ducts and eyelids. **Top**, Cross-sectional view of the upper eyelid. **Bottom**, The lacrimal secretory and drainage systems. (**Top**, From Dutton, J. J. (2011). The lacrimal systems. In J. J. Dutton (Ed.), *Atlas of clinical and surgical orbital anatomy* (2nd ed., Fig. 9.1, p. 165). Elsevier. **Bottom**, From Nguyen, J. (2017). Eyelid and lacrimal trauma. In A. Fay & P. J. Dolman (Eds.), *Diseases and disorders of the orbit and ocular adnexa* (Fig. 35.1, p. 645). Elsevier.)

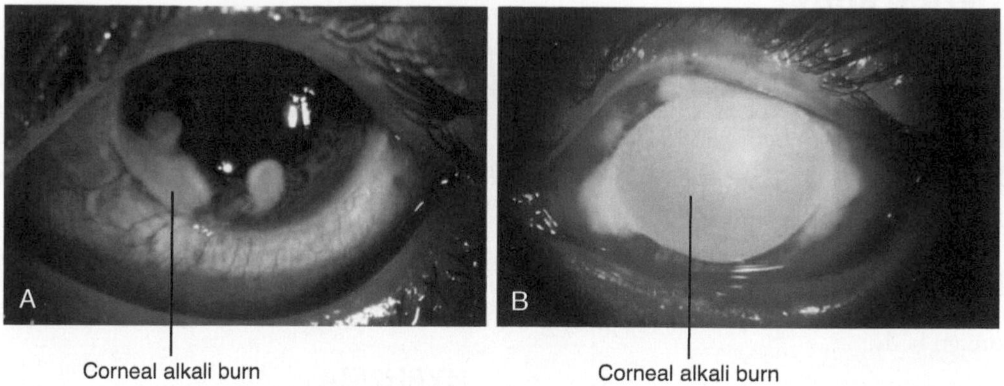

FIG. 142.2 **A.** Alkali burn demonstrating corneal burns and conjunctival injection on the day of the accident. **B.** Complete corneal tissue destruction 7 days after alkali burn. (From Kaiser, P. K., Friedman, N. J., & Pineda, R., II. (2004). *The Massachusetts Eye and Ear Infirmary illustrated manual of ophthalmology* (2nd ed., Fig. 5.5-6, p. 180). W. B. Saunders.)

irrigation. Check pH 5 to 10 minutes after irrigation. DO NOT attempt to neutralize by adding base/acid.
- Use a cotton applicator to sweep fornices and evert lids to remove any retained material.
- For minor burns, prescribe erythromycin ointment four times a day; a topical fluoroquinolone may be warranted for severe burns.
- Consult ophthalmology for all but minor burns. Most burns can be followed up in 24 to 48 hours, but more severe burns and those with tissue or visual acuity loss should be assessed by ophthalmology in the emergency department. If recommended by ophthalmology, prescribe prednisolone 1% ophthalmic for 1 week.

ULTRAVIOLET KERATITIS

General Principles

- Prolonged or excessive exposure to UV light, both natural (e.g., snow, water, altitude, or eclipses) and artificial (e.g., tanning beds, welder's instruments), induces an inflammatory response followed by a breakdown of corneal epithelium.
- Symptoms may not develop until after a latent asymptomatic period of up to 6 to 12 hours.

Clinical Presentation

- Patients present with eye pain, burning, foreign body sensation, excessive tearing, possible visual acuity loss, and blepharospasm. Pain should resolve with topical anesthetic; if it does not, one should evaluate for a deeper injury.

Diagnosis and Evaluation

- A slit lamp evaluation will demonstrate superficial punctate keratitis.

Treatment

- Treatment is supportive, focused mainly on pain control and may require oral medications. Mild oral opioids are often necessary at onset when pain is more severe. No evidence exists from clinical trials on the efficacy of various treatment options, although some clinicians do prescribe saline eye drops, a cycloplegic, and plus or minus topical antibiotic ointment.
- Simple cases of UV keratitis generally do not need ophthalmology follow-up, but those with intractable pain or visual acuity loss warrant an ophthalmology consult in the emergency department or within 24 hours.

CORNEAL ABRASION

General Principles

- When assessing corneal abrasions, it is important to document the timing of injury, substance/cause, and if the patient wears contact lenses.

Clinical Presentation

- Patients may present with foreign body sensation, tearing, eye pain, and photophobia. Visual acuity may be compromised if the defect is large or crosses the visual axis.

Diagnosis and Evaluation

- Note the size and location of the abrasion using fluorescein uptake under Woods or slit lamp.
- Evert the eyelids to ensure there is no retained foreign body; vertical or linear abrasions should raise concern for a retained foreign body.

Treatment

- Antibiotics: no evidence indicates that prophylactic antibiotics are beneficial, but they are often given for 3 to 5 days or until symptom-free for 24 hours. Commonly used regimens include ointments, such as erythromycin four times a day, which provide a protective barrier in addition to relieving discomfort; however, the ointment impairs vision while in the eye. Drops, such as polymyxin B/trimethoprim four times a day, are also often prescribed. Coverage for *Pseudomonas* with tobramycin or a fluoroquinolone is warranted in cases involving contact lens, fingernail injuries, and exposure to vegetable matter.
- No evidence supports patching or steroid application. The prescription of topical anesthetics is controversial, owing to a possible association with delayed epithelial healing, erosive keratopathy, and subsequent scarring.
- Contact lenses should not be used until healing is complete.

CORNEAL FOREIGN BODY

General Principles

- Although not always possible, it is important to describe the mechanism of injury (size, velocity, force, and substance and shape of the foreign body) and whether eye protection was used.

Clinical Presentation

- The presentation is similar to that of corneal abrasions, but there may also be blepharospasm. Deeper eye pain or visual acuity loss should raise concern for a retained intraocular foreign body.

Diagnosis and Evaluation

- Locate the foreign body using a slit lamp; assess the extent of injury and depth, evert eyelids, and inspect fornices (Fig. 142.3).
- High-velocity injuries may require computed tomography or ultrasound to rule out intracular involvement.

Treatment

- Irrigate the affected eye with sterile water or saline.
- If the foreign body is superficially embedded, under slit lamp guidance, use a cotton swab soaked in saline, or 25- to 27-gauge needle to attempt removal.
- Rust rings can be burred, especially if within the cornea. However, removal within 24 to 48 hours with referral to ophthalmology is preferred because the rust ring will have softened.
- Arrange ophthalmology follow-up within 24 to 48 hours.
- Consult ophthalmology emergently if a large area of visual axis is involved, an object is deeply embedded, or there are multiple foreign bodies.

TRAUMATIC IRITIS

General Principles

- Typically associated with other facial trauma, blunt orbital trauma induces spasm of the ciliary body and iris.
- Presentation is typically delayed by 2 days.

Clinical Presentation

- Patients may complain of a dull, throbbing ache with photophobia, tearing, and perilimbal erythema (ciliary flush).

Diagnosis and Evaluation

- Assess for direct and consensual photophobia, visual acuity loss, sluggish pupil, and perilimbal conjunctival injection. The cornea is clear without abrasion or ulcer.
- Classically, cell (white blood cells floating and appearing as dust specks) and flare (protein from inflamed blood vessels), owing to the increased permeability of inflamed uveal vessels, are seen in the anterior chamber on slit lamp examination.
- Rarely, in severe cases, the leukocytic exudate that precipitates from cells and flare can accumulate in dependent places and form a hypopyon.

Treatment

- Initiate steroid drops only in consultation with ophthalmology. Because traumatic injuries can lead to infection, and hypopyon can be present in both infection and other inflammatory conditions, it is best to leave this decision to ophthalmology. For example, trauma can introduce bacteria that lead to infection, thereby causing keratitis, uveitis, and endophthalmitis. Hypopyon can also be present in autoimmune inflammatory disorders, such as Behçet disease, inflammatory bowel disease, and so forth.
- Prescribe cycloplegics, such as homatropine 5% twice daily or cyclopentolate 2% three times daily.
- Ophthalmology follow-up within 24 to 48 hours should be arranged.

HYPHEMA

General Principles

- A hyphema is caused by an accumulation of blood in the anterior chamber, typically after blunt trauma, damaging vessels of the iris and/or ciliary body. This blood may present as a fluid layer or an area of blood tinge.
- It is important to ask about anticoagulant use, history of blood dyscrasias, sickle cell disease, and so forth.

Clinical Presentation

- Patients frequently present with pain and blurred or obstructed vision, depending on the level of the fluid layer. Worsening vision several days after trauma raises concern for a rebleed, continued bleeding, or another injury. Ciliary flush and a distorted pupillary shape may be present, as well as traumatic iritis. Concomitant open globe injury should be ruled out in the presence of traumatic hyphema.

Diagnosis and Evaluation

- Hyphemas are typically obvious on examination without magnification, but microhyphemas may only be seen with a slit lamp.
- Assess IOP, although an IOP increase may be delayed up to 3 days.

Treatment

- Avoid near vision work, and elevate head of bed. Cycloplegics are safe if globe rupture is excluded. Use topical steroids only with ophthalmology consultation.
- Admission is recommended for patients with coagulopathy, blood dyscrasias, sickle cell disease or trait, or if greater than 50% hyphema.
- If less than one-third of the anterior chamber is involved and the patient is reliable, the patient may follow-up as an outpatient in 24 hours. If greater than 50% hyphema *OR* 24 or more hours since injury *OR* elevated IOP, the risk for a rebleed 2 to 5 days later is increased.

RETROBULBAR HEMATOMA

General Principles

- This injury is most often caused by blunt trauma, but can occur spontaneously; it results in orbital compartment syndrome.
- Vision loss can occur within 60 to 120 minutes.

Clinical Presentation

- Patients present with pain, decreased visual acuity, swelling, and difficulty opening lids owing to the swelling.

Corneal Foreign Body Removal

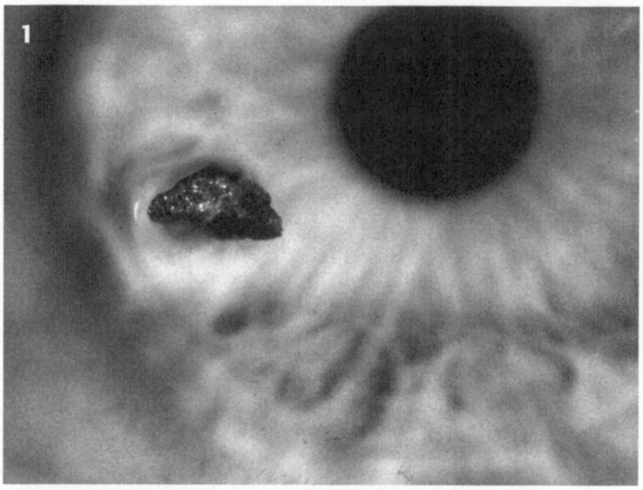

This embedded corneal FB is readily seen under slit lamp examination. A removal device (needle, spud, or bur drill) should be used for careful removal. A rust ring will remain if the FB has been there for only a few hours.

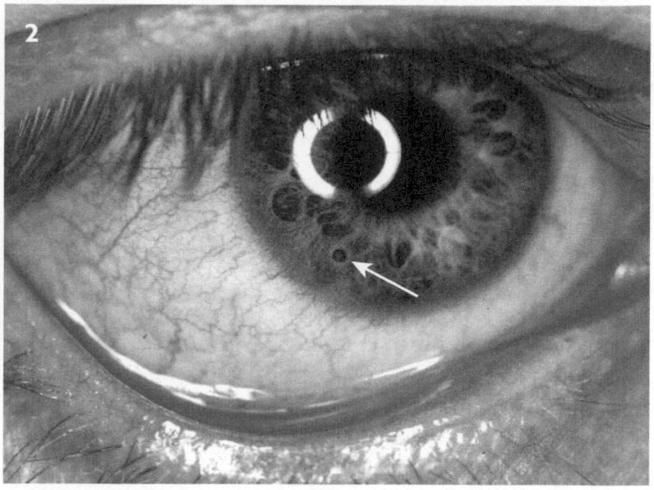

Rust rings *(arrow)* are retained FBs and are removed in a similar manner. Most rust rings should be removed, but there is no urgency. Small ones out of the line of sight may remain. A bur drill can be used for attempted removal, which if unsuccessful, can be reattempted in 24 hours. Alternatively, a small needle can be used to loosen the edges and then the ring scooped out. Both procedures will leave a corneal abrasion.

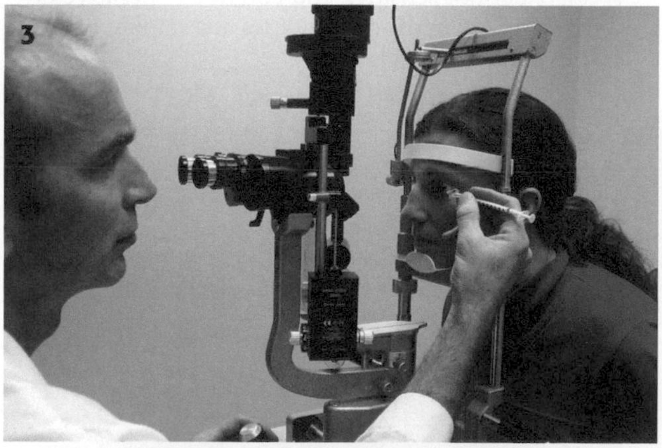

Under direct vision (not looking through the slit lamp), bring the syringe close to the eye while resting the hand on the patient's cheek. Be sure that the patient's forehead maintains continual contact with the crossbar on the slit lamp.

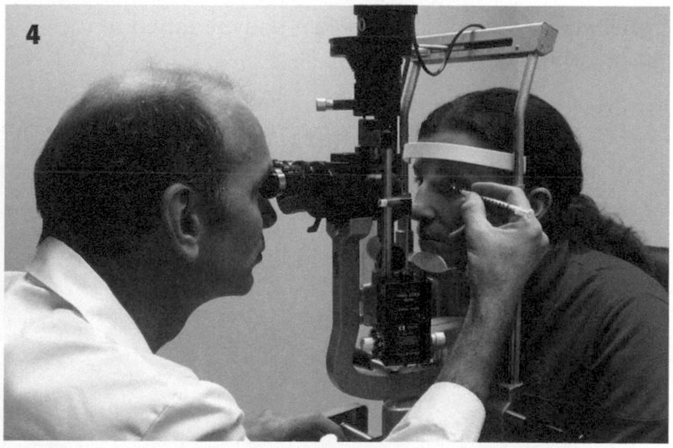

While looking through the slit lamp, bring the needle to the cornea and remove the FB.

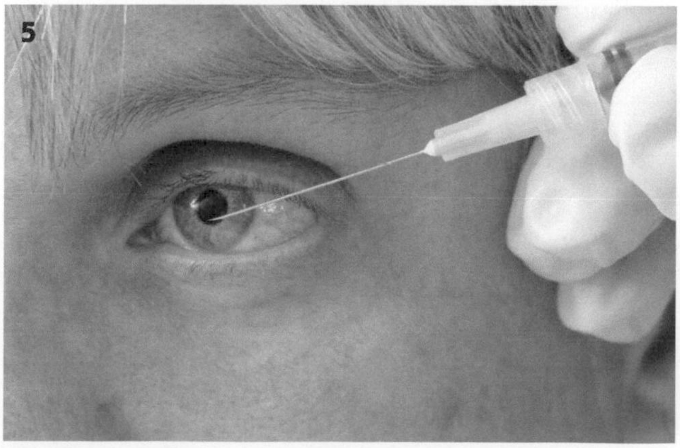

Hold the side of the instrument (drill bit or beveled edge of the needle) tangential to the cornea.

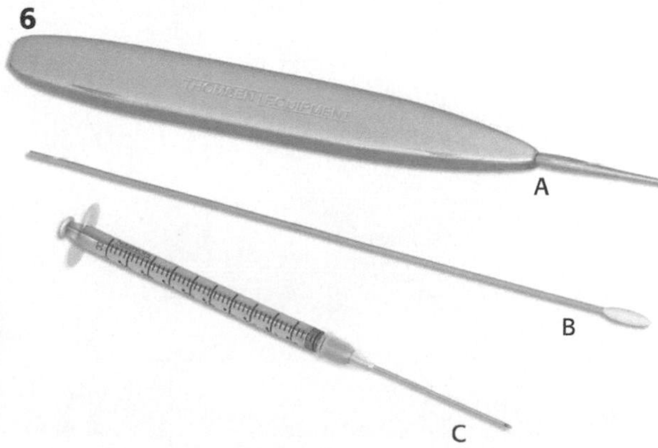

A variety of instruments may be used for FB removal, including an eye spud *(A)*, a cotton-tipped applicator *(B)*, and a 25- or 27-gauge needle on a tuberculin syringe *(C)*.

FIG. 142.3 Corneal foreign body (FB) removal. (From Knoop, K. J., & Dennis, W. R. (2019). Ophthalmologic procedures. In J. R. Roberts, C. B. Custalow, & T. W. Thomsen (Eds.), *Roberts and Hedges' clinical procedures in emergency medicine and acute care* (7th ed., p. 1315, Fig. 62.24). Elsevier.)

Diagnosis and Evaluation

- Proptosis with resistance to retropulsion, and a 360-degree subconjunctival hemorrhage may be present. Examination may demonstrate diminished visual acuity, loss of color vision, and an afferent pupil defect.
- This is a clinical diagnosis, and treatment should not be delayed for imaging.
- Measure baseline IOP.

Treatment

- Lateral canthotomy and cantholysis (Fig. 142.4).
  - Perform serial examinations and obtain an emergent ophthalmology consult.
  - Medical adjuncts that may be used include 20% mannitol 2 g/kg intravenously (IV), methylprednisolone 250 mg IV, or hydrocortisone 100 mg IV, and acetazolamide 500 mg IV.

GLOBE PENETRATION

General Principles

- Globe rupture: a globe rupture is defined by a full-thickness disruption in the outer membrane (sclera and/or cornea). It can be caused by a sudden increase in IOP from blunt trauma or, more commonly, penetrating trauma.
- Intraocular foreign body: foreign body retained in the globe itself.
- Intraorbital foreign body: retention of a foreign body in the orbital space, but outside the globe.

Clinical Presentation

- Presentation will depend on the mechanism and injury severity, but may include pain, diplopia or loss of vision, and tearing. The examination may demonstrate a distorted pupil, a dilated iris, extrusion of uveal tissue, 360-degree subconjunctival hemorrhage, lens dislocation, or afferent pupillary defect. It is important to describe the mechanism of injury, such as metal striking metal, glass breaking on face, and so forth, because the foreign body may be missed on imaging.

Diagnosis and Evaluation

- A thorough evaluation should be completed to inspect for evidence of lacerations to the cornea, conjunctiva, or sclera or foreign body that may suggest globe penetration. However, extensive manipulation of the globe should be deferred to ophthalmology if globe rupture is suspected (Fig. 142.5).
- Slit lamp: The examination may reveal hyphema, shallow anterior chamber, or lens dislocation, depending on the mechanism. Seidel sign (fluorescein streaming/leaking over area of laceration/penetration) is highly specific, but not sensitive and potentially negative or difficult to find with small injuries and minute foreign bodies entering the globe.

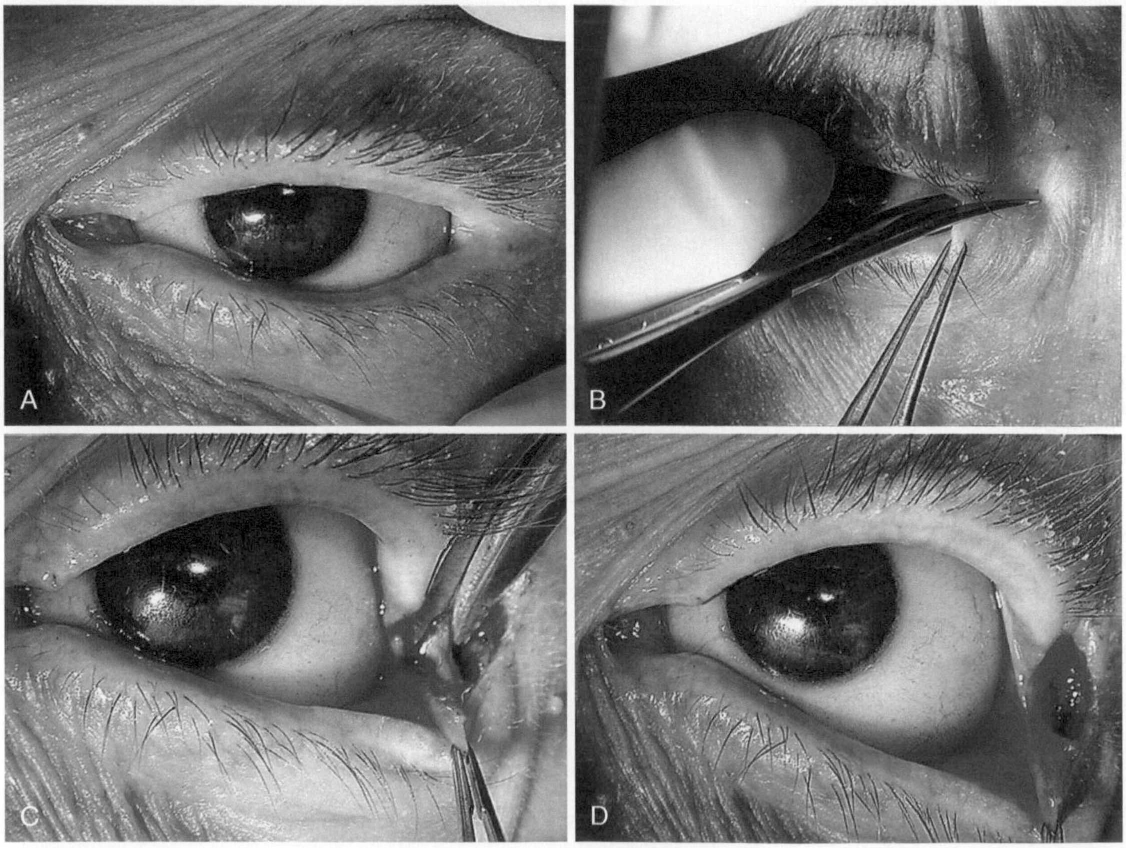

FIG. 142.4 Lateral canthotomy. **A**. Identifying the lateral canthus (*white arrow*). **B**. Crushing the lateral canthus with forceps. **C**. Cut the lateral canthus and retract the lower eyelid to expose the inferior crus. **D**. Cutting the inferior crus (cantholysis). (Reprinted from Ramakrishnan, V. R., & Palmer, J. N. (2010). Prevention and management of orbital hematoma. *Otolaryngologic Clinics of North America, 43*, 789–800, with permission.)

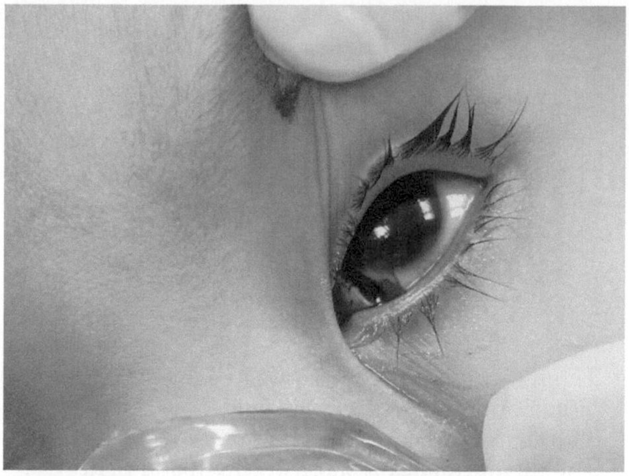

FIG. 142.5 Scleral laceration with penetrating globe injury. Note care being taken not to increase intraocular pressure (IOP) with examiner's fingers. (From Guluma, K., & Lee, J. E. (2018). Ophthalmology. In R. M. Walls, R. S. Hockberger, & M. Gausche-Hill (Eds.), *Rosen's emergency medicine: Concepts and clinical practice* (9th ed., pp. 790–819, Fig. 61.5). Elsevier.)

- Imaging: A noncontrast orbital computed tomography may reveal evidence of rupture (approximately 60% sensitive) or intraocular/orbital foreign body, although certain materials (e.g., wood) may be missed. Plain radiographs and ultrasound may also help to identify a foreign body.

Treatment

- DO NOT REMOVE if material/object is seen penetrating the globe or orbit.
- An emergent ophthalmology consult is indicated if globe penetration is suspected.
- Shield the affected eye and avoid any pressure or adherent dressings.
- Provide tetanus prophylaxis, if indicated, and administer antibiotics within 6 hours.
  - Adults: vancomycin plus third- or fourth-generation cephalosporin *OR* fluoroquinolone
  - Children: cefazolin plus gentamicin *OR* same as for adult if foreign body is present
  - If signs of infection or contaminated object, consider:
    - Vancomycin plus piperacillin/tazobactam *OR* ampicillin/sulbactam *OR* ceftriaxone and metronidazole
    - Vancomycin plus ciprofloxacin and metronidazole if penicillin- and cephalosporin-allergic

TRAUMATIC RETINAL DETACHMENTS

General Principles

- Retinal detachment in the setting of trauma is typically tractional, secondary to fibrocellular bands within the vitreous contracting and detaching the retina.
- It is important to determine if the macula is involved. If not, a more emergent ophthalmologic evaluation will be needed to save the patient's vision.

Clinical Presentation

- Immediately or shortly after trauma, patients may complain of floaters or flashes of light. As the retina separates, there may be visual acuity or visual field losses.

Diagnosis and Evaluation

- Visual acuity and visual fields should be assessed.
- On fundoscopy, a detachment will appear hazy gray and out of focus.
- Ocular ultrasound with maximum gain will reveal hyperechoic mobile membrane, often with a tethered membrane connected to the optic nerve sheath.

Treatment

- Consult ophthalmology for emergent versus urgent intervention. If discharged, follow-up should be within 24 to 48 hours.
- Prognosis depends on whether the macula is attached or not. If the macula is attached (not yet involved), then immediate ophthalmology consult is warranted.

SUGGESTED READINGS

Bowling, B., & Kanski, J. J. (2016). *Kanski's clinical ophthalmology: A systematic approach* (8th ed.) Elsevier.

Knoop, K. J., & Dennis, W. R. (2019). Ophthalmologic procedures. In J. R. Roberts, C. B. Custalow, & T. W. Thomsen (Eds.), *Roberts and Hedges' clinical procedures in emergency medicine and acute care* (7th ed., p. 1295–1337.e2). Elsevier.

Riviello, R. J. (2019). Otolaryngologic procedures. In J. R. Roberts, C. B. Custalow, & T. W. Thomsen (Eds.), *Roberts and Hedges' clinical procedures in emergency medicine and acute care* (7th ed., p. 1338–1383.e2). Elsevier.

CHAPTER **143** BOARD REVIEW

Pediatric Trauma and Fractures

SUPRIYA SHARMA, MD, and SHEETAL KHIYANI, MD

General Principles

The leading cause of death and disability in children each year, injury-related morbidity and mortality is a serious public health concern. Yearly, nearly one in six children require emergency department care for treatment of trauma-related injuries, and over 20,000 children die from their injuries. When caring for pediatric trauma patients, it is important for emergency providers to understand that special considerations must be made for their differences in anatomy, physiology, and emotional needs.

Mechanisms and Types of Injury

- Blunt trauma is the predominant mechanism of injury in children.
- Motor vehicle accidents account for the majority of trauma-related deaths in children, followed by drowning, house fires, homicides, and falls.
- It is important to consider child maltreatment in all trauma cases, especially those in infants younger than 12 months of age.

Unique Pediatric Characteristics and Considerations

Anatomic and Physiologic Considerations

- Children have a smaller body mass than adults.
  - Energy is transferred in higher concentration per unit of body area from objects or falls; thus, multisystem injury should be presumed.
- The larger body surface area-to-body mass ratio in children may lead to increased insensible fluid and heat losses.
- The head in pediatric patients is proportionately larger, resulting in a higher frequency of blunt brain injury.
- Children's skeletons are more flexible, so internal organ damage should be considered, even without the presence of an overlying fracture.
- It is important to remember that normal vital signs in children vary by age.

The Primary Survey

AIRWAY

- Establishing an airway in a pediatric trauma patient is critical; failure to do so is the most common cause of cardiac arrest in children.
- When establishing an airway in children, anatomic differences from adults must be taken into consideration.
  - The plane of the midface should be maintained parallel to the spine board to avoid passive flexion of the cervical spine and to obtain better visualization of the vocal cords.
  - The soft tissues of oropharynx are large, making visualization of the cords difficult.
  - The larynx and cords are anterior.
  - The infant trachea is short in length and right mainstem bronchus intubation can easily occur.
- The preferred method of obtaining definitive airway control is orotracheal intubation with direct visualization and cervical motion restriction.
  - Endotracheal tube size can be roughly calculated by the formula age/4 + 3.5 (cuffed tube).
  - Oral airways should only be inserted if the child's gag reflex is not intact and there should be no rotation of the device with insertion.
  - Needle cricothyroidotomy with jet insufflation should be used when adequate airway control cannot be established. Surgical cricothyroidotomy should only be performed in older children in whom the cricothyroid membrane is palpable, which usually occurs when greater than 12 years of age.

BREATHING

- Use pulse oximetry and end-tidal CO_2 monitoring to assess whether there is adequate oxygenation and ventilation, respectively
  - Signs of hypoxemia include:
    - Agitation
    - Altered mental status
    - Cyanosis
    - Poor end-organ function
    - Poor capillary refill
    - Desaturation on pulse oximetry
- Pediatric bag-mask is recommended for children under 30 kg to avoid barotrauma associated with using an adult bag-mask.
- Needle decompression should be performed over the top of the third rib in the midclavicular line when a pneumothorax is suspected.
  - Signs of tension pneumothorax in children are subtle and include:
    - Decreased breath sounds
    - Refractory hypotension
    - Refractory hypoxia

CIRCULATION

- Hypovolemic shock in children can present subtly, and should be suspected if any of the below are present.
  - Tachycardia
  - Weakening of peripheral pulses
  - Narrowing of pulse pressure less than 20 mm Hg
  - Skin mottling or clammy skin

- Cool extremities
- Decreased response to pain
- Children have an increased physiologic reserve.
  - Hypotension is a late sign of hypovolemic shock and results only when there is 30% or greater loss of circulating blood volume.
- The lower limit of normal systolic blood pressure is 70 plus twice the child's age in years until age 10 (when 90 mm Hg is used subsequently).
- Resuscitation traditionally has involved using up to three 20 mL/kg crystalloid boluses, followed by blood product administration.
  - Recent adult literature suggests that early intervention with blood products may improve patient outcomes.
  - Although pediatric literature is less clear, the 10th edition of Advanced Trauma Life Support (ATLS) has adapted the use of blood products for persistent instability following the initial 20 mL/kg of crystalloid infusion delivery.
  - For patients requiring massive transfusion (anticipated loss of 40 mL/kg of blood), a massive transfusion protocol is required, although no proven mortality benefit for children exists in the literature. Centers differ in protocol ratios, but typically this consists of 10 to 20 mL/kg of packed red blood cells and 10 to 20 mL/kg each of platelets and fresh frozen plasma, respectively.
  - Urine output is a reliable indicator of volume resuscitation in pediatric patients.
    - Normal urine output in infants is 1 to 2 mL/kg; in children, 1 mL/kg; and in adolescents, 0.5 mL/kg.
- Vascular access should be established early.
  - Percutaneous route is preferred.
  - If obtaining percutaneous access fails twice, use of intraosseous needle in the proximal tibia or distal femur is preferred.

DISABILITY

- Neurologic assessment should be performed using the Glasgow Coma Scale (GCS) and measurement of pupillary size.
  - The AVPU (*a*lert, *v*erbal, *p*ain, *u*nresponsive) scale (Table 143.1) may be substituted for the GCS to assess neurologic function.

EXPOSURE

- Complete exposure to identify injuries is critical; however, hypothermia can result quickly in the patient with prolonged exposure. Therefore, the child should be covered as soon as feasible after the examination.

TABLE 143.1 AVPU Scale for Assessing Level of Consciousness in Pediatric Patients

A	Alert: spontaneously opens eyes, will respond to voice, and will retain motor function
V	Verbal response: responds to verbal stimuli
P	Pain: Will respond with their eyes, voice, or movement with application of a pain stimulus
U	Unresponsive or unconscious if no response to voice or pain

The Secondary Survey

General Principles

- Components of the secondary survey include the following:
  - History (AMPLE history: *a*llergies, *m*edications, *p*ast medical and surgical history, *last* meal time, and *e*vents preceding injury)
  - Detailed head-to-toe physical examination
  - Laboratory and radiographic studies
- Reassessment of vital signs and any abnormalities found in the primary survey should be performed every 15 minutes.

Imaging Indications

Head Computed Tomography (CT) Scan

- PECARN head CT algorithm (or preferred algorithm) should be used to determine whether a patient requires a head CT.
- Indications for immediate head imaging are palpable skull deformity or basilar skull fracture, GCS less than 14, or inability to evaluate patient's mental status.

CT of the Cervical Spine

- Should be performed in those patients in whom clinical clearance is unable to be voluntarily performed, such as those with neck pain, high-risk motor vehicle collision, altered mental status, or focal neurologic deficits. NEXUS decision rules can likely be applied to children over 8 years of age; few children under this age were included in the study.

Chest/Abdominal Imaging

- If chest x-ray reveals a widened mediastinum, the patient should undergo CT angiography to look for aortic causes, although these are extremely rare in the pediatric population. Most chest pathology in children can be reasonably screened for on a routine chest radiograph.
- Abdominal CT scan, not focused abdominal sonography in trauma (FAST), is the gold-standard in defining abdominal injuries in children and should be performed when with any suspicion of intraabdominal injury.
- Positive FAST in the setting of hemodynamic instability is an indication to proceed directly to the operating room for exploration and management.

Pediatric Fractures

- Fractures account for about 10%–15% of all serious childhood injuries.
- Boys have a greater incidence of fractures. As compared with girls, boys have a 42% chance of having a fracture and girls have a 27% chance of having a fracture from birth to 16 years of age.
- Trauma from sports injuries account for most of the fractures, although non-accidental trauma needs to be considered (Table 143.2).

UNIQUE FACTORS OF PEDIATRIC BONE

- Children's bones have relatively more Haversian canals than do adult bones, making them more porous and susceptible to fractures.

TABLE 143.2 Frequency of Most Common Pediatric Fracture Types

Fracture Type	Percentage
Distal forearm	22.7
Hand, phalanges	18.9
Carpal-metacarpal	8.3
Clavicle	8.1
Ankle	5.5
Tibia, diaphysis	5.0
Tarsal-metatarsal	4.5
Foot, phalanges	3.4
Radius-ulna, diaphysis	3.4
Supracondylar region of the humerus	3.3
Proximal end of the humerus	2.2
Facial skeleton	2.1
Skull	1.8
Femur shaft	1.6

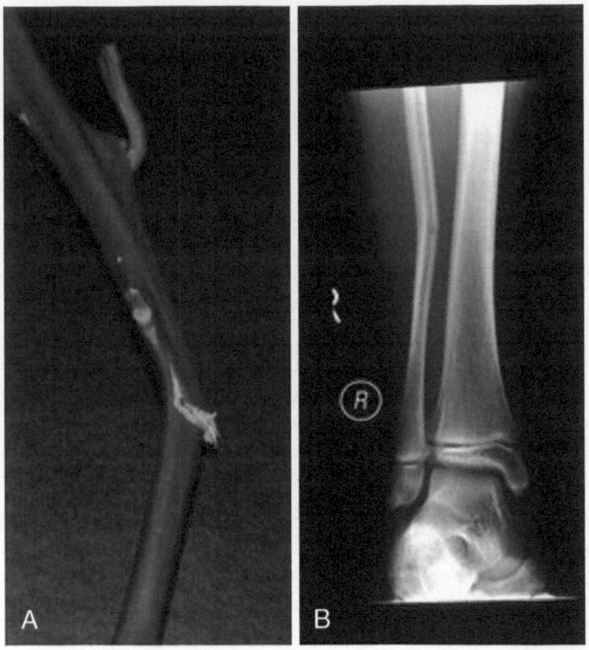

FIG. 143.2 Greenstick fracture.

- Periosteum is thicker and stronger in children, resulting in a cortical deformity, rather than a discontinuity, thereby reducing the incidence of displaced fractures.
- Pediatric bone also remodels more quickly than mature bone, promoting rapid healing, which may preclude the need for anatomic alignment and reduction.

UNIQUE FRACTURES SPECIFIC TO PEDIATRIC POPULATION:

- Buckle/torus fractures (Fig. 143.1)
  - Disruption of the cortex on the side of the compressive force, which appears as a bulge.
  - Mild or no angulation at the fracture site.
  - Stable fracture.
  - Most common site: distal radius at the junction of the metaphysis and diaphysis.
  - Treatment: removable splint for 3 to 4 weeks.

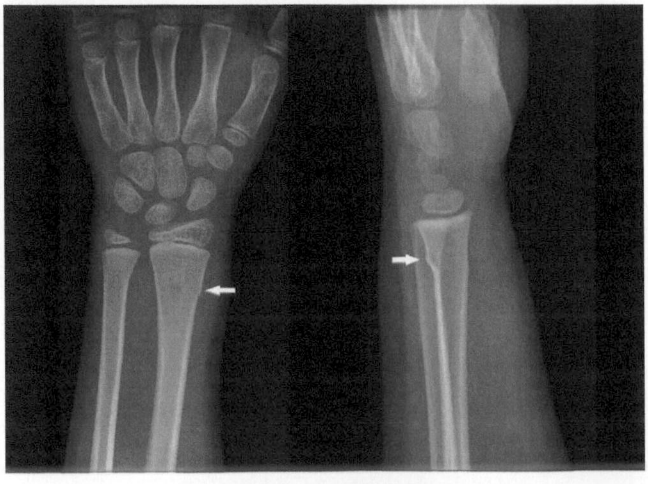
FIG. 143.1 Buckle fracture.

- Greenstick fractures (Fig. 143.2)
  - Disruption of the cortex and periosteum on the side of tension (convex side) with an intact periosteum and cortex on the side of compression (concave side).
  - Some degree of angulation is usually present.
  - Most common site: diaphysis of the radius, ulna, or fibula.
  - Treatment: acceptable angulation: immobilization with a cast.
  - Greater than acceptable angulation: closed reduction followed by immobilization with a cast.
  - Acceptable angulation on x-ray:
    - 0 to 5 years: lateral view: 20 to 25 degrees; antero-posterior (AP) view: less than 10 degrees.
    - 6 to 10 years: lateral view: 15 to 20 degrees; AP view: less than 5 degrees.
    - More than 10 years: lateral view: less than 10 degrees; AP view: 0 degree.
- Bowing/plastic fractures (Fig. 143.3)
  - No disruption of the cortex or periosteum.
  - Angulation is present.
  - Most common site: diaphysis of the ulna (most common) or fibula.
  - Treatment: acceptable angulation: immobilization with a cast.
  - Greater than acceptable angulation: closed reduction followed by immobilization with a cast.
  - Acceptable angulation on x-ray:
    - 0 to 5 years: lateral view: 20 to 25 degrees; AP view: less than 10 degrees.
    - 6 to 10 years: lateral view: 15 to 20 degrees; AP view: less than 5 degrees.
    - More than 10 years: lateral view: less than 10 degrees; AP view: 0 degree.
- Clinically the most important feature of children's bones is the presence of the growth plate (physis), the area of rapidly proliferating cells located between the

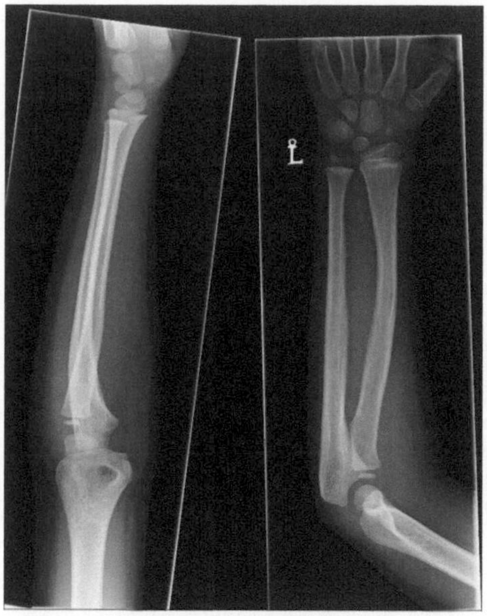

FIG. 143.3 Bowing fracture.

metaphysis and epiphysis of all long bones. Accounting for 20% to 35% of all pediatric fractures, growth plate injuries may occur at any age. However, they are most common during periods of rapid growth, peaking between the ages of 10 and 16 years, with boys more likely than girls to sustain the injury.

- Because the epiphysis provides the blood supply for the growth plate, any injury to the growth plate that also involves the epiphysis is likely to have impaired healing requiring more intensive treatment and follow up.
- Among the several classifications of growth plate fractures, the Salter-Harris system is used most widely and categorizes five fracture types (Fig. 143.4).
  - Type I: separating the epiphysis from the metaphysis, this fracture pattern occurs along the growth plate, rather than across it. Without any cortical break, radiographs often appear normal, and the diagnosis is made on clinical grounds (tenderness over a growth plate following an appropriate trauma).
  - Type II: a fracture along the growth plate, with an oblique extension through a piece of the metaphysis. This is the most common growth plate fracture and, as is the case with type I fractures, it has a good prognosis and generally does not require operative reduction.
  - Type III: a fracture through the growth plate that extends into the epiphysis and joint space.
  - Type IV: a fracture through the growth plate that extends into both the metaphysis and the epiphysis and into the joint space. Both type III and IV fractures threaten growth potential and articular integrity, thereby usually requiring open reduction and fixation.
  - Type V: a compression of the growth plate usually recognized only after the fact, when failure of growth is noted. This crush injury is the rarest type of fracture. It often requires surgical stabilization, immobilization, and a plan for management of growth arrest.

Clinical Presentation

- Irritability
- Pseudoparalysis (voluntary restriction of movement owing to pain)
- Refusal to bear weight
- Pain in the affected part

Physical Examination

- Deformity
- Point tenderness
- Swelling
- Erythema
- Decreased range of motion (younger child: position at rest and watch for spontaneous movement)

Diagnosis

- Radiographs, including joints above and below the suspected fracture.
- Anteroposterior and lateral views.
- Oblique views for growth plate injuries.
- Comparative views at times for Salter-Harris I and V fractures.
- The presence of swelling and point tenderness directly over a growth plate suggests a Salter I fracture, even in the absence of initial radiographic findings. Follow-up films may show periosteal changes that confirm the diagnosis.

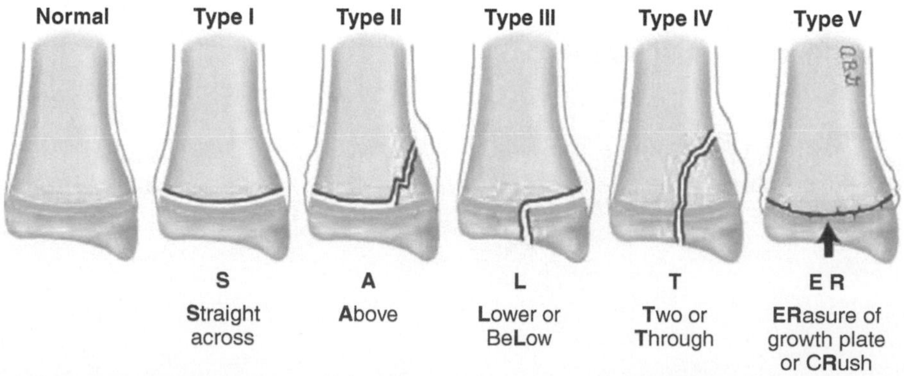

FIG. 143.4 Salter-Harris classification of physeal fractures. (Reproduced with permission from: Beutler A. General principles of fracture management: Bone healing and fracture description. In: UpToDate, Post TW (Ed.), UpToDate, Waltham, MA. Copyright © 2020 UpToDate, Inc. For more information visit www.uptodate.com.)

Treatment

- Pediatric fractures typically heal much more quickly than adult fractures. Compared with adults, children typically require shorter immobilization times, but malpositioned fragments become immovable much earlier than in adults. Whereas a clinician may have 8 to 10 days in which to detect and correct unacceptable fragment positions in an adult, the provider may have only 3 to 5 days in a young child and 5 to 7 days in an older child to do this.
- Remodeling with bone growth will often correct any malalignment.
- Children tolerate prolonged immobilization much better than adults; they rarely require physical therapy after immobilization.
- Advise to avoid collisions and contact activities for 2 to 4 weeks after discontinuing immobilization (growing bone is fibrous).
- Displaced fractures should be referred to orthopedics.

Evaluating Children with Fractures for Child Abuse

- Fractures are the second most common injury associated with child physical abuse; bruises are the most common injury.
- To identify child abuse as the cause of fractures, the physician must take into consideration the history, the age of the child, the location and type of fracture, the mechanism that causes the particular type of fracture, and the presence of other injuries.
- It is important to remember that even if a child has an underlying disorder or disability that could increase the likelihood of a fracture, the child may also have been abused. Children with disabilities and other special health-care needs are at increased risk of child abuse.
- Although some fracture types are highly suggestive of physical abuse, no pattern can exclude child abuse.
- When is a fracture suspicious for child abuse?

> - No history of injury
> - History of injury not plausible: mechanism described not consistent with injury
> - Inconsistent histories or changing histories provided by caregiver
> - Fracture in a nonambulatory child
> - Fracture of high specificity for child abuse (e.g., rib fractures)
> - Multiple fractures
> - Fractures of different ages
> - Other injuries suspicious for child abuse
> - Delay in seeking care for an injury

- Clinical and laboratory evaluation with imaging may help make the diagnosis of inflicted injuries.

> ***Specificity of Radiologic Findings in Infants and Toddlers***
>
> **High Specificity**
> - Classic metaphyseal lesions
> - Rib fractures, especially posteromedial
> - Scapular fractures
> - Spinous process fractures
> - Sternal fractures
>
> **Moderate Specificity**
> - Multiple fractures, especially bilateral
> - Fractures of different ages
> - Epiphyseal separations
> - Vertebral body fractures and subluxations
> - Digital fractures
> - Complex skull fractures
>
> **Common, but Low Specificity**
> - Subperiosteal new bone formation
> - Clavicular fractures
> - Long-bone shaft fractures
> - Linear skull fractures

SUGGESTED READINGS

American College of Surgeons. (2018). *Advanced trauma and life support* (10th ed.). American College of Surgeons.

George, M. P., & Bixby S. (2019). Frequently missed fractures in pediatric trauma. *Radiologic Clinics*, *57*, P843–P855.

Jones, C., Wolf, M., & Herman, M. (2017). Acute and chronic growth plate injuries. *Pediatrics in Review*, *38*, 129–138.

Tenenbein, M., Macias, C. G., Sharieff, G. Q., Yamamoto, L. G., & Schafermeyer, R. (2014). *Strange and Schafermeyer's pediatric emergency medicine* (5th ed.). McGraw-Hill.

CHAPTER 144

BOARD REVIEW

Trauma in Pregnancy

CASEY KREBS, MD, and BRADLEY CHAPPELL, DO, MHA, FACOEP

Traumatic injuries are the leading cause of non-obstetric morbidity and mortality in pregnant patients, involving nearly 8% of all pregnancies. Injury patterns and management of major trauma in pregnancy are affected by gestational age and related physiologic changes. In general, the management of pregnant trauma patients should mirror the standard care rendered to any non-pregnant patient, with a few additional considerations. Maintaining stable vital signs in the mother leads to optimal fetal outcomes.

General Principles

Multiple significant physiologic changes occur throughout pregnancy.

- Airway
  - There is potential for a more difficult airway owing to tissue edema and decreased oxygen reserve.
  - Pregnant patients are at an increased aspiration risk owing to decreased lower esophageal sphincter tone.
- Breathing
  - The pulmonary reserve and functional residual capacity are decreased owing to compression of the lungs by the diaphragm caused by the increased uterine size and subsequent amplified intraabdominal pressure.
  - As intraabdominal components shift upward with an enlarging gravid uterus, chest tubes should be placed one to two rib spaces higher than usual to avoid intraabdominal placement.
- Circulation
  - By the second trimester, the maternal heart rate generally increases 10 to 20 beats per minute, while the blood pressure decreases by 10 to 15 mm Hg.
  - The 20+ week uterus may compress the inferior vena cava (IVC), which can lead to supine hypotension. This can be easily mitigated by slightly turning the patient onto her left side or propping a backboard up with a rolled towel. The uterus may also be manually displaced to the left side during cardiopulmonary resuscitation.
  - By the third trimester, the blood volume may expand by as much as 45% without a significant change in the red blood cell counts, leading to a dilutional anemia.
  - Cardiac output increases to 50% above baseline, a result of a faster resting heart rate, lower systemic resistance, and an increase in blood volume with greater preload. Pregnant women can bleed 1 to 1.5 L, or 30%–35% of their blood volume, before showing signs of shock. At full term, the uterus receives approximately 20% of the total cardiac output, and injury can result in rapid exsanguination.
- Gestational age can be estimated by palpation and measurement (Fig. 144.1).
  - The uterus is at the pubic symphysis at 12 weeks; beyond this, it becomes an abdominal organ because it is no longer protected by the bony pelvis.
  - At 16 weeks, the uterus is halfway between the pubic symphysis and umbilicus.
  - By 20 weeks, the uterus should reach the umbilicus.
  - After 20 weeks, the gestational age in weeks is approximately equal to the distance in centimeters from the pubic symphysis to the uterine fundus.

Epidemiology

- Intimate partner violence is the leading cause of trauma in pregnancy (8,000 injuries per 100,000 live births each year). All pregnant women presenting for traumatic injuries should be screened for domestic violence. Other common causes of traumatic injuries in pregnancy are motor vehicle accidents (200 per 100,000 live births each year), falls (50 per 100,000 live births each year; even a ground level fall can compress the uterus, increasing the risk of abruption), burns, homicide, suicide, penetrating trauma, and toxic exposures.

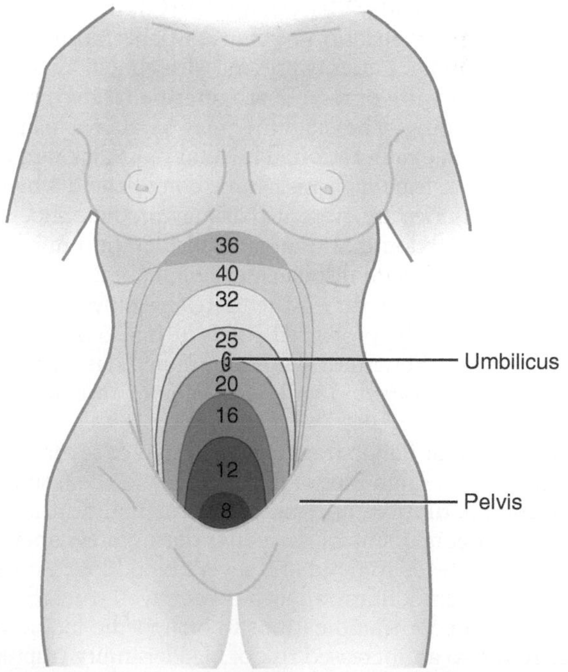

FIG. 144.1 Uterine size at different weeks of gestation. (From Kravis, T. C., & Warner, C. G. (Eds.). (1979). *Emergency medicine: A comprehensive review.* Aspen Publishers.)

- Because of ligament and tendon laxity, the most frequent injuries are orthopedic.
- An emergency department encounter is an excellent opportunity to provide education and reinforcement of safe behaviors. Seatbelts are always recommended because they decrease mortality; they should be worn low and snug over the anterior superior iliac spines. Airbags should be at least 10 cm away from the abdomen and should not be turned off.
- Pregnancy loss from traumatic injury, usually related to maternal hypotension, generally does not occur in the first trimester because the uterus is protected in the bony pelvis.
- Approximately 20% of pregnant trauma patients test positive on their urine drug screen. This is a moment for educational intervention.

Clinical Presentation

- Blunt abdominal trauma: Abdominal examination is less sensitive for peritoneal signs because guarding and rebound may be diminished. Abdominal pain is common following blunt abdominal trauma, but vaginal bleeding is not and should raise concern for placental abruption.
- Placental abruption: Often follows significant direct abdominal trauma, classically from a deceleration injury with shearing between the nonelastic placenta and uterus. Arterial bleeding dissects the placenta from the uterine wall, and the workup may reveal uterine tenderness, vaginal bleeding, or contractions. The second leading cause of traumatic fetal death (after maternal death), occurring in up to 5% of minor abdominal traumas, abruption should be suspected when severe contractions or shock is present.
- Uterine rupture: Although this typically occurs after multiple cesarean sections (C-sections) or during a trial of vaginal birth after C-section (VBAC), it is a rare but devastating complication of blunt or penetrating abdominal trauma. Patients present with shock, abnormal fetal heart tracing or fetal death, uterine tenderness, and vaginal bleeding. The examiner may be able to palpate fetal parts on examination. The fetal mortality rate is nearly 100%; the diagnosis can be complicated when multiple injuries are present that may produce shock.
- Penetrating abdominal trauma: Consideration must be given to the upward displacement of abdominal organs due to uterine growth. As the uterus becomes larger and moves outside the protected pelvis, it is also more likely to be injured. Penetrating uterine trauma has a high fetal mortality rate and will likely require an emergent C-section.
- Pelvic trauma: Pelvic fractures are a sign of severe trauma with a high rate of direct injury to the fetus, placental abruption, and maternal and fetal death. Venous engorgement in the pelvis during pregnancy potentially leads to rapid and severe blood loss. Angiography with embolization has not been well studied, but there are no contraindications to orthopedic fixation. There is also an increased risk of bladder injury (rupture), especially in the third trimester.
- Preterm labor: The diagnosis is based on cervical changes (effacement and dilatation over 3 cm), contractions on cardiotocography, and fetal fibronectin in vaginal secretions. Trauma increases the incidence of premature rupture of membranes, which can be diagnosed by pooling of fluid in the vaginal vault, ferning on microscopy, or nitrazine-positive secretions (indicating the presence of amniotic fluid).
- Burn patients: If the burns are over 50% of the total body surface area and the pregnancy is in the third trimester (week 28+), delivery may be indicated.

Diagnosis and Evaluation

- In prioritizing care of the two patients (mother and fetus), treating the mother always takes precedence because adequate resuscitation of the mother is the best predictor of good fetal outcomes. Blood flow to the uterus is not well autoregulated, and the fetus can be very sensitive to drops in maternal blood pressure or oxygenation. The benefits of early diagnosis and aggressive resuscitation outweigh potential risks of diagnostic imaging. No lifesaving diagnostic test or treatment should ever be withheld out of concern for potential fetal harm.
- Pelvic examination: A digital vaginal examination after 20 weeks is contraindicated until placenta previa is ruled out (via ultrasound) because it can provoke severe bleeding. Perform a sterile speculum examination to assess for bleeding, leakage of amniotic fluid, and cervical changes of labor.
- Laboratory studies
  - Complete blood cell count (mild leukocytosis and dilutional anemia are normal during pregnancy)
  - Basic metabolic panel, toxicology screen, lactate, and base deficit
  - Beta human chorionic gonadotropin (B-HCG), type and screen
  - D-dimer, fibrinogen, and fibrin split products to screen for abruption
  - Kleihauer-Betke test (if Rh-negative) detects fetal blood in the mother's circulation; however, this is neither sensitive nor specific for abruption, but it may indicate that additional doses of Rh immunoglobulin (beyond the standard 300 μg) are needed owing to significant fetal-maternal hemorrhage.
  - Pooling of yellowish-tinged amniotic fluid on speculum examination, blue (low pH) nitrazine test paper, and ferning on microscopic examination all suggest membrane rupture.
- Ultrasound
  - Screen the uterus during the FAST (*f*ocused *a*ssessment with *s*onography for *t*rauma) examination in pregnant women.
  - Ultrasound is highly insensitive (sensitivity is approximately only 25%) for abruption, especially when a retroplacental clot is present. Fetal cardiotocography demonstrating fetal distress is much more sensitive for detecting abruption.
  - A fetal anatomic ultrasound is indicated when suspecting blunt fetal injury, such as internal fetal bleeding, intracranial hemorrhage, or fractures.
- X-ray
  - Shield the uterus when possible; however, a single pelvic x-ray has very low ionizing radiation.

TABLE 144.1 Estimated Fetal Radiation Dose From Conventional Radiographic and Computed Tomography Examination

Imaging Study	Estimated Fetal Dose (mGy)*
RADIOGRAPHY	
Cervical spine (AP, lateral)	<0.001
Extremities	<0.001
Chest (PA, lateral)	0.002
Thoracic spine	0.003
Abdomen (AP) (21-cm patient thickness)	1
Abdomen (AP) (33-cm patient thickness)	3
Lumbar spine (AP, lateral)	1
COMPUTED TOMOGRAPHY	
Head	0
Chest (routine)	0.2
Chest (pulmonary embolism protocol)	0.2
Abdomen	4
Abdomen and pelvis	25
CT angiography of the aorta	34
CT angiography of the coronary arteries	0.1

AP, Anteroposterior; *CT,* computed tomography; *PA,* posteroanterior.
(From Raptis, C. A., Mellnick, V. M., Raptis, D. A., Kitchin, D., Fowler, K. J., Lubner, M., Bhalla, S., & Menias, C. O. (2014). Imaging of trauma in the pregnant patient. *Radiographics, 34*(3), 748–763.)

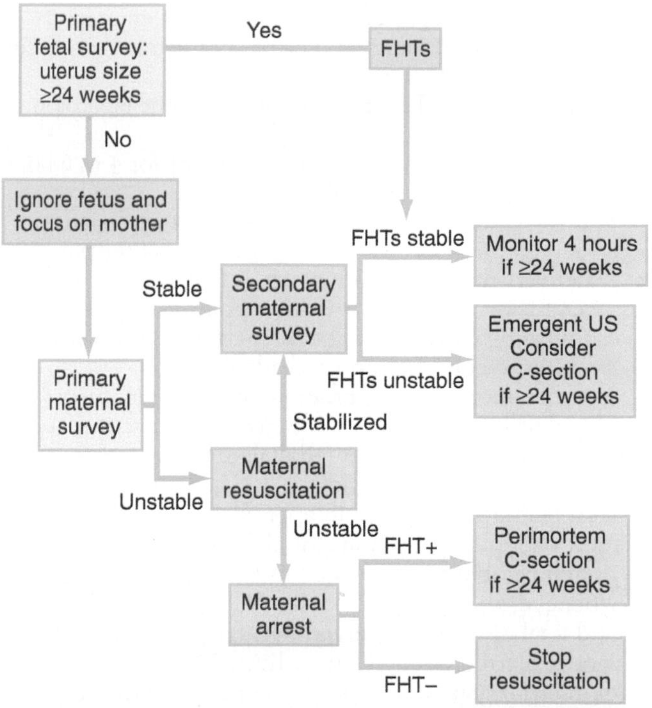

FIG. 144.2 Decision-making algorithm in emergency obstetric care. *C-section,* Cesarean section; *FHT,* fetal heart tone; *US,* ultrasonography. (From Dobiesz, V. A., & Robinson, D. W. (2018). Trauma in pregnancy. In R. M. Walls, R. S. Hockberger, & M. Gausche-Hill (Eds.), *Rosen's emergency medicine: Concepts and clinical practice* (9th ed., p. 2318, Fig. 182.1). Elsevier.)

- Computed tomography (CT)
  - The American College of Gynecology guidelines state that a single CT of the abdomen and pelvis in a pregnant patient is considered to be under the harmful dose of radiation to the fetus and should be performed with suspicion for clinically significant intraabdominal pathology. The fetus is most sensitive to radiation during organogenesis from 2 to 8 weeks and neural development during weeks 10 to 17.
  - Less than 50 mGy (absorbed radiation) is considered safe and not associated with adverse fetal malformations (a full-body CT scan approaches 26 mGy). The risk of childhood cancer increases by 0.05% over baseline risk of 0.2% to 0.3% with every 10 mGy. Individual institutions may have protocols to decrease the number of slices, thereby reducing the overall radiation exposure.
  - It is recommended that an informed consent process, discussing the risks and benefits of imaging options, occur prior to imaging (Table 144.1).
- Magnetic resonance imaging
  - Although very few data exist in trauma literature for pregnant patients, it may be a reasonable alternative in very stable patients.
- Fetal cardiotocography (toco)
  - Toco is indicated when the gestational age is over 22 weeks. If less than 22 weeks, the fetal heart rate (FHR) *should* be documented (normal FHR is 110 to 160).
  - Fetal distress may be the earliest signs of placental abruption and impending hemorrhagic shock in the mother. Fetal tachycardia or bradycardia, lack of beat-to-beat variability, and late decelerations often indicate hypoxia or maternal hypotension and may be indications for an emergent C-section by an obstetrician.
  - A minimum of 4 hours of monitoring after trauma is recommended. If contractions or other signs of uterine irritability are present, the fetal monitoring period is typically extended to at least 24 hours.
- Diagnostic peritoneal aspiration/lavage
  - If deemed necessary, this procedure should be performed from an open, suprapubic approach.

Treatment (Fig. 144.2)

- Resuscitation
  - Airway: Early intubation may be indicated for signs of respiratory compromise. A normal pCO_2 may be an early sign of impending respiratory failure because patients usually have a respiratory alkalosis. Be cognizant of the increased aspiration risk.
  - Breathing: Give supplemental oxygen, when indicated. The pregnant mother has decreased pulmonary reserve and this can result in rapid fetal hypoxia.
  - Circulation
    - Place the patient in the left lateral decubitus position to increase venous return if the uterus is above the umbilicus.
    - Aggressive fluid and blood resuscitation should be the mainstay because vasopressors may compromise fetal blood flow. Vasopressors should never be withheld if necessary for maternal support.

- Abruption: If suspected, always obtain an emergent obstetric consultation; fetal distress or demise can occur quickly.
- Uterine rupture: This requires an emergent laparotomy.
- Preterm labor
  - Monitor the baby via cardiotocography for 4 to 6 hours after the mother is stabilized.
  - If the gestational age is over 34 weeks with signs of preterm labor, admit the patient for potential delivery. If the gestational age is less than 34 weeks, admission for tocolysis is appropriate. Consider the following treatment options in conjunction with obstetric consultation (if available):
    - Betamethasone to promote fetal lung maturity;
    - Antibiotics if group B *Streptococcus* positive; and
    - Magnesium sulfate or terbutaline to slow contractions.
- Rh immunoglobulin (RhoGAM, Rhophylac): Maternal-fetal hemorrhage occurs in approximately 30% of pregnant patients with significant abdominal trauma. Rh immunoglobulin is indicated in Rh-negative patients whenever there is potential for mixing of maternal and fetal circulation (including vaginal spotting). It is most effective when given within 72 hours of trauma or abortion (spontaneous, threatened, or induced). The Kleihauer-Betke test can help direct the amount of Rh immunoglobulin necessary (50 μg treats less than 5 μL of hemorrhage, 300 μg covers approximately 30 μL of hemorrhage).
- Tetanus vaccine (Td and Tdap) is safe in pregnancy.
- Resuscitative hysterotomy (perimortem C-section): In the setting of sudden, witnessed maternal death with an estimated gestational age greater than 24 weeks (fundus above the umbilicus), a C-section should be performed by the most experienced available provider (preferably an obstetrician or surgeon) within 4 minutes of maternal death. The goal is delivery of the baby by post-arrest minute 5, which yields a neurologically intact infant approximately 70% of the time. To perform the C-section:
  - The skin incision is made from approximately 4 cm below the xiphoid to the pubis.
  - Bluntly dissect (fingers/scissors) to the uterus.
  - Make a small incision in the lower uterus.
  - Bluntly dissect the uterus vertically with scissors while protecting the baby with your nondominant hand.
  - After delivering the baby, clamp and cut the umbilical cord.
  - Deliver the placenta, pack the uterus with sterile towels, and staple the skin shut.
  - Continue the maternal resuscitation; delivery of the baby significantly improves the chances of a successful maternal resuscitation (by about 30%).
- Disposition: Monitor for 24 hours if any of the following are present: abdominal bruising or other abdominal injury, regular contractions (more than 1 every 10 minutes), vaginal bleeding, abnormal fetal heart tracing, abdominal or uterine pain, or coagulopathy (low platelets or fibrinogen).

SUGGESTED READINGS

Dobiesz, V. A., & Robinson, D. W. (2018). Trauma in pregnancy. In R. M. Walls, R. S. Hockberger, & M. Gausche-Hill (Eds.), *Rosen's emergency medicine: Concepts and clinical practice* (9th ed.). Elsevier.

Mendez Figueroa, H., Dahlke, J. D., Vrees, R. A., & Rouse, D. J. (2013). Trauma in pregnancy: An updated systematic review. *American Journal of Obstetrics and Gynecology, 209*(1), 1–10.

Smith, K., & Bryce, S. (2013). Trauma in the pregnant patient: An evidence-based approach to management. *Emergency Medicine Practice, 15*(4), 1–18.

CHAPTER 145

BOARD REVIEW

Orthopedic Trauma

JULIE ANDERSON, DO, and ADEDAMOLA OGUNNIYI, MD

Orthopedic trauma is a common reason for patients of all ages to present to the emergency department. A detailed history regarding the mechanism of injury, location of pain, changes in range of motion, and neurovascular status provide clues to the final diagnosis. Imaging is based on the history and physical examination, usually starting with standard radiographs and progressing to computed tomography (CT) or magnetic resonance imaging (MRI) for occult injuries or surgical planning. This chapter provides a review of upper and lower extremity orthopedic trauma and discusses the management of these conditions.

Basic Information

- A fracture is a disruption in the continuity of bone and covers a broad spectrum of injuries from nondisplaced stress fractures, to open, comminuted, or pathologic fractures.
- Patient age plays a role in which fractures for which they are more susceptible; for instance, Salter-Harris fractures occur in pediatric patients, whereas Tillaux avulsion fractures occur in adolescents.
- Fractures are described based on various criteria as highlighted in Table 145.1.

TABLE 145.1 *Fracture Terms and Descriptors*

Closed vs. open	Break in overlying skin indicates an open fracture. Open fractures may be classified by the Gustillo-Anderson Classification. • Type I and II: prophylaxis with a first generation cephalosporin (i.e., cefazolin) • Types IIIA–C: prophylaxis with both a first generation cephalosporin and an aminoglycoside (i.e., gentamicin) Tetanus vaccines should be updated for all open fractures
Displacement	Separation between proximal and distal fragment
Location	Proximal, mid-shaft, or distal. Anatomic bony reference points are used when able (for instance, a supracondylar fracture over the distal humerus).
Fracture line orientation	Transverse, oblique, spiral comminuted, segmental, torus, greenstick
Angulation	Direction and degree of the angle formed by the distal fragment
Joint disruption	Fracture-dislocations vs. fracture-subluxations

Upper Extremity Orthopedic Trauma

General Principles

- Upper extremity injuries are common emergency department orthopedic presentations, many of which can be successfully managed nonoperatively with splinting and active rehabilitation.
- Type of injury depends on the age of the patient and the mechanism of injury.
  - Children suffer buckle fractures or growth plate injuries, whereas young adults are susceptible to complete fractures or fracture-dislocations from high-energy mechanisms.
  - Elderly, osteoporotic patients may have fractures with low-energy mechanisms, such as ground-level falls.

Clinical Presentation

- Patients present with pain and swelling of the affected extremity.
- Deformity and ecchymosis may or may not be present, depending on the severity of the trauma.
- A detailed history is important, including handedness, and the reason for seeking care.
  - Acute trauma and high-energy mechanisms, such as falls from heights or motor vehicle crashes, should prompt a full trauma evaluation for associated injuries.

Diagnosis and Evaluation

- It is important to look for signs of injury, including deformity, swelling, and bruising. Examine closely for abrasions or lacerations, which may indicate an open fracture.
- Start the examination at the joint above the injury with the injured area palpated last.
- If no obvious deformity is seen, examine active and passive range of motion.
  - Rotation or "scissoring" should be assessed with suspected metacarpal fractures; tendon function should also be evaluated (Fig. 145.1) (White, Mackenzie, & Gray, 2016).
- A complete neurovascular examination is critical in all upper extremity injuries and should be documented before and after reduction or splinting.

Traumatic Injuries of the Hand

- Table 145.2 provides a summary of the various traumatic hand injuries.
- **Finger amputations** may be caused by blunt or penetrating trauma.
  - If the amputated fragment is available, it should be irrigated and wrapped in moist sterile gauze, placed in a bag with the bag subsequently placed in ice water.

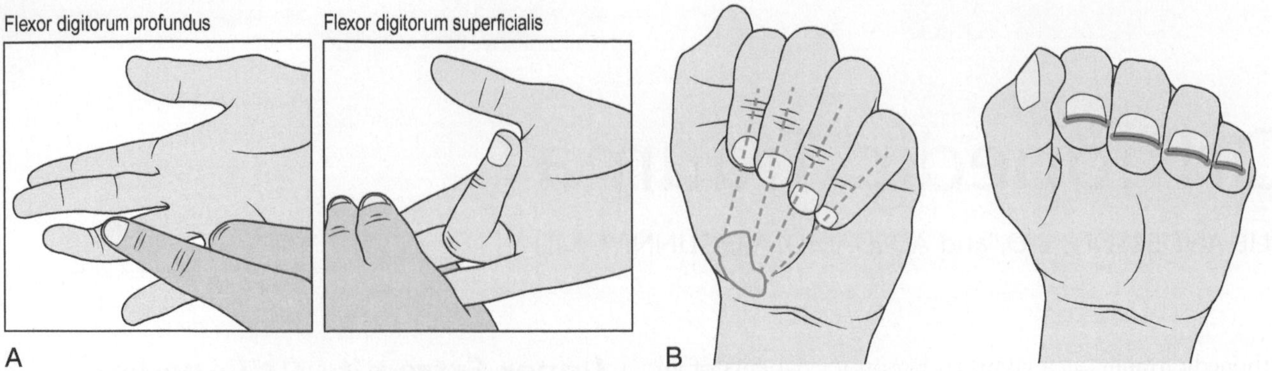

FIG. 145.1 Tendon and rotational assessment. (From White, T. O., Mackenzie, S. P., & Gray, A. J. (2016). *McRae's orthopaedic trauma and emergency fracture management.* (3rd ed., p. 266, Figs. 13.5 and 13.6). Churchill Pocketbooks, Elsevier Health Sciences.)

TABLE 145.2 ***Traumatic Injuries of the Hand***

Injury	Mechanism	Presentation	Treatment
Dorsal interphalangeal (DIP) joint dislocations	Direct blow	Pain and deformity; easily recognized on x-ray Mallet finger: flexion deformity at DIP with incomplete active extension at DIP	Mallet finger: full extension with a mallet splint (volar) for 3 weeks
Proximal interphalangeal (PIP) joint dislocations	Dorsal dislocations common: caused by hyperextension + direct blow Volar dislocations rare: caused by varus valgus stress + anterior force	Pain and deformity; easily recognized on x-ray	Closed reduction as above[a] Volar dislocations: treated with distraction, flexion and then pushing dorsally on the phalanx base
Metacarpophalangeal (MCP) joint dislocations	Forceful dorsiflexion with longitudinal impact	Pain and deformity, usually shortened and ulnar deviated in extension; easily recognized on x-ray	Usually require operating room for an entrapped volar plate[b] Closed reduction can be attempted with the wrist flexed and pressure applied to the proximal phalanx in a distal and volar direction.
Thumb carpometacarpal (CMC) dislocations	Axial force on flexed thumb	Pain, swelling, bruising over thenar eminence; usually demonstrated on anteroposterior and lateral x-rays (consider Roberts view)[c]	Reduction by flexion and abduction of the metacarpal, and applying pressure directed distally to the base of the proximal phalanx. Thumb spica splint
Thumb MCP ulnar collateral ligament (UCL) rupture (Gamekeeper or Skier's thumb)	Forced radial abduction of the thumb at the MCP joint, usually in associated with a fall (e.g., skiing with ski poles)	Impairs the ability to form a pincer grip, inability to resist adduction stress; tenderness over the UCL and clinical instability	Thumb spica splint. If more than 20-degree laxity, requires referral to a hand surgeon for definitive repair
Distal phalanx fractures	Often caused by crush injuries associated with subungual hematomas and nail bed lacerations	Deformity, pain and swelling; recognized on x-ray	A dorsal avulsion fracture of the base may result in mallet finger: treated with placement in a volar or hairpin splint extending beyond the DIP joint Nail bed trephination, depending on the size of the subungual hematoma
Proximal and middle phalanx fractures	Direct blow, crush injury, longitudinal traction (avulsion)	Pain and tenderness; examine closely for rotation of the digit (requires reduction)	Nondisplaced and stable: can be treated with buddy taping. Displaced: reduction is required (can use a pen as a fulcrum). Transverse, spiral midshaft fractures or intraarticular fractures: Gutter splint with the MCP joint flexed at 90 degrees, the PIP joint flexed at 20 degrees, and the DIP joint flexed at 10 degrees; often require surgical fixation

TABLE 145.2 *Traumatic Injuries of the Hand—cont'd*

Injury	Mechanism	Presentation	Treatment
Metacarpal (MC) fractures	Direct blow, most often after punching a hard surface. Fractures of the fourth or fifth MC neck (i.e., Boxer's fractures) are the most common.	Pain and tenderness; described based on involvement of head (most distal), neck, shaft, and base	Angulation more than 15 degrees in the second or third MC, 20 degrees in the fourth MC, 40 degrees in the fifth MC, requires reduction Ulnar gutter splints: for fractures of the fourth and fifth MC Radial gutter splints: for fractures of the second or third MC with the wrist extended to 20 degrees and the MCP joint flexed at 90 degrees
Thumb MC fractures	Axial force directed against a partially flexed metacarpal	Pain and tenderness; usually involve the base with intraarticular involvement (as either Bennett or Rolando fractures; see Fig. 145.2)	Thumb spica splint; often require operative repair, especially Rolando fractures

[a]Following successful reduction, it is important to assess the joint for stability and exclude a central slip injury. An irreducible joint may be from an entrapped volar plate, profundus tendon, or avulsion fracture, and requires immediate orthopedic evaluation.
[b]Irreducible joints are usually caused by "button-holing" of the metacarpal head between the flexor tendons and lumbricals with the entrapped plate potentially resulting in a visible dimple of the skin over the volar aspect of the joint. An operative open reduction is required.
[c]Roberts view: Anteroposterior view of the thumb taken with the hand rotated outwards (i.e., with the forearm in maximal pronation) and the dorsum of the thumb on the cassette for better visualization of the base of the thumb.

- Standard radiographs should be obtained, tetanus updated, and intravenous antibiotics administered for open fractures.
- Exposed bone may be trimmed back with a rongeur to below the level of the skin.
- Hand surgery should be contacted regarding possible reimplantation or revision amputation.
  - Indications for reimplantation include thumb amputations, amputations of multiple digits, amputation level between the metacarpophalangeal (MCP) and distal forearm, and amputations in children.
  - In general, amputations distal to the dorsal interphalangeal (DIP) are not amenable to reimplantation.
  - Other contraindications include crush injuries, prolonged ischemia time, severe contamination, advanced age, and poor health.

Traumatic Injuries of the Wrist

- The wrist is a complex joint composed of the distal radius, ulna, eight carpal bones and their associated ligaments.
  - The scaphoid is the most commonly fractured carpal bone, followed by the triquetrum.
- Evaluation of the wrist should include an examination for tenderness, range of motion, and neurovascular compromise.
- Posteroanterior (PA) and lateral wrist radiographs will reveal much of the pathology; however, it may be helpful to obtain scaphoid views (PA with maximal ulnar deviation) to identify scaphoid fractures; or carpal tunnel and oblique views, respectively, to delineate hook of hamate and pisiform fractures.
- Table 145.3 provides a summary of the traumatic injuries of the wrist, whereas Table 145.4 summarizes the traumatic injuries of the distal radius. Fig. 145.3 illustrates common distal forearm fractures.

TABLE 145.3 *Traumatic Injuries of the Wrist*

Classification	Injury and Mechanism	Presentation/Imaging	Treatment
Scapholunate dissociation	Forceful extension of the wrist	Wrist pain and swelling at the scapholunate joint. PA radiograph showing a space between the scaphoid and lunate greater than 3 mm.	Radial gutter splint or a thumb spica Prompt orthopedic referral
Perilunate dislocations	Hyperextension, ulnar deviation and intercarpal supination	Capitate is dislocated (usually dorsally), while the lunate remains aligned with the radius	Emergent consultation for closed reduction or surgical repair
Lunate dislocations	Hyperextension, ulnar deviation and intercarpal supination (lunate dislocates volar to the radius, but the capitate remains in anatomical position)	Lunate dislocation has a triangular shape on a posteroanterior radiograph ("piece of pie" sign) and on a lateral view, the "spilled teacup" sign	Emergent consultation for closed reduction or surgical repair
Carpal bone fractures	Falls, direct blow, crush injuries	Wrist pain and swelling often with normal x-ray	Conservative splinting and close outpatient follow-up

TABLE 145.4 *Distal Radius Fractures*

Injury	Mechanism	Presentation	Treatment
Colles fracture	Fall on an outstretched hand (FOOSH): extension injury with dorsal displacement of the distal radius	Classic "dinner fork" appearance on radiographs	Closed reduction and sugar tong splint; may require open reduction and internal fixation (ORIF).
Smith (reverse Colles) fracture	FOOSH or direct blow; supinated forearm with hand dorsiflexed	Volar displacement of distal radius without intraarticular involvement	Closed reduction and sugar tong splint; ORIF may be required.
Barton fracture	Extreme dorsiflexion + pronation flexion with volar displacement of the distal radius	Intraarticular and commonly involves the dorsal rim of the distal radius and fragmented bone; best seen on lateral radiographs	Closed reduction and sugar tong splint; ORIF may be required.
Radial styloid fractures	FOOSH or direct blow with force transmitted from the scaphoid to styloid (Hutchinson or Chauffer fracture)	Can produce carpal instability with scapholunate dissociation (up to 70% have extension injury to the scapholunate ligaments).	Sugar tong splint in mild flexion and ulnar deviation
Ulnar styloid fracture	FOOSH, direct blows	May result in radioulnar joint instability	Ulnar gutter splint with the wrist in neutral position and slight ulnar deviation

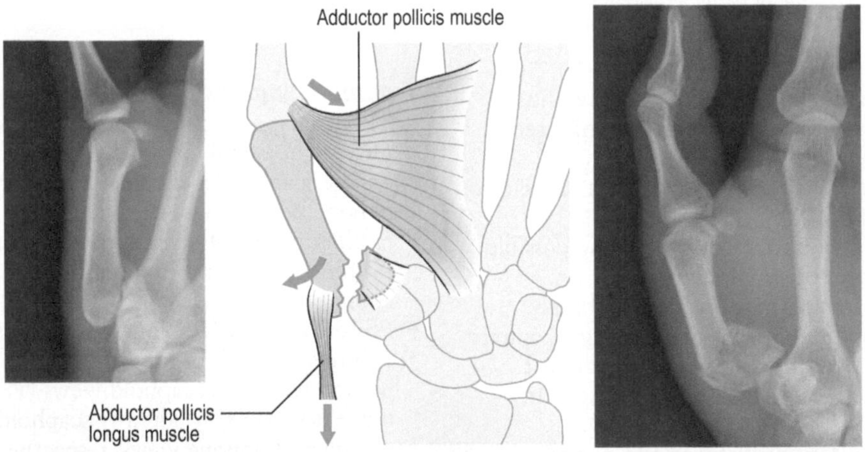

FIG. 145.2 Rolando and Bennett fractures. (From White, T. O., Mackenzie, S. P., & Gray, A. J. (2016). *McRae's orthopaedic trauma and emergency fracture management* (3rd ed., p. 276, Figs. 13.22 and 13.23). Churchill Pocketbooks, Elsevier Health Sciences.)

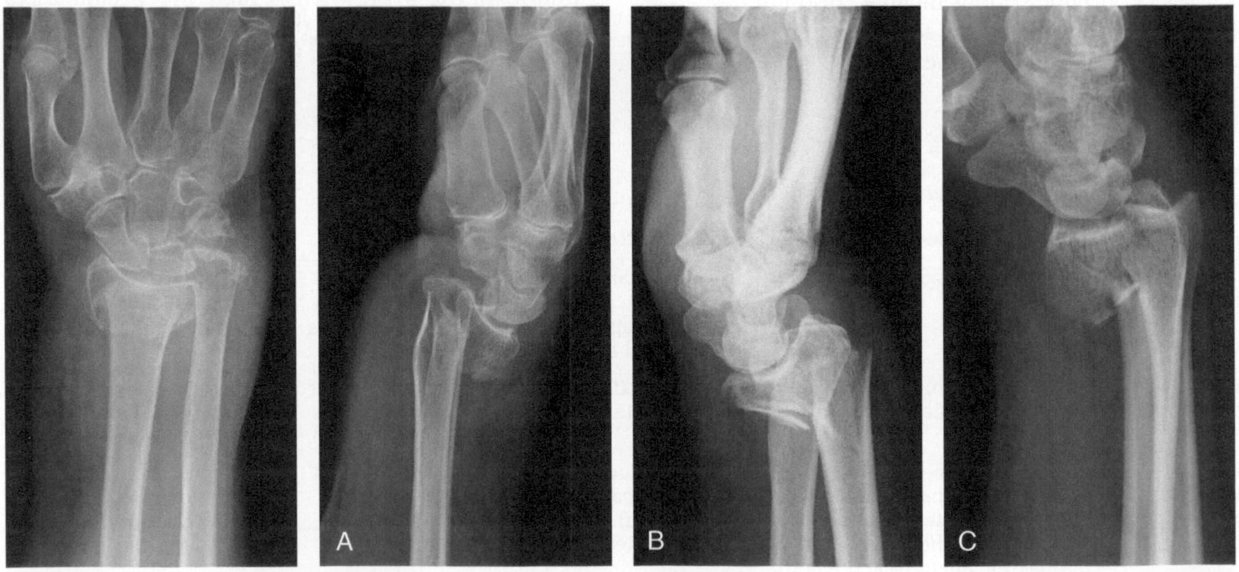

FIG. 145.3 Wrist fractures (Barton, Colles, and Smith fractures). (From White, T. O., Mackenzie, S. P., & Gray, A. J. (2016). *McRae's orthopaedic trauma and emergency fracture management* (3rd ed., pp. 235–236, Figs. 12.12–12.14). Churchill Pocketbooks, Elsevier Health Sciences.)

- Carpal fractures, especially scaphoid fractures, are susceptible to nonunion, and fractures of the scaphoid, lunate, or capitate are susceptible to avascular necrosis.
  - Scaphoid and lunate fractures are often not detected on plain radiographs, so emergency department diagnosis and treatment should be based on clinical findings with conservative thumb spica splinting and close outpatient follow-up.

Traumatic Injuries of the Forearm

- Forearm acts as a ring, with the radius and ulna rotating about each other for supination and pronation.
  - These bones are connected by ligaments, both proximally and distally, with the intraosseous membrane occupying the space between the radius and ulna.
- Forearm fractures are more common in men and represent the second most common site of open fractures (most common being the tibia).
- Evaluation should start with a complete examination for tenderness, open fractures, range of motion changes in supination and pronation, and neurovascular compromise.
- Radiographic examination should begin with anteroposterior (AP) and lateral views of the forearm, which includes the wrist and elbow, with a low threshold for adding views of both the wrist and elbow for better evaluation of injury patterns.
- Table 145.5 summarizes the traumatic injuries of the forearm with accompanying images in Fig. 145.4.

TABLE 145.5 *Traumatic Injuries of the Forearm*

Injury	Mechanism	Presentation	Treatment
Radial shaft fractures	Direct blow to radial shaft	Pain and tenderness along fracture site; careful examination of distal radioulnar joint	Nondisplaced, isolated fractures: closed reduction alone
Ulnar shaft fractures	Direct blow to the ulnar shaft ("nightstick" fracture)	Midshaft forearm tenderness	Nondisplaced fractures: long arm splint and close outpatient follow-up. Displaced fractures: temporized with a long arm splint and close orthopedic follow-up; may require ORIF
Monteggia fracture-dislocation (fracture of the proximal one-third of the ulna with a radial head dislocation)	Forceful pronation with external rotation (as in a fall)	Significant pain and swelling over the elbow; radiographs reveal disruption of the radiocapitellar line, with the apex of the ulna fracture pointing in the direction of the radial head dislocation	Definitive treatment by ORIF is usually required in adults.
Galeazzi fracture-dislocation (fracture of the middle and distal thirds of the radius with an associated distal radioulnar joint dislocation)	Fall on a hyperpronated hand	Localized tenderness and swelling over the distal radius; anteroposterior radiographs reveal widening of distal radioulnar joint space with dorsal displacement of the ulna on the lateral view.	Definitive treatment by ORIF is usually required in adults.

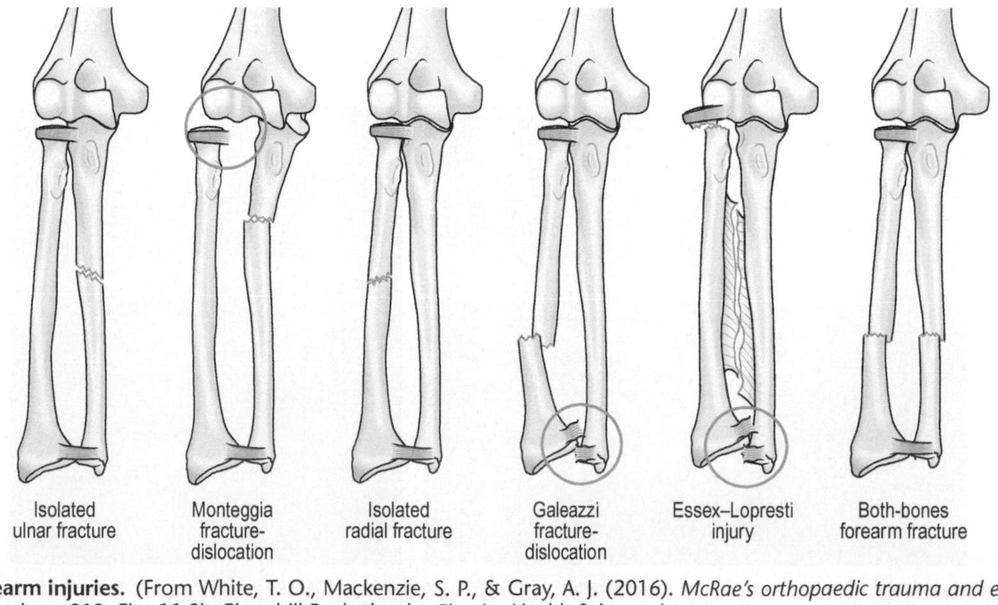

FIG. 145.4 Forearm injuries. (From White, T. O., Mackenzie, S. P., & Gray, A. J. (2016). *McRae's orthopaedic trauma and emergency fracture management* (3rd ed., p. 213, Fig. 11.3). Churchill Pocketbooks, Elsevier Health Sciences.)

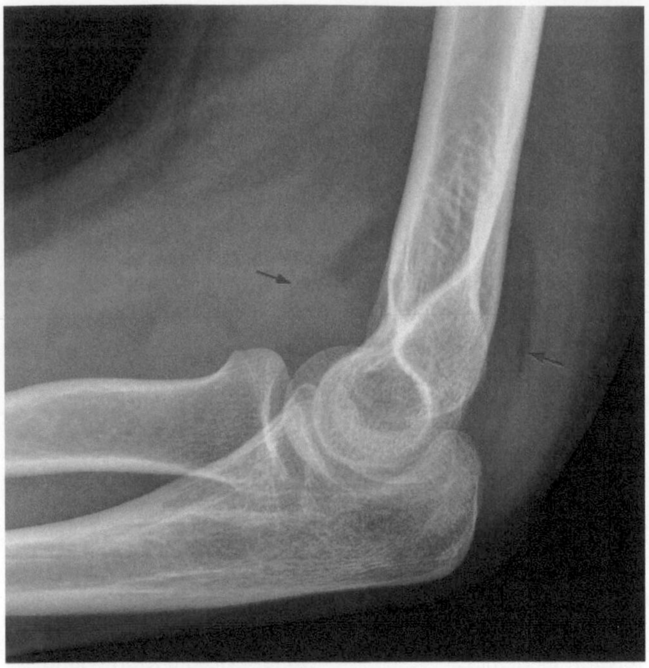

FIG. 145.5 Fat pad or "sail sign" (as depicted by the *red arrows*). (Courtesy https://en.wikipedia.org/wiki/Fat_pad_sign. Accessed November 16, 2019.)

Traumatic Injuries of the Elbow

- The elbow is a hinge joint composed of three articulations between the humerus, ulna, and radius.
- The distal humerus divides into two prominent epicondyles, medial and lateral, which provide tendinous attachments.
  - Between the two supracondylar ridges are two fossae: anteriorly is the coronoid fossa, and posteriorly is the olecranon fossa.
  - The anterior and posterior fossa are filled with fat pads, which, in the presence of a hemarthrosis, float out into the joint and become prominent on a lateral radiograph, known as the "sail sign," as illustrated in Fig. 145.5.
- **Elbow dislocations** most commonly occur as posterolateral dislocations. They usually occur in young adults during sporting or high-energy injuries. Recurrent dislocations are uncommon.
  - Elbow dislocations can be simple (without an associated fracture) or complex, involving a fracture.
  - Open dislocations, absence of a radial pulse before reduction, and polytrauma are all factors associated with brachial arterial injury.
  - Radiographs should be examined carefully for associated fractures and the "terrible triad," which consists of (1) elbow dislocation, (2) radial head fracture, and (3) coronoid process fracture, resulting in an unstable elbow (Fig. 145.6).
  - Simple elbow dislocations are relatively benign and are treated with closed reduction and splinting to 90 degrees.
    - Reduction techniques involve a combination of in-line traction to improve olecranon displacement, forearm supination to shift the coronoid under the trochlea, and elbow flexion with direct pressure on tip of olecranon.
  - Complex dislocations may require definitive operative repair.
- **Elbow fractures** may be defined as radial head, supracondylar, intercondylar, olecranon, or coronoid process fractures. A neurovascular examination is imperative because the complications are numerous.
  - Radial head and neck fractures are relatively common from fall-on-outstretched hand (FOOSH) injuries.
    - Abnormal fat pads, such as any posterior fat pad or a prominent anterior fat pad ("sail sign"), may be the only radiographic evidence of an injury. Disruption of the radiocapitellar line may be another clue to injury (especially in pediatrics).
  - Supracondylar fractures are most common in children.
    - Signs of Volkmann ischemic contracture, a dreaded complication of supracondylar fractures, include refusal to open the hand, pain with passive extension of the fingers, and forearm tenderness.
      - Most common nerve palsy in supracondylar fractures is anterior interosseous nerve (AIN)

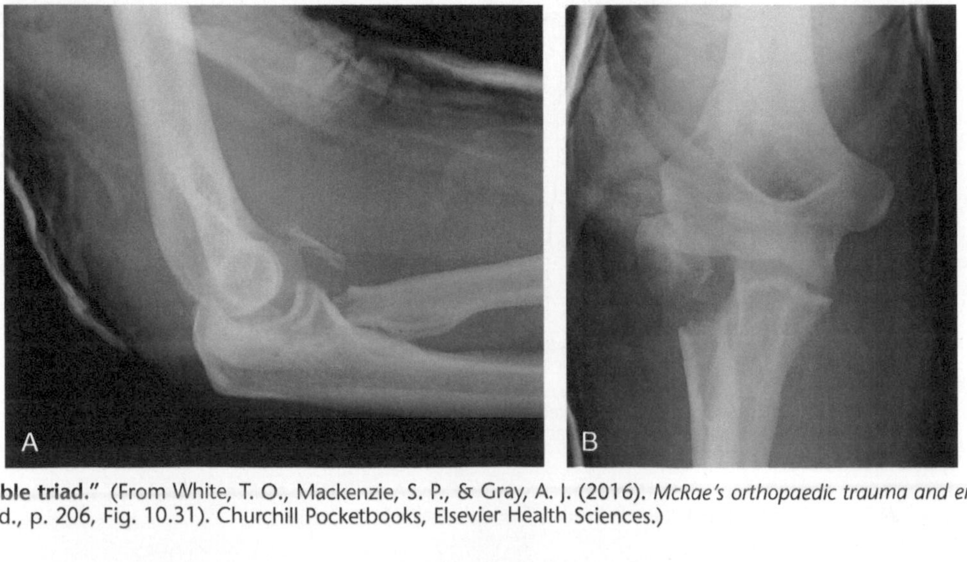

FIG. 145.6 "Terrible triad." (From White, T. O., Mackenzie, S. P., & Gray, A. J. (2016). *McRae's orthopaedic trauma and emergency fracture management* (3rd ed., p. 206, Fig. 10.31). Churchill Pocketbooks, Elsevier Health Sciences.)

neuropraxia, followed closely by radial nerve palsy.
  - Nondisplaced fractures with intact neurovascular status may be treated with splinting to 90 degrees elbow flexion with outpatient orthopedic follow-up within 1 week. Displaced fractures (type II or higher) will likely require closed reduction and percutaneous pinning or open reduction and internal fixation, and emergency department reduction and emergent orthopedic evaluation are warranted.
- Olecranon fractures are commonly caused by a direct fall onto the elbow with the proximal fragment displaced proximally by tension from the triceps.
- Olecranon fractures are frequently associated with ulnar nerve injury.
  - Nondisplaced fractures are treated with immobilization to 90 degrees elbow flexion with mobilization after 1 week. Displaced fractures may require closed reduction and close orthopedic follow-up because operative repair may be warranted.
- Coronoid process fractures are thought to be from hyperextension injuries, rarely occur in isolation, and are more commonly seen with posterior dislocations of the elbow.
  - Nondisplaced or minimally displaced fractures with a stable elbow joint may be treated with a brief period of immobilization followed by gradual mobilization. Any elbow instability or significantly displaced fracture patterns will require operative repair and emergent orthopedics consultation.

Traumatic Injuries of the Upper Arm

- Proximal humerus fractures represent almost half of all humerus fractures, with an increased incidence in females, thought to be due to differences in bone density.
- Patients with proximal humerus fractures have pain, swelling, tenderness, ecchymosis, and crepitance around the shoulder and upper arm. Range of motion is severely limited, and patients hold their arms against their chest wall.
- Radiographs confirm the diagnosis; the Neer classification divides the proximal humerus into four parts and is used to guide treatment.
- The axillary artery and nerve are most commonly affected, whereas the brachial plexus is affected infrequently.
- Nondisplaced or one-part proximal humerus fractures (displaced less than 1 cm or angulated less than 45 degrees) require only sling immobilization, ice, analgesics, and orthopedic referral.
- Humeral shaft fractures that are nondisplaced require a coaptation splint, hanging cast, or functional bracing.
- Multipart proximal humerus fractures, significantly displaced or angulated shaft fractures, open fractures, or neurovascular compromise require immediate orthopedic consultation.

Traumatic Injuries of the Acromioclavicular (AC) Joint

- Acromioclavicular joint dislocations typically follow a direct blow or fall onto the outer aspect of the shoulder.
- The injury is defined by the extent of ligamentous involvement and graded on a scale from I to VI based on the Rockwood classification (Table 145.6).
- Treatment involves sling and outpatient follow-up, except in the cases of neurovascular compromise, skin compromise, or Rockwood grade V to VI where immediate orthopedic consultation is required.

Traumatic Injuries of the Shoulder

- Shoulder dislocations are a common reason for presentation to the emergency department.
- These usually occur in young adult males engaged in contact sports, involving abduction and external rotation of the shoulder, forcing it beyond its stable range.
- Anterior dislocations are the most common, followed by posterior and inferior dislocations.
- Radiographs should be examined carefully for associated fractures, such as the Hill-Sachs and Bankart lesions.
  - A Hill-Sachs lesion is an impaction fracture of the posterior humeral head as it is compressed against the anterior glenoid after dislocation.
  - A bony Bankart lesion is a fracture of the anterior inferior glenoid.
  - For posterior dislocations, glenohumeral dislocations are most easily recognized in the axillary view, which may also demonstrate the reverse Hill-Sachs defect.
- Table 145.7 summarizes the various types of shoulder dislocations and their management.

TABLE 145.6 *Rockwood Classification of Acromioclavicular Injuries*

Classification	Ligaments	Radiographs	Treatment
Type I	AC ligament: sprain CC ligament: normal	Normal	Sling
Type II	AC ligament: torn CC ligament: sprain	AC joint disruption, increased CC distance less than 25% of contralateral	Sling
Type III	AC ligament: torn CC ligament: torn	Increased CC distance 25%–100% of contralateral	Controversial (operative repair vs. sling placement)
Type IV	AC ligament: torn CC ligament: torn	Clavicle displaced posteriorly into or through the trapezius muscle	Operative repair
Type V	AC ligament: torn CC ligament: torn	Increased CC distance more than 100% of contralateral	Operative repair
Type VI	AC ligament: torn CC ligament: torn	Inferior dislocation of lateral clavicle	Operative repair

AC, acromioclavicular; *CC*, coracoclavicular.

TABLE 145.7 *Traumatic Injuries of the Shoulder*

Injury	Mechanism	Presentation	Treatment
Anterior shoulder dislocation	Abduction with external rotation	Shoulder pain, a "squared-off" appearance of the shoulder	Closed reduction for all dislocations without humeral neck fractures and with or without an isolated tuberosity fracture; sling
Posterior shoulder dislocations	Direct blow to the anterior shoulder resulting in posterior translocation of humeral head Electric shock (e.g., lighning), convulsive mechanism (e.g., seizure), or injury while in position of adduction, flexion, and internal rotation	Arm held in adduction and internal rotation with severely limited abduction and inability to rotate externally	Closed reduction for all dislocations without a humeral neck fracture and with or without an isolated tuberosity fracture; sling
Inferior shoulder dislocation (luxatio erecta)	Forceful hyperabduction resulting in a locked inferior dislocation of the glenohumeral joint	Classic position with humerus locked in abduction and forward elevation (as if they are "asking a question")	Closed reduction for all dislocations without a humeral neck fracture and with or without an isolated tuberosity fracture; sling

Lower Extremity Orthopedic Trauma

General Principles

- Lower extremity injuries comprise a broad group of injuries involving the femur, knee, lower leg, ankle, and foot.
- Mechanisms may range from low-energy ankle sprains to high-energy motor vehicle collisions or a fall from a height.

Clinical Presentation

- Patients present with pain of the affected limb, decreased range of motion, gait changes, or inability to walk.
  - It is important to examine patients closely for neurovascular compromise and for wounds that may indicate open fractures.

Diagnosis and Evaluation

- Radiographs of the affected extremity should be obtained.
  - Consider obtaining imaging of the joint above and below the injury.
  - CT may also be required to identify occult fractures missed by plain radiographs (e.g., acetabular fractures or tibial plateau fractures).

Traumatic Injuries of the Foot

- The foot is divided into the hind foot, midfoot, and forefoot.
  - The Chopart joint separates the hind foot and midfoot, and the Lisfranc joint separates the midfoot and the forefoot.
- **Calcaneal fractures**: one of the most common hind foot injuries seen in the emergency department
  - Mechanism involves axial loading (i.e., high-energy mechanism, fall from height), and associated injuries such as a contralateral calcaneal fracture and/or lumbar compression fracture are common.
  - Radiographs of the foot (including dedicated calcaneal views) are indicated, but fractures may be subtle and can be missed.
    - On radiographs without clear evidence of fracture, Boehler angle can be measured (Fig. 145.7). An angle of less than 20 degrees is suggestive of a compression fracture.
    - CT may be required if suspicion is high and radiographs are unrevealing.
  - Treatment involves placement in a bulky Jones dressing and close orthopedic follow-up. Operative treatment remains controversial, but should be performed within 3 weeks of the injury, if indicated.
- **Midfoot injuries:** the midfoot is composed of five bones: navicular, cuboid, and medial, intermediate, and lateral cuneiforms.
  - Injuries around the tarsometatarsal joint and pain with torsion of the midfoot should raise suspicion for a Lisfranc injury (Fig. 145.8).
  - Lisfranc injuries are often associated with a fracture, especially at the base of the second metatarsal.

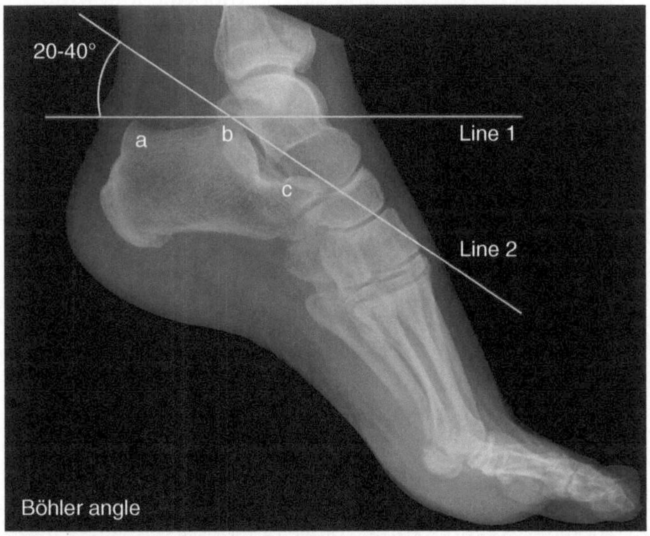

FIG. 145.7 **Boehler angle. Line 1:** Drawn between the most cephalic part of the posterior process of the calcaneus bone (**point a**) and the most cephalic point of the posterior facet of the calcaneus bone (**point b**). **Line 2:** Drawn between the most cephalic point of the posterior facet of the calcaneus bone (**point b**) and the highest point of the calcaneus bone articulating with the cuboid bone (**point c**). (Image and details courtesy https://litfl.com/bohler-angle/. Accessed November 16, 2019.)

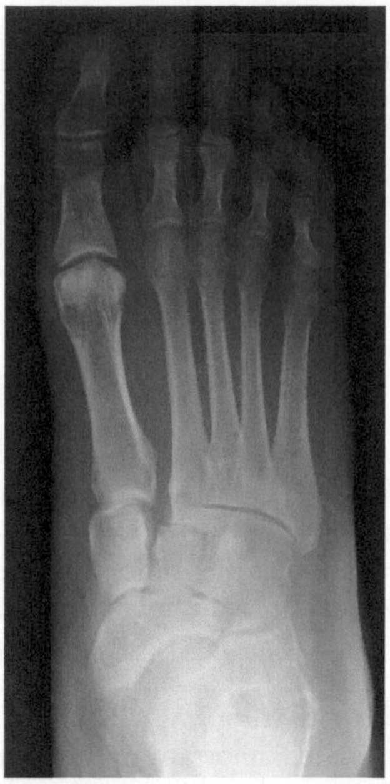

FIG. 145.8 Lisfranc injury. (From White, T. O., Mackenzie, S. P., & Gray, A. J. (2016). *McRae's orthopaedic trauma and emergency fracture management* (3rd ed., p. 544, Fig. 22.36). Churchill Pocketbooks, Elsevier Health Sciences.)

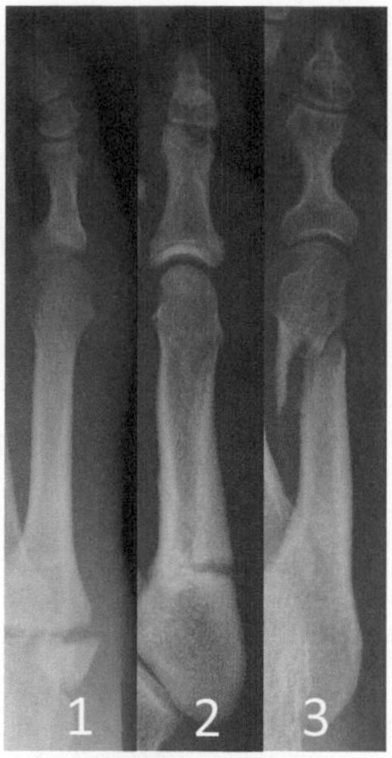

FIG. 145.9 Fifth metatarsal fracture zones. (From White, T. O., Mackenzie, S. P, & Gray, A. J. (2016). *McRae's orthopaedic trauma and emergency fracture management* (3rd ed., p. 547, Fig. 22.42). Churchill Pocketbooks, Elsevier Health Sciences.)

  - On radiographs, a gap more than 1 mm between the bases of the first and second metatarsal is considered unstable. Weight-bearing x-rays will assist in diagnosis of a Lisfranc injury. CT helps better delineate injury patterns.
  - These injuries require orthopedic consultation for definitive repair.
  - Isolated navicular, cuboid, and cuneiform injuries are rare and treated conservatively with a hard-sole shoe.
- **Metatarsal injuries:** metatarsal fractures of the forefoot are common.
  - Metatarsal fractures are described according to the fracture position, the affected metatarsal (1 to 5) and the location: base, shaft, neck, or head.
    - The exception to this is the fifth metatarsal, which is divided into three zones (Box 145.1 and Fig. 145.9).

Traumatic Injuries of the Ankle

- Ankle injuries are common; ankle pain is a common reason for seeking emergency department care.
- Anatomically, the ankle is most stable in dorsiflexion, when the wider anterior portion of the talus engages with the ankle mortise and allows for little movement.
- Overall, ligamentous injuries are far more common than fractures, but frequently coexist with fractures.
  - Ottawa Ankle Rules were developed to predict the likelihood of ankle fractures and reduce the number of radiographs obtained. Although validated in adults, these rules are not fully validated in school-aged children.
- **Posterior dislocations**, the most common ankle dislocations, occur with a backward force on the plantar-flexed foot.
  - This usually results in rupture of the tibiofibular ligaments or a lateral malleolus fracture.
  - Immediate reduction in the emergency department should be performed with assessment of neurovascular status followed by placement in a posterior short leg splint and an emergent orthopedics consultation.
- **Ankle fractures:** mechanism for ankle factures can be divided broadly into those caused by rotational forces and those secondary to axial loading.
  - Rotational forces, such as inversion, eversion, adduction, and abduction, result in injury to the distal tibia and fibula as well as ligamentous injuries.
    - Rotational ankle fractures are described by their involvement of malleoli: unimalleolar fracture, bimalleolar fracture (lateral and medial), and trimalleolar fractures (medial, lateral, and posterior).
  - Axial loading injuries result in fractures of the tibial plafond (pilon).
- Examination should begin with a complete history and physical examination followed by a detailed evaluation of the joint and neurovascular status.
- If radiographs are indicated, a complete ankle series (AP, mortise, and lateral) should be obtained.
  - Talar shift (Fig. 145.10) indicates an unstable fracture (disruption of primary stabilizers: medial malleolus or deltoid ligament).
  - Tibia and fibula radiographs may be obtained to identify proximal injury (i.e., Maisonneuve fractures). Stress views of the ankle can also be considered to assess for possible ligamentous injury.

BOX 145.1 ***Zones of Injury for Fifth Metatarsal Fractures***

Zone 1: Avulsion fracture of the fifth metatarsal tuberosity (Pseudo-Jones fracture)
Zone 2: Fracture of the intermetatarsal joint between the fourth and fifth metatarsals (Jones fracture)
Zone 3: Proximal diaphysis fractures; less common than fractures in zones 1 and 2

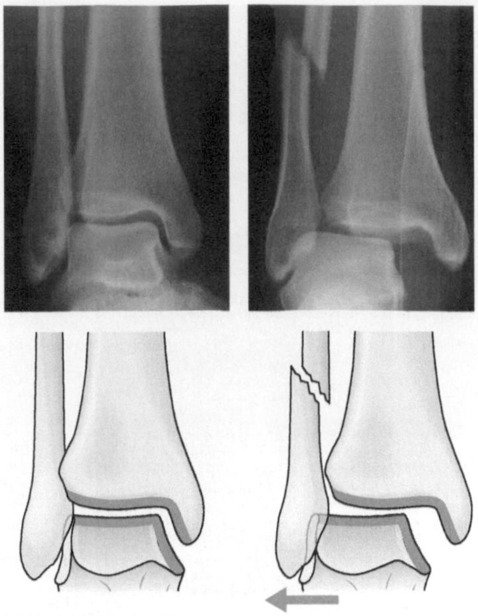

FIG. 145.10 **Talar shift.** (From White, T. O., Mackenzie, S. P., & Gray, A. J. (2016). *McRae's orthopaedic trauma and emergency fracture management* (3rd ed., p. 485, Fig. 21.18). Churchill Pocketbooks, Elsevier Health Sciences.)

- **Pilon fractures** are severe injuries to the ankle that are defined as intraarticular fractures of the plafond caused by an axial load.
  - The mechanism is usually a high-energy motor vehicle crash or fall from height.
  - Any obvious deformity on examination should be immediately reduced.
    - CTs are required for preoperative planning and to evaluate the fracture fragments.
- Treatment of ankle fractures depends on the stability of the ankle joint; examples are provided in Table 145.8.
  - Stable fractures are treated nonoperatively and unstable fractures are treated operatively.
  - Stable fractures should be splinted (e.g., posterior short-leg splint), and the patient provided with crutches and referred for orthopedic evaluation within 1 week.
  - Emergent orthopedic evaluation is indicated for open fractures, unstable ankle fractures, and neurovascular compromise.

Traumatic Injuries of the Knee and Lower Leg

- Lower leg fractures often follow sporting injuries and falls.
- Because the tibia is more subcutaneous, tibial fractures are usually apparent on arrival at the emergency department as an obvious deformity or open fracture.

TABLE 145.8 ***Examples of Stable and Unstable Ankle Fractures***

Stable	Unstable
Isolated lateral malleolus fractures, with no medial fracture or deltoid ligament rupture Isolated avulsion fractures of the tip of the fibula (Weber A) Isolated fractures of the medial malleolus	Bimalleolar fractures Trimalleolar fracture High fibular fractures (Weber C – suprasyndesmotic and Maisonneuve fractures)

- Table 145.9 describes the various lower leg fractures, the mechanisms of injury, imaging, and management.
- **Patellar dislocations** result in pain, swelling, and deformity of the knee, with patients often reporting a sensation of feeling their knee "go out."
  - Mechanisms of injury
    - Powerful contraction of the quadriceps with sudden flexion and external rotation of the tibia on the femur (most common mechanism for lateral patellar dislocations)
    - Direct trauma/blow with the knee in flexion (less common)
  - These injuries will often spontaneously reduce in the field, but patients may have a positive patellar apprehension test on examination.
    - Of note, tearing of the joint capsule can also occur.
    - Multidirectional instability of the knee, which should not occur with a simple patellar dislocation, should raise the suspicion for a spontaneously reduced knee dislocation.
      - It is critically important to differentiate correctly between a patellar dislocation and a posterior knee dislocation because there is a significant risk of vascular compromise with the latter condition.
  - AP and lateral radiographs should be obtained to assess for fractures.
  - Reduction of lateral patellar dislocations can be performed by placing the patient supine with the hip in flexion, putting gentle pressure on the patella in the medial direction while extending the knee.
  - Management involves knee immobilization (ideally with J braces around the kneecap to help keep the patella in its proper position during movement), and orthopedic follow-up.
    - Intraarticular, horizontal, and superior dislocations often require operative repair.
- **Knee (tibiofemoral) dislocations** are classified by the position of the tibia in relation to the femur and are considered orthopedic emergencies owing to the high risk of neurovascular injury, specifically popliteal artery injury (peroneal nerve injury can also occur).
  - Patients present with knee pain and associated swelling, although a joint effusion may be absent because tears in the joint capsule allow for blood to extend to soft tissues.
  - Mechanism of injury
    - Anterior (40%): hyperextension
    - Posterior (33%): high energy (motor vehicle crash, fall from height) resulting from direct force applied to tibia with knee in flexion, with 15%–20% resulting in open dislocations
    - Lateral (18%) and medial (4%) dislocations also occur and can be in combination with anterior and posterior dislocations.
  - Imaging
    - AP and lateral x-rays are usually adequate, but there should be a low threshold to obtain a CT angiography and vascular surgery consultation owing to the high incidence of concurrent neurovascular injuries, especially with contralateral differences in ankle-brachial indices.

TABLE 145.9 *Lower Leg Fractures*

Injury	Mechanism	Imaging	Complications	Treatment
Femoral condyles	Axial load injury or direct blow to distal femur	AP and lateral radiographs; consider CT to evaluate intraarticular fracture and better view of Hoffa fracture	Risk of injury to popliteal artery	Nondisplaced: knee brace, NWB, outpatient follow-up Displaced: operative repair
Patellar fracture	Direct blow or forceful quadriceps contraction	AP, lateral, sunrise radiographs	Osteonecrosis, stiffness	Nondisplaced with intact extensor mechanism: knee brace with weight bearing, outpatient follow-up Displaced with disrupted extensor mechanism or severely comminuted: operative repair
Tibial spine fracture	Rapid deceleration or hyperextension/ rotation of the knee	AP, lateral, oblique, ± intercondylar view (notch view)	Hemarthrosis, ACL injury (attached to medial spine)	Nondisplaced or incomplete fractures: knee extension brace, outpatient orthopedics within 1 week Displaced or complete: early referral for operative repair
Tibial plateau fracture	Varus/valgus load with axial load that compresses the femoral condyle into the tibia	AP, lateral, oblique radiographs. CT important to identify articular depression and comminution. Note: lipohemarthrosis indicates an occult fracture	Meniscal tears, ACL injuries, compartment syndrome, vascular injury more common in Schatzker IV fracture-dislocations	Nondisplaced, unilateral fracture: knee immobilizer, NWB, orthopedic follow-up within 1 week Depression of articular surface: early orthopedic consult for operative repair

ACL, anterior cruciate ligament; *CT*, computed tomography; *NWB*, non–weight bearing; *AP*, anteroposterior.

- In contrast to patellar dislocations, knee dislocations generally require definitive surgery for primary repair of ligaments and menisci.

Traumatic Injuries of the Pelvis, Hip, and Femur

- The bony and ligamentous attachments of the pelvis form a stable ring with the acetabulum connecting to the hip and proximal femur.
- The presentation for patients with pelvic, hip, and femur injuries varies from ambulatory patients with localized pain to hemodynamically unstable polytrauma patients.
  - Ambulatory patients may localize pain to their groin, hip, or upper leg.
- Examination should begin by observing the affected limb for shortening, rotation, or deformities, followed by palpation, assessment of neurovascular status, and range-of-motion testing.
  - Patients with injuries from traumatic mechanisms should undergo a complete trauma survey for associated injuries.
  - Hemodynamically unstable patients should be evaluated for alternative sources of bleeding.
- Pelvic fractures are frequently associated with hemorrhage and other injuries.
  - Airway, breathing, and circulation should be addressed first, and the patient appropriately resuscitated before evaluating the extremities.
- Passive hip rotation is often painful in hip and acetabular fractures, but well-tolerated in ramus fractures. Similarly, axial loading is painful in hip fractures, but better tolerated in ramus fractures.
  - Comfortable active range-of-motion testing usually excludes a hip or acetabular fracture.
- Obtain standard AP pelvis radiographs in patients with suspected pelvic injury.
  - In unstable trauma patients, this allows for emergent assessment for bony injury in patients who require more emergent resuscitation and stabilization.
  - Three radiographs are required for complete evaluation of the pelvic ring: AP, inlet, and outlet views.
  - CT of the pelvis is commonly acquired as part of the polytrauma evaluation and may replace the plain radiographs because CT is superior for identifying pelvic and acetabular fractures and evaluating for pelvic ring stability.
    - However, it is still helpful to obtain the plain radiographs first because prompt pelvic binder placement may be indicated if an "open book" fracture is identified.
- Pelvic fractures include fracture patterns with disruption of the pelvic ring, single fractures without disruption of the pelvic ring (Table 145.10), and acetabular fractures.
  - Young and Burgess classification (Fig. 145.11) describes fracture patterns with a disrupted pelvic ring based on the vector of the disrupting force and degree of displacement.
  - The forces are broadly divided into AP compression (force applied from the front), lateral compression (side-on impact), and vertical shear (upward movement of the hemipelvis in relation to the sacrum, often the result of landing from a height on to one leg).
  - Pelvic fractures may be initially stabilized with pelvic binding.
    - The goal of a pelvic binder is to compress the pelvic volume and to stop/minimize hemorrhage.

TABLE 145.10 *Fractures of the Pelvis*

Fracture	Mechanism	Treatment
Iliac wing	Direct blow, usually lateral to medial	Usually nonoperative if nondisplaced: analgesics, non–weight bearing, orthopedic follow-up in 1 to 2 weeks Displaced fractures may require operative repair
Single ramus or pubis or ischium	Elderly: fall, direct trauma; stress fracture in younger patients	Nonoperative: analgesics, protected weight bearing (crutches, canes), donut ring cushion, orthopedic follow-up in 1 to 2 weeks
Ischium body	Fall in sitting position	Nonoperative: analgesics, bed rest, weight bearing as tolerated (crutches, canes), orthopedic follow-up in 1 to 2 weeks
Sacral fracture	Fall or direct trauma	Usually nonoperative: analgesics, bed rest, weight bearing as tolerated (crutches, canes), orthopedic follow-up in 1 to 2 weeks. Immediate consultation indicated for displaced fractures or neurologic deficits.
Coccygeal fracture	Fall in sitting position	Nonoperative: analgesics, stool softeners, weight bearing as tolerated (crutches, canes), donut ring cushion, Sitz baths, orthopedic follow-up in 2 weeks
Anterior superior iliac spine (ASIS)	Forceful Sartorius contraction	Nonoperative: analgesics, bed rest for 3 to 4 weeks with hip flexed and abducted, weight bearing as tolerated (crutches, canes), orthopedic follow-up in 1 to 2 weeks
Anterior inferior iliac spine (AIIS)	Forceful rectus femoris contraction	Nonoperative: analgesics, bed rest for 3 to 4 weeks with hip flexed, weight bearing as tolerated (crutches), orthopedic follow-up in 1 to 2 weeks
Ischial tuberosity	Forceful hamstring contraction	Nonoperative: analgesics, bed rest for 3 to 4 weeks in extension and external rotation, weight bearing as tolerated (crutches, canes), orthopedic follow-up in 1 to 2 weeks

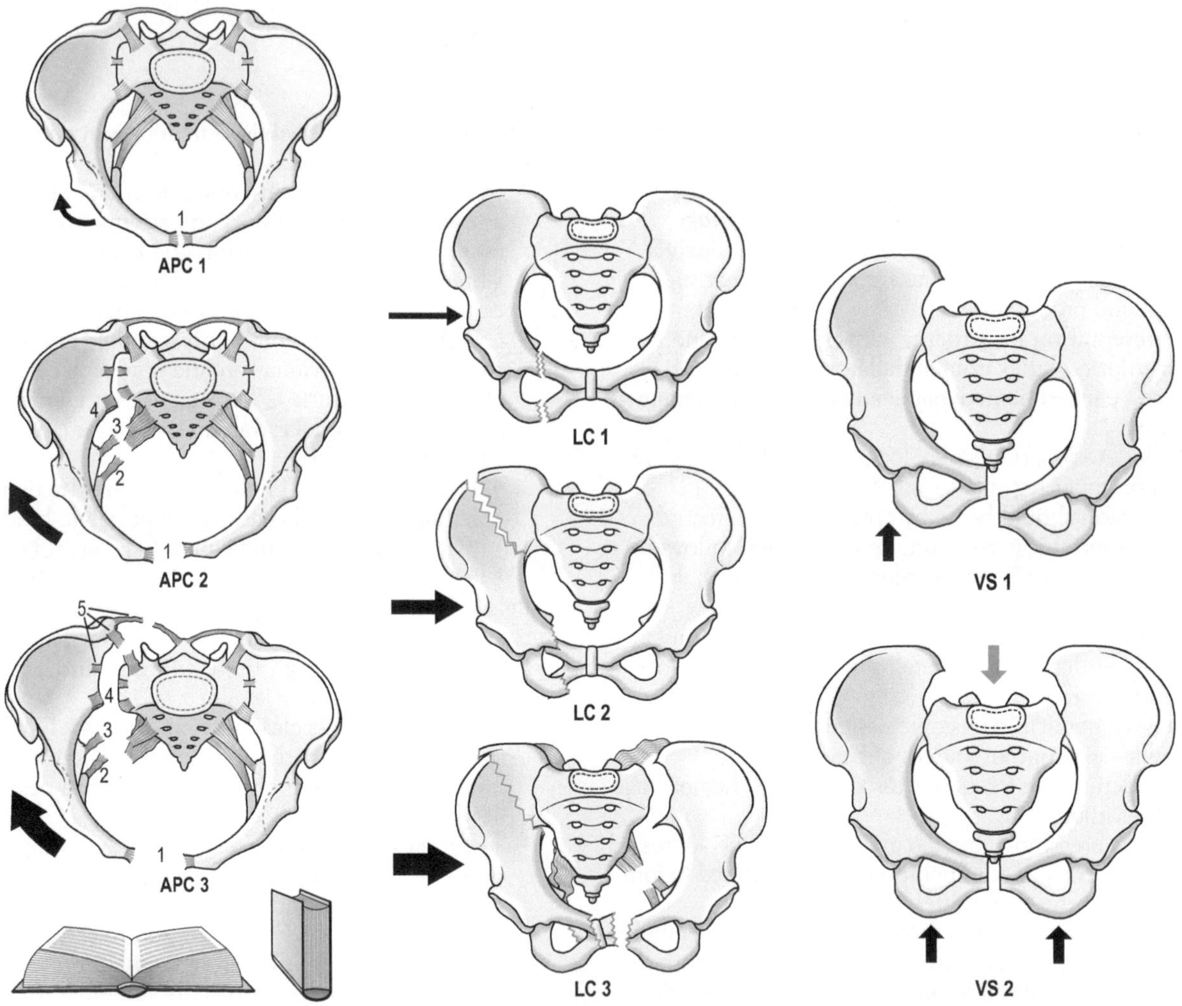

FIG. 145.11 Young and Burgess classification (VS, vertical shear; LC, lateral compression; APC, anteroposterior compression). (From White, T. O., Mackenzie, S. P., & Gray, A. J. (2016). *McRae's orthopaedic trauma and emergency fracture management* (3rd ed., pp. 330–331, Figs. 15.9, 15.10. and 15.12). Churchill Pocketbooks, Elsevier Health Sciences.)

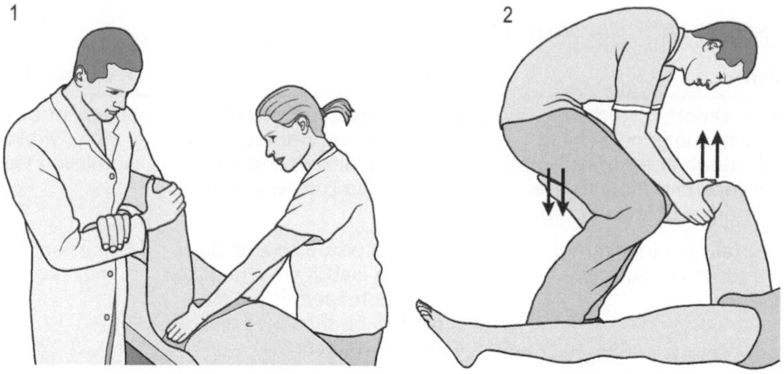

FIG. 145.12 The Allis maneuver. (From White, T. O., Mackenzie, S. P., & Gray, A. J. (2016). *McRae's orthopaedic trauma and emergency fracture management* (3rd ed., p. 376, Fig. 17.37). Churchill Pocketbooks, Elsevier Health Sciences.)

These are recommended in AP compression fractures (or "open book" pelvic fractures) and may not be useful in other pelvic fractures.
    - For adequate compression of the pelvic ring, pelvic binders should be placed at the level of the greater trochanter.
  - Hemorrhage from pelvic fractures may be treated with pelvic embolization, external fixation, or operative repair.
- **Acetabular fractures** are commonly seen with hip dislocations.
  - Standard AP pelvis radiograph and Judet views can help identify the fracture pattern, although CT is more sensitive and can assist with preoperative planning.
  - Acetabular fractures require hospital admission and orthopedic consultation.
    - Nondisplaced fractures may be treated conservatively, but displaced fractures require early open reduction and internal fixation.
- **Hip dislocations** may be anterior or posterior, and commonly result after high-speed motor vehicle crashes.
  - Approximately 90% of hip dislocations are posterior and may be associated with acetabular fractures.
    - On examination, the extremity is shortened, internally rotated, and adducted.
    - With anterior dislocations, the extremity is held in abduction and external rotation.
  - Dislocation of a hip prosthesis usually results from a position of flexion and internal rotation, such as when pulling on shoes or rising from a low seat. The majority of these dislocations are also posterior.
  - Imaging should start with radiographs of the hip and pelvis; further evaluation of the acetabulum and femur may be done with Judet views or CT.
  - Native hip dislocations are orthopedic emergencies and should be reduced within 6 hours owing to a higher incidence of avascular necrosis with delay.
    - The Allis maneuver is one of the most common methods for hip reduction (Fig. 145.12).
- **Proximal femur/hip fractures:** the vast majority of hip fractures occur in elderly patients with osteoporosis after a ground-level fall.
  - Younger patients may present with hip fractures after high-energy trauma or avulsion injuries from forceful muscle contraction.
  - Initial radiographs of the pelvis and hip should be obtained; however, a CT or MRI may be required for occult fractures.
  - Common proximal femur and hip injuries are summarized in Table 145.11, along with the mechanisms of injury, imaging, and treatment.
- **Femoral shaft fractures:** fractures of the femoral shaft are most common in younger patients secondary to high-energy trauma.
  - Patients often present with a shortened limb, pain, swelling, and deformity.
  - A prompt evaluation of neurovascular status should be performed.
  - Owing to the high-energy mechanism, a complete trauma survey should be performed for other injuries.
  - Femoral shaft fractures should be treated with traction and splinting.
  - Open fractures require IV antibiotics, copious irrigation, and operative repair. Tetanus vaccine should also be updated/given.
  - These patients should be admitted to the trauma service or orthopedic service for definitive treatment.

REFERENCE

White, T. O., Mackenzie, S. P., & Gray, A. J. (2016). *McRae's orthopaedic trauma and emergency fracture management* (3rd ed.). Churchill Pocketbooks, Elsevier Health Sciences.

SUGGESTED READINGS

Arnold, C., Fayos, Z., Bruner, D., Arnold, D., Gupta, N., & Nusbaum, J. (2017). Managing dislocations of the hip, knee, and ankle in the emergency department. *Emergency Medicine Practice, 19*, 1–2.

Fiechtl, J. F., & Gibbs, M. A. (2010). An evidence-based approach to managing injuries of the pelvis and hip in the emergency department. *Emergency Medicine Practice, 12*(12).

Pescatore, R., & Nyce, A. (2017). Managing shoulder injuries in the emergency department: Fracture, dislocation, and overuse. *Emergency Medicine Practice, 20*, 1–28.

TABLE 145.11 *Proximal Femur and Hip Injuries*

Injury	Mechanism	Presentation	Treatment
Femoral head dislocation	Anterior dislocation: forced abduction with the femoral head tearing through anterior capsule Posterior dislocation: blow to the knee with hip and knee flexed	Limb shortened and externally rotated (anterior dislocation); shortened, flexed, and internally rotated (posterior dislocation)	Emergent closed reduction of the dislocation (within 6 hours from time of injury) Admission with orthopedic consultation
Femoral neck fracture	Low-impact falls in elderly; high-energy trauma in younger patients	Ranges from pain with ambulation to an inability to ambulate, often in osteoporotic patients. Limb may be shortened and externally rotated.	Admission with orthopedics consult; may require operative repair
Greater trochanteric fracture	Direct trauma in elderly; avulsion fracture from contraction of gluteus medius in younger patients	Usually ambulatory with pain with palpation or abduction	Analgesics with weight bearing as tolerated with gait aids (crutches, cane, walker) Orthopedic follow-up in 1 to 2 weeks If displaced more than 1 cm, may require operative repair
Lesser trochanteric fracture	Adolescents: avulsion owing to forceful contraction of iliopsoas Adults: pathologic fracture	Usually ambulatory, pain with flexion or rotation	Analgesics with weight bearing as tolerated; orthopedic follow-up in 1 to 2 weeks. Admission for pathologic fractures
Intertrochanteric fracture	Falls and high-energy trauma	Severe pain, swelling, limb shortened and externally rotated, nonambulatory	Admission with orthopedics consult for operative repair
Subtrochanteric fracture	Falls and high-energy trauma; may also be pathologic	Severe pain, ecchymosis, limb shortened, abducted, externally rotated, nonambulatory	Admission with orthopedics consult for operative repair

SECTION EIGHTEEN

BOARD REVIEW

Procedures and Skills

CHAPTER 146

BOARD REVIEW

Airway Management

SARAH LOPEZ, MD, MBA, and ALEXANDER GARRETT, MD

General Principles

- Airway management is one of the foundational skills of emergency medicine, and must be mastered and practiced with repeated hands-on experience to provide care to the critically ill patient.
- It is estimated that a minimum number of 57 endotracheal intubations are necessary to achieve 90% proficiency, and this number does not address continuing practice out of residency.
- Airway and breathing are part of the initial "ABCs" in assessing any emergency patient. The significant morbidity and mortality associated with prolonged hypoxia make the establishment of a protected, well-ventilated airway essential to caring for the critically ill.
- A common mistake during preparation for intubation is failure to perform a difficult airway evaluation, which all emergency doctors should do when assessing the airway. LEMON (*l*ook, *e*valuate with 3-3-2 rule, *M*allampati score, *o*bstruction, *n*eck mobility) and BOOTS (*b*eard, *o*ld, *o*bese, *t*oothless, *s*noring) are useful for predicting difficult airways/laryngoscopy and difficult bag-mask ventilations, respectively. It is also necessary to recognize when a step in the algorithm has failed, and when to proceed to the next step.
- Fundamental airway management techniques (Box 146.1)
- Sample advanced airway management algorithm (Fig. 146.1)
- Sample failed/difficult airway algorithm (Fig. 146.2)

BOX 146.1 *Fundamental Airway Management Techniques*

Oxygen Delivery
Nasal cannula, simple mask, non-rebreather mask
Noninvasive positive pressure ventilation (NPPV): BPAP/CPAP/High-flow nasal cannula
Bag-mask ventilation

Airway Adjuncts
Oropharyngeal/Nasopharyngeal airways
LMA/ILMA
Combitube/King tube

Direct Laryngoscopy
Mac/Miller blade
Bougie

Video-Assisted Laryngoscopy
Glidescope, McGrath, C-MAC

Flexible Bronchoscopy/Fiberoptic

Nasotracheal
Blind/Laryngoscopic/Fiberoptic

Cricothyrotomy
Surgical airway, needle method

BPAP, bilevel positive airway pressure ventilation; *CPAP*, continuous positive airway pressure ventilation; *LMA*, laryngeal mask airway; *ILMA*, intubating laryngeal mask airway.

Indications

POSITIONING, HEAD-TILT, JAW THRUST

- Angle and position will determine vocal cord exposure.
- Concern for upper airway obstruction
- Poor bag-mask ventilation

NASAL CANNULA, SIMPLE MASK, NON-REBREATHER

- Hypoxemia
- Respiratory distress
- Hemodynamic insufficiency
- CO poisoning
- Preoxygenation

NONINVASIVE POSITIVE PRESSURE VENTILATION (NIPPV)

- BPAP (*b*ilevel *p*ositive *a*irway *p*ressure ventilation), CPAP (*c*ontinuous *p*ositive *a*irway *p*ressure ventilation), HFNC (*h*igh-*f*low *n*asal *c*annula)
  - Failure of medical management or anticipation of an increased need for respiratory support despite maximal medical therapy. NIPPV provides positive end-expiratory pressure (PEEP) support and can reduce the work of breathing.
  - Chronic obstructive pulmonary disease/asthma exacerbations
  - Hypercapnic respiratory failure
- HFNC: may provide similar benefits to BPAP and CPAP methods (e.g., generation of PEEP, reduction of dead space ventilation, and reduced work of breathing). This is a good option to try in patients with contraindications to BPAP/CPAP because of mask fit, anxiety, claustrophobia, or altered mental status.

BAG-MASK VENTILATION

- Preoxygenation
- Ventilation in anticipation of establishing a definitive airway

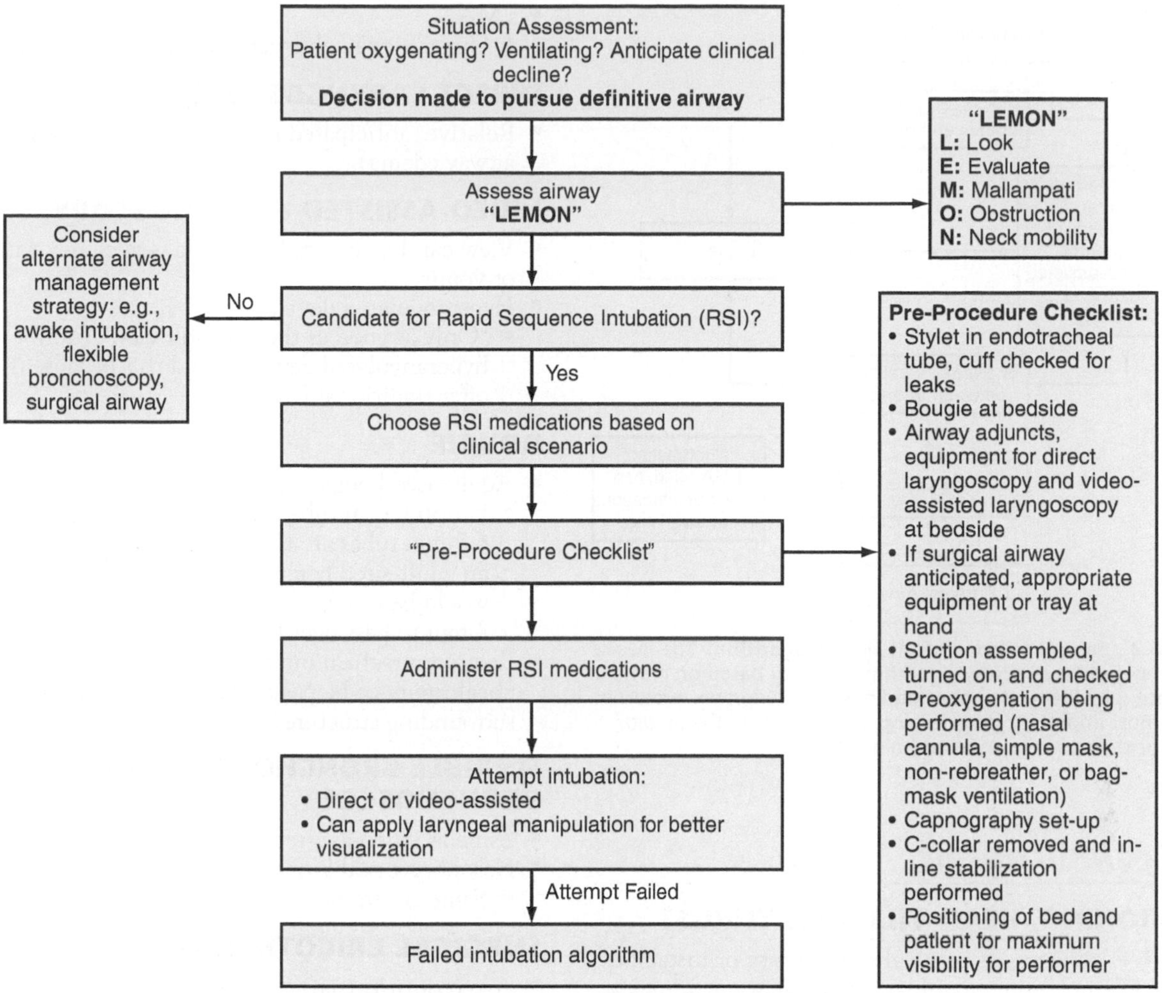

FIG. 146.1 Sample endotracheal intubation with the rapid sequence induction (RSI) pathway algorithm. This pathway demonstrates important preparation steps and checklists before performing endotracheal intubation via RSI. Examples of patients not appropriate for RSI include those for whom you predict poor success with bag-mask ventilation, or those with significant airway compromise (e.g., angioedema, Ludwig angina).

- Use in between failed intubation attempts.

AIRWAY ADJUNCTS

- Oropharyngeal and nasopharyngeal airways, laryngeal mask airway (LMA)/intubating laryngeal mask airway (ILMA)
  - Difficult ventilation (rescue ventilation)
  - Concern for upper airway obstruction
  - Use with bag-mask ventilation to increase effectiveness.
- LMA/ILMA
  - Facilitate blind intubation in a difficult airway; rescue for failed intubation.

DIRECT LARYNGOSCOPY (DL)

- Need for definitive airway
  - Failure to ventilate, failure to oxygenate, inability to protect airway, anticipated clinical course, altered/combative patient who requires imaging or procedure

VIDEO-ASSISTED LARYNGOSCOPY (VL)

- Educational settings (instructor can see what the trainee sees)
- Hyperangulated device (e.g., Glidescope, C-MAC with D-blade attachment)
  - Difficult airway, strict c-spine precautions
- DL/VL device (e.g., C-MAC with traditional [Macintosh or Miller] blade)
  - Same technique as traditional DL, but with possibility for video-assisted views

BOUGIE

- First-pass intubation success rate with direct laryngoscopy may be higher, especially for providers who frequently utilize the bougie.
- Used on anticipated difficult airway with limited visibility (blood, emesis, airway edema/trauma) and should be part of a back-up plan for any airway.

FLEXIBLE BRONCHOSCOPY/FIBEROPTIC BRONCHOSCOPY

- Distorted anatomy (angioedema, mass, abscess, trauma, burns)

CRICOTHYROTOMY

- Inability to establish a definitive airway or adequately ventilate ("can't intubate, can't oxygenate")

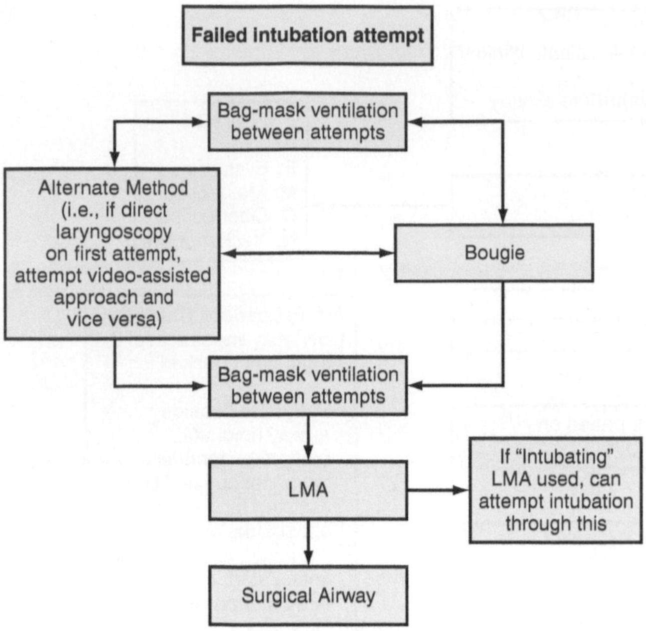

FIG. 146.2 Sample failed/difficult airway algorithm. The specific steps in one's difficult airway algorithm may vary based on provider experience, provider preferences, and hospital equipment/protocols. What is most important is to develop a systematic pathway with defined next steps to take if a technique fails.

Contraindications

POSITIONING, HEAD-TILT, JAW THRUST

- Relative: concern for cervical spine injury or instability
  - For example, rheumatoid arthritis, Down syndrome, trauma

NASAL CANNULA, SIMPLE MASK, NON-REBREATHER

- Relative: chronic CO_2 retainer with O_2 saturation greater than 90% (unless utilized for preoxygenation)

NIPPV

- Altered patient
- Inability to synchronize with device or manage secretions/protect airway
- Inability to fit mask properly (facial deformities, facial hair)
- Recent sinus/airway surgery
- Extremis (need for emergent definitive airway)

BAG-MASK VENTILATION

- Inability to achieve adequate mask seal
  - For example, significant facial hair, dentures/edentulous patient, facial trauma

AIRWAY ADJUNCTS

- Nasopharyngeal
  - Maxillofacial trauma, concern for basilar skull fracture
- Oropharyngeal
  - Awake patient, intact gag reflex
- LMA
  - Upper airway obstruction, edema, or distortion

DIRECT LARYNGOSCOPY

- Relative: anticipated limited visualization (trauma or airway edema)

VIDEO-ASSISTED LARYNGOSCOPY

- View can be obscured if camera gets cloudy with blood or vomit.
- Hyperangulated device
  - "Only as good as the camera's view" (non-hyperangulated devices avoid this because they still offer traditional DL view.)

BOUGIE

- Adult-sized bougie
  - Endotracheal tube (ETT) smaller than 6.0 mm; 6.0-mm tubes are the smallest that can pass over an adult-sized bougie. An alternative in this patient would be to use a pediatric bougie (smallest ETT 4 mm to pass over bougie).
- Relative: tracheal injury: a bougie may exacerbate a tracheal injury or be passed through a tracheal defect into surrounding structures.

FLEXIBLE BRONCHOSCOPY/FIBEROPTIC BRONCHOSCOPY

- Same as video-assisted
- Nasopharyngeal bronchoscopy
  - Same contraindications to nasopharyngeal airway

SURGICAL CRICOTHYROTOMY

- Age (controversial)
  - Needle cricothyrotomy may be preferentially performed in children under the age of 12 owing to anatomic differences. In children, the cricothyroid membrane is narrower, possibly increasing the risk of permanent laryngeal damage during a surgical cricothyrotomy.

Equipment/Supplies

THE BASICS

- Any room set up to care for critically ill patients should have these items inside or close at hand, at a minimum.
  - Oxygen delivery
    - O_2 hookup or O_2 tanks
    - Nasal cannula, simple mask, non-rebreather mask
    - Bag-valve mask
  - Suction
    - Canister, tubing, suction device (e.g., Yankauer or DuCanto tip)

AIRWAY TRAY/CART

- Should include the equipment necessary for the most common steps in the airway algorithm, arranged in a logical, standardized order to minimize wasted time in acute airway situations.

- Syringes
  - 10 cc for inflating endotracheal tube cuffs
  - 35 cc or larger for inflating LMAs and removing extraglottic devices (e.g., King Laryngeal Tube, Combitube) placed by emergency medical services; balloons are larger than endotracheal tube (ETT) cuffs.
- Adjuncts
  - Oropharyngeal/nasopharyngeal airways, various sizes
  - LMA/ILMA, various sizes (can use down to 34 weeks post-conceptual age preterm infants who are >1500 g)
- Direct laryngoscopy
  - Laryngoscope handle
  - Blades
    - Macintosh and Miller blades, various sizes, tested with handle for proper function
  - Endotracheal tubes, various sizes, with cuffs tested for leaks
    - Use the formula "(Age/4) + 4" for pediatric uncuffed ETT estimated size.
    - Subtract 0.5 mm for cuffed pediatric tubes.
    - Cuffed tubes are recommended in infants and children over uncuffed tubes. Attention should be paid to cuff pressure to avoid pressure-related injury.
  - Bougie
  - Capnography
    - Color-change (semiquantitative) capnometry, waveform capnography

VIDEO LARYNGOSCOPY

- Hyperangulated device
  - Glidescope with Glidescope-specific blades and associated hyperangulated stylet
  - C-MAC with D-blade attachment and associated hyperangulated stylet
- DL/VL device
  - C-MAC with Macintosh or Miller blade attachments

FLEXIBLE BRONCHOSCOPY/FIBEROPTIC BRONCHOSCOPY

- Fiberoptic scopes: reusable or disposable

CRICOTHYROTOMY

- Most hospitals have prearranged surgical airway trays. However, the most basic requirements for a cricothyrotomy are a scalpel, a bougie, and an endotracheal tube.
  - Scalpel
  - Tracheal hook/retractors
  - Hemostats, forceps
  - Bougie
  - Tracheostomy tube (common adult size: 6 Shiley)/endotracheal tube (size 6 ETT)
    - Confirm bougie fits well before initiating cricothyroidotomy.
  - Transtracheal jet ventilation set-up (for children younger than 12 years)
    - 12- to 14-gauge angiocath
    - 3-cc syringe full of saline (aspirate while advancing until bubbles are seen in saline to confirm tracheal placement)
    - ETT adaptor (7.0)
    - Ventilation source

Complications/Pitfalls

POSITIONING, HEAD-TILT, JAW THRUST

- Theoretic
  - Cervical spine injury in cases of c-spine instability
- Pitfall
  - Poor positioning technique (i.e., atlantooccipital overextension causing "epiglottis camouflage")
- Failure to recognize need to position the patient with head-tilt and/or jaw-thrust

NASAL CANNULA, SIMPLE MASK, NON-REBREATHER

- Over-oxygenation of chronic CO_2 retainer leading to decreased respiratory drive and subsequent hypercapnic respiratory failure. If using as a preoxygenation method prior to intubation, this is not a concern.

NIPPV

- Aspiration
- Decreased cardiac output secondary to increased intrathoracic pressure

BAG-MASK VENTILATION

- Gastric insufflation
- Aspiration

AIRWAY ADJUNCTS

- Nasopharyngeal
  - Nasal trauma, epistaxis, insertion through the cribriform plate in cases of basilar skull fracture
- Oropharyngeal
  - Aspiration

DIRECT LARYNGOSCOPY

- Complications
  - Prolonged hypoxemia, esophageal placement/aspiration, inadequate tracheal placement, bradycardia, dental trauma/aspiration
- Pitfalls
  - Inadequate preoxygenation, prolonged intubation attempts, inability to recognize difficult airway/need to move to the next step in the algorithm, dental/lip trauma, inadequate positioning/preparation

BOUGIE

- Not having one at hand

VIDEO-ASSISTED LARYNGOSCOPY/FLEXIBLE BRONCHOSCOPY

- Pitfalls
  - Poor visualization secondary to vomitus/secretions/blood, inadequate suctioning
- Only as good as your camera's view; lack of experience

- Nasopharyngeal bronchoscopy
  - Same as nasopharyngeal airway

CRICOTHYROTOMY

- Unable to recognize landmarks
- Bleeding, soft-tissue placement
- Pitfalls
  - Inability to recognize a difficult airway situation that may require a surgical airway (angioedema, significant trauma)
  - Not having equipment ready
  - Delay in committing to proceeding with surgical airway

SUGGESTED READINGS

Driver, B. E., Prekker, M. E., Klein, L. R., Reardon, R. F., Miner, J. R., Fagerstrom, E. T., Cleghorn, M. R., McGill, J. W., & Cole, J. B. (2018). Effect of use of a bougie vs endotracheal tube and stylet on first-attempt intubation success among patients with difficult airways undergoing emergency intubation: A randomized clinical trial. *Journal of the American Medical Association, 319*(21), 2179–2189.

Frerk, C., Mitchell, V. S., Mcnarry, A. F., Mendonca, C., Bhagrath, R., Patel, A., O'Sullivan, E. P., Woodall, N. M., Ahmad, I., & Difficult Airway Society intubation guidelines working group (2015). Difficult airway society 2015 guidelines for management of unanticipated difficult intubation in adults. *British Journal of Anaesthesia, 115*(6), 827–848.

Roberts, J. R., Custalow, C. B., & Thomsen, T. W. (2019). *Roberts and Hedges' clinical procedures in emergency medicine and acute care* (7th ed.). Elsevier.

Cardiac Arrest (Adult, Pediatric, Neonate), ROSC

KATIE REBILLOT, DO, and BRITTNEY MULL, MD, MPH

Cardiopulmonary arrest is the absence of mechanical cardiac activity in the setting of pulselessness, unresponsiveness, and apnea or agonal breathing. In-hospital cardiac arrests have shown better outcomes overall, compared with out-of-hospital events. Approximately 70% to 90% of individuals with out-of-hospital cardiac arrest die before arriving to the hospital. Whereas cardiac arrest is commonly secondary to a primary cardiac event in adults, hypoxia or shock is the most common cause of pediatric arrest.

General Principles

- Cardiac arrest rhythms
  - Shockable: Early defibrillation of shockable rhythms is associated with an increased likelihood of return of spontaneous circulation (ROSC) and survival to out-of-hospital discharge. Defibrillation should occur within 3 minutes of a witnessed cardiac arrest.
    - Pulseless ventricular tachycardia (pVT)
    - Pulseless ventricular fibrillation (VF)
  - Not shockable
    - Pulseless electrical activity (PEA)
    - Asystole: associated with extremely poor survival
- Cardiopulmonary resuscitation (CPR): Chest compressions generate critical blood flow to provide oxygen to the heart and brain during cardiac arrest. Optimal CPR is performed as follows:
  - Compression rate of 100 to 120 with adequate compression depth (2 to 2.4 in for adults and one-third depth of chest for prepubescent children) and complete chest recoil between compressions
  - Minimize interruptions in compressions.
  - Avoid excessive ventilation (decreased venous return and cerebral perfusion pressure).
  - End-tidal CO_2 greater than 10 mm Hg
  - Manual or mechanical CPR
- Airway and breathing: CPR should not be delayed for basic or advanced airway management. However, the airway should be secured promptly if the cardiac arrest is thought to be secondary to hypoxic respiratory arrest.
- Ventilation and compression rates for neonates, pediatric patients, and adults can be found in Table 147.1.
- Reversible causes of cardiac arrest
  - Hypoxia
  - Hypothermia
  - Hydrogen ion (acidosis)
  - Hypo/Hyperkalemia
  - Hypovolemia
  - Tension pneumothorax
  - Tamponade, cardiac
  - Toxins
  - Thrombosis, pulmonary
  - Thrombosis, cardiac
- Basic approach to adult cardiac arrest can be found in Fig. 147.1.

Neonatal and Pediatric Cardiac Arrest

PEDIATRIC RESUSCITATION

- Airway and breathing should be prioritized, because pediatric arrest is usually caused by hypoxia or shock.

TABLE 147.1 *Ventilation and Compression Rates for Neonates, Pediatric Patients, and Adults*

		Neonate	Pediatric	Adult
Ventilation	Rate (breaths/min)	40–60 breaths/min to maintain HR >100	8–10 breaths/min	8–10 breaths/min
Compression	Position	Lower half of sternum using two-thumb encircling hands technique (most effective) or two-finger anterior technique	Heel of hand placed over lower half of sternum	Heel of hand placed over lower half of sternum
	Depth	⅓ depth of chest	⅓ depth of chest	2.5 inches
	Rate	90/min	100/min	100/min
	Compression to Ventilation Ratio	3:1	15:2	30:2
	Defibrillation	Use pediatric pads 2–4 J/kg	Use pediatric pads 2–4 J/kg	Use adult pads 120–200 J (biphasic)

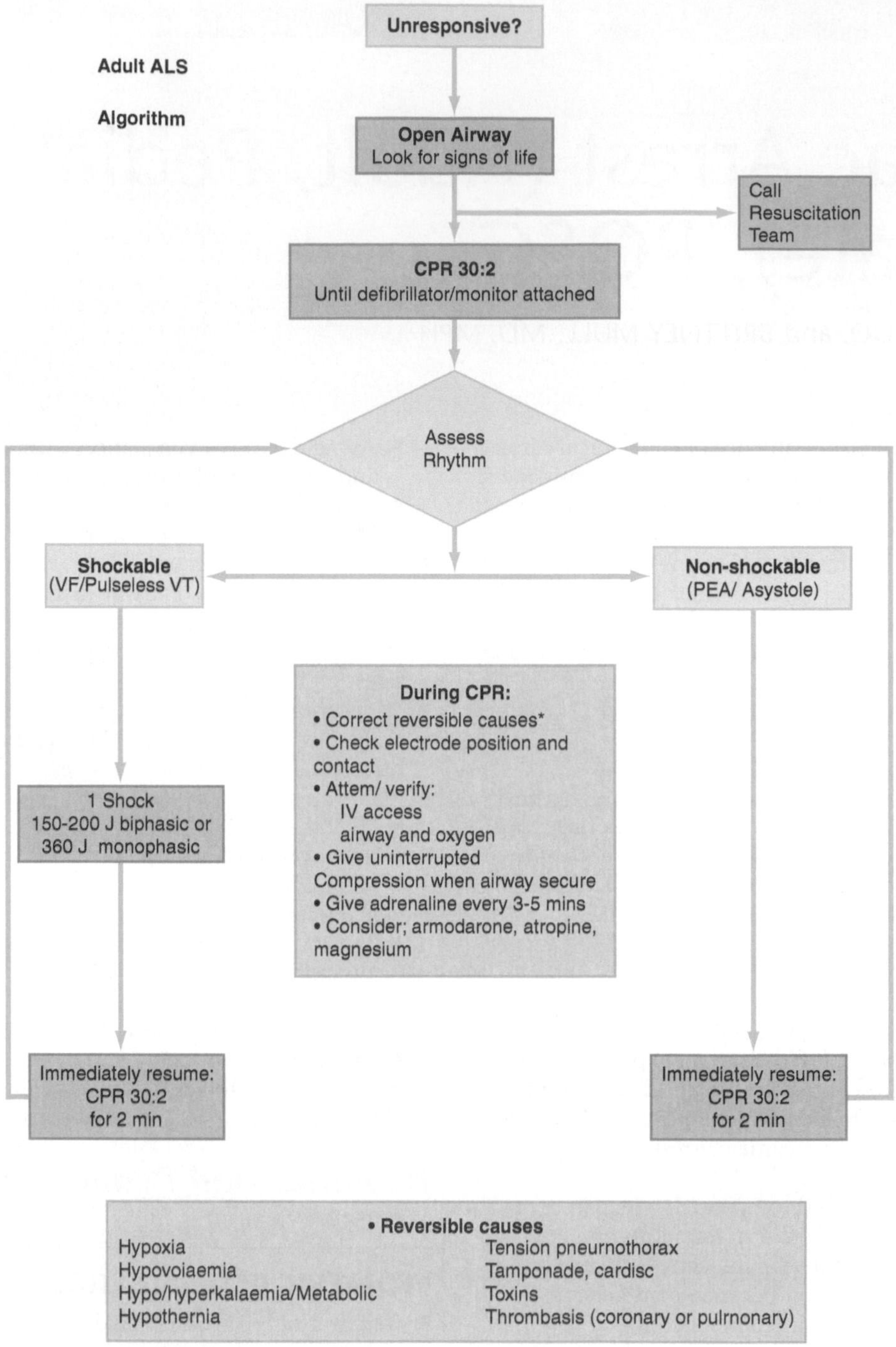

FIG. 147.1 Adult cardiac arrest algorithm. *CPR,* cardiopulmonary resuscitation; *ET,* endotracheal; *IO,* intraosseous; *IV,* intravenous; *PEA,* pulseless electrical activity; *P etco 2,* partial pressure of end-tidal carbon dioxide; *pVT,* pulseless ventricular tachycardia; *VF,* ventricular fibrillation. (Reprinted from Nolan, J. P., Deakin, C. D., Soar, J., Böttiger, B. W., & Smith, G. (2005). European Resuscitation Council guidelines for resuscitation 2005. Section 4. Adult advanced life support. *Resuscitation, 67*(suppl 1), S39–S86.)

- Basic approach to pediatric cardiac arrest can be found in Fig. 147.2.
- Vascular access: intravenous > intraosseous (IO) > endotracheal
- IO access
  - The preferred site of IO needle placement for infants and children younger than 6 years is the proximal tibia (Fig. 147.3A). The distal tibia and femur may also be used (Fig. 147.3B and C).
  - IO insertion at proximal tibia
    - Cleanse insertion site with antiseptic solution.
    - Option to anesthetize the skin and periosteum if the patient is conscious
    - IO needle should be inserted 1 to 3 cm distal to the tibial tuberosity and over the medial aspect of the tibia.
    - Confirmation of position
      - Aspiration of blood or marrow contents (not always reliable). If unable to aspirate contents,

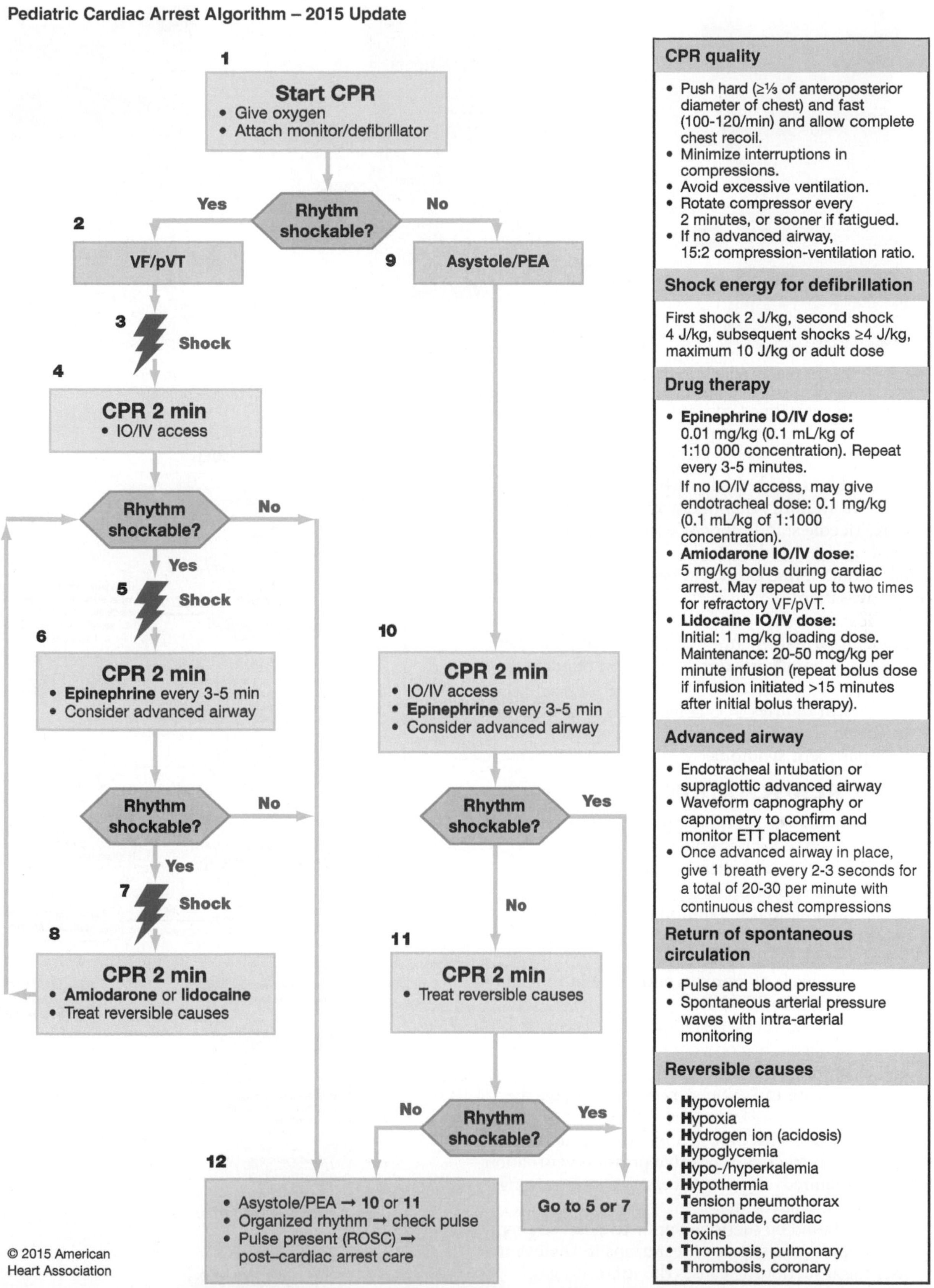

FIG. 147.2 The American Heart Association (AHA) guidelines algorithm for management of infants and children in cardiopulmonary arrest. *CPR,* Cardiopulmonary resuscitation; *ETT,* endotracheal tube; *IO/IV,* intraosseous/intravenous; *PEA,* pulseless electrical activity; *ROSC,* return of spontaneous circulation; *VF/pVT,* ventricular fibrillation/pulseless. (From Easter, J. S., & Scott, H. F. (2018). Pediatric resuscitation. In R. M. Walls, R. S. Hockberger, & M. Gausche-Hill (Eds.), *Rosen's emergency medicine: Concepts and clinical practice* (9th ed., pp. 2020–2031.e2, Fig. 163.1). Elsevier.

147

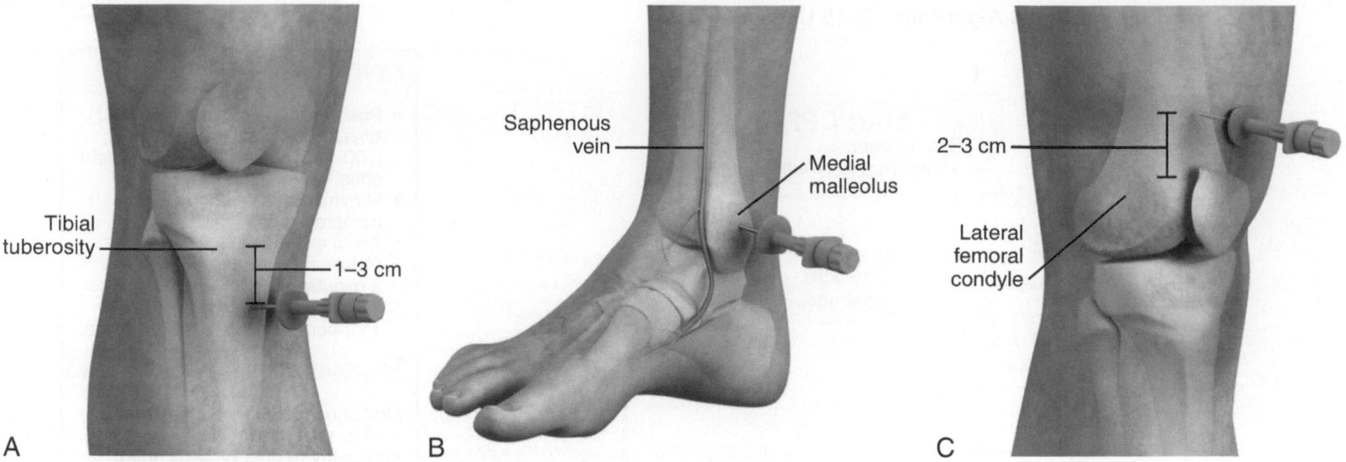

FIG. 147.3 Intraosseous needle insertion sites. **A**, Proximal tibia, **B**, medial malleolus, and **C**, distal femur. (From Deitch, K. (2019). Intraosseous infusion. In J. R. Roberts, C. B. Custalow, & T. W. Thomsen (Eds.), *Roberts and Hedges' clinical procedures in emergency medicine and acute care* (7th ed., pp. 461–475, Fig. 25.7). Elsevier.)

but able to flush easily without surrounding soft tissue swelling, then likely in correct position
    - IO needle stands upright without support.
  - Flush and secure IO
- Fluids should infuse easily without evidence of swelling or extravasation.
- Complications
  - Inadequate placement, including incomplete penetration of bony cortex or penetration of posterior cortex
  - Epiphyseal injuries
  - Infection
  - Compartment syndrome

NEONATAL RESUSCITATION

- Most term infants with good respiratory effort and good tone do not need resuscitation.
- The most important and effective step in neonatal resuscitation is ventilation of the lungs.
- Initial steps and basic resuscitation are shown in Fig. 147.4.
  - Dry and stimulate the infant.
  - Warm with towels or blankets and place in radiant warmer (36.5°C to 37.5°C).
    - If less than 32 weeks' gestation, place body of infant in plastic bag or wrap to reduce conductive and evaporative heat loss.
  - Position neonate in "sniffing" position to open the airway.
  - Clear secretions with bulb syringe or wall suction if airway is obstructed or positive pressure ventilation (PPV) is required; avoid unnecessary suction owing to the risk of bradycardia.
    - Mouth should be suctioned prior to nose, so that the oropharynx is clear of secretions in the event that nasal suctioning causes the infant to gasp.
    - Meconium-stained amniotic fluid is no longer an indication for aggressive deep suctioning or routine intubation in nonvigorous infants and the provider should follow the normal neonatal resuscitation pathway.

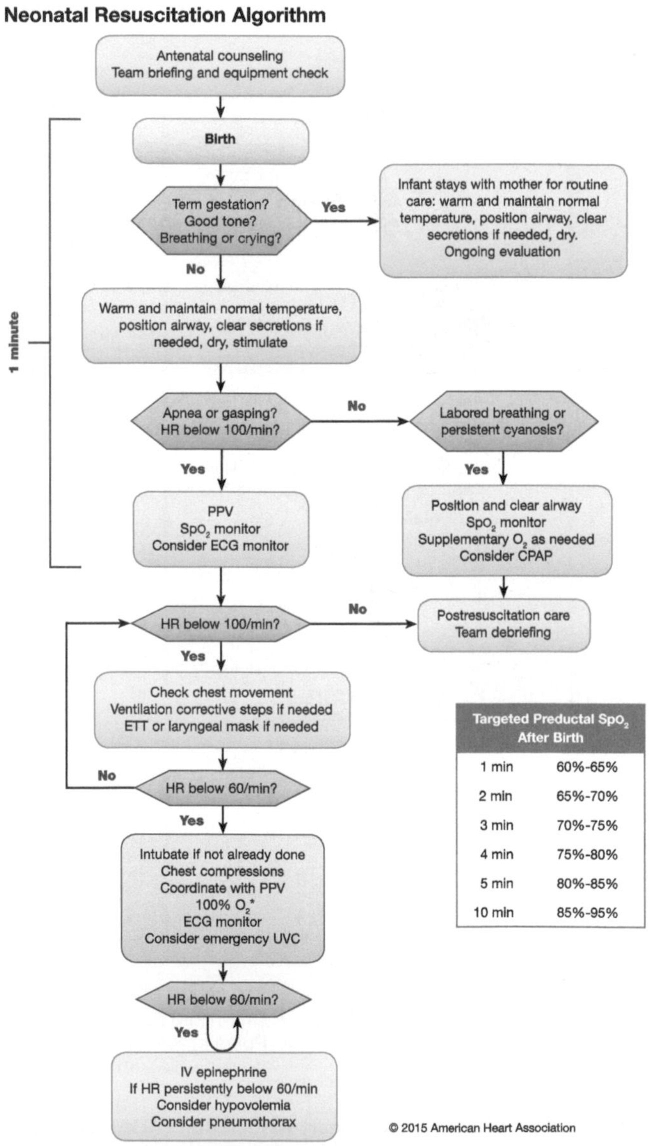

FIG. 147.4 Neonatal resuscitation algorithm. (From Brady, J. M., & Kamath-Rayne, B. D. (2020). Neonatal resuscitation and delivery room emergencies. In R. M. Kliegman, J. W. St. Geme III, N. J. Blum, S. S. Shah, R. C. Tasker, K. M. Wilson, & R. E. Behrman (Eds.), *Nelson textbook of pediatrics* (21st ed., Fig. 121.2). Elsevier.)

- Assess respiratory effort and heart rate (HR) every 30 seconds.
  - After initial 30 seconds: if apneic or HR fewer than 100 beats/min
    - Attach SpO_2 monitor to right hand for preductal oxygen saturation measurement and initiate electroencephalographic (ECG) monitoring.
    - Begin assisted PPV with a bag valve mask at 20/5 cm H_2O delivering 40 to 60 breaths/min attached to oxygen blender at 21% for term infants and 21%–30% for preterm infants (100% oxygen should be avoided if possible in preterm infants owing to its detrimental toxic effects).
  - Recheck after 30 seconds.
    - If infant begins spontaneously breathing or HR more than 100 beats/min with improvement in tone and color, may discontinue oxygen and PPV
    - If infant remains apneic or HR less than 100 beats/min after 30 seconds of effective PPV
      - Correct ventilation techniques using MRSOPA:
        - Mask adjustment
        - Reposition airway
        - Suction mouth and nose
        - Open mouth
        - Pressure increase by 5 to 10 cm H_2O (max 40 cm H_2O)
        - Airway alternative
      - If PPV corrective measures do not improve HR or respirations, consider intubation.
      - Oxygen saturation is a poor marker, because it does not reach 85% to 95% until 10 minutes of life.
      - If HR less than 60 beats/min, intubate first, increase supplemental oxygen to 100% and begin chest compressions.
    - Recheck after 30 seconds.
      - If HR more than 60 beats/min, discontinue chest compressions and titrate oxygen to SpO_2 more than 90%.
      - If HR less than 60 beats/min, increase FiO2, obtain intravenous (IV) (I UV line is now considered) or IO access (consider umbilical vein catheter if difficult access) and consider drug therapy.
- Umbilical vein catheterization (Fig. 147.5): the umbilical vein may be used for short-term central venous access in neonates.
- Drug therapy: epinephrine, glucose, normal saline bolus (10 mL/kg over 5 to 10 minutes; rapid infusions of large volumes have been associated with intraventricular hemorrhage).

147

Medications

- **Epinephrine**: First-line medication
  - Shown to increase coronary and cerebral perfusion pressures during CPR, but does not appear to improve neurologically intact survival.
  - Class: natural catecholamine, adrenergic agonist, sympathomimetic
  - Mechanism of action
    - Binds to alpha- and beta-adrenergic receptors
    - Increases heart rate and force of contraction

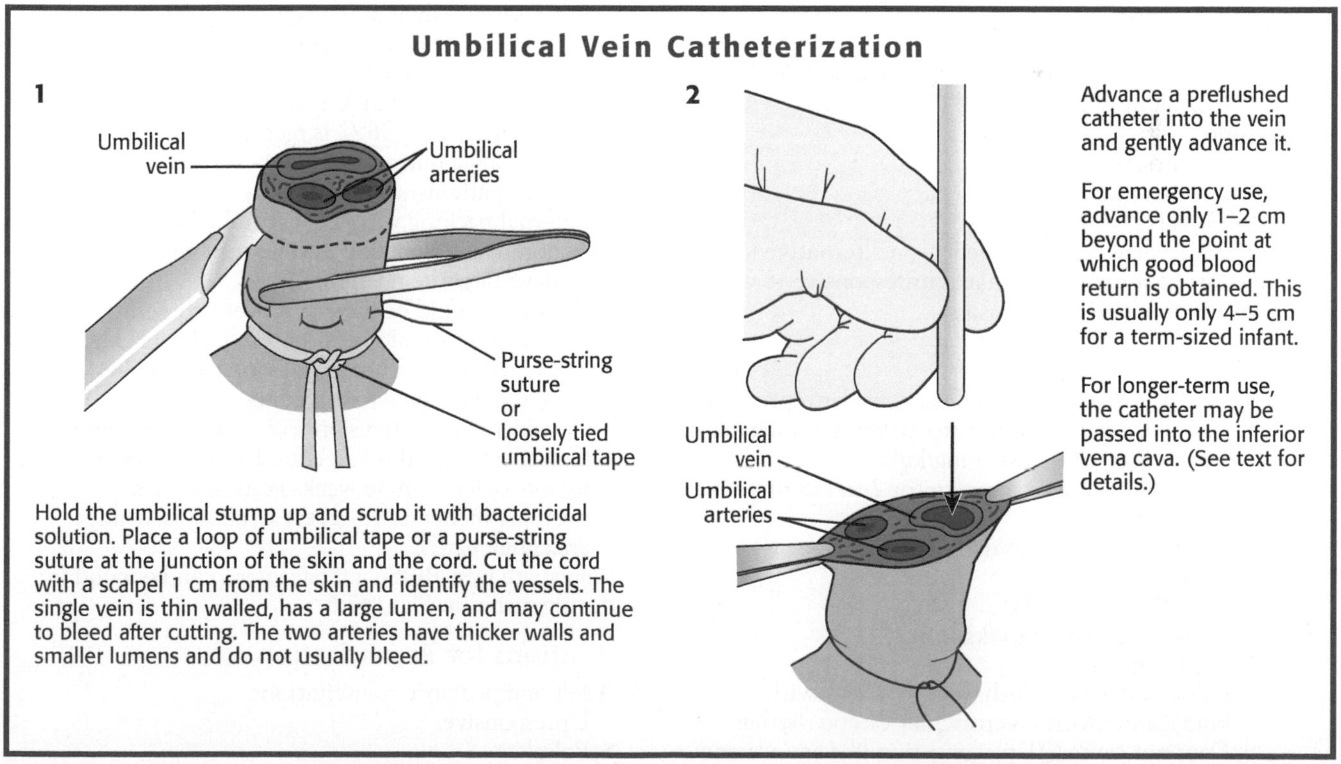

Umbilical Vein Catheterization
1
Umbilical vein
Umbilical arteries
Purse-string suture or loosely tied umbilical tape
Hold the umbilical stump up and scrub it with bactericidal solution. Place a loop of umbilical tape or a purse-string suture at the junction of the skin and the cord. Cut the cord with a scalpel 1 cm from the skin and identify the vessels. The single vein is thin walled, has a large lumen, and may continue to bleed after cutting. The two arteries have thicker walls and smaller lumens and do not usually bleed.
2
Umbilical vein
Umbilical arteries
Advance a preflushed catheter into the vein and gently advance it.
For emergency use, advance only 1–2 cm beyond the point at which good blood return is obtained. This is usually only 4–5 cm for a term-sized infant.
For longer-term use, the catheter may be passed into the inferior vena cava. (See text for details.)

FIG. 147.5 Umbilical vein catheterization (From Santillanes, G., & Claudius, I. (2019). Pediatric vascular access and blood sampling techniques. In J. R. Roberts, C. B. Custalow, & T. W. Thomsen (Eds.), *Roberts and Hedges' clinical procedures in emergency medicine and acute care* (7th ed., pp. 353–376, Fig. 19.14). Elsevier.)

- Vasoconstriction
- Relaxation of bronchial smooth muscle
- Indication: cardiac arrest: pVT, VF, PEA, asystole
- Dosage
  - IV/IO concentration 1:10,000
  - Endotracheal concentration: 1:1,000
  - Repeat every 3 to 5 minutes, as needed
  - Adult
    - IV/IO: 1 mg
    - Endotracheal: 2.5 mg
    - Postcardiac arrest: continuous infusion of 0.1 to 0.5 μg/kg/min infusion titrated to response
  - Pediatric
    - IV/IO: 0.01 mg/kg (maximum single dose 1 mg)
    - Endotracheal: 0.1 mg/kg
  - Neonate
    - IV/IO: 0.01 to 0.03 mg/kg
    - Endotracheal: 0.05 to 0.1 mg/kg
- Amiodarone
  - Class III antiarrhythmic
  - Mechanism of action
    - Inhibits K^+ channels, thereby prolonging repolarization
    - Depresses automaticity of SA and AV nodes
    - Slows conduction through AV node and accessory pathway of Wolff-Parkinson-White
    - Inhibits alpha- and beta-adrenergic receptors
    - Coronary and peripheral vasodilator
  - Indication: May be used for pVT/VF that is unresponsive to CPR, defibrillation, and vasopressor therapy
  - Dosage
    - Adult: pVT/VF: bolus of 300 mg IV/IO, may be followed by a second bolus of 150 mg IV/IO.
    - Pediatric: 5 mg/kg, repeat up to 15 mg/kg (maximum dose 300 mg)
  - Considerations
    - May cause hypotension, bradycardia, and AV block
    - May prolong PR, QRS, and QT interval
- Lidocaine
  - Class Ib antiarrhythmic
  - Mechanism of action
    - Inhibits Na^+ ion channels
  - Indication: may be considered as an alternative to amiodarone for pVT/VF that is unresponsive to CPR, defibrillation, and vasopressors
  - Dosage
    - Adult
      - IV/IO: 1 to 1.5 mg/kg bolus; consider repeat dose (0.5 to 0.75 mg/kg) at 5- to 10-minute intervals (maximum total dose 3 mg/kg)
      - Endotracheal: 2 to 3 mg/kg (or 2 to 2.5 times the IV dose)
      - Infusion: 1 to 4 mg/min
    - Pediatric
      - IV/IO/ETT: 1 mg/kg
      - Infusion: 20 to 50 μg/kg/min
    - Considerations
      - Lidocaine may be lethal for a patient with bradycardia with a ventricular escape rhythm.
      - Does not cause QT prolongation like amiodarone.
- Magnesium
  - Mechanism of action: shortens QT interval and terminates torsades de pointes
  - Indication: polymorphic ventricular tachycardia with prolonged QT interval (e.g., torsades de pointes)
  - Dosage
    - Adult: 1 to 2 g IV diluted in 10 mL D5W IV/IO infused over 15 minutes
    - Pediatric: 25 to 50 mg/kg IV/IO (maximum dose 2 g)
  - Considerations: Routine use of magnesium is not recommended in adult cardiac arrest, but should be given for torsades de pointes.
- Glucose
  - Dosage: 0.5 to 1 g/kg IV/IO
    - Adult: D50W 1 mL/kg
    - Pediatric: D25W 2 mL/kg
    - Neonate: D10W 5 mL/kg
- Medications that can be given via the endotracheal route can be remembered by the mnemonic LANE: lidocaine, atropine, naloxone, and epinephrine.

Return of Spontaneous Circulation (ROSC) and Post-Cardiac Arrest Therapy:

- ROSC is the resumption of an organized cardiac electrical rhythm AND palpable central pulses.
- Optimize ventilation and oxygenation, with a focus on maintaining normal oxygen levels (avoiding hyperoxia/hypoxia).
- Treat hypotension
  - First-line: intravenous fluid boluses up to 3 L
    - If unresponsive, proceed to vasoactive agents.
  - Second-line: vasoactive agents
    - Electrocardiogram: patients with ST elevation myocardial infarction on post-ROSC electrocardiogram should be considered for emergency percutaneous coronary intervention or thrombolytics.
    - Targeted temperature management: target temperature of 32°C to 36°C is recommended to improve neurologic outcomes in post-ROSC, comatose adult patients.
  - External packing with ice, central cooling catheters, or noninvasive cooling devices may be used to achieve target temperature.
  - Sedation should be used to prevent shivering.
  - Temperature should be monitored with bladder or central cooling catheter, or esophageal probe.
- Postresuscitation care for neonates
  - Consider glucose infusion to avoid hypoglycemia.
  - Consider induced therapeutic hypothermia for infants older than 36 weeks gestation with evolving moderate-to-severe hypoxic-ischemic encephalopathy.
- Immediate post-ROSC management can be found in the algorithm in Fig. 147.6.

Indications for Resuscitation

- Adult and pediatric resuscitation
  - Unresponsive
  - Pulseless
  - Apnea or agonal/gasping respirations
- Neonatal resuscitation
  - Apnea

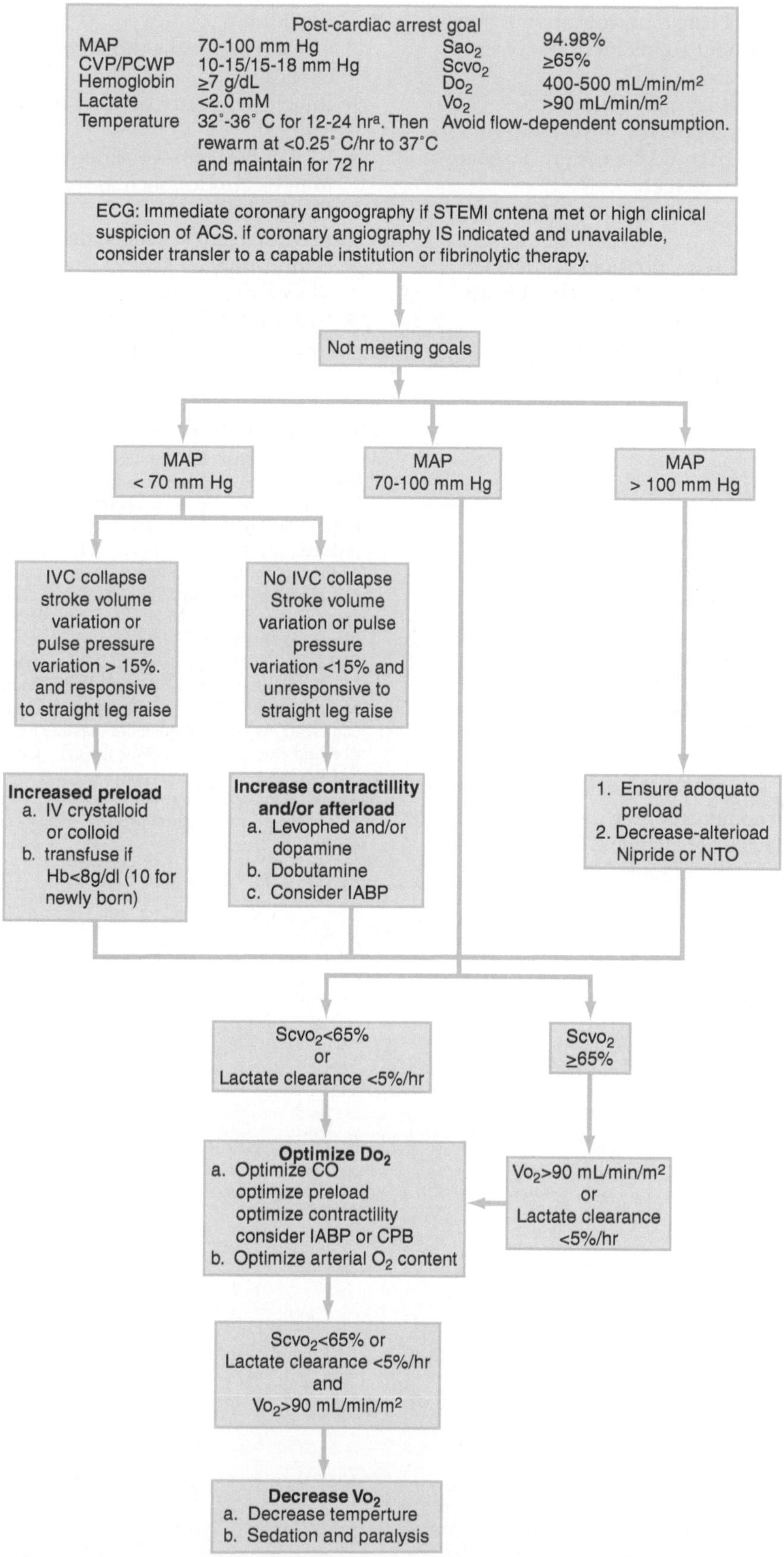

FIG. 147.6 Adult immediate post-cardiac arrest care algorithm. *AMI,* Acute myocardial infarction; *ECG,* electrocardiogram; *Fio$_2$,* fraction of inspired oxygen; *IO,* intraosseous; *IV,* intravenous; *PETCO$_2$,* partial pressure of end-tidal carbon dioxide; *SBP,* systolic blood pressure; *SpO$_2$,* pulse oximeter oxygen saturation; *STEMI,* ST-segment elevation myocardial infarction. (Reprinted from Kurz, M. C., & Neumar, R. W. (2018). Adult resuscitation. In R. M. Walls, R. S. Hockberger, & M. Gausche-Hill (Eds.), *Rosen's emergency medicine: Concepts and clinical practice* (9th ed., pp. 85–95.e2). Elsevier.)

- Heart rate less than 100 beats/min: initiate positive pressure ventilation without supplemental oxygen and consider advanced airway.
- Heart rate less than 60 beats/min: initiate chest compressions and consider epinephrine; if resuscitation started and HR still less than 60 beats/min, intubate and provide supplemental oxygen.

Contraindications

- Patient has documentation (e.g., physician orders for life-sustaining treatments [POLST] form) that clearly states **DO NOT RESUSCITATE.**
- Successful resuscitation would be futile owing to obvious signs of irreversible death (e.g., decapitation, rigor mortis).

Equipment/Supplies

- Resuscitation team and ancillary technicians
- Airway equipment and waveform capnography
- Defibrillator

Complications/Pitfalls

- Chest compression
  - Inadequate position, depth, rate, or recoil
  - Rescuer fatigue
  - Overventilation
  - Frequent and/or prolonged interruption
  - Delayed initiation of compression owing to mechanical chest compression device deployment
- Defibrillation
  - Chest hair: ideally should be shaved prior to application of pads
  - Injury to operator or other members of the resuscitation team
  - Risk of fire: remove patient from potential fire risk from electrodes, such as wet clothing
  - Dysrhythmia
- Post cardiac arrest syndrome
  - Brain injury
  - Myocardial dysfunction
  - Systemic ischemia/reperfusion response
  - Persistent precipitating cause

SUGGESTED READINGS

de Caen, A. R., Maconochie, I. K., Aickin, R., Atkins, D. L., Biarent, D., Guerguerian, A. M., Kleinman, M. E., Kloeck, D. A., Meaney, P. A., Nadkarni, V. M., Ng, K.-C., Nuthall, G., Reis, A. G., Shimizu, N., Tibballs, J., & Pintos, R. V. (2015). Part 6: Pediatric basic life support and pediatric advanced life support: 2015 International consensus on cardiopulmonary resuscitation and emergency cardiovascular care science with treatment recommendations. *Circulation, 132*(16 Suppl. 1), S177–S203.

Neumar, R. W., Shuster, M., Callaway, C. W., Gent, L. M., Atkins, D. L., Bhanji, F., Brooks, S. C., de Caen, A. R., Donnino, M. W., Ferrer, J. M. E., Kleinman, M. E., Kronick, S. L., Lavonas, E. J., Link, M. S., Mancini, M. E., Morrison, L. J., O'Connor, R. E., Samson, R. A., Schexnayder, S. M., … Hazinski, M. F. (2015). Part 1: Executive summary: 2015 American Heart Association guidelines update for cardiopulmonary resuscitation and emergency cardiovascular care. *Circulation, 132*(18 Suppl. 2), S315–S367.

Sawyer, T., Umoren, R. A., & Gray, M. M. (2016). Neonatal resuscitation: Advances in training and practice. *Advances in Medical Education and Practice*, 8, 11–19.

Central and Intraosseous Lines

CHINWE ONU, MD, and JASMIN ENGLAND, MD, FAAP

Vascular access is essential for resuscitation and critical care management of patients in the emergency department. This chapter covers central venous and intraosseous access. Peripherally inserted central catheters are not discussed in this chapter.

Central Venous Access

- Sites of insertion using the Seldinger technique include the internal jugular, subclavian, and femoral veins.
- Ultrasound-guided insertion has better outcomes than the landmark-guided approach.
- Chest radiograph must be obtained to confirm internal jugular and subclavian vein catheter placement and to rule out pneumothorax.
- Site of central line insertion depends on experience level and purpose of the line.
  - Subclavian has lowest infection risk, but may be difficult to access during chest compressions. The subclavian site should be avoided for hemodialysis because of a high incidence (15%–50%) of subclavian vein stenosis and thrombosis, which compromises future permanent ipsilateral upper extremity arteriovenous hemodialysis access.
- Triple-lumen catheters can be used for patients requiring multiple ports for multiple medications, but this catheter has slower infusion rates.
- A single-lumen percutaneous introducer sheath is appropriate for large-volume resuscitation such as in hemorrhagic shock.
- Hemodialysis dual-lumen catheters are used for dialysis or plasmapheresis.

Indications in the Emergency Department

- Rapid volume resuscitation, administering long-term peripherally incompatible drugs, transvenous cardiac pacemakers.

Contraindications

- Infection over the placement site, anatomic venous obstruction (thrombosis).
- Relative contraindications: coagulopathy (for the subclavian site since pressure cannot be applied), distortion of landmarks, prior vessel injury, combative patient.

Equipment

- Catheter size and depth (Table 148.1).
- Kits usually contain sterile drape, chlorhexidine, 1% lidocaine, syringe and small-gauge needles, syringe and 18-gauge needle, guidewire, #11 blade scalpel, venodilator, single or multilumen catheter and clamps, suture with straight or curved needle, needle driver, and sterile dressing.
- Additionally, obtain sterile protective gear (gown, hair cover, mask and gloves), antimicrobial wound dressings, sterile saline flushes, sterile caps for lumen ports, sterile ultrasound probe cover (if using ultrasound guidance).

Complications

- Pneumothorax or hemothorax (more common with subclavian lines)

TABLE 148.1 *Central and Intraosseous Access Size and Depth*[a]

	PEDIATRIC AGE				
	0-6 mo (size)	**≤2 y (size)**	**3–6 y (size)**	**≥7 y (size)**	**Adult (7–13.5 Fr) (depth)**
Internal jugular	3 Fr	3 Fr	4 Fr	4–5 Fr	13–15 cm deep
Subclavian	3 Fr	3 Fr	4 Fr	4–5 Fr	12–17 cm deep
Supraclavicular	3 Fr	3 Fr	4 Fr	4–5 Fr	14–18 cm deep
Femoral	3 Fr	3–4 Fr	4–5 Fr	5–8 Fr	24–25 cm deep
Intraosseous[b] (15-gauge needle)	Pink (15 mm)	Pink	Pink	Pink or blue (25 mm)	Blue or yellow (45 mm: only for adult humerus or thick tissue)

[a]Catheter size in French or intraosseous needle length (millimeters) are based on age. Depths for pediatric central lines can be estimated using 0.07 × height (cm) for the left internal jugular vein, 0.08 × height (cm) for the left subclavian vein, and 0.06 × height (cm) for the right internal jugular vein, although this has not been validated. Femoral lines can be estimated by the distance from insertion site to pubic bone to xiphoid process.
[b]Example given with colors from the Arrow EZ-IO device (Teleflex, Morrisville, NC); colors may vary by manufacturer.

- Arterial puncture and dilation
- Hematoma
- Bloodstream infection (least common with subclavian lines)
- Venous thrombosis or air embolism
- Bleeding
- Arrhythmia from guidewire insertion
- Pseudoaneurysm

Intraosseous Access

For intraosseous access (IO), sites of insertion include the proximal tibia, distal tibia, proximal humerus in adults, distal femur in children, and pelvic anterior superior iliac spine.

Indications in the Emergency Department

- Immediate vascular access when intravenous access is not readily available. Blood used for type and cross, chemistry, and blood gas. Poor correlation with sodium, potassium (due to hemolysis), bicarbonate, and calcium. Do not use for complete blood cell count.

Contraindications

- Osteoporosis, underlying osteomyelitis or fractured bone, osteogenesis imperfecta, recent IO in same location, overlying skin infection or defect such as a burn.

Equipment

- IO insertion device, IO needle and extension set, chlorhexidine, saline flush, preservative-free lidocaine (see Table 148.1).

Complications

- Compartment syndrome, osteomyelitis (rare), skin necrosis, fracture, fat or bone marrow embolism.

SUGGESTED READINGS

Castro, D., Martin Lee, L. A. M., & Bhutta, B. S. (2020). Femoral vein central venous access. [Updated June 28, 2020]. In *StatPearls* [Internet]. Retrieved from https://www.ncbi.nlm.nih.gov/books/NBK459255/

Graham, A. S., Ozment, C., Tegtmeyer, K., Lai, S., & Braner, D. A. V. (2007). Videos in clinical medicine. Central venous catheterization. *The New England Journal of Medicine, 356*(21), e21. doi:10.1056/NEJMvcm055053

Miller, J. H., & Moake, M. (2017). Procedures. In L. Kahl & H. Hughes (Eds.), *The Harriet Lane handbook* (21st ed., pp. 30–72). Elsevier.

Cardiovascular Procedures

CINDY D. CHANG, MD, and JAMES T. NIEMANN, MD

Pericardiocentesis

Indication

- Cardiac tamponade is a life-threatening hemodynamic compromise caused by a pericardial effusion.
  - Clinical manifestations include hypotension, narrow pulse pressure, pulsus paradoxus, distended neck veins, and muffled heart sounds.
  - Classically, the electrocardiogram (ECG) shows sinus tachycardia, low-voltage QRS complexes ($\leq$5 mm amplitude in the limb leads and $\leq$10 mm in the precordial leads), and electrical alternans (beat-to-beat variation in QRS amplitude) (Fig. 149.1).
  - Focused ultrasound typically shows right ventricular and/or right atrial "collapse" during diastole (Fig. 149.2).

Contraindications

- No absolute contraindications exist in the setting of life-threatening tamponade.

Procedure

- Elevate head of bed to 30 to 45 degrees.
- If possible, maintain a sterile technique with chlorhexidine. Use lidocaine for local anesthesia if the patient is alert.
- Select an approach for pericardiocentesis and perform under ultrasound guidance (if available) to visualize needle entering the pericardial space. Attach an 18-gauge spinal needle of 7–9 cm (adults) or 20-gauge spinal needle (children) to a large-volume syringe.
  - Subcostal (subxiphoid)—preferred approach
    - Insert and advance the needle 1 cm below the left xiphocostal angle and advance it toward the left shoulder at a 45-degree angle.
  - Parasternal
    - Advance the needle over the fifth or sixth rib right next to the sternal margin. If too lateral, may injure the internal thoracic vessels. Best performed under ultrasound guidance.
- Aspirate and stop advancing the needle once fluid is aspirated.
- With the needle stationary, aspirate as much fluid as possible. Removal of even a small amount of fluid (30 to 50 mL) usually results in hemodynamic improvement. If serous or serosanguinous fluid is aspirated, it is unlikely that the needle has penetrated a cardiac cavity. Because nontraumatic pericardial effusions do not reaccumulate rapidly, the needle can be removed at this point if hemodynamic improvement is noted.

Electrical Alternans in Pericardial Tamponade

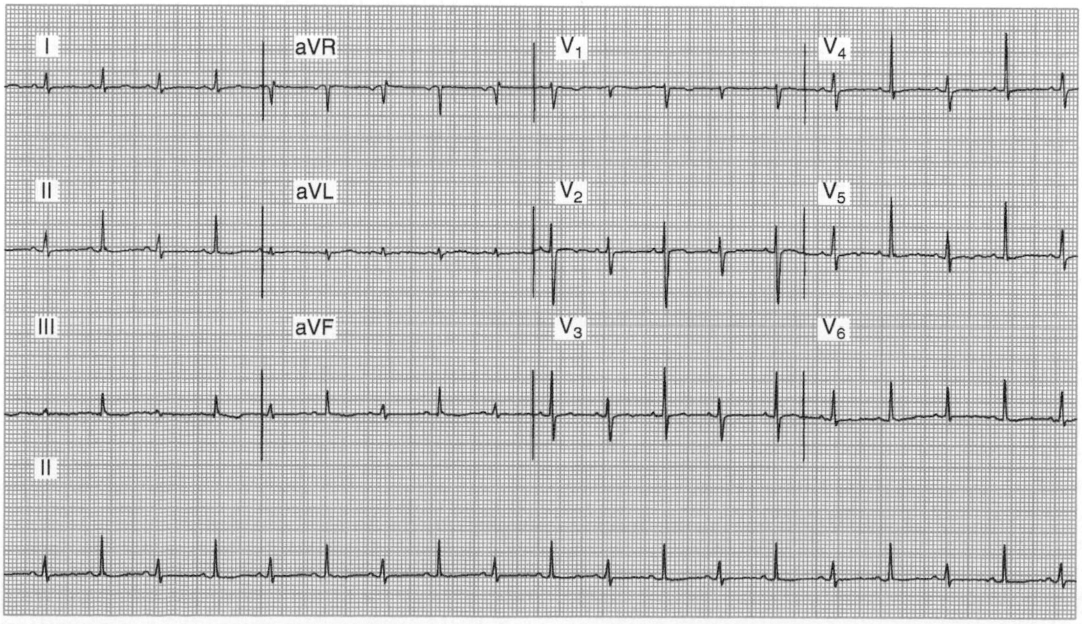

FIG. 149.1 Electrical alternans caused by a large pericardial effusion, showing beat-to-beat alternation in the QRS amplitude and axis, owing to the "swinging" motion of the heart. (From Goldberger, A. L. Goldberger, Z. D., & Shvilkin, A. (Eds.) (2018). *Goldberger's clinical electrocardiography: A simplified approach* (9th ed., Fig. 12.3). Elsevier.)

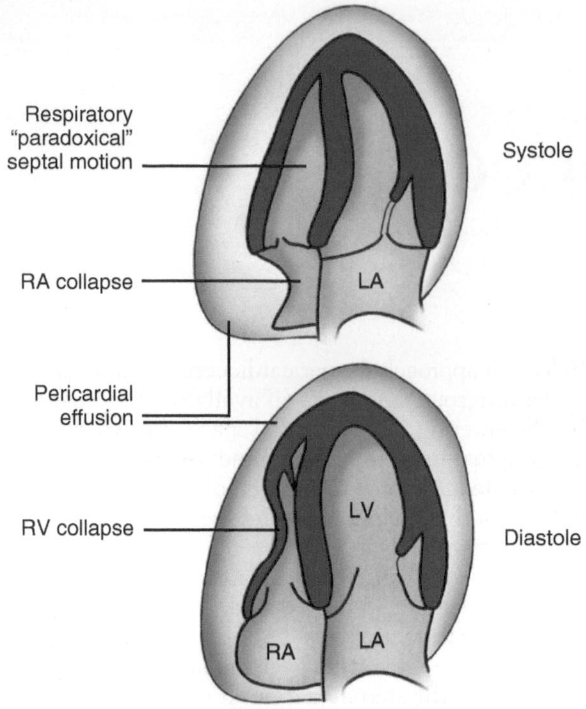

FIG. 149.2 Pericardial effusion with tamponade physiology, showing RA (right atrial, top) and RV (right ventricular, bottom) collapse. (From Otto, C. M. (2018). *Textbook of clinical echocardiography* (6th ed., Fig. 10.12). Elsevier.)

- If rapid reaccumulation is expected or if removal of a larger volume of fluid is required to improve hemodynamics, the Seldinger technique can be used to place a pigtail catheter in the pericardial space.
- Advance the pigtail over the guidewire and remove guidewire.
- Aspirate pericardial fluid.
- Secure the drain with sutures and place a sterile dressing over the puncture site.

Temporary Cardiac Pacing

Indication

- Bradyarrhythmia with hemodynamic instability unresponsive to pharmacologic interventions (atropine, epinephrine, and/or norepinephrine).

Contraindications

- No absolute contraindications exist.

Procedure

Transcutaneous Pacing

- Place adhesive electrode patches on the chest in the apical and left parasternal location, or in an anterior and posterior alignment. Body hair may need to be shaved to achieve direct skin contact. Attach electrodes to cardiac monitor with pacing capability.
- Set initial pacing rate to 60 to 70 beats/min.
- Set current to 25 mA and increase by 5 to 10 mA until palpation reveals an increase in pulse rate and a paced QRS complex and T wave are seen after each pacer stimulus artifact or "spike." During transcutaneous pacing, the pacer "spike" may mimic a QRS complex or obscure it. If clear T waves are observed after each "spike," ventricular capture has occurred. Always confirm with palpation.
- Significant patient discomfort is expected at higher stimulus currents (e.g., more than 60 to 70 mA). Sedation and analgesia will be required.

Transvenous Pacing

- Achieve central venous access through either the right internal jugular or left subclavian vein using the Seldinger technique and secure the introducer sheath.
- Introduce transvenous pacing catheter (5 Fr) and advance until it is in the right ventricular apex and in contact with the right ventricular endocardium. If available, monitor and confirm with ultrasound.
- Secure transvenous pacing catheter onto the patient's skin.
- Connect the transvenous pacing lead to the pacemaker generator. Attach the + and – electrodes of the pacing catheter to the + and – poles on the pacemaker generator.
- Set initial pacing rate to 60 to 70 beats/min.
- Set current to minimal output to 5 mA and incrementally increase by 2 to 5 mA until a QRS and T wave complex is seen after each pacer spike. Sensitivity should be set at a level needed to inhibit artificial pacing if spontaneous QRS complexes occur. With sensitivity function enabled, the pacing mode is VVI.

Synchronized Cardioversion

Indication

- Hemodynamically unstable tachyarrhythmias
  - Atrial fibrillation
  - Atrial flutter
  - Other supraventricular tachycardias (SVT), such as atrioventricular (AV) node reentrant tachycardia, AV reentrant tachycardia, atrial tachycardia
  - Ventricular tachycardia with a pulse

Contraindication

- Successful cardioversion of atrial fibrillation or flutter carries a significant risk of thromboembolism if the tachyarrhythmia has persisted for more than 48 hours. In such cases, urgent rate control is preferred in hemodynamically stable patients.

Procedure

- Patient should have continuous cardiorespiratory monitoring with blood pressure, pulse, pulse oximetry, $EtCO_2$, and cardiac telemetry. Have supplemental oxygen and intubation equipment available in case of any respiratory complications.
- Place pads in anterior-posterior orientation, away from implanted devices, if possible. Connect pads to defibrillator.
- If the patient is conscious, consider administering fentanyl (1 μg/kg) for pain and using etomidate (0.15 mg/kg) or propofol (1 mg/kg) for moderate sedation.
- Select appropriate energy (biphasic waveform defibrillator) in adults.

- Atrial fibrillation: 120 to 200 J
- Atrial flutter: 50 to 100 J
- Supraventricular tachycardia: 50 to 100 J
- Ventricular tachycardia with a pulse: 100 J

- Select synchronized mode, ensure R or S wave is larger than T wave, and that the indicator is above each beat on the monitor screen. If not, select another lead until parameters are met.
- Cardiovert the patient by holding the shock button until a shock is delivered.
- Atrial flutter, SVT owing to reentry, and VT typically respond to one to two shocks.

SUGGESTED READINGS

Hayes, D. (2019). *Temporary cardiac pacing*. UpToDate.
Heffner, A. (2019). *Emergency pericardiocentesis*. UpToDate.

SUGGESTED VIDEO

Fitch, M. T., Nicks, B. A., Pariyadath, M., McGinnis, H. D., & Manthey, D. E. (2012). Emergency pericardiocentesis. *The New England Journal of Medicine*, 366, e17. *Transcutaneous pacing*. Available at: https://vimeo.com/23461387.

CHAPTER 150

BOARD REVIEW

Wound Management

RYAN DEVIVO, DO, MS, and WENDY C. COATES, MD

Wound Evaluation and Preparation

- Obtaining a detailed medical history, the mechanism of injury, the setting in which a wound occurred, and tetanus immunization status are crucial for initial evaluation of wounds.
- Wound care decisions are affected by both injury-related factors (risk of foreign body, neurovascular injuries) as well as host factors for suboptimal outcomes (e.g., immunocompromised, peripheral vascular disease, diabetes mellitus, or structural defects that welcome bacterial seeding, such as damaged or prosthetic heart valves).
- Risk for damage to other structures should be assessed and evaluated with a careful physical examination.
- An appropriately anesthetized, bloodless field will allow for optimal evaluation.
- Notable characteristics include anatomic location, length, and depth. Wounds may need to be probed or even extended to evaluate extent and depth.
- Postinjury edema may cause wounds to reapproximate and appear more superficial than they truly are.
- For extremities and digits especially, the appendage may have been in a different state of tension when the wound was sustained, so all structures should be moved through their entire range of motion to assess for tendon, ligament, and nerve injuries.
- Assessing regional and distal vascular supply with pulse checks and capillary refill is crucial for high-force/velocity injuries or those that are deeply penetrating.

General Principles

Wound Infection Risk Factors

- In general, wounds should be closed within 12 hours, but clinicians must consider all risk factors prior to deciding on optimal closure timing (e.g., bite wounds within 8 hours).
- Lacerations of the face and scalp may be closed up to 24 hours or more, given a low infection rate of approximately 4%, secondary to robust vasculature.
- Certain populations, such as those with diabetes, HIV/AIDS, and those on immunosuppressants, chemotherapy or long-term steroids, are at higher risk for wound infection and poor wound healing. These issues may affect timing of repair, technique, and after-care.
- Location of wound impacts associations with infection. Leg and thigh wounds have highest risk of around 20%; arms and torso have a 10% risk. Blunt or crush injuries are at higher risk than most fine-cut lacerations. Missile-type injuries, such as bullet wounds, damage surrounding tissue that may take days to become apparent.
- Contaminated wounds with devitalized tissue have an extremely high infection risk. Saliva and feces have bacterial concentrations that exceed the concentration needed to produce infection (generally 10^5 CFU/cm^2 of organisms).
- Presence of any foreign material reduces the wound's resistance to infection.

Evaluation for Foreign Body

- Foreign bodies may be discovered after wound exploration in approximately 78% of cases.
- Imaging may assist in assessment, but identification is limited by material, size, and density.
  - A computed tomography scan will identify most foreign bodies, but it should be a last resort owing to expense and radiation risk.
  - Ultrasound may also be of clinical utility, but it is often difficult to interpret images in the setting of infection, air, or edema.
  - Plain radiograph utility depends on adequacy of views and density of the material and adjacent tissues. Metal is visible in most cases, whereas glass greater than 1 mm thick is identified in 75% of cases. Wood and organic material are not radiopaque; soft-tissue views demonstrating radiolucent shadows or displacement of surrounding structures suggest the presence of foreign body.

Anesthesia

- Anesthesia facilitates evaluation of wounds free of pain, and conditions for proper skin and wound preparation prior to repair or dressing.
- Lidocaine 1% is the most widely used anesthetic.
  - Generally safe and effective when dosed properly with rapid onset.
  - Duration of action: 20 to 60 minutes for local, and 75 to 120 minutes for regional blocks; effect may be prolonged by addition of epinephrine, up to 2 to 6 hours.
  - Dose: 3 to 5 mg/kg, or 5 to 7 mg/kg dose when combined with epinephrine.
- Bupivacaine's effects last 4 to 8 hours longer than lidocaine, but has a somewhat longer onset of action.
  - Dose: 2.5 mg/kg or 3.5 mg/kg when combined with epinephrine.
  - Care should be taken to prevent intravascular injection because cardiac arrest has been reported.

- Epinephrine
  - May delay healing and increase risk of infection in nonviable tissue or high-risk wounds.
  - Safety of epinephrine in digits, genitals, ears, and nose repairs still controversial.
  - Phentolamine and/or topical nitroglycerin mitigate ischemia due to vasoconstriction, but patients with peripheral vascular disease, Raynaud phenomenon or disease should be screened prior to using epinephrine-containing products.
- Topical anesthesia
  - Effective in pediatrics and wounds where injections distort tissue and loss of landmarks, which impacts proper repair
  - TAC (*t*etracaine 0.5%, 1:2000 epinephrine [*a*drenaline], and 11% *c*ocaine): widely used and shown to be effective at half-dose; reaches toxic levels when applied to heavily contaminated wounds and mucous membranes, especially in children, and should be avoided in these cases
  - LET (*l*idocaine 1%–4%, *e*pinephrine 1:1000 to 1:2000, and *t*etracaine 0.5%–2%): increasingly popular and equally effective as TAC, without toxicity from cocaine; usually effective within 30 minutes.
- Allergy to anesthetic agents
  - Uncommon, especially to esters, but also rare for amides
  - Methylparaben, a preservative used in multidose vials, is the more likely cause of allergy to amides.
  - Cardiac lidocaine and single-dose vials can be substituted if concern for amide allergy, because these are free of preservatives.

Skin Preparation

- Povidone-iodine (Betadine) or chlorhexidine (Hibiclens)
  - May be used to disinfect surrounding intact skin structures
  - Not to be used on the wound itself; may delay wound healing and increase infection
  - Povidine-iodine effective against gram-positive and gram-negative bacteria, viruses, and fungi whereas
  - Chlorhexidine has less gram-negative activity and unclear effect on viruses.
  - Simple soap and water is effective in combination with the wound irrigation.
- Avoid hair getting trapped within the wound; may cause foreign body reaction and increase infection risk.
- Apply petroleum-based product to displace hair from the wound for better visualization.
- Not necessary to remove hair to properly assess, evaluate, and repair a wound
- Razors increase the rate of infection; damage proximal hair follicle and provide entry point for bacteria.
- Eyebrow hairs should never be trimmed because of cosmetic issues and slow growth.

Wound Preparation

- Irrigation is the most important step (Fig. 150.1); dislodges bacteria and microscopic foreign bodies.
- For wound cleansing and irrigation, tap water is equivalent to normal saline and sterile water regarding infection rates and cosmesis.
- Antiseptic substances are toxic to wounds and may increase infection rate.
- Iodine-containing compounds prevent collagen synthesis.
- Irrigation with 15 psi of continuous pressure is superior to flooding the wound with running water.
- Antiseptic solution may be detrimental to wound healing and increase the risk of infection.
- Extreme pressures above 50 psi may cause soft-tissue damage and impair wound healing.
- An 18-gauge needle and 30 mL syringe can produce an adequate stream of irrigation.
- Never scrub wound bed vigorously; this may damage surrounding viable tissue.
- Debridement
  - Debride wound edges that are necrotic.
  - If large defect after debridement, allow wound to heal by secondary intention and schedule for delayed plastics revision.
  - Risk of debridement, especially on extremities (less so on trunk): a debrided wound may be under a higher tension, create a larger scar, and lead to nonunion.

Approach to Wound Closure

- Physician judgment is best method for deciding on the closure plan, or lack thereof. The first step is deciding whether the wound should be closed and, if so, when. Three main options are available.

Primary closure

- Closure at the time of initial evaluation.

Delayed primary closure

- Employed when closure is not possible within ideal postinjury period (12 hours; 24 hours for face/scalp), or for a bite wound.
- Day 1—irrigate wound; apply a nonadherent dressing to prevent wound edges from touching; and prescribe antibiotic (e.g., cephalexin, amoxicillin/clavulanate).
- Day 3—close the wound if healthy and noninfected after anesthesia and irrigation.

Secondary intention

- Typically for those wounds where patient delayed seeking care
- Leave wound open after wound preparation and dressing.
- Relatively contraindicated for wounds whose edges have already granulated, unless a qualified practitioner can adequately debride the wound edges to create a clean tissue surface
- Location, shape, size, depth, and, most importantly, tension must be assessed prior to deciding on proper closure technique and materials
- Reduction of dead space by placing deep sutures, or judiciously undermining the superficial tissue from the deeper tissues, can help ameliorate tension.
- Use meticulous technique when undermining to minimize compromising vascular supply to the wound.
- Multilayer closure with sutures should be used in wounds under tension; alternatives include the horizontal mattress technique or using a deep absorbable suture to eliminate tension, followed by epidermal closure with strips or tissue adhesive.

Wound Cleansing: Mechanical Scrubbing and Irrigation

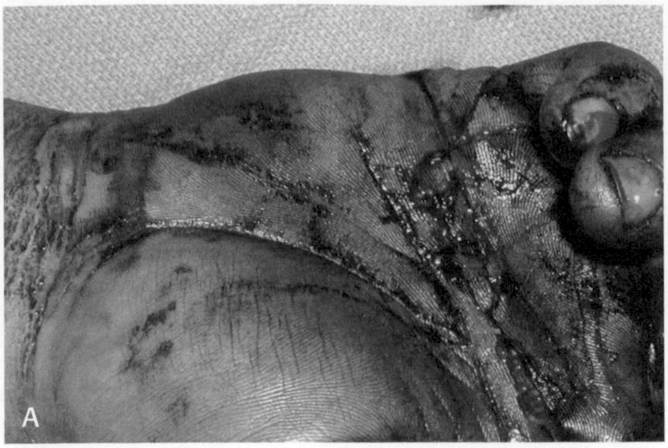

Grossly contaminated wounds such as this need to be thoroughly cleansed prior to repair, by mechanical scrubbing and/or irrigation.

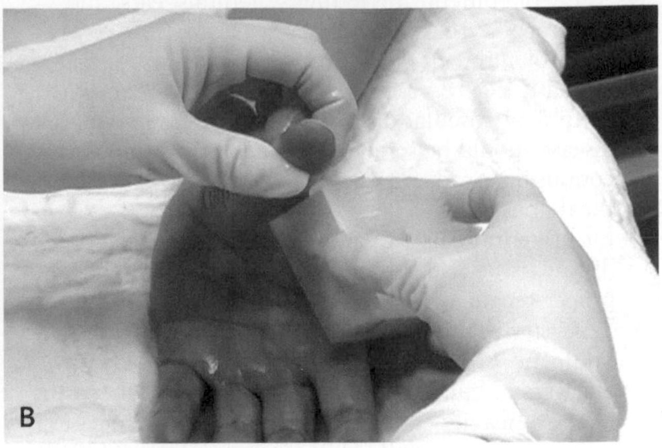

Reserve mechanical scrubbing for wounds contaminated with significant amounts of bacteria or foreign material. Use a fine-pore sponge (e.g., 90 pores/inch) to minimize tissue abrasion.

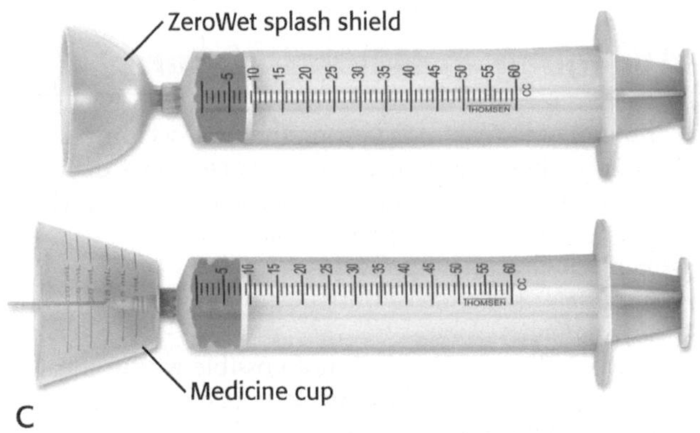

Top, ZeroWet splash shield attached to the end of a syringe. The shield is held near or against the skin and protects the user from splashes from the high-pressure laminar flow nozzle. *Bottom*, a makeshift splash protector can be made from a medication cup.

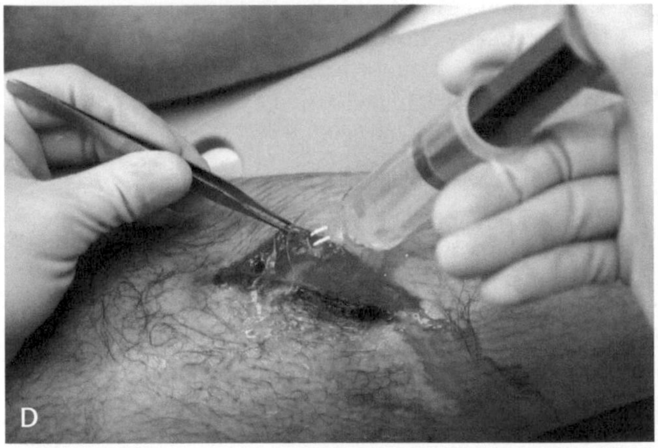

Use of the ZeroWet device. Note that the clinician is holding the laceration open with forceps to allow irrigation of the deep structures.

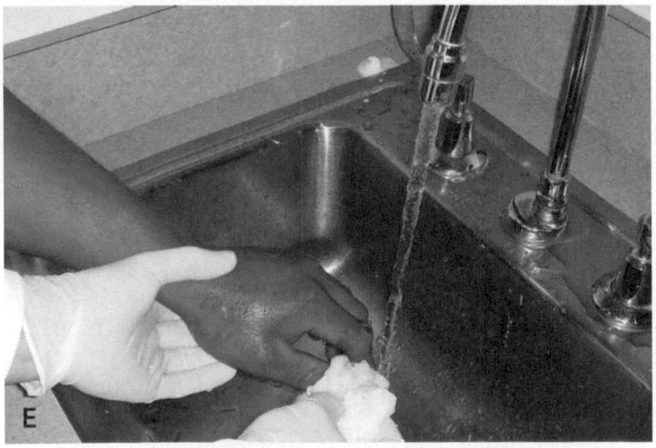

Tap water and nonsterile gloves are commonly used to copiously irrigate wounds of the extremities by taking advantage of the volume and force parameters from the faucet. Anesthetize lacerations before cleaning. Be mindful of the potential for the patient to faint.

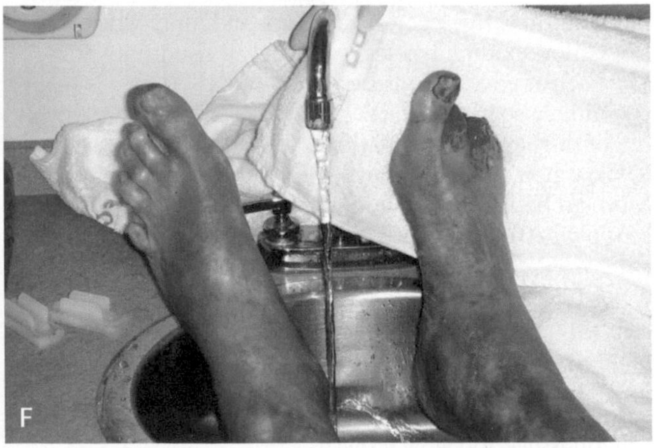

For foot wounds, the patient is placed on a stretcher and wheeled to the sink.

FIG. 150.1 Wound preparation and exploration. (From Lammers, R. L., & Aldy, K. M. (2019). Principles of wound management. In J. R. Roberts, C. B. Custalow, & T. W. Thomsen (Eds.), *Roberts and Hedges' clinical procedures in emergency medicine and acute care* (7th ed., pp. 621–654, Fig. 34.5). Elsevier.)

- Approximate all nonlinear wounds with viable edges, to relieve tension and facilitate natural scarring; the half-buried mattress suture technique may be helpful.

TISSUE ADHESIVE

- Indicated for small, superficial linear wounds that are not under tension
- Can be used for scalp wounds with hair apposition technique
- Compound polymerizes on contact with moisture
- Gram-positive antimicrobial effect
- Less tensile strength than sutures over first 3 to 4 days, but comparable cosmetic outcomes.
- Adhesive sloughs off in 5 to 10 days.
- Petroleum-containing substances dissolve tissue adhesive; do not apply to wounds postoperatively. However, these may be helpful to remove the compound, if necessary.
- *Equipment:* 2-octylcyanoacrylate (Dermabond) and N-butyl-2-cyanoacrylate (Indermil)
- *Technique:* Hold wound edges together with forceps or gloved fingers.
  - Each compound has explicit directions for optimal application.
  - Dermabond: expel contents from the applicator and apply to the approximated wound, extending 5 to 10 mm from each side of wound in 3 to 4 layers. Hold edges for at least 1 minute. Apply wound closure strips when dry, if necessary.
- *Contraindications:* Infection, deep wounds, high-tension regions, poor hemostasis, hairy areas (except hair apposition technique for scalp), poorly approximated wound edges, eyelids
- *Complications:* burning sensation from heat of polymerization
  - Adhesive can fracture if manipulated, if petroleum is applied, or if immersed in water.

STAPLES

- Indicated for superficial scalp wounds, extremities, and trunk wounds. Cosmetic outcomes are somewhat worse than meticulous sutures, but rates of healing, infection, and dehiscence are comparable.
- *Equipment:* A variety of devices is available.
- *Technique:* Evert edges on own or with the help of an assistant using forceps or thumb/forefinger. Stapling a flat wound will result in inversion. Avoid pressing too deeply to the center of the wound to prevent ischemia to staple loop. Dress wound appropriately when completed.
- *Contraindications:* Do not use on cosmetically important areas, such as the face, neck, and hand. Do not place prior to computed tomography or magnetic resonance imaging if anticipated.
- *Complications:* Inversion if done on flat wound. May produce a more pronounced scar in patients who scar easily (e.g., keloid formers).

SUTURE METHODS

- Certain methods may have advantages for specific wounds or wound locations.
- Routine suturing supplies include sutures, needle drivers, tissue forceps, suture scissors, sterile gloves, and drapes.
- Needle driver use:
  - Grasp the loaded needle driver with the palm of the dominant hand.
  - Place an index finger along the closed needle driver pointing toward the needle, using the palm to open and close the driver, as needed. This allows for ease of rotation while suturing, but if unable to accomplish this, the thumb and ring fingers can be placed within the needle driver rings.
  - Insert needle at 90 degrees to the skin to allow for optimal wound edge eversion.
  - Pass the needle through one side and reinsert into the dermis of the opposing side of the wound or from side to side in one pass, depending on provider comfort and wound amenability.
  - Care should be taken to assure that the suture depth and distance from the wound are symmetric (Fig. 150.2).

Simple Interrupted Sutures

- Most commonly practiced method in the emergency department
- Appropriate for most wounds with low infection rates with optimal cosmetic outcomes (Fig. 150.3)
- If one suture becomes infected, it can be removed without having to disrupt the entire closure.
- *Technique:*
  - While holding the needle at a 90-degree angle to the skin surface, penetrate through to the dermis, advancing through to the opposite side of the laceration.
  - Ensure both sides of wounds are at the same level.
  - Using an instrument tie, perform a surgeon's knot with an initial double throw, followed by sequential single throws in opposite directions.
  - For cosmetic purposes, place sutures at symmetric and parallel intervals.
- *Contraindications:* Any general contraindication to wound repair or patient refusal
- *Complications:*
  - May leave suture marks
  - May cause ischemia to wound
  - May increase infection risk if suture tied too tightly
  - May result in dehiscence and worse scarring if wound edges are not everted

Continuous (Running) Sutures

- Appropriate for closing wounds under little to no tension, are clean, linear, and low infection risk
- Strength is evenly distributed across the suture line.
- Sutures may be placed within the dermis (subcuticular) or externally.
- *Technique (External):*
  - First, place an interrupted stitch at one end of wound, only cutting the free tail end.
  - Hold the thread partially taut with the nondominant hand, pass the needle in a spiral pattern, gently pulling the wound until it approximates with each pass
  - Place the last loop adjacent to the end of the wound and use the last loop as the tail for tying the knot.
  - A locking technique can be used along more irregular wounds, if desired.
  - Applying subcuticular sutures may further reduce tension and decrease scarring and stitch marks.

General Suturing Technique

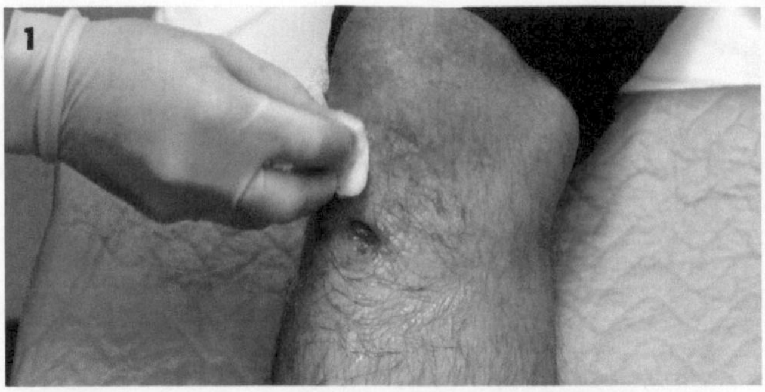

Cleanse the skin surrounding the wound with an antiseptic such as chlorhexidine or povidone-iodine. Avoid introducing antiseptic into the wound because it may be toxic to tissue.

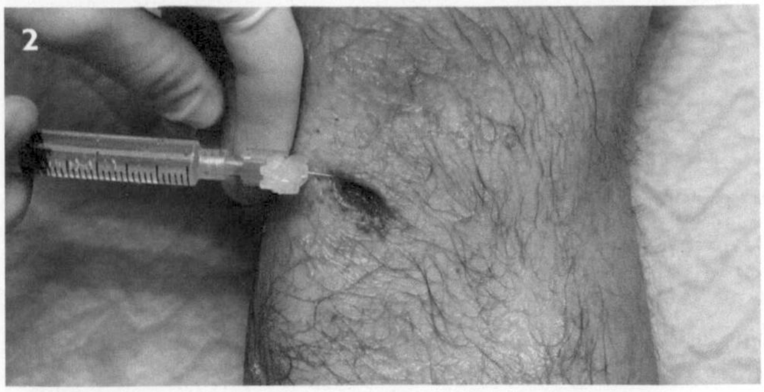

Anesthetize the wound prior to exploration and irrigation. Introduce the needle through the wound (as opposed to through the epidermis).

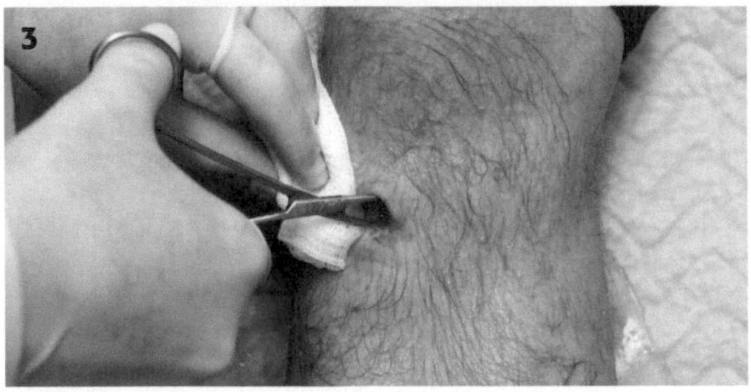

Explore the wound to exclude the presence of foreign bodies, gross contamination, or injuries to deep structures. Débride grossly contaminated or devitalized tissue.

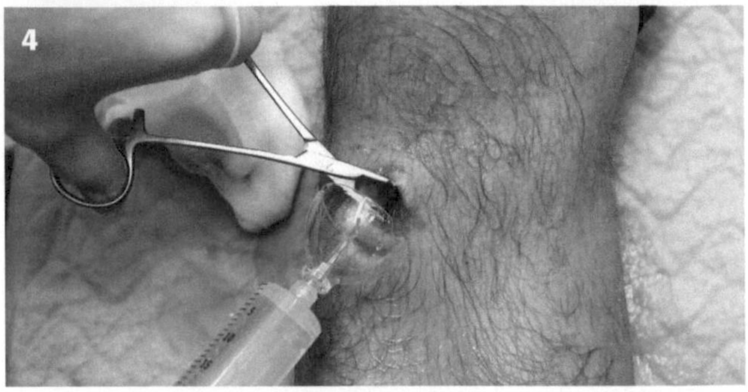

Irrigate the wound thoroughly until it is visibly clean. Use of a large syringe with a splash guard is ideal. Retract the wound edges with an instrument to facilitate thorough irrigation.

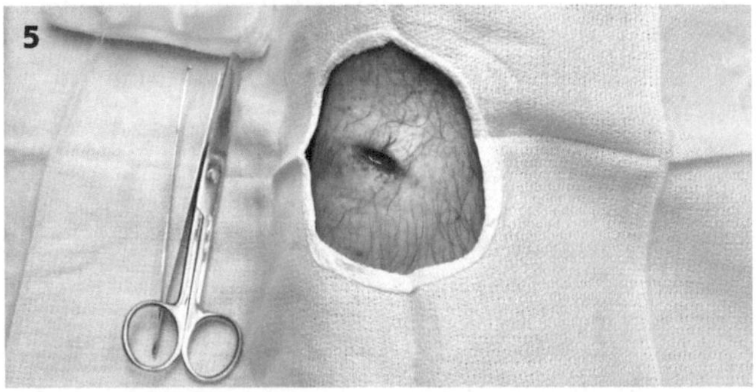

Apply a sterile drape, gather the instruments, and ensure that the field is appropriately lit.

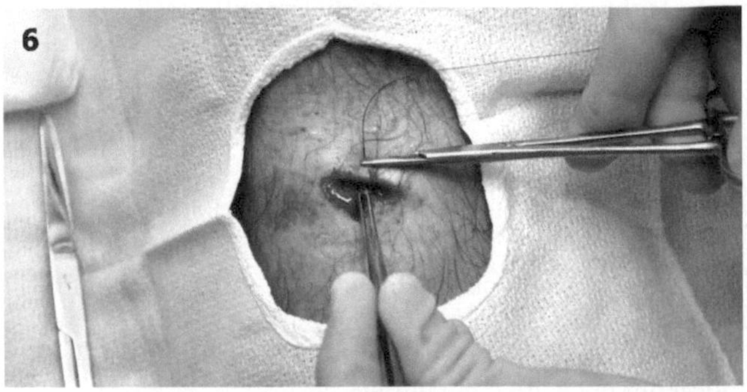

Place the first suture at the center of the wound so that it bisects the laceration into two equal segments.

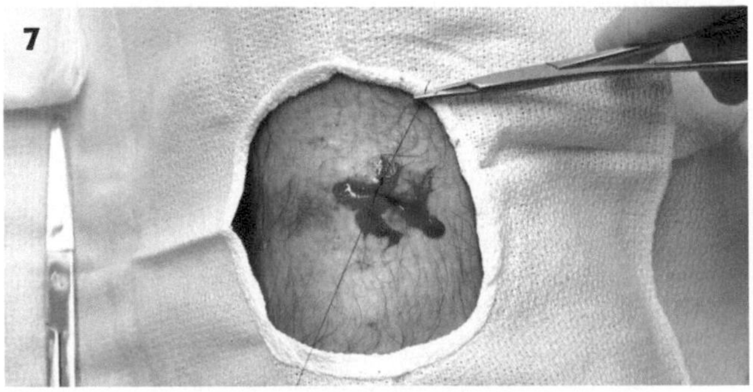

Tie the knot. The first throw should be a double throw (i.e., surgeon's knot) to prevent it from loosening. Place an additional three (single) throws and then cut the sutures while leaving 1- to 2-cm tails.

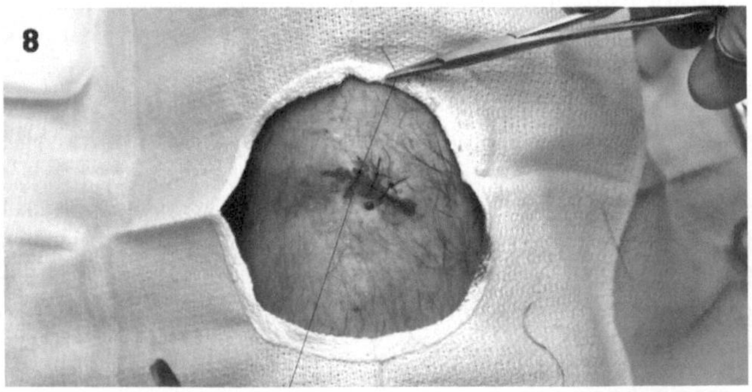

Continue to place additional sutures by further bisecting each segment of the laceration. After the last stitch has been placed, cleanse the area and apply an appropriate dressing.

FIG. 150.2 General suturing technique. (From Lammers, R. L., & Scrimshaw, L. E. (2019). Principles of wound closure. In J. R. Roberts, C. B. Custalow, & T. W. Thomsen (Eds.), *Roberts and Hedges' clinical procedures in emergency medicine and acute care* (7th ed., pp. 655–707, Fig. 35.17). Elsevier.)

Simple Interrupted Sutures

1

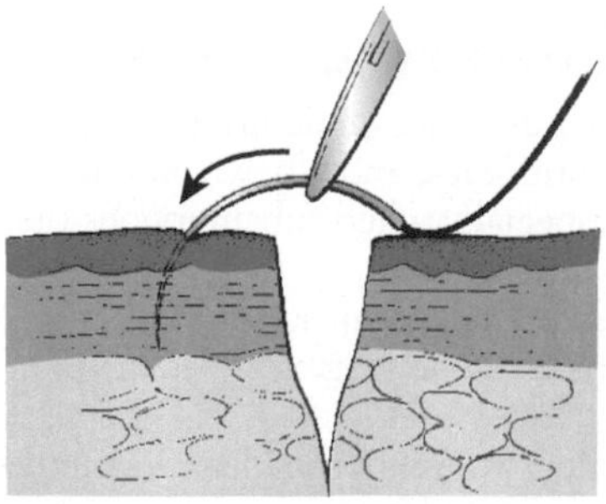

Hold the needle pointing downward by excessively pronating the wrist so that the needle tip initially moves farther from the laceration as the needle penetrates deeper into the skin. Drive the needle tip downward and away from the cut edge into the subcutaneous layer.

2

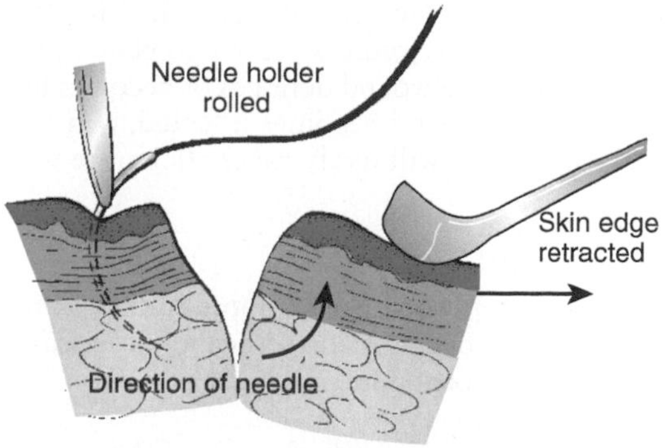

Advance the needle into the laceration. The needle tip is directed toward the opposite side at the same level by rolling the needle holder. The arc of the needle pathway is controlled by retracting the skin edge. This method incorporates more tissue within the stitch in the deeper layers of the wound than at the surface. As an alternative, if a small needle is used in thick skin or the distance across the wound is great, the needle can be removed from the first side, remounted on the needle holder, and advanced to the opposite side.

3

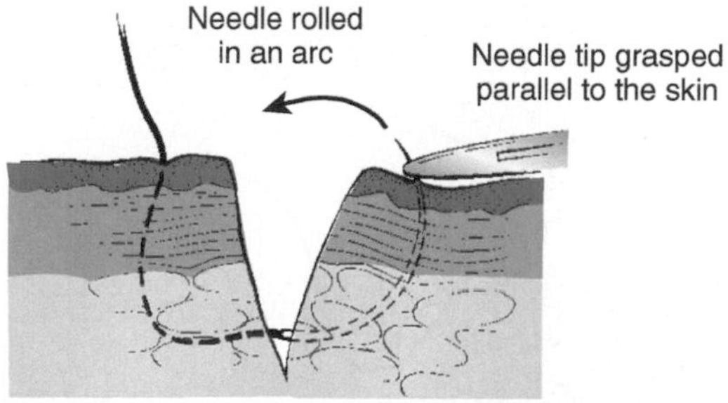

Advance the needle upward toward the surface so that it exits at the same distance from the wound edge as on the contralateral side of the wound. Grasp the needle behind the tip and roll it out in the arc of the needle.

4

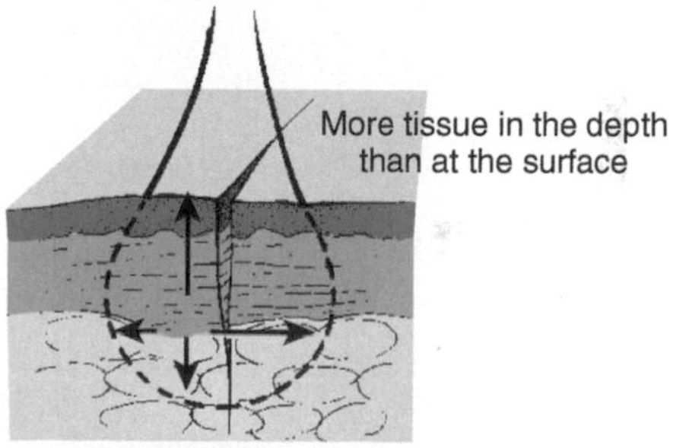

The final position, with more tissue in the depth than in the surface. The distance from each exit of the suture to the laceration is half the depth of the dermis.

5

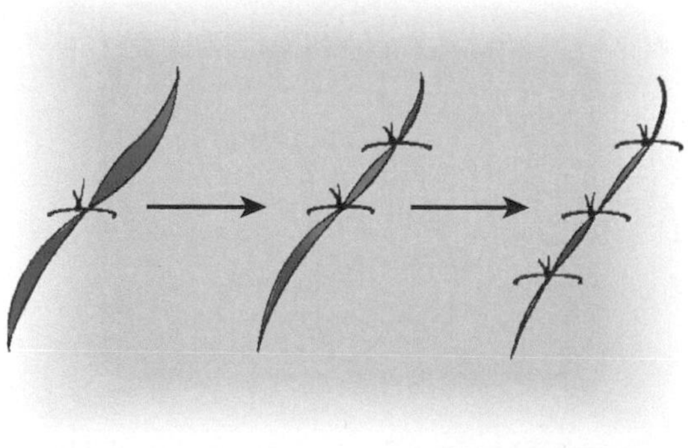

Close the surface of the wound in segments rather than from one end. Place the first suture in the center of the wound for a straight suture line.

6

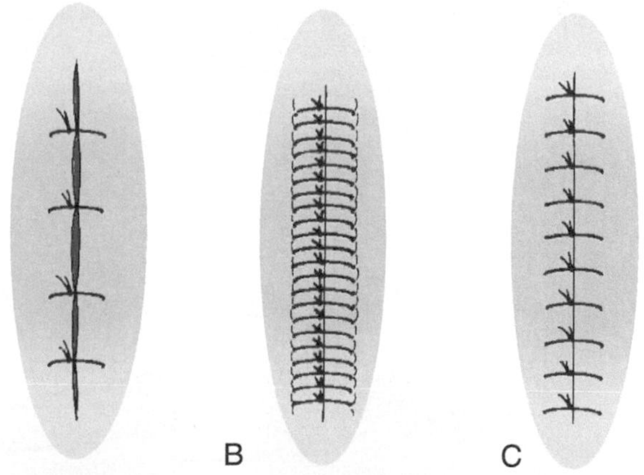

A, Too few stitches used. Note the gaping between the sutures. **B**, Too many stitches used. **C**, Correct number of stitches used for a wound under an average amount of tension.

FIG. 150.3 Simple interrupted suture technique. (Steps 1–4, From Kaplan, E. N., & Hentz, V. R. (1984). *Emergency management of skin and soft tissue wounds: An illustrated guide* (p. 86). Little, Brown. Reproduced by permission.)

150

- *Contraindications:*
  - Do not use to close wounds overlying joints or mobile body areas
  - Do not use to close wounds at high risk of infection, because the entire closure will have to be removed if any portion of the wound dehisces or becomes infected.
- *Complications:* If wound becomes infected, cutting even a single suture loop will likely cause the entire wound to fall open.

Vertical Mattress

- Indicated for deep wounds with loose surface skin to promote wound edge eversion, especially in areas where deep sutures are contraindicated (Fig. 150.4)
- *Technique:*
  - Pass the needle through both sides of the wound similar to a simple interrupted suture.
  - Next, insert the needle extremely close to the wound from the side where the initial suture exited, passing superficially to the original side of the wound.
  - Apply surgeon's knot.
- *Contraindications:*
  - Avoid in areas with a high risk for infection, tension, and ischemia or when cosmesis is of concern, such as the face.
- *Complications:*
  - Can result in "railroad track"-like marks.
  - Edge necrosis of the wound and deeper tissue ischemia may occur, especially if tied too tightly.

Horizontal Mattress and Corner Stitch

- Indicated for wounds under moderate (not high) tension, including palms and soles, and where some level of eversion is desired, especially when subcutaneous tissue is limited
- A half-buried technique, or corner stitch, can be used for wounds that contain a flap (Fig. 150.5).
- *Technique:*
  - Pass the needle through both sides of wound similar to a simple interrupted suture.
  - At the exit site of the initial pass, move distally along the wound and reinsert the needle at the point where the next simple interrupted stitch would have been placed, exiting the wound on the opposing side, parallel to the first insertion site and tie the two ends with an instrument tie.
  - For the corner stitch, insert the needle away from the apex of the non-flap portion of the wound. Exit through the mid-dermis and then, while everting the

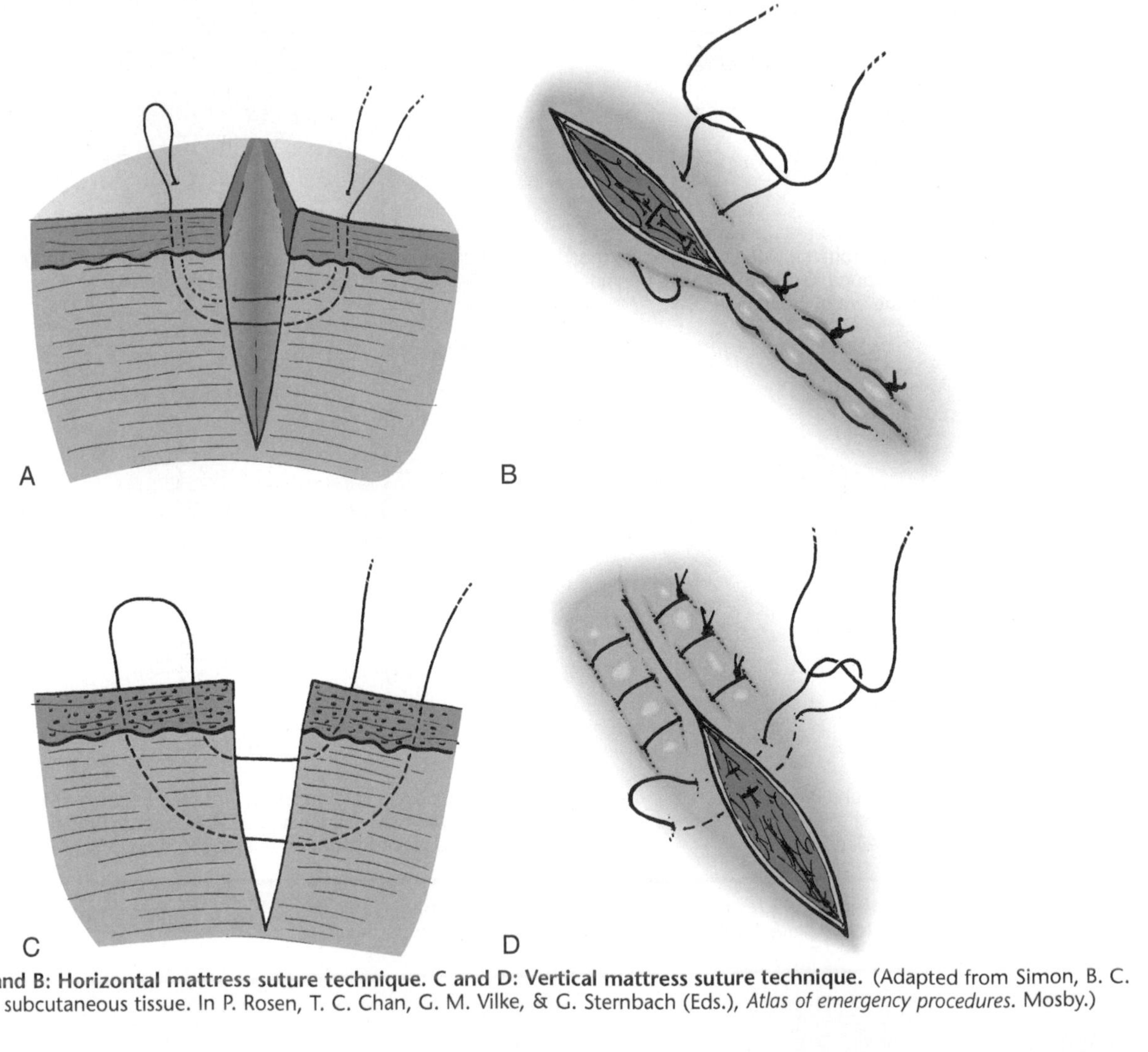

FIG. 150.4 A and B: Horizontal mattress suture technique. C and D: Vertical mattress suture technique. (Adapted from Simon, B. C. (2001). Skin and subcutaneous tissue. In P. Rosen, T. C. Chan, G. M. Vilke, & G. Sternbach (Eds.), *Atlas of emergency procedures*. Mosby.)

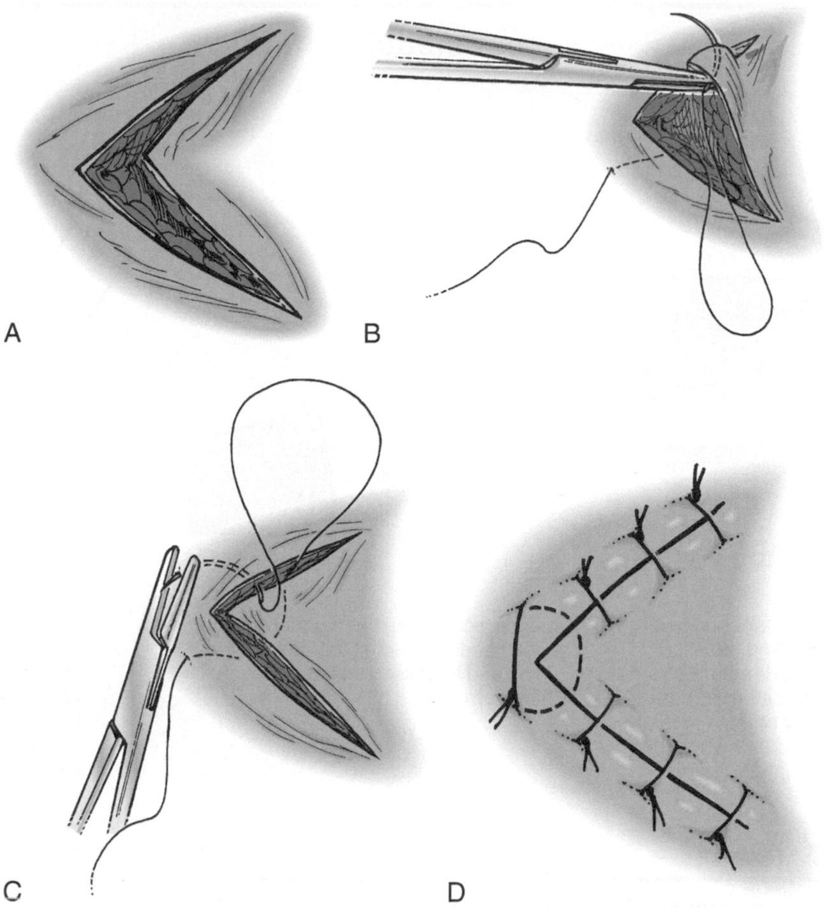

FIG. 150.5 Corner stitch technique. (Adapted from Simon, B. C. (2001). Skin and subcutaneous tissue. In P. Rosen, T. C. Chan, G. M. Vilke, & G. Sternbach (Eds.), *Atlas of emergency procedures*. Mosby.)

flap, pass the suture through and through the dermis of the flap at the same depth.
  - Reinsert the needle equidistant from the apex of the non-flap portion of the dermal layer, exiting through the skin and tying the knot similar to above.
  - Tie the stitch on intact skin, not over the corner of the flap.
  - Avoid blanching the flap when pulling taut.
- *Contraindications:*
  - Avoid in areas with a high risk for infection or ischemia or when cosmesis is of concern, such as the face.
- *Complications:*
  - Can result in more suture marks and increase the potential for scarring.
  - Edge necrosis of the wound may occur owing to ischemia within the suture loops.
  - For corner stitches, the distal tip may not be viable, resulting in poor healing, especially if the wound is pulled too taut.
  - Inform patient about the high likelihood of flap necrosis.

Intradermal (Deep) Sutures

- Indicated for wounds with significant depth or tension, or those wounds where reducing tension as much as possible will benefit cosmesis (Fig. 150.6).
- *Technique:*
  - Using absorbable sutures, bury the knot by placing the needle deep and then exiting more superficially through the dermis layer, followed by reinsertion in reverse manner on the opposite side.
  - This method prevents the knot from spitting through the superficial wound margins.
  - Close the epidermis with wound closure strips, simple interrupted nonabsorbable sutures, tissue adhesive, etc.

DRESSINGS

- Choose dressings based on the type of wound, location, and risk for infection.
- Dressings should have a non-adherent surface, be permeable to gases for enhanced epithelialization in the presence of oxygen, and absorb some fluid to prevent maceration, but prevent desiccation.
- The simplest dressing for wounds is a transparent film or impregnated gauze.
- Hydrogels can be used for extremely dry wounds because they provide moisture.
- Foam dressings are made of sponge-like materials and absorb more fluid, which may be useful in wounds at risk of producing large volumes of fluid.
- Facial wounds can be dressed with a simple adhesive bandage (Band-Aid) or a thin layer of ointment.

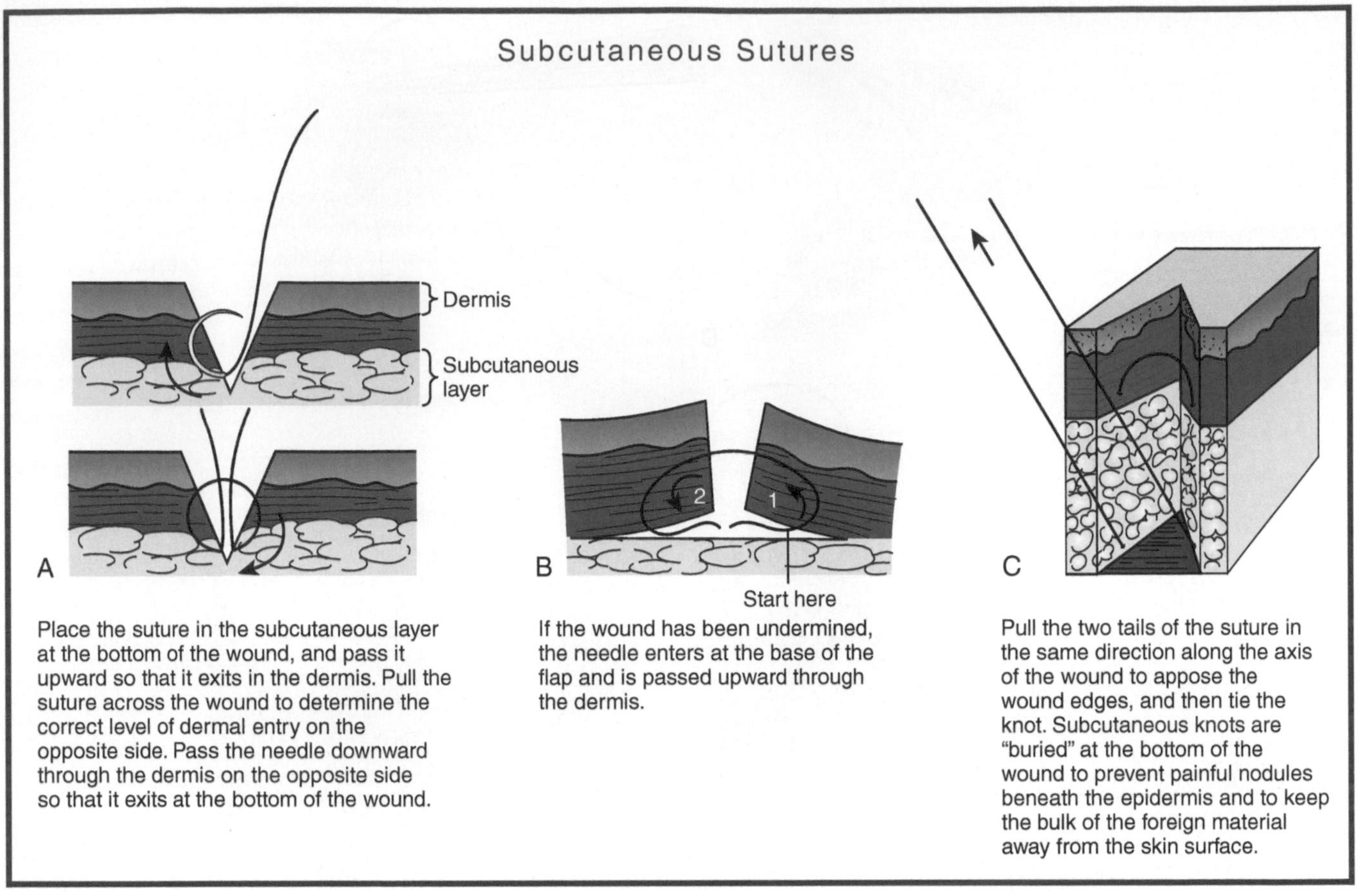

Subcutaneous Sutures
Dermis
Subcutaneous layer
A
Place the suture in the subcutaneous layer at the bottom of the wound, and pass it upward so that it exits in the dermis. Pull the suture across the wound to determine the correct level of dermal entry on the opposite side. Pass the needle downward through the dermis on the opposite side so that it exits at the bottom of the wound.
2
1
B
Start here
If the wound has been undermined, the needle enters at the base of the flap and is passed upward through the dermis.
C
Pull the two tails of the suture in the same direction along the axis of the wound to appose the wound edges, and then tie the knot. Subcutaneous knots are "buried" at the bottom of the wound to prevent painful nodules beneath the epidermis and to keep the bulk of the foreign material away from the skin surface.

FIG. 150.6 Subcutaneous deep sutures. (From Lammers, R. L., & Scrimshaw, L. E. (2019). Principles of wound closure. In J. R. Roberts, C. B. Custalow, & T. W. Thomsen (Eds.), *Roberts and Hedges' clinical procedures in emergency medicine and acute care* (7th ed., pp. 655–707, Fig. 35.25). Elsevier.)

- Splint or immobilize wounds close to joint or in areas of tension to prevent dehiscence, poor wound healing, and poor cosmetic outcomes.

WOUND CARE INSTRUCTIONS

1. Daily cleansing to remove accumulating debris: tap water will do, but diluted hydrogen peroxide may be used as well.
2. If on an extremity, elevate. A splint may be used if needed. Immobilization should remain until suture removal.
3. Monitor for signs of infection, including redness, worsening pain or swelling, fever, purulent discharge or lymphangitic spread.
4. Wounds can be reevaluated by providers on an individual basis. Heavily contaminated wounds and those at risk of poor healing should be reevaluated in 48 hours, others can be reevaluated on an individual basis.
5. **Suture Removal** (Fig. 150.7)
   a. Face: 3 to 5 days (replace with wound closure strips)
   b. Arm and trunk: 7 to 10 days

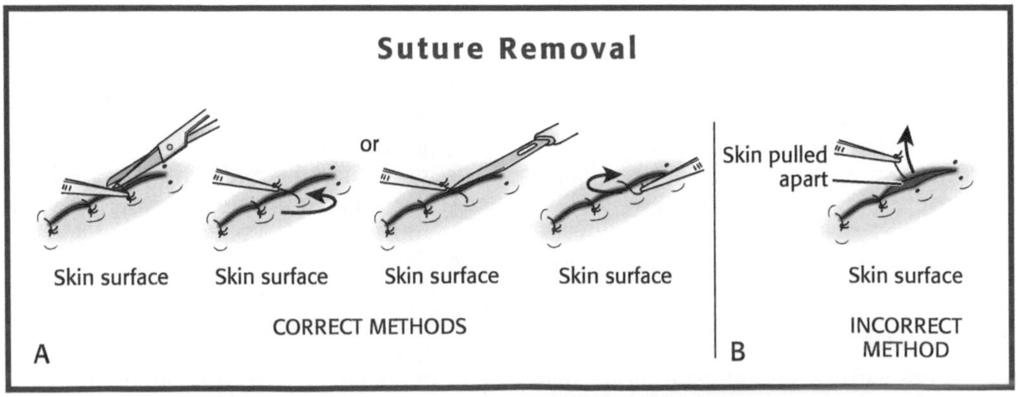

FIG. 150.7 Suture removal. (From Lammers, R. L., & Aldy, K. M. (2019). Principles of wound management. In J. R. Roberts, C. B. Custalow, & T. W. Thomsen (Eds.), *Roberts and Hedges' clinical procedures in emergency medicine and acute care* (7th ed., pp. 621–654, Fig. 34.21). Elsevier.)

c. Legs: 10 to 14 days
d. Scalp: 14 days
e. Joints and plantar foot: 14 days

Antibiotic Prophylaxis

- Not typically recommended for most wounds, although immunocompromised patients and heavily contaminated non-bite wounds may benefit in certain circumstances.
- Consider antibiotics for crush injuries because they produce significant tissue damage.
  - Crush wounds should be considered for delayed primary closure.
  - In patients with wounds involving joints or open fractures, timely antibiotic administration has proven to be beneficial.
  - Wounds involving open fractures should receive antibiotics for 72 hours, at minimum, and the regimen should include a cephalosporin, such as cefazolin or equivalent (clindamycin can be used in allergic patients), with or without an antibiotic with gram-negative coverage if the wound is heavily contaminated.
- The following special scenarios typically are not amenable to primary closure, but closure may be indicated in specific circumstances:
  - ***Cat bites:***
    - Due to their deep extending, puncture-like wounds, which are difficult to irrigate and debride completely
    - 10%–40% of cat bites are estimated to become infected.
    - Organisms typically include *Staphylococcus* and *Streptococcus* species, and most often, *Pasteurella multocida*, which is present in 70% of cats' normal oral flora.
    - Amoxicillin/clavulanate for 7 days should provide coverage.
    - Alternative regimens include trimethoprim/sulfamethoxazole and metronidazole or a fluoroquinolone and metronidazole.
  - ***Dog bites:***
    - Typically larger, tearing injuries that allow appropriate irrigation and debridement, unlike cat wounds, and have less risk of infection (Fig. 150.8B).
    - Antibiotic prophylaxis is controversial.
    - Multiple individual studies found no benefit, but a pooled study did find some statistical benefit.
    - Regimens recommended are the same as for those of cat bites, because the organisms are similar.
    - Safe to close dog bites to the face (after irrigation) to achieve better cosmetic outcomes, because facial lacerations typically are low risk for infection owing to their robust vascular and lymph supply.
    - A randomized trial also showed that dog bites closed within 8 hours (when also given amoxicillin/clavulanate) had a similar infection risk to all emergency department lacerations.
  - ***Hand bites:***
    - Wounds of the metacarpophalangeal joints should be considered human bite wounds or "fight bites" until proven otherwise (Fig. 150.8A).
    - Carefully inspect for joint space involvement and, if involved, aggressive irrigation with possible debridement in the operating room may be required.
    - Organisms include *Streptococcus* and *Staphylococcus* species as well as *Eikenella corrodens*, highly resistant to clindamycin, first-generation cephalosporins, and macrolides, and *Bacteroides* species.
    - Prophylaxis and/or treatment can be performed with the above regimens. With any bite wound, if there is bone or joint involvement, orthopedics should be consulted emergently in the emergency department for recommendations on further management and consideration for washout in the operating room.
    - Most "fight bites" should be left open for either secondary intention or delayed closure, given their propensity for infection.
  - ***Puncture wounds of the foot:***
    - Infection rate reported close to 15% despite their benign appearing nature (Fig. 150.8C).
    - Most occur on the plantar surface of the distal half of the foot and are frequently caused by *Pseudomonas* species.

150

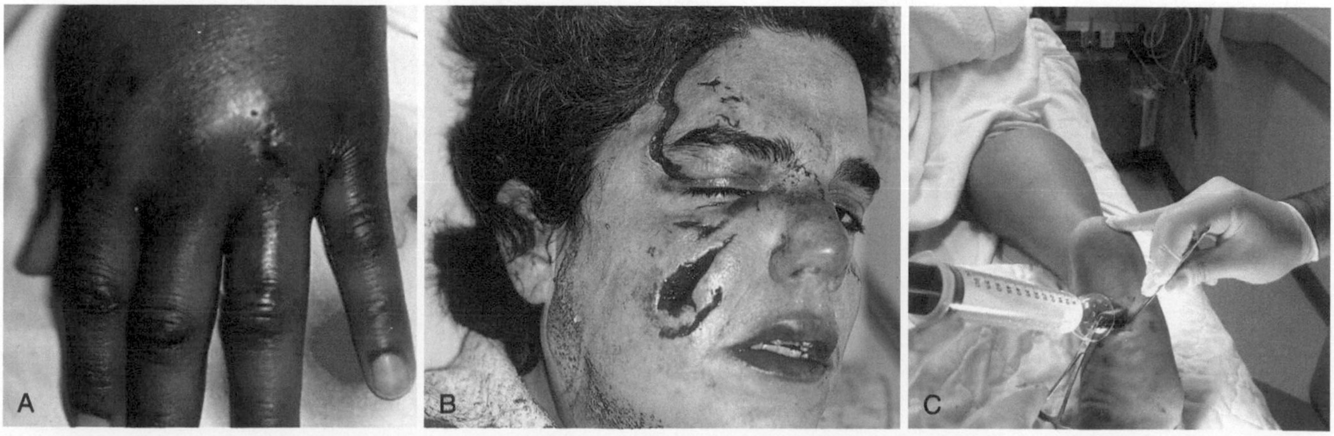

FIG. 150.8 Bite wounds from (**A**) human (fight bite), (**B**) dog, and (**C**) stepping on an object. (From Lammers, R. L., & Aldy, K. M. (2019). Principles of wound management. In J. R. Roberts, C. B. Custalow, & T. W. Thomsen (Eds.), *Roberts and Hedges' clinical procedures in emergency medicine and acute care* (7th ed., pp. 621–654, Fig. 34.15). Elsevier.)

- Many are seen after an object passes through a shoe, sandal, etc. into the foot.
- Those likely to be caused by *Pseudomonas aeruginosa* require some degree of prophylaxis, which can include ciprofloxacin for 7 days.
- Treated with an antibiotic agent that covers typical skin bacteria, such as cephalexin, dicloxacillin, or clindamycin.
- If there is concern for methicillin-resistant *Staphylococcus aureus*, consider using trimethoprim/sulfamethoxazole or doxycycline.
- These wounds typically do not require closure.

Tetanus Immunization Status

- Consider tetanus prophylaxis in all wounds, regardless of mechanism, depth, or severity.
- Of tetanus wounds, 40% occur in small wounds and/or in patients with no recollection of how the injury was sustained.
- Higher risk: age > 50 with waning immunity, immigrants from countries where vaccinations are not required are at highest risk.
- Typical incubation period for tetanus is 1 to 3 weeks, but ranges from a few days to 5 weeks.
- Immunization can be considered even days or weeks after the injury.
- If fully immunized (at least three injections in lifetime) and less than 5 years with documentation or reliable history, no tetanus prophylaxis is warranted. All others should receive Tdap or Td 0.5 mL intramuscularly once.
- Administer tetanus immunoglobulin to any patient with incomplete or absent vaccination.
- Providing up to 4 weeks of antibodies, immunoglobulin can be administered simultaneously, but at a different site than Tdap.

CHAPTER **151** BOARD REVIEW

Point-of-Care Ultrasound in the Emergency Department

JOSEPH FRIEDRICH, MD, and JACKIE SHIBATA, MD, MS

Point-of-care ultrasound (POCUS) is a bedside imaging modality that facilitates rapid diagnosis and aids treatment decisions for a vast array of organ systems. This chapter reviews basic orientation and a selection of common POCUS studies.

Basics of an Ultrasound Image

- The ultrasound probe emits high-frequency sound waves (more than 20,000 Hz) and analyzes the returning echoes to create a grayscale representation seen in two-dimensional mode imaging. Fig. 151.1 provides a basic overview of orientation, echogenicity, depth, and gain.

Common Point-of-Care Ultrasound Scans

RIGHT UPPER QUADRANT ULTRASOUND

- The right upper quadrant (RUQ) POCUS has high sensitivity and specificity to diagnose biliary pathology, such as acute cholecystitis or cholelithiasis (Fig. 151.2).

KIDNEY AND BLADDER

- Kidney and bladder POCUS examinations are primarily performed to assess hydronephrosis (Fig. 151.3) and postvoid residual bladder volumes to aid diagnosis of postrenal azotemia, acute kidney injury, mechanical obstruction, or neurologic dysfunction. Kidney and bladder POCUS can also guide and confirm urinary catheter placement.

FOCUSED ASSESSMENT WITH SONOGRAPHY IN TRAUMA (FAST)

- This widely used systematic ultrasound assessment can identify intraabdominal bleeding and pericardial effusion following blunt or penetrating trauma. In unstable patients who have sustained blunt trauma, a positive FAST facilitates direct transfer to the operating room without further diagnostic imaging. The extended FAST (eFAST) adds evaluation of the lungs and can rule out pneumothorax and hemothorax (Fig. 151.4 and Table 151.1).

FOCUSED ECHOCARDIOGRAPHY

- Application of basic cardiac sonography (Fig. 151.5) in the emergency department allows clinicians to evaluate for the following: (1) global cardiac function to assess whether the heart is hypodynamic or hyperdynamic, (2) the presence of pericardial fluid and tamponade physiology, and (3) right ventricular strain, indicative of acute pulmonary embolism. Focused echocardiography generally includes the four views summarized in Table 151.2;

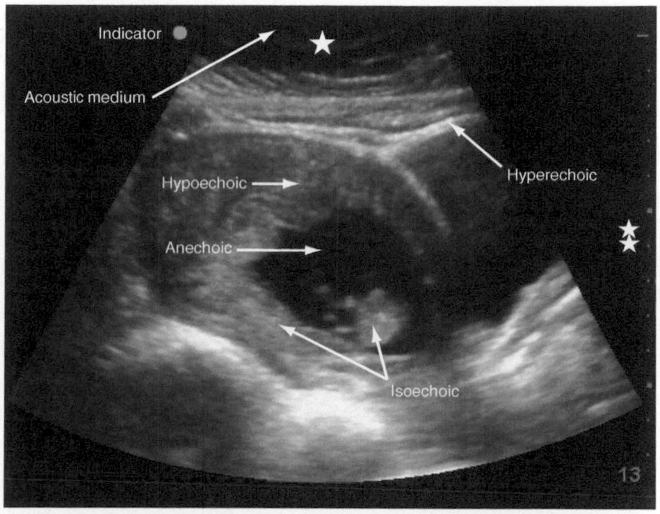

FIG. 151.1 The Basics: Orientation, Echogenicity, Depth, and Gain *Acoustic medium:* Ultrasound gel, or water bath, act as acoustic mediums to enhance images. Echogenic structures, such as bones, stones, and tendons, appear bright on ultrasound. *Hyperechoic:* Bright or white appearance of anterior bladder wall (fetal skull is also hyperechoic). *Anechoic:* Fluids such as amniotic fluid, blood, or urine lack echoes and appear black. *Hypoechoic:* The myometrium is less bright than surrounding structures. *Isoechoic:* The fetal pole and endometrium are isoechoic because they have similar brightness. *Gain*, which refers to the brightness of the overall image, can be adjusted; decreasing gain will darken the image. *Green dot:* The indicator is on the top left of the screen. By convention, the indicator on the probe is generally directed to the patient's right (transverse) or toward the patient's head (longitudinal). In this image, the probe indicator is oriented longitudinally, toward the patient's head, depicting a sagittal cut through the bladder and uterus with an intrauterine pregnancy visualized. Note that the uterine fundus is superior to the bladder, because the fundus is closer to the left side or indicator side of the image. The top of the image corresponds to structures closest to the ultrasound probe; skin (*star*) can be visualized closest to the probe while the fetal pole is much deeper. The hatch marks (*double star*) each indicate 1 cm of depth and can be adjusted. The depth in this image is 13 cm. Identification of a yolk sac or fetal pole (as depicted above) with POCUS can rule in an intrauterine pregnancy, making coexistence of an ectopic pregnancy very unlikely in nonassisted pregnancies.

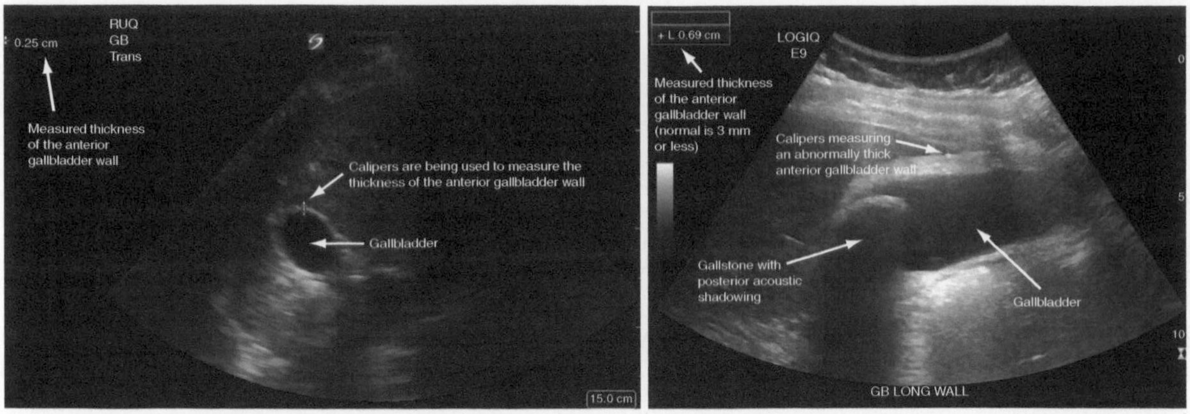

FIG. 151.2 Right upper quadrant ultrasound: Normal gallbladder versus cholecystitis. The gallbladder (GB) is a well-defined, anechoic fluid-filled structure adjacent to liver parenchyma. Low-frequency probes, such as phased array (*left*) or curvilinear (*right*), can be used to image the GB. This transverse GB (*left*) shows no signs of cholecystitis: no stones, the wall is less than 3 mm, no pericholecystic fluid or wall edema is visualized and no sonographic Murphy sign (tenderness with pressure applied by the probe while directly visualizing GB) is documented. Complete fanning through transverse and longitudinal GB planes can aid in visualization of hidden gallstones. The longitudinal GB (*right*) shows a gallstone, a large hyperechoic structure with posterior shadowing near the GB neck. Caliper measurement reveals a thickened anterior GB wall suggestive of inflammation or cholecystitis. The GB wall can also appear thickened after meals owing to contraction or in conditions with hepatic congestion. Do not measure the posterior wall, which displays posterior acoustic enhancement artifact. Wall thickening or presence of stones alone do not confirm cholecystitis, but each additional finding increases diagnostic certainty.

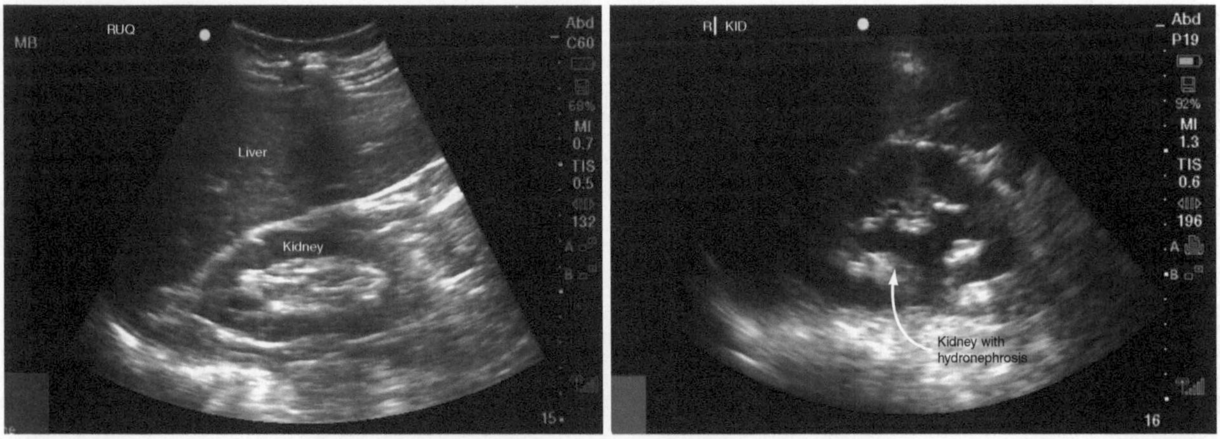

FIG. 151.3 Normal kidney versus hydronephrosis. Normal kidneys have a central hyperechoic renal pelvis (*left*), whereas hydronephrosis, or dilation of the collecting system, has centralized anechoic fluid (*right*). Color Doppler mode placed over the anechoic area can be used to differentiate hydronephrosis (no flow) from renal vessels (positive color flow).

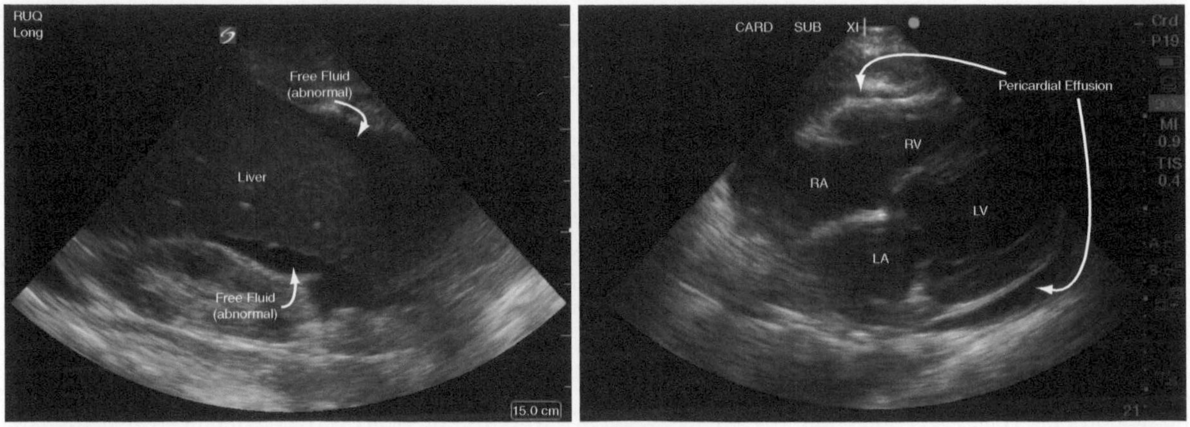

FIG. 151.4 Positive FAST examination. In this RUQ view (*left*), free fluid (FF) is seen in both the Morrison pouch, the potential space between the liver and the kidney, as well as around the liver tip. Any amount of FF noted on a FAST examination is considered positive. A FAST examination can detect as little as 100 mL of FF. In this subxiphoid view (*right*), a pericardial effusion (*arrows*) can be seen anterior to the heart, between the right ventricle and the liver, and posteriorly (deep to the left ventricle). *FAST,* Focused assessment with sonography in trauma; *RUQ,* right upper quadrant; *RV,* right ventricle, *RA,* right atrium; *LV,* left ventricle; *LA,* left atrium

TABLE 151.1 *eFAST*

Ultrasound scan name	Extended focused assessment with sonography in trauma (eFAST)
Indications	Blunt or penetrating trauma, concern for intraabdominal hemorrhage, hypotension, pneumothorax, hemothorax, tamponade, breathing "B" and circulatory "C" assessment in trauma
Relevant anatomy and structures visualized	Heart, kidneys, liver, spleen, bladder and pelvis, bilateral lungs
Probe	Low frequency, e.g. curvilinear abdominal probe or cardiac phased array probe
How to do the scan	• Subcostal view: evaluate for pericardial effusion or tamponade. • Right upper quadrant (RUQ): search the hepatorenal recess, also known as the Morrison pouch (potential space between liver and kidney) and the area around the liver tip for the presence of free fluid (FF) seen as anechoic collections tracking around abdominal structures. • Left upper quadrant (LUQ): evaluate the splenodiaphragmatic recess and splenorenal recess for the presence of FF. • Pelvis: evaluate space around the urinary bladder in both sagittal and axial plane to evaluate for the presence of FF. • Lungs: check most anterior portion of lungs for lung sliding. Check lung bases for hemothorax by translating cephalad 1 to 2 rib spaces after evaluating RUQ and LUQ.
Findings suggestive of pathology	Pericardial effusion: fluid around heart Abdominal or pelvic hemorrhage: any abdominal FF Hemothorax: fluid above the diaphragm or a spine sign Pneumothorax: lack of lung sliding or visualization of lung point
Pearls or pitfalls	• In patients with a known history of cirrhosis or ascites, a FAST study may be falsely positive. • FAST has high specificity and low sensitivity for clinically significant intraabdominal hemorrhage.

TABLE 151.2 *Focused Echocardiography Windows*

View	Evaluate	General Approach
Parasternal long axis	Global function Chamber sizes Pericardial effusion	Visual estimation, E-point septal separation Normal RV-to-LVOT-to-LA ratio is approximately 1:1:1 Anechoic collection surrounding heart, often anterior to descending aorta
Parasternal short axis	Global function Chamber sizes Pericardial effusion	Visual estimation, fractional shortening "D" sign or flat intraventricular septum suggests RV enlargement or strain Anechoic collection, circumferential when large
Apical four chamber	Global function Chamber sizes Pericardial effusion	Visual estimation, Simpson method, calculations for stroke volume and cardiac output Normal RV-to-LV ratio 0.6:1; RV enlargement if 1:1 or greater Anechoic collection within pericardium
Subcostal or subxiphoid	Pericardial effusion Chamber sizes Inferior vena cava (IVC)	First visualized superior to liver, anterior to RV RV enlargement if RV-to-LV ratio 1:1 or greater Evaluate for fluid tolerance (collapsing IVC walls) *vs.* obstruction (plump, no respirophasic variation)

RV, Right ventricle; *LVOT,* left ventricular outflow tract; *LV,* left ventricle.

however, many more cardiac windows, calculations, and measurements can be utilized to assess the heart.

ABDOMINAL AORTA ULTRASOUND

- Abdominal aortic ultrasound (Fig. 151.6) allows visualization of the size and structure of the aorta to evaluate for abdominal aortic aneurysm (high specificity and sensitivity) or aortic dissection (high specificity).

EVALUATING FOR DEEP VENOUS THROMBOSIS

- Deep vein thrombosis (DVT) and pulmonary embolism must not be missed by an emergency physician. Compression ultrasound (Fig. 151.7) allows the clinician to rule out DVT with high sensitivity.

LUNG ULTRASOUND

- Lung POCUS facilitates rapid diagnosis and targeted treatment for patients with acute respiratory distress. Fig. 151.8 shows commonly encountered lung artifacts.

Procedural Use of POCUS in the Emergency Department

- In addition to identifying pathology, POCUS is a common procedural aid in the emergency department for placement and confirmation of peripheral and central venous access, thoracostomy tubes, urinary catheters, and transvenous pacemakers. It can also be used to guide peripheral nerve blocks, incision and drainage, foreign body removal, paracentesis, and lumbar punctures.

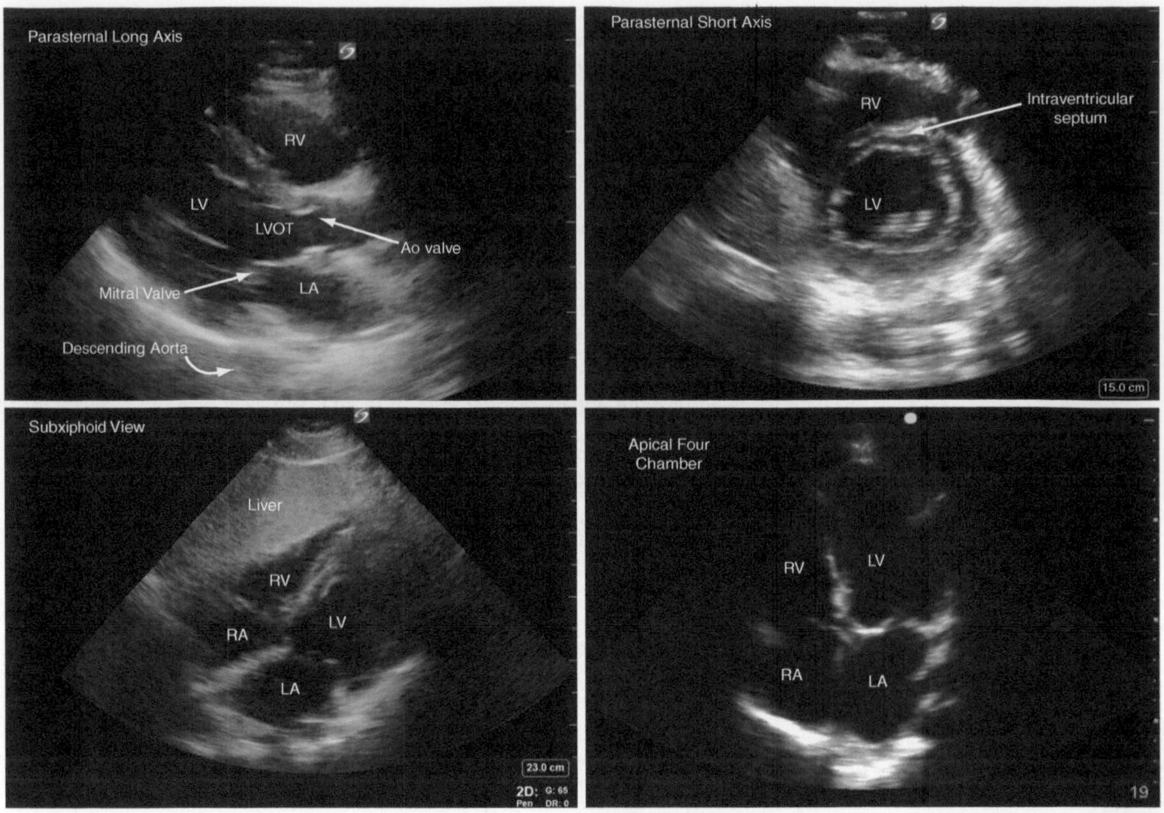

FIG. 151.5 Focused echocardiography windows. These are four common echocardiographic views to evaluate global cardiac function, presence of pericardial effusion, and presence of right-sided heart strain. See Table 151.2 for details regarding each window. *Ao,* Aortic; *LA,* left atrium; *LV,* left ventricle; *LVOT,* left ventricular outflow tract; *RA,* right atrium; *RV,* right ventricle

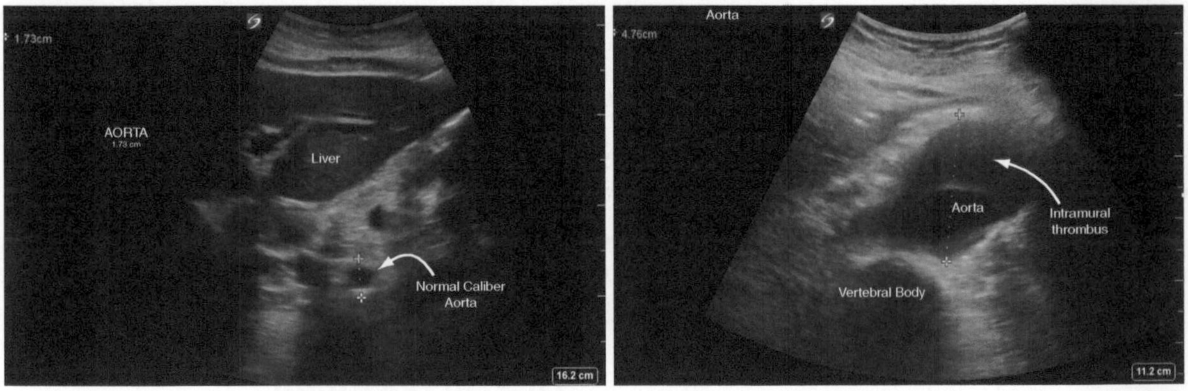

FIG. 151.6 Normal aorta versus abdominal aortic aneurysm (AAA). The aorta can be visualized from the subxiphoid region to the iliac bifurcation. In this normal study (*left*), calipers measure the transverse diameter of the aorta, from outside the anterior aortic wall to outside of the posterior wall to assess for aneurysm (diameter greater than 3 cm). To avoid underestimation, include intramural thrombus when measuring aortic diameter as seen in this AAA (*right*). Longitudinal views facilitate identification of saccular aneurysms. Abdominal girth and bowel gas commonly obscure the aorta. Bending the knees and application of deep, steady pressure help displace bowel gas.

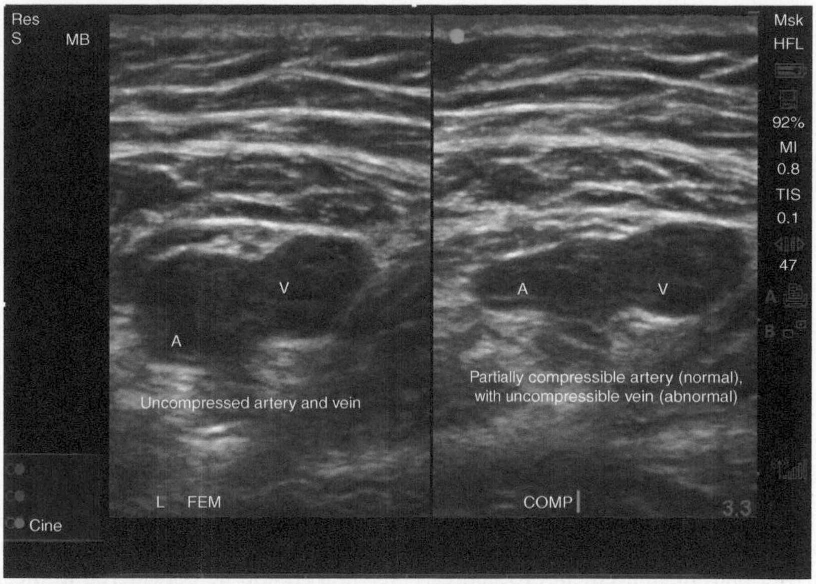

FIG. 151.7 Deep venous thrombosis (DVT). This common femoral vein DVT is identified by the inability to compress the vein (*right*). Sufficient pressure is applied to partially compress the artery (*right*) when compared with the uncompressed artery (*left*). This amount of pressure should easily collapse the vein; however, this vein remains incompressible (*right*) and suggests the presence of a DVT. Note that a vein without a DVT may appear incompressible when the probe is not perpendicular to the vessel, a common pitfall that can be avoided by adjusting the angle of the probe and reapplying pressure to compress the vessel. DVTs may also reveal lack of flow with color Doppler mode. Identification of enlarged lymph nodes may suggest infection rather than DVT as a cause for asymmetric lower extremity presentations.

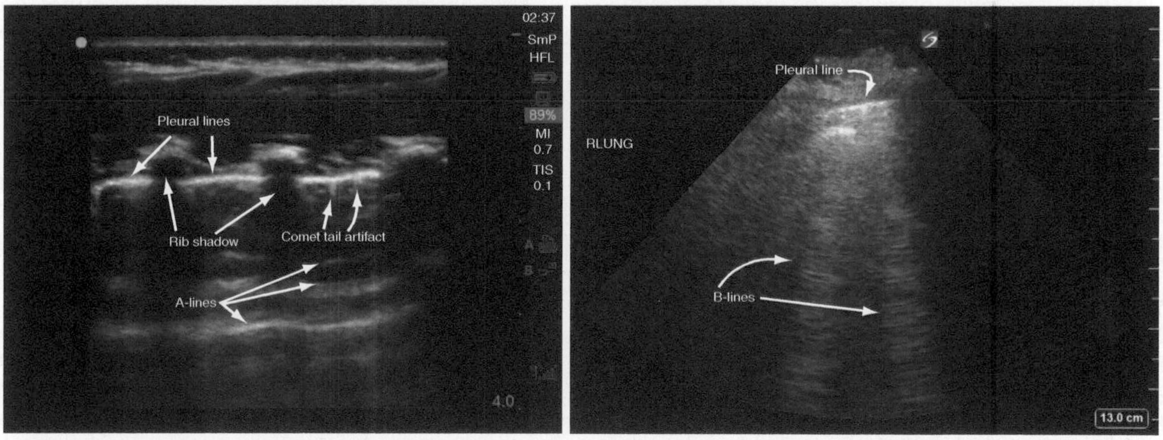

FIG. 151.8 Lung ultrasound. Interpretation of lung ultrasound requires understanding artifacts, because air poorly conducts sound waves. The pleural line is where the visceral pleura slides along the parietal pleura with respiration. This hyperechoic line is located just deep to the ribs; lung sliding to rule out pneumothorax is visualized here. A-lines (*left*) or horizontal hyperechoic lines parallel and deep to the pleural line are reverberation artifacts that signify the presence of air. These will be seen in normal lung, pneumothorax, asthma, and chronic obstructive pulmonary disease. B-lines (*right*) are seen when interstitial fluid is present, such as pulmonary edema, pneumonia, or contusions. B-lines appear like searchlights, originate at the pleural line, and stretch to the bottom of the screen, erasing A-lines. They must be differentiated from comet tails (a normal artifact arising from the pleura), which do not stretch as deeply and do not erase A-lines. Increasing image depth will differentiate comet tail artifacts from B-lines.

SUGGESTED READINGS

Carmody, K. A., Moore, C. L., & Feller-Kopman, D. (2011). *Handbook of critical care and emergency ultrasound*. McGraw-Hill Medical.

Dawson, M., & Mallen, M. (2013). *Introduction to bedside ultrasound Volume 1 & Volume 2*. Emergency Ultrasound Solutions, iBooks.

Zedu Ultrasound Training Solutions. *#FOAMus Free Ultrasound e-Books*. Available at: https://www.ultrasoundtraining.com.au/foamus/foamus-free-ebooks. Accessed on May 29, 2019.

Analgesia and Procedural Sedation

MICHAEL GHERMEZI, MD, MS, and YIJU TERESA LIU, MD

General Principles

- Pain is the most common complaint encountered in the emergency department.
- Patients experience further pain from medical procedures performed frequently in emergency care.
- Analgesia provides adequate control of acute or chronic pain with variable effects on mental status.
- Approach to analgesia is multimodal, including nonpharmacologic and pharmacologic interventions. Nonpharmacologic treatments include patient-centered communication, physical interventions, ice or heat, topical coolant sprays, and relaxation or mind-body therapies. Pharmacologic interventions include systemic analgesia, local analgesia, trigger point injections, and regional anesthesia (e.g., nerve blocks).
- Procedural sedation and analgesia (PSA) is a technique involving the delivery of a combination of analgesic and sedative or dissociative agents, with the goal of inducing a transient depressed level of consciousness and simultaneously controlling pain. Notably, this procedure reduces pain and discomfort without compromising cardiorespiratory function, improving overall patient and provider experience. Traditionally, PSA provides pain relief and sedation during urgent/emergent procedures.
- There are five levels of achieved sedation depths frequently cited in the medical literature, representing a dynamic continuum:
  - *Minimal sedation:* anxiolysis with normal but slowed response to verbal stimuli (midazolam, fentanyl, or low-dose ketamine)
  - *Moderate sedation:* depressed level of consciousness with purposeful response to motor/verbal stimuli (propofol, etomidate, or ketamine)
  - *Dissociative sedation:* profound analgesia and amnesia with preservation of cardiopulmonary stability (ketamine)
  - *Deep sedation:* depressed level of consciousness with purposeful response after repeated/painful stimulation (propofol, etomidate, ketamine/propofol mixture)
  - *General anesthesia:* loss of consciousness and not arousable; absence of airway reflexes

Indications for the Procedure

- Indications for analgesia depend on chief complaint and patient population.
- Systemic analgesia (e.g., acetaminophen, nonsteroidal antiinflammatory agents, low-dose ketamine, and opioids) is the most common form of pain management and should be considered in most circumstances.
- Local anesthesia provides a sensory block without motor deficits and is indicated in simple procedures including laceration repair, wound care, and abscess incision and drainage.
- Trigger point injections can be very effective and are safe in treating musculoskeletal pain (e.g., muscle spasms) and headaches.
- Regional anesthesia (nerve block) is typically used for large abscesses, complex lacerations, fractures, and dislocations. This method can induce transient paralysis with analgesia, facilitating the performance of procedures. Additionally, nerve blocks provide a safe alternative to systemic opioid analgesia in elderly patients.
- Regional anesthesia and PSA have similar indications, but sometimes PSA is preferred when multiple anatomic regions are involved or when patient amnesia is desirable.

Contraindications

- Other than drug allergies, there are no absolute contraindications to analgesia and PSA. Nerve blocks may limit the neurovascular examination, and caution should be exercised when considering related pathologies (e.g., compartment syndrome, crush injury, acute vascular injury).
- An increased risk of PSA complications may exist in patients with underlying systemic disease, patients at the extremes of age, patients with potential intubation or ventilation difficulty, and patients undergoing higher depths of sedation.
- Preprocedure focused history and physical examination are required to determine medical comorbidities, medications, allergies, prior experiences with analgesia/PSA, fasting state, and potentially difficult airways or hemodynamic compromise.
- PSA should not be delayed in patients in the emergency department based on fasting time. Please refer to the toxicology chapters (Chapter 121. Local Anesthetics and Chapter 132. Cellular Asphyxiants) for further information regarding side effects and contraindications of various local and systemic analgesics.

TABLE 152.1 *Guidelines for Maximum Doses of Commonly Used Anesthetic Agents*[a]

Agent	Without Epinephrine (mg/kg)	With Epinephrine (mg/kg)
Lidocaine HCl	3–5	7
Mepivacaine HCl	8	7[b]
Bupivacaine HCl[c]	1.5	3

[a]All maximum doses should be reduced by 20%–25% in very young, old, and very sick patients.
[b]Epinephrine adds to the potential cardiac toxicity of this drug.
[c]Not recommended for children younger than 12 years.
From Miner, J. R., & Burton, J. H. (2018). Pain management. In R. M. Walls, R. S. Hockberger, & M. Gausche-Hill (Eds.), *Rosen's emergency medicine: Concepts and clinical practice* (9th ed., pp. 34–51). Elsevier.

BOX 152.1 *Equipment for Procedural Sedation and Analgesia*

High-flow oxygen source
Suction
Airway management equipment
Monitoring equipment
–Pulse oximeter
–Cardiac monitor and defibrillator
–Blood pressure monitor
–Capnography
Vascular access equipment
Reversal agents
Resuscitation drugs
Adequate staff (per hospital guidelines)

From Godwin, S. A. (2018). Procedural sedation and analgesia. In R. M. Walls, R. S. Hockberger, & M. Gausche-Hill (Eds.), *Rosen's emergency medicine: Concepts and clinical practice* (9th ed., pp. 52–61). Elsevier.

Equipment/Supplies

- When performing local anesthesia, trigger point injections, or regional anesthesia, calculate the appropriate volume and concentration of drug used (Table 152.1).
- Equipment should be available including syringes, needles, skin-cleansing agents (such as alcohol, chlorhexidine, or povidone-iodine swabs), gauze, clean gloves and drape, ultrasound equipment if indicated, and patient monitoring equipment for PSA (e.g., pulse oximetry, cardiac monitoring).
- Complications of systemic analgesia and PSA include allergic reactions, airway complications (e.g., laryngospasm), drug overdoses, and respiratory or cardiopulmonary arrest.
- Supportive equipment should be readily available at bedside to deal with these life-threatening complications (Box 152.1). The selection of pharmacologic agents should be considered on an individual basis. Each agent may have various routes of administration, onset of action, duration, advantages, and adverse effects. To provide analgesia and perform PSA safely, each provider must be familiar with medication doses, onset of action, and effects (Tables 152.2–152.4).

SUGGESTED READINGS

Godwin, S. A. (2018). Procedural sedation and analgesia. In R. M. Walls, R. S. Hockberger, & M. Gausche-Hill (Eds.), *Rosen's emergency medicine: Concepts and clinical practice* (9th ed., pp. 52–61). Elsevier.

Godwin, S. A., Burton, J. H., Gerardo, C. J., Hatten, B. W., Mace, S. E., Silvers, S. M., Fesmire, F. M., & American College of Emergency Physicians. (2014). Clinical policy: Procedural sedation and analgesia in the emergency department. *Annals of Emergency Medicine, 63*(2), 247–258.

Miner, J. R., & Burton, J. H. (2018). Pain management. In R. M. Walls, R. S. Hockberger, & M. Gausche-Hill (Eds.), *Rosen's emergency medicine: Concepts and clinical practice* (9th ed., pp. 34–51). Elsevier.

Tintinalli, J. E., Stapczynski, J. S., Ma, O. J., Yealy, D. M., Meckler, G. D., & Cline, D. M. (Eds.). (2016). *Tintinalli's emergency medicine: A comprehensive study guide* (8th ed., Section 5, Chapters 35–38, pp. 231–263). McGraw-Hill Education.

TABLE 152.2 *Characteristics of Common Local Anesthetic Agents*

Agent	Potency (Lipid Solubility)	Duration of Action (min)	Onset	Comments
Tetracaine	8	180–600	Slow	Topical for ophthalmic use
Lidocaine	3	90–200	Rapid	Most commonly used agent; 1.5 times as toxic as procaine
Mepivacaine	2.4	120–240	Very rapid	Less potent and less toxic than lidocaine
Bupivacaine	8	180–600	Intermediate	Long-acting agent used in infiltration and blocks

From Miner, J. R., & Burton, J. H. (2018). Pain management. In R. M. Walls, R. S. Hockberger, & M. Gausche-Hill (Eds.), *Rosen's emergency medicine: Concepts and clinical practice* (9th ed., pp. 34–51). Elsevier.

TABLE 152.3 Procedural Sedation and Analgesia Agents: Recommended Adult Starting Doses

Agent	Class	Main Effect	Route of Administration	Usual Starting Dose
Fentanyl	Opioid	Analgesia	IV	1 μg/kg
Morphine	Opioid	Analgesia	IV	0.1 mg/kg
Midazolam	Benzodiazepine	Sedation, amnesia	IV	0.05 mg/kg
Ketamine	Phencyclidine derivative	Dissociation, analgesia, sedation, amnesia	IV IM	Low-dose: 0.3 mg/kg Dissociative dose: 1–2 mg/kg Dissociative dose: 4–5 mg/kg
Etomidate	Imidazole derivative	Sedation, amnesia	IV	0.15 mg/kg
Propofol	Alkylphenol derivative	Sedation, amnesia, antiemetic	IV	0.5–1 mg/kg
Ketofol	Ketamine-propofol combination	Sedation, dissociation, amnesia, analgesia	IV	Ketamine-propofol: 1:1 mixture. Initial dose of 0.75 mg/kg over 15–30 s; repeat at half-dose with 0.375 mg/kg after 1–3 min until desired sedation
Dexmedetomidine	α_2 –Adrenergic agonist	Analgesia, sedation	IV	1 μg/kg over 10 min, then 0.2–0.7 μg/kg/hr

IM, intramuscular; *IV*, intravenous.
From Godwin, S. A. (2018). Procedural sedation and analgesia. In R. M. Walls, R. S. Hockberger, & M. Gausche-Hill (Eds.), *Rosen's emergency medicine: Concepts and clinical practice* (9th ed., pp. 52–61). Elsevier.

TABLE 152.4 Procedural Sedation and Analgesia Agents: Benefits and Adverse Effects

Agent	Route(s) of Administration	Onset (min)	Duration (min)	Advantages	Adverse Effects
Fentanyl	IV, transmucosal	1–2 10–30	30–40 60–120	Rapid onset Short duration Decreased histamine release Minimal CV effects	Respiratory depression Rigid chest syndrome
Morphine	IV	10	240–360	Longer lasting	Hypotension Respiratory depression
Midazolam	IV IM Oral Rectal, intranasal	1–2 10–15 15–30 10–30 10–15	30–60 60–120 60–90 60–90 45–60	Rapid onset Short duration Easy to titrate Multiple routes	Respiratory depression
Ketamine	IV IM Oral Rectal, intranasal	1 5 30–45 5–10 5–10	15 15–30 120–240 15–30 30–120	Airway reflexes maintained No respiratory depression Predictable	Emergence phenomena Emesis Laryngospasm
Etomidate	IV	<1	5–10	Rapid onset Short duration Minimal CV effects Cerebroprotective	Respiratory depression Myoclonus Adrenal suppression
Propofol	IV	<1	8–10	Rapid onset Short duration Antiemetic Cerebroprotective	Respiratory depression Hypotension Injection pain
Ketofol	IV	1-3	10–15	Rapid onset Reduction in repeat dosing Reduction in emesis	Recovery agitation Respiratory depression Increased HR
Dexmedetomidine	IV	10–15 after initial loading infusion	5–8 half life; 2-h terminal elimination	Rapid onset Short duration Minimal ventilator effects	Bradycardia Hypotension

CV, cardiovascular; *HR*, heart rate; *IM*, intramuscular; *IV*, intravenous.
From Godwin, S. A. (2018). Procedural sedation and analgesia. In R. M. Walls, R. S. Hockberger, & M. Gausche-Hill (Eds.), *Rosen's emergency medicine: Concepts and clinical practice* (9th ed., pp. 52–61). Elsevier.

SECTION NINETEEN

BOARD REVIEW

Other

CHAPTER **153** BOARD REVIEW

Negotiation, Conflict Management, and Violence in the Emergency Department

MARK MOROCCO, MD, and ASHLEY VUONG, MD, MA

Definition of Workplace Violence

- Workplace violence is defined by the Occupational Safety and Health Administration (OSHA) as "violence or the threat of violence against workers" and can occur both in and out of the workplace. Violence can range from threats to verbal abuse to physical assault.

Statistics

- In a 2018 survey of emergency medicine physicians, 72.4% reported that they experienced some form of violence in the emergency department.
  - 38.1% reported that they experienced physical assault, an increase from 28.1% in 2005.
  - 21.9% frequently felt fearful that they would be a victim of violence, an increase from 9.4% in 2005.
  - 8.1% felt that they were constantly fearful of being a victim of violence, an increase from 1.2% in 2005.
  - With the rise of social media, 6.3% also reported threats of violence over social media.
- Workplace violence also affects the hospital workforce. Of physicians, 71% reported that they personally witnessed others being assaulted while they were at work.
- Many physicians believe that the threat of violence is greatest when caring for psychiatric patients, patients who are intoxicated, or patients with drug-seeking behavior.
- 96% of female emergency physicians and 80% of male emergency physicians reported that a patient made inappropriate comments or unwanted advances toward them.
- Of the emergency physicians who were injured as the result of an assault, 44% reported being hit or slapped and almost one-third reported getting punched, kicked, or spit upon.
- Also, 97% reported that a patient was the one who committed the assault, whereas 28% reported that they had been assaulted by a patient's family member or friend.
- Workplace violence often occurs in the setting of patient or family member agitation. Causes of agitation include the following:
  - Agitation is defined as "a state of excessive psychomotor activity accompanied by increased tension and irritability."
    - Agitation can be caused by both psychiatric *and* medical conditions.
    - Multiple agitation assessments are available (e.g., Overt Agitation Severity Scale, Overt Aggression Scale, Behavioral Activity Rating Scale [BARS]), and one is not recommended over another. However, the BARS is simple, reliable, and easy to use. Thus, it is helpful in assessments made by all staff (Table 153.1).
  - In an emergent medical setting, obtaining vital signs, chief complaint, and a brief history can help triage and identify causes of agitation, which aid in determining a life-threatening cause of agitation (Table 153.2).
  - O_2 saturation and blood glucose should be checked on every patient.
  - Conditions that may cause agitation include the following:
    - Head trauma
    - Encephalitis, meningitis, or other infection

TABLE 153.1 *Behavioral Activity Rating Scale*

1	Difficult or unable to rouse
2	Asleep but responds normally to verbal or physical contact
3	Drowsy, appears sedated
4	Quiet and awake (normal level of activity)
5	Signs of overt (physical or verbal) activity, calms down with instructions
6	Extremely or continuously active, not requiring restraint
7	Violent, requires restraint

(From Swift, R. H., Harrigan, E. P., Cappelleri, J. C., Kramer, D., & Chandler, L. P. (2002). Validation of the Behavioural Activity Rating Scale (BARS): A novel measure of activity in agitated patients. *Journal of Psychiatric Research, 36*(2), 87–95. doi:10.1016/s0022-3956(01)00052-8. PMID: 11777497.)

TABLE 153.2 Symptoms That May Indicate a Medical Problem

Symptoms	Signs
Memory loss, disorientation	Abnormal vital signs
Severe headache	Overt trauma
Muscle stiffness or weakness	Unequal pupils
Heat intolerance	Slurred speech
Unintentional weight loss	Dyscoordination
Psychosis (new onset/late age)	Seizures
Difficulty breathing	Focal neurologic findings
Known psychiatric illness, but new or unusual presentation	Waxing/waning attention or consciousness

(From Nordstrom, K., Zun, L. S., Wilson, M. P., Stiebel, V., Ng, A. T., Bregman, B., & Anderson, E. L. (2012). Medical evaluation and triage of the agitated patient: Consensus statement of the American Association for Emergency Psychiatry Project BETA Medical Evaluation Workgroup. *Western Journal of Emergency Medicine, 13*(1), 3–10. doi:10.5811/westjem.2011.9.6863)

- Encephalopathy
- Environmental exposure
- Metabolic derangement
- Hypoxia
- Thyroid disease
- Seizure (postictal)
- Toxic levels of medications
- Intoxication from recreational drugs/alcohol
- Psychotic disorders
- Mania
- Depression
- Anxiety

De-escalation Techniques

- The use of verbal de-escalation methods rather than the use of traditional methods of treating agitated patients (i.e., physical restraints and chemical sedation) leads to better outcomes for both patients and staff. Using verbal de-escalation techniques is less demeaning to patients. The use of physical or chemical restraints reinforces the idea that violence is necessary to resolve conflict, whereas verbal de-escalation techniques prevent unwanted physical injury of staff and patient by avoiding physical confrontation. Furthermore, patients placed in physical restraints are more likely to end up admitted to a psychiatry hospital *and* have a longer length of stay.

VERBAL NEGOTIATION

- "10 domains of verbal de-escalation"
  - Respect personal space.
  - Do not be provocative.
  - Establish verbal contact.
  - Be concise.
  - Identify wants and feelings.
  - Listen closely to what the patient is saying.
  - Agree to agree or disagree.
  - Lay down the law and set clear limits.
  - Offer choices and optimism.
  - Debrief the patient and staff.

TYPES OF AGGRESSION

- Determining the type of aggression a patient is exhibiting can help formulate the best way to de-escalate the situation.
  - Instrumental aggression
    - Describes the use of violence (or threats of violence) as a means of manipulation to get what an individual wants; not emotionally driven
    - Combat instrumental aggression by using nonspecific counter-offers to the threat.
      - Example: if a patient threatens to hurt someone if they do not get what they want, a suggested response is, "I don't think that's a good idea." If elaboration is prompted, a subsequent response would be, "let's not go that far and find out."
  - Fear-driven aggression
    - Occurs when a patient wants to avoid getting hurt and may attack *first* in order to prevent getting hurt
    - Combat fear-driven aggression by providing the patient with plenty of space and avoiding any show of force or intimidation that may provoke retaliation. Slowly decreasing the pace of the conversation can help calm the patient.
  - Irritable aggression comes in two forms:
    - Violations of boundaries
      - Occurs in patients who have had their boundaries violated and are using anger to regain self-worth
      - These patients want to be validated in their anger. The best way to de-escalate this situation is by validating their feelings (not their response) and responding that you would like to hear more once they have calmed down.
      - A "broken record" approach can be effective, because patients may need to go through the loop of understanding and calming numerous times before complying.
    - Chronically angry
      - Occurs in patients who are chronically angry and are waiting for something to set them off in order to release internal pressure. Such patients often will make unrealistic demands and use them as an excuse to "go off" when they are not met.
      - They often seek to create fear and confusion. The best way to de-escalate the situation is by not giving them the emotional response they are seeking and removing all nonessential persons from the area.
      - A provider can set firm limits, offer choices other than violence, and remain firm in offering only those choices once the patient calms down.

CHEMICAL/PHARMACOLOGIC RESTRAINTS

- In cases where verbal de-escalation fails, providers may have no choice but to turn to chemical/pharmacologic restraints. Traditional methods of subduing patients include the use of haloperidol, midazolam, lorazepam, and the "B52" (the combination of Benadryl [diphenhydramine], haloperidol, and lorazepam). However, patients have differing needs and careful consideration should be put into determining the best medication(s) for sedation.

TABLE 153.3 *First-Line Choices for Sedation of the Acutely Agitated Patient*

Violent Patient	Intoxication with CNS Stimulant	Intoxication with CNS Depressant	Known Psychotic Disorder	Cooperative Patient
Droperidol 2.5–5 mg IM/IV	Lorazepam 2–4 mg IM/IV	Haloperidol 2.5–10 mg IM/IV	Haloperidol 2.5–10 mg IM/IV	Lorazepam 2–4 mg PO
Midazolam 2.5–5 mg IM/IV	Midazolam 2.5–5 mg IM/IV	Droperidol 2.5–5 mg IM/IV	Droperidol 2.5-5 mg IM/IV	Risperidone 2 mg PO
Midazolam 2.5–5 mg + Droperidol 2.5–5 mg IM/IV	Haloperidol 5 mg IM/IV + Lorazepam 2 mg IM/IV		Haloperidol 5 mg IM/IV + Lorazepam 2 mg IM/IV	Olanzapine 5–10 mg PO
Haloperidol 5 mg IM/IV + Lorazepam 2 mg IM/IV			Ziprasidone 20 mg IM	
			Olanzapine 10 mg IM	

IM, intramuscularly; *IV,* intravenously; *PO,* orally.

(Reproduced with permission from: Moore, G., & Pfaff, J. A. Assessment and emergency management of the acutely agitated or violent adult. In: UpToDate, Post, T. W. (Ed.). Copyright © 2020 UpToDate, Inc. For more information visit www.uptodate.com.)

TABLE 153.4 *Comparison of IM Treatment Options*

Medication	Typical Dose	Max Single Dose	Repeat Dosing	Max Adult Dose/24hrs	Time to Onset	Time to Peak Cp	Half-life (hours)
Lorazepam	1–2 mg	4 mg	0.5 hour	12 mg	20–30 min	1–3 hr	14
Haloperidol lactate	5–10 mg	10 mg	1 hour	40 mg	30–60 min	20 min	20
Chlorpromazine[1,2]	25–50 mg	100 mg	2 hours	400 mg	–	1–4 hr	2–30
Ziprasidone[2]	10 mg 20 mg	20 mg	2 hours 4 hours	40 mg	15 min	1 hr	2–5
Olanzapine[2,3]	10 mg	10 mg	2 hours[3]	30 mg	15–45 min	15–45 min	30

[1]IM chlorpromazine is not recommended for the management of acute agitation. There are significant risks of QTc prolongation, hypotension, reduction in seizure threshold, a slow onset of effect, and risk of local irritation at the injection site.
[2]Reconstitution required before administration.
[3]Monitor for orthostatic hypotension prior to administration of repeat dosing.
Source: Texas Health and Human Services

- Although the use of second-generation (atypical) antipsychotics to control agitation in the emergency department has not been widely studied, some evidence indicates that it has equivalent efficacy to first-generation antipsychotics in calming patients with a psychiatric basis of agitation. Furthermore, patients prefer the use of second-generation antipsychotics, because they have reported fewer side effects.

PHYSICAL RESTRAINTS

- Seclusion and physical restraints are a method of last resort to be used when verbal de-escalation fails to calm a patient.
  - Seclusion
    - Seclusion is the physical confinement of patients to an area where they are physically prevented from leaving.
    - Seclusion may be an effective way to decrease environmental stimulation and reduce agitation. However, seclusion should not be used if a patient is or may become hemodynamically unstable, suicidal, or self-injurious.
  - Restraints
    - Physical restraints are a method of purposeful restriction of freedom of bodily movement.
    - Physical restraints must be used as a humane tactic in order to prevent self-injurious behavior, harm to others, or owing to the threat of significant damage or disruption of the environment.
- Restraints should never be used for convenience or punishment and should be removed as soon as possible.
- Appropriate pharmacologic treatment should accompany the application of restraints, as noted in Tables 153.3, 153.4, and Table 153.5.

Infrastructure to Promote Safety

- Reducing harm to both patients and hospital staff is essential for safe and effective care. Whereas hospitals have begun to increase security measures by adding more security guards, cameras, and visitor screening protocols, 49% of polled emergency medicine physicians believe that more can be done.
- Patient agitation is dangerous for hospital staff and other patients in the emergency department. By providing services that help create a safe environment, physicians and staff will, in turn, feel safer when using verbal de-escalation techniques rather than rushing to use physical and chemical restraints, resulting in better overall care for all patients.

TABLE 153.5 *Comparison of Oral Agents for Acute Agitation*

Medication	Typical Dose	Repeat Dosing (hours)	Max Adult Dose/24hrs	Estimated Time of Onset (minutes)	Time to Peak Cp (hours)	Half-life (hours)
Lorazepam	1–2 mg	2	10 mg	20–30	2	12
Haloperidol	5–10 mg	1	40 mg	30	2–6	14–37
Chlorpromazine[1]	25–50 mg	X	2000 mg	X	2.8	6
Ziprasidone[2]	20–40 mg	X	240 mg	X	6–8	7
Olanzapine ODT	5–10 mg	2	30 mg	≤ 60	6	30
Risperidone m-tab Risperidone soln.[3]	1–2 mg 1–2 mg	2	8 mg	X ≤ 60	~1	20

X, Not studied as a treatment for acute agitation and aggression.
[1]Chlorpromazine is expressed as having limited, poor, and outdated data as treatment for acute agitation.
[2]Oral ziprasidone absorption is significantly decreased without administration with a meal (250–500 calories).
[3]When given in combination with IM lorazepam.
Source: Texas Health and Human Services

SUGGESTED READINGS

Fishkind, A. (2002). Calming agitation with words, not drugs: 10 commandments for safety. *Current Psychiatry, 1*(4), 32–39. Available at: http://www.currentpsychiatry.com/pdf/0104/0104_Fishkind.pdf.

Nordstrom, K., Zun, L. S., Wilson, M. P., Stiebel, V., Ng, A. T., Bregman, B., & Anderson, E. L. (2012). Medical evaluation and triage of the agitated patient: Consensus statement of the American Association for Emergency Psychiatry Project BETA medical evaluation workgroup. *Western Journal of Emergency Medicine, 13*(1), 3–10. doi:10.5811/westjem.2011.9.6863.

Richmond, J. S., Berlin, J. S., Fishkind, A. B., Holloman, G. H., Jr., Zeller, S. L., Wilson, M. P., Rifai, M. A., & Ng, A. T. (2012). Verbal de-escalation of the agitated patient: consensus statement of the American Association for Emergency Psychiatry Project BETA De-escalation Workgroup. *Western Journal of Emergency Medicine, 13*(1), 17–25. doi:10.5811/westjem.2011.9.6864.

Medical Errors, Error Disclosure, and Delivering Bad News

JESSA BAKER, MD, and ANGELIQUE CAMPEN, MD, FACEP

Medical Errors

- Many studies suggest that most medical errors resulting in patient harm occur as the result of communication failures, especially during transitions of care between providers. Quality improvement and patient safety initiatives have prioritized the reduction of errors by implementing a standard approach to patient handoffs.
  - Overseeing this process is the Joint Commission, whose mission is to "improve the safety and quality of patient care through performance improvement" in acute care hospitals.
  - The World Health Organization (WHO) considers the prevention of hand-off errors as high of a priority in patient safety as is hand hygiene, and recommends standardization to reduce human error (Fig. 154.1).
  - The Accreditation Council of Graduate Medical Education (ACGME), the governing body that oversees accreditation of all graduate medical training programs, states that residency programs are required to monitor all trainees (i.e., interns, residents, fellows) for competence in hand-off communication.

COMMUNICATION STRATEGIES TO REDUCE RISK OF ERROR

- With the goal of reducing medical errors, several strategies have been developed to improve communication between providers.
  - Facilitate an effective hand-off
    - Goal: create a shared understanding of the patient through verbal communication, written communication, and transfer of professional responsibility.
  - System-based strategies: standardized hand-off formats
    - IPASS: *i*llness severity, *p*atient summary, *a*ction list, *s*ituational awareness and contingency planning, and *s*ynthesis by receiver
      - Associated with a 30% reduction in preventable adverse events
    - SBAR: *s*ituation, *b*ackground, *a*ssessment, *r*ecommendation
      - Used frequently in nursing hand-offs
    - Customize hand-offs for high-risk patients
      - Current literature supports that the risk of a failed hand-off is higher when patients are clinically

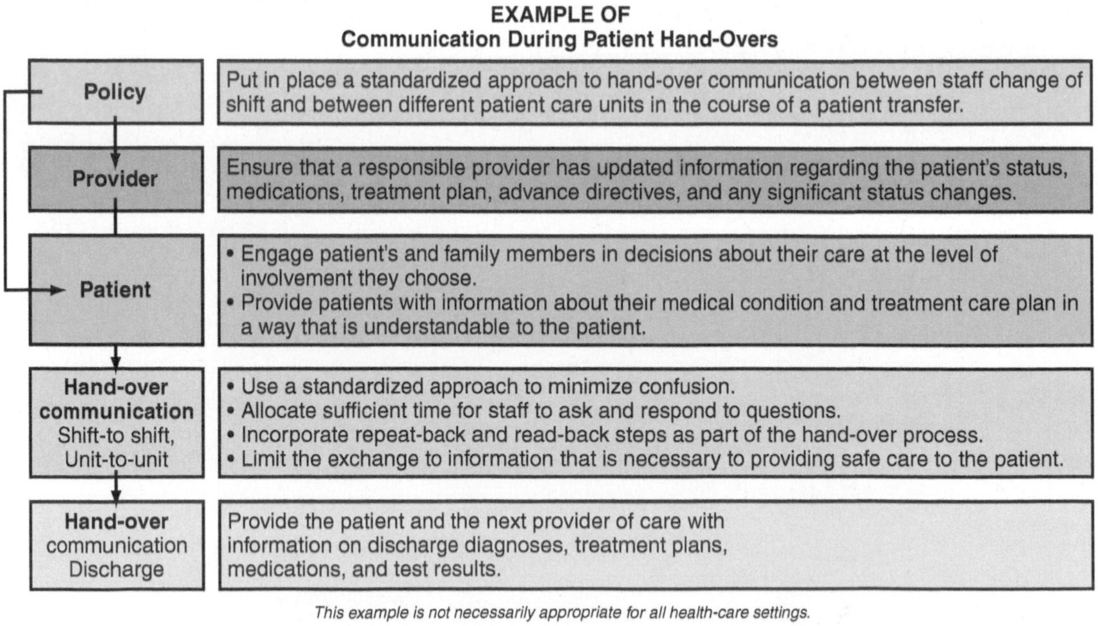

EXAMPLE OF
Communication During Patient Hand-Overs
Policy
Put in place a standardized approach to hand-over communication between staff change of shift and between different patient care units in the course of a patient transfer.
Provider
Ensure that a responsible provider has updated information regarding the patient's status, medications, treatment plan, advance directives, and any significant status changes.
Patient
• Engage patient's and family members in decisions about their care at the level of involvement they choose.
• Provide patients with information about their medical condition and treatment care plan in a way that is understandable to the patient.
Hand-over communication Shift-to shift, Unit-to-unit
• Use a standardized approach to minimize confusion.
• Allocate sufficient time for staff to ask and respond to questions.
• Incorporate repeat-back and read-back steps as part of the hand-over process.
• Limit the exchange to information that is necessary to providing safe care to the patient.
Hand-over communication Discharge
Provide the patient and the next provider of care with information on discharge diagnoses, treatment plans, medications, and test results.
This example is not necessarily appropriate for all health-care settings.

FIG. 154.1 Communication During Patient Hand-Overs. (From Communication During Patient Hand-Overs. (2007). World Health Organization: Patient Safety Solutions. Vol. 1, Solution 3.)

unstable, transferring locations, and transferring services/care teams.
- Sender-based strategies
  - Focus verbal hand-off on the most important items (i.e., pertinent medical history, key events, and interventions during medical evaluation, and so forth).
  - Emphasize tasks to be completed (i.e., to-do list).
  - Relay anticipatory guidance (i.e., if-then statements).
  - Check for receiver understanding.
- Receiver-based strategies
  - Receiver must confirm thorough comprehension of information.
  - Use of read-back: allows sender to ensure that information has been appropriately received.
  - Actively listen (i.e., note-taking, asking questions).

ADDITIONAL SOURCES OF ERROR

- The nomenclature of look-alike and sound-alike medications (i.e., hydrocodone and oxycodone, nicardipine and nimodipine, hydralazine and hydroxyzine, Celebrex [celecoxib] and Celexa [citalopram], and so forth) is a major source of medical error when dispensing medications. Whereas many inadvertent medication errors have not been reported to cause significant patient harm, some poor outcomes have resulted in patient hospitalization, and can be fatal. The Institute for Safe Medication Practices maintains a list of common look-alike and sound-alike medications. This institute recommends a strategy for reducing medication error: include indications for medications.
- Other common sources of medication error are in the right patient, timing, dosage, and route of administration. Despite risk- and error-reduction efforts, medication errors remain a serious safety issue today. In-house pharmacy personnel and infusion pumps offer safeguards to miscalculations, but are not immune to implementation and human error. Current practice models (Tall Man lettering, bar code technology, single-use packaging, provider-patient and provider-provider communication) should be implemented, and in conjunction with upcoming prediction model tools, will assist in reducing the frequency of potentially lethal medical errors.

Error Disclosure

- Physicians have traditionally shied away from discussing errors with patients, in part out of fear of precipitating consequences (litigation), but also owing to discomfort and unfamiliarity with how to approach this type of discussion. However, today, the disclosure of errors and adverse events is endorsed by a broad range of organizations. When a medical error is revealed, health-care providers are encouraged to follow standardized and established guidelines for disclosing this information to the affected patient. The disclosure of medical error "aligns with the ethical principle of patient autonomy that is important in modern-day health care."
  - The American Medical Association (AMA) Code of Medical Ethics Opinion 8.121: "Physicians must offer professional and compassionate concern toward patients who have been harmed, regardless of whether the harm was caused by a health care error. An expression of concern need not be an admission of responsibility. When patient harm has been caused by an error, physicians should offer a general explanation regarding the nature of the error and the measures being taken to prevent similar occurrences in the future. Such communication is fundamental to the trust that underlies the patient–physician relationship and may help reduce the risk of liability."
- Joint Commission standard RI. 1.2.2: "Patients and, when appropriate, their families are informed about the outcomes of care, including unanticipated outcomes."
  - Indicates involvement of both physician and hospital in disclosure of treatment outcomes, both when favorable and when adverse
  - Does not require expressed admission or apology
- American College of Emergency Physicians (ACEP) recommendations:
  - "Emergency physicians should provide prompt and truthful information to patients or their representatives about their medical conditions and treatments. If, after careful review of all available relevant information, emergency physicians determine that a medical error has occurred during their care of a patient in the ED, they or an appropriate designee should inform the patient in a timely manner that an error has occurred and provide information about the error and its consequences, following institutional and practice group policies and considering applicable state statutes on this subject. If the patient is incapacitated and therefore unable to receive this information, emergency physicians or an appropriate designee should provide the information to the patient's representative."
  - Disclosure of errors should include an apology to show respect for the patient.
    - Institutional or practice group policies should be followed.
    - Apology may be offered by the emergency physician, another member of the patient's health-care team, or an officer of the institution.
  - For adverse events where it is unclear whether an error occurred versus an unavoidable complication, an emergency physician or designee should inform the patient or representative that the event is being examined and that further information will be provided when available.
  - To overcome obstacles with error disclosure, ACEP recommends the following initiatives:
    - "Health care institutions should develop and implement policies and procedures for identifying and responding to medical errors, including continuous quality improvement systems and procedures for disclosing significant errors to patients."
    - "Medical educators should develop and provide specific instruction to trainees at all levels on identifying and preventing medical errors and on communicating truthfully and sensitively with patients or their representatives about errors."

- "States should enact legislation that makes apology statements by physicians related to disclosure of medical errors inadmissible in malpractice actions."

Delivering Bad News

- The delivery of bad news is a highly sensitive topic that all physicians must face. Effective communication between the provider, the patient, and his/her family can ameliorate the task of sharing unwanted outcomes. Although the task of delivering bad news is never easy, there are several techniques that providers can employ to assist in these challenging conversations. The SPIKES six-step protocol developed by Buckman and colleagues is commonly used in emergency medicine.
  - S: Setting up the interview
    - Review pertinent medical facts before entering the room.
    - Create a quiet space and set aside adequate time.
    - Introduce yourself to family members, make eye contact, sit at patient/family level.
    - Offer a medical interpreter for those with limited English proficiency.
    - Offer available religious services (i.e., hospital chaplain).
  - P: Assess the patient's Perception
    - Before you tell, ask.
    - Use open-ended questions, such as "What do you understand about your medical condition so far?" or "What have other doctors told you thus far?"
  - I: Obtaining the patient's Invitation
    - Discuss information disclosure.
    - If patients do not want to know details, offer to answer questions they may have and/or if they wish for another family member to receive more detailed information.
  - K: Giving Knowledge and information to the patient.
    - Provide a warning, "I'm sorry to tell you that…"
    - Praise the family for seeking medical care, administrating CPR, calling EMS, and so forth.
    - Communicate at the comprehension and vocabulary level of the patient.
    - Avoid using medical jargon and terminology ("spread" instead of "metastasized").
    - Avoid excessive bluntness.
    - Provide information in small chunks, and check in periodically for understanding.
  - E: Addressing the patient's Emotions with Empathic responses (Table 154.1)
    - Provide an empathic response.

TABLE 154.1 *Examples of Empathic, Exploratory, and Validating Responses*

Empathic Statements	Exploratory Questions	Validating Responses
"I can see how upsetting this is to you."	"How do you mean?"	"I can understand why you felt that way."
"I can tell you weren't expecting to hear this."	"Tell me more about it."	"I guess anyone might have that same reaction."
"This is very difficult for me also."	"Could you tell me what you're worried about?"	"It appears that you've thought through things very well."

(From Baile, W. F., Buckman, R., Lenzi, R., Glober, G., Beale, E. A., & Kudelka, A. P. (2000). SPIKES—A six-step protocol for delivering bad news: Application to the patient with cancer. *Oncologist, 5*, 302–311.)

    - Allow the patient and/or family time to process the information.
    - Be prepared for varying emotional responses.
    - Utilize resources (i.e., social work, religious personnel) to provide support.
    - Provide the patient and/or family time to respond.
    - If emotions are not clearly expressed, ask an exploratory question.
    - Validate that the patient and/or family's feelings are normal and to be expected.
  - S: Strategy and Summary
    - Ask the patient and/or family members if they are ready to discuss the next steps.
    - Outline next steps (i.e., treatment plan/options, consultation, postmortem options).
- Understand specific goals that the patients and their families have: symptom control, best possible treatment, continuity of care.

SUGGESTED READINGS

American College of Emergency Physicians. (Revised 2017). Disclosure of medical errors. Available at: https://www.acep.org/patient-care/policy-statements/disclosure-of-medical-errors/.

Baile, W. F., Buckman, R., Lenzi, R., Glober, G., Beale, E. A., & Kudelka, A. P. (2000). SPIKES—A six-step protocol for delivering bad news: Application to the patient with cancer. Available at: https://www.mdanderson.org/documents/education-training/project-echo/10%2027%2016%20ECHO-PACA%20SPIKES.pdf.

National Institute of Medicine. (1999). *To err is human: Building a safer health system*. National Academies Press.

CHAPTER **155** BOARD REVIEW

Capacity, Consent, & AMA

ANGELIQUE CAMPEN, MD, FACEP, and CLAUDIE BOLDUC, MD, MPH

Ethical medical practice is predicated on four core principles: beneficence, nonmaleficence, justice, and autonomy.

- Beneficence connotes that health-care providers intend to provide the best care and treatment to their patients.
- Nonmaleficence is the active avoidance of any act that may cause harm to a patient.
- Justice states that there should be an element of fairness in all actions and decisions.
- Autonomy implies that a patient has the right to either accept or refuse medical treatment.

In medical decision-making, a physician may offer suggestions and advisement based on medical literature and evidence, but a patient's autonomous decision should be free of persuasion and coercion. The application of these principles is universally accepted and applied by physicians in their medical decision-making conversations with patients.

Capacity

Capacity is the basis for informed consent. Patients exhibit medical decision-making capacity once they demonstrate an understanding of the situation; appreciate the risks, alternatives, and consequences of a proposed treatment or intervention; process the information; and communicate their decision (Box 155.1). Although capacity may be relatively apparent and intuitively gathered by a physician's interaction with a patient, a formal capacity evaluation should be considered if a patient's medical decision-making ability is in question. Additionally, the provider should be familiar with factors (i.e., age, education level, language barrier) that may contribute to the impairment of decision-making (Box 155.2). In summary, the structure of a medical decision-making discussion addresses the following four points.

1. *Understanding*: Does the patient understand the facts about the medical condition as well as the risks and benefits of a proposed treatment?
2. *Appreciation*: Does the patient appreciate that these facts apply to this given situation?
3. *Reasoning*: Is the patient applying the facts against his or her own set of values and preferences to make a decision based in logic congruent with those values?
4. *Communication*: Is the patient able to communicate his or her choice clearly?

Once it is deemed that a patient has decision-making capacity, it is the responsibility of the clinician to provide the medical evidence surrounding the presentation, address concerns that the patient may have, and facilitate the completion of the medical decision.

BOX 155.1 *Questions to Ask Patients to Facilitate the Determination of Decision-Making Capacity*

The ability to communicate a choice:

- Have you decided what you want to do?
- We have discussed many things; have you made a decision?

The ability to understand relevant information as it is communicated:

- What is your understanding of your medical condition?
- What are the possible diagnostic tests or treatments of your condition?
- What are some of the risks of the options that we have discussed?
- How likely is it that you will have a bad outcome?
- What could happen if you choose to do nothing at this time?

The ability to appreciate the significance of the information to one's own individual circumstances:

- Why do you think your doctor has recommended this specific test or treatment for you?
- Do you think that the recommended test or treatment is the best option for you?
- Why do you think that this is the best option for you at this time?
- What do you think will happen if you accept (or refuse) this option?

The ability to use reasoning to arrive at a specific choice:

- Why have you chosen the option that you did?
- What factors influenced your decision?
- What weight did you give to these different factors?
- How do you balance the positives and negatives (or risks and benefits)?

Reprinted from Heller, D. B. (2013). Informed consent and assessing decision-making capacity in the emergency department. In *Emergency Medicine*, ed 2. Adams, J. G. (Ed.). Saunders.

If a physician has identified a lack of medical decision-making capacity, the next step is to determine if the patient has a legal document expressing his or her wishes, either referenced from specific instructions (i.e., living will, advanced directive) or through the identification of a preferred surrogate decision-maker (i.e., health care power of attorney). If a patient has neither a legal document nor a health care power of attorney, the next-of-kin may serve as a surrogate decision-maker, and consent can be obtained from this individual. It is important to establish that the surrogate decision-maker is applying the patient's values and preferences in the decision-making process. Certain states have codified a next-of-kin hierarchy. The universally

BOX 155.2 When Capacity Is at Issue

If any of the "red flag" situations exist or if there are other reasons to have heightened concern regarding a patient's decision-making capacity, the emergency physician (EP) should take care to document the following elements carefully:

- Whether the patient exhibits each of the elements of decision-making capacity
- The patient's medical condition
- The proposed treatment or procedure and its necessity
- The urgent or emergency nature of the proposed treatment or procedure
- Actions by the EP to maximize patient capacity
- Actions by the EP to minimize impediments to patient capacity
- Availability and involvement of family members or surrogate decision makers
- Psychiatric consultation when obtained

Reprinted from Heller, D. B. (2013). Informed consent and assessing decision-making capacity in the emergency department. In *Emergency Medicine*, ed 2. Adams, J. G. (Ed.). Saunders.

accepted progression is a patient's spouse, adult children, parents, adult siblings, and the nearest relative thereafter. In the absence of a surrogate decision-maker, providers are enabled to involve hospital counsel (i.e., administrator on-call, ethics committee) to finalize medical decisions, keeping the patient's best interest in mind. Once a patient's medical condition has stabilized, a guardian may be appointed to help make legal decisions if the patient is expected to lack decision-making capacity indefinitely.

Considerations in Decision-Making Capacity

NEUROCOGNITIVE DISORDERS

- Dementia is one of the most common causes of impaired capacity. However, a patient who is diagnosed with a neurocognitive disorder is not automatically precluded from decision-making. In fact, patients with an Mini-Mental State Exam (MMSE) greater than 24 have been shown to retain the ability to understand and appreciate information and are not considered limited in this ability. With progressive disorders, however, capacity needs to be reassesed at regular intervals.

PSYCHIATRIC DISORDERS

- Within the *Diagnostic and Statistical Manual of Mental Disorders* of psychiatric disorders, schizophrenia has been found to have the biggest impact on decision-making capacity. This is more profound in patients with more severe cognitive impairments or negative symptoms (i.e., apathy, lack of emotion, poor social functioning), whereas symptoms consistent with major depressive disorder have less of an impact on decision-making capacity.

In 2015, Boetgger and colleagues reviewed 300 psychiatric consultations for decision-making capacity assessment and found that 37% of people with substance abuse disorders lacked this capacity compared with only 17% of those with mood disorders. In comparison, this was less than the 54% who lacked decision-making capacity in the neurocognitive disorders population.

CAPACITY VS. COMPETENCE

- Capacity and competence are often incorrectly interchanged. Capacity is both dynamic over time and task-specific. In other words, someone's capacity can change. Competence, on the other hand, is a static and legal identification of a patient's global capacity and ability to manage his or her own affairs. For example, a patient with a progressive neurocognitive disorder can legally be deemed to lack competence, whereas individuals with acute delirium can lack capacity to make an immediate decision regarding their medical treatment plan, but may regain capacity upon reassessment of their cognitive status.

Consent

Informed consent is an integral component of communication between a provider and his or her patient. Medical informed consent is an ethical and legal responsibility that physicians use as a foundation for decision-making in simple and complex medical scenarios. All physicians have a moral and legal obligation to offer treatment only with consent, because the converse (treatment without consent) may be considered battery and have legal ramifications. The American College of Emergency Physicians' Code of Ethics reaffirms the importance of informed consent, stating that "adult patients with decision-making capacity have a right to accept or refuse recommended health care, and physicians have a concomitant duty to respect their choices."

Informed consent requires two conditions: (1) the patient possesses decision-making capacity and (2) the patient is making a voluntary choice. Therefore, in addition to assessing capacity, the physician must also ensure that the patient is both adequately informed and free of coercion or undue influence. To meet these latter requirements, the physician is responsible for providing two key pieces of information: material facts and disclosures.

Material facts include all facts considered relevant to aid in the patient's medical decision-making process:

- Differential diagnosis, how it was developed, and its implications
- Description of the proposed treatment or procedure
- Risks and benefits of the proposed treatment or procedure
- Alternative treatment options, along with their risks and benefits
- The risk(s) associated with refusal of treatment and prognosis if the treatment is or is not accepted

Important risks and benefits to disclose include common minor complications (i.e., bleeding during laceration repair) and major complications, such as permanent disability or death, even if these are rare.

Disclosures include:

- Physician's ability to perform the procedure and, if asked, success rates experienced
- Any financial conflicts that may cloud the physician's medical judgment

Certain states' legal systems have additionally mandated that a physician must disclose his/her own relevant medical background, including substance abuse or human immunodeficiency virus (HIV) status.

The provider performing a medical procedure must be the same person obtaining the written consent. A provider may choose to delegate obtaining consent to another member of the health-care team (nurse, resident, attending physician), but doing so does not transfer the legal responsibility of the provider performing the procedure.

Some states have specific requirements regarding written consent. Where written consent is not codified by law, verbal consent is considered legally binding. However, a verbal agreement, even with strict documentation, offers a weaker evidence of consent if the process is later challenged. Medicare mandates that consent forms are obtained for all nonemergent procedures, including those performed in the emergency department. At minimum, a written form should contain the name of the person who obtained the consent; the performing provider; information about the risks, benefits, and alternatives that were disclosed; and that the patient had an opportunity to ask questions.

Two important exceptions to informed consent that the emergency physician should be aware of: emergency exception and public health imperative.

An *emergency exception* is one in which emergency physicians are exempt from the aforementioned process to provide care to a critically ill patient. In this case scenario, assessing for decision-making capacity, obtaining formal consent, identifying legal documents or surrogate decision-makers may delay time-sensitive treatment(s) resulting in serious harm or death. Therefore, in following with *primum non nocere*, the emergency physician can, and should, provide emergency care without formal consent. The basis for this exception is *implied* consent, which posits that a reasonable person with decision-making capacity would, in most situations, consent to lifesaving interventions in an emergency.

A *public health imperative* states that individual autonomy can be restricted against a patient's own will in situations where the public good must take precedence. Important applications of the public health imperative include patients with high-risk communicable diseases (i.e., tuberculosis, measles) and patients with mental illness who pose a danger to themselves or to others.

CONSENT INVOLVING MINORS

- A minor is defined as a person younger than 18 years of age. In most clinical scenarios, a minor presenting with a medical condition and requesting treatment, requires parental consent. However, the exceptions to this include life-threatening emergencies, specific circumstances (see below), emancipated minors, and situations in which a parent has been convicted or accused of committing sexual assault or violence against the minor.

Emergency Exception

In an emergency, a minor should receive treatment and procedures performed which may be lifesaving, without delay. Once medically stable, a parental or guardianship consent is required. When circumstances do not allow, the provider may document a concurrent opinion of another provider agreeing with the need to perform the procedure urgently.

Specific Circumstances. Several exceptions grant minors the ability to consent as adults. These exceptions include the following:

- Mature minor: older than 14 years of age, mature enough to express capacity for beneficial treatment of relatively low risk
- Sexually transmitted infections (STIs): older than 12 years of age, covers testing and treatment of STIs in all states (HIV may be an exception)
- Prenatal/pregnancy: approximately two-thirds of states allow pregnant minors to consent for prenatal care and for treatment of their child.
- Mental health and substance abuse: nearly all states allow minors to access treatment for mental health and substance abuse services without parental consent.
- Sexual or physical abuse: evaluation and treatment are permitted without parental consent under the emergency exception.
- Please note: state laws regarding minor care vary widely; review state-specific laws and regulations as necessary.

Minor's Interests Not Protected. When a parent or legal guardian lacks capacity or disagrees with the recommendation of seeking and obtaining medical treatment based on religious or moral ground, placing the patient at risk of life-threatening illness or outcome, the physician's judgment may override the decision-making of the parent. Emergent stabilization should be undertaken, as necessary. In instances where treatment of the minor violates the wishes of a guardian with capacity but may cause harm to the patient, consider seeking hospital administrative counsel before proceeding.

Against Medical Advice (AMA)

Against medical advice (AMA) refers to the formal recognition of a competent patient's choice to decline further medical care and leave the hospital prior to, or against the physician's recommended clinical endpoint. Every year in the United States, approximately 1%–2% of all emergency department visits (as high as 6% in disadvantaged inner city populations) result in a patient leaving AMA. Subsequently, patients who leave the hospital AMA are associated with a 10% increase in adjusted relative risk of 30-day mortality as compared with routine patient discharges.

Given the prevalence of and the risks associated with AMA discharges, providers should make every attempt to encourage patients to stay for the duration of their medical evaluation. The population of patients who are at higher risk of signing out AMA include those who are male, undomiciled, lack medical insurance, and patients with substance abuse disorders, psychiatric illness, or HIV.

Once a patient expresses interest in leaving AMA, Levy and colleagues suggest three requirements of a well-executed AMA process.

- Capacity assessment
  - When patients sign out AMA, they are exercising their right to refuse care under the principle of self-determination. It is the provider's responsibility to formally assess a patient's decision-making capacity at that specific place and time.

- Adequate disclosure
  - It is imperative that the provider have a discussion with the patient about the risks and benefits of leaving AMA. This discussion is like that of informed consent and should include all material facts, ensure comprehension by the patient (free of limitations), and ensure voluntariness (free of coercion). The discussion must also include disclosure of other therapeutic alternatives and the specific risks of leaving, including death, where applicable. In order to limit the risks for vulnerable populations, the physician should stress that, although this encounter is closing with an AMA release, the patient has every right to return for medical care at any time. Using threats or false statements such as "your insurer will not pay for this if you leave AMA" further discourages vulnerable patients from seeking the care they need (and is incorrect).
- Proper documentation
  - Proper documentation includes the following key elements: the patient's decision-making capacity, any and all risks that were disclosed, patient's understanding of the risk(s), the patient's decision, and both the patient and the provider's signatures.

There is discordance in medical literature about the formalization of the AMA process through signed forms, and whether it provides liability protection for the provider, especially in high-risk and vulnerable populations. Levy and colleagues argue that properly executed AMA discharges do provide significant legal protection from liability risks. When a patient elopes (leaves AMA without informing the medical team), the emergency physician should make a good faith effort to locate and contact the patient. Regardless of the AMA process or the conditions of the patient leaving, thorough documentation reflecting the above points is essential.

SUGGESTED READING

Marco, C. A., Brenner, J. M., Krauss, C. K., McGrath, N. A., & Derse, A. R. (2017). Refusal of emergency medical treatment: Case studies and ethical foundations. *Annals of Emergency Medicine, 70*(5), 696–703.

Palliative Care, Advance Directives, and Hospice

JAMES J. MURPHY JR., MD, MPH, and PAMELA L. DYNE, MD

Palliative Care

General Principles

- Most patients present to the emergency department (ED) with a chief complaint relating to a painful symptom. An important subset of patients with this chief complaint also suffer from life-limiting or terminal illnesses. Palliative care is a specialty focused on providing relief from unnecessary suffering in these chronic conditions through symptom relief—pain, nausea, air hunger, anxiety, and terminal agitation—separate from any life-prolonging efforts. For patients who present to the ED nearing the end of life with advanced directives that do not include aggressive attempts at resuscitation and those who are enrolled in a hospice program, it is imperative for emergency physicians to be skilled in swiftly recognizing these symptoms to provide patients with relief. Establishing a patient's goals of care, identifying any reversible causes of their symptoms, and aggressively treating with a titration of appropriate medications improves the quality of care delivered and the patient's experience.

PAIN HISTORY

Nociceptive Pain

- Somatic: transmitted by myelinated fibers with rapid transmission of pain impulses and discrete localization of pain
- Visceral: transmitted by fewer myelinated fibers that transmit diffuse, poorly localized symptoms (e.g., cramping)
- *Neuropathic pain*: develops from neurotoxic effects of chemotherapy or other drugs, metabolic or microvascular conditions, such as diabetes or HIV, or by direct invasion of neural tissue from neoplastic tissue. Perceived as tingling, burning, numbness, hypersensitivity, or allodynia.
- Note: Terminal cancer—a common palliative care diagnosis—can often cause pain that is a combination of all pain types. For *example*, a pancreatic mass directly invading pleura (somatic), causing a bowel obstruction (visceral), and directly invading neurovascular structures (neuropathic) requires a multimodal approach to analgesia to manage all facets of the pain produced.

Pain Severity

- Measuring in the verbal patient: Visual analog scale, numerical rating scale, Wong-Baker FACES scale, and verbal rating scale
- Measuring in the nonverbal patient: Pain Assessment in Advanced Dementia or Critical Care Pain Observation Tool
- Reassessment: Frequent for symptomatic relief, adverse effects, and over-sedation (i.e., every 15 minutes until adequate analgesia achieved, and then every 4 hours)

Previous Analgesic Experience

- What medications have or have not previously been effective?
- Calculate the patient's daily dose of opiates, if receiving outpatient therapy, in morphine equivalents.
- Consider history of prior opiate or alcohol use disorder to help gauge tolerance.

Pain Goals

- What symptoms are most distressing to the patient?
- What are tolerable side effects?
  - Degree of sedation tolerable is an important question. Some patients prefer to remain 100% alert and oriented to say their goodbyes near the end of life, whereas others may elect for symptomatic relief at the expense of consciousness.
    - **Palliative sedation**, usually achieved via intravenous benzodiazepines, can be used with patient consent for complete symptomatic relief for the sole purpose of alleviating suffering from intractable symptoms.

TREATING ACUTE EXACERBATIONS OF CHRONIC PAIN

Routes

- Intravenous (IV) is preferred for in-hospital management of pain crisis, given ability to titrate medications quickly.
- Subcutaneous is an available route in patients for whom establishing IV access would cause more distress.
- Intranasal administration (i.e., fentanyl 1.5–2 μg/kg every 1–2 hours or benzodiazepines) may also be considered in patients with difficult or no IV access.
- Buccal or transdermal delivery are also considerations for some medications (i.e., fentanyl formulations available).
- Oral (PO) and rectal routes are less commonly used in the acute care setting.

Medication Choice

- Select a therapeutic agent based on patient characteristics (i.e., vital signs, patient's goals of care, hepatic and renal function) and prior patient experience.
  - Morphine is often the initial opiate used in palliative care.
    - Avoid in renal failure because of the risk of accumulation of toxic metabolites.
  - Hydromorphone and fentanyl have safer pharmacokinetic profiles in patients with liver and/or kidney dysfunction.
  - Fentanyl is often a preferred short-acting choice, and has fewer effects on blood pressure.

Onset of Action

- Fentanyl has a quick onset of action (5 minutes), which allows for more rapid titration to relief.
- Morphine and hydromorphone reach peak effect in 15 minutes IV, 30 minutes subcutaneously, and 1 hour PO.

Starting Dose

- Opiate-tolerant: Consider patients as such if they take at least morphine PO 60 mg/day, oxycodone PO 40 mg/day, hydromorphone PO 8 mg/day, or fentanyl transdermal 25 μg/h. In an acute pain crisis that is not manageable with a home regimen, start with an initial IV dose equivalent to their home PO dose, or start with a bolus that is 10% of their 24-hour equianalgesic dose (Table 156.1).
- Opiate-naive: Initiate treatment at a lower therapeutic dose, and titrate appropriately.
  - *Titration*: Reassess frequently for pain relief and serious side effects (i.e., apnea). For example, monitor every 5 minutes with fentanyl or every 15 minutes with morphine or hydromorphone. Continue to monitor and titrate until pain is either acceptably relieved or side effects are intolerable. If pain is not relieved but limited by side effects, consider converting to a different opiate and/or adding adjuvant medications. It is reasonable to consult palliative care or a pain specialist as well.
  - *Rotating opiates*: If pain is adequately relieved but use is limited by side effects, reduce equianalgesic dose of new opiate by 25%–50% to account for incomplete cross-tolerance. If pain is still not adequately controlled, do not reduce dose.
  - *Reversal*: Reversal is rarely necessary in palliative patients, but providers should be aware of signs to look for such as hypoventilation, oversedation, malignant arrhythmia.
- Naloxone 0.04 mg IV may be administered every few minutes and titrated to effect.
  - Note: aggressive naloxone administration may lead to a sympathomimetic crisis.

Adjuvants: Aid in controlling pain without increasing opiate dosage and thereby reduce undesired side effects, and provide a multimodal analgesic approach.

- Nonsteroidal antiinflammatory drugs: consider renal and hepatic function, particularly effective for visceral and inflammatory pain.
- Acetaminophen: Consider hepatic function, utilized routinely to reduce opiate needs.
- Ketamine: Subdissociative ketamine dosages do not require cardiopulmonary monitoring; has the advantage of analgesia without respiratory drive depression.
  - General dosing: 0.1–0.3 mg/kg IV loading dose over 15–30 minutes, followed by 0.1–0.3 mg/kg per hour infusion
- Gabapentin, tricyclic antidepressants: Useful for neuropathic pain, but only available PO
- Steroids: Option for inflammatory pain, especially if a patient is unable to tolerate nonsteroidal antiinflammatory drugs, commonly administered in patients with spinal or nerve compression, bony metastases

TABLE 156.1 *Equianalgesic Opiate Dosing*

Opiate	Parenteral (mg)	Oral (mg)
Morphine	10	30
Oxycodone	N/A	20–30
Hydromorphone	1.5	7.5
Fentanyl	0.1 (100 μg)	N/A (cannot directly interconvert transdermal, buccal fentanyl dosing)

N/A, not applicable.

Other Symptoms and Their Treatment

- Air hunger: Dyspnea at the end of life can be distressing to the patient and family members present. It can be managed with opiates and anxiolytics, as well as scopolamine patches or glycopyrrolate to reduce secretions. Relief can also be provided by general respiratory supportive measures, such as bronchodilators, supplementary oxygen if indicated, and a fan with cool mist directed toward the face.
- Anxiety: An initial approach involves comfort measures: a calming room with family or caregivers present if the patient desires, minimizing unnecessary interruptions, lighting adjustment (bright or dim, as desired), and minimizing sounds (comfort mode for monitors, turn off in-room beeping). Treating pain can also help to reduce anxiety because patients are often anxious about continued or worsening pain, and inadequate treatment of future pain. Finally, benzodiazepines may be used in addition to these environmental measures.
- Nausea: Unless contraindicated (i.e., prolonged QTc), antiemetics such as ondansetron or metoclopramide may be used.

Advanced Directives

General Principles

- Goals-of-care conversations are essential in the ED, where many patients enter the hospital for the first time, and can present in extremis, warranting invasive lifesaving interventions. Although some laws and terminology are state-specific, the overarching goal is to verify goals of care with the patient. When the patient is unable to express their wishes, a designated health care proxy or medical decision maker, or a prepared legal memorandum is accepted. A well-informed discussion about the patient's prognosis, including the limitations of resuscitation, are essential components of an informed decision between a provider and the patient and/or health care proxy.

Hospice

General Principles

- Hospice care is a holistic program that provides care for terminally ill patients in the last 6 months of their lives. Although programs are designed to minimize hospitalizations and ED visits, some patients may present with new concerns (i.e., fracture after fall, altered mental status from infection) not directly related to their terminal diagnosis. Patients may also present if they, or a family member, changes their mind regarding treatment or simply because of anxiety from terminal pain, air hunger, or other symptoms. As with all patients, it is important to establish goals of care early, carefully weigh the burden:benefit ratio of invasive testing, and treat accordingly. Continuing home pain medications is appropriate, especially in opiate-dependent patients who have the potential to go into benzodiazepine or opiate withdrawal in the ED. If home medication lists are not readily available, contact the patient's home hospice agency, where staff are usually available 24 hours a day, 7 days a week.

SUGGESTED READINGS

Desandre, P. L., & Chandrasekaran, E. B. (n.d.). Pain at the end of life. In R. Strayer, S. Motov, & L. Nelson (Eds.), *Management of pain and procedural sedation in acute care* [open access online book]. https://painandpsa.org/endoflife/.

Moryl, N., Coyle, N., & Foley, K. M. (2008). Managing an acute pain crisis in a patient with advanced cancer. *Journal of the American Medical Association, 299*(12), 1457–1467. doi:10.1001/jama.299.12.1457.

CHAPTER **157**

BOARD REVIEW

Health Insurance Portability and Accountability Act (HIPAA)

ANGELIQUE CAMPEN, MD, FACEP, and CLAUDIE BOLDUC, MD, MPH

Maintaining patient privacy and confidentiality is legally required and of utmost importance in the ethical practice of medicine. These tenets form the foundation of trust between the physician and the patient. However, in the delivery of high-quality health care practices, protected health information (PHI) must also be readily accessible to different providers. With this in mind, the U.S. Department of Health and Human Services (HHS) released the *Standards for Privacy of Individually Identifiable Health Information* ("Privacy Rule") in 2000, with the goal of protecting patient privacy rights and ensuring the safe transfer of PHI. The rules were formulated to reflect the obligations outlined in the 1996 Health Insurance Portability and Accountability Act (HIPAA).

General Principles and Definitions

- **Covered Entities**: health plans, providers, clearinghouses, business associates
- **Protected Health Information (PHI):** any individually identifiable health information that includes demographic data, relating to the individual's past, present, or future physical or mental condition; health care services rendered; or any payment thereof. Except as outlined in the Privacy Rule below, PHI may not be used without prior consent from a patient.
- **De-identified Health Information:** health information that does not provide any basis to identify an individual, and can be used or disclosed without restriction.
- **Minimum Necessary Standard:** a covered entity must make reasonable efforts to use, disclose, and request only the minimal amount of information needed.
- **Use of PHI:** HIPAA allows covered entities to use PHI, without prior authorizations for daily health care operations, treatment, and billing. PHI may be accessed and utilized without explicit patient authorization, under specific circumstances (Table 157.1).
- **Permitted PHI disclosures:** in certain situations, a patient's individual rights are superseded by the needs of the public. Under HIPAA, there are 12 national priorities for which the use of PHI is permitted without the written consent of a patient (Box 157.1).
- **Mandated reporting** varies by state, but generally includes:
  - Child abuse or neglect (all states)
  - Elder abuse or neglect (most states)
  - Domestic partner violence (few states); occasionally dependent on whether there was use of a deadly weapon or bodily injury
  - Injury by a deadly weapon or criminal act, such as a stab or gun shot wound (most states)
  - Driving impairment (i.e., epilepsy, neurocognitive or visual impairment) (some states)
  - Contagious diseases under national surveillance; reporting is mandated by the U.S. federal government.

TABLE 157.1 ***PHI Use by Covered Entities Without Prior Authorization Allowed Under HIPAA***

Treatment	Direct provision of care Care management Coordination of care Consultations Discussions with primary care providers Referrals
Operations	Quality improvement activities Employee evaluation Credentialing Auditing and compliance programs Business administration
Payment	Billing third-party payers Health plan activities for determination or provision of benefits Clearinghouse activities

BOX 157.1 ***The 12 National Priorities for Which PHI May Be Used Without Written Authorization***

1. Required by law
2. Public health activities
3. Reporting abuse, neglect, or domestic violence
4. Health oversight activities
5. Judicial and administrative proceedings
6. Law enforcement purposes
7. Decedents
8. Cadaveric organ, eye, and tissue donation
9. Research (occasionally)
10. Serious threat to health or safety
11. Essential government functions
12. Worker's compensation

A list of these diseases is provided on the Centers for Disease Control and Prevention website.

- **Patient Rights to PHI:** HIPAA regulations state that patients must receive a notice of privacy practices informing them of their own rights in relation to their PHI, which include the following:
  - Access to their PHI in their preferred format
  - Request that amendments be made to their PHI records
  - Request for additional restrictions on the use of their PHI by covered entities
  - A complete accounting of disclosures made from their PHI

This does not imply that the emergency physician providing care is required to provide his or her patient with this information. In most hospital settings the release of PHI will be handled by the medical records department.

- **Law Enforcement Rights to PHI:** the transfer of PHI with law enforcement officials requires the patient's consent, except as listed below. HIPAA allows the release of PHI in the following circumstances:
  - Judicially issued warrant, subpoena, or court order
  - Limited PHI (name, address, date of birth, Social Security number, blood type, type of injury, date of service, and a description of physical traits) can be released to aid law enforcement officials in the identification of a suspect, fugitive, material witness, or missing person.
  - If the victim of a crime is unable to consent, a provider may release PHI to law enforcement officials if doing so is deemed to be in the patient's best interest.
- Unauthorized Release of PHI:
  - The release of patient information to family members or friends may be permitted with the patient's informal permission (verbal or written).
  - The accessing or release of PHI of a patient for whom you are not the treating provider is unlawful and may result in criminal penalties.

157

SUGGESTED READINGS

HIPAA Social Media Rules. https://www.hipaajournal.com/hipaa-social-media/

Moskop, J. C., Marco, C. A., Larkin, G. L., Geiderman, J. M., & Derse, A. R. (2005). From Hippocrates to HIPAA: Privacy and confidentiality in emergency medicine – Part II: Challenges in the emergency department. *Annals of Emergency Medicine*, 45(1), 60–67.

CHAPTER **158**

BOARD REVIEW

Billing, Coding, and Reimbursement

CATHERINE WEAVER, MD, and JESSA BAKER, MD

Medical records coding allows for standardized billing and reimbursement. The American Medical Association maintains a list of current procedure terminology (CPT) codes, which is the basis of evaluation and management (E/M) levels used to bill patients for medical services. Centers for Medicare & Medicaid Services created a coding system to assign an E/M level for different elements included in the chart. Reimbursement for medical services is based on relative value units (RVUs), which are designed to standardize physician payments and are assigned to CPT codes, including E/M levels. RVU calculations include work done in a visit (time spent, expertise required, intensity of patient care), practice expense (overhead, expenses), and professional liability insurance.

Evaluation and Management Levels

General Principles

- E/M levels range from level 1 (lowest) to level 5 (highest) (Table 158.1). The levels are determined by interventions that occur during a visit; however, coding to the appropriate level depends on three elements: (1) history, (2) physical examination, and (3) medical decision-making. Most emergency department visits are billed as E/M levels 3–5.

Level 1

- **Possible interventions:** no medications or treatments, asymptomatic prescription refill request, uncomplicated dressing change, straightforward D/C (discharge) instructions.
- **Examples:** uncomplicated insect bite, PPD test, uncomplicated suture removal.

Level 2

- **Possible interventions:** emergency department point-of-care tests, visual acuity, urine clean-catch test, bandage or sling application, procedure preparation (minor laceration, incision and drainage), simple D/C instructions.
- **Examples:** localized skin rash or lesion, minor injuries without workup, minor problems without workup or prescription (i.e., viral illness, toothache, isolated urinary frequency).

Level 3

- **Possible interventions:** emergency medical services arrival, nebulizer (one), single test (laboratory test, electrocardiogram, radiograph), oral medication, Foley catheter placement, cervical spine precautions, routine psychiatric clearance, procedure preparation (joint aspiration, simple fracture), moderately complex D/C instructions.
- **Examples:** minor head injury, foreign body in the eye, fever responsive to antipyretics, gastroenteritis without intravenous (IV) treatment, conditions requiring prescription (i.e., streptococcal pharyngitis ["strep throat"], cystitis).

Level 4

- **Possible interventions:** two diagnostic tests (laboratory tests, electrocardiogram, radiograph), multiple radiographs,

TABLE 158.1 *Chart Elements by Evaluation and Management Level*

E/M Level	HISTORY				PHYSICAL EXAMINATION			MDM			
	Type	HPI	ROS	PMFS	Type	'95 Systems	'97 Bullets	Type	Dx/Tx	Data	Risk
1	PF	1–3	0	0	PF	1	1–5	SF	Min	Min	Min
2	EPF	1–3	1	0	EPF	2-4	6–11	LC	Lim	Lim	Low
3								MC	Mult	Mod	Med
4	Detailed	4	2-9	1/3	Detailed	5-7	12+ bullets in 2+ systems				
5	Comp	4	10+	2/3	Comp	8+	9+ systems with 2+ bullets	HC	Ext	Ext	High

Comp, comprehensive; *E/M*, evaluation and management; *Dx/Tx*, diagnosis/treatment; *EPF*, expanded problem-focused; *Ext*, extensive; *HC*, high complexity; *HPI*, history of present illness; *LC*, low complexity; *Lim*, limited; *MC*, moderate complexity; *MDM*, medical decision-making; *Med*, medium; *Min*, minimal; *Mod*, moderate; *Mult*, multiple; *PF*, problem-focused; *PMFS*, past medical/surgical, family, and social history; *ROS*, review of systems; *SF*, straightforward.

special imaging (computed tomography, magnetic resonance imaging, ultrasonography), cardiac monitoring, nebulizer (two), IV infusions, nasogastric tube, more than one reassessment, psychotic patient (not suicidal), procedure preparation (eye irrigation, bladder irrigation, pelvic examination), complex D/C instructions.
- **Examples:** assault with multiple injuries, fall from height, headache or gastroenteritis requiring IV intervention, pneumonia, asthma, pyelonephritis, uncomplicated pelvic inflammatory disease.

Level 5

- **Possible interventions:** frequent monitoring, more than two diagnostic tests, blood product administration, supplemental oxygen via facemask, nebulizers (more than two), moderate sedation, procedure preparation (central line, gastric lavage, lumbar puncture, paracentesis), cooling/heating blanket, extended social work, sexual assault examination with specimen, restraints, 1:1 observation, critical care time <30 minutes.
- **Examples:** headache requiring computed tomography/lumbar puncture, acute stroke, status asthmaticus, infection requiring IV antibiotics, any extensive workup, most admissions.

Chart Elements

Chart elements are also outlined in Table 158.1.

History

- Chief complaint clearly presented.
- History of present illness (HPI): location, quality, severity, duration, timing, context, modifying factors, associated signs and symptoms.
- Review of systems (ROS): constitutional, eye, ear/nose/mouth/throat, cardiovascular, respiratory, gastrointestinal, genitourinary, musculoskeletal, integumentary, neurologic, psychiatric, endocrine, hematologic/lymphatic, allergy/immunology.
- Past medical/surgical, family, and social history (PFSH).
  - Past medical/surgical history: illnesses, injuries, surgeries, hospitalizations, immunizations.
  - Family history: health status, hereditary diseases, deaths.
  - Social history: tobacco/alcohol/drug use, employment, marital status, sexual history, education, living situation.
- Lowest-scoring element (HPI, ROS, PFSH) determines E/M level.
  - Underdocumentation can limit E/M level and lead to significant revenue loss.
- If patient's circumstance limits acquisition of history, add qualifier describing limitation (e.g., intubation, altered mental status, dementia, etc.) and source of collateral information.

Physical Examination

Body areas and organ systems: constitutional, eyes, ears/nose/mouth/throat, neck, cardiovascular, respiratory, chest, gastrointestinal, genitourinary, musculoskeletal, skin, neurologic, psychiatric, hematologic/immunologic/lymphatic.

Medical Decision-Making

General Principles

- Coding for medical decision-making (MDM) evaluates the complexity of data (i.e., tests ordered, other sources) and considers risks of complications, morbidity, and mortality associated with problem(s) and management options. The charted progress notes and interpretation of data also factor into the MDM. This is arguably the most important section of the chart.

  Three key elements are considered.
- Complexity of diagnostic and management options
  - Typically scored based on Marshfield Clinic scoring tool (Tables 158.2 and 158.3)
- Description and interpretation of data obtained and reviewed (Table 158.4)
  - Score calculated based on testing, interpretation, and record review (Table 158.5)

158

TABLE 158.2 Marshfield Clinic Scoring Tool

Problem and Course	Number	× Points
Self-limited or minor problem (any course)	0–2	1 each
Established problem (stable or improving)	Any number	1 each
Established problem (worsening)	Any number	2 each
New problem, no additional workup planned	0–1	3
New problem, additional workup planned	Any number	4 each

Summation of points applied to Table 158.3 to determine evaluation and management level.

TABLE 158.3 Evaluation and Management Medical Decision-Making Complexity

No. of Problem Points	No. of Diagnostic and Management Options
1	Minimal
2	Limited
3	Multiple
≥4	Extensive

TABLE 158.4 Scoring for Data Reviewed

Data Reviewed	Points
Laboratory tests	1
Radiology (except cardiac catheterization and echocardiography)	1
Medical tests[a]	1
Discuss tests with performing physician	1
Independent review of image, tracing, specimen	2
Decision to obtain old records	1
Review and summary of old records	2

[a]Electrocardiogram, catherization, echocardiography, pulmonary function tests.
Summation of points applied to Table 158.5 to determine evaluation and management level.

TABLE 158.5 *Evaluation and Management Medical Decision-Making Data Review*

Total Data Points	Complexity of Data Reviewed
1	Minimal or none
2	Limited
3	Moderate
≥ 4	Extensive

- Risk to patient from underlying pathology, required testing, and intervention (Table 158.6)

Critical Care Time

- According to the CPT definition, a critical illness is a condition that impairs one or more vital organ system(s) "such that there is a high probability of imminent or life-threatening deterioration in the patient's condition." Critical care (CC) time is the cumulative time "spent engaged in work directly related to the individual patient's care" with interventions requiring "highly complex decision-making to assess, manipulate, and support vital organ system functions." Billing categories include the first 30–74 minutes and each additional 30-minute interval. CC time <30 minutes is automatically billed at level 5.
- **Bundled in CC time:** cardiac output measurements, imaging interpretation, venous and arterial blood gases, nasogastric tube placement, transcutaneous pacing, ventilator management, peripheral vascular access.
- **Excluded from CC time (procedures billed separately):** cardiopulmonary resuscitation, intubation, central line placement, tube thoracostomy, transvenous pacer placement, electrocardiogram interpretation.

SUGGESTED READINGS

Carter, K., Dawson, B., Brewer, K., & Lawson, L. (2009). RVU ready? Preparing emergency medicine resident physicians in documentation for an incentive-based work environment. *Academic Emergency Medicine*, *16*(5), 423–428.

Takacs, M., & Stilley, J. (2015). Billing and coding shift for emergency medicine residents: A win-win-win proposition. *Annals of Emergency Medicine*, *66*(4), S60.

TABLE 158.6 *Evaluation and Management Medical Decision-Making Risk Levels*

Risk	Presenting Problems (With Examples)	Diagnostics Examples	Management Examples
Minimal	Self-limited/minor (at most 1 problem): insect bite, common cold	Laboratory tests, XR, EKG, US	Rest, bandage
Low	Acute, uncomplicated: simple sprain, cystitis, ≥2 self-limited problems	Imaging with contrast, ABG	Minor surgery, IV fluids, over-the-counter medications, PT/OT
Moderate	Acute with systemic symptoms: pyelonephritis, pneumonia, colitis Acute, complicated injury: head injury with loss of consciousness New diagnosis with uncertain prognosis: breast mass Chronic with exacerbation: COPD, CHF	Lumbar puncture, thoracentesis, paracentesis	Prescription drug, reduction and splinting, IV fluids with additives
High	Threat to life of bodily function: MI, PE, respiratory distress, suicidality, altered mental status, polytrauma, peritonitis, acute renal failure Chronic illness w/ severe exacerbation		IV controlled substances, drug therapy requiring monitoring, DNR decision

ABG, arterial blood gas; *CHF*, chronic heart failure; *COPD*, chronic obstructive pulmonary disease; *DNR*, do not resuscitate; *EKG*, electrocardiogram; *IV*, intravenous; *MI*, myocardial infarction; *PE*, pulmonary embolism; *PT/OT*, physical therapy/occupational therapy; *US*, ultrasonography; *XR*, radiograph.

CHAPTER **159** BOARD REVIEW

Conflicts of Interest, and Resource Stewardship

MARK MOROCCO, MD, and ASHLEY VUONG, MD, MA

Conflicts of Interest

General Principles

- A conflict of interest is "a set of circumstances that creates a risk that professional judgment or actions regarding a primary interest will be unduly influenced by a secondary interest." In medicine the primary interest is providing the highest quality of care for patients. The details that are not directly related to patient care are considered secondary interests. Emergency physicians (EPs) seek to focus only on their primary interest, but are exposed to multiple sources of secondary interests that may lead to conflicts of interest.

Sources and Examples of Conflict of Interest

- Industry influences (pharmaceutical companies, devices, biotechnology, technology, etc.)
  - Example: A pharmaceutical representative provides samples of a new drug to be given to indigent patients while providing lunch to providers.
- Economic influences include payment incentives, reimbursement
  - Example: A research study gives the physician a gift card for every patient enrolled during overnight hours when research staff is unavailable.
- Nonpatient personal and professional relationships
  - Example: A colleague's spouse suggests additional imaging studies be added to the workup for convenience and "completeness."
- Research
  - Example: A reputable journal publishes an article supporting a link between an accepted treatment and a rare complication/disease. Should you stop using the treatment?
- Academic and professional requirements
  - Example: A multicenter study funded by the makers of a controversial treatment offers site investigator positions to academic physicians who require publications for promotion.
- Prestige
  - Example: An institution partners with a professional sports team and requires physicians to provide treatment priority to the organization's personnel and players.
- Conflicts of interest are pervasive and inevitable. To avoid potential pitfalls, it is important for physicians to be aware of potential conflicts of interest that may steer decision-making. Physicians must be flexible in their approach to patient care to ensure that care is focused solely on providing benefit to the patient, rather than on secondary interests (especially those of the treating physician).

Resource Stewardship

General Principles

- Stewardship is the "careful and responsible management of something entrusted to one's care." EPs are uniquely qualified and situated as stewards of health care. Because EPs care for *all* patients at any time of day or night, regardless of a patient's ability to pay, EPs act as the gateway and gatekeeper to the hospital and most health care resources. It is important that EPs recognize and embrace this responsibility to allocate finite resources to patients who need them.
- The cost of health care in the United States totaled \$3.3 trillion in 2016.
- Health care costs continue to remain above the rate of economic growth, and national health care expenditures took up 17.9% of the country's gross domestic product.
- To determine which patients receive what treatment or test, EPs must weigh a number of factors:
  - What is the pretest probability of a considered illness? Is the test result likely to change treatment of the patient?
  - What is the risk of the test? Is it reasonable when balanced with the benefit?
  - Although EPs do not perform a cost analysis to guide diagnostic testing and emergent treatment, they should be aware of the costs as well as the risks of testing and interventions.
    - For example, computed tomography scans are expensive, and the risk—including radiation exposure and contrast administration—is not negligible.
- Health care resources are limited commodities and EPs cannot practice as if the health care system has infinite time, resources, or money. Every decision and treatment that a physician makes is associated with a cost. It is important to consider that there may be another person who requires medical attention, emergent treatments can be expensive, and therapies carry risk and expense. EPs have a unique responsibility and training to deter-

mine what care is emergently necessary, while keeping the patient's best interest as their primary responsibility. It is equally important to recognize what is not appropriate care that is unnecessary, costly, and only marginally beneficial.

SUGGESTED READINGS

Committee on Conflict of Interest in Medical Research, Education, and Practice, Board on Health Science Policy, Institute of Medicine of the National Academies. (2009). Principles for identifying and assessing conflicts of interest. In B. Lo & M. J. Field (Eds.), *Conflict of interest in medical research, education, and practice* (pp. 44–61). National Academies Press.

Geiderman, J. M., Iserson, K. V., Marco, C. A., Jesus, J., & Venkat, A. (2017). Conflicts of interest in emergency medicine. *Academic Emergency Medicine, 24*(12), 1517–1526. doi:10.1111/acem.1325

Thompson, D. F. (1993). Understanding financial conflicts of interest. *The New England Journal of Medicine, 329*, 573–576.

Risk: Liability, Litigation, and Malpractice Insurance

HANNAH SPUNGEN, MD, MPH, and MALKEET GUPTA, MD, MS

Liability and Insurance

- **Malpractice** is legally considered a form of negligence, which involves four components: a duty to act, a breach of that duty, harm suffered by the patient, and a causal relationship between the latter two elements.
- Typically requires that a plaintiff's attorney establish that a standard of care was not met, or that the actions of the accused were not consistent with how a reasonable physician might have acted in the same situation.
- Most malpractice cases involve expert testimony on both sides, which theoretically helps the court to establish the relevant standard of care.
- Malpractice is a source of **liability**, or financial risk, that physicians assume by practicing medicine. By virtue of presenting to the emergency department, patients establish a fiduciary relationship with the attending emergency physician, and therefore have the reasonable expectation that any emergent medical condition they may have will be treated appropriately.
- If a diagnostic error, delay in care, or other contingency arises wherein a patient suffers an adverse outcome, it is not uncommon for patients and/or their estates to seek recompense through a malpractice lawsuit, although in practice, very few of these cases (approximately 4% of those that go to trial) are decided in favor of the plaintiff.
- If a physician has transferred risk to an insurance company by virtue of purchasing a medical professional liability insurance (MPLI) policy, and the policy applies to the specific time and nature of the incident in question, the insurance company is responsible for paying both **indemnity**, or the dollar amount awarded to the plaintiff, and (usually) the cost of litigation for the physician, regardless of the lawsuit outcome (Box 160.1).
- Traditionally, many MPLI policies fell under the category of "**occurrence**" policies, wherein the physician was covered against claims arising from incidents occurring during a specified time period, regardless of the date the claim was filed. The distinction becomes relevant because the amount of time a plaintiff has to file a claim in MPLI cases can extend up to or even beyond 20 years after the incident takes place, thus adding to the amount of time for which the insurance company is liable.

BOX 160.1 *Common Malpractice Terms*

Indemnity: The payment that an insurance company makes to a plaintiff in the course of settling a claim
Occurrence: A form of coverage wherein the insurance company is liable for any incident occurring while the policy is in effect, regardless of when a claim is brought
Claims-made: A more common form of MPLI coverage where the insurance company is liable only for incidents that occur and are reported while the policy is in effect
Tail coverage: An extension of a claims-made policy that provides coverage for incidents that occurred while the policy was in effect, but are reported after the policy expires

- However, in response to a changing insurance marketplace climate in recent years, these types of policies have fallen out of favor. For insurers to turn profits from an increasingly litigious society, most current MPLI policies take the form of "**claims-made**" policies, wherein a physician is covered only for incidents provided the incident *and* the claim filed both occur while the physician's MPLI policy remains active. In other words, even if a physician has an active policy when an incident occurs for which they are sued, the insurance company will not cover any costs if the physician subsequently changes jobs or otherwise terminates their policy in between the incident occurring and the time of claim filing. For this reason, many physicians nowadays choose to purchase "**tail coverage**," which generally covers any claims originating from the time during which the policy was active but filed after its expiration. The period of tail coverage, and the exact terms thereof, vary widely by the specific type of policy and insurance company.

Litigation in the Emergency Department

- Many emergency medicine providers deal with litigation at some point in their careers; by one estimate, emergency physicians have a 7.5% annual risk of litigation, although emergency medicine indemnity payments tend to be lower than average across specialties. In one recent study of 11,529 emergency department related claims, emergency physicians represented only 19% of the primary defendants (as opposed to consultants or hospital systems).

- High-risk diagnoses frequently involved in malpractice claims include missed acute myocardial infarction, appendicitis, and intracranial hemorrhage. Lower-risk but commonly missed diagnoses also make up a substantial portion of malpractice claims, and most common among these are missed fractures.
- In addition to specific diagnoses, certain provider characteristics have been found to share associations with litigation risk. Remarkably, provider communication skills seem to be more important than the degree of adverse outcome in determining the likelihood that a case will progress to litigation.

Litigation and Provider Well-being

- For many physicians, involvement in the litigation process can be an emotionally trying experience. Not only are lawsuits financially costly, but the duration of a case can extend up to 4 or more years. Particularly in cases that involve unexpected adverse outcomes, this can be re-traumatizing for the physician every time the case details are revisited. Anger, anxiety, and depression are all extremely common among physicians undergoing litigation stress. Somatic symptoms are also common.
- It is often helpful for individuals being sued to seek counsel and support from other physicians who have themselves been involved in the litigation process, for both practical advice and normalization of an experience that is sometimes unavoidable in the practice of medicine. Professional counseling or therapy can also be beneficial during this intensely stressful period.

SUGGESTED READINGS

American College of Emergency Physicians Medical Legal Committee, & Rice, M. W. (2007). Medical professional liability insurance (Information Paper). https://www.acep.org/globalassets/uploads/uploaded-files/acep/clinical-and-practice-management/resources/medical-legal/mplipaperapril04.pdf

American College of Emergency Physicians Medical Legal Committee, Syzek, T., Andrew, L., Freund, N., Bibb, J., & Sullivan, D. (2004). So you have been sued! (Resource Document). https://www.acep.org/globalassets/uploads/uploaded-files/acep/clinical-and-practice-management/resources/medical-legal/so-you-have-been-sued.pdf

Shapiro, R., Simpson, D., & Lawrence, S. (1989). A survey of sued and nonsued physicians and suing patients. *Archives of Internal Medicine*, *149*(10), 2190–2196.

Strauss, R. W., & Mayer, T. A. (2014). *Strauss and Mayer's emergency department management* (pp. xxiii, 760). McGraw-Hill Education/Medical.

CHAPTER 161

Quality Improvement and Root Cause Analysis

HANNAH SPUNGEN, MD, MPH, and MALKEET GUPTA, MD, MS

The Institute of Medicine (IOM) defines health-care quality as "the degree to which health care services for individuals and populations increase the likelihood of desired health outcomes and are consistent with current professional knowledge." Physicians and health-care systems are increasingly being evaluated on the quality of care that they deliver, sometimes with financial implications.

History of the Quality Movement

- Systematic improvements in health care started as early as the 19th century through hygiene-related interventions.
- Some of the most influential contributors to the current philosophy of quality improvement (QI) have come from non–health-care sectors.
- W. Edwards Deming was a prolific statistician who published extensively on the importance of controlling process variation to achieve consistent desirable outcomes. He primarily focused on manufacturing, famously transforming the layout and workflow within a Toyota plant with such astounding success that his methods were quickly adopted throughout the industry. He relied heavily on the concept of Plan-Do-Check-Act cycles.
- Many other frameworks initially developed for manufacturing have become widely used in health care QI, including Six Sigma, Lean, and Structure-Process-Outcome (Box 161.1).
- Using these manufacturing principles, Dr. Avedis Donabedian, a physician and professor of public health at the University of Michigan, developed a novel framework for examining the quality of health care through the analysis of **structure** (physical surroundings) and **process** (sequences of steps or events) in addition to **outcomes**.

From Quality Assurance to Quality Improvement

- Building upon Donabedian's work, the IOM released two seminal reports—*To Err Is Human* (1999) and *Crossing the Quality Chasm* (2001)—that catapulted the QI discipline into a broader public consciousness with its startling conclusions about the prevalence of preventable error across health-care settings.

BOX 161.1 *Examples of Well-Used Quality Improvement Frameworks in Health Care*

Plan-Do-Check-Act (PDCA): Also known as Plan-Do-Study-Act, this is a strategy based on the scientific method, wherein a hypothesis is tested, data are generated, and outcomes are analyzed. The cyclic aspect emphasizes the need to continually evaluate the impact of policy changes implemented in the "act" phase.

Six Sigma: Six Sigma refers to the degree of process variation deemed acceptable in high-reliability organizations such as aeronautics. A process with a variation rate of 6σ (six sigma) will result in 99.99967% standardization. Although helpful for highly predictable situations (e.g., hernia repair), Six Sigma is not always an appropriate framework for use in the emergency department, where patient presentations and illnesses are highly variable.

DMAIC: DMAIC stands for Define, Measure, Analyze, Improve, Control. It is the primary methodology used by Six Sigma (see above) and can be loosely conceptualized as a more comprehensive version of the PDCA sequence.

Lean: Lean is a methodology pioneered by Toyota that involves eliminating all sources of waste (of both material and labor) to achieve low levels of process variability.

Structure-Process-Outcome: Donabedian's approach to quality improvement that emphasizes the use of benchmarks other than pure outcome to gauge quality, allowing for a more nuanced focus on the determinants thereof.

- This caused a shift from what had previously been termed "quality assurance," wherein an implicit culture of blame led organizations to target the mistakes of individual providers, to a more holistic focus on systems-level interventions—in other words, focusing on how humans function within the built environment and hierarchies of their workplaces.
- The IOM reports delineated six core tenets of high quality care: safety, effectiveness, patient-centeredness, timeliness, efficiency, and equity. Using these reports as a springboard, health care systems across the country began to standardize their QI efforts. In 2002, the Joint Commission and the Centers for Medicare & Medicaid Services both initiated programs to require hospitals to provide performance data. Subsequently, these data have become increasingly available to the public and linked

to reimbursement, a trend that has furthered hospital systems' interest in QI.

Root Cause Analysis

- Patient safety is perhaps the most discussed of the six IOM areas of focus for quality improvement, given that its failures tend to be the most devastating. The language to describe potential or actual error-related adverse outcomes, also known as patient safety events, has been formalized by the Joint Commission.
- The most serious of these, also known as a sentinel event, is defined as a patient safety event that causes either death, permanent harm, or severe temporary harm necessitating lifesaving intervention on the patient's behalf.
- These are events that should be reported and, per Joint Commission requirements, must be subjected to a root cause analysis (RCA) to identify the systems-level failings that precipitated it, in the interest of avoiding a similar outcome in the future.
- Echoing the quality discipline's shift from the individual-centered quality assurance models to a more systems-centered approach, the goal of the RCA is to identify systems-level failings rather than to ascribe personal blame.
- Creating a culture of blame in health-care settings, as in other industries, tends to decrease error reporting, which in turn perpetuates the failings that led to the sentinel event in the first place.
- Reason's Swiss cheese model is often used as an analogy illustrative of the process by which sentinel events occur: rather than a single "hole," or weakness, directly causing the event, a series of failings (or "holes") occur on multiple levels that happen to align. Under this framework, the blame for the sentinel event rests not on any one individual's failing but on the series of systems-level events that aligned in an unfortunate coincidence to produce an adverse outcome.
- By identifying and minimizing the specific contributory weaknesses, RCA seeks to help foster more robust systems that are less prone to overlapping (and potentially fatal) weaknesses.

SUGGESTED READINGS

American College of Emergency Physicians Medical Legal Committee, Syzek, T., Andrew, L., Freund, N., Bibb, J., & Sullivan, D. (2004). So you have been sued! (Resource Document). https://www.acep.org/globalassets/uploads/uploaded-files/acep/clinical-and-practice-management/resources/medical-legal/so-you-have-been-sued.pdf

Andrew Taylor, R., Venkatesh, A., Parwani, V., Chekijian, S., Shapiro, M., Oh, A., Harriman, D., Tarabar, A., & Ulrich, A. (2018). Applying advanced analytics to guide emergency department operational decisions: A proof-of-concept study examining the effects of boarding. *American Journal of Emergency Medicine*, 36(9), 1534–1539.

Asplin, B. R., Magid, D. J., Rhodes, K. V., Solberg, L. I., Lurie, N., & Camargo, C. A., Jr. (2003). A conceptual model of emergency department crowding. *Annals of Emergency Medicine*, *42*(2), 173–180.

Gupta, M. (2014). Happy meals for everyone? *Annals of Emergency Medicine*, 64(6), 609–611.

Institute of Medicine (U. S.) Committee on Quality of Health Care in America. (2001). *Crossing the quality chasm: A new health system for the 21st century* (pp. xx, 337). National Academies Press.

Prentice, J. C., Frakt, A. B., & Pizer, S. D. (2016). Metrics that matter. *Journal of General Internal Medicine*, *31*(Suppl. 1), 70–73.

Strauss, R. W., & Mayer, T. A. (2014). *Strauss and Mayer's emergency department management* (pp. xxiii, 760). McGraw-Hill Education/Medical.

Welch, S. J., Asplin, B. R., Stone-Griffith, S., Davidson, S. J., Augustine, J., & Schuur, J. (2011). Emergency department operational metrics, measures and definitions: Results of the second performance measures and benchmarking summit. *Annals of Emergency Medicine*, 58(1), 33–40.

Operational Metrics and Patient Satisfaction

HANNAH SPUNGEN, MD, MPH, and MALKEET GUPTA, MD, MS

Dramatic growth of the quality improvement movement in recent years has necessitated the development of a formal set of tools and language to measure value and quality in health care.

Operational metrics is the "umbrella term" for the collection and analysis of quantitative data that can be used to draw conclusions that guide the structure and function of health-care delivery, whether in ambulatory clinics, inpatient wards, or the emergency department (ED).

Emergency Department–Specific Metrics

- Asplin and colleagues developed a widely used conceptual model for operations management to address crowding in the ED involving three components: input, throughput, and output.
- Using this model as a lens to evaluate ED patient flow in a broader sense, specific targets for measurement can be identified. These target areas are then used for myriad purposes: to guide potential interventions, as benchmarks to compare ED characteristics against a national average, and to help analyze individual provider performance. Commonly used ED operational metrics are listed in Table 162.1.

System-Level Implications

- The Joint Commission and the Centers for Medicare & Medicaid Services now require hospitals to track and report specific ED metrics. These include door-to-thrombolytic time for qualifying stroke patients, median time from arrival to ED to first electrocardiogram for ST-elevation myocardial infarction patients, time to troponin, and time to pain management in long-bone fractures, to name a few.
- In recognition of the strain that patient boarding places upon the entire hospital throughput, the Joint Commission

TABLE 162.1 *Types of ED Operational Metrics*

Metric Type	Description	Examples
Operating characteristics	Allows comparison of ED function to other EDs with similar population demographics	Annual ED census Acuity by Emergency Severity Index scale Admission rate ICU admission rate Percent pediatric visits Percent geriatric visits
Interval metrics	Allows granular analysis of ED throughput and rapid identification of bottleneck areas	Arrival to provider time ("door to doc") ED length of stay Provider to data-ready time Provider to subspecialist consult time Data-ready to decision time Decision to departure time
Proportion metrics	Related to patient satisfaction, sometimes used as a proxy of overall care quality	Left without being seen rate Left against medical advice Left before treatment complete rate (includes "eloped") Complaint ratio per 1000 visits
Utilization metrics	Number of "emergency service units" of a given resource; by convention, expressed in units per 100 ED visits	ECGs/CT scans/other imaging modalities Medication dosages Psychiatric consultations Subspecialist consultations

CT, Computed tomography; *ECGs*, electrocardiograms; *ED*, emergency department; *ICU*, intensive care unit.

also now requires hospitals to measure and set goals for mitigating patient boarding in the ED with buy-in from multiple stakeholders, including hospital and community behavioral health leadership. Because these data are publicly reported, and because there can be financial implications of failing to meet specific quality standards, health-care systems are understandably focused on improving these metrics.

Provider-Level Implications

- In addition to systems-level data, granular data on provider-specific metrics are also being collected.
- Examples of provider-level metrics include number of patients seen per provider per hour, provider-specific lengths of stay, and frequency of computed tomography scan utilization.
- Degree of transparency and the specific areas of focus for provider-specific metrics vary by organization. There is a general trend toward tying at least some portion of physician reimbursement to these types of metrics.

Patient Satisfaction

- The Institute of Medicine has identified patient satisfaction as one of six core areas of quality measurement.
- Although no specific federal reimbursement schemes are tied to ED patient satisfaction scores, emergency physicians' performances are nonetheless being scrutinized closely.
- Proponents of the patient satisfaction movement contend that improving patient satisfaction scores is an intrinsically worthy exercise and that higher scores correlate with a host of other desirable outcomes tied to quality of care.

Limitations of Metrics Gathering and Analysis

- Despite the widespread adoption of operational metrics as quality improvement tools, the collection, analysis, and dissemination of these data sometimes lacks the methodologic rigor to be truly statistically meaningful.
- Most ED satisfaction survey data currently used reflect only the opinions of a narrow subset of discharged patients, and thus are subject to significant response bias. Moreover, patient expectations do not always coincide with best medical practices, which is problematic for the physician whose performance evaluation is linked to survey data.
  - For instance, patients with chronic low back pain may be dissatisfied with an emergency provider's refusal to refill a narcotic prescription or obtain magnetic resonance imaging, even when neither is indicated.
- Some argue that overreliance on patient satisfaction surveys may influence provider behavior in the form of overprescribing and overuse of testing resources in the interest of meeting patient expectations as opposed to employing best medical practices.

SUGGESTED READINGS

American College of Emergency Physicians Medical Legal Committee, Syzek, T., Andrew, L., Freund, N., Bibb, J., & Sullivan, D. (2004). So you have been sued! (Resource Document). https://www.acep.org/globalassets/uploads/uploaded-files/acep/clinical-and-practice-management/resources/medical-legal/so-you-have-been-sued.pdf

Andrew Taylor, R., Venkatesh, A., Parwani, V., Chekijian, S., Shapiro, M., Oh, A., Harriman, D., Tarabar, A., & Ulrich, A. (2018). Applying advanced analytics to guide emergency department operational decisions: A proof-of-concept study examining the effects of boarding. *American Journal of Emergency Medicine*, *36*(9), 1534–1539.

Asplin, B. R., Magid, D. J., Rhodes, K. V., Solberg, L. I., Lurie, N., & Camargo, C. A., Jr. (2003). A conceptual model of emergency department crowding. *Annals of Emergency Medicine*, *42*(2), 173–180.

INDEX

Page numbers followed by "*f*" indicate figures, "*t*" indicate tables, and "*b*" indicate boxes.

D

E

N

O

P

T

U